## Third
## Edition
Revised and Expanded

# Acute Coronary
# Syndromes

# Third Edition
## Revised and Expanded

# Acute Coronary Syndromes

Edited by **Eric J. Topol**

The Cleveland Clinic Foundation
Cleveland, Ohio, U.S.A.

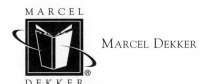

MARCEL DEKKER                    NEW YORK

**Library of Congress Cataloging-in-Publication Data**
A catalog record for this book is available from the Library of Congress.

**ISBN: 0-8247-5795-5**

This book is printed on acid-free paper.

**Headquarters**
Marcel Dekker, 270 Madison Avenue, New York, NY 10016, U.S.A.
tel: 212-696-9000; fax: 212-685-4540

**Distribution and Customer Service**
Marcel Dekker, Cimarron Road, Monticello, New York 12701, U.S.A.
tel: 800-228-1160; fax: 845-796-1772

**World Wide Web**
http://www.dekker.com

The publisher offers discounts on this book when ordered in bulk quantities. For more information, write to Special Sales/Professional Marketing at the headquarters address above.

Current printing (last digit):

10   9   8   7   6   5   4   3   2   1

**PRINTED IN THE UNITED STATES OF AMERICA**

# Preface

This book was the first of its kind and the first to be called *Acute Coronary Syndromes* when it was published in 1998. Since the first edition of this book was published, our understanding of the biologic basis of acute coronary syndromes has been greatly enhanced. While the process of arterial inflammation was acknowledged as important at that time, recent work has provided considerable insight on the specific genes and proteins that drive atherosclerotic plaque disruption. Beyond the biologic basis of the clinical syndrome, there continues to be intensive, rigorous clinical investigation in the field to provide the evidence for improving care. One of the most significant developments since the last edition was published has been the full validation of the use of early coronary revascularization as the preferred strategy to manage patients with acute coronary syndromes.

While progress is being made, there are sobering aspects of the campaign to prevent and improve management of acute coronary syndromes. While the population is graying at an accelerated rate, the incidence of the disease is compounded by the ''diabesity'' epidemic. Nearly 70% of Americans are obese or overweight, and now evidence has mounted that this profound public health epidemic has reached global proportions. Furthermore, the population is at the nadir of physical activity, which not only contributes to the obesity problem but independently adds risk of developing acute coronary syndromes. Accordingly, the incidence and prevalence of this condition is on the rise despite our better biologic understanding and improvements in therapy.

In this third edition, seven new chapters have been added to fulfill the objective of providing the most comprehensive and up-to-date panoramic view of the field. Now that specific genes have been identified, a chapter dedicated to the genomics of acute myocardial infarction is incorporated. One of the most important advances in recent years has been the use of protein biomarker measurements, such as the impressive body of data for brain natiuretic peptide and its pro-peptide. A chapter that hones in on this is included in the new edition and emphasis is placed throughout the book on the other useful biomarkers that include Troponin, C-reactive protein, and myeloperoxidase. A sweep across the data for the new arterial inflammatory markers is the subject of a new, dedicated chapter.

Now that we have seen validation for early percutaneous coronary intervention, the need for specialized centers of excellence, akin to trauma centers, has been raised. A new chapter that presents the case for these regional centers of excellence is an important component of this edition. At the time of coronary revascularization, there is a significant limitation of providing normal coronary blood flow. This is typically due to arterial inflammation and embolization of microparticulate atheromatous debris or thrombus, and the microcirculation or "watershed zone" is the problematic zone. A chapter that features concerns about improving microcirculatory perfusion in the coronary bed is a new dimension of the book. The other major trend in recent years that deserves highlighting is the appreciation that diabetes, and the metabolic syndrome, is a cardiovascular entity. Patients with diabetes or the metabolic syndrome have excessive risk of developing acute coronary syndromes, and particular high adverse outcomes once this condition arises. Thus, it is pivotal for the practitioner to recognize the importance of diabetes, and a new chapter delves into this pressing issue.

A particularly frustrating aspect of acute myocardial infarction management is that considerable damage to the myocardium has already occurred at the time of the patient's initial presentation. The topic of cardiogenic shock and Killip Class III, which carry a dreadful diagnosis, is now fully covered in a new chapter, as well as the most exciting new therapy, which has a chance to regenerate myocardium and involves the use of pluripotent stem cells. A chapter has been added to feature the biology of and review the initial data on stem cell therapy for acute myocardial infarction.

Many of the leading investigators of the field have contributed to this project and I remain deeply indebted for their willingness to cull their insights and expertise into this new edition. In the 32 chapters, 45 authors from around the world have come together to refine the only dedicated book that exists in this field. As the Editor, I am deeply thankful to all of the authors for their timely submission of high quality manuscripts that assured the fine makeup of this monograph, and to all of the production team at Marcel Dekker for their supportive effort. In particular, I would like to acknowledge the Managing Editor, Ms. Donna Wasiewicz-Bressan at the Cleveland Clinic Foundation. We hope that this book will serve as a useful resource for all clinicians, including cardiologists, internists, nurses, and paraprofessional staff, who are engaged in caring for patients with acute coronary syndromes. If the book promotes better understanding and care of these patients, we have again achieved our primary objective.

*Eric J. Topol*

# Contents

# Contents

# Contributors

**Ramtin Agah**   University of Utah, Salt Lake City, Utah, U.S.A.

**Arman T. Askari**   University Hospitals of Cleveland and Case Western Reserve University, Cleveland, Ohio, U.S.A.

**Eric R. Bates**   University of Michigan, Ann Arbor, Michigan, U.S.A.

**Kevin J. Beatt**   Hammersmith Hospital, London, England

**Richard C. Becker**   Duke University Medical Center, Durham, North Carolina, U.S.A

**Peter Berger**   Duke University Medical Center Duke Clinical Research Institute, Durham, North Carolina, U.S.A.

**Deepak L. Bhatt MD**   The Cleveland Clinic Foundation, Cleveland, Ohio, U.S.A.

**Andra L. Blomkalns**   University of Cincinnati College of Medicine and University Hospital, Cincinatti, Ohio, U.S.A.

**Sorin J. Brener**   The Cleveland Clinic Foundation, Cleveland, Ohio, U.S.A.

**Vladimir Dzavik**   University of Toronto, Toronto, Canada

**Eric L. Eisenstein**   Duke University Medical Center, Durham, North Carolina, USA

**Erling Falk**   Aarhus University Hospital, Denmark

**Farzin Fath-Ordoubadi**   Hammersmith Hospital, London, England

**Ole Frøbert**   University of Aarhus, Denmark

**Gary S. Francis**    The Cleveland Clinic Foundation, Cleveland, Ohio, U.S.A.

**W. Brian Gibler**    Department of Emergency Medicine, University of Cincinnati College of Medicine and University Hospital, Cincinnati, Ohio, U.S.A.

**Hitinder S. Gurm**    The Cleveland Clinic Foundation, Cleveland, Ohio, U.S.A

**Hans-Henrik Tilsted Hansen**    Department of Cardiology, S. Aalborg University Hospital, Denmark

**Stanley L. Hazen**    The Cleveland Clinic Foundation, Cleveland, Ohio, U.S.A.

**Judith S. Hochman**    Harold Snyder Family Professor of Cardiology, New York University, New York, U.S.A.

**James G. Jollis**    Duke University Medical Center, Durham, North Carolina, U.S.A

**Samir R. Kapadia**    The Cleveland Clinic Foundation, Cleveland, Ohio, U.S.A.

**Dean J. Kereiakes**    The Carl and Edyth Lindner Center for Research and Education, Ohio Heart Health Center, Ohio State University, Ohio, U.S.A.

**Philippe L. L'Allier**    Montreal Heart Institute, Montreal, Canada

**Michael A. Lincoff**    The Cleveland Clinic Foundation, Cleveland, Ohio, U.S.A.

**Koon-Hou Mak**    National Heart Centre, Singapore

**Daniel B. Mark**    Duke University Medical Center, Durham, North Carolina, USA,

**Michael Miller**    University of Maryland School of Medicine, Baltimore, Maryland, U.S.A.

**David J. Moliterno**    University of Kentucky, Lexington, Kentucky, U.S.A.

**Debabrata Mukherjee**    University of Michigan, Ann Arbor, Michigan, U.S.A.

**L. Kristin Newby**    Duke University Medical Center, Durham, North Carolina, U.S.A.

**Steven E. Nissen**    The Cleveland Clinic Foundation, Cleveland, Ohio, U.S.A.

**Marc S. Penn**    The Cleveland Clinic Foundation, Cleveland, Ohio, U.S.A.

**Thomas A. Pezzella**    University of Massachusetts Medical School, Worcester, Massachusetts, U.S.A

**Louise Pilote**    McGill University Health Centre, Montreal, Quebec, Canada

**Jacqueline Saw**    The Cleveland Clinic Foundation, Cleveland, Ohio, U.S.A.

**Mehdi H. Shishehbor**    The Cleveland Clinic Foundation, Cleveland, Ohio, U.S.A.

**Peter Sinnaeve**  Gasthuisberg University Hospital, Leuven, Belgium

**Steven R. Steinhubl**  Associate Professor of Medicine, University of Kentucky, Lexington, Kentucky, U.S.A

**W. H. Wilson Tang**  The Cleveland Clinic Foundation, Cleveland, Ohio, U.S.A.

**Eric J. Topol**  The Cleveland Clinic Foundation, Cleveland, Ohio, U.S.A

**Murat E. Tuzcu**  The Cleveland Clinic Foundation, Cleveland, Ohio, U.S.A.

**Frans Van de Werf**  Gasthuisberg University Hospital, Leuven, Belgium

**Robert A. Vogel**  University of Maryland School of Medicine, Baltimore, Maryland, U.S.A.

**Albrecht Vogt**  Medizinische Klinik II Klinikum Kassel, Kassel, Germany

**Michael H. Yen**  The Cleveland Clinic Foundation, Cleveland, Ohio, U.S.A.

# Third
# Edition
## Revised and Expanded

# Acute Coronary
# Syndromes

# 1
# Coronary Artery Inflammation

**Deepak L. Bhatt, MD**
*The Cleveland Clinic Foundation*
*Cleveland, Ohio, U.S.A.*

## INTRODUCTION

In the 1980s, the role of the thrombus in acute coronary syndromes (ACS) was elucidated. It was realized in the 1990s that the platelet was of particular importance in arterial thrombosis [1]. Now, it has become clear that arterial inflammation is a major player in initiating plaque rupture and also predisposes to recurrent ischemic events in both the short and long term [2]. Indeed, the platelet itself has emerged as an inflammatory cell. These basic science insights are of direct relevance to clinicians caring for patients with acute coronary syndromes.

Coronary arterial inflammation is widespread in acute coronary syndromes [3]. Such inflammation leads to endothelial dysfunction, plaque progression, and ultimately plaque rupture and thrombosis (Figure 1). This underlying inflammatory process is linked not only to solitary plaque rupture but also to multiple plaque rupture [4]. While multiple ruptured plaques have been detected by angiography for years, angiography is an insensitive tool for such detection. Indeed, the prevalence of multiple plaque rupture increases with the use of intravascular ultrasound, with even greater detection rates seen on angioscopy. Corresponding to a greater prevalence of ruptured plaques is a greater prevalence of elevated inflammatory markers [3]. While some degree of systemic inflammation is induced by myocardial necrosis, local production of inflammatory mediators by ruptured plaque is also important [5].

Therefore, both systemic and local arterial inflammation predisposes to acute coronary syndromes and participates in the pathogenesis. Measurement of inflammatory markers helps further risk stratify patients beyond mere characterization of clinical risk factors. Novel imaging modalities are helping further characterize the inflammatory process as it pertains to atherosclerotic disease. Existent therapies are being evaluated for their anti-inflammatory potential and specific therapies are being developed to target inflammation in cardiovascular diseases. Progress in understanding the genetic underpinnings of inflammation will further add to our appreciation of the role of inflammation in acute coronary syndromes.

## ROLE OF INFLAMMATION IN ACS

A number of different cell types participate in the process that leads to arterial inflammation. White blood cells, such as neutrophils, macrophages, and T cells, obviously are key

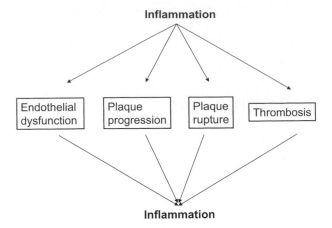

**Figure 1** Inflammation leads to endothelial dysfunction, plaque progression, plaque erosion and rupture, and thrombosis. These events themselves lead to further inflammatory marker/mediator release, leading to a dangerous cycle that may cause recurrent ischemic events.

components of any inflammatory process. They produce a variety of proinflammatory mediators (Figure 2). The endothelium also produces various adhesion molecules that facilitate the binding of white blood cells and initiate the local arterial inflammatory process, rather than what was previously conceived as consisting of inert cells. Adipocytes also produce proinflammatory molecules that promulgate the inflammatory state. The liver participates in this production cycle as well. Platelets are also inflammatory cells, perhaps most relevant to inflammation that occurs in the setting of acute coronary syndromes.

## The Platelet as Inflammatory Cell

While the role of the platelet in thrombotic syndromes is now firmly established, what has become clear is that the platelet is also an inflammatory cell. Numerous inflammatory mediators are secreted by activated platelets. Perhaps the most interesting of these is CD40, a transmembrane glycoprotein that belongs to the tumor necrosis factor (TNF) receptor superfamily. CD40 appears to be a potent mediator of interaction between diverse cell types, including endothelial cells, smooth muscle cells, macrophages, T cells, and platelets (Figure 3) [6,7]. Indeed, the majority of soluble CD40 ligand (sCD40L) is produced by activated platelets. Platelets, via CD40, have been shown to be capable of inducing dendritic cell maturation, B-cell isotype switching, and augmentation of T cell function [8]. With regards to thrombosis, CD40L interacts with the GPIIb/IIIa receptors to help stabilize arterial thrombi [9]. Exposure of platelets to high shear stress results in the translocation of CD40 to the surface [10].

ACS patients with elevated levels of soluble CD40 have a worse prognosis, with a significantly increased risk of death or myocardial infarction (MI) compared with ACS patients without elevated levels. Furthermore, it is these ACS patients with elevated CD40 that are most likely to benefit from the intravenous glycoprotein (GP) IIb/IIIa inhibitor abciximab [11]. Ex vivo work demonstrated that the adenosine diphosphate (ADP) receptor antagonist clopidogrel suppressed production of CD40 by platelets, a property that was not shared by aspirin in that study [12]. Preliminary work has found that pretreatment

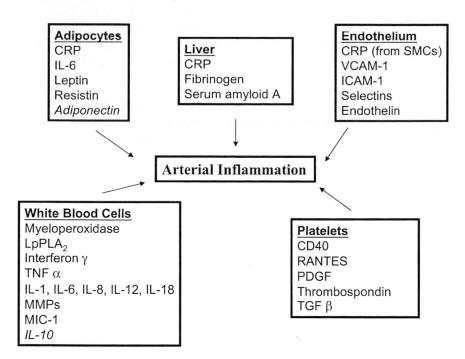

Figure 2    There are several inflammatory mediators from various sources that participate in arterial inflammation. Numerous different cell types participate in the process of arterial inflammation. In the context of arterial inflammation, most of these mediators are viewed as deleterious. However, the ones in italics are believed to be beneficial. CRP, C-reactive protein; ICAM, intercellular cell adhesion molecule; IL, interleukin; LpPLA$_2$, lipoprotein-associated phospholipase A$_2$; MIC-1, macrophage inhibitory cytokine-1; MMP, matrix metalloproteinase; PDGF, platelet derived growth factor; RANTES, regulated on activation normally T-cell express and secreted; SMCs, smooth muscle cells; TGF, transforming growth factor; TNF, tumor necrosis factor; VCAM, vascular cell adhesion molecule.

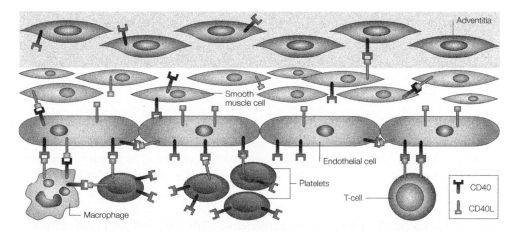

Figure 3    The role of CD40 in mediating diverse cell–cell interactions. (From Ref. 6)

with clopidogrel in patients prior to percutaneous coronary intervention (PCI) blunts the production of CD40 by platelets [13]. In fact, a substantial proportion of benefit of GPIIb/IIIa inhibitors and ADP receptor antagonists may be due to their ability to diminish production of sCD40L.

CD40 appears to have a role in restenosis as well. Patients with increased preprocedural levels of sCD40L have higher rates of 6-month restenosis [14]. Furthermore, preprocedural sCD40 levels also correlate with monocyte chemoattractant protein-1 (MCP-1) generation and adhesion molecule expression [14]. In the setting of heart failure, platelets express more CD40, with correspondingly higher levels found in more advanced degrees of New York Heart Association defined heart failure [15]. Notably, in this study of heart failure, aspirin did not appear to have an effect on CD40 expression. In the setting of carotid artery stenting, abciximab reduced sCD40L, but interestingly, so did emboli protection filters [16]. This latter finding supports the premise that embolization leads to platelet activation and inflammation, and while intravenous GPIIb/IIIa blockade is beneficial to mitigate the consequences of embolization, preventing embolization in the first place would likely be even better, especially so in ACS lesions.

Oxidized LDL leads to increased expression of CD40L in a variety of cell types [17]. However, treatment with statins diminishes this response to oxidized LDL. Furthermore, statin treatment decreases levels of sCD40L as well. Perhaps, then, the purported antithrombotic effect of statins is in part mediated via reductions in sCD40L [18].

Just as CD40 appears to be a bad player in ACS and percutaneous coronary intervention (PCI), the same holds true for bypass surgery. Patients placed on cardiopulmonary bypass have been found to have elevation of sCD40L derived from platelets [19]. Potentially, platelet CD40L release is responsible for some of the adverse thrombotic and inflammatory sequelae of cardiopulmonary bypass.

Levels of CD40 expression on platelets of patients with Kawasaki disease are higher than seen in febrile controls [20]. The extent of CD 40 expression has been found to correlate with the presence of coronary artery lesions [20]. The administration of intravenous immunoglobulin significantly decreased the expression of CD40L in patients with Kawasaki disease.

The knowledge gained by study of the CD40 pathway is of relevance to fields outside cardiovascular medicine as well. For example, patients with inflammatory bowel disease have elevated levels of sCD40L in proportion to the extent of mucosal inflammation [21]. This increase in soluble CD40L was paralleled by an increase in the platelet surface expression and release of CD40L. It was hypothesized that the transit of platelets through an inflamed mucosal microvasculature resulted in platelet activation, though it is intriguing to think that platelets as inflammatory cells may actually play a part in the pathogenesis of Crohn's disease and ulcerative colitis [22].

Via CD40, glycoprotein IIb/IIIa receptors, ADP receptors, and other pathways, the interrelation of inflammation and platelet-driven thrombosis has been established and serves as a target for further discovery and therapeutic manipulation.

## Inflammatory Cells

Inflammatory cells participate in multiple beneficial tasks, such as protecting the body from bacteria and viruses. However, if atherosclerosis is viewed as an invading pathogen, the inflammatory cascade may be activated in an ultimately maladaptive fashion.

## Infection

The immune system may play a role in atherosclerosis. The T helper Type 1 (Th1) response appears to promote the development of atherosclerosis, while inhibiting this response appears to suppress atherosclerosis [23]. While a direct role of infection in atherosclerosis remains a possibility, more likely, infection leads to inflammation that predisposes to plaque rupture. Epidemiological evidence supports a link between antecedent upper respiratory infection and ischemic events. Furthermore, influenza vaccination appears to decrease the risk of ischemic syndromes and decrease the risk in demographic populations at risk, it makes sense to provide vaccination. Human immunodeficiency virus (HIV) infection increases the risk of premature atherosclerosis. Patients receiving highly active antiretroviral therapy (HAART) are predisposed to lipid abnormalities and the metabolic syndrome, conditions associated with arterial inflammation. Whether HIV directly increases atherogenesis or whether it is some of the medications such as HAART that are used to treat HIV or both remains to be sorted out.

## Periodontal Disease

Periodontal infection appears to be associated with an increased incidence of cardiovascular disease, even after controlling for age, medical comorbidity, and socioeconomic status [24]. The associations hold true for MI, stroke, and peripheral arterial disease [25,26]. For example, greater degrees of tooth loss due to periodontitis are associated with greater degrees of carotid plaque [27]. More extensive periodontal disease is also associated with elevated levels of C-reactive protein (CRP) and endothelial dysfunction as assessed by brachial flow-mediated dilation [28,29]. Periodontitis also elevates other inflammatory markers such as interleukin-6 (IL-6) [30]. However, it is unclear if the systemic inflammatory response is directly due to the infection itself or, rather, the low-grade chronic inflammation that may be coexistent. In either case, a recommendation for appropriate dental hygiene and care remains prudent. Large-scale randomized trials to assess whether more intensive efforts at eradication of gingival plaque may benefit coronary plaque are in the planning stages. A pilot study testing this concept, Periodontal Intervention in Cardiac Events (PAVE), is already under way.

## Systemic Disease Causing Arterial Inflammation

Systemic disorders may predispose to an inflammatory state. Obesity is one of the strongest determinants of elevated CRP. Across the spectrum of body mass index (BMI), higher weight is associated with higher levels of CRP and IL-6 [31]. Regardless of whether obesity is defined by BMI, waist circumference, waist to hip ratio, or other means, there is a striking correlation between overweight and inflammation. Abdominal adiposity in particular seems to promote inflammation, perhaps due to cytokine production by adipocytes. Similarly, metabolic syndrome and diabetes lead to CRP elevation. Hypothyroidism has been linked with elevated CRP levels [32]. Renal dysfunction has been associated with increased levels of CRP and IL-6 in multiple studies [33,34]. This may explain to some extent why patients with renal dysfunction have such a grim cardiovascular prognosis. Inflammation in rheumatological diseases, such as systemic lupus erythematosus and rheumatoid arthritis, may, in part, explain the excess cardiovascular risk seen with these disease states [35].

## MARKERS AND MEDIATORS OF INFLAMMATION

Numerous markers of inflammation have been described, and most have associated data supporting their roles as mediators of inflammation as well (Table 1).

**Table 1**   Markers/Mediators of Inflammation

C-reactive protein (CRP)
CD40L
P-selectin
Matrix metalloproteinases (MMPs)
Vascular cell adhesion molecule (VCAM)
Intercellular cell adhesion molecule (ICAM)
Interleukin-1 receptor antagonist
Interleukin-6
Tumor necrosis factor (TNF) α
Interferon γ
Interleukin-18
Monocyte chemoattractant protein-1 (MCP-1)
Macrophage colony stimulating factor (M-CSF)
Macrophage inhibitory cytokine-1 (MIC-1)
White blood cell count (WBC)
Myeloperoxidase
Nitrotyrosine
Asymmetric dimethylarginine (ADMA)
Serum amyloid A
Lipoprotein-associated phospholipase A2 (LpPLA2)
Pregnancy-associated plasma protein A (PAPP-A)
Tissue factor
Heat shock proteins
Neopterin

## CRP—A Potent Marker of Risk

Of the available inflammatory markers, high-sensitivity C-reactive protein (hs-CRP) is the only one ready for clinical prime time [36,37]. In particular, in acute coronary syndromes, hs-CRP is well validated [38]. For example, in a study by Zairis et al, elevation of CRP on admission in patients with ST segment elevation MI was associated with higher likelihood of incomplete ST segment resolution with fibrinolysis, in-hospital mortality, and 3-year cardiac mortality [39]. In patients with non-ST elevation MI (NSTEMI) ACS, elevated CRP predicts a higher risk for mortality [40]. This even holds true in patients with normal troponin values. CRP predicts adverse outcomes, including mortality, after successful PCI (Figure 4) [41]. Impressively, CRP elevation is associated with sudden cardiac death [42]. Patients who died suddenly with plaque rupture or plaque erosion were found to have not only higher levels of CRP in postmortem sera, but also greater immunohistochemical staining intensity for CRP in the plaque itself [42]. In the setting of surgery for carotid stenosis, elevated CRP levels were associated with unstable plaque, as defined by the presence of macrophages and T cells in plaque, as well as with stenoses that were symptomatic [43]. CRP levels predict the development of diabetes mellitus [44]. Elevation of CRP more recently has been shown to predict the future development of hypertension [45]. Thus, in multiple studies in an assortment of clinical situations spanning the continuum of risk, CRP independently predicts adverse outcomes. While prospective data regarding the ability of a CRP-guided approach to therapy are desirable, until such time as those data are accrued, CRP measurement, including serially, can help guide intensity of therapy, whether lifestyle or pharmaceutical based [2,46]. Of course, in the

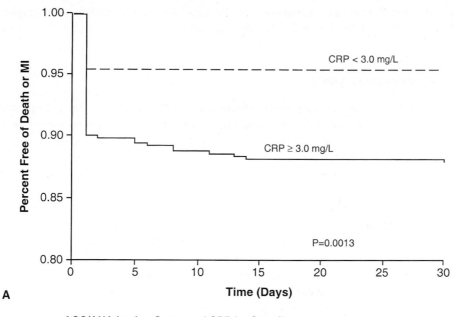

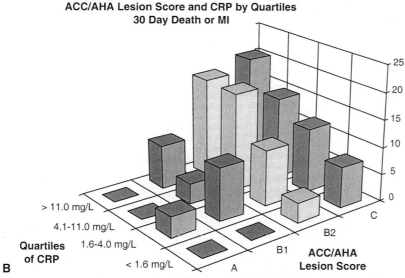

**Figure 4** (**A**) The high-sensitivity C-reactive protein (CRP) is a potent, independent predictor of risk in patients undergoing percutaneous coronary intervention (PCI). (**B**) The ability of high-sensitivity CRP protein to predict death or myocardial infarction (MI) after percutaneous coronary intervention is incremental to the angiographic risk, as assessed by the American College of Cardiology/American Heart Association (ACC/AHA) lesion score (From Ref. 41)

future, other markers or sets of markers may be developed that complement or surpass hs-CRP as a risk stratification tool or therapeutic target.

## CRP—A Pathogenic Entity

Beyond its role as a proven marker of inflammation, CRP appears to be a direct and indirect pathogen. It is found in atherosclerotic intima, but not in normal intima [47]. Numerous adverse effects of CRP have now been described (Table 2). CRP stabilizes plasminogen activator inhibitor-1 (PAI-1) mRNA and leads to increased PAI-1 expression by endothelial cells [48]. In contradistinction, CRP causes down-regulation of endothelial nitric oxide synthase (eNOS) mRNA synthesis by adversely affecting mRNA stability [49]. CRP is known to activate complement, especially in patients with acute coronary syndromes, potentially leading to plaque destabilization [50,51]. It also promotes opsonization and uptake of low-density lipoprotein (LDL) by the CRP CD32 receptor on macrophages [52]. CRP induces chemotaxis of monocytes to the intima via its interaction with the CRP receptor on monocytes [53]. CRP activates the deleterious nuclear factor-kappa B signal transduction pathway in endothelial cells [54]. Thus, CRP simultaneously promotes endothelial dysfunction, inflammation, plaque instability, and thrombosis, all particularly undesirable in patients with, or at risk for, acute coronary syndromes.

## White Blood Cell Count

Even the lowly white blood cell count (WBC) appears to be a potent prognosticator of risk. WBC is a rather crude measurement of inflammation by modern standards. Nevertheless, there is a vast body of data that supports the ability of WBC to contribute to risk stratification across the spectrum of ACS and PCI [55–58]. The benefit of revascularization in patients with ACS is most pronounced in those with evidence of heightened inflammation as assessed by the WBC (Figure 5) [55]. Even in those patients with ACS within the normal range of WBC, higher WBC levels are associated with worse outcomes.

**Table 2**   Multiple Modes of Action of C-Reactive Protein Have Been Described, Illustrating Its Role Not Only as a Risk Marker but an Actual Mediator of Risk (47)

| |
|---|
| Facilitates LDL cholesterol uptake by macrophages |
| Oxidizes LDL cholesterol |
| Activates complement |
| Induces production of tissue factor in monocytes |
| Recruits monocytes into the arterial wall |
| Blunts endothelial reactivity |
| Stabilizes plasminogen activator inhibitor-1 (PAI-1) mRNA |
| Decreases endothelial nitric oxide synthase expression |
| Increases expression of cell adhesion molecules |
| Activates nuclear factor-kappa B |

LDL, low-density lipoprotein

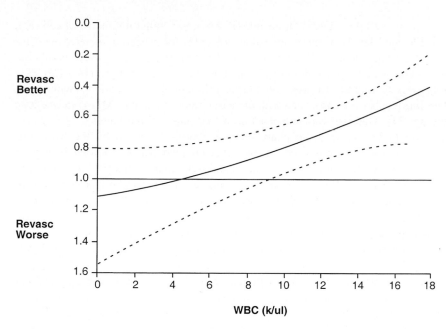

**Figure 5** Patients with acute coronary syndromes (ACS) with higher white blood cell counts (WBC) derive greater benefit from revascularization (Revasc). The six-month mortality risk ratio (with 95% confidence intervals) is depicted as a function of in-hospital revascularization. (From Ref. 55)

In the setting of carotid stenting, it has been observed that patients with higher levels of baseline WBC are more likely to embolize during the procedure [59]. Thus, two key processes in the pathogenesis of ACS, inflammation and embolization, appear linked. Perhaps, patients with elevated WBC have more comorbidities and an elevated WBC is an epiphenomenon. However, it is plausible that the elevated WBC directly participates in the genesis of the increased risk. Neutrophils have a direct role in promoting plaque rupture [60]. More recently, work on myeloperoxidase suggests a deleterious role in cardiovascular disease for this protein found in leukocytes.

Myeloperoxidase has a key role in innate host defense by generating reactive oxidant species. However, elevated levels appear to be associated with a higher risk of ACS and possibly also with adverse ventricular remodeling after myocardial infarction [61]. High numbers of macrophages expressing myeloperoxidase are found in ruptured plaque in ACS, though the macrophages in fatty streaks do not appear to express significant amounts of myeloperoxidase [62]. Furthermore, serum levels of myeloperoxidase are potent predictors of risk [63,64]. Thus, myeloperoxidase expression may be one mechanism by which activated white blood cells lead to worse outcomes.

Neopterin is a marker of macrophage activation. Patients with myocardial infarction and unstable angina have much higher levels of neopterin than those with chronic stable angina [65,66]. In patients with ACS, higher neopterin levels occur in association with more complex lesion morphology on coronary angiography [67,68]. Higher levels of neopterin, as well as other inflammatory markers, are found in patients with diminished renal function [69]. Patients treated with statins have lower levels of neopterin [70].

Selectins such as E-selectin and P-selectin help mediate cell adhesion. P-selectin, for example, facilitates platelet–neutrophil interactions [71]. Vascular cell adhesion molecule

(VCAM-1) and intercellular adhesion molecule (ICAM-1) are other regulators of cell–cell interactions. Elevated levels of these adhesion molecules have been associated with increased risk of cardiac events [72]. Exposure to CRP significantly increases endothelial expression of cell adhesion molecules [73]. Monocyte chemoattractant protein-1 (MCP-1) causes monocytes to migrate to areas of arterial inflammation. In patients with ACS, elevated baseline levels were associated with increased rates of death or MI in intermediate term follow-up [74]. This risk was independent of troponin or CRP levels.

Serum amyloid A is an acute phase reactant that is produced by the liver, just as CRP and fibrinogen are produced by the liver in response to various biological stressors. It also appears to predict risk of future cardiovascular events [75]. Lipoprotein-associated phospholipase A[2] has been shown to predict cardiovascular risk in hyperlipidemic men. However, a large study of healthy women did not corroborate the independent value of this test when LDL cholesterol and CRP were also measured [76]. Pregnancy-associated plasma protein (PAPP-A) is a metalloproteinase that has been found to be elevated in acute coronary syndromes. It appears to correlate with levels of CRP also [77].

Matrix metalloproteinases (MMPs) produced by WBC degrade the extracellular matrix and thus may contribute to plaque rupture. Levels of MMP-9 have also been found to be higher in patients with a history of MI compared with controls [78]. In fact, levels of CRP and MMP-9 correlate with one another in patients with acute coronary syndromes, chronic coronary artery disease, and controls [79]. Tissue inhibitors of matrix metalloproteinases (TIMPs) counter the effects of MMPs, so higher levels are thought to be beneficial.

## Interleukins

Interleukins are cytokines that mediate diverse functions in cell-to-cell communication. Predominantly, interleukins are viewed as causing inflammatory reactions in infection, autoimmune diseases, rheumatological disease, and, most recently, also in atherosclerosis [80]. Different interleukins have pro- and anti-inflammatory activities.

Elevated levels of IL-6 were found to be an independent marker for an increased risk of death in the Fragmin and Fast Revascularization During Instability in Coronary Artery Disease II (FRISC-2) trial of acute coronary syndrome patients [81]. Additionally, those patients with elevated IL-6 levels derived a significant mortality benefit from randomization to an early invasive strategy. This is qualitatively similar to the findings from Platelet Glycoprotein IIb/IIIa in Unstable Angina: Receptor Suppression Using Integrilin Therapy (PURSUIT) in which patients with an elevated WBC were most likely to derive benefit from an invasive approach [55]. Even in healthy men, elevated baseline levels of IL-6 predict an increased risk of myocardial infarction in the future [82]. IL-6 levels and CRP levels do correlate, but it does appear that they still confer independent contributions to evaluating risk [82].

IL-10 appears to have a protective effect on arteries. Patients with unstable angina have significantly lower levels of IL-10 than patients with chronic stable angina [83,84]. In a murine apo E knockout model, IL-10 deficiency increased LDL cholesterol levels, MMP and tissue factor expression, the Th1 response, and plaque size [85]. IL-10 reduces the expression of MMP-9 and increases the production of TIMP, potentially leading to a plaque-stabilizing effect [86]. Furthermore, there appears to be an interaction with CRP, such that patients with unstable angina with an elevated level of CRP were found to be somewhat protected from ischemic events if their IL-10 level is also increased [87]. Thus, there appears to be a delicate balance between pro- and anti-inflammatory forces, what has been labeled the "Yin and Yang of inflammation" [88]. Purposeful overexpression of IL-10 may prove to be useful therapeutically, assuming that counter-regulatory mechanisms do not immediately negate such attempts [89].

In a prospective study of 1229 patients with stable or unstable angina, elevated levels of IL-18 were found to increase the risk of death [90]. In the Prospective Epidemiological Study of Myocardial Infarction (PRIME), 10,600 healthy European males were followed for 5 years and the rate of subsequent coronary events was determined [91]. Elevated levels of IL-18 at baseline increased the risk of subsequent coronary events in a manner independent to CRP, IL-6, and fibrinogen. CRP has been demonstrated to increase production of IL-18, while IL-10 decreases its production [92].

## Heat Shock Proteins

Autoimmunity to heat shock proteins (HSP) has been hypothesized to contribute to atherosclerosis. Immunoreactivity against HSP has been associated with increased carotid and femoral intima-media thickness (IMT) [93]. Higher levels of antibodies to HSP-65 have been correlated with retinopathy in diabetic patients [94]. Nasal vaccination of LDL receptor-deficient mice with HSP-65 reduced the size of aortic plaques, as well as their macrophage and T cell content [95]. At the same time, HSP vaccination increased IL-10 expression. Induction of oral tolerance with HSP-65 has also been demonstrated to suppress plaque progression in a murine model [96].

## Oxidative Stress and Inflammation

Markers of oxidative stress may also reflect ongoing arterial inflammation. Nitrotyrosine is a marker of protein modification by nitric oxide-derived oxidants. Levels on nitrotyrosine are higher in people with coronary artery disease than in controls [97]. Asymmetric dimethylarginine (ADMA) is an endogenous inhibitor of nitric oxide synthase. A study of patients undergoing hemodialysis found that elevated levels of ADMA correlated with worsening carotid IMT, and that there was an interaction between ADMA and CRP with regards to atheroma progression [98]. Thus, any measurement of inflammatory status will likely need to incorporate markers of oxidative stress in order to give a complete profile of the state of arterial health.

## Measurement of Multiple Markers—The Future

A multimarker approach to risk stratification in ACS is likely to be a higher yield risk stratification tool than measurement of isolated markers. Incorporation of inflammatory markers, such as hs-CRP, markers of embolization and myocardial necrosis such as troponin, and markers of hemodynamic stress, such as B-type natriuretic peptide (BNP), has been shown to provide incremental risk prognostication [99]. In the Global Use of Strategies To Open occluded arteries IV (GUSTO-IV) trial of ACS patients, troponin and CRP both predicted 30-day mortality, but only troponin predicted 30-day risk of MI. Therefore, it does appear that different markers may predict different components of risk at various time-points. Incorporation of even more inflammatory markers should be better still, though this will need to be tested prospectively. Systemic Inflammation Evaluation in patients with non-ST segment elevation acute coronary syndromes (SIESTA) is one such study that will prospectively assess the value of a battery of markers, including CRP, WBC, fibrinogen, BNP, neopterin, interleukins 6, 8, 10 and

18, TNF, E-selectin, endothelin-1, tissue factor, VCAM-1, ICAM-1, PAPP-A, troponin and creatine kinase-MB, in risk prognostication in patients of Mediterranean origin [100]. Studies such as this will be necessary to determine what the incremental value is of newer markers of inflammation.

## NOVEL METHODS TO DETECT ARTERIAL INFLAMMATION

While serum markers of inflammation appear to be most practical, current markers do suffer somewhat from a lack of specificity. An alternative approach to detect arterial inflammation involves going directly to the source—the artery. Technologies to detect inflammation at the plaque level are being developed and tested. For example, intravascular thermography involves using a catheter-thermistor apparatus to measure temperature of coronary plaque. Several studies now support that there is heterogeneity of plaque temperature, likely representing underlying inflammation [101]. Indeed, temperature of coronary plaque appears to correlate with CRP measured peripherally in the blood [102]. The Percutaneous Assessment of Regional and Acute Coronary Hot Unstable plaques by Thermographic Evaluation (PARACHUTE) trial will perform intracoronary thermography on patients with acute coronary syndromes and follow their outcomes. In the future, if techniques can be developed to reliably identify which plaques are prone to rupture, these plaques can be targeted for intervention. Theoretically, plaques that are "hot," even if nonflow limiting, may be treated with a drug-eluting stent or some other modality to mechanically "seal" the plaque, preventing its rupture, superimposed thrombosis, and subsequent ischemia or vessel occlusion.

Virtual histology is another modality that may be useful to determine plaque composition and determine which plaques are rich with inflammatory cells and lipids and likely to rupture. Using radiofrequency backscatter obtained from intravascular ultrasound imaging, it is possible to determine whether a region of plaque is composed of calcium, lipid, or fibrous elements. Combining virtual histology with thermography may lend even further insight into plaque behavior.

While invasive techniques allow precise, localized measurements, they are not, by their invasive nature, appropriate for screening techniques, but, rather, are of potential use only for those patients already in the catheterization laboratory. Magnetic resonance imaging (MRI) is rapidly improving in its degree of image resolution. With its ability to image plaque and characterize its constituents, it may allow us to visualize arterial inflammation that elevated inflammatory markers would suggest. For example, a study of patients with carotid atherosclerosis who underwent high resolution MRI were categorized as either having or not having an intra-plaque lipid pool [103]. Levels of sCD40L were significantly higher in patients with intraplaque lipid, though they did not reflect the diameter stenosis. Thus, CD40 may reflect which plaques are more prone to rupture.

Similarly, elevation of inflammatory markers appears to correlate with carotid IMT, providing further evidence that plaque burden and inflammation are connected [104,105]. CRP, WBC, fibrinogen, VCAM-1, and ICAM-1 are all elevated in those with greater carotid IMT. Simultaneous measurement of inflammatory markers and use of noninvasive imaging modalities may enable us to understand just what component of risk each test measures. Very likely, these forms of risk assessment will be complementary [106].

## THERAPIES TO TARGET INFLAMMATION

Existing therapies for cardiovascular disease have been shown additionally to have anti-inflammatory effects (Table 3). It is not clear in all cases that the anti-inflammatory action

**Table 3**  Existing Drugs that May Target Inflammation

Statins
PPAR γ agonists
Niacin
Fibrates
Ezetimibe
ACE inhibitors
ARBs
Beta-blockers
Aspirin (dose-dependent effect?)
Clopidogrel
Heparin
Enoxaparin
Intravenous GP IIb/IIIa inhibitors
COX-2 inhibitors
NSAIDS
Steroids

PPAR, peroxisome proliferator-activated receptor; ACE, angiotensin converting enzyme; ARBs, angiotensin receptor blockers; GP, glycoprotein; COX, cyclo-oxygenase; NSAIDS, nonsteroidal antiinflammatory drugs

is the dominant or even a minor mode of benefit. Nevertheless, the appreciation that available therapies have anti-inflammatory properties allows us to further explore the role of inflammation in cardiovascular disease and attempt to modify the associated risk.

## Antithrombotic Medications

Perhaps most relevant to a discussion of ACS are therapies that target thrombosis and inflammation simultaneously.

## Aspirin

Several moieties that are important in the thrombotic cascade are also active participants in the inflammatory cascade, and vice versa. Thus, agents conventionally viewed as anti-thrombotic appear to have anti-inflammatory activity. The role of aspirin in ACS is incontrovertible. This benefit is largely due to an antiplatelet effect. Data on an anti-inflammatory effect of aspirin, in doses used for prevention of events in coronary artery disease, have been conflicting [107–109]. Certainly, data from the Physicians' Health Study support that for primary prevention the largest benefit of aspirin is in those with elevated CRP levels [110].

## Glycoprotein IIb/IIIa Intravenous Inhibitors

All the glycoprotein IIb/IIIa inhibitors have been shown to have an anti-inflammatory effect. Abciximab (Centocor, Malvern, PA) was the first agent shown to be able to blunt the rise in inflammatory markers that normally occurs with percutaneous coronary intervention [111]. However, patients with baseline elevation of CRP do not appear to derive any greater benefit from abciximab [112]. This is in contradistinction to CD40 elevation, which does predict benefit from intravenous GPIIb/IIIa inhibitors. All three commercially available intravenous GPIIb/IIIa inhibitors at concentrations sufficient to lead to platelet inhibition suppress CD40 release [113]. Interestingly, levels of intravenous GPIIb/IIIa inhibitors that are subtherapeutic for platelet inhibition can lead to paradoxical platelet activation. Perhaps, this is the mechanism by which oral glycoprotein IIb/IIIa inhibitors were found to be detrimental [114,115]. Platelet adhesion via the GPIIb/IIIa receptor leads to up-regulation of CD40L and induces MMP-2 and MMP-9 proteolytic activity; in theory, this mechanism could contribute to plaque instability and potentially may explain some of the long-term benefits seen with short-term intravenous GPIIb/IIIa inhibition [116].

### Adenosine Diphosphate Receptor Antagonists

Clopidogrel pretreatment prior to PCI has been shown to have its greatest benefit in patients in the highest quartile of baseline CRP (Figure 6) [117]. This suggests, though does not prove, a specific anti-inflammatory benefit. It could be that CRP is serving as a surrogate marker for risk and that clopidogrel is simply of greater benefit in higher risk patients. To address this question, investigators compared the rise in hs-CRP that occurs following PCI between patients either pretreated or not pretreated with clopidogrel [6]. A significant reduction in CRP levels was found in those patients who were clopidogrel pretreated. While this was not a randomized study, the significant differences persisted after multivariate adjustment. A study of patients with acute stroke also suggested that therapy with clopidogrel was associated with a reduction in CRP levels [118].

A small ex vivo study of healthy volunteers showed that clopidogrel significantly diminished CD40 release in response to stimulation with ADP, while aspirin did not [12]. This observation was corroborated in a larger study of patients undergoing PCI in which

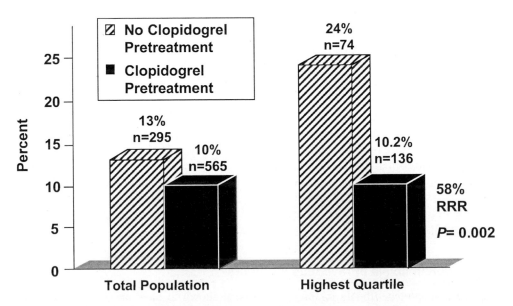

**Figure 6**  The benefit of clopidogrel pretreatment in patients undergoing percutaneous coronary intervention (PCI) is most robust in those within the highest quartile of baseline high sensitivity C-reactive protein (CRP). (From Ref. 117)

clopidogrel pretreatment markedly diminished expression of CD40 [13]. Reductions in other inflammatory markers were also noted in this study. Clopidogrel has also been observed to diminish the extent of interactions between platelets and leukocytes [119].

The Clopidogrel for High Atherothrombotic Risk and Ischemic Stabilization, Management, and Avoidance (CHARISMA) trial will prospectively assess the impact of clopidogrel plus aspirin versus placebo plus aspirin in a population of patients with a history of atherothrombotic events or at risk for atherothrombosis [120]. An inflammatory marker substudy is being performed in which multiple markers are being measured at baseline and on follow-up. The majority of patients will be receiving statins, so CHARISMA will allow a prospective evaluation of the incremental effect of long-term therapy with clopidogrel on inflammatory markers, including hs-CRP and CD40.

## Anticoagulation

Heparin has long been appreciated to have anti-inflammatory properties. Its anti-inflammatory effects are at least in part mediated by blocking P-selectin and L-selectin mediated cell adhesion [121]. Chemical modification of heparin may allow its anti-inflammatory properties to be maximized, while its anticoagulant properties are minimized [121]. Enoxaparin has been shown to lower CRP and von Willebrand Factor levels when compared with dalteparin (or unfractionated heparin) in acute coronary syndromes in the Attribution Randomisee enoxaparine/heparine/dalteparine pour evaluer les Marqueurs d' Activation cellulaire Dans l' Angor instable (ARMADA) study [122]. This suggests that within the class of low-molecular weight heparins, there may be important differences between specific agents. These biological differences may account for the differing levels of clinical efficacy observed with the various low-molecular weight heparins, with apparent superiority of enoxaparin. Thrombin may also function as an inflammatory mediator [123]. Thus, direct thrombin inhibitors such as bivalirudin may also have anti-inflammatory potential.

## Medical Therapy for Inflammation

Beyond antithrombotic therapy, a number of other classes of medications appear to have anti-inflammatory effect and may be pertinent to the management of patients with acute coronary syndromes.

## Statins

Certainly, statins have been shown to have an anti-inflammatory effect. As a class, they have been shown to lower levels of CRP. For the most part, this effect seems independent of their lipid lowering activity [124–126]. This may explain part of their benefit observed even in patients with low levels of cholesterol. Alternatively, it may just be that CRP and LDL cholesterol measurement in concert more accurately reflects the level of oxidized LDL, the more proximate cause of plaque instability and atherosclerotic disease progression. Oxidized LDL binds to CRP [127]. In fact, antibodies to oxidized LDL cholesterol predict worse cardiovascular prognosis [128]. However, some studies do show that the reductions in CRP and LDL are in fact correlated [129]. It does appear that higher doses of statins do lower CRP more than lower doses [130]. Ongoing trials will determine whether this differential effect on inflammatory markers translates into reductions in clinical events.

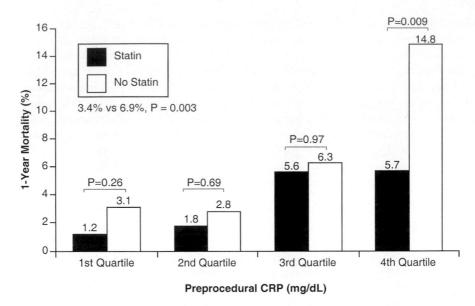

**Figure 7** The mortality benefit of statin pretreatment is most apparent in patients with elevated levels of baseline high-sensitivity C-reactive protein (CRP) (From Ref. 132)

In the setting of PCI, there is evidence that statin pretreatment in associated with improved outcomes, including lower mortality (Figure 7) [131]. Furthermore, this benefit is largely confined to patients with baseline elevation of hs-CRP [132]. This benefit, if real, could not be due to a lipid-lowering effect, but rather must be due to a relatively rapid anti-inflammatory effect. The CRP-lowering effect of statins is measurable within one week of starting therapy [129]. In the setting of ACS, this would support rapid initiation of statin therapy [133]. Regardless of a mortality benefit, starting statin therapy in the inpatient setting is likely to enhance long-term compliance, with no obvious downside to this strategy [134].

The Justification for the Use of Statins in Primary Prevention—an Intervention Trial Evaluating Rosuvastatin (JUPITER) study is randomizing 15,000 healthy patients without markedly elevated cholesterol (LDL cholesterol $<$ 130 mg/dL) but with elevated CRP (hs-CRP $>$ 2 mg/L) levels to either rosuvastatin 20 mg/day or placebo for 3 to 4 years [47,135]. This study will likely validate the use of statins in patients with elevated CRP as a criterion to initiate therapy in a primary prevention population.

## Other Lipid-Lowering Therapy

Therapy classified as lipid-lowering appears to have an anti-inflammatory effect in general. Ezetimibe lowers CRP levels in an incremental manner when added to statin therapy [136,137]. Niacin, when given with a statin, also appears to lower CRP levels [138]. Fibrates, which function as nuclear receptor peroxisome proliferator-activated receptor (PPAR) a agonists, lower CRP levels. Fibrates have been demonstrated to reduce IL-1 induced hepatocyte synthesis of CRP [139]. Decreases in fibrinogen, IL-6, and TNF have also been reported with fibrate therapy [140,141]. Decreases in CRP with fibrates have been correlated with improvements in endothelial dysfunction [142].

## Peroxisome Proliferator-Activated Receptor γ Agonists

PPAR γ agonists, such as the thiazolidinedione rosiglitazone, have been demonstrated to lower levels of hs-CRP, as well as MMP-9, in patients with diabetes mellitus [143]. Even in patients without diabetes mellitus but with coronary artery disease, treatment with rosiglitazone has been found to reduce levels of CRP, E-selectin, von Willebrand Factor, and fibrinogen [144]. PPAR γ agonists inhibit expression of VCAM-1 and ICAM-1 by cultured activated endothelial cells and also prevent monocyte cells from homing to atherosclerotic plaque in an apo-E-deficient murine model [145]. The role of rosiglitazone in patients with the metabolic syndrome in patients undergoing PCI is being investigated in the PPAR γ agonists for the Prevention of Adverse Events following Percutaneous Revascularization (PPAR) trial. As part of PPAR, inflammatory markers and carotid IMT are being compared between rosiglitazone and placebo treated patients.

## Angiotensin Blockade

Angiotensin converting enzyme inhibitors (ACE-I) have been found to have beneficial effects in patients with vascular disease or at high risk for developing it [146]. These benefits have, at times, seemed out of proportion to their blood lowering effects [146]. However, the data set showing that ACE-I lower markers of inflammation is not as large as one might expect [147]. Ongoing work from the European trial on reduction of cardiac events with perindopril in stable coronary artery disease (EUROPA) will examine whether ACE-I really has an effect on inflammation [148]. Angiotensin receptor blockers (ARB) have been shown to lower inflammatory markers including CRP, though more confirmatory studies are necessary [149].

## Nonsteroidal anti-inflammatory drugs

Nonsteroidal anti-inflammatory drugs (NSAIDS) obviously have anti-inflammatory effects. Whether these may provide cardiovascular benefit has not been very thoroughly studied. The clinical data regarding the cardiovascular benefit or detriment of cyclo-oxygenase-2 (COX-2) inhibitors are conflicting [150]. COX-2 inhibitors are, of course, anti-inflammatory agents. COX-2 is up-regulated in atherosclerosis. A 2-week cross-over study of 14 patients with severe coronary artery disease on aspirin and statins found that celecoxib lowered levels of hs-CRP [151]. However, in a randomized, double-blinded placebo controlled trial of 60 patients with angiographic coronary artery disease taking low dose aspirin, it did not appear that rofecoxib had any effect on inflammatory markers, including hs-CRP [152]. On the other hand, the Nonsteroidal Anti-inflammatory Drugs in Unstable Angina Treatment-2 (NUT-2) pilot study found a lower rate of ischemic events in 60 patients who were randomized to 30 days of meloxicam, in addition to therapy with aspirin and heparin [153]. Thus, there are data and plausible explanations for why COX-2 inhibitors may be either pro- or anti-inflammatory with regards to arterial pathology and, perhaps, there may be significant heterogeneity amongst the different COX-2 inhibitors. This conundrum can only be resolved with adequately powered clinical trials of COX-2 inhibitors versus placebo in patients with cardiovascular disease.

## Steroids

Steroids are known to produce many deleterious side effects. Nevertheless, they are anti-inflammatory, so one might expect that their short-term use may have some beneficial cardiovascular effect. Indeed, the Immunosuppressive Therapy for the Prevention of Restenosis after Coronary Artery Stent Implantation (IMPRESS) trial provides such evidence [154]. After undergoing successful stenting, 83 patients with elevated levels of CRP ($>$ 5mg/L) measured 72 hours after their procedure were randomized to 45 days of oral prednisone or placebo. There was a dramatic reduction in 6-month restenosis (7% vs. 33%, p $=$ 0.001) and late loss (0.39 mm vs. 0.85 mm, p $=$ 0.001). If replicated, this may provide a very cost-effective method to reduce restenosis rates with bare metal stents. Beyond that, the IMPRESS trial validates the importance of post-procedural inflammation in patients undergoing PCI.

### Hormone Replacement Therapy

Hormone replacement therapy (HRT) raises levels of CRP [155,156]. Cessation of HRT would, therefore, be expected to reduce CRP levels, and given the absence of cardiovascular benefit of hormone replacement therapy in randomized clinical trials (and indeed a suggestion of detriment), there is no good reason to recommend it for the prevention of cardiovascular disease.

### Antibiotics

As infections have been hypothesized to play a role in atherosclerotic syndromes, antibiotics have been tested to see if they have a beneficial role. Additionally, certain antibiotics may have anti-inflammatory effects separate from their bacteriocidal or bacteriostatic effects. To date, large trials of antibiotics have not shown a reduction in ischemic events, at least not in the dosing regimens and durations studied [157,158].

### Designer Antiinflammatory Agents

Therapies designed to target inflammation specifically are being tested, though they are still in rather preliminary stages of development [159]. One such approach is blockade of the MCP-1 receptor CCR2 on monocytes [160]. Such a blockade reduced neointimal hyperplasia after stenting in a primate model. However, a blockade of neutrophil CD18 was necessary to prevent neointimal hyperplasia after balloon angioplasty in this same model.

Recombinant immunoglobulin soluble P-selectin glycoprotein ligand has been shown to block P-selectin in a porcine model of balloon injury [161]. There is a significant resultant decrease in neointimal hyperplasia and infiltration of macrophages into the area of balloon injury. Immunohistochemistry revealed a significant decrease in TNF $\alpha$ and IL-1 $\beta$. This resulted in a significant increase in luminal area.

### Lifestyle Modification—The Natural Anti-inflammatory

Lifestyle modification may also lower levels of CRP (Table 4). Weight loss has been associated with lowering of inflammatory markers. Exercise can also lower CRP levels. Dieting can lower CRP levels. Fish oil and murine n-3 polyunsaturated fatty acids may lower CRP levels [162]. Perhaps this explains some of the associations between fish oil intake and reductions in sudden cardiac death. Long-term vitamin E and vitamin C supplementation has not been found to lower serum markers of inflammation, paralleling the clinical trials, which have failed to show cardiovascular benefit of these supplements [163,164]. Smoking cessation can lower levels of CRP. Air pollution appears to raise

**Table 4**  Lifestyle Measures that May
Decrease Inflammation

---

Weight loss
Diet
Exercise
n-3 polyunsaturated fatty acids
Smoking cessation
Moderate alcohol intake
Nonuse of hormone replacement therapy
Combating depression
Reducing exposure to air pollution

---

levels of CRP [165]. Moderate alcohol intake is also associated with lower CRP levels compared to than no or occasional alcohol intake [166,167]. The J-shaped relationship between amount of alcohol intake and outcome may, in part, be explained by levels of inflammatory markers [168]. Though preliminary, evidence is also emerging that depressed mood may contribute to CRP elevation [169,170]. More work is needed in this area to ensure that confounding variables are not responsible for this association. Regardless, prior to discharge of the patient with acute coronary syndromes, healthy diet, exercise, weight loss, psychological state, and other lifestyle issues must be addressed to improve patient well-being, decrease future ischemic risk, and, also, combat arterial inflammation.

## GENOMICS OF INFLAMMATION

While the role of inflammation in acute coronary syndromes is now indisputable, the next step in this line of scientific inquiry is the elaboration of the genes that control the production of inflammatory mediators. The first steps in this greater level of understanding have come from the study of single nucleotide polymorphisms (SNPs). For example, Berger and colleagues have demonstrated that CRP levels (as well as fibrinogen levels) are influenced by polymorphisms in the IL-1 gene [171]. Similarly, SNPs of the 3' untranslated region of the CRP gene affect basal CRP levels, as well as levels after stimuli, such as CABG [172]. A polymorphism of the CRP intron has been found to influence CRP levels [173]. Polymorphisms in the IL-6 promoter gene also affect CRP levels [174]. Thus, a component of CRP variability is definitely due to genetic influences.

A specific SNP of the IL-6 promoter gene increases the risk of developing postoperative atrial fibrillation [175]. Patients with atrial fibrillation have higher levels of IL-6 postoperatively and potentially there is a genetic predisposition to the development of atrial fibrillation. IL-6 has been found to be a determinant of outcome in ACS and perhaps patients with this SNP are also more susceptible to complications such as recurrent ischemia—such hypotheses are ripe for testing.

SNPs in the promoter region of the IL-10 gene may affect levels of IL-10 production and may influence the development of disease. A study of dialysis patients found that the risk of cardiovascular events was increased almost threefold if patients carried a particular allele responsible for low levels of IL-10 [176]. Further work on SNPs of the IL-10 gene will likely lead to a deeper appreciation of the role of genetics and inflammation [177]. A functional SNP that results in lower levels of myeloperoxidase activity has been identi-

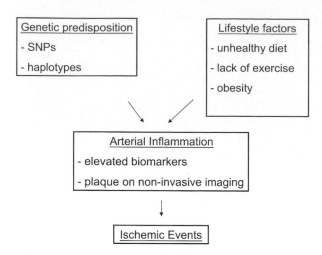

**Figure 8** The interaction between genetics and lifestyle, leading first to subclinical arterial inflammation, then to overt ischemic events. SNP, single nucleotide polymorphism.

fied. In patients with end stage renal disease, this SNP has been associated with a lower prevalence of cardiovascular disease [178].

While the study of SNPs is useful, combinations of polymorphisms, or haplotypes, are of potentially greater importance. For example, an association with restenosis after femoropopliteal angioplasty has been described with SNPs of the IL-1 β gene and a variable number tandem repeat polymorphism in intron 2 of the IL-1 receptor antagonist gene in combination [179].

In the Los Angeles Atherosclerosis Study, investigators found a significant increase in carotid IMT in carriers of two variant 5-lipoxygenase promoter alleles [180,181]. The 6% of the population that carried the variant genes had a significant increase in carotid IMT, and also had a doubling in CRP levels. Interestingly, a diet high in arachidonic acid increased the propensity to carotid plaque progression in patients with the variant alleles, while n-3 fatty acid intake diminished the impact of the variant genotype. Thus, evidence is starting to emerge linking genetic predispositions to arterial inflammation with abnormalities seen by noninvasive plaque imaging modalities, potentially allowing tailoring of dietary recommendations and ultimately individualized medical therapy (Figure 8).

## CONCLUSION

The role of inflammation in acute coronary syndromes is now beyond dispute. While cardiologists were initially resistant to the concept that coronary artery disease is largely a disorder of arterial inflammation, several lines of converging evidence now support this paradigm. Numerous inflammatory markers have proven useful to augment our ability to risk stratify patients who present with acute coronary syndromes. Likely, in the future, panels of inflammatory markers will be assayed with point of care testing at the time of patient presentation. Beyond an incremental ability to risk stratify, these markers may enable specific application of therapies to patients with particular ''inflammatory profiles.'' Ultimately, the genetic basis of arterial inflammation will be unraveled, allowing even greater precision of risk stratification and individualization of therapy.

# REFERENCES

1. Bhatt DL, Topol EJ. Current role of platelet glycoprotein IIb/IIIa inhibitors in acute coronary syndromes. JAMA; 2000;284:1549-1558.

2. Bhatt DL, Topol EJ. Need to test the arterial inflammation hypothesis. Circulation; 2002; 106:136-40.

3. Buffon A, Biasucci LM, Liuzzo G, D'Onofrio G, Crea F, Maseri A. Widespread coronary inflammation in unstable angina. N Engl J Med; 2002;347:5-12.

4. Rioufol G, Finet G, Ginon I, Andre-Fouet X, Rossi R, Vialle E, Desjoyaux E, Convert G, Huret JF, Tabib A. Multiple atherosclerotic plaque rupture in acute coronary syndrome: a three-vessel intravascular ultrasound study. Circulation; 2002;106:804-8.

5. Cusack MR, Marber MS, Lambiase PD, Bucknall CA, Redwood SR. Systemic inflammation in unstable angina is the result of myocardial necrosis. J Am Coll Cardiol; 2002;39:1917-23.

6. Bhatt DL, Topol EJ. Scientific and therapeutic advances in antiplatelet therapy. Nat Rev Drug Discov; 2003;2:15-28.

7. Henn V, Slupsky JR, Grafe M, Anagnostopoulos I, Forster R, Muller-Berghaus G, Kroczek RA. CD40 ligand on activated platelets triggers an inflammatory reaction of endothelial cells. Nature; 1998;391:591-4.

8. Elzey BD, Tian J, Jensen RJ, Swanson AK, Lees JR, Lentz SR, Stein CS, Nieswandt B, Wang Y, Davidson BL, Ratliff TL. Platelet-mediated modulation of adaptive immunity. A communication link between innate and adaptive immune compartments. Immunity; 2003; 19:9-19.

9. Andre P, Prasad KS, Denis CV, He M, Papalia JM, Hynes RO, Phillips DR, Wagner DD. CD40L stabilizes arterial thrombi by a beta3 integrin-dependent mechanism. Nat Med; 2002; 8:247-52.

10. Tamura N, Yoshida M, Ichikawa N, Handa M, Ikeda Y, Tanabe T, Handa S, Goto S. Shear-induced von Willebrand factor-mediated platelet surface translocation of the CD40 ligand. Thromb Res; 2002;108:311-5.

11. Heeschen C, Dimmeler S, Hamm CW, van den Brand MJ, Boersma E, Zeiher AM, Simoons ML. Soluble CD40 ligand in acute coronary syndromes. N Engl J Med; 2003;348:1104-11.

12. Hermann A, Rauch BH, Braun M, Schror K, Weber AA. Platelet CD40 ligand (CD40L)-sub-cellular localization, regulation of expression, and inhibition by clopidogrel. Platelets; 2001; 12:74-82.

13. Quinn M, Bhatt DL, Zidar F, Vivekananthan D, Chew DP, Ellis SG, Plow E, EJ T. Effect of clopidogrel pretreatment on inflammatory marker expression in patients undergoing percutaneous coronary intervention. American Journal of Cardiology; 2004;93:679-84.

14. Cipollone F, Ferri C, Desideri G, Paloscia L, Materazzo G, Mascellanti M, Fazia M, Iezzi A, Cuccurullo C, Pini B, Bucci M, Santucci A, Cuccurullo F, Mezzetti A. Preprocedural level of soluble CD40L is predictive of enhanced inflammatory response and restenosis after coronary angioplasty. Circulation; 2003;108:2776-82.

15. Stumpf C, Lehner C, Eskafi S, Raaz D, Yilmaz A, Ropers S, Schmeisser A, Ludwig J, Daniel WG, Garlichs CD. Enhanced levels of CD154 (CD40 ligand) on platelets in patients with chronic heart failure. Eur J Heart Fail; 2003;5:629-37.

16. Kopp CW, Steiner S, Nasel C, Seidinger D, Mlekusch I, Lang W, Bartok A, Ahmadi R, Minar E. Abciximab reduces monocyte tissue factor in carotid angioplasty and stenting. Stroke; 2003;34:2560-7.

17. Schonbeck U, Gerdes N, Varo N, Reynolds RS, Horton DB, Bavendiek U, Robbie L, Ganz P, Kinlay S, Libby P. Oxidized low-density lipoprotein augments and 3-hydroxy-3- methyl-glutaryl coenzyme A reductase inhibitors limit CD40 and CD40L expression in human vascular cells. Circulation; 2002;106:2888-93.

18. Cipollone F, Mezzetti A, Porreca E, Di Febbo C, Nutini M, Fazia M, Falco A, Cuccurullo F, Davi G. Association between enhanced soluble CD40L and prothrombotic state in hypercholesterolemia: effects of statin therapy. Circulation; 2002;106:399-402.

19. Nannizzi-Alaimo L, Rubenstein MH, Alves VL, Leong GY, Phillips DR, Gold HK. Cardiopul-monary bypass induces release of soluble CD40 ligand. Circulation; 2002;105:2849-54.

20. Wang CL, Wu YT, Liu CA, Lin MW, Lee CJ, Huang LT, Yang KD. Expression of CD40 ligand on CD4+ T-cells and platelets correlated to the coronary artery lesion and disease progress in Kawasaki disease. Pediatrics; 2003;111:E140-7.

21. Danese S, Katz JA, Saibeni S, Papa A, Gasbarrini A, Vecchi M, Fiocchi C. Activated platelets are the source of elevated levels of soluble CD40 ligand in the circulation of inflammatory bowel disease patients. Gut; 2003;52:1435-41.

22. Danese S, de la Motte C, Sturm A, Vogel JD, West GA, Strong SA, Katz JA, Fiocchi C. Platelets trigger a CD40-dependent inflammatory response in the microvasculature of inflammatory bowel disease patients. Gastroenterology; 2003;124:1249-64.

23. Mallat Z, Gojova A, Brun V, Esposito B, Fournier N, Cottrez F, Tedgui A, Groux H. Induction of a regulatory T cell type 1 response reduces the development of atherosclerosis in apolipo-protein E-knockout mice. Circulation; 2003;108:1232-7.

24. Janket SJ, Baird AE, Chuang SK, Jones JA. Meta-analysis of periodontal disease and risk of coronary heart disease and stroke. Oral Surg Oral Med Oral Pathol Oral Radiol Endod; 2003;95:559-69.

25. Joshipura KJ, Hung HC, Rimm EB, Willett WC, Ascherio A. Periodontal disease, tooth loss, and incidence of ischemic stroke. Stroke; 2003;34:47-52.

26. Hung HC, Willett W, Merchant A, Rosner BA, Ascherio A, Joshipura KJ. Oral health and peripheral arterial disease. Circulation; 2003;107:1152-7.

27. Desvarieux M, Demmer RT, Rundek T, Boden-Albala B, Jacobs DR, Jr, Papapanou PN, Sacco RL. Relationship between periodontal disease, tooth loss, and carotid artery plaque: the Oral Infections and Vascular Disease Epidemiology Study (INVEST). Stroke; 2003;34: 2120-5.

28. Slade GD, Ghezzi EM, Heiss G, Beck JD, Riche E, Offenbacher S. Relationship between periodontal disease and C-reactive protein among adults in the Atherosclerosis Risk in Com-munities study. Arch Intern Med; 2003;163:1172-9.

29. Amar S, Gokce N, Morgan S, Loukideli M, Van Dyke TE, Vita JA. Periodontal disease is associated with brachial artery endothelial dysfunction and systemic inflammation. Arte-rioscler Thromb Vasc Biol; 2003;23:1245-9.

30. Loos BG, Craandijk J, Hoek FJ, Wertheim-van Dillen PM, van der Velden U. Elevation of systemic markers related to cardiovascular diseases in the peripheral blood of periodontitis patients. J Periodontol; 2000;71:1528-34.

31. Rexrode KM, Pradhan A, Manson JE, Buring JE, Ridker PM. Relationship of total and abdominal adiposity with CRP and IL-6 in women. Ann Epidemiol; 2003;13:674-82.

32. Christ-Crain M, Meier C, Guglielmetti M, Huber PR, Riesen W, Staub JJ, Muller B. Elevated C-reactive protein and homocysteine values: cardiovascular risk factors in hypothyroidism? A cross-sectional and a double-blind, placebo-controlled trial. Atherosclerosis; 2003;166: 379-86.

33. Panichi V, Migliori M, De Pietro S, Taccola D, Bianchi AM, Giovannini L, Norpoth M, Metelli MR, Cristofani R, Bertelli AA, Sbragia G, Tetta C, Palla R. C-reactive protein and interleukin-6 levels are related to renal function in predialytic chronic renal failure. Nephron; 2002;91:594-600.

34. Shlipak MG, Fried LF, Crump C, Bleyer AJ, Manolio TA, Tracy RP, Furberg CD, Psaty BM. Elevations of inflammatory and procoagulant biomarkers in elderly persons with renal insufficiency. Circulation; 2003;107:87-92.

35. Roman MJ, Shanker BA, Davis A, Lockshin MD, Sammaritano L, Simantov R, Crow MK, Schwartz JE, Paget SA, Devereux RB, Salmon JE. Prevalence and correlates of accelerated atherosclerosis in systemic lupus erythematosus. N Engl J Med; 2003;349:2399-406.

36. Shishehbor MH, Bhatt DL, Topol EJ. Using C-reactive protein to assess cardiovascular disease risk. Cleve Clin J Med; 2003;70:634-40.

37. Pearson TA, Mensah GA, Alexander RW, Anderson JL, Cannon RO, 3rd, Criqui M, Fadl YY, Fortmann SP, Hong Y, Myers GL, Rifai N, Smith SC, Jr, Taubert K, Tracy RP, Vinicor

F. Markers of inflammation and cardiovascular disease: application to clinical and public health practice: A statement for healthcare professionals from the Centers for Disease Control and Prevention and the American Heart Association. Circulation; 2003;107:499-511.

38. Blake GJ, Ridker PM. C-reactive protein and other inflammatory risk markers in acute coronary syndromes. J Am Coll Cardiol.; 2003;41:37S-42S.

39. Zairis MN, Manousakis SJ, Stefanidis AS, Papadaki OA, Andrikopoulos GK, Olympios CD, Hadjissavas JJ, Argyrakis SK, Foussas SG. C-reactive protein levels on admission are associated with response to thrombolysis and prognosis after ST-segment elevation acute myocardial infarction. Am Heart J; 2002;144:782-9.

40. Morrow DA, Rifai N, Antman EM, Weiner DL, McCabe CH, Cannon CP, Braunwald E. C-reactive protein is a potent predictor of mortality independently of and in combination with troponin T in acute coronary syndromes: a TIMI 11A substudy. Thrombolysis in Myocardial Infarction. J Am Coll Cardiol; 1998;31:1460-5.

41. Chew DP, Bhatt DL, Robbins MA, Penn MS, Schneider JP, Lauer MS, Topol EJ, Ellis SG. Incremental prognostic value of elevated baseline C-reactive protein among established markers of risk in percutaneous coronary intervention. Circulation; 2001;104:992-7.

42. Burke AP, Tracy RP, Kolodgie F, Malcom GT, Zieske A, Kutys R, Pestaner J, Smialek J, Virmani R. Elevated C-reactive protein values and atherosclerosis in sudden coronary death: association with different pathologies. Circulation; 2002;105:2019-23.

43. Alvarez Garcia B, Ruiz C, Chacon P, Sabin JA, Matas M. High-sensitivity C-reactive protein in high-grade carotid stenosis: risk marker for unstable carotid plaque. J Vasc Surg; 2003; 38:1018-24.

44. Thorand B, Lowel H, Schneider A, Kolb H, Meisinger C, Frohlich M, Koenig W. C-reactive protein as a predictor for incident diabetes mellitus among middle-aged men: results from the MONICA Augsburg cohort study, 1984- 1998. Arch Intern Med; 2003;163:93-9.

45. Sesso HD, Buring JE, Rifai N, Blake GJ, Gaziano JM, Ridker PM. C-reactive protein and the risk of developing hypertension. Jama; 2003;290:2945-51.

46. Bhatt DL, Topol EJ. The arterial inflammation hypothesis. Arch Intern Med; 2002;162:2249-51.

47. Ridker PM. Rosuvastatin in the primary prevention of cardiovascular disease among patients with low levels of low-density lipoprotein cholesterol and elevated high-sensitivity C-reactive protein: rationale and design of the JUPITER trial. Circulation; 2003;108:2292-7.

48. Devaraj S, Xu DY, Jialal I. C-reactive protein increases plasminogen activator inhibitor-1 expression and activity in human aortic endothelial cells: implications for the metabolic syndrome and atherothrombosis. Circulation; 2003;107:398-404.

49. Verma S, Wang CH, Li SH, Dumont AS, Fedak PW, Badiwala MV, Dhillon B, Weisel RD, Li RK, Mickle DA, Stewart DJ. A self-fulfilling prophecy: C-reactive protein attenuates nitric oxide production and inhibits angiogenesis. Circulation; 2002;106:913-9.

50. Yasojima K, Schwab C, McGeer EG, McGeer PL. Generation of C-Reactive Protein and Complement Components in Atherosclerotic Plaques. Am J Pathol; 2001;158:1039-1051.

51. Hoffmeister HM, Ehlers R, Buttcher E, Kazmaier S, Szabo S, Beyer ME, Steinmetz A, Seipel L. Comparison of C-reactive protein and terminal complement complex in patients with unstable angina pectoris versus stable angina pectoris. Am J Cardiol; 2002;89:909-12.

52. Zwaka TP, Hombach V, Torzewski J. C-reactive protein-mediated low density lipoprotein uptake by macrophages : implications for atherosclerosis. Circulation; 2001;103:1194-7.

53. Torzewski M, Rist C, Mortensen RF, Zwaka TP, Bienek M, Waltenberger J, Koenig W, Schmitz G, Hombach V, Torzewski J. C-reactive protein in the arterial intima: role of C-reactive protein receptor-dependent monocyte recruitment in atherogenesis. Arterioscler Thromb Vasc Biol; 2000;20:2094-9.

54. Verma S, Badiwala MV, Weisel RD, Li SH, Wang CH, Fedak PW, Li RK, Mickle DA. C-reactive protein activates the nuclear factor-kappaB signal transduction pathway in saphenous vein endothelial cells: Implications for atherosclerosis and restenosis. J Thorac Cardiovasc Surg; 2003;126:1886-91.

55. Bhatt DL, Chew DP, Lincoff AM, Simoons ML, Harrington RA, Ommen SR, Jia G, Topol EJ. Effect of revascularization on mortality associated with an elevated white blood cell count in acute coronary syndromes. Am J Cardiol; 2003;92:136-140.

56. Yen MH, Bhatt DL, Chew DP, Harrington RA, Newby LK, Ardissino D, Werf FV, White JA, Moliterno DJ, Topol EJ. Association between admission white blood cell count and one-year mortality in patients with acute coronary syndromes. Am J Med; 2003;115:318-21.

57. Gurm HS, Bhatt DL, Lincoff AM, Tcheng JE, Kereiakes DJ, Kleiman NS, Jia G, Topol EJ. Impact of preprocedural white blood cell count on long term mortality after percutaneous coronary intervention: insights from the EPIC, EPILOG, and EPISTENT trials. Heart; 2003; 89:1200-4.

58. Gurm HS, Bhatt DL, Gupta R, Ellis SG, Topol EJ, Lauer MS. Preprocedural white blood cell count and death after percutaneous coronary intervention. Am Heart J; 2003;146:692-8.

59. Aronow HD, Shishebor MH, Davis DA. White blood cell count predicts microembolic Doppler signals during carotid stenting: a link between inflammation and embolization. Circulation; 2002;106:II-577.

60. Naruko T, Ueda M, Haze K, van der Wal AC, van der Loos CM, Itoh A, Komatsu R, Ikura Y, Ogami M, Shimada Y, Ehara S, Yoshiyama M, Takeuchi K, Yoshikawa J, Becker AE. Neutrophil infiltration of culprit lesions in acute coronary syndromes. Circulation; 2002;106: 2894-900.

61. Askari AT, Brennan ML, Zhou X, Drinko J, Morehead A, Thomas JD, Topol EJ, Hazen SL, Penn MS. Myeloperoxidase and plasminogen activator inhibitor 1 play a central role in ventricular remodeling after myocardial infarction. J Exp Med; 2003;197:615-24.

62. Sugiyama S, Okada Y, Sukhova GK, Virmani R, Heinecke JW, Libby P. Macrophage myeloperoxidase regulation by granulocyte macrophage colony-stimulating factor in human atherosclerosis and implications in acute coronary syndromes. Am J Pathol; 2001;158:879-91.

63. Baldus S, Heeschen C, Meinertz T, Zeiher AM, Eiserich JP, Munzel T, Simoons ML, Hamm CW. Myeloperoxidase serum levels predict risk in patients with acute coronary syndromes. Circulation; 2003;108:1440-5.

64. Brennan ML, Penn MS, Van Lente F, Nambi V, Shishehbor MH, Aviles RJ, Goormastic M, Pepoy ML, McErlean ES, Topol EJ, Nissen SE, Hazen SL. Prognostic value of myeloperoxidase in patients with chest pain. N Engl J Med; 2003;349:1595-604.

65. Smith DA, Zouridakis EG, Mariani M, Fredericks S, Cole D, Kaski JC. Neopterin levels in patients with coronary artery disease are independent of Chlamydia pneumoniae seropositivity. Am Heart J; 2003;146:69-74.

66. Auer J, Berent R, Labetanig E, Eber B. Serum neopterin and activity of coronary artery disease. Heart Dis; 2001;3:297-301.

67. Garcia-Moll X, Coccolo F, Cole D, Kaski JC. Serum neopterin and complex stenosis morphology in patients with unstable angina. J Am Coll Cardiol; 2000;35:956-62.

68. Gurfinkel EP, Scirica BM, Bozovich G, Macchia A, Manos E, Mautner B. Serum neopterin levels and the angiographic extent of coronary arterial narrowing in unstable angina pectoris and in non-Q-wave acute myocardial infarction. Am J Cardiol; 1999;83:515-8.

69. Pecoits-Filho R, Heimburger O, Barany P, Suliman M, Fehrman-Ekholm I, Lindholm B, Stenvinkel P. Associations between circulating inflammatory markers and residual renal function in CRF patients. Am J Kidney Dis; 2003;41:1212-8.

70. Walter RB, Fuchs D, Weiss G, Walter TR, Reinhart WH. HMG-CoA reductase inhibitors are associated with decreased serum neopterin levels in stable coronary artery disease. Clin Chem Lab Med; 2003;41:1314-9.

71. Ikeda H, Ueyama T, Murohara T, Yasukawa H, Haramaki N, Eguchi H, Katoh A, Takajo Y, Onitsuka I, Ueno T, Tojo SJ, Imaizumi T. Adhesive interaction between P-selectin and sialyl Lewis(x) plays an important role in recurrent coronary arterial thrombosis in dogs. Arterioscler Thromb Vasc Biol; 1999;19:1083-90.

72. Ridker PM, Buring JE, Rifai N. Soluble P-selectin and the risk of future cardiovascular events. Circulation; 2001;103:491-5.

73. Pasceri V, Willerson JT, Yeh ET. Direct proinflammatory effect of C-reactive protein on human endothelial cells. Circulation; 2000;102:2165-8.

74. de Lemos JA, Morrow DA, Sabatine MS, Murphy SA, Gibson CM, Antman EM, McCabe CH, Cannon CP, Braunwald E. Association between plasma levels of monocyte chemoattractant

protein-1 and long-term clinical outcomes in patients with acute coronary syndromes. Circulation; 2003;107:690-5.

75. Ridker PM, Hennekens CH, Buring JE, Rifai N. C-reactive protein and other markers of inflammation in the prediction of cardiovascular disease in women. N Engl J Med; 2000; 342:836-43.

76. Blake GJ, Dada N, Fox JC, Manson JE, Ridker PM. A prospective evaluation of lipoprotein-associated phospholipase A(2) levels and the risk of future cardiovascular events in women. J Am Coll Cardiol; 2001;38:1302-6.

77. Beaudeux JL, Burc L, Imbert-Bismut F, Giral P, Bernard M, Bruckert E, Chapman MJ. Serum plasma pregnancy-associated protein A: a potential marker of echogenic carotid atherosclerotic plaques in asymptomatic hyperlipidemic subjects at high cardiovascular risk. Arterioscler Thromb Vasc Biol; 2003;23:e7-10.

78. Ferroni P, Basili S, Martini F, Cardarello CM, Ceci F, Di Franco M, Bertazzoni G, Gazzaniga PP, Alessandri C. Serum metalloproteinase 9 levels in patients with coronary artery disease: a novel marker of inflammation. J Investig Med; 2003;51:295-300.

79. Nomoto K, Oguchi S, Watanabe I, Kushiro T, Kanmatsuse K. Involvement of inflammation in acute coronary syndromes assessed by levels of high-sensitivity C-reactive protein, matrix metalloproteinase-9 and soluble vascular-cell adhesion molecule-1. J Cardiol; 2003;42:201-6.

80. Maksimowicz-McKinnon K, Bhatt DL, Calabrese LH. Recent advances in vascular inflammation: C-reactive protein and other inflammatory biomarkers. Curr Opin Rheumatol; 2004;16: 18-24.

81. Lindmark E, Diderholm E, Wallentin L, Siegbahn A. Relationship between interleukin 6 and mortality in patients with unstable coronary artery disease: effects of an early invasive or noninvasive strategy. Jama; 2001;286:2107-13.

82. Ridker PM, Rifai N, Stampfer MJ, Hennekens CH. Plasma concentration of interleukin-6 and the risk of future myocardial infarction among apparently healthy men. Circulation; 2000; 101:1767-72.

83. Smith DA, Irving SD, Sheldon J, Cole D, Kaski JC. Serum levels of the antiinflammatory cytokine interleukin-10 are decreased in patients with unstable angina. Circulation; 2001; 104:746-9.

84. Anguera I, Miranda-Guardiola F, Bosch X, Filella X, Sitges M, Marin JL, Betriu A, Sanz G. Elevation of serum levels of the anti-inflammatory cytokine interleukin-10 and decreased risk of coronary events in patients with unstable angina. Am Heart J; 2002;144:811-7.

85. Caligiuri G, Rudling M, Ollivier V, Jacob MP, Michel JB, Hansson GK, Nicoletti A. Interleukin-10 deficiency increases atherosclerosis, thrombosis, and low-density lipoproteins in apolipoprotein E knockout mice. Mol Med; 2003;9:10-7.

86. Waehre T, Halvorsen B, Damas JK, Yndestad A, Brosstad F, Gullestad L, Kjekshus J, Froland SS, Aukrust P. Inflammatory imbalance between IL-10 and TNFalpha in unstable angina potential plaque stabilizing effects of IL-10. Eur J Clin Invest; 2002;32:803-10.

87. Heeschen C, Dimmeler S, Hamm CW, Fichtlscherer S, Boersma E, Simoons ML, Zeiher AM. Serum level of the antiinflammatory cytokine interleukin-10 is an important prognostic determinant in patients with acute coronary syndromes. Circulation; 2003;107:2109-14.

88. Bhatt DL, Mills R. The yin and yang of arterial inflammation. J Am Coll Cardiol; 2004;44: 50-2.

89. Pinderski LJ, Fischbein MP, Subbanagounder G, Fishbein MC, Kubo N, Cheroutre H, Curtiss LK, Berliner JA, Boisvert WA. Overexpression of interleukin-10 by activated T lymphocytes inhibits atherosclerosis in LDL receptor-deficient Mice by altering lymphocyte and macrophage phenotypes. Circ Res; 2002;90:1064-71.

90. Blankenberg S, Tiret L, Bickel C, Peetz D, Cambien F, Meyer J, Rupprecht HJ. Interleukin-18 is a strong predictor of cardiovascular death in stable and unstable angina. Circulation; 2002;106:24-30.

91. Blankenberg S, Luc G, Ducimetiere P, Arveiler D, Ferrieres J, Amouyel P, Evans A, Cambien F, Tiret L. Interleukin-18 and the risk of coronary heart disease in European men: the Prospec-

tive Epidemiological Study of Myocardial Infarction (PRIME). Circulation; 2003;108:2453-9.

92. Yamaoka-Tojo M, Tojo T, Masuda T, Machida Y, Kitano Y, Kurosawa T, Izumi T. C-reactive protein-induced production of interleukin-18 in human endothelial cells: a mechanism of orchestrating cytokine cascade in acute coronary syndrome. Heart Vessels; 2003;18:183-7.

93. Knoflach M, Kiechl S, Kind M, Said M, Sief R, Gisinger M, van der Zee R, Gaston H, Jarosch E, Willeit J, Wick G. Cardiovascular risk factors and atherosclerosis in young males: ARMY study (Atherosclerosis Risk-Factors in Male Youngsters). Circulation; 2003;108:1064-9.

94. Weitgasser R, Lechleitner M, Koch T, Galvan G, Muhlmann J, Steiner K, Hoppichler F. Antibodies to heat-shock protein 65 and neopterin levels in patients with type 1 diabetes mellitus. Exp Clin Endocrinol Diabetes; 2003;111:127-31.

95. Maron R, Sukhova G, Faria AM, Hoffmann E, Mach F, Libby P, Weiner HL. Mucosal administration of heat shock protein-65 decreases atherosclerosis and inflammation in aortic arch of low-density lipoprotein receptor-deficient mice. Circulation; 2002;106:1708-15.

96. Harats D, Yacov N, Gilburd B, Shoenfeld Y, George J. Oral tolerance with heat shock protein 65 attenuates Mycobacterium tuberculosis-induced and high-fat-diet-driven atherosclerotic lesions. J Am Coll Cardiol; 2002;40:1333-8.

97. Shishehbor MH, Aviles RJ, Brennan ML, Fu X, Goormastic M, Pearce GL, Gokce N, Keaney JF, Jr, Penn MS, Sprecher DL, Vita JA, Hazen SL. Association of nitrotyrosine levels with cardiovascular disease and modulation by statin therapy. JAMA; 2003;289:1675-80.

98. Zoccali C, Benedetto FA, Maas R, Mallamaci F, Tripepi G, Malatino LS, Boger R. Asymmetric dimethylarginine, C-reactive protein, and carotid intima-media thickness in end-stage renal disease. J Am Soc Nephrol; 2002;13:490-6.

99. Sabatine MS, Morrow DA, de Lemos JA, Gibson CM, Murphy SA, Rifai N, McCabe C, Antman EM, Cannon CP, Braunwald E. Multimarker approach to risk stratification in non-ST elevation acute coronary syndromes: simultaneous assessment of troponin I, C-reactive protein, and B-type natriuretic peptide. Circulation; 2002;105:1760-3.

100. Kaski JC, Cruz-Fernandez JM, Fernandez-Berges D, Garcia-Moll X, Martin Jadraque L, Mostaza J, Lopez Garcia-Aranda V, Gonzalez Juanatey JR, Castro Beiras A, Martin Luengo C, Alonso Garcia A, Lopez-Bescos L, Marcos Gomez G. [Inflammation markers and risk stratification in patients with acute coronary syndromes: design of the SIESTA Study (Systemic Inflammation Evaluation in Patients with non-ST segment elevation Acute coronary syndromes)]. Rev Esp Cardiol; 2003;56:389-95.

101. Stefanadis C, Diamantopoulos L, Vlachopoulos C, Tsiamis E, Dernellis J, Toutouzas K, Stefanadi E, Toutouzas P. Thermal heterogeneity within human atherosclerotic coronary arteries detected in vivo: A new method of detection by application of a special thermography catheter. Circulation; 1999;99:1965-71.

102. Stefanadis C, Diamantopoulos L, Dernellis J, Economou E, Tsiamis E, Toutouzas K, Vlachopoulos C, Toutouzas P. Heat production of atherosclerotic plaques and inflammation assessed by the acute phase proteins in acute coronary syndromes. J Mol Cell Cardiol; 2000;32:43-52.

103. Blake GJ, Ostfeld RJ, Yucel EK, Varo N, Schonbeck U, Blake MA, Gerhard M, Ridker PM, Libby P, Lee RT. Soluble CD40 ligand levels indicate lipid accumulation in carotid atheroma: an in vivo study with high-resolution MRI. Arterioscler Thromb Vasc Biol; 2003;23:e11-4.

104. Magyar MT, Szikszai Z, Balla J, Valikovics A, Kappelmayer J, Imre S, Balla G, Jeney V, Csiba L, Bereczki D. Early-onset carotid atherosclerosis is associated with increased intima-media thickness and elevated serum levels of inflammatory markers. Stroke; 2003;34:58-63.

105. Papagianni A, Kalovoulos M, Kirmizis D, Vainas A, Belechri AM, Alexopoulos E, Memmos D. Carotid atherosclerosis is associated with inflammation and endothelial cell adhesion molecules in chronic haemodialysis patients. Nephrol Dial Transplant; 2003;18:113-9.

106. Cao JJ, Thach C, Manolio TA, Psaty BM, Kuller LH, Chaves PH, Polak JF, Sutton-Tyrrell K, Herrington DM, Price TR, Cushman M. C-reactive protein, carotid intima-media thickness,

and incidence of ischemic stroke in the elderly: the Cardiovascular Health Study. Circulation; 2003;108:166-70.

107. Feng D, Tracy RP, Lipinska I, Murillo J, McKenna C, Tofler GH. Effect of short-term aspirin use on C-reactive protein. J Thromb Thrombolysis; 2000;9:37-41.

108. Ikonomidis I, Andreotti F, Economou E, Stefanadis C, Toutouzas P, Nihoyannopoulos P. Increased proinflammatory cytokines in patients with chronic stable angina and their reduction by aspirin. Circulation; 1999;100:793-8.

109. Feldman M, Jialal I, Devaraj S, Cryer B. Effects of low-dose aspirin on serum C-reactive protein and thromboxane B2 concentrations: a placebo-controlled study using a highly sensitive C-reactive protein assay. J Am Coll Cardiol; 2001;37:2036-41.

110. Ridker PM, Cushman M, Stampfer MJ, Tracy RP, Hennekens CH. Inflammation, aspirin, and the risk of cardiovascular disease in apparently healthy men. N Engl J Med; 1997;336: 973-9.

111. Lincoff AM, Kereiakes DJ, Mascelli MA, Deckelbaum LI, Barnathan ES, Patel KK, Frederick B, Nakada MT, Topol EJ. Abciximab suppresses the rise in levels of circulating inflammatory markers after percutaneous coronary revascularization. Circulation; 2001;104:163-7.

112. Lenderink T, Boersma E, Heeschen C, Vahanian A, de Boer MJ, Umans V, van den Brand MJ, Hamm CW, Simoons ML. Elevated troponin T and C-reactive protein predict impaired outcome for 4 years in patients with refractory unstable angina, and troponin T predicts benefit of treatment with abciximab in combination with PTCA. Eur Heart J; 2003;24:77-85.

113. Nannizzi-Alaimo L, Alves VL, Phillips DR. Inhibitory effects of glycoprotein IIb/IIIa antagonists and aspirin on the release of soluble CD40 ligand during platelet stimulation. Circulation; 2003;107:1123-8.

114. Chew DP, Bhatt DL, Sapp S, Topol EJ. Increased mortality with oral platelet glycoprotein IIb/IIIa antagonists: A meta-analysis of phase III multicenter randomized trials. Circulation; 2001;103:201-206.

115. Chew DP, Bhatt DL. Oral glycoprotein IIb/IIIa antagonists in coronary artery disease. Curr Cardiol Rep; 2001;3:63-71.

116. May AE, Kalsch T, Massberg S, Herouy Y, Schmidt R, Gawaz M. Engagement of glycoprotein IIb/IIIa (alpha(IIb)beta3) on platelets upregulates CD40L and triggers CD40L-dependent matrix degradation by endothelial cells. Circulation; 2002;106:2111-7.

117. Chew DP, Bhatt DL, Robbins MA, Mukherjee D, Roffi M, Schneider JP, Topol EJ, Ellis SG. Effect of clopidogrel added to aspirin before percutaneous coronary intervention on the risk associated with C-reactive protein. Am J Cardiol; 2001;88:672-4.

118. Cha JK, Jeong MH, Lee KM, Bae HR, Lim YJ, Park KW, Cheon SM. Changes in platelet p-selectin and in plasma C-reactive protein in acute atherosclerotic ischemic stroke treated with a loading dose of clopidogrel. J Thromb Thrombolysis; 2002;14:145-50.

119. Klinkhardt U, Graff J, Harder S. Clopidogrel, but not abciximab, reduces platelet leukocyte conjugates and P-selectin expression in a human ex vivo in vitro model. Clin Pharmacol Ther; 2002;71:176-85.

120. Bhatt DL, Topol EJ. The Rationale and Design of the CHARISMA Trial. Am Heart J 2004:; In :press.

121. Wang L, Brown JR, Varki A, Esko JD. Heparin's anti-inflammatory effects require glucosamine 6-O-sulfation and are mediated by blockade of L- and P-selectins. J Clin Invest; 2002; 110:127-36.

122. Montalescot G, Bal-dit-Sollier C, Chibedi D, Collet JP, Soulat T, Dalby M, Choussat R, Cohen A, Slama M, Steg PG, Dubois-Rande JL, Metzger JP, Tarragano F, Guermonprez JL, Drouet L. Comparison of effects on markers of blood cell activation of enoxaparin, dalteparin, and unfractionated heparin in patients with unstable angina pectoris or non-ST-segment elevation acute myocardial infarction (the ARMADA study). Am J Cardiol; 2003;91:925-30.

123. Cirino G, Cicala C, Bucci MR, Sorrentino L, Maraganore JM, Stone SR. Thrombin functions as an inflammatory mediator through activation of its receptor. J Exp Med; 1996;183:821-7.

124. Ridker PM, Rifai N, Pfeffer MA, Sacks F, Braunwald E. Long-term effects of pravastatin on plasma concentration of C-reactive protein. The Cholesterol and Recurrent Events (CARE) Investigators. Circulation; 1999;100:230-5.

125. Ridker PM, Rifai N, Lowenthal SP. Rapid reduction in C-reactive protein with cerivastatin among 785 patients with primary hypercholesterolemia. Circulation; 2001;103:1191-1193.

126. Albert MA, Danielson E, Rifai N, Ridker PM. Effect of statin therapy on C-reactive protein levels: the pravastatin inflammation/CRP evaluation (PRINCE): a randomized trial and cohort study. Jama; 2001;286:64-70.

127. Miller YI, Chang MK, Binder CJ, Shaw PX, Witztum JL. Oxidized low density lipoprotein and innate immune receptors. Curr Opin Lipidol; 2003;14:437-45.

128. Bayes B, Pastor MC, Bonal J, Junca J, Hernandez JM, Riutort N, Foraster A, Romero R. Homocysteine, C-reactive protein, lipid peroxidation and mortality in haemodialysis patients. Nephrol Dial Transplant; 2003;18:106-12.

129. Ansell BJ, Watson KE, Weiss RE, Fonarow GC. hsCRP and HDL Effects of Statins Trial (CHEST): Rapid Effect of Statin Therapy on C-Reactive Protein and High-Density Lipoprotein Levels A Clinical Investigation. Heart Dis; 2003;5:2-7.

130. van de Ree MA, Huisman MV, Princen HM, Meinders AE, Kluft C. Strong decrease of high sensitivity C-reactive protein with high-dose atorvastatin in patients with type 2 diabetes mellitus. Atherosclerosis; 2003;166:129-35.

131. Chan AW, Bhatt DL, Chew DP, Quinn MJ, Moliterno DJ, Topol EJ, Ellis SG. Early and sustained survival benefit associated with statin therapy at the time of percutaneous coronary intervention. Circulation; 2002;105:691-6.

132. Chan AW, Bhatt DL, Chew DP, Reginelli J, Schneider JP, Topol EJ, Ellis SG. Relation of inflammation and benefit of statins after percutaneous coronary interventions. Circulation; 2003;107:1750-1756.

133. Aronow HD, Topol EJ, Roe MT, Houghtaling PL, Wolski KE, Lincoff AM, Harrington RA, Califf RM, Ohman EM, Kleiman NS, Keltai M, Wilcox RG, Vahanian A, Armstrong PW, Lauer MS. Effect of lipid-lowering therapy on early mortality after acute coronary syndromes: an observational study. Lancet; 2001;357:1063-8.

134. Aronow HD, Novaro GM, Lauer MS, Brennan DM, Lincoff AM, Topol EJ, Kereiakes DJ, Nissen SE. In-hospital initiation of lipid-lowering therapy after coronary intervention as a predictor of long-term utilization: a propensity analysis. Arch Intern Med; 2003;163:2576-82.

135. Ridker PM. High-sensitivity C-reactive protein and cardiovascular risk: rationale for screening and primary prevention. Am J Cardiol; 2003;92:17K-22K.

136. Sager PT, Melani L, Lipka L, Strony J, Yang B, Suresh R, Veltri E. Effect of coadministration of ezetimibe and simvastatin on high-sensitivity C-reactive protein. Am J Cardiol; 2003;92:1414-8.

137. Ballantyne CM, Houri J, Notarbartolo A, Melani L, Lipka LJ, Suresh R, Sun S, LeBeaut AP, Sager PT, Veltri EP. Effect of ezetimibe coadministered with atorvastatin in 628 patients with primary hypercholesterolemia: a prospective, randomized, double-blind trial. Circulation; 2003;107:2409-15.

138. Kashyap ML, McGovern ME, Berra K, Guyton JR, Kwiterovich PO, Harper WL, Toth PD, Favrot LK, Kerzner B, Nash SD, Bays HE, Simmons PD. Long-term safety and efficacy of a once-daily niacin/lovastatin formulation for patients with dyslipidemia. Am J Cardiol; 2002;89:672-8.

139. Kleemann R, Gervois PP, Verschuren L, Staels B, Princen HM, Kooistra T. Fibrates down-regulate IL-1-stimulated C-reactive protein gene expression in hepatocytes by reducing nuclear p50-NFkappa B-C/EBP-beta complex formation. Blood; 2003;101:545-51.

140. Rizos E, Kostoula A, Elisaf M, Mikhailidis DP. Effect of ciprofibrate on C-reactive protein and fibrinogen levels. Angiology; 2002;53:273-7.

141. Jonkers IJ, Mohrschladt MF, Westendorp RG, van der Laarse A, Smelt AH. Severe hypertriglyceridemia with insulin resistance is associated with systemic inflammation: reversal with bezafibrate therapy in a randomized controlled trial. Am J Med; 2002;112:275-80.

142. Malik J, Melenovsky V, Wichterle D, Haas T, Simek J, Ceska R, Hradec J. Both fenofibrate and atorvastatin improve vascular reactivity in combined hyperlipidaemia (fenofibrate versus atorvastatin trial–FAT). Cardiovasc Res; 2001;52:290-8.

143. Haffner SM, Greenberg AS, Weston WM, Chen H, Williams K, Freed MI. Effect of rosiglitazone treatment on nontraditional markers of cardiovascular disease in patients with type 2 diabetes mellitus. Circulation; 2002;106:679-84.

144. Sidhu JS, Cowan D, Kaski JC. The effects of rosiglitazone, a peroxisome proliferator-activated receptor-gamma agonist, on markers of endothelial cell activation, C-reactive protein, and fibrinogen levels in non-diabetic coronary artery disease patients. J Am Coll Cardiol; 2003; 42:1757-63.

145. Pasceri V, Wu HD, Willerson JT, Yeh ET. Modulation of vascular inflammation in vitro and in vivo by peroxisome proliferator-activated receptor-gamma activators. Circulation; 2000; 101:235-8.

146. Yusuf S, Sleight P, Pogue J, Bosch J, Davies R, Dagenais G. Effects of an angiotensin-converting-enzyme inhibitor, ramipril, on cardiovascular events in high-risk patients. The Heart Outcomes Prevention Evaluation Study Investigators. N Engl J Med; 2000;342:145-53.

147. Hernandez-Presa MA, Bustos C, Ortego M, Tunon J, Ortega L, Egido J. ACE inhibitor quinapril reduces the arterial expression of NF-kappaB- dependent proinflammatory factors but not of collagen I in a rabbit model of atherosclerosis. Am J Pathol; 1998;153:1825-37.

148. PERTINENT–perindopril-thrombosis, inflammation, endothelial dysfunction and neurohormonal activation trial: a sub-study of the EUROPA study. Cardiovasc Drugs Ther; 2003;17: 83-91.

149. Dandona P, Kumar V, Aljada A, Ghanim H, Syed T, Hofmayer D, Mohanty P, Tripathy D, Garg R. Angiotensin II receptor blocker valsartan suppresses reactive oxygen species generation in leukocytes, nuclear factor-kappa B, in mononuclear cells of normal subjects: evidence of an antiinflammatory action. J Clin Endocrinol Metab; 2003;88:4496-501.

150. Mukherjee D, Nissen SE, Topol EJ. Risk of cardiovascular events associated with selective COX-2 inhibitors. JAMA; 2001;286:954-9.

151. Chenevard R, Hurlimann D, Bechir M, Enseleit F, Spieker L, Hermann M, Riesen W, Gay S, Gay RE, Neidhart M, Michel B, Luscher TF, Noll G, Ruschitzka F. Selective COX-2 inhibition improves endothelial function in coronary artery disease. Circulation; 2003;107: 405-9.

152. Title LM, Giddens K, McInerney MM, McQueen MJ, Nassar BA. Effect of cyclooxygenase-2 inhibition with rofecoxib on endothelial dysfunction and inflammatory markers in patients with coronary artery disease. J Am Coll Cardiol; 2003;42:1747-53.

153. Altman R, Luciardi HL, Muntaner J, Del Rio F, Berman SG, Lopez R, Gonzalez C. Efficacy assessment of meloxicam, a preferential cyclooxygenase-2 inhibitor, in acute coronary syndromes without ST-segment elevation: the Nonsteroidal Anti-Inflammatory Drugs in Unstable Angina Treatment-2 (NUT-2) pilot study. Circulation; 2002;106:191-5.

154. Versaci F, Gaspardone A, Tomai F, Ribichini F, Russo P, Proietti I, Ghini AS, Ferrero V, Chiariello L, Gioffre PA, Romeo F, Crea F. Immunosuppressive Therapy for the Prevention of Restenosis after Coronary Artery Stent Implantation (IMPRESS Study). J Am Coll Cardiol; 2002;40:1935-42.

155. Ridker PM, Hennekens CH, Rifai N, Buring JE, Manson JE. Hormone replacement therapy and increased plasma concentration of C- reactive protein. Circulation; 1999;100:713-6.

156. Manns PJ, Williams DP, Snow CM, Wander RC. Physical activity, body fat, and serum C-reactive protein in postmenopausal women with and without hormone replacement. Am J Human Biol; 2003;15:91-100.

157. Muhlestein JB, Anderson JL, Carlquist JF, Salunkhe K, Horne BD, Pearson RR, Bunch TJ, Allen A, Trehan S, Nielson C. Randomized secondary prevention trial of azithromycin in patients with coronary artery disease: primary clinical results of the ACADEMIC study. Circulation; 2000;102:1755-60.

158. O'Connor CM, Dunne MW, Pfeffer MA, Muhlestein JB, Yao L, Gupta S, Benner RJ, Fisher MR, Cook TD. Azithromycin for the secondary prevention of coronary heart disease events: the WIZARD study: a randomized controlled trial. Jama; 2003;290:1459-66.

159.  Bhatt DL. Inflammation and restenosis - is there a link? . Am Heart J; 2004;147:945-7.
160.  Horvath C, Welt FG, Nedelman M, Rao P, Rogers C. Targeting CCR2 or CD18 inhibits experimental in-stent restenosis in primates: inhibitory potential depends on type of injury and leukocytes targeted. Circ Res; 2002;90:488-94.
161.  Wang K, Zhou Z, Zhou X, Tarakji K, Topol EJ, Lincoff AM. Prevention of intimal hyperplasia with recombinant soluble P-selectin glycoprotein ligand-immunoglobulin in the porcine coronary artery balloon injury model. J Am Coll Cardiol; 2001;38:577-82.
162.  Madsen T, Skou HA, Hansen VE, Fog L, Christensen JH, Toft E, Schmidt EB. C-reactive protein, dietary n-3 fatty acids, and the extent of coronary artery disease. Am J Cardiol; 2001; 88:1139-42.
163.  Bruunsgaard H, Poulsen HE, Pedersen BK, Nyyssonen K, Kaikkonen J, Salonen JT. Long-term combined supplementations with alpha-tocopherol and vitamin C have no detectable anti-inflammatory effects in healthy men. J Nutr; 2003;133:1170-3.
164.  Engler MM, Engler MB, Malloy MJ, Chiu EY, Schloetter MC, Paul SM, Stuehlinger M, Lin KY, Cooke JP, Morrow JD, Ridker PM, Rifai N, Miller E, Witztum JL, Mietus-Snyder M. Antioxidant vitamins C and E improve endothelial function in children with hyperlipidemia: Endothelial Assessment of Risk from Lipids in Youth (EARLY) Trial. Circulation; 2003; 108:1059-63.
165.  Brook RD, Brook JR, Rajagopalan S. Air pollution: the "Heart" of the problem. Curr Hypertens Rep; 2003;5:32-9.
166.  Albert MA, Glynn RJ, Ridker PM. Alcohol consumption and plasma concentration of C-reactive protein. Circulation; 2003;107:443-7.
167.  Sierksma A, van der Gaag MS, Kluft C, Hendriks HF. Moderate alcohol consumption reduces plasma C-reactive protein and fibrinogen levels; a randomized, diet-controlled intervention study. Eur J Clin Nutr; 2002;56:1130-6.
168.  Chrysohoou C, Panagiotakos DB, Pitsavos C, Skoumas J, Toutouza M, Papaioannou I, Toutouzas PK, Stefanadis C. Effects of chronic alcohol consumption on lipid levels, inflammatory and haemostatic factors in the general population: the 'ATTICA' Study. J Cardiovasc Risk; 2003;10:355-61.
169.  Danner M, Kasl SV, Abramson JL, Vaccarino V. Association between depression and elevated C-reactive protein. Psychosom Med; 2003;65:347-56.
170.  Ladwig KH, Marten-Mittag B, Lowel H, Doring A, Koenig W. Influence of depressive mood on the association of CRP and obesity in 3205 middle aged healthy men. Brain Behav Immun; 2003;17:268-75.
171.  Berger P, McConnell JP, Nunn M, Kornman KS, Sorrell J, Stephenson K, Duff GW. C-reactive protein levels are influenced by common IL-1 gene variations. Cytokine; 2002;17: 171-4.
172.  Brull DJ, Serrano N, Zito F, Jones L, Montgomery HE, Rumley A, Sharma P, Lowe GD, World MJ, Humphries SE, Hingorani AD. Human CRP Gene Polymorphism Influences CRP Levels: Implications for the Prediction and Pathogenesis of Coronary Heart Disease. Arterioscler Thromb Vasc Biol; 2003;23:2063-9.
173.  Szalai AJ, McCrory MA, Cooper GS, Wu J, Kimberly RP. Association between baseline levels of C-reactive protein (CRP) and a dinucleotide repeat polymorphism in the intron of the CRP gene. Genes Immun; 2002;3:14-9.
174.  Ferrari SL, Ahn-Luong L, Garnero P, Humphries SE, Greenspan SL. Two promoter polymorphisms regulating interleukin-6 gene expression are associated with circulating levels of C-reactive protein and markers of bone resorption in postmenopausal women. J Clin Endocrinol Metab; 2003;88:255-9.
175.  Gaudino M, Andreotti F, Zamparelli R, Di Castelnuovo A, Nasso G, Burzotta F, Iacoviello L, Donati MB, Schiavello R, Maseri A, Possati G. The -174G/C interleukin-6 polymorphism influences postoperative interleukin-6 levels and postoperative atrial fibrillation. Is atrial fibrillation an inflammatory complication? Circulation; 2003;108 Suppl 1:II195-9.
176.  Girndt M, Kaul H, Sester U, Ulrich C, Sester M, Georg T, Kohler H. Anti-inflammatory interleukin-10 genotype protects dialysis patients from cardiovascular events. Kidney Int; 2002;62:949-55.

177.   Lio D, Scola L, Crivello A, Colonna-Romano G, Candore G, Bonafe M, Cavallone L, Marchegiani F, Olivieri F, Franceschi C, Caruso C. Inflammation, genetics, and longevity: further studies on the protective effects in men of IL-10 -1082 promoter SNP and its interaction with TNF-alpha -308 promoter SNP. J Med Genet; 2003;40:296-9.

178.   Pecoits-Filho R, Stenvinkel P, Marchlewska A, Heimburger O, Barany P, Hoff CM, Holmes CJ, Suliman M, Lindholm B, Schalling M, Nordfors L. A functional variant of the myeloperoxidase gene is associated with cardiovascular disease in end-stage renal disease patients. Kidney Int Suppl 2003:S172-6.

179.   Marculescu R, Mlekusch W, Exner M, Sabeti S, Michor S, Rumpold H, Mannhalter C, Minar E, Wagner O, Schillinger M. Interleukin-1 cluster combined genotype and restenosis after balloon angioplasty. Thromb Haemost; 2003;90:491-500.

180.   Dwyer JH, Allayee H, Dwyer KM, Fan J, Wu H, Mar R, Lusis AJ, Mehrabian M. Arachidonate 5-Lipoxygenase Promoter Genotype, Dietary Arachidonic Acid, and Atherosclerosis. N Engl J Med; 2004;350:29-37.

181.   De Caterina R, Zampolli A. From Asthma to Atherosclerosis – 5-Lipoxygenase, Leukotrienes, and Inflammation. N Engl J Med; 2004;350:4-7.

# 2
# Genetic Basis of Acute Coronary Syndromes

**Ramtin Agah**
*University of Utah*
*Salt Lake City, Utah, U.S.A.*

**Eric Topol**
*The Cleveland Clinic Foundation*
*Cleveland, Ohio, U.S.A.*

## INTRODUCTION

A significant component of the attributable risk of coronary heart disease is due to genetic predisposition unrelated to known risk factors [1]. Despite tremendous success in the past several decades in identifying (and modifying) risk factors associated with coronary heart disease, little progress has been made in identifying the specific genetic susceptibility factors associated with the disease. However, with recent advances in high-throughput genotyping, molecular genetics, and sequencing of the first draft of the human genome, our understanding of the genetic basis of coronary disease will advance significantly in the coming decade.

Although coronary artery disease (CAD) and myocardial infarction (MI) have traditionally been conceived along the same continuum, clinically we have begun to appreciate that MI may not be a predefined outcome of atherosclerosis in the majority of patients. For instance, serum markers for inflammation can dissect out-patients at high risk of events from low-risk patients despite similar degree of obstructive disease [2–6]. The dichotomy of atherosclerosis from MI can potentially be explained through their distinct pathophysiology. On one hand, atherosclerosis can be delineated as one of continuing arterial injury spanning several decades. On the other hand, MI is considered a discrete event, as a culmination of hemodynamic, inflammatory, and extracellular matrix hemostatic factors leading to plaque rupture and activation of platelets and the coagulation pathway. Although there are numerous genes that participate in both processes, the contribution of each gene to either process can be different. As such, from a genetic standpoint, the pathophysiology and, hence, the inherited risk for these two processes can be separated into two, as shown in Figure 1. In this chapter we would primarily focus on the genetic susceptibility for MI.

## MENDELIAN VS. NON-MENDELIAN GENETICS IN MI

Both atherosclerosis and MI are considered complex genetic traits. The term ''complex trait'' refers to any phenotype that does not exhibit the classic Mendelian recessive or

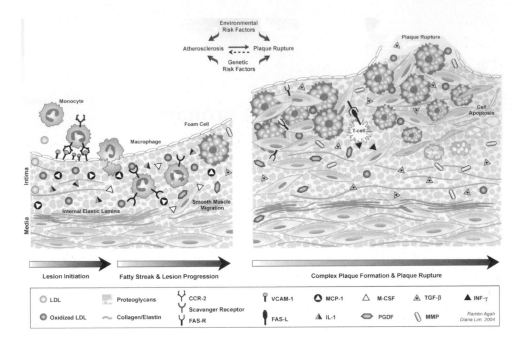

**Figure 1**  Dichotomy in the pathogenesis of myocardial infarction (MI) from atherosclerosis; an interaction between various genetic and environmental risk factors.

dominant inheritance pattern attributable to a single gene locus. The complexities arise when the simple relationship between genotype and phenotype breaks down, either because of the same genotype resulting in different phenotype (due to chance, environment, or interactions with other genes) or different genotypes resulting in the same phenotype [7,8]. Although complex diseases tend to cluster within families, they do not segregate in a Mendelian fashion; furthermore, most susceptibility alleles are neither necessary nor sufficient to cause disease and only confer a modest to moderate increase in risk.

Therefore, as a complex genetic trait, the overwhelming number of patients with myocardial infarction do not demonstrate traditional Mendelian inheritance pattern for the disease. There are some rare syndromes with Mendelian pattern of inheritance characterized by many clinical features including MI (Table 1); none has been solely associated with MI. To date, the only exception to this has been our recent report of a deletion in the gene encoding the cardiac transcription factor MEF-2A (myocyte enhancer factor): carriers of this deletion have complete penetrance for MI in their lifetime, but no other significant constellation of findings [9].

In most patients with MI, multiple genes and environmental influences interact in the manifestation of myocardial infarction [8]. Accordingly, the evaluation of any single gene in this context will only produce an assessment of relative risk (RR) for developing the condition. To discover these susceptibility genes, the adopted genetic approaches can be broadly categorized into two: linkage analysis versus candidate gene association studies [10–12]. We shall briefly discuss both techniques and summarize potential culprit genes associated with MI using each technique.

## METHODS OF GENE DETECTION

Linkage analysis is based on the premise that a common ancestral mutation is responsible for the disease of interest in the pedigree under study [7]. Hence, affected individuals

**Table 1**  Genetic Disorders with Mendelian Pattern of Inheritance and Myocardial Infarction as One of the Phenotypic Features

| Syndrome | Clinical profile *beyond* MI phenotype | Mendelian Inheritance Pattern |
|---|---|---|
| Fibromuscular dysplasia of arteries (OMIM 135580) | Aortic dissection, claudication, stroke, hypertension, MI | Autosomal dominant |
| Hutchinson-Gilford Progeris Syndrome (OMIM 176670) | Growth retardation, microganthia, premature CAD, congestive heart failure, early death (age 13), MI | Autosomal dominant 1q23 (Lamin A/C) |
| Snedden Syndrome (OMIM 182410) | Livido reticularis, noninflammatory arteriopathy, CVA, MI | Autosomal dominant |
| Cerebrotendinous Xanthomattosis (OMIM 213700) | Juvenile cataracts, respiratory insufficiency, osteoporosis, tendon and tuberous xanthoma, dementia, cerebral ataxia, mental retardation, MI | Autosomal recessive 2q35, Cytochrome P450 formA1 |
| Arterial calcification, generalized, of infancy (OMIM 208000) | Coronary artery calcification, early death (6 months of age), MI | Autosomal recessive, 6q |
| Arteriosclerosis, Severe Juvenile (OMOM 208060) | Early onset medial calcification, short stature, hypertension, MI | Autosomal recessive |
| Fabry Disease (OMIM 301500) | Retarded growth, corneal dystrophy, left ventricular hypertrophy, autonomic dysfunction, seizures, stroke, renal failure, mitral valve disease, MI | X-linked recessive, Xq22 Alpha-galactosidaseA |
| MEF-2A (OMIM 600660) | Coronary artery disease | Autosomal dominant, 15q26, MEF-2a |

OMIM, Online Mendelian Inheritance in Man—a database of human genetic disorders (from Ref. 144); MI, myocardial infarction; CAD, Coronary artery disease; CVA, Cerebrovascular accident; MEF-2A,.

share alleles in a chromosomal region that contains the susceptibility gene more often than would be expected by chance alone. This deviation from random inheritance of the culprit allele in the affected individuals can be discerned as linkage. This approach does not require *a priori* knowledge of the location of the culprit gene in the genome, but rather is a systematic analysis of the whole genome, or what is more commonly called a genome-wide scan.

Linkage analysis (and genome-wide scans) has traditionally been used to identify culprit susceptibility genes in monogenic traits with high phenotypic penetrance. To overcome these limitations and accommodate environmental and/or polygenic nature of complex diseases such as MI, several variations of the traditional linkage approach have been adopted—the so-called mixed models (i.e., allele sharing methods such as sib–pair analysis) [7]. Recently, they have been used successfully to identify susceptibility genes for many complex disease traits such as Chron's disease, asthma, stroke, and schizophrenia [13–16]. Still, the application of genome-wide scans in complex genetic traits, such as MI, is limited by the following issues:

- Most genome-wide scans can only pinpoint the susceptibility gene, at best, to within a several-hundred-thousand base pair region in the genome. By and large, the difficulty has been pinpointing the exact gene variation in this vast region responsible for the disease.

- Incomplete penetrance—despite genetic susceptibility, younger patients in the pedigree may not manifest the disease.
- Overlap can exist with other loci known to be associated with established risk factors for CHD, such as hypertension, diabetes, and dyslipidemia [17–21]. This will limit the ability to identify *de novo* genetic pathways associated with disease. This is especially true if the phenotypic inclusion criterion is atherosclerosis rather than MI.
- If multiple families are used in the analysis, different families in the cohort can have different single-gene predisposition that may attenuate the contribution of any single loci in the overall cohort [17,22].

In spite of these limitations, 5 groups have successfully used genome wide scans to identify a number of linkage peaks associated with MI as shown in Table 2 [9,17,23–25].

A chromosomal linkage peak for MI has been identified on the short arm of chromosome 6, 6p21. Over 50 different diseases have been associated with markers and/or genes in this chromosomal region, likely due to residence of the major histocompatibility complex (MHC) genes and genes involved in immunity [26–35] in this area. Initially this region was linked to coronary calcification in a cohort of Caucasian patients with clinical hypertension [36]. Subsequently, a more recent study using a high density map of single nucleotide polymorphisms has identified two gene variants in the lymphotoxin-$\alpha$ in this region associated with increased risk of MI in the Japanese population [37].

A second chromosomal region of interest is 1p34-36. Initially, Yamada et al., using a case-control study of sporadic (nonfamilial) MI, reported an association between a variation in connexin 37 gene (encoding an endothelial gap junction protein) located in this chromosomal region and risk of MI in a Japanese cohort of male patients [38]. More recently, Topol et al., using a genome wide scan of 428 predominantly Caucasian families with premature myocardial infarction, have discovered a linkage peak with a marker in this same chromosomal region with a logarithm of the odds ratio (LOD) of 11.7 [25]. Further studies are currently under way to establish if connexin-37 gene or a different potential culprit gene in this region is responsible for MI in this Caucasian cohort.

Lastly, in a single family with preponderance of MI across three generations, Topol et al. have used a genome-wide scan and successfully identified a region in chromosome 15-q26 linked to MI [9]. Subsequently, using direct sequencing of candidate genes in the region, they discovered a 21 base-pair deletion in the MEF-2A gene, a cardiac transcription factor, associated with MI in this family. Initial reports do not support this mutation to

**Table 2**  Studies Using Genome-Wide Scans to Identify Susceptibility Loci Associated with Myocardial Infarction

| Cohort | Chromosomal locations | References |
|---|---|---|
| North Eastern Indian Families (99) | 16p13 | (23) |
| Australian Sib-Pairs (61) | 2q36–37 | (24) |
| Western European Families (513) | 14q | (17) |
| Caucasians Families (428) | 1p34–36 | (25) |
| A single Caucasian pedigree | 15q26 (MEF-2A gene) | (9) |

MEF-2A, myocyte enhancer factor

be present in significant frequency in the general population; but other, more common allelic variation of MEF-2A gene may be linked to MI and are currently under investigation. Interestingly, this large pedigree represents an autosomal dominant Mendelian inheritance pattern and complete penetrance for MI in their life time with no other significant constellation of findings (Table 1). As in other complex diseases, elucidation of a causative Mendelian gene may be especially helpful in unraveling related genes that do not follow a classic Mendelian inheritance pattern.

## CANDIDATE GENE APPROACHES

The association studies are case-controlled studies comparing the frequency of a genetic variation, often a single nucleotide-polymorphism (SNP), in individuals with the phenotype compared with a control group [7,39]. This approach is independent of the mechanism of the inheritance of the gene and can be performed as a population-based study versus family-based studies in linkage analysis.

Most studies to identify genes associated with MI to date have used association studies. Despite hundreds of such publications and reports of various susceptibility alleles for MI, there have been very few gene variants that have endured validation in repeat studies. The major limitation in most of these reports (likely responsible for lack of reproducibility) is study design [40]. Some of these issues are delineated below:

- Control group—As with any case-control study, the lack of an adequate control group can be a major pitfall. Beyond traditional matching for age and sex, close attention has to be given to matching other clinical and environmental factors that may influence and interact with the culprit gene. Furthermore, as various ethnic groups have substantially different frequency of any one polymorphism, the case and control groups have to be closely matched for racial makeup to avoid population stratification [41]. Furthermore, controls in coronary disease are especially problematic because CAD is a late onset disease, which may be asymptomatic, and may require coronary angiography to define a suitable unaffected individual.

- Phenotypic definition—Lack of a consistent definition for the clinical phenotype may alter the findings. For instance, MI has been defined using serum blood tests, hospital discharge diagnosis, angiographic finding, and autopsy results in various studies [42–45]. This lack of consistency in phenotypic definition can lead to loss of sensitivity and inability to compare the findings from one study to another.

- Sample size—Most studies have used a cohort of several hundred patients; hence, based on common allele frequencies (0.1 to 0.5), they have the ability to detect risk ratio ranging between 2.0–4.0 [46]. This can lead to false negative results, especially with genetic variations that have small affects (risk ratio < 2.0). Furthermore, as most studies report only positive findings without correction for multiple comparisons after testing many candidate SNPs, the potential for false positive results is high.

- Gene-environment interactions—A restrictive allele may only affect gene expression under certain environmental conditions; unless these environmental influences are known and accounted for, the ability to discern an association with a specific phenotype will diminish. As such, elucidation of gene-environment interactions may be a key to unraveling the roles of candidate genes in complex phenotypes such as MI [47].

With these limitations in mind, Table 3 summarizes case-control studies of SNPs that have been reported to be an associated with MI. From an organizational standpoint, these

**Table 3**   Genetic Variations Associated with Myocardial Infarction Using Candidate Gene Approaches

| Platelet surface proteins and enzymes | GPIIIa/Pla2 | −/+ | (45, 50–52, 59, 69, 72, |
|---|---|---|---|
| | GPIbα/VNTR | + | 145–149) |
| | GP1bα/HPA-2 | −/+ | (150) |
| | GP Ia/C807T | −/+ | (69, 150) |
| | TSP- I/A8831G | + | (45, 151–153) |
| | HRG/A-G | + | (59) |
| | Prost. Syn C1117A | + | (59) |
| | PAF/V279F | + | (154) |
| | | | (63) |
| Clotting factors | Fact. V/G1691A | −/+ | (44, 45, 59, 69, 72, 75, 76, 78, |
| | Fact. VII/R353Q | −/+ | 155, 156) |
| | Fact.XIII/V34L | −/+ | (65, 67, 157) |
| | Prothrom./G20210A | −/+ | (43, 45, 66, 77, 91) |
| | PAI-1/4G-5G | −/+ | (43–45, 59, 68, 69, 71–74, 76, |
| | PAI-2/u5C-G | + | 78, 155) |
| | PAI-2/u4C-G | + | (38, 45, 51, 66, 69, 88–90, 155) |
| | PAI-2/u1A-G | + | (59) |
| | Throm. Syn./-386T-G | + | (59) |
| | Thrombomd./C1418T | + | (59) |
| | Thrombomd/G-33A | + | (158) |
| | Thrombpoit/A5713G | + | (159) |
| | Fibrinogen/BCL-1 | −/+ | (160) |
| | Fibrinogen/G-455A | | (161) |
| | | | (70, 80) |
| | | | (45, 80, 82, 162) |
| Cytokines, Inflammatory factors | Phospholip. γ1/T-C | + | (59) |
| | CD14/C-260T | −/+ | (163, 164) (165) |
| | CD14/T-159C | + | (166) |
| | IL-1/RN | −/+ | (167–170) |
| | IL-6/G-174C | −/+ | (171) (172–174) |
| | Thrombopo./G5713A | + | (104) |
| | TNF-α/ G-308A | −/+ | (175, 176) |
| Adhesion molecules | P-selectin/ T715P | −/+ | (59, 124, 177) (125) |
| | P-selectin/ S290N | + | (123) |
| | P-selectin/ N562D | + | (123) |
| | E-selectin/S128R | + | (178) |
| | PECAM-1/V125L | + | (179) |
| | PECAM-1/N563S | + | (179) |
| | PECAM-1/G670R | + | (179) |
| | ICAM/W478R | + | (178) |
| Matrix regulating proteins | MMP-3/5A6A | + | (81, 130) (38, 131) |
| | MMP-9/C-1562T | −/+ | (42, 135) |
| | TGF-B1/T29C | + | (180–182) |
| | Thrombosp II/T-G | + | (59, 183) |
| | Thrombosp IV/G-C | + | (59, 183) |
| Endothelial function | ACE/I-D | −/+ | (94, 95, 99, 100, 184–186) |
| | AT1 Rec./A1166C | −/+ | (98 99, 100) |
| | Angiotensin/T235M | −/+ | (99, 100, 186) |
| | eNOS/Int4 | −/+ | (187–189) |

*(Continued)*

**Table 3** Continued

| | | | |
|---|---|---|---|
| | eNOS/G298A | + | (188, 190) |
| | eNOS/T-786C | + | (191) |
| | ANP/T2238C | + | (192) |
| Lipid metabolism | LDL R.P./G-T | + | (59) |
| | ApoE/ϵ4 | + | (193) |
| | ApoE/G-1219T | + | (102) |
| | ApoA PNR/-1373 | + | (110) |
| | PON1/G192A | −/+ | (106, 194) (195–197) |
| | CETP/Taq1b | −/+ | (104) (117, 119, 198) |
| | ApoB/SP-D | + | (199) |
| | OLR1/G501C | + | (200) |
| Systemic risk factors | MTHFRp677/C-T | −/+ | (45, 59, 69, 72, 201–204) |
| | Met. Synthase | + | (205) |
| | α2-adrenergic rec./dd | + | (206) |
| | β2adrenergic rec/E27 | + | (59, 207) |
| | p22$^{phox}$/C242T | + | (38) |
| | Glycop. PC-1/K121Q | + | (208) |
| | GSTM1/del | + | (209) |
| | NADH/A518C | + | (210) |
| | Connexin 37/C1019T | + | (38) |
| | Annexin IV/C-T | + | (53) |
| | Annexin V/C-1T | + | (211) |

GP, Glycoprotein; Thromposp., Thrombospondin; HRG, histidine-rich glycoprotein; Prost. Syn., Prostacyclin Synthase; PAF-ah, platelet activating factor acetylhydrolase; Fact., Factor; PAI, Plasminogen activator inhibitor; Prothrom., Prothrombin; Throm. Syn., thromboxane synthase; thrombomd., thrombomodulin; thrombopoit., thrombopoietin; phospholip., phospholipase; IL, interlukin; MMP, matrix metalloproteinase; TGF,,Transforming growth factor; ACE, angiotensin converting enzyme; AT1 Rec., Angiotensin II type I receptor; NOS, nitiric oxide synthase; ANP, atrial natriuretic peptide; MTHFR, Methylenetetrahydrofolate reducatse; Met., methionine; LDL, low-density lipoprotein; B.C.T., binding cassette transporter; PON, Paraxonase; CETP, cholesteryl ester transfer protein; rec., receptor; IL1-RN, IL-1 receptor antagonist.

gene variants can broadly be divided into eight categories of genes. As some genes may have functions that overlap several of these categories, this canvas should only be used as a general framework. A limited discussion of some of the more relevant SNPs associated with MI in each group is presented later.

## PLATELET SURFACE PROTEINS AND ENZYMES

Formation of platelet thrombi at the site of plaque rupture is the pathological culprit for the clinical presentation of MI. The platelet surface proteins, in their roles in initiating this cascade of events, have successfully been targeted in recent therapeutic interventions of patients with ACS. Central among these proteins is the glycoprotein (GP) IIb-IIIa receptor involved in fibrinogen binding. Several SNPs in both the GPIIb and GPIIIa molecules have been reported; most notable is the PLA (protein leucine 33) polymorphism in codon 196 (T → C) of GPIIIa molecule. Although there is no well-established relationship between this polymorphism and the level of protein expression or activity, there have been reports suggesting that this polymorphism may affect platelet fibrinogen binding and aggregation [48,49]. Numerous studies have linked this polymorphism to a variety of clinical conditions including unstable angina, myocardial infarction, stroke, coronary and carotid atherosclerosis, postangioplasty restenosis, in-stent thrombosis, and abdominal aneurysm [50–58]. Unfortunately, despite PLA allele's obvious appeal, no consistent association has been found in the large case-controlled and prospective studies between the presence of this polymorphism and risk of MI so far.

Other platelet proteins of interest include the thrombospondin (TSP) gene. A variation in the calcium binding motif of TSP-1 (D700S) has been shown to be a risk factor for MI in at least one report [59]. A second validation study has shown that this polymorphism affects calcium binding capacity and the secondary structure of the TSP-1 protein [60]

Platelet activating factor (PAF) is an inflammatory phospholipids with chemo attractant and leukocyte activation properties [61]. Activation of PAF via acetylhydrolase (PAF-AH) has been shown to be a marker of ACS [62]. A functional mutation of this gene (present primarily in the Japanese population), causing an amino acid substitution at position 279 (V279F), has been associated with multiple disease processes including asthma, stroke, and MI [61,63].

## COAGULATION AND FIBRINOLYSIS

Gene variants in thrombotic factors have been extensively studied as potential culprits in predisposition to MI. Since increased levels of certain coagulation factors have been shown to lead to an increase risk of MI (Northwick Park Heart Study [64]), multiple studies have attempted to demonstrate an association between the SNPs in genes involved in the thrombotic pathway and their protein level [65–67]. A focus of investigation has been SNPs in the 5' upstream or the 3' downstream region of these genes that may affect their expression [68–71]. We shall discuss some of the more comprehensively studied variants among these genes.

The gene variants in factor V, A506G, and factor II, G20210A, have both been shown to affect protein activity and protein levels, respectively. Furthermore, both of these mutations have been shown to be a risk factor for venous thrombosis. Despite the functional affect of these mutations and their established role in venous thrombosis, no role for these gene variants has been convincingly demonstrated for patients with MI; however, a modest role in increasing risk of MI in the low-risk group (specifically young patients) cannot be ruled out [43–45,71–78].

Fibrinogen levels have also been shown to be an important risk factor for both atherosclerosis and MI [79]. A gene variant in the promoter region of the fibrinogen gene, G-455A, has been shown to increase expression of the gene [80,81]. However, a direct link has not been made between this gene variant and the clinical phenotype of MI [82]. A possible explanation could be the modest effect of this gene variant on expression level (less than 20% increase) [70]. Alternatively, as there are several reports establishing an interaction between environmental factors such as smoking, chronic infection (i.e., periodontal disease), and enhanced expression of fibrinogen in the carrier of this gene variant, the influence of gene–environment interaction may need to be assessed in validating the influence of these gene variants on risk of MI [83,84].

The plasminogen activator inhibitor-1 (PAI-1) serum level has also been shown to be a risk factor for many clinical conditions including MI, restenosis, successful fibrinolysis, survival post-MI, restenosis, and clotting postangioplasty [85,86]. A guanine insertion/deletion polymorphism in the promoter region of the PAI-1 gene has been reported to increase the protein expression [87]. Several studies attempting to link this genotype with the risk of MI have produced conflicting results with no uniform consensus [37,38,59,88–90].

Lastly, some studies have suggested a protective role from MI in carriers of the mutation Val34Leu in factor XIII—although the results have not been uniform [45,66,77,91]. Due to proximity of this mutation to the thrombin cleavage site, it has been suggested that the Leucine substitution in this position may enhance factor XIII activation by thrombin but paradoxically decrease activation in patients on aspirin—as a potential protective effect [92].

## ENDOTHELIAL FUNCTION

Possibly the single-most studied gene variant in cardiovascular disease is an intron 16 insertion/deletion (I/D) polymorphism in the angiotensin-converting enzyme (ACE) gene. Individuals with the double deletion (DD) genotype have been shown to have higher plasma levels of ACE [93]. As first reported by Cambien, patients homozygote for the DD allele have a modest increased risk for MI, with relative increased risk of 1.1 [94]. This initial finding was subsequently confirmed in a cohort of 10,000 patients by Kearny [95]. The importance of this gene variant appears to be more significant in patients considered at low risk of MI (increased relative risk of 3.2) [94]. Since ACE inhibition is important in treatment of many disease processes including vascular disease, left ventricular hypertrophy, cardiac remodeling, and hypertension, several studies have attempted to uncover a pharmacogenomic role for ACE I/D allele and response to ACE-inhibition without success [96,97].

Another point of interest with respect to this gene variant is the possible interaction of this allele with both the upstream substrate and downstream receptor as a possible example of gene–gene interactions in manifestation of the allelic phenotype. A study by Tiert and coworkers has shown an interaction between the ACE I/D polymorphism and another genetic variant in its receptor, AT-1 A1666C [98]. The presence of each individual variant resulted in only a modest increased risk of MI, but the presence of both variants together resulted in a synergistic interaction with increased relative risk of 3-4. Another study by Fomicheva et al. has suggested an additive interaction between the ACE I/D polymorphism and the M235T SNP in the upstream substrate of the angiotensinogen gene [99]. A small study in a second cohort of 142 patients with premature myocardial infarction (age < 55) has confirmed a synergistic interaction between ACE I/D and presence of either the AT-1 A1666C or M235T polymorphism and risk of MI [100].

## LIPID METABOLISM

Early studies of families with premature atherosclerosis focused on rare mutations in genes involved in cholesterol transport and uptake leading to discovery of rare monogenic traits. However, studies of the more common variant of these gene and newly discovered genes involved in cholesterol metabolism have taken up recent attention [101]. In the majority of these studies, the specific SNP is linked to the intermediate phenotype, cholesterol profile [102–107]. However, some studies have also shown a direct association between the gene variants and clinical disease such as atherosclerosis and are more relevant to our discussion of MI [102–104,108,109].

Some of the candidate genes that have been studied so far include apolipoprotein E (ApoE), lipoprotein lipase, lipoprotein receptor-related protein, ApoB, Oxidized low-density lipoprotein receptor (OLR), ApoA, Paraxonase (PON), and genes involved in reverse cholesterol transport including cholesterol ester transfer protein (CETP) [102–104,107,108,110,111]. The most extensively studied among these genes is the ApoE [112,113]. A variant of this gene, with an allelic frequency of 15% in the Caucasian population, the ApoE4, has been linked to premature atherosclerosis, decreased longevity, stroke, Alzheimer's disease, and MI [112–116]. Furthermore, even though an effect of this gene variant on intermediate phenotypes, increasing low-density lipoprotein (LDL) level has been established, the effect of this gene variant on disease manifestation does not appear to be limited to its effect on the LDL level [113].

The CETP gene variant (Taq1b), involved in cholesterol ester transfer, is another example of a functional mutation in the lipid regulatory genes. This gene variant has been correlated with both enzyme activity and the intermediate phenotype high-density lipoprotein (HDL) level [104]. Several studies have further linked this gene variant with the clinical phenotype atherosclerosis and MI [104,117]. Of interest is the apparent gene–environment interaction in manifestation of the effect of this SNP variant; specifically, the synergistic association between alcohol consumption and HDL levels in carriers of this SNP [118,119]. Furthermore, at least one study relates a selective benefit of Pravastatin in abolishing progression of atherosclerosis only in carriers of this gene variant [104]. If validated, a diagnostic test for this SNP may have future pharmacogenomic application.

## CYTOKINES

In the past decade, inflammation has been established as the key underlying mechanism for plaque stability [120]. Despite recent data establishing a strong link between multiple inflammatory markers and risk of MI, the data establishing a link between variant alleles in these inflammatory genes and risk of MI has not been forthcoming [2–6]. A potential explanation may lay in the fact that there are strong environmental influences (rather than genetic influences) on expression of these genes in the setting of ACS; hence, the paucity of data linking genetic variants in these genes with risk of MI. However, at least in terms of one well-validated inflammatory marker, C-reactive protein, there is strong evidence for significant heritability [121]. An alternative explanation is the potential complex nature of interactions of the various cytokines in the setting of ACS, precluding a simple straight-forward association as sought thus far. Further studies looking more extensively at gene variants of other cytokines, their receptors, coactivators, and potential interaction between these alleles on risk for events may shed more light on this issue.

## ADHESION MOLECULES

Adhesion molecules involved in cell–cell signaling and interaction play a key role in recruitment of the inflammatory cell into the atherosclerotic plaque [122]. A gene variant of interest in this group is the SNP in the coding sequence of P-selectin gene leading to an amino acid substitution in position 715 (T715P). This gene variant has been associated with the intermediate phenotype (lower soluble forms of P-selectin) and also with protection from MI [123–125]. So far, the protective effect of this polymorphism has been validated in two different ethnic groups [123,124].

## MATRIX REGULATING PROTEINS

A prerequisite for plaque rupture is matrix degradation. As our understanding of the molecular mechanism of atherosclerosis has advanced, we now understand that the plaque undergoes remodeling through an ongoing tug-of-war between matrix degrading enzymes and matrix stabilizing factors [126]. A key enzyme in this process, shown to be present in complex plaque and specifically around the fibrous cap (the vulnerable portion of the plaque), is the matrix metalloproteinase-3 (MMP-3) [126]. A polymorphism in the promoter region of MMP-3 has been shown to affect its expression [127]. This polymorphism has been linked to increase risk for atherosclerosis, coronary aneurysm, and myocardial infarction [38,128–131]. Of note, this association with MI has been consistently validated in several large studies with various ethnic cohorts; furthermore, two separate studies have shown that there is a synergistic interaction between smoking and attributable risk of this allele [38,131–133]. The underlying mechanism for this genetic–environmental interaction is yet to be elucidated.

Elevated serum MMP-9 levels have been reported to be an associated risk of myocardial infarction [134,135]. An SNP in the promoter region of this enzyme, C-1562T, has also been shown to affect its expression [134,136]. Although several studies suggest that this SNP affects clinical phenotype of atherosclerosis, coronary aneurysm, and presence of complex plaque in autopsy studies, no direct association with MI has yet been made [42,136–139).

## OTHER SYSTEMIC FACTORS

Among these genes, two are noteworthy due to the rigorous approach used by the investigators to discover their association to MI. Yamada et al., using a cohort of 2819 Japanese patients with myocardial infarction, conducted a two-phase study [38]. In the first phase of the study they screened 112 SNPs in 909 subjects to identify candidate SNPs with potential association with MI. Thirty-seven SNPs were selected from phase I for validation using 2000 subjects in the second phase of the study. At completion of phase II of the study, a polymorphism in connexin 37 and another polymorphism in p22$^{Phox}$ genes were significantly associated with MI in men. Of note, these associations were only seen in the male subjects, as two other SNPs (MMP-3 5A-1171/6A and PAI-1 4G-668/5G) were found to be associated with MI in the female subjects. This gender dichotomy can likely be due to significant difference in clinical characteristics of the male vs. female subjects in the screening part of the study. Both these finds are awaiting validation in other studies and potentially other cohorts with different ethnicity.

## FUTURE DIRECTIONS

*Diagnosis & Primary Prevention: who should be screened?* The key caveat here lies in the magnitude of the susceptibilities. As most common gene variants associated with MI discovered to date seem to have a modest effect on increasing patient's risk for MI (relative risk < 2), universal screening of patients at risk does not seem justified at this point.

However, the number of ''common'' gene variants associated with myocardial infarction would likely increase in the next 5 years. If so, one can conceive of an ''MI gene chip'' where, in one setting, a patient can be screened for all gene variants known to be associated with increased risk of MI. However, to undertake such a ''global'' genetic risk assessment, we have to be able to take into account combinatorial affect of various alleles and environmental risk factors. The studies looking at gene–gene interactions and gene–environment interactions are critical to this issue [140–142]. Several small studies to date have begun to address this issue of interaction between environment and the risk associated with a specific variant allele [98,99]. Lastly, the advantage of such screening becomes of value and ethically justifiable only if preventive measures are deemed effective in modifying patient risk.

As we address these complex issues in the future, eventually the process of screening patients at risk for MI will transition from research labs to commercial availability.

## THERAPY AND SECONDARY PREVENTION: PHARMACOGENOMICS

Would there be any role in genetic screening of patients who have already suffered an MI? The answer will likely be yes.

First, information from such screening may become part of routine secondary risk stratification algorithms to identify patients for further invasive workup and intervention based on the level of "genetic risk." A relevant example is the present application of genetic screening for factor-V Lieden mutation in secondary-prevention clinical algorithms in patients with deep venous thrombosis. Also the individual's offspring could benefit from aggressive preventive measures if a particular gene is diagnosed and transmitted.

Furthermore, the genetic screening for various alleles responsible for heritable risk of MI may enable us to identify a specific gene(s) affecting a particular pathway(s) as the culprit mechanism in an individual patient. Customization of secondary preventive measures could be more directly (and aggressively) targeted to that pathway to achieve maximum risk modification. For instance, a patient with genetic predisposition for MI due to aspirin resistance because of a defect in the prostacyclin synthase gene would benefit from a different approach in risk modification than a patient requiring risk modification due to a genetic defect affecting expression of the angiotensin-converting enzyme gene.

Lastly, most clinical trials have shown that patients can have diverse therapeutic response to the same clinical regimen. A significant component of this variation is due to pharmacogenetic differences leading to individual drug metabolism and activity. Pharmacogentic differences are often 10-fold and can be as high as 40-fold between the highest and lowest individual in any given population [41]. To achieve therapeutic response in most drug trials, the "highest" tolerable range of a compound is used in order to overcome this large pharamcogenomic variation. As such, adverse drug reactions, due in large part to this interindividual variability in drug response, ranks between the fourth and sixth leading cause of death in the United States [143]. With a more rational understanding of the individual genetic response to various drugs, a more individualized drug–dose regimen can be tailored to achieve the maximum therapeutic response with minimal adverse response.

## CONCLUSIONS

At the present time, the significant heritable risk of MI is just beginning to be defined. With recent advances in tools used to search, characterize, and decipher the genome, our ability to dissect the complex genetic traits of MI has significantly improved. Of note is the impact of the availability of the template of the human genome and high throughput genotyping. With these tools in hand, present approaches using either association studies or linkage analysis (and likely hybrids of the two techniques) will significantly improve our ability to test genome-wide susceptibility loci with lower genotype risk ratio. Furthermore, we will be able to gradually discern gene–gene interactions and gene–environment interactions as a rational complement to the emerging field of proteomics.

In the not-too-distant future we may be able to routinely risk stratify patients based on their genetic makeup: both in the primary and secondary setting. Furthermore, with discovery of these culprit genes, we will likely uncover new pathways involved in disease manifestation as potential new specific targets for therapy. It is envisioned that someday the ultimate effect in ACS—preventing the events—will be facilitated by wide-scale use of genetic detection and individualized lifestyle and, if needed, pharmacotherapy.

## REFERENCES

1. Sorensen TI, Nielsen GG, Andersen PK, Teasdale TW. Genetic and environmental influences on premature death in adult adoptees. N Engl J Med 1988;318(12):727-32.

2. Heeschen C, Dimmeler S, Hamm CW, van den Brand MJ, Boersma E, Zeiher AM, Simoons ML. Soluble CD40 ligand in acute coronary syndromes. N Engl J Med 2003;348(12):1104-11.

3. Heeschen C, Dimmeler S, Hamm CW, Fichtlscherer S, Boersma E, Simoons ML, Zeiher AM. Serum level of the antiinflammatory cytokine interleukin-10 is an important prognostic determinant in patients with acute coronary syndromes. Circulation 2003;107(16):2109-14.

4. Damas JK, Waehre T, Yndestad A, Otterdal K, Hognestad A, Solum NO, Gullestad L, Froland SS, Aukrust P. Interleukin-7-mediated inflammation in unstable angina: possible role of chemokines and platelets. Circulation 2003;107(21):2670-6.

5. de Lemos JA, Morrow DA, Sabatine MS, Murphy SA, Gibson CM, Antman EM, McCabe CH, Cannon CP, Braunwald E. Association between plasma levels of monocyte chemoattractant protein-1 and long-term clinical outcomes in patients with acute coronary syndromes. Circulation 2003;107(5):690-5.

6. Chew DP, Bhatt DL, Robbins MA, Penn MS, Schneider JP, Lauer MS, Topol EJ, Ellis SG. Incremental prognostic value of elevated baseline C-reactive protein among established markers of risk in percutaneous coronary intervention. Circulation 2001;104(9):992-7.

7. Lander ES, Schork NJ. Genetic dissection of complex traits. Science 1994;265(5181):2037-48.

8. Risch NJ. Searching for genetic determinants in the new millennium. Nature 2000;405(6788):847-56.

9. Wang L, Fan C, Topol SE, Topol EJ, Wang Q. Mutation of MEF2A in an inherited disorder with features of coronary artery disease. Science 2003;302(5650):1578-81.

10. Terwilliger JD, Weiss KM. Linkage disequilibrium mapping of complex disease: fantasy or reality? Curr Opin Biotechnol 1998;9(6):578-94.

11. Weiss KM, Terwilliger JD. How many diseases does it take to map a gene with SNPs? Nat Genet 2000;26(2):151-7.

12. Talmud PJ, Humphries SE. Genetic polymorphisms, lipoproteins and coronary artery disease risk. Curr Opin Lipidol 2001;12(4):405-9.

13. Blouin JL, Dombroski BA, Nath SK, Lasseter VK, Wolyniec PS, Nestadt G, Thornquist M, Ullrich G, McGrath J, Kasch L, Lamacz M, Thomas MG, Gehrig C, Radhakrishna U, Snyder SE, Balk KG, Neufeld K, Swartz KL, DeMarchi N, Papadimitriou GN, Dikeos DG, Stefanis CN, Chakravarti A, Childs B, Pulver AE, al et. Schizophrenia susceptibility loci on chromosomes 13q32 and 8p21. Nat Genet 1998;20(1):70-3.

14. Laitinen T, Daly MJ, Rioux JD, Kauppi P, Laprise C, Petays T, Green T, Cargill M, Haahtela T, Lander ES, Laitinen LA, Hudson TJ, Kere J. A susceptibility locus for asthma-related traits on chromosome 7 revealed by genome-wide scan in a founder population. Nat Genet 2001;28(1):87-91.

15. Gretarsdottir S, Sveinbjornsdottir S, Jonsson HH, Jakobsson F, Einarsdottir E, Agnarsson U, Shkolny D, Einarsson G, Gudjonsdottir HM, Valdimarsson EM, Einarsson OB, Thorgeirsson G, Hadzic R, Jonsdottir S, Reynisdottir ST, Bjarnadottir SM, Gudmundsdottir T, Gudlaugsdottir GJ, Gill R, Lindpaintner K, Sainz J, Hannesson HH, Sigurdsson GT, Frigge ML, Kong A, Gudnason V, Stefansson K, Gulcher JR. Localization of a susceptibility gene for common forms of stroke to 5q12. Am J Hum Genet 2002;70(3):593-603.

16. Rioux JD, Silverberg MS, Daly MJ, Steinhart AH, McLeod RS, Griffiths AM, Green T, Brettin TS, Stone V, Bull SB, Bitton A, Williams CN, Greenberg GR, Cohen Z, Lander ES, Hudson TJ, Siminovitch KA. Genomewide search in Canadian families with inflammatory bowel disease reveals two novel susceptibility loci. Am J Hum Genet 2000;66(6):1863-70.

17.  Broeckel U, Hengstenberg C, Mayer B, Holmer S, Martin LJ, Comuzzie AG, Blangero J, Nurnberg P, Reis A, Riegger GA, Jacob HJ, Schunkert H. A comprehensive linkage analysis for myocardial infarction and its related risk factors. Nat Genet 2002;30(2):210-4.

18.  Pajukanta P, Cargill M, Viitanen L, Nuotio I, Kareinen A, Perola M, Terwilliger JD, Kempas E, Daly M, Lilja H, Rioux JD, Brettin T, Viikari JS, Ronnemaa T, Laakso M, Lander ES, Peltonen L. Two loci on chromosomes 2 and X for premature coronary heart disease identified in early- and late-settlement populations of Finland. Am J Hum Genet 2000;67(6):1481-93.

19.  Pajukanta P, Nuotio I, Terwilliger JD, Porkka KV, Ylitalo K, Pihlajamaki J, Suomalainen AJ, Syvanen AC, Lehtimaki T, Viikari JS, Laakso M, Taskinen MR, Ehnholm C, Peltonen L. Linkage of familial combined hyperlipidaemia to chromosome 1q21-q23. Nat Genet 1998; 18(4):369-73.

20.  Berg K, Pedersen JC. Genetic risk factors coronary heart disease. Scand J Clin Lab Invest Suppl 1990;202:82-5.

21.  Klos KL, Kardia SL, Ferrell RE, Turner ST, Boerwinkle E, Sing CF. Genome-wide linkage analysis reveals evidence of multiple regions that influence variation in plasma lipid and apolipoprotein levels associated with risk of coronary heart disease. Arterioscler Thromb Vasc Biol 2001;21(6):971-8.

22.  Hixson JE, Blangero J. Genomic searches for genes that influence atherosclerosis and its risk factors. Ann N Y Acad Sci 2000;902:1-7.

23.  Francke S, Manraj M, Lacquemant C, Lecoeur C, Lepretre F, Passa P, Hebe A, Corset L, Yan SL, Lahmidi S, Jankee S, Gunness TK, Ramjuttun US, Balgobin V, Dina C, Froguel P. A genome-wide scan for coronary heart disease suggests in Indo- Mauritians a susceptibility locus on chromosome 16p13 and replicates linkage with the metabolic syndrome on 3q27. Hum Mol Genet 2001;10(24):2751-65.

24.  Harrap SB, Zammit KS, Wong ZY, Williams FM, Bahlo M, Tonkin AM, Anderson ST. Genome-wide linkage analysis of the acute coronary syndrome suggests a locus on chromosome 2. Arterioscler Thromb Vasc Biol 2002;22(5):874-8.

25.  Topol EJ. Genome-wide linkage analysis of familial, premature myocardial infarction identifies novel susceptibility loci. Circulation 2003;108(17):IV-49.

26.  Barille-Nion S, Barlogie B, Bataille R, Bergsagel PL, Epstein J, Fenton RG, Jacobson J, Kuehl WM, Shaughnessy J, Tricot G. Advances in biology and therapy of multiple myeloma. Hematology (Am Soc Hematol Educ Program) 2003: ;:248-78.

27.  Jones DE, Donaldson PT. Genetic factors in the pathogenesis of primary biliary cirrhosis. Clin Liver Dis 2003;7(4):841-64.

28.  Kelly JA, Moser KL, Harley JB. The genetics of systemic lupus erythematosus: putting the pieces together. Genes Immun 2002;3 Suppl 1:S71-85.

29.  Capon F, Dallapiccola B, Novelli G. Advances in the search for psoriasis susceptibility genes. Mol Genet Metab 2000;71(1-2):250-5.

30.  Chistyakov DA, Savost'anov KV, Turakulov RI, Nosikov VV. Genetic determinants of Graves disease. Mol Genet Metab 2000;71(1-2):66-9.

31.  Todd JA, Farrall M. Panning for gold: genome-wide scanning for linkage in type 1 diabetes. Hum Mol Genet 1996;5 Spec No:1443-8.

32.  Jordanova ES, Philippo K, Giphart MJ, Schuuring E, Kluin PM. Mutations in the HLA class II genes leading to loss of expression of HLA-DR and HLA-DQ in diffuse large B-cell lymphoma. Immunogenetics 2003;55(4):203-9.

33.  Tait KF, Gough SC. The genetics of autoimmune endocrine disease. Clin Endocrinol (Oxf) 2003;59(1):1-11.

34.  Coraddu F, Lai M, Mancosu C, Cocco E, Sawcer S, Setakis E, Compston A, Marrosu MG. A genome-wide screen for linkage disequilibrium in Sardinian multiple sclerosis. J Neuroimmunol 2003;143(1-2):120-3.

35.  Seidl S, Kaufmann H, Drach J. New insights into the pathophysiology of multiple myeloma. Lancet Oncol 2003;4(9):557-64.

36.  Lange LA, Lange EM, Bielak LF, Langefeld CD, Kardia SL, Royston P, Turner ST, Sheedy 2nd PF, Boerwinkle E, Peyser PA. Autosomal genome-wide scan for coronary artery calcifica-

tion loci in sibships at high risk for hypertension. Arterioscler Thromb Vasc Biol 2002;22(3): 418-23.

37. Ozaki K, Ohnishi Y, Iida A, Sekine A, Yamada R, Tsunoda T, Sato H, Hori M, Nakamura Y, Tanaka T. Functional SNPs in the lymphotoxin-alpha gene that are associated with susceptibility to myocardial infarction. Nat Genet 2002;32(4):650-4.

38. Yamada Y, Izawa H, Ichihara S, Takatsu F, Ishihara H, Hirayama H, Sone T, Tanaka M, Yokota M. Prediction of the risk of myocardial infarction from polymorphisms in candidate genes. N Engl J Med 2002;347(24):1916-23.

39. Johnson GC, Todd JA. Strategies in complex disease mapping. Curr Opin Genet Dev 2000; 10(3):330-4.

40. Winkelmann BR, Hager J. Genetic variation in coronary heart disease and myocardial infarction: methodological overview and clinical evidence. Pharmacogenomics 2000;1(1):73-94.

41. Nebert DW, Menon AG. Pharmacogenomics, ethnicity, and susceptibility genes. Pharmacogenomics J 2001;1(1):19-22.

42. Pollanen PJ, Karhunen PJ, Mikkelsson J, Laippala P, Perola M, Penttila A, Mattila KM, Koivula T, Lehtimaki T. Coronary artery complicated lesion area is related to functional polymorphism of matrix metalloproteinase 9 gene: an autopsy study. Arterioscler Thromb Vasc Biol 2001;21(9):1446-50.

43. Butt C, Zheng H, Randell E, Robb D, Parfrey P, Xie YG. Combined carrier status of prothrombin 20210A and factor XIII-A Leu34 alleles as a strong risk factor for myocardial infarction: evidence of a gene-gene interaction. Blood 2003;101(8):3037-41.

44. Tanis BC, Bloemenkamp DG, van den Bosch MA, Kemmeren JM, Algra A, van de Graaf Y, Rosendaal FR. Prothrombotic coagulation defects and cardiovascular risk factors in young women with acute myocardial infarction. Br J Haematol 2003;122(3):471-8.

45. No evidence of association between prothrombotic gene polymorphisms and the development of acute myocardial infarction at a young age. Circulation 2003;107(8):1117-22.

46. Risch N, Merikangas K. The future of genetic studies of complex human diseases. Science 1996;273(5281):1516-7.

47. Tiret L. Gene-environment interaction: a central concept in multifactorial diseases. Proc Nutr Soc 2002;61(4):457-63.

48. Feng D, Lindpaintner K, Larson MG, Rao VS, O'Donnell CJ, Lipinska I, Schmitz C, Sutherland PA, Silbershatz H, D'Agostino RB, Muller JE, Myers RH, Levy D, Tofler GH. Increased platelet aggregability associated with platelet GPIIIa PlA2 polymorphism: the Framingham Offspring Study. Arterioscler Thromb Vasc Biol 1999;19(4):1142-7.

49. Michelson AD, Furman MI, Goldschmidt-Clermont P, Mascelli MA, Hendrix C, Coleman L, Hamlington J, Barnard MR, Kickler T, Christie DJ, Kundu S, Bray PF. Platelet GP IIIa Pl(A) polymorphisms display different sensitivities to agonists. Circulation 2000;101(9): 1013-8.

50. Weiss EJ, Bray PF, Tayback M, Schulman SP, Kickler TS, Becker LC, Weiss JL, Gerstenblith G, Goldschmidt-Clermont PJ. A polymorphism of a platelet glycoprotein receptor as an inherited risk factor for coronary thrombosis. N Engl J Med 1996;334(17):1090-4.

51. Ridker PM, Hennekens CH, Schmitz C, Stampfer MJ, Lindpaintner K. PIA1/A2 polymorphism of platelet glycoprotein IIIa and risks of myocardial infarction, stroke, and venous thrombosis. Lancet 1997;349(9049):385-8.

52. Carter AM, Ossei-Gerning N, Wilson IJ, Grant PJ. Association of the platelet Pl(A) polymorphism of glycoprotein IIb/IIIa and the fibrinogen Bbeta 448 polymorphism with myocardial infarction and extent of coronary artery disease. Circulation 1997;96(5):1424-31.

53. Aleksic N, Juneja H, Folsom AR, Ahn C, Boerwinkle E, Chambless LE, Wu KK. Platelet Pl(A2) allele and incidence of coronary heart disease: results from the Atherosclerosis Risk In Communities (ARIC) Study. Circulation 2000;102(16):1901-5.

54. Garg UC, Arnett DK, Folsom AR, Province MA, Williams RR, Eckfeldt JH. Lack of association between platelet glycoprotein IIb/IIIa receptor PlA polymorphism and coronary artery disease or carotid intima-media thickness. Thromb Res 1998;89(2):85-9.

55. Garcia-Ribes M, Gonzalez-Lamuno D, Hernandez-Estefania R, Colman T, Pocovi M, Delgado-Rodriguez M, Garcia-Fuentes M, Revuelta JM. Polymorphism of the platelet glycoprotein IIIa gene in patients with coronary stenosis. Thromb Haemost 1998;79(6):1126-9.

56. Bottiger C, Kastrati A, Koch W, Mehilli J, von Beckerath N, Dirschinger J, Gawaz M, Schomig A. Polymorphism of platelet glycoprotein IIb and risk of thrombosis and restenosis after coronary stent placement. Am J Cardiol 1999;84(9):987-91.

57. Mikkelsson J, Perola M, Kauppila LI, Laippala P, Savolainen V, Pajarinen J, Penttila A, Karhunen PJ. The GPIIIa Pl(A) polymorphism in the progression of abdominal aortic atherosclerosis. Atherosclerosis 1999;147(1):55-60.

58. Goldschmidt-Clermont PJ, Cooke GE, Eaton GM, Binkley PF. PlA2, a variant of GPIIIa implicated in coronary thromboembolic complications. J Am Coll Cardiol 2000;36(1):90-3.

59. Topol EJ, McCarthy J, Gabriel S, Moliterno DJ, Rogers WJ, Newby LK, Freedman M, Metivier J, Cannata R, O'Donnell CJ, Kottke-Marchant K, Murugesan G, Plow EF, Stenina O, Daley GQ. Single nucleotide polymorphisms in multiple novel thrombospondin genes may be associated with familial premature myocardial infarction. Circulation 2001;104(22): 2641-4.

60. Hannah BL, Misenheimer TM, Annis DS, Mosher DF. A polymorphism in thrombospondin-1 associated with familial premature coronary heart disease causes a local change in conformation of the Ca2 + -binding repeats. J Biol Chem 2003;278(11):8929-34.

61. Tjoelker LW, Stafforini DM. Platelet-activating factor acetylhydrolases in health and disease. Biochim Biophys Acta 2000;1488(1-2):102-23.

62. Packard CJ, O'Reilly DS, Caslake MJ, McMahon AD, Ford I, Cooney J, Macphee CH, Suckling KE, Krishna M, Wilkinson FE, Rumley A, Lowe GD. Lipoprotein-associated phospholipase A2 as an independent predictor of coronary heart disease. West of Scotland Coronary Prevention Study Group. N Engl J Med 2000;343(16):1148-55.

63. Yamada Y, Ichihara S, Fujimura T, Yokota M. Identification of the G994–> T missense in exon 9 of the plasma platelet-activating factor acetylhydrolase gene as an independent risk factor for coronary artery disease in Japanese men. Metabolism 1998;47(2):177-81.

64. Meade TW, Mellows S, Brozovic M, Miller GJ, Chakrabarti RR, North WR, Haines AP, Stirling Y, Imeson JD, Thompson SG. Haemostatic function and ischaemic heart disease: principal results of the Northwick Park Heart Study. Lancet 1986;2(8506):533-7.

65. Iacoviello L, Di Castelnuovo A, De Knijff P, D'Orazio A, Amore C, Arboretti R, Kluft C, Benedetta Donati M. Polymorphisms in the coagulation factor VII gene and the risk of myocardial infarction. N Engl J Med 1998;338(2):79-85.

66. Kohler HP, Stickland MH, Ossei-Gerning N, Carter A, Mikkola H, Grant PJ. Association of a common polymorphism in the factor XIII gene with myocardial infarction. Thromb Haemost 1998;79(1):8-13.

67. Doggen CJ, Manger Cats V, Bertina RM, Reitsma PH, Vandenbroucke JP, Rosendaal FR. A genetic propensity to high factor VII is not associated with the risk of myocardial infarction in men. Thromb Haemost 1998;80(2):281-5.

68. Rosendaal FR, Siscovick DS, Schwartz SM, Psaty BM, Raghunathan TE, Vos HL. A common prothrombin variant (20210 G to A) increases the risk of myocardial infarction in young women. Blood 1997;90(5):1747-50.

69. Ardissino D, Mannucci PM, Merlini PA, Duca F, Fetiveau R, Tagliabue L, Tubaro M, Galvani M, Ottani F, Ferrario M, Corral J, Margaglione M. Prothrombotic genetic risk factors in young survivors of myocardial infarction. Blood 1999;94(1):46-51.

70. Zito F, Di Castelnuovo A, Amore C, D'Orazio A, Donati MB, Iacoviello L. Bcl I polymorphism in the fibrinogen beta-chain gene is associated with the risk of familial myocardial infarction by increasing plasma fibrinogen levels. A case-control study in a sample of GISSI-2 patients. Arterioscler Thromb Vasc Biol 1997;17(12):3489-94.

71. Smiles AM, Jenny NS, Tang Z, Arnold A, Cushman M, Tracy RP. No association of plasma prothrombin concentration or the G20210A mutation with incident cardiovascular disease: results from the Cardiovascular Health Study. Thromb Haemost 2002;87(4):614-21.

72. Araujo F, Santos A, Araujo V, Henriques I, Monteiro F, Meireles E, Moreira I, David D, Maciel MJ, Cunha-Ribeiro LM. Genetic risk factors in acute coronary disease. Haemostasis 1999;29(4):212-8.

73. Arruda VR, Siquiera LH, Chiaparini LC, Coelho OR, Mansur AP, Ramires A, Annichino-Bizzacchi JM. Prevalence of the prothrombin gene variant 20210 G –> A among patients with myocardial infarction. Cardiovasc Res 1998;37(1):42-5.

74. Ridker PM, Hennekens CH, Miletich JP. G20210A mutation in prothrombin gene and risk of myocardial infarction, stroke, and venous thrombosis in a large cohort of US men. Circulation 1999;99(8):999-1004.

75. Rosendaal FR, Siscovick DS, Schwartz SM, Beverly RK, Psaty BM, Longstreth WT Jr, Raghunathan TE, Koepsell TD, Reitsma PH. Factor V Leiden (resistance to activated protein C) increases the risk of myocardial infarction in young women.. Blood 1997;89(8):2817-21.

76. Doggen CJ, Cats VM, Bertina RM, Rosendaal FR. Interaction of coagulation defects and cardiovascular risk factors: increased risk of myocardial infarction associated with factor V Leiden or prothrombin 20210A. Circulation 1998;97(11):1037-41.

77. Endler G, Mannhalter C. Polymorphisms in coagulation factor genes and their impact on arterial and venous thrombosis. Clin Chim Acta 2003;330(1-2):31-55.

78. Rallidis LS, Belesi CI, Manioudaki HS, Chatziioakimidis VK, Fakitsa VC, Sinos LE, Laoutaris NP, Apostolou TS. Myocardial infarction under the age of 36: prevalence of thrombophilic disorders. Thromb Haemost 2003;90(2):272-8.

79. Danesh J, Collins R, Appleby P, Peto R. Association of fibrinogen, C-reactive protein, albumin, or leukocyte count with coronary heart disease: meta-analyses of prospective studies. Jama 1998;279(18):1477-82.

80. Behague I, Poirier O, Nicaud V, Evans A, Arveiler D, Luc G, Cambou JP, Scarabin PY, Bara L, Green F, Cambien F. Beta fibrinogen gene polymorphisms are associated with plasma fibrinogen and coronary artery disease in patients with myocardial infarction. The ECTIM Study. Etude Cas-Temoins sur l'Infarctus du Myocarde. Circulation 1996;93(3):440-9.

81. Ye S, Watts GF, Mandalia S, Humphries SE, Henney AM. Preliminary report: genetic variation in the human stromelysin promoter is associated with progression of coronary atherosclerosis. Br Heart J 1995;73(3):209-15.

82. Tybjaerg-Hansen A, Agerholm-Larsen B, Humphries SE, Abildgaard S, Schnohr P, Nordestgaard BG. A common mutation (G-455-> A) in the beta-fibrinogen promoter is an independent predictor of plasma fibrinogen, but not of ischemic heart disease. A study of 9,127 individuals based on the Copenhagen City Heart Study. J Clin Invest 1997;99(12):3034-9.

83. Gardemann A, Schwartz O, Haberbosch W, Katz N, Weiss T, Tillmanns H, Hehrlein FW, Waas W, Eberbach A. Positive association of the beta fibrinogen H1/H2 gene variation to basal fibrinogen levels and to the increase in fibrinogen concentration during acute phase reaction but not to coronary artery disease and myocardial infarction. Thromb Haemost 1997; 77(6):1120-6.

84. Schmidt H, Schmidt R, Niederkorn K, Horner S, Becsagh P, Reinhart B, Schumacher M, Weinrauch V, Kostner GM. Beta-fibrinogen gene polymorphism (C148->T) is associated with carotid atherosclerosis: results of the Austrian Stroke Prevention Study. Arterioscler Thromb Vasc Biol 1998;18(3):487-92.

85. Hamsten A, Wiman B, de Faire U, Blomback M. Increased plasma levels of a rapid inhibitor of tissue plasminogen activator in young survivors of myocardial infarction. N Engl J Med 1985;313(25):1557-63.

86. De Lorenzo F, Xiao H, Kakkar VV. Prognostic role of plasminogen-activator-inhibitor-1 (PAI-1) levels in treatment with streptokinase of patients with acute myocardial infarction. Clin Cardiol 2000;23(12):877-8.

87. Burzotta F, Di Castelnuovo A, Amore C, D'Orazio A, Di Bitondo R, Donati MB, Iacoviello L. 4G/5G promoter PAI-1 gene polymorphism is associated with plasmatic PAI- 1 activity in Italians: a model of gene-environment interaction. Thromb Haemost 1998;79(2):354-8.

88. Eriksson P, Kallin B, van 't Hooft FM, Bavenholm P, Hamsten A. Allele-specific increase in basal transcription of the plasminogen- activator inhibitor 1 gene is associated with myocardial infarction. Proc Natl Acad Sci U S A 1995;92(6):1851-5.

89. Anderson JL, Muhlestein JB, Habashi J, Carlquist JF, Bair TL, Elmer SP, Davis BP. Lack of association of a common polymorphism of the plasminogen activator inhibitor-1 gene with coronary artery disease and myocardial infarction. J Am Coll Cardiol 1999;34(6):1778-83.

90. Doggen CJ, Bertina RM, Cats VM, Reitsma PH, Rosendaal FR. The 4G/5G polymorphism in the plasminogen activator inhibitor-1 gene is not associated with myocardial infarction. Thromb Haemost 1999;82(1):115-20.

91. Wartiovaara U, Perola M, Mikkola H, Totterman K, Savolainen V, Penttila A, Grant PJ, Tikkanen MJ, Vartiainen E, Karhunen PJ, Peltonen L, Palotie A. Association of FXIII Val34Leu with decreased risk of myocardial infarction in Finnish males. Atherosclerosis 1999;142(2):295-300.

92. Undas A, Sydor WJ, Brummel K, Musial J, Mann KG, Szczeklik A. Aspirin alters the cardioprotective effects of the factor XIII Val34Leu polymorphism. Circulation 2003;107(1):17-20.

93. Rigat B, Hubert C, Alhenc-Gelas F, Cambien F, Corvol P, Soubrier F. An insertion/deletion polymorphism in the angiotensin I-converting enzyme gene accounting for half the variance of serum enzyme levels. J Clin Invest 1990;86(4):1343-6.

94. Cambien F, Poirier O, Lecerf L, Evans A, Cambou JP, Arveiler D, Luc G, Bard JM, Bara L, Ricard S, al et. Deletion polymorphism in the gene for angiotensin-converting enzyme is a potent risk factor for myocardial infarction. Nature 1992;359(6396):641-4.

95. Keavney B, McKenzie C, Parish S, Palmer A, Clark S, Youngman L, Delepine M, Lathrop M, Peto R, Collins R. Large-scale test of hypothesised associations between the angiotensin-converting-enzyme insertion/deletion polymorphism and myocardial infarction in about 5000 cases and 6000 controls. International Studies of Infarct Survival (ISIS) Collaborators.. Lancet 2000;355(9202):434-42.

96. Zee RY, Solomon SD, Ajani UA, Pfeffer MA, Lindpaintner K. A prospective evaluation of the angiotensin-converting enzyme D/I polymorphism and left ventricular remodeling in the 'Healing and Early Afterload Reducing Therapy' study. Clin Genet 2002;61(1):21-5.

97. Matsubara M, Suzuki M, Fujiwara T, Kikuya M, Metoki H, Michimata M, Araki T, Kazama I, Satoh T, Hashimoto J, Hozawa A, Ohkubo T, Tsuji I, Katsuya T, Higaki J, Ogihara T, Satoh H, Imai Y. Angiotensin-converting enzyme I/D polymorphism and hypertension: the Ohasama study. J Hypertens 2002;20(6):1121-6.

98. Tiret L, Bonnardeaux A, Poirier O, Ricard S, Marques-Vidal P, Evans A, Arveiler D, Luc G, Kee F, Ducimetiere P, al et. Synergistic effects of angiotensin-converting enzyme and angiotensin-II type 1 receptor gene polymorphisms on risk of myocardial infarction. Lancet 1994;344(8927):910-3.

99. Fomicheva EV, Gukova SP, Larionova-Vasina VI, Kovalev YR, Schwartz EI. Gene-gene interaction in the RAS system in the predisposition to myocardial infarction in elder population of St. Petersburg (Russia). Mol Genet Metab 2000;69(1):76-80.

100. Petrovic D, Zorc M, Kanic V, Peterlin B. Interaction between gene polymorphisms of renin-angiotensin system and metabolic risk factors in premature myocardial infarction. Angiology 2001;52(4):247-52.

101. Humphries SE, Ordovas JM. Genetics and atherosclerosis: broadening the horizon. Atherosclerosis 2001;154(3):517-9.

102. Lambert JC, Brousseau T, Defosse V, Evans A, Arveiler D, Ruidavets JB, Haas B, Cambou JP, Luc G, Ducimetiere P, Cambien F, Chartier-Harlin MC, Amouyel P. Independent association of an APOE gene promoter polymorphism with increased risk of myocardial infarction and decreased APOE plasma concentrations-the ECTIM study. Hum Mol Genet 2000;9(1):57-61.

103. Brazier L, Tiret L, Luc G, Arveiler D, Ruidavets JB, Evans A, Chapman J, Cambien F, Thillet J. Sequence polymorphisms in the apolipoprotein(a) gene and their association with lipoprotein(a) levels and myocardial infarction. The ECTIM Study. Atherosclerosis 1999; 144(2):323-33.

104. Kuivenhoven JA, Jukema JW, Zwinderman AH, de Knijff P, McPherson R, Bruschke AV, Lie KI, Kastelein JJ. The role of a common variant of the cholesteryl ester transfer protein gene in the progression of coronary atherosclerosis. The Regression Growth Evaluation Statin Study Group. N Engl J Med 1998;338(2):86-93.

105. Lutucuta S, Ballantyne CM, Elghannam H, Gotto AM Jr, Marian AJ. Novel polymorphisms in promoter region of atp binding cassette transporter gene and plasma lipids, severity, progression, and regression of coronary atherosclerosis and response to therapy. Circ Res 2001; 88(9):969-73.

106. Turban S, Fuentes F, Ferlic L, Brugada R, Gotto AM, Ballantyne CM, Marian AJ. A prospective study of paraoxonase gene Q/R192 polymorphism and severity, progression and regression of coronary atherosclerosis, plasma lipid levels, clinical events and response to fluvastatin. Atherosclerosis 2001;154(3):633-40.

107. Holmer SR, Hengstenberg C, Mayer B, Doring A, Lowel H, Engel S, Hense HW, Wolf M, Klein G, Riegger GA, Schunkert H. Lipoprotein lipase gene polymorphism, cholesterol subfractions and myocardial infarction in large samples of the general population. Cardiovasc Res 2000;47(4):806-12.

108. Brousseau T, Arveiler D, Cambou JP, Evans AE, Luc G, Fruchart JC, Cambien F, Amouyel P. Familial defective apolipoprotein B-100 and myocardial infarction. The ECTIM study. Etude Cas-Temoins de l'Infarctus du Myocarde. Atherosclerosis 1995;116(2):269-71.

109. Ballantyne CM, Herd JA, Stein EA, Ferlic LL, Dunn JK, Gotto AM Jr, Marian AJ. Apolipoprotein E genotypes and response of plasma lipids and progression-regression of coronary atherosclerosis to lipid-lowering drug therapy. J Am Coll Cardiol 2000;36(5):1572-8.

110. Volkova MV, Vasina VI, Fomicheva EV, Schwartz EI. Comparative analysis of apo(a) gene alleles: distribution of pentanucleotide repeats in position -1373 and C/T transition in position +93 among patients with myocardial infarction and a control group in St. Petersburg, Russia. Biochem Mol Med 1997;61(2):208-13.

111. Imai Y, Morita H, Kurihara H, Sugiyama T, Kato N, Ebihara A, Hamada C, Kurihara Y, Shindo T, Oh-hashi Y, Yazaki Y. Evidence for association between paraoxonase gene polymorphisms and atherosclerotic diseases. Atherosclerosis 2000;149(2):435-42.

112. Wilson PW, Schaefer EJ, Larson MG, Ordovas JM. Apolipoprotein E alleles and risk of coronary disease. A meta-analysis. Arterioscler Thromb Vasc Biol 1996;16(10):1250-5.

113. Eichner JE, Dunn ST, Perveen G, Thompson DM, Stewart KE, Stroehla BC. Apolipoprotein E polymorphism and cardiovascular disease: a HuGE review. Am J Epidemiol 2002;155(6):487-95.

114. Roses AD, Saunders AM. APOE is a major susceptibility gene for Alzheimer's disease. Curr Opin Biotechnol 1994;5(6):663-7.

115. Eichner JE, Kuller LH, Orchard TJ, Grandits GA, McCallum LM, Ferrell RE, Neaton JD. Relation of apolipoprotein E phenotype to myocardial infarction and mortality from coronary artery disease. Am J Cardiol 1993;71(2):160-5.

116. de Andrade M, Thandi I, Brown S, Gotto A Jr, Patsch W, Boerwinkle E. Relationship of the apolipoprotein E polymorphism with carotid artery atherosclerosis. Am J Hum Genet 1995;56(6):1379-90.

117. Eiriksdottir G, Bolla MK, Thorsson B, Sigurdsson G, Humphries SE, Gudnason V. The -629C>A polymorphism in the CETP gene does not explain the association of TaqIB polymorphism with risk and age of myocardial infarction in Icelandic men. Atherosclerosis 2001;159(1):187-92.

118. Corbex M, Poirier O, Fumeron F, Betoulle D, Evans A, Ruidavets JB, Arveiler D, Luc G, Tiret L, Cambien F. Extensive association analysis between the CETP gene and coronary heart disease phenotypes reveals several putative functional polymorphisms and gene-environment interaction. Genet Epidemiol 2000;19(1):64-80.

119. Fumeron F, Betoulle D, Luc G, Behague I, Ricard S, Poirier O, Jemaa R, Evans A, Arveiler D, Marques-Vidal P, al et. Alcohol intake modulates the effect of a polymorphism of the cholesteryl ester transfer protein gene on plasma high density lipoprotein and the risk of myocardial infarction. J Clin Invest 1995;96(3):1664-71.

120. Libby P. Molecular bases of the acute coronary syndromes. Circulation 1995;91(11):2844-50.

121. Pankow JS, Folsom AR, Cushman M, Borecki IB, Hopkins PN, Eckfeldt JH, Tracy RP. Familial and genetic determinants of systemic markers of inflammation: the NHLBI family heart study. Atherosclerosis 2001;154(3):681-9.

122. Cybulsky MI, Iiyama K, Li H, Zhu S, Chen M, Iiyama M, Davis V, Gutierrez-Ramos JC, Connelly PW, Milstone DS. A major role for VCAM-1, but not ICAM-1, in early atherosclerosis. J Clin Invest 2001;107(10):1255-62.

123.  Tregouet DA, Barbaux S, Escolano S, Tahri N, Golmard JL, Tiret L, Cambien F. Specific haplotypes of the P-selectin gene are associated with myocardial infarction. Hum Mol Genet 2002;11(17):2015-23.

124.  Kee F, Morrison C, Evans AE, McCrum E, McMaster D, Dallongeville J, Nicaud V, Poirier O, Cambien F. Polymorphisms of the P-selectin gene and risk of myocardial infarction in men and women in the ECTIM extension study. Etude cas-temoin de l'infarctus myocarde. Heart 2000;84(5):548-52.

125.  Carter AM, Anagnostopoulou K, Mansfield MW, Grant PJ. Soluble P-selectin levels, P-selectin polymorphisms and cardiovascular disease. J Thromb Haemost 2003;1(8):1718-23.

126.  Galis ZS, Sukhova GK, Lark MW, Libby P. Increased expression of matrix metalloproteinases and matrix degrading activity in vulnerable regions of human atherosclerotic plaques. J Clin Invest 1994;94(6):2493-503.

127.  Ye S, Eriksson P, Hamsten A, Kurkinen M, Humphries SE, Henney AM. Progression of coronary atherosclerosis is associated with a common genetic variant of the human stromelysin-1 promoter which results in reduced gene expression. J Biol Chem 1996;271(22):13055-60.

128.  Gnasso A, Motti C, Irace C, Carallo C, Liberatoscioli L, Bernardini S, Massoud R, Mattioli PL, Federici G, Cortese C. Genetic variation in human stromelysin gene promoter and common carotid geometry in healthy male subjects. Arterioscler Thromb Vasc Biol 2000;20(6):1600-5.

129.  Ye S, Watts GF, Mandalia S, Humphries SE, Henney AM. Preliminary report: genetic variation in the human stromelysin promoter is associated with progression of coronary atherosclerosis. Br Heart J 1995;73(3):209-15.

130.  Terashima M, Akita H, Kanazawa K, Inoue N, Yamada S, Ito K, Matsuda Y, Takai E, Iwai C, Kurogane H, Yoshida Y, Yokoyama M. Stromelysin promoter 5A/6A polymorphism is associated with acute myocardial infarction. Circulation 1999;99(21):2717-9.

131.  Beyzade S, Zhang S, Wong YK, Day IN, Eriksson P, Ye S. Influences of matrix metalloproteinase-3 gene variation on extent of coronary atherosclerosis and risk of myocardial infarction. J Am Coll Cardiol 2003;41(12):2130-7.

132.  Humphries SE, Martin S, Cooper J, Miller G. Interaction between smoking and the stromelysin-1 (MMP3) gene 5A/6A promoter polymorphism and risk of coronary heart disease in healthy men. Ann Hum Genet 2002;66(Pt 5-6):343-52.

133.  Liu PY, Chen JH, Li YH, Wu HL, Shi GY. Synergistic effect of stromelysin-1 (matrix metallo-proteinase-3) promoter 5A/6A polymorphism with smoking on the onset of young acute myocardial infarction. Thromb Haemost 2003;90(1):132-9.

134.  Blankenberg S, Rupprecht HJ, Poirier O, Bickel C, Smieja M, Hafner G, Meyer J, Cambien F, Tiret L. Plasma concentrations and genetic variation of matrix metalloproteinase 9 and prognosis of patients with cardiovascular disease. Circulation 2003;107(12):1579-85.

135.  Zhang B, Ye S, Herrmann SM, Eriksson P, de Maat M, Evans A, Arveiler D, Luc G, Cambien F, Hamsten A, Watkins H, Henney AM. Functional polymorphism in the regulatory region of gelatinase B gene in relation to severity of coronary atherosclerosis. Circulation 1999; 99(14):1788-94.

136.  Zhang B, Henney A, Eriksson P, Hamsten A, Watkins H, Ye S. Genetic variation at the matrix metalloproteinase-9 locus on chromosome 20q12.2-13.1. Hum Genet 1999;105(5):418-23.

137.  Morgan AR, Zhang B, Tapper W, Collins A, Ye S. Haplotypic analysis of the MMP-9 gene in relation to coronary artery disease. J Mol Med 2003;81(5):321-6.

138.  Lamblin N, Bauters C, Hermant X, Lablanche JM, Helbecque N, Amouyel P. Polymorphisms in the promoter regions of MMP-2, MMP-3, MMP-9 and MMP-12 genes as determinants of aneurysmal coronary artery disease. J Am Coll Cardiol 2002;40(1):43-8.

139.  Cho HJ, Chae IH, Park KW, Ju JR, Oh S, Lee MM, Park YB. Functional polymorphism in the promoter region of the gelatinase B gene in relation to coronary artery disease and restenosis after percutaneous coronary intervention. J Hum Genet 2002;47(2):88-91.

140.  Moore JH, Williams SM. New strategies for identifying gene-gene interactions in hypertension. Ann Med 2002;34(2):88-95.

141. Thomas DC. Design of gene characterization studies: an overview. J Natl Cancer Inst Monogr 1999;(26):17-23.

142. Goldstein AM, Andrieu N. Detection of interaction involving identified genes: available study designs. J Natl Cancer Inst Monogr 1999;(26):49-54.

143. Lazarou J, Pomeranz BH, Corey PN. Incidence of adverse drug reactions in hospitalized patients: a meta-analysis of prospective studies. Jama 1998;279(15):1200-5.

144. http://wwwncbinlmnihgov/entrez/queryfcgi?db=OMIM.

145. Senti M, Aubo C, Bosch M, Pavesi M, Pena A, Masia R, Marrugat J. Platelet glycoprotein IIb/IIIa genetic polymorphism is associated with plasma fibrinogen levels in myocardial infarction patients. The REGICOR Investigators. Clin Biochem 1998;31(8):647-51.

146. Herrmann SM, Poirier O, Marques-Vidal P, Evans A, Arveiler D, Luc G, Emmerich J, Cambien F. The Leu33/Pro polymorphism (PlA1/PlA2) of the glycoprotein IIIa (GPIIIa) receptor is not related to myocardial infarction in the ECTIM Study. Etude Cas-Temoins de l'Infarctus du Myocarde. Thromb Haemost 1997;77(6):1179-81.

147. Zotz RB, Winkelmann BR, Nauck M, Giers G, Maruhn-Debowski B, Marz W, Scharf RE. Polymorphism of platelet membrane glycoprotein IIIa: human platelet antigen 1b (HPA-1b/PlA2) is an inherited risk factor for premature myocardial infarction in coronary artery disease. Thromb Haemost 1998;79(4):731-5.

148. Durante-Mangoni E, Davies GJ, Ahmed N, Ruggiero G, Tuddenham EG. Coronary thrombosis and the platelet glycoprotein IIIA gene PLA2 polymorphism. Thromb Haemost 1998; 80(2):218-9.

149. Samani NJ, Lodwick D. Glycoprotein IIIa polymorphism and risk of myocardial infarction. Cardiovasc Res 1997;33(3):693-7.

150. Gonzalez-Conejero R, Lozano ML, Rivera J, Corral J, Iniesta JA, Moraleda JM, Vicente V. Polymorphisms of platelet membrane glycoprotein Ib associated with arterial thrombotic disease. Blood 1998;92(8):2771-6.

151. Corral J, Gonzalez-Conejero R, Rivera J, Ortuno F, Aparicio P, Vicente V. Role of the 807 C/T polymorphism of the alpha2 gene in platelet GP Ia collagen receptor expression and function—effect in thromboembolic diseases. Thromb Haemost 1999;81(6):951-6.

152. Santoso S, Kunicki TJ, Kroll H, Haberbosch W, Gardemann A. Association of the platelet glycoprotein Ia C807T gene polymorphism with nonfatal myocardial infarction in younger patients. Blood 1999;93(8):2449-53.

153. Croft SA, Hampton KK, Sorrell JA, Steeds RP, Channer KS, Samani NJ, Daly ME. The GPIa C807T dimorphism associated with platelet collagen receptor density is not a risk factor for myocardial infarction. Br J Haematol 1999;106(3):771-6.

154. Nakayama T, Soma M, Saito S, Honye J, Yajima J, Rahmutula D, Kaneko Y, Sato M, Uwabo J, Aoi N, Kosuge K, Kunimoto M, Kanmatsuse K, Kokubun S. Association of a novel single nucleotide polymorphism of the prostacyclin synthase gene with myocardial infarction. Am Heart J 2002;143(5):797-801.

155. Boekholdt SM, Bijsterveld NR, Moons AH, Levi M, Buller HR, Peters RJ. Genetic variation in coagulation and fibrinolytic proteins and their relation with acute myocardial infarction: a systematic review. Circulation 2001;104(25):3063-8.

156. Ridker PM, Hennekens CH, Lindpaintner K, Stampfer MJ, Eisenberg PR, Miletich JP. Mutation in the gene coding for coagulation factor V and the risk of myocardial infarction, stroke, and venous thrombosis in apparently healthy men. N Engl J Med 1995;332(14):912-7.

157. Lane A, Green F, Scarabin PY, Nicaud V, Bara L, Humphries S, Evans A, Luc G, Cambou JP, Arveiler D, Cambien F. Factor VII Arg/Gln353 polymorphism determines factor VII coagulant activity in patients with myocardial infarction (MI) and control subjects in Belfast and in France but is not a strong indicator of MI risk in the ECTIM study. Atherosclerosis 1996;119(1):119-27.

158. Tsujita Y, Kinoshita M, Tanabe T, Iwai N. Role of a genetic variation in the promoter of human thromboxane synthase gene in myocardial infarction. Atherosclerosis 2000;153(1): 261-2.

159. Norlund L, Holm J, Zoller B, Ohlin AK. A common thrombomodulin amino acid dimorphism is associated with myocardial infarction. Thromb Haemost 1997;77(2):248-51.

160. Park HY, Nabika T, Jang Y, Kwon HM, Cho SY, Masuda J. Association of G-33A polymorphism in the thrombomodulin gene with myocardial infarction in Koreans. Hypertens Res 2002;25(3):389-94.

161. Webb KE, Martin JF, Hamsten A, Eriksson P, Iacoviello L, Gattone M, Donati MB, Di Castelnuovo A, Erusalimsky J, Humphries SE. Polymorphisms in the thrombopoietin gene are associated with risk of myocardial infarction at a young age. Atherosclerosis 2001;154(3): 703-11.

162. Yu Q, Safavi F, Roberts R, Marian AJ. A variant of beta fibrinogen is a genetic risk factor for coronary artery disease and myocardial infarction. J Investig Med 1996;44(4):154-9.

163. Shimada K, Watanabe Y, Mokuno H, Iwama Y, Daida H, Yamaguchi H. Common polymorphism in the promoter of the CD14 monocyte receptor gene is associated with acute myocardial infarction in Japanese men. Am J Cardiol 2000;86(6):682-4, A8.

164. Zee RY, Lindpaintner K, Struk B, Hennekens CH, Ridker PM. A prospective evaluation of the CD14 C(-260)T gene polymorphism and the risk of myocardial infarction. Atherosclerosis 2001;154(3):699-702.

165. Shimada K, Watanabe Y, Mokuno H, Iwama Y, Daida H, Yamaguchi H. Common polymorphism in the promoter of the CD14 monocyte receptor gene is associated with acute myocardial infarction in Japanese men. Am J Cardiol 2000;86(6):682-4, A8.

166. Unkelbach K, Gardemann A, Kostrzewa M, Philipp M, Tillmanns H, Haberbosch W. A new promoter polymorphism in the gene of lipopolysaccharide receptor CD14 is associated with expired myocardial infarction in patients with low atherosclerotic risk profile. Arterioscler Thromb Vasc Biol 1999;19(4):932-8.

167. Manzoli A, Andreotti F, Varlotta C, Mollichelli N, Verde M, van de Greef W, Sperti G, Maseri A. Allelic polymorphism of the interleukin-1 receptor antagonist gene in patients with acute or stable presentation of ischemic heart disease. Cardiologia 1999;44(9):825-30.

168. Iacoviello L, Donati MB, Gattone M. Possible different involvement of interleukin-1 receptor antagonist gene polymorphism in coronary single vessel disease and myocardial infarction. Circulation 2000;101(18):E193.

169. Zee RY, Lunze K, Lindpaintner K, Ridker PM. A prospective evaluation of the interleukin-1 receptor antagonist intron 2 gene polymorphism and the risk of myocardial infarction. Thromb Haemost 2001;86(5):1141-3.

170. Momiyama Y, Hirano R, Taniguchi H, Nakamura H, Ohsuzu F. Effects of interleukin-1 gene polymorphisms on the development of coronary artery disease associated with Chlamydia pneumoniae infection. J Am Coll Cardiol 2001;38(3):712-7.

171. Georges JL, Loukaci V, Poirier O, Evans A, Luc G, Arveiler D, Ruidavets JB, Cambien F, Tiret L. Interleukin-6 gene polymorphisms and susceptibility to myocardial infarction: the ECTIM study. Etude Cas-Temoin de l'Infarctus du Myocarde. J Mol Med 2001;79(5-6):300-5.

172. Basso F, Lowe GD, Rumley A, McMahon AD, Humphries SE. Interleukin-6 -174G>C polymorphism and risk of coronary heart disease in West of Scotland coronary prevention study (WOSCOPS). Arterioscler Thromb Vasc Biol 2002;22(4):599-604.

173. Nauck M, Winkelmann BR, Hoffmann MM, Bohm BO, Wieland H, Marz W. The interleukin-6 G(-174)C promoter polymorphism in the LURIC cohort: no association with plasma interleukin-6, coronary artery disease, and myocardial infarction. J Mol Med 2002;80(8):507-13.

174. Jenny NS, Tracy RP, Ogg MS, Luong le A, Kuller LH, Arnold AM, Sharrett AR, Humphries SE. In the elderly, interleukin-6 plasma levels and the -174G>C polymorphism are associated with the development of cardiovascular disease. Arterioscler Thromb Vasc Biol 2002;22(12): 2066-71.

175. Bernard V, Pillois X, Dubus I, Benchimol D, Labouyrie JP, Couffinhal T, Coste P, Bonnet J. The -308 G/A tumor necrosis factor-alpha gene dimorphism: a risk factor for unstable angina. Clin Chem Lab Med 2003;41(4):511-6.

176. Herrmann SM, Ricard S, Nicaud V, Mallet C, Arveiler D, Evans A, Ruidavets JB, Luc G, Bara L, Parra HJ, Poirier O, Cambien F. Polymorphisms of the tumour necrosis factor-alpha gene, coronary heart disease and obesity. Eur J Clin Invest 1998;28(1):59-66.

177. Herrmann SM, Ricard S, Nicaud V, Mallet C, Evans A, Ruidavets JB, Arveiler D, Luc G, Cambien F. The P-selectin gene is highly polymorphic: reduced frequency of the Pro715 allele carriers in patients with myocardial infarction. Hum Mol Genet 1998;7(8):1277-84.

178. Yoshida M, Takano Y, Sasaoka T, Izumi T, Kimura A. E-selectin polymorphism associated with myocardial infarction causes enhanced leukocyte-endothelial interactions under flow conditions. Arterioscler Thromb Vasc Biol 2003;23(5):783-8.

179. Sasaoka T, Kimura A, Hohta SA, Fukuda N, Kurosawa T, Izumi T. Polymorphisms in the platelet-endothelial cell adhesion molecule-1 (PECAM-1) gene, Asn563Ser and Gly670Arg, associated with myocardial infarction in the Japanese. Ann N Y Acad Sci 2001;947:259-69; discussion 269-70.

180. Syrris P, Carter ND, Metcalfe JC, Kemp PR, Grainger DJ, Kaski JC, Crossman DC, Francis SE, Gunn J, Jeffery S, Heathcote K. Transforming growth factor-beta1 gene polymorphisms and coronary artery disease. Clin Sci (Lond) 1998;95(6):659-67.

181. Cambien F, Ricard S, Troesch A, Mallet C, Generenaz L, Evans A, Arveiler D, Luc G, Ruidavets JB, Poirier O. Polymorphisms of the transforming growth factor-beta 1 gene in relation to myocardial infarction and blood pressure. The Etude Cas-Temoin de l'Infarctus du Myocarde (ECTIM) Study. Hypertension 1996;28(5):881-7.

182. Yokota M, Ichihara S, Lin TL, Nakashima N, Yamada Y. Association of a T29->C polymorphism of the transforming growth factor- beta1 gene with genetic susceptibility to myocardial infarction in Japanese. Circulation 2000;101(24):2783-7.

183. Boekholdt SM, Trip MD, Peters RJ, Engelen M, Boer JM, Feskens EJ, Zwinderman AH, Kastelein JJ, Reitsma PH. Thrombospondin-2 polymorphism is associated with a reduced risk of premature myocardial infarction. Arterioscler Thromb Vasc Biol 2002;22(12):e24-7.

184. Lindpaintner K, Pfeffer MA, Kreutz R, Stampfer MJ, Grodstein F, LaMotte F, Buring J, Hennekens CH. A prospective evaluation of an angiotensin-converting-enzyme gene polymorphism and the risk of ischemic heart disease. N Engl J Med 1995;332(11):706-11.

185. Agerholm-Larsen B, Nordestgaard BG, Steffensen R, Sorensen TI, Jensen G, Tybjaerg-Hansen A. ACE gene polymorphism: ischemic heart disease and longevity in 10,150 individuals. A case-referent and retrospective cohort study based on the Copenhagen City Heart Study. Circulation 1997;95(10):2358-67.

186. Katsuya T, Koike G, Yee TW, Sharpe N, Jackson R, Norton R, Horiuchi M, Pratt RE, Dzau VJ, MacMahon S. Association of angiotensinogen gene T235 variant with increased risk of coronary heart disease. Lancet 1995;345(8965):1600-3.

187. Ichihara S, Yamada Y, Fujimura T, Nakashima N, Yokota M. Association of a polymorphism of the endothelial constitutive nitric oxide synthase gene with myocardial infarction in the Japanese population. Am J Cardiol 1998;81(1):83-6.

188. Hibi K, Ishigami T, Tamura K, Mizushima S, Nyui N, Fujita T, Ochiai H, Kosuge M, Watanabe Y, Yoshii Y, Kihara M, Kimura K, Ishii M, Umemura S. Endothelial nitric oxide synthase gene polymorphism and acute myocardial infarction. Hypertension 1998;32(3):521-6.

189. Wang XL, Sim AS, Badenhop RF, McCredie RM, Wilcken DE. A smoking-dependent risk of coronary artery disease associated with a polymorphism of the endothelial nitric oxide synthase gene. Nat Med 1996;2(1):41-5.

190. Hingorani AD, Liang CF, Fatibene J, Lyon A, Monteith S, Parsons A, Haydock S, Hopper RV, Stephens NG, O'Shaughnessy KM, Brown MJ. A common variant of the endothelial nitric oxide synthase (Glu298− >Asp) is a major risk factor for coronary artery disease in the UK. Circulation 1999;100(14):1515-20.

191. Nakayama M, Yasue H, Yoshimura M, Shimasaki Y, Ogawa H, Kugiyama K, Mizuno Y, Harada E, Nakamura S, Ito T, Saito Y, Miyamoto Y, Ogawa Y, Nakao K. T(-786)-> C mutation in the 5'-flanking region of the endothelial nitric oxide synthase gene is associated with myocardial infarction, especially without coronary organic stenosis. Am J Cardiol 2000; 86(6):628-34.

192. Gruchala M, Ciecwierz D, Wasag B, Targonski R, Dubaniewicz W, Nowak A, Sobiczewski W, Ochman K, Romanowski P, Limon J, Rynkiewicz A. Association of the ScaI atrial natri-

uretic peptide gene polymorphism with nonfatal myocardial infarction and extent of coronary artery disease. Am Heart J 2003;145(1):125-31.

193. Gerdes LU, Gerdes C, Kervinen K, Savolainen M, Klausen IC, Hansen PS, Kesaniemi YA, Faergeman O. The apolipoprotein epsilon4 allele determines prognosis and the effect on prognosis of simvastatin in survivors of myocardial infarction : a substudy of the Scandinavian simvastatin survival study. Circulation 2000;101(12):1366-71.

194. Gardemann A, Philipp M, Hess K, Katz N, Tillmanns H, Haberbosch W. The paraoxonase Leu-Met54 and Gln-Arg191 gene polymorphisms are not associated with the risk of coronary heart disease. Atherosclerosis 2000;152(2):421-31.

195. Sen-Banerjee S, Siles X, Campos H. Tobacco smoking modifies association between Gln-Arg192 polymorphism of human paraoxonase gene and risk of myocardial infarction. Arterioscler Thromb Vasc Biol 2000;20(9):2120-6.

196. Senti M, Tomas M, Marrugat J, Elosua R. Paraoxonase1-192 polymorphism modulates the nonfatal myocardial infarction risk associated with decreased HDLs. Arterioscler Thromb Vasc Biol 2001;21(3):415-20.

197. Senti M, Aubo C, Tomas M. Differential effects of smoking on myocardial infarction risk according to the Gln/Arg 192 variants of the human paraoxonase gene. Metabolism 2000; 49(5):557-9.

198. Liu S, Schmitz C, Stampfer MJ, Sacks F, Hennekens CH, Lindpaintner K, Ridker PM. A prospective study of TaqIB polymorphism in the gene coding for cholesteryl ester transfer protein and risk of myocardial infarction in middle-aged men. Atherosclerosis 2002;161(2): 469-74.

199. Gardemann A, Ohly D, Fink M, Katz N, Tillmanns H, Hehrlein FW, Haberbosch W. Association of the insertion/deletion gene polymorphism of the apolipoprotein B signal peptide with myocardial infarction. Atherosclerosis 1998;141(1):167-75.

200. Tatsuguchi M, Furutani M, Hinagata J, Tanaka T, Furutani Y, Imamura S, Kawana M, Masaki T, Kasanuki H, Sawamura T, Matsuoka R. Oxidized LDL receptor gene (OLR1) is associated with the risk of myocardial infarction. Biochem Biophys Res Commun 2003;303(1):247-50.

201. Schmitz C, Lindpaintner K, Verhoef P, Gaziano JM, Buring J. Genetic polymorphism of methylenetetrahydrofolate reductase and myocardial infarction. A case-control study. Circulation 1996;94(8):1812-4.

202. Adams M, Smith PD, Martin D, Thompson JR, Lodwick D, Samani NJ. Genetic analysis of thermolabile methylenetetrahydrofolate reductase as a risk factor for myocardial infarction. Qjm 1996;89(6):437-44.

203. Schwartz SM, Siscovick DS, Malinow MR, Rosendaal FR, Beverly RK, Hess DL, Psaty BM, Longstreth WT Jr, Koepsell TD, Raghunathan TE, Reitsma PH. Myocardial infarction in young women in relation to plasma total homocysteine, folate, and a common variant in the methylenetetrahydrofolate reductase gene. Circulation 1997;96(2):412-7.

204. van Bockxmeer FM, Mamotte CD, Vasikaran SD, Taylor RR. Methylenetetrahydrofolate reductase gene and coronary artery disease. Circulation 1997;95(1):21-3.

205. Hyndman ME, Bridge PJ, Warnica JW, Fick G, Parsons HG. Effect of heterozygosity for the methionine synthase 2756 A–>G mutation on the risk for recurrent cardiovascular events. Am J Cardiol 2000;86(10):1144-6, A9.

206. Snapir A, Heinonen P, Tuomainen TP, Alhopuro P, Karvonen MK, Lakka TA, Nyyssonen K, Salonen R, Kauhanen J, Valkonen VP, Pesonen U, Koulu M, Scheinin M, Salonen JT. An insertion/deletion polymorphism in the alpha2B-adrenergic receptor gene is a novel genetic risk factor for acute coronary events. J Am Coll Cardiol 2001;37(6):1516-22.

207. Sala G, Di Castelnuovo A, Cuomo L, Gattone M, Giannuzzi P, Iacoviello L, De Blasi A. The E27 beta2-adrenergic receptor polymorphism reduces the risk of myocardial infarction in dyslipidemic young males. Thromb Haemost 2001;85(2):231-3.

208. Endler G, Mannhalter C, Sunder-Plassmann H, Schillinger M, Klimesch A, Exner M, Kapiotis S, Meier S, Kunz F, Raiger E, Huber K, Wagner O, Sunder-Plassmann R. The K121Q polymorphism in the plasma cell membrane glycoprotein 1 gene predisposes to early myocardial infarction. J Mol Med 2002;80(12):791-5.

209. Wilson MH, Grant PJ, Kain K, Warner DP, Wild CP. Association between the risk of coronary artery disease in South Asians and a deletion polymorphism in glutathione S-transferase M1. Biomarkers 2003;8(1):43-50.

210. Mukae S, Aoki S, Itoh S, Sato R, Nishio K, Iwata T, Katagiri T. Mitochondrial 5178A/C genotype is associated with acute myocardial infarction. Circ J 2003;67(1):16-20.

211. Gonzalez-Conejero R, Corral J, Roldan V, Martinez C, Marin F, Rivera J, Iniesta JA, Lozano ML, Marco P, Vicente V. A common polymorphism in the annexin V Kozak sequence (-1C>T) increases translation efficiency and plasma levels of annexin V, and decreases the risk of myocardial infarction in young patients. Blood 2002;100(6):2081-6.

# 3

# Plaque Rupture: Pathoanatomical and Biomechanical Considerations

**Ole Frøbert**
*Department of Cardiology,*
*University of Aarhus, Denmark*

**Hans-Henrik Tilsted Hansen and Erling Falk**

## INTRODUCTION

Atherosclerosis in the coronary arteries is a very common autopsy finding, even in people not suffering from ischemic heart disease [1]. Although ischemic heart disease is the leading cause of death in the industrialized countries [2], more persons live with coronary atherosclerosis than die of it. Therefore, the key question is not why atherosclerosis develops but, rather, why a quiescent atherosclerotic plaque, after years of indolent growth, suddenly ruptures and becomes highly thrombogenic—the life-threatening event responsible for the great majority of the acute coronary syndromes (ACS)[3,4].

The risk of plaque rupture is related to intrinsic properties within a plaque (its vulnerability) that predispose it to rupture and extrinsic forces acting on the plaque (rupture triggers) that may precipitate rupture if the plaque is vulnerable [3]. This chapter will review possible mechanisms responsible for the sudden conversion of a quiescent atherosclerotic plaque to a rapidly progressing and highly thrombogenic lesion.

## MATURE ATHEROSCLEROTIC PLAQUES

The distribution of atherosclerotic lesions is not random. Plaques tend to evolve at places of low shear stress and a high degree of flow oscillation—typically on the outer wall of bifurcations, along the inner wall of curved segments, and proximal to myocardial bridging [1,5–8]. The diversity of atherosclerosis in different organs should be seen in light of the fact that smooth muscle cells (SMC) are locally derived from individual organ parenchyma during embryogenesis in contrast to the embryonic endothelium that invades the organ [9]. Although atherogenesis starts in early childhood, it takes decades to develop the mature plaques responsible for clinical diseases such as ischemic heart disease, ischemic stroke, aortic aneurysm, and claudication. As the name *atherosclerosis* implies, mature plaques

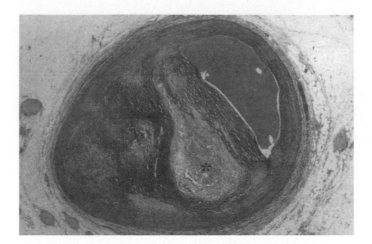

**Figure 1** Athersclerosis is characterized by two main components: atheromatous "gruel" and sclerotic tissue. The atheromatous component (*asterisk*) is lipid-rich and dangerous because it softens plaques, making them vulnerable to rupture with subsequent thrombosis. The sclerotic collagen-rich component is, as here, usually the most voluminous plaque component. Sclerosis, however, is rather innocuous; it may in fact, be good because it conveys stability to the lesion. (From Ref. 3. Copyright 1995, the American Heart Association

consist typically of two main components: soft, lipid-rich *atheromatous* "gruel" and hard, collagen-rich *sclerotic* tissue (Figure 1). The sclerotic component (fibrous tissue), by far, is usually the most voluminous component of the plaque, constituting greater than 70% of an average stenotic coronary plaque [3]. Sclerosis, however, is relatively innocuous because fibrous tissue appears to stabilize plaques, protecting them against rupture. In contrast, the usually less voluminous atheromatous component is the most dangerous component because the soft, lipid-rich gruel destabilizes plaques, making them vulnerable to rupture.

The lipid-rich core within a plaque is devoid of supporting collagen, avascular, hypocellular (except at the periphery of the core), and rich in extracellular lipids and soft-like gruel [3]. Macrophage foam cells surround the core, ceroid and macrophage specific CD68 antigen, and indicators of oxidant stress (F2-Isoprostanes and hydroxyeicosatetraenoic acids), but not SMC actin, are found within the gruel [10–12]. This suggests that the death of lipid-laden macrophages contributes to gruel formation and thereby to core enlargement, which is why the core has been called "the graveyard of dead macrophages" [10,13]. Another explanation of core formation is direct lipid trapping of low-density lipoproteins (LDL) in the extracellular space of the arterial intima as a result of binding between transcytosed LDL and glycosaminoglycans, collagen, and fibrinogen [14–17]. The relative contribution of cell necrosis vs. direct lipid trapping in the development of the lipid-rich core is not clear.

## Plaque Size and Composition

Several pathoanatomical studies indicate that the lipid-rich atheromatous component enlarges with plaque growth, but the variability is great [3]. One study revealed no significant correlation between the size of a plaque and its composition [18], while more recent studies indicate that lipid core size, medial atrophy, internal elastic lamina rupture, and macrophage burden are all determinants of plaque vulnerability [19,20]. Expansive remodelling, the fact that the external elastic membrane area at the lesion site is increased compared to a proximal reference site, is more often observed in culprit lesions whereas constrictive remodelling is more often observed with stable angina [21–23]. Increased plaque thrombogenicity rather than increased vulnerability represents an alternative explanation for the clinical observation that severely obstructive plaques are more prone to occlude and/or become culprit for myocardial infarction than less obstructive plaques [24–28].

## Risk Factors and Plaque Composition

There is a remarkable and poorly understood variability in the way plaques evolve, and it is unclear how the various risk factors for clinical disease influence the development, composition, and vulnerability of atherosclerotic plaques. Age, male sex, hypercholesterolemia, hypertension, smoking, and diabetes correlate with the coronary plaque burden (extent of ''plaquing'') found at autopsy [29–32], and there is an increase in calcification with age and possibly male sex [33]. Fibrous tissue constitute the most voluminous component of mature coronary plaques, regardless of individual risk factors [3]. In autopsy studies, cigarette smoking is more often associated with acute coronary thrombosis than with stable plaque development [34,35]. High total cholesterol to high-density lipoprotein (HDL) cholesterol ratio in men [34] and total cholesterol in women [35] were, in one study, associated with plaque rupture, and age greater than 50 years was associated with vulnerable plaques in women [35]. The association between plasma cholesterol levels and plaque rupture was, however, not confirmed in a subsequent large autopsy series [36]. An ultrasound study found that echo-lutency of carotid plaques was associated with high plasma levels of triglyceride-rich lipoproteins, which might predict a particularly vulnerable lipid-rich plaque type [37].

## PLAQUE VULNERABILITY

Plaques containing a soft, lipid-rich core are vulnerable to rupture, i.e., the fibrous cap separating the core from the lumen may disintegrate, tear, or break, whereby the highly thrombogenic gruel is suddenly exposed to the flowing blood. Such ruptured plaques are found beneath about 75% of the thrombi responsible for ACS [38–42]. Beneath the remaining thrombi, superficial plaque erosions without frank rupture (no deep injury) are usually found, often in combination with a severe atherosclerotic stenosis [38–40,43,44].

Pathoanatomical studies have identified three major determinants of a plaque's vulnerability to rupture: (a) size and consistency of the lipid-rich core, (b) thickness of the fibrous cap covering the core, and (c) inflammation and repair processes within the cap [45].

## Atheromatous Core

The size and consistency of the lipid-rich core vary greatly and are critical for the stability of individual lesions. Gertz and Roberts reported the composition of plaques in 5-mm segments from 17 infarct-related arteries examined postmortem and found much larger cores in the 39 segments with plaque rupture than in the 229 segments with intact surface (32% and 5–12% of plaque area, respectively) [46]. In aortic plaques, Davies et al. found a similar relation between core size and plaque rupture, and they identified a critical threshold; intact aortic plaques containing a core occupying less than 40% of the plaque were considered particularly vulnerable and at high risk of rupture and thrombosis [47].

The consistency of the core depends on lipid composition and temperature; it is usually soft, like toothpaste, at room temperature postmortem, and is even softer at body temperature in vivo. The semifluid cholesteryl esters soften plaques whereas the solid crystalline cholesterol has the opposite effect [48,49]. Lipid-lowering therapy is expected to deplete plaque lipid, with an overall reduction in cholesteryl esters (liquid and mobile) and a relative increase in crystalline cholesterol (solid and inert), theoretically resulting in a stiffer and more stable plaque [48–50].

## Cap Thickness

Fibrous caps vary widely in thickness, cellularity, matrix, strength, and stiffness, but they are often thinnest (and macrophage infiltrated) at their shoulder regions, where rupture most frequently occurs [38]; the thinner the cap is, the greater risk of rupture [51–53]. Loss of cells and calcification in fibrous caps are associated with increased stiffness [54], although calcification per se does not increase fibrous cap stress or decrease mechanical stability [55].

## Cap Inflammation and Repair

Autopsy studies have shown that ruptured fibrous caps usually are heavily infiltrated by macrophage foam cells that are activated, indicating ongoing inflammation at the site of plaque rupture [39,40,56–58) (Figure 2). For eccentric plaques, the shoulder regions are sites of predilection for both active inflammation and rupture [38,59,60], and in vitro mechanical testing of aortic fibrous caps indicates that foam cell infiltration indeed weakens caps locally, reducing their tensile strength [61]. These postmortem findings have been confirmed by studies of plaque tissue retrieved by atherectomy. Coronary culprit lesions responsible for acute coronary syndromes contain significantly more macrophages [28,62] and neutrophils [63] than lesions responsible for stable angina pectoris. Also, lipoprotein(s) appears to be more massively engaged in coronary plaques from unstable than stable angina patients [64]. Lipid-rich, rupture-prone plaques have an increased microvessel density and express increased levels of endothelial adhesion molecules (intercellular cell adhesion molecule [ICAM-1], vascular cell adhesion molecule [VCAM-1], PECAM, E-Selectin) [65], an increase in inducible nitric oxide synthase [66] and increased expression of angiotensin II [67] compared with stable fibrous plaques. CD40 ligand, an immunoregulatory signaling molecule previously considered restricted to activated CD4 + T lymphocytes, is coexpressed with its receptor CD40 on vascular endothelial cells, SMCs, and macrophages in human atherosclerotic lesions in situ [68] and elevation of CD40 ligand serum levels indicates an increased risk of cardiovascular events [69].

Macrophages are capable of degrading extracellular matrix by phagocytosis or by secreting proteolytic enzymes such as plasminogen activators and a family of matrix metalloproteinases (matrix metalloproteinase (MMPs): collagenases, gelatinases, and stromelysins) that may weaken the fibrous cap, predisposing it to rupture [70]. There is apparently no link to loci encoding for tissue inhibitors of MMPs in early coronary artery disease [71], but, in diabetic patients, the receptor for advanced glycation end products (RAGE) is overexpressed in plaque macrophages, which might contribute to plaque destabilization [72]. Thermal heterogeneity in coronary and carotid plaques indicates heat released by activated macrophages [73,74]. Oxidized LDL, in combination with tumor necrosis factor (TNF-alpha), increases MMP production in macrophages [75,76] and decreases tissue inhibitor of metalloproteinase-1 (TIMP-1) [75]. Activated mast cells are also present in ruptured caps [77], and they secrete powerful proteolytic enzymes such as tryptase [78] and chymase that can activate pro-MMPs secreted by other cells. Their number, however, is rather small in comparison with macrophages [79]. Furthermore, increased immunoreac-

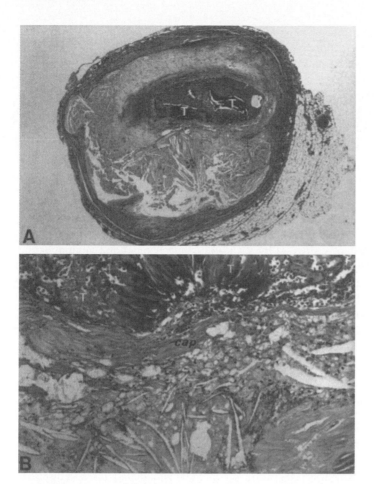

**Figure 2** (A) A severely stenotic vulnerable plaque containing a huge atheromatous core (asterisk) that is separated from the narrowed lumen by only a think fibrous cap. The lumen contains a nonoccluding thrombus (**T**). (**B**) Higher magnification of the plaque thrombus interface reveals that the fibrous cap beneath the thrombus is very thin and heavily foam-cell infiltrated, indicating ongoing disease activity. The cap was ruptured nearby (the actual rupture site is not represented in this section), explaining why a luminal thrombus has evolved. (From Ref. 80a. Copyright 1992, the American Heart Association.)

tivity of the nonlysosomal ubiquitin protein degradation pathway has been found colocalized with macrophages and T cells in high-risk coronary plaques [80].

Collagen is the main component of fibrous caps responsible for their tensile strength. Collagen is synthesized by vascular SMCs and it is likely that interferon γ produced by T lymphocytes decrease the ability of the SMCs to express the interstitial collagen genes in lipid-rich plaques [81]. Ruptured caps contain fewer SMCs and less collagen than intact caps [39,47,79,82,83]. Hypercholesterolemia is associated with local collagen degradation and plaque weakening [84]. Human monocyte-derived macrophages grown in culture are capable of degrading cap collagen and express MMP-1 (interstitial collagenase) and induce MMP-2 (gelatinolytic) activity in the culture medium [85]. Several studies have now identified MMPs in human coronary plaques [86–88]. Monocytes/macrophages could also play a detrimental role after plaque rupture, promoting thrombin generation and luminal thrombosis via tissue factor expression [89–93].

A number of infectious agents have been suggested to play an active role in the development of cardiovascular diseases, particularly *Chlamydia pneumoniae* [94], but also herpes-viruses (including cytomegalovirus) and *Helicobacter pylori* [45,95,96]. Chlamydia contains lipopolysaccharide and heat shock protein 60, which are well-known strong inducers of many enzymes, among others MMPs [97]. Chlamydia also reduces cap thickness in plaques from ApoE double knockout mice [98]. A possible interplay between infectious agents and development of atherosclerotic plaques may be driven by T helper type 1 lymphocytes [99].

## RUPTURE TRIGGERS

Coronary plaques are constantly stressed by a variety of mechanical and hemodynamic forces that may precipitate or "trigger" rupture of vulnerable plaques [100,101]. Stresses imposed on plaques are usually concentrated at the weak points discussed previously, namely at points where the fibrous cap is thinnest and tearing most frequently occurs [51]. In theory, mechanical forces may act in the three principal directions: the circumferential, the longitudinal, and the radial. The following discussion will review the literature with respect to these principal directions and will also consider shear, fatigue, and plaque configuration.

### Circumferential Deformation

Stretching of the coronary artery wall results in a systolic-diastolic change in the circumferential length of about 10% in normal compliant arteries [100]. The stiffness apparently increases with age [102,103], but there is no clear-cut relation between the degree of atherosclerosis and arterial stiffness [104–106]. As could be anticipated, the less diseased arcs of the arterial wall are stretched more than diseased, often calcified arcs of the wall [23,106–109]. The stress gradient in these zones—which usually coincide with the shoulder region of the plaque—from uneven circumferential stretching of the wall could partly explain why rupture frequently takes place here. In a population-based finite element analysis it was shown that the area of greatest stress in coronary atherosclerosis above 20 years of age is at the shoulder region of the plaque and that age was strongly correlated with shoulder stress [110]; these findings have been confirmed by in vivo angioplasty data [111].

A promising add-on to intravascular ultrasound, termed intravascular elastography, measures local circumferential strain as an indicator of the local compliance of tissue [109,112]. In vitro this method has demonstrated a high sensitivity and specificity to detect vulnerable plaques, a high correlation between strain in vulnerable plaques and the amount of macrophages, and an inverse relation between the amount of SMCs and strain [113].

Pharmacologically, reduction in peak systolic circumferential coronary artery wall stress was more effective with the beta-blocker esmolol than the dihydropyridine calcium–antagonist nicardipine [114].

### Longitudinal Deformation

The cyclic longitudinal stretching of the coronary arteries with each heartbeat imposes equal tensile forces on the entire arterial wall where the direction of the deformation is in parallel with the artery. Where the artery curves, the deformation is nonparallel relative to the course of the artery, and some parts of the arterial wall are stretched more than others. At points of bending, some parts of the wall may even be in compression while the opposite segments are in tension. Angiographically, the angle of flexion during systole (an assessment of both longitudinal stretching and bending) is higher in lesions which subsequently progressed than in lesions which do not progress [115], and von Mises stresses—a measure predicting material failure—are higher within the subendothelium along the inner walls of curvatures compared to the outer walls [115]. Plaque surface deformations are more likely to be of equal orientation and magnitude in asymptomatic carotid plaques compared with symptomatic plaques that demonstrated inherent plaque movement [20].

## Radial Deformation

Compressive forces acting from the lumen in the radial direction alone are unlikely to lead to plaque rupture. Lee et al. [54] applied uniaxial compression to atherosclerotic plaques from human abdominal aortas in order to study plaque stiffness. They were unable to produce evidence of fracture despite increases in stress to more than 20 atm. The authors explained the failure of the plaques to fracture from the fact that the specimens were not under circumferential or longitudinal tension in the testing apparatus.

In theory, plaque rupture may also occur in the opposite direction—from the plaque into the lumen. With high-grade stenosis, a diseased artery may experience negative instead of positive transmural pressure around the stenotic region because of accelerated velocities in the throat of the stenosis [116]. In a two-dimensional finite element model, Aoki and Ku [117] could demonstrate that the lateral edge of a stenotic cap may be subjected to high concentrations of compressive stresses. The stresses further increase with collapse of compliant stenoses, causing bending deformation from buckling of the wall.

Vasospasm has been suspected of "blowing" the fibrous cap off the plaque into the lumen [118,119]. There is frequent coexistence of vasospasm and plaque rupture [120], but it is believed that the latter most often gives rise to the former rather than the other way around [120,121]. Kaski and coworkers [122] found that drug-induced spasms seldom gave rise to myocardial infarction. By contrast, Noboyoshi et al. [123] found a strong positive correlation between ergonovine-induced coronary spasm and subsequent plaque progression, with or without infarct development.

Hemorrhage from fragile vasa vasorum into the plaque has been suggested to cause plaque rupture [124,125]. The vasa vasorum blood flow has been shown to be up to ten times as high in the coronary arteries of atherosclerotic monkeys compared with normal monkeys [126]. It seems unlikely that the pressure generated by bleeding from capillary size vessels should exceed intracoronary blood pressure [127], but intraplaque microhemorrhages could initiate platelet and erythrocyte phagocytosis, iron deposition, macrophage activation, and foam cell formation [128].

## Shear Stress

In atherogenesis, unsteady blood flow characteristics (turbulence and recirculation) rather than the magnitude of shear stress per se is considered the major determinant of hemodynamically induced endothelial cell turnover [129,130] and thereby, possibly, endothelial injury. Whereas the influence from shear stress on atherosclerotic lesion development is well accepted, it has been questioned whether shear alone may rupture a stenotic plaque [46,101]. A study of carotid plaques demonstrated that low-shear areas downstream of plaques contain more SMC's and less macrophages than upstream, high-shear areas, where less SMCs, more macrophages, and more plaque ruptures are found [83].

Shear stresses are generally considered an order of magnitude smaller than the stresses imposed on the plaque by the blood pressure [101], but the stress in the cell membrane of an endothelial cell may be extremely high because of shear [131]. In stenotic regions, shear stress may shave the endothelium away [132], giving rise to plaque erosion rather than plaque rupture. However, it is important to realize that two vessels with identical percent stenosis but differences in plaque morphologies may have dramatically different flow fields. Wall shear stress increases significantly in the presence of plaque valleys and surface irregularities [133].

## Fatigue and Turbulence

A stress may accentuate weaknesses in a material if applied repeatedly, in the same way that a wire may eventually be broken by repetitive bending [23,51]. Fatigue failure is proportional to the number of stress cycles, the stress amplitude, and the mean stress [134]. Fluttering of coronary stenoses between collapse and patency [117] and turbulent pressure fluctuations just distal to the stenoses fatigue areas of the plaque surface promote plaque rupture [135].

The frequency of the applied stress, in terms of oscillating pressure, also changes the mechanical properties of a plaque [136]. Regardless of the type of plaque (cellular, hypocellular, calcified), fibrous caps increase in stiffness with the frequency (0.5 to 2.0 Hz) of the applied stress [54]. Increased stiffness has also been found in model atherosclerotic lipid pools with increasing frequency of stress ranging from 0.1 to 3 Hz [48]. One of the patho-anatomical consequences of the stiffness of plaque tissue may be that in stiff, calcified fibrous caps rupture may occur abruptly (as in a piece of glass), whereas cellular caps may fracture more gradually or be more ductile [101].

## ONSET OF CLINICAL DISEASE

Onset of ACS does not occur at random; a great fraction appears to be "triggered" by external factors or conditions [2,137,138]. Myocardial infarction occurs at increased frequency in the morning [137,139–143], on Mondays [143,144], during winter months [145–148], and during emotional stress [149–152] and vigorous exercise [149,153–155]. The pathophysiological mechanisms responsible for the nonrandom and apparently often-triggered onset of infarction are unknown but probably related to: (a) *plaque rupture*, most likely caused by surges in sympathetic activity with a sudden increase in blood pressure, pulse rate, heart contraction, and coronary blood flow; (b) *thrombosis*, occurring on previously ruptured or intact plaques when the systemic thrombotic tendency is high because of platelet hyperaggregability, hypercoagulability, and/or impaired fibrinolysis; (c) *vasoconstriction*, occurring locally around a coronary plaque or generally [3]; and (d) *systemic mechanisms*. Plaque instability is not just a focal process, but occurs widespread in the coronary tree as documented by angiography [156], angioscopy [157], intravascular ultrasound [158], and by measurement of neutrophil myeloperoxidase content in the cardiac circulation in patients with unstable angina, regardless of the location of the culprit stenosis [159].

## PLAQUE RUPTURE: CLINICAL MANIFESTATIONS

Plaque rupture is common and probably asymptomatic in the great majority of cases; only when a flow-limiting thrombus evolves does plaque rupture manifest itself clinically

[3,160]. Autopsy data indicate that 9% of "normal" healthy persons have asymptomatic ruptured plaques in their coronary arteries, increasing to 22% in persons with diabetes or hypertension [161]. Many persons who die of ischemic heart disease harbour both thrombosed and nonthrombosed ruptured plaques in their coronary arteries [156,162–164]. In two studies of 47 and 83 persons who died of coronary atherosclerosis, 103 and 211 ruptured plaques, respectively, were identified [40,41]. In 142 men who died of sudden coronary death, 61% had healed plaque ruptures, which, by the authors, was interpreted as a form of wound healing that results in increased percent stenosis [165]. Additional plaques are frequently found adjacent to the culprit lesions in patients undergoing percutaneous coronary intervention, with a higher prevalence of ulceration in patients with acute myocardial infarction vs. stable coronary presentation [166].

The most feared consequence of coronary plaque rupture is luminal thrombosis. The clinical presentation and outcome depend on the location, severity, and duration of myocardial ischemia. A nonocclusive or transiently occlusive thrombus most frequently underlies primary unstable angina with pain at rest and myocardial infarction without ST-elevation, whereas a more stable and occlusive thrombus is most frequently seen in ST-elevation infarction—overall, modified by vascular tone and available collateral flow [167]. The lesion responsible for out-of-hospital cardiac arrest or sudden death is often similar to that of unstable angina: a ruptured plaque with superimposed nonocclusive thrombosis [162,168,169]. It is noteworthy that many coronary arteries apparently occlude silently without causing myocardial infarction, probably because of a well-developed collateral circulation at the time of occlusion [25,170,171].

## CONCLUSION

Coronary atherosclerosis is a common and often harmless finding. However, various mechanisms may convert a stable atherosclerotic plaque into a rapidly progressing and highly thrombogenic lesion causing unstable angina, myocardial infarction, and/or sudden death. The risk of plaque rupture is related to plaque vulnerability and rupture triggers. The composition of the plaque, the location, and the different mechanical forces acting on it probably play a more important role for rupture than the size of the plaque. Rupture tends to occur in plaques with a large lipid-rich core and a thin overlying cap at locations weakened by inflammation and at points of stress concentrations. However, plaques with similar characteristics may have different clinical presentations because of blood thrombogenicity (vulnerable blood) or myocardial susceptibility to develop fatal arrhythmia (vulnerable myocardium), which recently led to the introduction of the term "cardiovascular vulnerable patient" for subjects with high likelihood of developing cardiac events in the near future [172,173]. Identification of cardiovascular vulnerable patients will be a future challenge for the health care system.

## REFERENCES

1. Enos WF, Holmes RH, Beyer J. Coronary disease among United States soldiers killed in action in Korea. JAMA 1953;152:1090–1093.
2. Muller JE, Abela GS, Nesto RW, Tofler GH. Triggers, acute risk factors and vulnerable plaques: the lexicon of a new frontier. J Am Coll Cardiol 1994;23(3):809–813.
3. Falk E, Shah PK, Fuster V. Coronary plaque disruption. Circulat 1995;92(3):657–671.
4. Farb A, Tang AL, Burke AP, Sessums L, Liang Y, Virmani R. Sudden coronary death. Frequency of active coronary lesions, inactive coronary lesions, and myocardial infarction. Circulat 1995;92(7):1701–1709.

5.  Ge J, Erbel R, Gorge G, Haude M, Meyer J. High wall shear stress proximal to myocardial bridging and atherosclerosis: intracoronary ultrasound and pressure measurements. Br Heart J 1995;73(5):462–465.

6.  Ku DN, Giddens DP, Zarins CK, Glagov S. Pulsatile flow and atherosclerosis in the human carotid bifurcation. Positive correlation between plaque location and low oscillating shear stress. Arteriosclerosis 1985;5(3):293–302.

7.  Asakura T, Karino T. Flow patterns and spatial distribution of atherosclerotic lesions in human coronary arteries. Circ Res 1990;66(4):1045–1066.

8.  Kimura BJ, Russo RJ, Bhargava V, McDaniel MB, Peterson KL, DeMaria AN. Atheroma morphology and distribution in proximal left anterior descending coronary artery: in vivo observations. J Am Coll Cardiol 1996;27:825–831.

9.  Schwartz SM, Heimark RL, Majesky MW. Developmental mechanisms underlying pathology of arteries. Physiol Rev 1990;70(4):1177–1209.

10. Ball RY, Stowers EC, Burton JH, Cary NR, Skepper JN, Mitchinson MJ. Evidence that the death of macrophage foam cells contributes to the lipid core of atheroma. Atherosclerosis 1995;114(1):45–54.

11. Mallat Z, Nakamura T, Ohan J, Leseche G, Tedgui A, Maclouf J, Murphy RC. The relationship of hydroxyeicosatetraenoic acids and F2-isoprostanes to plaque instability in human carotid atherosclerosis. The Journal of Clinical Investigation 1999;103:421–427.

12. Pratico D, Iuliano L, Mauriello A, Spagnoli L, Lawson JA, Rokach J, Maclouf J, Violi F, Fitzgerald GA. Localization of distinct F2-isoprostanes in human atherosclerotic lesions. The Journal of Clinical Investigation 1997;100:2028–2034.

13. Geng YJ, Libby P. Evidence for apoptosis in advanced human atheroma. Colocalization with interleukin-1 beta-converting enzyme [see comments]. Am J Pathol 1995;147(2):251–266.

14. Guyton JR, Klemp KF. Development of the atherosclerotic core region. Chemical and ultra-structural analysis of microdissected atherosclerotic lesions from human aorta. Arterioscler Thromb 1994;14(8):1305–1314.

15. Witztum JL. The oxidation hypothesis of atherosclerosis [see comments]. Lancet 1994; 344(8925):793–795.

16. Guyton JR, Klemp KF. Transitional features in human atherosclerosis. Intimal thickening, cholesterol clefts, and cell loss in human aortic fatty streaks. Am J Pathol 1993;143(5): 1444–1457.

17. Okura Y, Brink M, Itabe H, Scheidegger KJ, Kalangos A, Delafontaine P. Oxidized low-density lipoprotein is associated with apoptosis of vascular smooth muscle cells in human atherosclerotic plaques. Circulat 28-11-2000;102(22):2680–2686.

18. Mann JM, Davies MJ. Vulnerable plaque. Relation of characteristics to degree of stenosis in human coronary arteries. Circulat 1996;94:928–931.

19. Burke AP, Kolodgie FD, Farb A, Weber D, Virmani R. Morphological predictors of arterial remodeling in coronary atherosclerosis. Circulat 22-1-2002;105(3):297–303.

20. Moreno PR, Purushothaman KR, Fuster V, O'Connor WN. Intimomedial interface damage and adventitial inflammation is increased beneath disrupted atherosclerosis in the aorta: implications for plaque vulnerability. Circulat 28-5-2002;105(21):2504–2511.

21. Schoenhagen P, Ziada KM, Kapadia SR, Crowe TD, Nissen SE, Tuzcu EM. Extent and direction of arterial remodeling in stable versus unstable coronary syndromes : an intravascular ultrasound study. Circulat 15-2-2000;101(6):598–603.

22. von Birgelen C, Klinkhart W, Mintz GS, Papatheodorou A, Herrmann J, Baumgart D, Haude M, Wieneke H, Ge J, Erbel R. Plaque distribution and vascular remodeling of ruptured and nonruptured coronary plaques in the same vessel: an intravascular ultrasound study in vivo. J Am Coll Cardiol 1-6-2001;37(7):1864–1870.

23. Takano M, Mizuno K, Okamatsu K, Yokoyama S, Ohba T, Sakai S. Mechanical and structural characteristics of vulnerable plaques: analysis by coronary angioscopy and intravascular ultrasound. J Am Coll Cardiol 2001;38(1):99–104.

24. Giroud D, Li JM, Urban P, Meier B, Rutishauer W. Relation of the site of acute myocardial infarction to the most severe coronary arterial stenosis at prior angiography [see comments]. Am J Cardiol 1992;69(8):729–732.

25. Alderman EL, Corley SD, Fisher LD, Chaitman BR, Faxon DP, Foster ED, Killip T, Sosa JA, Bourassa MG. Five-year angiographic follow-up of factors associated with progression of coronary artery disease in the Coronary Artery Surgery Study (CASS). CASS Participating Investigators and Staff. J Am Coll Cardiol 1993;22(4):1141–1154.

26. Chen L, Chester MR, Redwood S, Huang J, Leatham E, Kaski JC. Angiographic stenosis progression and coronary events in patients with 'stabilized' unstable angina [see comments]. Circulat 1995;91(9):2319–2324.

27. Ambrose JA, Tannenbaum MA, Alexopoulos D, Hjemdahl Monsen CE, Leavy J, Weiss M, Borrico S, Gorlin R, Fuster V. Angiographic progression of coronary artery disease and the development of myocardial infarction. J Am Coll Cardiol 1988;12(1):56–62.

28. Kotani J, Mintz GS, Castagna MT, Pinnow E, Berzingi CO, Bui AB, Pichard AD, Satler LF, Suddath WO, Waksman R, Laird JR, Kent KM, Weissman NJ. Intravascular ultrasound analysis of infarct-related and non-infarct-related arteries in patients who presented with an acute myocardial infarction. Circulat 17-6-2003;107(23):2889–2893.

29. Natural history of aortic and coronary atherosclerotic lesions in youth. Findings from the PDAY Study. Pathobiological Determinants of Atherosclerosis in Youth (PDAY) Research Group. Arterioscler Thromb 1993;13(9):1291–1298.

30. Solberg LA, Strong JP. Risk factors and atherosclerotic lesions: a review of autopsy studies. Arteriosclerosis 1983;3:187–198.

31. Reed DM, Strong JP, Resch J, Hayashi T. Serum lipids and lipoproteins as predictors of atherosclerosis: an autopsy study. Arteriosclerosis 1989;9:560–564.

32. Robertson WB, Strong JP. Atherosclerosis in persons with hypertension and diabetes mellitus. Lab.Invest 1968;18:538–551.

33. Devries S, Wolfkiel C, Fusman B, Bakdash H, Ahmed A, Levy P, Chomka E, Kondos G, Zajac E, Rich S. Influence of age and gender on the presence of coronary calcium detected by ultrafast computed tomography. J Am Coll Cardiol 1995;25:76–82.

34. Burke AP, Farb A, Malcom GT, Liang Y, Smialek J, Virmani R. Coronary risk factors and plaque morphology in men with coronary disease who died suddenly. The New England Journal of Medicine 1997;336:1276–1282.

35. Burke AP, Farb A, Malcom GT, Liang Y, Smialek J, Virmani R. Effect of risk factors on the mechanism of acute thrombosis and sudden coronary death in women. Circulat 1998;97:2110–2116.

36. Kojima S, Nonogi H, Miyao Y, Miyazaki S, Goto Y, Itoh A, Daikoku S, Matsumoto T, Morii I, Yutani C. Is preinfarction angina related to the presence or absence of coronary plaque rupture? Heart 2000;83(1):64–68.

37. Grønholdt MM, Nordestgaard BG, Wiebe BM, Wilhjelm JE, Sillesen H. Echo-lutency of computerized ultrasound images of carotid atherosclerotic plaques are associated with increased levels of triglyceride-rich lipoproteins as well as increased plaque lipid content. Circulat 1998;97:34–40.

38. Richardson PD, Davies MJ, Born GVR. Influence of plaque configuration and stress distribution on fissuring of coronary atherosclerotic plaques. Lancet 1989;2:941–944.

39. van der Wal AC, Becker AE, van der Loos CM, Das PK. Site of intimal rupture or erosion of thrombosed coronary atherosclerotic plaques is characterized by an inflammatory process irrespective of the dominant plaque morphology [see comments]. Circulat 1994;89(1):36–44.

40. Falk E. Plaque rupture with severe pre-existing stenosis precipitating coronary thrombosis. Characteristics of coronary atherosclerotic plaques underlying fatal occlusive thrombi. Br Heart J 1983;50(2):127–134.

41. Frink RJ. Chronic ulcerated plaques: new insights into the pathogenesis of acute coronary disease. J Invasive Cardiol 1994;6:173–185.

42. Arbustini E, Dal Bello B, Morbini P, Burke AP, Bocciarelli M, Specchia G, Virmani R. Plaque erosion is a major substrate for coronary thrombosis in acute myocardial infarction. Heart 1999;82(3):269–272.

43. Farb A, Burke AP, Tang AL, Liang Y, Mannan P, Smialek J, Virmani R. Coronary plaque erosion without rupture into a lipid core. A frequent cause of coronary thrombosis in sudden coronary death. Circulat 1996;93:1354–1363.

44. Davies MJ. Stability and instability: two faces of coronary atherosclerosis. The Paul Dudley White Lecture 1995. Circulat 1996;94:2013–2020.

45. Ross R. Atherosclerosis--an inflammatory disease [see comments]. N Engl J Med 1999; 340(2):115–126.

46. Gertz SD, Roberts WC. Hemodynamic shear force in rupture of coronary arterial atherosclerotic plaques [editorial]. Am J Cardiol 1990;66(19):1368–1372.

47. Davies MJ, Richardson PD, Woolf N, Katz DR, Mann J. Risk of thrombosis in human atherosclerotic plaques: role of extracellular lipid, macrophage, and smooth muscle cell content. Br Heart J 1993;69(5):377–381.

48. Loree HM, Tobias BJ, Gibson LJ, Kamm RD, Small DM, Lee RT. Mechanical properties of model atherosclerotic lesion lipid pools. Arterioscler Thromb 1994;14(2):230–234.

49. Small DM. George Lyman Duff memorial lecture. Progression and regression of atherosclerotic lesions. Insights from lipid physical biochemistry. Arteriosclerosis 1988;8(2):103–129.

50. Wagner WD, St. Clair RW, Clarkson TB, Connor JR. A study of atherosclerosis regression in Macaca mulatta: III. Chemical changes in arteries from animals with atherosclerosis induced for 19 months and regressed for 48 months at plasma cholesterol concentrations of 300 or 200 mg/dl. Am J Pathol 1980;100(3):633–650.

51. Cheng GC, Loree HM, Kamm RD, Fishbein MC, Lee RT. Distribution of circumferential stress in ruptured and stable atherosclerotic lesions. A structural analysis with histopathological correlation. Circulat 1993;87:1179–1187.

52. Loree HM, Kamm RD, Stringfellow RG, Lee RT. Effects of fibrous cap thickness on peak circumferential stress in model atherosclerotic vessels. Circ Res 1992;71(4):850–858.

53. Dhume AS, Soundararajan K, Hunter WJ, Agrawal DK. Comparison of vascular smooth muscle cell apoptosis and fibrous cap morphology in symptomatic and asymptomatic carotid artery disease. Ann Vasc Surg 2003;17(1):1–8.

54. Lee RT, Grodzinsky AJ, Frank EH, Kamm RD, Schoen FJ. Structure-dependent dynamic mechanical behavior of fibrous caps from human atherosclerotic plaques. Circulat 1991;83(5): 1764–1770.

55. Huang H, Virmani R, Younis H, Burke AP, Kamm RD, Lee RT. The impact of calcification on the biomechanical stability of atherosclerotic plaques. Circulat 27-2-2001;103(8):1051–1056.

56. Constantinides P. Plaque fissures in human coronary thrombosis. Journal of Atherosclerosis Research 1966;6:1–17.

57. Friedman M. The coronary thrombus: its origin and fate. Hum Pathol 1971;2:81–128.

58. Pasterkamp G, Schoneveld AH, van der Wal AC, Hijnen D, van Wolveren WJA, Plomp S, Teepen HLJM, Borst C. Inflammation of the atherosclerotic cap and shoulder of the plaque is a common and locally observed feature in unruptured plaques of femoral and coronary arteries. Arterioscler Thromb Vasc Biol 1999;19:54–58.

59. Johnson Tidey RR, McGregor JL, Taylor PR, Poston RN. Increase in the adhesion molecule P-selectin in endothelium overlying atherosclerotic plaques. Coexpression with intercellular adhesion molecule-1. Am J Pathol 1994;144(5):952–961.

60. Poston RN, Haskard DO, Coucher JR, Gall NP, Johnson Tidey RR. Expression of intercellular adhesion molecule-1 in atherosclerotic plaques. Am J Pathol 1992;140:665–673.

61. Lendon CL, Davies MJ, Born GV, Richardson PD. Atherosclerotic plaque caps are locally weakened when macrophages density is increased. Atherosclerosis 1991;87(1):87–90.

62. Moreno PR, Falk E, Palacios IF, Newell JB, Fuster V, Fallon JT. Macrophage infiltration in acute coronary syndromes. Implications for plaque rupture. Circulat 1994;90(2):775–778.

63. Naruko T, Ueda M, Haze K, van der Wal AC, van der Loos CM, Itoh A, Komatsu R, Ikura Y, Ogami M, Shimada Y, Ehara S, Yoshiyama M, Takeuchi K, Yoshikawa J, Becker AE. Neutrophil infiltration of culprit lesions in acute coronary syndromes. Circulat 3-12-2002; 106(23):2894–2900.

64. Dangas G, Mehran R, Harpel PC, Sharma SK, Marcovina SM, Dube G, Ambrose JA, Fallon JT. Lipoprotein(a) and inflammation in human coronary atheroma: association with the severity of clinical presentation. J Am Coll Cardiol 1998;32:2035–2042.

65. de Boor OJ, van der Wal AC, Teeling P, Becker AE. Leucocyte recruitment in rupture prone regions of lipid-rich plaques: a prominent role for neovascularization? Cardiovasc.Res 1999; 41:443–449.

66. Behr-Roussel D, Rupin A, Sansilvestri-Morel P, Fabiani JN, Verbeuren TJ. Histochemical evidence for inducible nitric oxide synthase in advanced but non-ruptured human atherosclerotic carotid arteries. Histochem J 2000;32(1):41–51.

67. Schieffer B, Schieffer E, Hilfiker-Kleiner D, Hilfiker A, Kovanen PT, Kaartinen M, Nussberger J, Harringer W, Drexler H. Expression of angiotensin II and interleukin 6 in human coronary atherosclerotic plaques: potential implications for inflammation and plaque instability. Circulat 28-3-2000;101(12):1372–1378.

68. Mach F, Schonbeck U, Sukhova GK, Bourcier T, Bonnefoy JY, Pober JS, Libby P. Functional CD40 ligand is expressed on human vascular endothelial cells, smooth muscle cells, and macrophages: implications for CD40-CD40 ligand signaling in atherosclerosis. Proc Natl Acad Sci U.S.A 4-3-1997;94(5):1931–1936.

69. Heeschen C, Dimmeler S, Hamm CW, van den Brand MJ, Boersma E, Zeiher AM, Simoons ML. Soluble CD40 ligand in acute coronary syndromes. N Engl J Med 20-3-2003;348(12): 1104–1111.

70. Matrisian LM. The matrix degrading metalloproteinases. Bioessays 1992;14:455–463.

71. Dorsch MF, Barrett JA, Lawrance RA, Maqbool A, Durham NP, Ellis S, Samani NJ, Bishop T, Ball SG, Balmforth AJ, Hall AS. Premature coronary artery disease shows no evidence of linkage to loci encoding for tissue inhibitors of matrix metalloproteinases. J Hum Genet 19-9-2003.

72. Cipollone F, Iezzi A, Fazia M, Zucchelli M, Pini B, Cuccurullo C, De Cesare D, De Blasis G, Muraro R, Bei R, Chiarelli F, Schmidt AM, Cuccurullo F, Mezzetti A. The receptor RAGE as a progression factor amplifying arachidonate-dependent inflammatory and proteolytic response in human atherosclerotic plaques: role of glycemic control. Circulat 2-9-2003;108(9): 1070–1077.

73. Casscells W, Hathorn B, David M, Krabach T, Vaughn WK, McAllister HA, Bearman G, Willerson JT. Thermal detection of cellular infiltrates in living atherosclerotic plaques: possible implications for plaque rupture and thrombosis. Lancet 1996;347:1447–1449.

74. Stefanadis C, Diamantopoulos L, Vlachopoulos C, Tsiamis E, Dernellis J, Toutouzas K, Stefanadi E, Toutouzas P. Thermal heterogeneity within human atherosclerotic coronary arteries detected in vivo: A new method of detection by application of a special thermography catheter. Circulat 1999;99(15):1965–1971.

75. Xu XP, Meisel SR, Ong JM, Kaul S, Cercek B, Rajavashisth TB, Sharifi B, Shah PK. Oxidized low-density lipoprotein regulates matrix metalloproteinase-9 and its tissue inhibitor in human monocyte-derived macrophages. Circulat 2-3-1999;99(8):993–998.

76. Ardans JA, Economou AP, Martinson JM, Zhou M, Wahl LM. Oxidized low-density and high-density lipoproteins regulate the production of matrix metalloproteinase-1 and -9 by activated monocytes. J. Leukoc. Biol 2002;71(6):1012–1018.

77. Kaartinen M, van der Wal AC, van der Loos CM, Piek JJ, Koch KT, Becker AE, Kovanen PT. Mast cell infiltration in acute coronary syndromes: implications for plaque rupture. J Am Coll Cardiol 1998;32:606–612.

78. Filipiak KJ, Tarchalska-Krynska B, Opolski G, Rdzanek A, Kochman J, Kosior DA, Czlonkowski A. Tryptase levels in patients after acute coronary syndromes: the potential new marker of an unstable plaque? Clin.Cardiol 2003;26(8):366–372.

79. Kovanen P, Kaartinen M, Paavonen T. Infiltrates of activated mast cells at the site of coronary atheromatous erosion or rupture in myocardial infarction. Circulat 1995;92:1084–1088.

80. Herrmann J, Edwards WD, Holmes DR, Shogren KL, Lerman LO, Ciechanover A, Lerman A. Increased ubiquitin immunoreactivity in unstable atherosclerotic plaques associated with acute coronary syndromes. J Am Coll Cardiol 4-12-2002;40(11):1919–1927.

80a. Falk EWhy do plaques rupture? Circulat 1992;86(Suppl. III):30–42.

81. Libby P. Molecular bases of the acute coronary syndromes. Circulat 1995;91(11):2844–2850.

82. Burleigh MC, Briggs AD, Lendon CL, Davies MJ, Born GV, Richardson PD. Collagen types I and III, collagen content, GAGs and mechanical strength of human atherosclerotic plaque caps: span-wise variations. Atherosclerosis 1992;96(1):71–81.

83. Dirksen MT, van der Wal AC, van den Berg FM, van der Loos CM, Becker AE. Distribution of inflammatory cells in atherosclerotic plaques relates to the direction of flow. Circulat 1998; 98:2000–2003.

84.  Rekhter MD, Hicks GW, Brammer DW, Hallak H, Kindt E, Chen J, Rosebury WS, Anderson MK, Kuipers PJ, Ryan MJ. Hypercholesterolemia causes mechanical weakening of rabbit atheroma : local collagen loss as a prerequisite of plaque rupture. Circ Res 7-1-2000;86(1): 101–108.

85.  Shah PK, Falk E, Badimon JJ, Fernandez Ortiz A, Mailhac A, Villareal Levy G, Fallon JT, Regnstrom J, Fuster V. Human monocyte-derived macrophages induce collagen breakdown in fibrous caps of atherosclerotic plaques. Potential role of matrix- degrading metalloproteinases and implications for plaque rupture. Circulat 1995;92(6):1565–1569.

86.  Galis ZS, Sukhova GK, Lark MW, Libby P. Increased expression of matrix metalloproteinases and matrix degrading activity in vulnerable regions of human atherosclerotic plaques. The Journal of Clinical Investigation 1994;94(6):2493–2503.

87.  Brown DL, Hibbs MS, Kearney M, Loushin C, Isner JM. Identification of 92-kD gelatinase in human coronary atherosclerotic lesions. Association of active enzyme synthesis with unstable angina. Circulat 1995;91(8):2125–2131.

88.  Henney AM, Wakeley PR, Davies MJ, Foster K, Hembry R, Murphy G, Humphries S. Localization of stromelysin gene expression in atheroscleotic plaques by in situ hybridization. Proc Natl Acad Sci U.S.A 1991;88:8154–8158.

89.  Wilcox JN, Smith KM, Schwartz SM, Gordon D. Localization of tissue factor in the normal vessel wall and in the atherosclerotic plaque. Proc Natl Acad Sci U.S.A 1989;86(8): 2839–2843.

90.  Palabrica T, Lobb R, Furie BC, Aronovitz M, Benjamin C, Hsu YM, Sajer SA, Furie B. Leukocyte accumulation promoting fibrin deposition is mediated in vivo by P-selectin on adherent platelets. Nature 1992;359:848–851.

91.  Jude B, Agraou B, McFadden EP, Susen S, Bauters C, Lepelley P, Vanhaesbroucke C, Devos P, Cosson A, Asseman P. Evidence for time-dependent activation of monocytes in the systemic circulation in unstable angina but not in acute myocardial infarction or in stable angina. Circulat 1994;90:1662–1668.

92.  Leatham EW, Bath PMV, Tooze JA, Camm AJ. Increased tissue factor expression in coronary disease. Br Heart J 1995;73:10–13.

93.  Moreno PR, Bernadi VH, López-Cuéllar J, Murcia AM, Palacios IF, Gold HK, Mehran R, Sharma SK, Nemerson Y, Fuster V, Fallon JT. Macrophages, smooth muscle cells, and tissue factor in unstable angina. Implications for cell-mediated thrombogenicity in acute coronary syndromes. Circulat 1996;94:3090–3097.

94.  Muhlestein JB, Hammond EH, Carlquist JF, Radicke E, Thomson MJ, Karagounis LA, Woods ML, Anderson JL. Increased incidence of Chlamydia species within the coronary arteries of patients with symptomatic atherosclerotic versus other forms of cardiovascular disease. J Am Coll Cardiol 1996;27:1555–1561.

95.  Danesh J, Collins R, Peto R. Chronic infections and coronary heart disease: is there a link? [see comments]. Lancet 1997;350(9075):430–436.

96.  Libby P, Egan D, Skarlatos S. Roles of infectious agents in atherosclerosis and restenosis: an assessment of the evidence and need for future research. Circulat 1997;96(11):4095–4103.

97.  Kol A, Sukhova GK, Lichtman AH, Libby P. Chlamydial heat shock protein 60 localizes in human atheroma and regulates macrophage tumor necrosis factor-alpha and matrix metalloproteinase expression. Circulat 1998;98(4):300–307.

98.  Ezzahiri R, Stassen FR, Kurvers HA, van Pul MM, Kitslaar PJ, Bruggeman CA. Chlamydia pneumoniae infection induces an unstable atherosclerotic plaque phenotype in LDL-receptor, ApoE double knockout mice. Eur.J.Vasc.Endovasc.Surg 2003;26(1):88–95.

99.  Benagiano M, Azzurri A, Ciervo A, Amedei A, Tamburini C, Ferrari M, Telford JL, Baldari CT, Romagnani S, Cassone A, D'Elios MM, Del Prete G. T helper type 1 lymphocytes drive inflammation in human atherosclerotic lesions. Proc Natl Acad Sci U.S.A 27-5-2003;100(11): 6658–6663.

100. Lee RT, Kamm RD. Vascular mechanics for the cardiologist. J Am Coll Cardiol 1994;23: 1289–1295.

101. MacIsaac AI, Thomas JD, Topol EJ. Toward the quiescent coronary plaque. J Am Coll Cardiol 1993;22(4):1228–1241.

102. Alfonso F, Macaya C, Goicolea J, Hernandez R, Segovia J, Zamorano J, Bañuelos C, Zarco P. Determinants of coronary compliance in patients with coronary artery disease: An intravascular ultrasound study. J Am Coll Cardiol 1994;23:879–884.

103. Shimazu T, Hori M, Mishima M, Kitabatake A, Kodama K, Nanto S, Inoue M. Clinical assessment of elastic properties of large coronary arteries: pressure-diameter relationship and dynamic incremental elastic modulus. Int.J.Cardiol 1986;13(1):27–45.

104. Pynadath TI, Mukherjee DP. Dynamic mechanical properties of atherosclerotic aorta. A correlation between the cholesterol ester content and the viscoelastic properties of atherosclerotic aorta. Atherosclerosis 1977;26:311–318.

105. Newman DL, Gosling RG, Bowden NL. Changes in aortic distensibility and area ratio with the development of atherosclerosis. Atherosclerosis 1971;14:231–240.

106. Frøbert O, Schiønning J, Gregersen H, Baandrup U, Petersen JAK, Bagger JP. Impaired human coronary artery distensibility by atherosclerotic lesions: a mechanical and histological investigation. Int.J.Exp.Path 1997;78:421–428.

107. Isner JM, Rosenfield K, Losordo DW, Rose L, Langevin RE, Razvi S, Kosowsky BD. Combination balloon-ultrasound imaging catheter for percutaneous transluminal angioplasty. Validation of imaging, analysis of recoil, and identification of plaque fracture. Circulat 1991;84(2): 739–754.

108. Baptista J, di Mario C, Ozaki Y, Escaned J, Gil R, de Feyter P, Roelandt JR, Serruys PW. Impact of plaque morphology and composition on the mechanisms of lumen enlargement using intracoronary ultrasound and quantitative angiography after balloon angioplasty. Am J Cardiol 1996;77(2):115–121.

109. de Korte CL, Cespedes EI, van der Steen AFW, Pasterkamp G, Bom N. Intravascular ultrasound elastography: assessment and imaging of elastic properties of diseased arteries and vulnerable plaque. Eur J Ultrasound 1998;7:219–224.

110. Veress AI, Cornhill JF, Herderick EE, Thomas JD. Age-related development of atherosclerotic plaque stress: a population-based finite-element analysis. Coronary Artery Disease 1998;9: 13–19.

111. Ohayon J, Teppaz P, Finet G, Rioufol G. In-vivo prediction of human coronary plaque rupture location using intravascular ultrasound and the finite element method. Coron Artery Dis 2001; 12(8):655–663.

112. Cespedes EI, de Korte CL, Van Der Steen AF, von Birgelen C, Lancee CT. Intravascular elastography: principles and potentials. Semin.Interv.Cardiol 1997;2(1):55–62.

113. Schaar JA, de Korte CL, Mastik F, Strijder C, Pasterkamp G, Boersma E, Serruys PW, Van Der Steen AF. Characterizing Vulnerable Plaque Features With Intravascular Elastography. Circulat 27-10-2003.

114. Williams MJ, Low CJ, Wilkins GT, Stewart RA. Randomised comparison of the effects of nicardipine and esmolol on coronary artery wall stress: implications for the risk of plaque rupture. Heart 2000;84(4):377–382.

115. Stein PD, Hamid MS, Shivkumar K, Davis TP, Khaja F, Henry JW. Effects of cyclic flexion of coronary arteries on progression of atherosclerosis. Am J Cardiol 1994;73(7):431–437.

116. Tang D, Yang C, Kobayashi S, Ku DN. Steady flow and wall compression in stenotic arteries: a three-dimensional thick-wall model with fluid-wall interactions. J Biomech Eng 2001; 123(6):548–557.

117. Aoki T, Ku DN. Collapse of diseased arteries with eccentric cross section. J Biomech 1993; 26(2):133–142.

118. Leary T. Coronary spasm as a possible factor in producing sudden death. Am Heart J 1934; 10:338–344.

119. Lin CS, Penha PD, Zak FG, Lin JC. Morphodynamic interpretation of acute coronary thrombosis, with special reference to volcano-like eruption of atheromatous plaque caused by coronary artery spasm. Angiology 1988;39(6):535–547.

120. Bogaty P, Hackett D, Davies G, Maseri A. Vasoreactivity of the culprit lesion in unstable angina [see comments]. Circulat 1994;90(1):5–11.

121. Lam JY, Chesebro JH, Steele PM, Badimon L, Fuster V. Is vasospasm related to platelet deposition? Relationship in a porcine preparation of arterial injury in vivo. Circulat 1987; 75(1):243–248.

122. Kaski JC, Tousoulis D, McFadden E, Crea F, Pereira WI, Maseri A. Variant angina pectoris. Role of coronary spasm in the development of fixed coronary obstructions. Circulat 1992; 85(2):619–626.

123. Nobuyoshi M, Tanaka M, Nosaka H, Kimura T, Yokoi H, Hamasaki N, Kim K, Shindo T, Kimura K. Progression of coronary atherosclerosis: is coronary spasm related to progression? J Am Coll Cardiol 1991;18(4):904–910.

124. Barger AC, Beeuwkes R3, Lainey LL, Silverman KJ. Hypothesis: vasa vasorum and neovascularization of human coronary arteries. A possible role in the pathophysiology of atherosclerosis. N Engl J Med 1984;310(3):175–177.

125. Paterson JC. Capillary rupture with intimal hemorrhage as a causative factor in coronary thrombosis. Arch Pathol 1938;25:474–487.

126. Williams JK, Armstrong ML, Heistad DD. Vasa vasorum in atherosclerotic coronary arteries: responses to vasoactive stimuli and regression of atherosclerosis. Circ Res 1988;62(3): 515–523.

127. Jiang JP, Feldman CL, Stone PH. Models of the intracoronary pathogenesis of acute coronary heart disease  Willich SN , Muller JE, Eds. Triggering of acute coronary syndromes. Implications for prevention, Kluwer Academic Publishers. 1996(15):237–257.

128. Kockx MM, Cromheeke KM, Knaapen MW, Bosmans JM, De Meyer GR, Herman AG, Bult H. Phagocytosis and macrophage activation associated with hemorrhagic microvessels in human atherosclerosis. Arterioscler Thromb Vasc Biol 1-3-2003;23(3):440–446.

129. Davies PF, Tripathi SC. Mechanical stress mechanisms and the cell. An endothelial paradigm. Circ Res 1993;72(2):239–245.

130. Davies PF, Remuzzi A, Gordon EJ, Dewey CF, Gimbrone MA. Turbulent fluid shear stress induces vascular endothelial cell turnover in vitro. Proc Natl Acad Sci U.S.A 1986;83(7): 2114–2117.

131. Fung YC. Biomechanics: motion, flow, stress, and growth. New York: Springer-Verlag New York Inc, 1990.

132. Gertz SD, Uretzky G, Wajnberg RS, Navot N, Gotsman MS. Endothelial cell damage and thrombus formation after partial arterial constriction: relevance to the role of cornary aretry spasm in the pathogenesis of myocardial infarction. Circulat 1981;63:476–486.

133. Stroud JS, Berger SA, Saloner D. Influence of stenosis morphology on flow through severely stenotic vessels: implications for plaque rupture. J Biomech 2000;33(4):443–455.

134. Bank AJ, Versluis A, Dodge SM, Douglas WH. Atherosclerotic plaque rupture: a fatigue process? Med.Hypotheses 2000;55(6):480–484.

135. Loree HM, Kamm RD, Atkinson CM, Lee RT. Turbulent pressure fluctuations on surface of model vascular stenoses. Am J Physiol 1991;261(3 Pt 2):H644–50.

136. Bergel DH. The dynamic elastic properties of the arterial wall. J.Physiol 1961;156:458–469.

137. Muller JE, Tofler GH, Stone PH. Circadian variation and triggers of onset of acute cardiovascular disease [see comments]. Circulat 1989;79(4):733–743.

138. Willich SN, Maclure M, Mittleman MA, Arntz HR, Muller JE. Sudden cardiac death: support for a role of triggering in causation. Circulat 1993;87:1442–1450.

139. Goldberg RJ, Brady P, Muller JE, Chen ZY, de Groot M, Zonneveld P, Dalen JE. Time of onset of symptoms of acute myocardial infarction. Am J Cardiol 1990;66(2):140–144.

140. Quyyumi AA, Panza JA, Diodati JG, Lakatos E, Epstein SE. Circadian variation in ischemic threshold. A mechanism underlying the circadian variation in ischemic events. Circulat 1992; 86(1):22–28.

141. Kono T, Morita H, Nishina T, Fujita M, Hirota Y, Kawamura K, Fujiwara A. Circadian variations of onset of acute myocardial infarction and efficacy of thrombolytic therapy. J Am Coll Cardiol 1996;27:774–778.

142. Willich SN, Collins R, Peto R, Linderer T, Sleight P, Schröder R. ISIS-2 (Second International Study of Infarct Survival) Collaborative Group. Morning peak in the incidence of myocardial infarction: experience in the ISIS-2 trial. Eur Heart J 1992;13:594–598.

143. Gnecchi-Ruscone T, Piccaluga E, Guzzeti S, Contini M, Montano N, Nicolis E. Morning and Monday: critical periods for the onset of acute myocardial infarction: the GISSI 2 Study experience. Eur Heart J 1994;15:882–887.

144. Willich SN, Lowel H, Lewis M, Hormann A, Arntz HR, Keil U. Weekly variation of acute myocardial infarction. Increased Monday risk in the working population. Circulat 1994;90(1): 87–93.

145. Ornato JP, Siegel L, Craren EJ, Nelson N. Increased incidence of cardiac death attributed to acute myocardial infarction during winter. Coron Artery Dis 1990;1:199–203.

146. Douglas AS, al Sayer H, Rawles JM, Allan TM. Seasonality of disease in Kuwait. Lancet 1991;337:1393–1397.

147. Kloner RA, Poole KW, Perritt RL. When throughout the year is coronary death most likely to occur? A 12-year population-based analysis of more than 220 000 cases. Circulat 1999; 100:1630–1634.

148. Spencer FA, Goldberg RJ, Becker RC, Gore JM. Seasonal distribution of acute myocardial infarction in the second National Registry of Myocardial Infarction. J Am Coll Cardiol 1998; 31(6):1226–1233.

149. Gabbay FH, Krantz DS, Kop WJ, Hedges SM, Klein J, Gottdiener JS, Rozabski A. Triggers of myocardial ischemia during daily life in patients with coronary artery disease: Physical and mental activities, anger and smoking. J Am Coll Cardiol 1996;27:585–592.

150. Mittleman MA, Maclure M, Sherwood JB, Mulry RP, Tofler GH, Jacobs SC, Friedman R, Benson H, Muller JE. Triggering of acute myocardial infarction by episodes of anger. Circulat 1995;92:1720–1725.

151. Leor J, Poole K, Kloner R. Sudden cardiac death triggered by an earthquake. The New England Journal of Medicine 1996;334:413–419.

152. Brown DL. Disparate effects of the 1989 Loma Prieta and 1994 Northridge earthquakes on hospital admissions for acute myocardial infarction: importance of superimposition of triggers [see comments]. Am Heart J 1999;137(5):830–836.

153. Mittleman MA, Maclure M, Tofler GH, Sherwood JB, Goldberg RJ, Muller JE. Triggering of acute myocardial infarction by heavy physical exertion. Protection against triggering by regular exertion. Determinants of Myocardial Infarction Onset Study Investigators [see comments]. N Engl J Med 1993;329(23):1677–1683.

154. Willich SN, Lewis M, Löwel H, Arntz HR, Schubert F, Schröder R. Physical exertion as a trigger of acute myocardial infarction. The New England Journal of Medicine 1993;329: 1684–1690.

155. Burke AP, Farb A, Malcom GT, Liang Y, Smialek J, Virmani R. Plaque rupture and sudden death related to exertion in men with coronary artery disease. Journal of the American Medical Association 1999;281:921–926.

156. Goldstein JA, Demetriou D, Grines CL, Pica M, Shoukfeh M, O'Neill WW. Multiple complex coronary plaques in patients with acute myocardial infarction. N Engl J Med 28-9-2000; 343(13):915–922.

157. Uchida Y, Nakamura F, Tomaru T, Morita T, Oshima T, Sasaki T, Morizuki S, Hirose J. Prediction of acute coronary syndromes by percutaneous coronary angioscopy in patients with stable angina. Am Heart J 1995;130(2):195–203.

158. Rioufol G, Finet G, Ginon I, Andre-Fouet X, Rossi R, Vialle E, Desjoyaux E, Convert G, Huret JF, Tabib A. Multiple atherosclerotic plaque rupture in acute coronary syndrome: a three-vessel intravascular ultrasound study. Circulat 13-8-2002;106(7):804–808.

159. Buffon A, Biasucci LM, Liuzzo G, D'Onofrio G, Crea F, Maseri A. Widespread coronary inflammation in unstable angina. N Engl J Med 4-7-2002;347(1):5–12.

160. Mann J, Davies MJ. Mechanisms of progression in native coronary artery disease: role of healed plaque disruption. Heart 1999;82(3):265–268.

161. Davies MJ, Bland JM, Hangartner JR, Angelini A, Thomas AC. Factors influencing the presence or absence of acute coronary artery thrombi in sudden ischaemic death. Eur Heart J 1989;10(3):203–208.

162. Davies MJ, Thomas A. Thrombosis and acute coronary-artery lesions in sudden cardiac ischemic death. The New England Journal of Medicine 1984;310:1137–1140.

163. ElFawal MA, Berg GA, Wheatley DJ, Harland WA. Sudden coronary death in Glasgow: nature and frequency of acute coronary lesions. Br Heart J 1987;57:329–335.

164. Qiao JH, Fishbein MC. The severity of coronary atherosclerosis at sites of plaque rupture with occlusive thrombus. J Am Coll Cardiol 1991;17:1138–1142.

165. Burke AP, Kolodgie FD, Farb A, Weber DK, Malcom GT, Smialek J, Virmani R. Healed plaque ruptures and sudden coronary death: evidence that subclinical rupture has a role in plaque progression. Circulat 20-2-2001;103(7):934–940.

166. Schoenhagen P, Stone GW, Nissen SE, Grines CL, Griffin J, Clemson BS, Vince DG, Ziada K, Crowe T, Apperson-Hanson C, Kapadia SR, Tuzcu EM. Coronary plaque morphology and frequency of ulceration distant from culprit lesions in patients with unstable and stable presentation. Arterioscler Thromb Vasc Biol 1-10-2003;23(10):1895–1900.

167. Fuster V, Lewis A. Conner Memorial Lecture: Mechanisms leading to myocardial infarction: insights from studies of vascular biology. Circulat 1994;90:2126–2146.

168. Lo Y SA, Cutler JE, Blake K, Wright AM, Kron J, Swerdlow CD. Angiographic coronary morphology in survivors of cardiac arrest. Am Heart J 1988;115:781–785.

169. Fuster V, Badimon L, Cohen M, Ambrose JA, Badimon JJ, Chesebro J. Insights into the pathogenesis of acute ischemic syndromes. Circulat 1988;77:1213–1220.

170. Danchin NIs myocardial revascularisation for tight coronary stenoses always necessary? Lancet 1993;342:224–225.

171. Bissett JK, Ngo WL, Wyeth RP, Matts JP. and the POSCH Group. Angiographic progression to total coronary occlusion in hyperlipidemic patients after acute myocardial infarction. Am J Cardiol 1990;66:1293–1297.

172. Naghavi M, Libby P, Falk E, Casscells SW, Litovsky S, Rumberger J, Badimon JJ, Stefanadis C, Moreno P, Pasterkamp G, Fayad Z, Stone PH, Waxman S, Raggi P, Madjid M, Zarrabi A, Burke A, Yuan C, Fitzgerald PJ, Siscovick DS, de Korte CL, Aikawa M, Airaksinen KE, Assmann G, Becker CR, Chesebro JH, Farb A, Galis ZS, Jackson C, Jang IK, Koenig W, Lodder RA, March K, Demirovic J, Navab M, Priori SG, Rekhter MD, Bahr R, Grundy SM, Mehran R, Colombo A, Boerwinkle E, Ballantyne C, Insull W, Schwartz RS, Vogel R, Serruys PW, Hansson GK, Faxon DP, Kaul S, Drexler H, Greenland P, Muller JE, Virmani R, Ridker PM, Zipes DP, Shah PK, Willerson JT. From vulnerable plaque to vulnerable patient: a call for new definitions and risk assessment strategies: Part II. Circulat 14-10-2003; 108(15):1772–1778.

173. Naghavi M, Libby P, Falk E, Casscells SW, Litovsky S, Rumberger J, Badimon JJ, Stefanadis C, Moreno P, Pasterkamp G, Fayad Z, Stone PH, Waxman S, Raggi P, Madjid M, Zarrabi A, Burke A, Yuan C, Fitzgerald PJ, Siscovick DS, de Korte CL, Aikawa M, Juhani Airaksinen KE, Assmann G, Becker CR, Chesebro JH, Farb A, Galis ZS, Jackson C, Jang IK, Koenig W, Lodder RA, March K, Demirovic J, Navab M, Priori SG, Rekhter MD, Bahr R, Grundy SM, Mehran R, Colombo A, Boerwinkle E, Ballantyne C, Insull W, Schwartz RS, Vogel R, Serruys PW, Hansson GK, Faxon DP, Kaul S, Drexler H, Greenland P, Muller JE, Virmani R, Ridker PM, Zipes DP, Shah PK, Willerson JT. From vulnerable plaque to vulnerable patient: a call for new definitions and risk assessment strategies: Part I. Circulat 7-10-2003; 108(14):1664–1672.

# 4

# Embolization As a Pathological Mechanism

**Deepak L. Bhatt and Eric J. Topol**
*Department of Cardiovascular Medicine*
*The Cleveland Clinic Foundation*
*Cleveland, Ohio, U.S.A.*

## INTRODUCTION

Spontaneous plaque rupture is the central event in the pathogenesis of acute coronary syndromes (ACS). Similarly, iatrogenic plaque rupture is induced in the cardiac catheterization laboratory during percutaneous coronary intervention. Plaque rupture leads to superimposed platelet adhesion, aggregation, and thrombus formation. Subsequent embolization of atherothrombotic material rich in platelets can lead to microvascular obstruction and dysfunction, and, ultimately, to myocardial necrosis (Figure 1). The real frequency and clinical significance of such distal embolization has only recently been appreciated. While other etiologies of microvascular obstruction such as tissue inflammation or edema exist, embolization has been increasingly recognized as having a major role in this process. Therapies that prevent embolization or minimize its impact in creating microvasculature obstruction are in evolution. Embolization and microvascular obstruction have a significant impact during both coronary interventional procedures and ACS. However, the impact and importance of distal embolization was first established for percutaneous coronary intervention. Initially, embolization was believed to be of little consequence unless it was manifest angiographically. Accumulating evidence has revealed that embolization is not as benign a process as interventional cardiologists would like to believe. Using an emboli capture device in routine stent and balloon coronary revascularization procedures, Yadav and colleagues have shown that all patients undergoing coronary intervention have evidence of atheroembolic material [1]. This observation provides a basis for interpretation of much of the pivotal data in the field.

## PERIPROCEDURAL CREATINE KINASE ELEVATION

Measurement of periprocedural cardiac enzyme levels has provided insight into the occurrence of distal embolization. Even in the absence of clinically manifest myocardial necrosis, periprocedural cardiac enzyme elevation is associated with adverse long-term outcomes, including cardiac death [2–4]. There is a gradient of risk, with larger degrees of creatine kinase (CK) elevation being associated with a progressively worse prognosis.

**New Paradigm for Acute Coronary Syndromes**

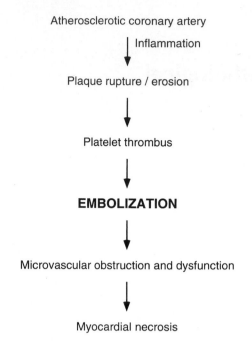

**Figure 1**   Pathogenesis of acute coronary syndromes, highlighting the importance of distal embolization.

Initially, the importance of so-called ''infarctlets'' was debated within the interventional cardiology community. However, the Evaluation of Platelet IIb/IIIa Inhibition for Prevention of Ischemic Complications (EPIC) 3-year data conclusively demonstrate the importance of periprocedural myocardial infarction (MI) and the long-term benefit of the glycoprotein IIb/IIIa inhibitor abciximab [5]. In EPIC, the all-cause mortality for patients increased as a function of periprocedural creatine kinase elevation. At a creatine kinase elevation five times the upper limit of normal, the risk of death more than doubles. Only part of this elevated risk of death is attributable to death within thirty days of the periprocedural creatine kinase elevation, with the rest of the deaths occurring later, as can be appreciated from the EPIC survival curves (Figure 2). Other studies have corroborated the importance of even minimal cardiac enzyme elevation [6,7]. The Evaluation of Platelet IIb/IIIa Inhibitor for Stenting (EPISTENT) data show a reduction not only in periprocedural MI but also in 1-year all-cause mortality in patients treated with abciximab compared with placebo [8]. Thus, agents that reduce embolization and prevent periprocedural MI ultimately also reduce mortality. The benefit of glycoprotein IIb/IIIa inhibitors in decreasing periprocedural MI, immediate ischemic complications, and long-term mortality supports the importance of distal embolization as a pathological entity, worthy of recognition and prevention.

## ATHERECTOMY

Atherectomy is perhaps the ultimate in vivo model of distal embolization. Calcific ather-oemboli have been documented in patients who have died after rotational atherectomy [9]. Rotational atherectomy can also result in large amounts of creatine kinase elevation.

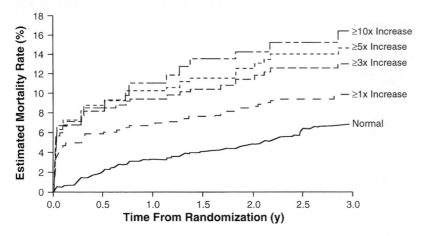

**Figure 2** Long-term prognostic value of periprocedural creatine kinase elevation from the 3-year EPIC data. Mortality rises for patients with 1-fold to 10-fold increases in periprocedural creatine-kinase (CK) levels as compared with patients without CK elevation. (From Ref. 5)

Braden et al. showed that abciximab can decrease the magnitude of creatine kinase elevation, and even its incidence [10]. Rotational atherectomy often leads to transient perfusion defects on radionuclide imaging (Figure 3), though abciximab markedly decreases such hypoperfusion [11]. Interestingly, the patients who had elevation in cardiac enzymes associated with the procedure had larger perfusion defects than the patients without such injury. Again, distal embolization leads to ischemia, but antiplatelet therapy ameliorates the response of the microvasculature to the shower of atherothrombotic gruel.

Of note, directional coronary atherectomy (DCA) has the highest risk of periprocedural MI, compared with rotablation, stenting, or balloon [12,13]. The Coronary Angioplasty Versus Excisional Atherectomy Trial (CAVEAT) trial found that DCA was associated with a higher rate of ischemic complications than percutaneous transluminal coronary angioplasty (PTCA) [14]. Directional atherectomy also caused significantly more non–Q-wave MI than did PTCA in the EPIC trial [15]. The rate of non–Q-wave MI was 9.6% for DCA compared with 4.9% for PTCA, but use of abciximab in the DCA patients reduced the rate from 15.4% for placebo to 4.5% with treatment. Thus, much of the excess risk of DCA, due to platelet aggregation and embolization, can be minimized by abciximab use.

## VEIN GRAFT EMBOLIZATION

The phenomenon of "no reflow," the lack of adequate blood flow despite epicardial patency, has been a perpetual concern with saphenous vein graft intervention. The embolization of atherothrombotic debris is widely accepted as responsible for no reflow. On histopathological examination, balloon angioplasty has been shown to be capable of causing extensive plaque rupture [16]. This plaque rupture results in atheroembolization into the microvasculature. Percutaneous intervention of aged, degenerated atherosclerotic vein grafts is particularly plagued by such distal embolization [17] Atherectomy, as in native vessels, is especially prone to embolization. The CAVEAT II trial showed that the combination of directional coronary atherectomy and vein graft intervention was also associated with adverse outcomes [18]. In the subset of patients from the EPIC trial who underwent vein graft intervention, 18% had distal embolization.

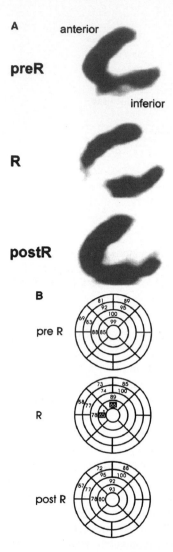

**Figure 3** **(A)** Transient apical perfusion defect after rotational atherectomy of the left anterior descending artery (LAD), as identified by single-photon emission computed tomography (SPECT) imaging. Images were obtained before (preR), during (R), and 2 days after (postR) atherectomy. **(B)** Polar maps of the left ventricle of the same patient show relative tracer uptake values in the LAD territory. The highlighted regions indicate significantly reduced perfusion. (From Ref. 11)

Abciximab treatment decreased this rate to 2%. This reduction in distal embolization translated into a reduction in non–Q-wave MI.

An interesting observation was made by Trono et al. in a study of patients undergoing percutaneous intervention of saphenous vein grafts [19]. Autopsies of two patients who died revealed multiple atherosclerotic emboli to the distal epicardial coronary artery supplied by the vein graft upon which intervention was performed. This, of course, is not surprising. More importantly, there were multiple infarcts of varying ages, including some that clearly occurred prior to the time of intervention. Therefore, akin to the embolization caused by intervention, spontaneous embolization can occur in vein grafts as well.

Transluminal extraction atherectomy, initially proposed as a solution to distal embolization, is itself associated with a high rate of embolization [20]. Furthermore, in patients who had distal embolization, the in-hospital mortality rate was 18.5% vs. 3.0% in those without distal embolization. Interestingly, a small study of transluminal extraction atherectomy for occluded vein grafts revealed that abciximab dramatically reduced the incidence of embolization, again highlighting the relevance of platelet aggregation to this process [21].

While atherectomy is not a solution for distal embolization in vein grafts, and in fact contributes to the problem, other technologies have been developed to either capture or filter vein graft debris created at the site of intervention and prevent migration downstream into the microvasculature. In 21 out of 23 vein graft interventions, Webb et al. were able to retrieve particulate matter [22]. The average size of the atheromatous particles was 240 by 83 microns. A randomized trial of saphenous vein graft intervention demonstrated a significant reduction in ischemic complications in those patients where a balloon occlusion emboli protection device was utilized [23]. Subsequently, a randomized trial of vein graft intervention showed that a filter-based emboli protection device was at least as good as an occlusion balloon [24]. Emboli protection devices have been incorporated into all the trials of carotid stenting. Similar emboli protection devices are being tested in the setting of acute myocardial infarction, potentially creating a marriage of mechanical and pharmacological therapies for prevention of embolization in ACS.

## CORONARY ARTERY BYPASS GRAFTING

That atheroembolism can occur during bypass surgery has long been appreciated by cardiothoracic surgeons. In fact, it may occur on a much larger scale than with percutaneous intervention. Keon et al. described thirteen cases of fatal perioperative myocardial infarction [25]. Five of the cases involved emboli that originated from ulcerative atherosclerotic lesions in the aortic root at the site of the vein graft ostia. Embolization from coronary endarterectomy sites occurred in two cases. Two cases were due to mechanical disruption of plaque in the major epicardial coronary arteries during surgery. An additional four cases occurred during repeat bypass procedures and resulted from dislodgment of atheroma from previous vein grafts while they were being manipulated. If routine measurement of cardiac enzyme myocardial band (MB) fractions were performed following surgery, the true incidence of distal embolization with microvascular obstruction could be appreciated. However, this practice was abandoned a number of years ago, owing to concerns of spurious laboratory results not reflective of actual myocardial necrosis [4,26–28]. Recently, there has been a resurgence of interest in periprocedural cardiac enzyme measurement. The Guard During Ischemia Against Necrosis (GUARDIAN) trial demonstrated a relationship between CK elevation greater than 10x ULN and 6-month mortality [29]. However, the authors did not find the same sort of stepped relationship that occurs across the spectrum of CK elevation in de novo plaque rupture seen in ACS patients. Potentially, with a longer-term follow-up, there would have been an association even with lower rates of CK rise.

## THROMBOLYTIC THERAPY

The provocation of distal embolization, just as with percutaneous intervention, can also occur after thrombolytic therapy. An autopsy study from the Mayo Clinic examined 32 patients who died within three weeks of either balloon angioplasty or thrombolytic therapy [30]. Microemboli were seen in 81% of the patients. The majority of emboli were either thrombotic or atheromatous. The presence of emboli was significantly correlated with the development of new electrocardiographic abnormalities, new myocardial infarction, or extension of prior myocardial infarction after the procedure. The authors speculate that, in the living, recurrent ischemia can be due to microembolization. An earlier report had also provided histological evidence that thrombolytic therapy can lead to distal embolization of thrombus [31]. In addition, thrombolytic therapy can actually create a prothrombotic milieu. For example, activated platelets are capable of secreting plasminogen activator inhibitor-1 [32]. Catheter-directed ultrasound thrombolysis is another possible therapy that is being investigated for thrombus dissolution [33,34]. However, as a stand-alone technique, it is unlikely that it will eliminate the problem of distal embolization of thrombus entirely, as embolization has been documented to occur with this device [35]. It would seem that any device that has to be put into a diseased artery before being used or activated will always have a liability.

Thus, the wealth of data from the percutaneous coronary intervention literature supports the mechanistic importance of distal embolization and the value of minimizing its impact on the microvasculature. Furthermore, these data provide a conceptual framework for understanding spontaneous embolization that occurs during ACS.

## Embolization During Acute Coronary Syndromes

In the setting of ACS, just as with percutaneous coronary intervention, distal embolization occurs and glycoprotein (GP) IIb/IIIa inhibitors improve outcomes [36]. Numerous studies have documented the beneficial impact on death or MI that GPIIb/IIIa inhibitors have in ACS [37–40]. Much of the benefit of GPIIb/IIIa inhibitors can be attributed to the effects they have on the occurrence of platelet embolization, as well as the microvasculature's response to this embolic burden (Table 1).

## Platelet Embolization

A seminal contribution to the understanding of embolization in ACS was made by Davies et al. in an autopsy study of 90 patients who suffered sudden cardiac death [41]. Thirty percent of the patients had platelet aggregates found in small intramyocardial vessels (Figure 4). In patients with unstable angina before death, 44.4% were found to have such

**Table 1**  Mechanisms of Myocyte Necrosis Due to Distal Embolization

---

Thrombosis
  Platelet aggregation
  Thrombin generation
Inflammation
  Release of cytokines
  Recruitment of monocytes and neutrophils
  Apoptosis
Vasoconstriction
  Endothelial dysfunction
  Vasoactive amines, thromboxane $A_2$, serotonin
Compromised collateral flow
  Infarct expansion

---

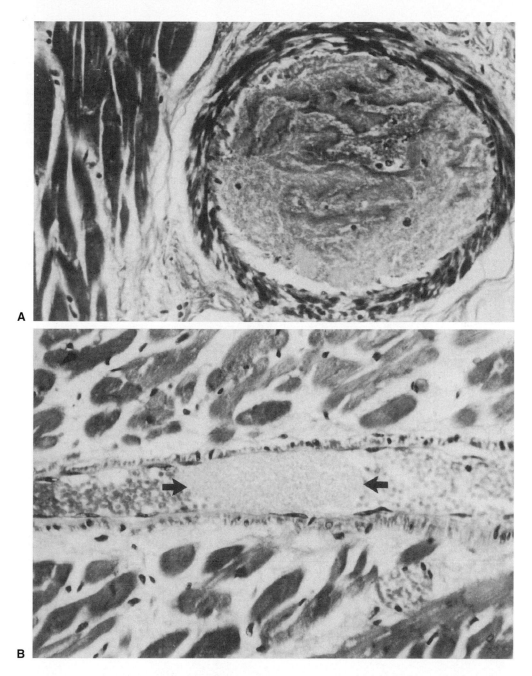

**Figure 4** Deposition of platelet aggregates in the microvasculature, occupying the entire lumen of an intramyocardial artery, in cross section (**A**) and in longitudinal section (**B**). (From Ref. 41)

platelet aggregates. Those patients with platelet emboli were much more likely to have multifocal microscopic necrosis involving the entire ventricular wall. The platelet aggregates were present in the myocardial territory subserved by an epicardial artery containing a ruptured plaque with overlying thrombus. Similarly, in a study of patients who died of acute MI, 79% had platelet emboli found in the microcirculation (Figure 5) [42]. Another

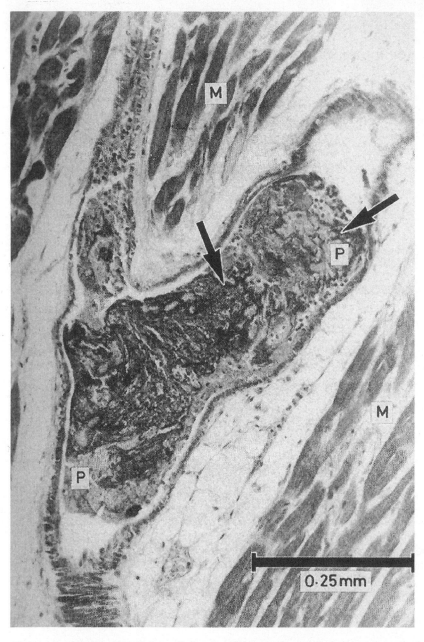

**Figure 5** Intramyocardial arteriole containing a microembolus composed of platelets and fibrin. The *arrows* show fibrin strands forming islands of platelets; *P* represents platelets; *M*, myocardium. (From Ref. 42)

autopsy study of 25 patients with sudden death revealed that 81% had epicardial thrombi with a layered structure, composed of thrombus material of differing ages [43]. This important finding implies periodic growth of the epicardial thrombus, which was accompanied by intermittent fragmentation and embolization of thrombus in 73% of the cases, resulting in occlusion of small intramyocardial arteries with associated microscopic infarcts. Furthermore, during acute MI, platelet microthrombi are not just confined to the infarct-related artery, but can be found in the circulation and are associated with infarct extension [44]. Platelet and thrombin microthrombi are not found in normal hearts, only in patients with cardiac disease [45]. In addition, platelet aggregation and embolization can lower the threshold for ventricular fibrillation [46]. Thus, platelet embolization not only occurs, but also can lead to infarction of myocardial cells and even trigger sudden death.

Further indirect evidence of the importance of microvascular obstruction due to platelet aggregates comes from an analysis of patients with angiographically ''insignificant'' coronary artery disease in PURSUIT [47]. Those patients presenting with acute coronary syndromes with less than 50% stenosis in any epicardial vessel nevertheless appeared to have modest benefit from eptifibatide therapy. Potentially, platelet embolization from the site of a ruptured plaque is minimized by GPIIb/IIIa blockade.

## ROLE OF THE ENDOTHELIUM

Concomitant endothelial dysfunction further aggravates the situation created by platelet embolization. Endothelial expression of P-selectin, capable of binding platelets and leukocytes, is upregulated distal to severe epicardial stenoses [48]. In addition, endothelial integrity as assessed by electron microscopy can be disrupted. A study by Mutin et al. found circulating endothelial cells in patients with acute MI and unstable angina, but not those with stable angina or in controls [49]. It is also known that endothelial microparticles have both adhesive properties and procoagulant effects [50]. Thus, embolization of endothelial cells in ACS does occur and can lead to further platelet activation and aggregation in the microvasculature, ultimately leading to obstruction and myocardial necrosis. An interesting hypothesis to explain part of the benefit of abciximab, in addition to its properties as GPIIb/IIIa inhibitor, is its ability to bind the vitronectin receptor. This integrin is heavily expressed on activated endothelial cells. Potentially, by binding to this receptor on endothelial cells, endothelial microparticles are unable to bind to other tissue elements in the microvasculature.

## INFLAMMATION AND EMBOLIZATION

Inflammation and embolization are intimately intertwined. The inflamed artery contributes to plaque erosion, rupture, and the potential for subsequent distal embolization. The embolization of friable microparticulate atherosclerotic material, with or without platelet thrombus, likely promotes further inflammation. The CD40 ligand on activated platelets causes endothelial cells to express adhesion molecules and to secrete chemokines that attract leukocytes [51]. Compared with control patients and those with stable angina, patients with unstable angina have elevated levels of CD40 ligand, both in its soluble and membrane-bound forms [52]. Of note, the ADP receptor antagonist clopidogrel appears to have a potent role in suppressing CD40 [53]. Similarly, patients with ACS who have elevated levels of soluble CD40 are those that are most likely to derive benefit from abciximab [54]. Activated platelets can also cause endothelial cells to express tissue factor, generating a prothrombotic milieu [55]. Platelet-leukocyte adhesion can occur via interaction between P-selectin on platelets and sialyl Lewis(x) on leukocytes [56,57]. Compared with controls, patients with ACS have higher levels of platelet microparticles and greater degrees of platelet-leukocyte interaction [58]. In patients with acute MI, platelet-leukocyte adhesion is increased, leading to induction of IL-1 beta, IL-8, and MCP-1 and activation of nuclear factor-kappa B [59]. Thus, platelet embolization in ACS induces an inflammatory response that can lead to formation of a multicellular plug, composed of platelets, neutrophils, and endothelial cells, capable of occluding microvascular flow [60].

Prevention of platelet activation seems to be paramount in halting this deleterious cascade of events. However, it would be naïve to assume that the antiplatelet effect produced by GPIIb/IIIa therapy is the only operative mechanism. Abciximab binds to several other receptors in addition to the platelet GPIIb/IIIa receptor. It binds to the leukocyte integrin MAC-1, preventing binding of fibrinogen and intercellular adhesion molecule-1 (ICAM-1) [61]. Abciximab also binds to the vitronectin receptor and can lead to further reductions in thrombin generation, independent of the effects on GPIIb/IIIa inhibition [62]. Blockade of the vitronectin receptor has other important biological effects and has resulted in a decrease in neointimal proliferation in animal models of arterial injury [63]. Vitronectin can mediate platelet attachment to activated endothelium in the plasma of patients with acute MI undergoing reperfusion [64]. This nonspecific binding of abciximab to multiple receptors, in addition to promoting an antiplatelet and antithrombotic effect, produces simultaneous blockade of endothelial cells and leukocytes as well. These other actions may translate into further improvements in microvascular flow, beyond the improvements exclusively due to antiplatelet effects. Supportive of this premise, abciximab appears to blunt the rise in CRP that otherwise occurs with percutaneous coronary intervention [65]. However, abciximab does not appear to be of specific benefit in patients with elevated baseline levels of CRP [66]. Recent data from the carotid stent literature suggest that patients with elevated levels of baseline white blood cell count, a surrogate marker of inflammation, are those who are most likely to have embolization occur during their procedure [67]. Thus, the relationship between inflammation and embolization is quite complex and our understanding is in its infancy.

## MICROVASCULAR FUNCTION

Superimposed thrombus formation in the setting of distal embolization of atheromatous material further contributes to microvascular flow obstruction by triggering a cascade of biochemical events. Platelet activation and aggregation and vascular tone are intimately linked [68]. Coronary stenosis and associated endothelial injury with subsequent platelet aggregation, dislodgment and distal embolization lead to the now well-recognized phenomenon of cyclic flow variation [69]. Measures that reduce platelet aggregation reduce cyclic flow variation. This has been demonstrated for nitric oxide production [70], thrombin inhibition [71], and ADP receptor blockade [72].

Release of substances, such as vasoactive amines, from activated platelets leads to vasoconstriction and microcirculatory abnormalities. Intense microvascular constriction can occur due to release of such factors from platelets [73]. Prostaglandin production can cause vasoconstriction [74]. Platelet activating factor can be released by either platelets or neutrophils and can lead to vasoconstriction in coronary arterioles [75,76]. Thromboxane $A_2$ and serotonin, released from activated platelets, are potent vasoconstrictors [32]. Thrombin, the production of which is accelerated by aggregated platelets, can also cause vasoconstriction [77]. Agents that reverse this vasoconstriction, induced by multiple agonists, are potentially therapeutic in this situation. Taniyama et al. showed that intracoronary verapamil at the time of primary PTCA leads to further improvements in microvascular flow [78]. Similarly, Ito et al. demonstrated that intravenous nicorandil, an adenosine triphosphate-sensitive potassium channel opener, further improves microvascular flow after apparently successful PTCA [79]. Impaired flow even in non-culprit arteries during acute myocardial infarction has been demonstrated with the corrected TIMI frame count [80]. Even with successful angioplasty of the culprit artery, flow in all arteries is still reduced compared to normal, likely due, at least in part, to abnormalities of microvascular flow [81]. In addition to its effects on microvascular function, embolization may also compromise collateral flow and contribute to infarct expansion.

## EMBOLIZATION IN DIABETIC PATIENTS

Diabetic patients with ACS have a higher rate of adverse outcomes [82–86]. While this is due to multiple factors, diabetics are prone to distal embolization and particularly ill-suited to deal with its consequences. Diabetics have hyperreactivity of their platelets [87], making them more likely to adhere to the endothelium under conditions of shear stress [88]. Their platelets are more prone to spontaneous aggregation [89]. Even the prediabetic state is associated with increased platelet activation [90]. Diabetics with unstable angina are much more likely to have ulcerated plaque and intracoronary thrombus, as documented by angioscopy [91]. Therefore, they are at much higher risk of embolization into the microvasculature. Their microvasculature is often diffusely diseased and dysfunctional, as reflected by a diminished coronary flow reserve [92,93], and an embolic shower is less likely to be tolerated and more likely to lead to microvascular obstruction and myocardial necrosis. Furthermore, the diabetic state leads to a heightened tendency for platelet-leukocyte interaction to occur [94]. These findings may help explain the remarkable benefit of abciximab in reducing the increased rate of mortality in diabetic patients undergoing percutaneous coronary intervention [95]. Thus, diabetic patients are particularly prone to distal embolization and more likely to suffer adverse clinical consequences as a result, but, fortunately, therapy with abciximab can attenuate the adverse effect of embolization on their microvasculature.

## MEASUREMENT OF EMBOLIZATION WITH TROPONINS

Troponin measurement is a sensitive indicator of distal embolization and resultant myocardial cellular damage [96]. Troponins are found in myocytes in the troponin-tropomyosin complex. Troponins are much more sensitive than CK-MB at detecting myocardial damage and are useful in risk-stratifying patients with ACS [97–99]. Elevated troponin levels are associated with an increased rate of adverse outcomes. This holds true even when the creatine kinase level is not elevated above normal limits. Hamm et al. reported on the value of troponins in risk-stratifying patients with acute coronary syndromes and showed their usefulness in allocating patients to intravenous antiplatelet therapy in the c7E3 Fab Antiplatelet Therapy in Unstable Refractory Angina (CAPTURE) trial (Figure 6A and B) [100]. In fact, troponin elevation appears to be a more powerful tool for risk stratification and selection of patients for abciximab therapy than angiography in patients with unstable angina [101]. In the Platelet Receptor Inhibition in Ischemic Syndrome Management (PRISM) trial as well, both troponin T and I were found to identify the group of patients with unstable angina who derived maximum benefit from GPIIb/IIIa blockade with tirofiban [102,103] (Figure 6C and D). While the CAPTURE data documented the value of

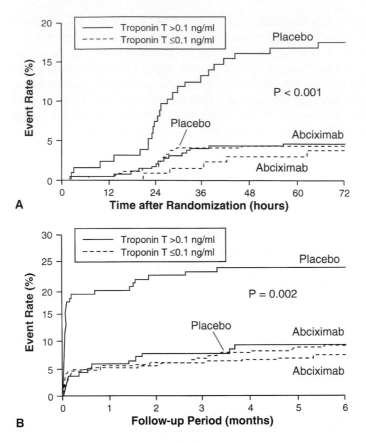

**Figure 6** Data from the C7E3 Fab Antiplatelet Therapy in Unstable Refractory Angina (CAPTURE) trial, showing the benefit of abciximab in reducing death and nonfatal MI in patients who are troponin positive in the initial 72 hours after randomization (**A**) and during 6 months of follow-up (**B**). (From Ref. 100) The Platelet Receptor Inhibition in Ischemic Syndrome Management (PRISM) trial likewise showed a reduction in death and MI in patients who were troponin positive

troponin measurement in risk stratification in a relatively high-risk cohort of patients, the PRISM analysis extended this finding to a lower-risk cohort. In PRISM, tirofiban treatment in patients with positive troponins resulted in a significant decrease in mortality, both in patients who were medically managed and in those who subsequently underwent revascularization. In addition, the Fragmin and Fast Revascularization during Instability in Coronary Artery disease (FRISC) trial found that both troponin and C-reactive protein, a marker of inflammation, were independently able to predict cardiac death in a multivariable model [104]. In FRISC II, long-term treatment with the low molecular weight heparin dalteparin in troponin positive patients with unstable angina was also found to decrease cardiac events [105]. Thus, measurement of troponins as a marker of distal embolization allows detection of levels of myocardial damage not previously possible. Measurements of inflammation such as C-reactive protein or CD40 appear to add additional prognostic value. Furthermore, such information allows targeting of intravenous antiplatelet therapy or antithrombotic therapy to those patients most likely to have distal embolization.

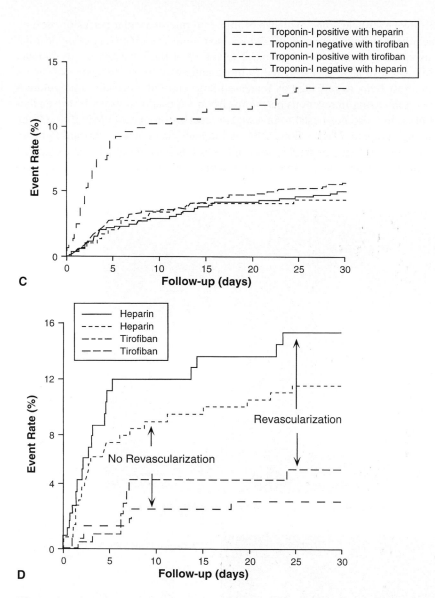

**Figure 6** (**C**). This reduction was seen both in patients treated medically and with revascularization (**D**). (From Ref. 101)

## IMAGING THE IMPACT OF EMBOLIZATION

Rapid evolution of imaging technology has allowed visualization of the importance of distal embolization on the microvasculature. Both contrast echocardiography and magnetic resonance imaging are expanding our appreciation of embolization. Coronary flow measurements have also refined our understanding of microvasular function.

## CONTRAST ECHOCARDIOGRAPHY

Initially, Ito et al. used intracoronary myocardial contrast echocardiography to study acute MI patients before and after revascularization [106]. A sizable proportion of patients with TIMI 3 flow nevertheless had evidence of impaired microvascular perfusion, despite adequate epicardial patency; these patients did not have significant recovery of myocardial function as assessed by the ejection fraction. The ability of the left ventricle to remodel after acute MI was also adversely affected in those patients without adequate reflow on myocardial contrast echo, as reflected by increased left ventricular end-diastolic volumes [107]. Contrast echo using intravenous perfluorocarbon-exposed sonicated dextrose albumin microbubbles has also been used to investigate reperfusion in acute MI [108]. Of the patients with angiographic TIMI 3 flow, 29% had defects on contrast echocardiography (see Figure 7). While the patients with reflow on contrast echocardiography had a significant decrease in end-systolic volume index, those with no reflow had a significant increase

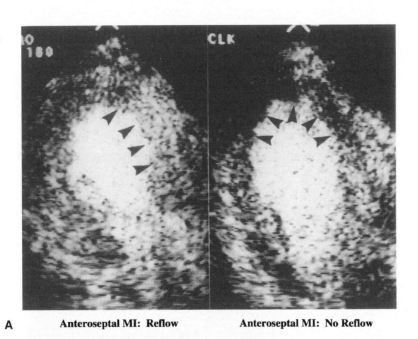

A          **Anteroseptal MI: Reflow**                **Anteroseptal MI: No Reflow**

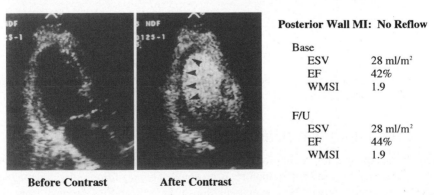

**Posterior Wall MI: No Reflow**

Base
   ESV          28 ml/m²
   EF           42%
   WMSI         1.9

F/U
   ESV          28 ml/m²
   EF           44%
   WMSI         1.9

B      **Before Contrast**            **After Contrast**

**Figure 7**  Contrast echocardiograms in two patients with restored epicardial flow in the LAD, one showing reflow and the other showing no reflow during anteroseptal myocardial infarction (MI) (**A**). In this patient with an acute left circumflex artery infarction, despite Thrombolysis in Myocardial Infarction (TIMI) 3 flow on angiography, a microvascular perfusion defect as assessed by contrast echocardiography is seen in the posterior wall (**B**). (From Ref. 108)

in this parameter. Determination of microvascular integrity by contrast echocardiography was also found useful for predicting subsequent clinical events [109]. Myocardial contrast echo is, thus, poised to transition from being a research tool to being a clinically relevant method to assess embolization and microvascular flow.

## MAGNETIC RESONANCE IMAGING

Advances in magnetic resonance imaging (MRI) technology have also occurred at a rapid pace. Much like contrast echo, MRI can quantify microvascular obstruction and compares favorably with histopathologic methods (see Figure 8) [110]. MRI can quantify microvascular obstruction after MI and correlates well with radioactive microsphere blood flow measurements [111]. A study of 44 patients with acute MI by Wu et al. examined cardiovascular outcomes at two years [112]. Patients classified as having microvascular obstruction had a significantly higher rate of cardiovascular events than those without, 45% versus 9%. Importantly, even after adjusting for infarct size, microvascular obstruction remained a statistically significant prognostic marker of complications. Among the 17 patients returning for follow-up MRI at 6 months, the presence of microvascular obstruction was associated with both fibrous scar formation and left ventricular remodeling. Therefore, although TIMI 3 flow on angiography has been the gold standard for reperfusion therapy, newer imaging modalities have conclusively demonstrated that TIMI 3 flow alone is not sufficient for demonstration of adequate tissue level perfusion. Furthermore, inadequate tissue perfusion leads to impaired left ventricular remodeling and function, as well as higher rates of cardiovascular events.

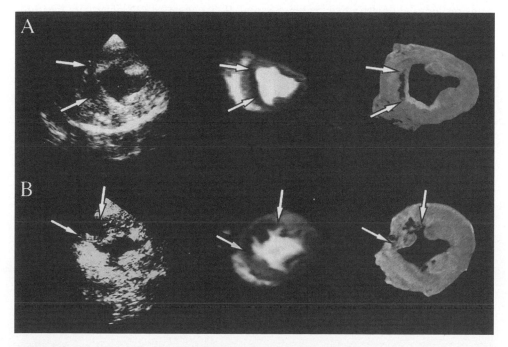

**Figure 8** MRI showing two examples of microvascular obstruction and correlation with contrast echocardiography or postmortem thioflavin-S staining. (From Ref. 110)

## ELECTROCARDIOGRAM ST-SEGMENT RESOLUTION

While sophisticated imaging methodologies have been developed, the full potential of the standard electrocardiogram (ECG) has still not been exhausted. Electrocardiographic resolution of ST-segment elevation appears to be a powerful method to detect epicardial patency as well as tissue level reperfusion [113–115]. Greater than or equal to 70% ST-segment resolution in patients with acute MI identified those who had preserved left ventricular function measured one week later [116]. Continuous ST-segment monitoring may provide a method to detect successful reperfusion or reocclusion [117–119]. ST segment resolution may also provide insight into cyclic flow variation [120]. The correlation of ST segment resolution with myocardial contrast echo is excellent [121]. After either chemical or mechanical reperfusion, ST-segment resolution is able to provide important prognostic information [122]. An analysis of the TIMI 14 data examined the percent ST-resolution in patients with angiographically demonstrated TIMI 3 flow [123]. Patients who received abciximab in addition to reduced dose tPA had significantly greater ST-segment resolution than patients who received standard tPA, 69% complete resolution versus 44%, p = 0.0002. Thus, ECG ST-segment resolution may be the gold standard to detect reperfusion at the tissue level and to identify therapies that enhance microvascular flow.

## PREVENTING EMBOLIZATION—CLINICAL RELEVANCE

Potentially, impaired microvascular perfusion could be due to factors other than distal embolization, such as reperfusion injury, edema, or inflammation. While it is likely that the mechanism is multifactorial, there is direct evidence that therapies that target platelet aggregation (and possibly endothelial and neutrophil adhesion) improve tissue level perfusion. In an elegant analysis of patients undergoing stent implantation for acute MI, Neumann et al. demonstrated that abciximab, in addition to its known beneficial effect on epicardial patency, improves microvascular perfusion [124]. Compared with heparin, patients randomized to abciximab had higher peak flow velocity on Doppler wire measurements (see Figure 9). Furthermore, the improvement in tissue level perfusion was associated with favorable left ventricular function, as the abciximab treated group had a higher ejection fraction than the heparin treated group, 62% versus 56%, p = 0.003.

In an analysis of patients who received either thrombolytic therapy or primary angioplasty for a first time acute MI, Agati et al. assessed microvascular perfusion via intracoro-

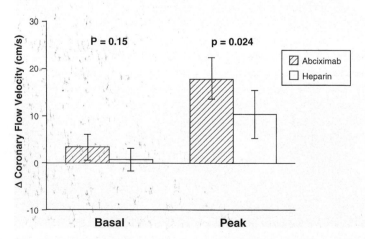

**Figure 9** Differences in basal and peak coronary flow velocity for abciximab versus placebo. (From Ref. 124)

**Table 2** Markers to Detect Embolization and Their Ability to Predict Outcome

| Condition | Primary Marker(s) of Embolization | Outcome |
|---|---|---|
| Percutaneous Coronary Intervention | CK-MB | +++ |
| Unstable Angina | Troponin | ++++ |
| Acute MI | ECG ST Resolution | ++++ |
| | Contrast Echo | ++ |
| | MRI | ++ |

CK-MB, creatine kinase myocardial band; ECG, electrocardiagram; MI, myocardial infarction; MRI, magnetic resonance imaging.

nary injection of sonicated microbubbles [125]. In the subset of patients with TIMI 3 flow at one month, a perfusion defect occurred in 72% of the patients who received tPA versus 31% of the patients who received primary angioplasty, p = 0.00001. The wall motion score index at one month was also significantly better in the patients treated with angioplasty. Again, improvements in tissue level reperfusion translate into improved ventricular function. Furthermore, tissue level reperfusion can be enhanced by both pharmacological therapy with GPIIb/IIIa inhibition and by mechanical reperfusion therapy.

Recent data from the Transplantation of Progenitor Cells and Regeneration Enhancement in Acute Myocardial Infarction (TOPCARE-AMI) trial suggest that intracoronary infusion of either bone marrow- or circulating blood-derived progenitor cells can lead to near normalization of infarct artery coronary flow reserve over a four month period [126,127]. Thus, in the MI patient in whom substantial embolization has already occurred, infusion of progenitor cells may promote neovascularization and allow myocardial salvage.

## CONCLUSION

The great frequency with which embolization occurs is only now being appreciated. Filter devices that capture embolic debris, troponin measurements, and newer imaging modalities have each demonstrated that embolization is common and results in significant myocardial damage. Clearly, these recent data have shifted the focus in ACS from merely ensuring epicardial patency to reestablishing adequate microvascular perfusion. Methods of measuring embolization will continue to be refined (Table 2). Distal embolization is the major contributor to microvascular obstruction in the setting of ischemia, operating via a number of intertwined cellular and biochemical pathways. Successful mechanical, catheter-based approaches, as well as pharmacological approaches, have been developed to prevent embolization. However, the future lies in combining both of these previously divergent philosophies of reperfusion, and such efforts are underway with promising initial results. Thus, therapies that decrease embolization are effective in improving both short- and long-term outcomes of patients with ACS and represent a major advance in the field of cardiovascular medicine.

## REFERENCES

1. Yadav JS, Grube E, Rowold S, Kirchof N, Sedgewick J, Topol EJ. Detection and characterization of emboli during coronary intervention. Circulation 1999;100:1–780.
2. Abdelmeguid AE, Topol EJ. The myth of the myocardial "infarctlet" during percutaneous coronary revascularization procedures. Circulation 1996;94:3369–3375.

3.  Abdelmeguid AE, Topol EJ, Whitlow PL, Sapp SK, Ellis SG. Significance of mild transient release of creatine kinase-MB fraction after percutaneous coronary interventions. Circulation 1996;94:1528–1536.

4.  Califf RM, Abdelmeguid AE, Kuntz RE, Popma JJ, Davidson CJ, Cohen EA, Kleiman NS, Mahaffey KW, Topol EJ, Pepine CJ, Lipicky RJ, Granger CB, Harrington RA, Tardiff BE, Crenshaw BS, Bauman RP, Zuckerman BD, Chaitman BR, Bittl JA, Ohman EM. Myonecrosis after revascularization procedures. J Am Coll Cardiol 1998;31:241–251.

5.  Topol EJ, Ferguson JJ, Weisman HF, Tcheng JE, Ellis SG, Kleiman NS, Ivanhoe RJ, Wang AL, Miller DP, Anderson KM, Califf RM. Long-term protection from myocardial ischemic events in a randomized trial of brief integrin beta-3 blockade with percutaneous coronary intervention. EPIC Investigator Group. Evaluation of Platelet IIb/IIIa Inhibition for Prevention of Ischemic Complication. JAMA 1997;278:479–484.

6.  Simoons ML, van den Brand M, Lincoff M, Harrington R, van der Wieken R, Vahanian A, Rutsch W, Kootstra J, Boersma E, Califf RM, Topol E. Minimal myocardial damage during coronary intervention is associated with impaired outcome. Eur Heart J 1999;20:1112–1119.

7.  Kong TQ, Davidson CJ, Meyers SN, Tauke JT, Parker MA, Bonow RO. Prognostic implication of creatine kinase elevation following elective coronary artery interventions. JAMA 1997;277:461–466.

8.  Topol EJ, Mark DB, Lincoff AM, Cohen E, Burton J, Kleiman N, Talley D, Sapp S, Booth J, Cabot CF, Anderson KM, Califf RM. Outcomes at 1 year and economic implications of platelet GPIIb/IIIa blockade in patients undergoing coronary stenting: results from a multi-centre randomised trial. EPISTENT Investigators. Evaluation of Platelet IIb/IIIa Inhibitor for Stenting. Lancet 1999;354:2019–2024.

9.  Farb A, Roberts DK, Pichard AD, Kent KM, Virmani R. Coronary artery morphologic features after coronary rotational atherectomy: insights into mechanisms of lumen enlargement and embolization. Am Heart J 1995;129:1058–1067.

10. Braden GA, Applegate RJ, Young TM, Love WW, Sane DC. Abciximab decreases both the incidence and magnitude of creatine kinase elevation during rotational atherectomy. J Am Coll Cardiol 1997;29:499A.

11. Koch KC, vom Dahl J, Kleinhans E, Klues HG, Radke PW, Ninnemann S, Schulz G, Buell U, Hanrath P. Influence of a platelet GPIIb/IIIa receptor antagonist on myocardial hypoperfusion during rotational atherectomy as assessed by myocardial Tc-99m sestamibi scintigraphy. J Am Coll Cardiol 1999;33:998–1004.

12. Abdelmeguid AE, Ellis SG, Sapp SK, Whitlow PL, Topol EJ. Defining the appropriate threshold of creatine kinase elevation after percutaneous coronary interventions. Am Heart J 1996;131:1097–1105.

13. Kini A, Kini S, Marmur JD, Bertea T, Dangas G, Cocke TP, Sharma SK. Incidence and mechanism of creatine kinase-MB enzyme elevation after coronary intervention with different devices. Catheter Cardiovasc Interv 1999;48:123–129.

14. Topol EJ, Leya F, Pinkerton CA, Whitlow PL, Hofling B, Simonton CA, Masden RR, Serruys PW, Leon MB, Williams DO, et al. A comparison of directional atherectomy with coronary angioplasty in patients with coronary artery disease. The CAVEAT Study Group. N Engl J Med 1993;329:221–227.

15. Lefkovits J, Blankenship JC, Anderson KM, Stoner GL, Talley JD, Worley SJ, Weisman HF, Califf RM, Topol EJ. Increased risk of non-Q wave myocardial infarction after directional atherectomy is platelet dependent: evidence from the EPIC trial. Evaluation of c7E3 for the Prevention of Ischemic Complications. J Am Coll Cardiol 1996;28:849–855.

16. Saber RS, Edwards WD, Holmes DR, Vlietstra RE, Reeder GS. Balloon angioplasty of aortocoronary saphenous vein bypass grafts: a histopathologic study of six grafts from five patients, with emphasis on restenosis and embolic complications. J Am Coll Cardiol 1988; 12:1501–1509.

17. Mak KH, Challapalli R, Eisenberg MJ, Anderson KM, Califf RM, Topol EJ. Effect of platelet GPIIb/IIIa receptor inhibition on distal embolization during percutaneous revascularization of aortocoronary saphenous vein grafts. EPIC Investigators. Evaluation of IIb/IIIa platelet

receptor antagonist 7E3 in Preventing Ischemic Complications. Am J Cardiol 1997;80: 985–988.

18. Lefkovits J, Holmes DR, Califf RM, Safian RD, Pieper K, Keeler G, Topol EJ. Predictors and sequelae of distal embolization during saphenous vein graft intervention from the CAVEAT-II trial. Coronary Angioplasty Versus Excisional Atherectomy Trial. Circulation 1995;92: 734–740.

19. Trono R, Sutton C, Hollman J, Suit P, Ratliff NB. Multiple myocardial infarctions associated with atheromatous emboli after PTCA of saphenous vein grafts. A clinicopathologic correlation. Cleve Clin J Med 1989;56:581–584.

20. Moses JW, Moussa I, Popma JJ, Sketch MH, Yeh W. Risk of distal embolization and infarction with transluminal extraction atherectomy in saphenous vein grafts and native coronary arteries. NACI Investigators. New Approaches to Coronary Interventions. Catheter Cardiovasc Interv 1999;47:149–154.

21. Sullebarger JT, Dalton RD, Nasser A, Matar FA. Adjunctive abciximab improves outcomes during recanalization of totally occluded saphenous vein grafts using transluminal extraction atherectomy. Catheter Cardiovasc Interv 1999;46:107–110.

22. Webb JG, Carere RG, Virmani R, Baim D, Teirstein PS, Whitlow P, McQueen C, Kolodgie FD, Buller E, Dodek A, Mancini GB, Oesterle S. Retrieval and analysis of particulate debris after saphenous vein graft intervention. J Am Coll Cardiol 1999;34:468–475.

23. Baim DS, Wahr D, George B, Leon MB, Greenberg J, Cutlip DE, Kaya U, Popma JJ, Ho KK, Kuntz RE. Randomized trial of a distal embolic protection device during percutaneous intervention of saphenous vein aorto-coronary bypass grafts. Circulation 2002;105: 1285–1290.

24. Stone GW, Rogers C, Hermiller J, Feldman R, Hall P, Haber R, Masud A, Cambier P, Caputo RP, Turco M, Kovach R, Brodie B, Herrmann HC, Kuntz RE, Popma JJ, Ramee S, Cox DA. Randomized comparison of distal protection with a filter-based catheter and a balloon occlusion and aspiration system during percutaneous intervention of diseased saphenous vein aorto-coronary bypass grafts. Circulation 2003;108:548–553.

25. Keon WJ, Heggtveit HA, Leduc J. Perioperative myocardial infarction caused by atheroembolism. J Thorac Cardiovasc Surg 1982;84:849–855.

26. McGregor CG, Muir AL, Smith AF, Miller HC, Hannan WJ, Cameron EW, Wheatley DJ. Myocardial infarction related to coronary artery bypass graft surgery. Br Heart J 1984;51: 399–406.

27. Roberts AJ, Combes JR, Jacobstein JG, Alonso DR, Post MR, Subramanian VA, Abel RM, Brachfeld N, Kline SA, Gay WA. Perioperative myocardial infarction associated with coronary artery bypass graft surgery: improved sensitivity in the diagnosis within 6 hours after operation with 99mTc-glucoheptonate myocardial imaging and myocardial-specific isoenzymes. Ann Thorac Surg 1979;27:42–48.

28. Warren SG, Wagner GS, Bethea CF, Roe CR, Oldham HN, Kong Y. Diagnostic and prognostic significance of electrocardiographic and CPK isoenzyme changes following coronary bypass surgery: correlation with findings at one year. Am Heart J 1977;93:189–196.

29. Gavard JA, Chaitman BR, Sakai S, Stocke K, Danchin N, Erhardt L, Gallo R, Chi E, Jessel A, Theroux P. Prognostic significance of elevated creatine kinase MB after coronary bypass surgery and after an acute coronary syndrome: results from the GUARDIAN trial. J Thorac Cardiovasc Surg 2003;126:807–813.

30. Saber RS, Edwards WD, Bailey KR, McGovern TW, Schwartz RS, Holmes DR. Coronary embolization after balloon angioplasty or thrombolytic therapy: an autopsy study of 32 cases. J Am Coll Cardiol 1993;22:1283–1288.

31. Menke DM, Jordan MD, Aust CH, Storer W, Waller BF. Histologic evidence of distal coronary thromboembolism. A complication of acute proximal coronary artery thrombolysis therapy. Chest 1986;90:614–616.

32. Lefkovits J, Topol EJ. Role of platelet inhibitor agents in coronary artery disease. In: Topol EJ, Ed. Textbook of Interventional Cardiology. 3rd ed.. Philadelphia: W. B. Saunders Company, 1999:3–24.

33. Rosenschein U, Bernstein JJ, DiSegni E, Kaplinsky E, Bernheim J, Rozenzsajn LA. Experimental ultrasonic angioplasty: disruption of atherosclerotic plaques and thrombi in vitro and arterial recanalization in vivo. J Am Coll Cardiol 1990;15:711–717.

34. Rosenschein U, Roth A, Rassin T, Basan S, Laniado S, Miller HI. Analysis of coronary ultrasound thrombolysis endpoints in acute myocardial infarction (ACUTE trial). Results of the feasibility phase. Circulation 1997;95:1411–1416.

35. Rosenschein U, Gaul G, Erbel R, Amann F, Velasguez D, Stoerger H, Simon R, Gomez G, Troster J, Bartorelli A, Pieper M, Kyriakides Z, Laniado S, Miller HI, Cribier A, Fajadet J. Percutaneous transluminal therapy of occluded saphenous vein grafts: can the challenge be met with ultrasound thrombolysis? Circulation 1999;99:26–29.

36. Kong DF, Califf RM, Miller DP, Moliterno DJ, White HD, Harrington RA, Tcheng JE, Lincoff AM, Hasselblad V, Topol EJ. Clinical Outcomes of Therapeutic Agents That Block the Platelet GPIIb/IIIa Integrin in Ischemic Heart Disease. Circulation 1998;98:2829–2835.

37. PURSUIT Investigators. Inhibition of platelet GPIIb/IIIa with eptifibatide in patients with acute coronary syndromes. Platelet GPIIb/IIIa in Unstable Angina: Receptor Suppression Using Integrilin Therapy. N Engl J Med 1998;339:436–443.

38. Bhatt DL, Topol EJ. Current role of platelet GPIIb/IIIa inhibitors in acute coronary syndromes. JAMA 2000;284:1549–1558.

39. PRISM Investigators. A comparison of aspirin plus tirofiban with aspirin plus heparin for unstable angina. Platelet Receptor Inhibition in Ischemic Syndrome Management (PRISM) Study. N Engl J Med 1998;338:1498–1505.

40. PRISM-PLUS Investigators. Inhibition of the platelet GPIIb/IIIa receptor with tirofiban in unstable angina and non-Q-wave myocardial infarction. Platelet Receptor Inhibition in Ischemic Syndrome Management in Patients Limited by Unstable Signs and Symptoms (PRISM-PLUS). N Engl J Med 1998;338:1488–1497.

41. Davies MJ, Thomas AC, Knapman PA, Hangartner JR. Intramyocardial platelet aggregation in patients with unstable angina suffering sudden ischemic cardiac death. Circulation 1986; 73:418–427.

42. Frink RJ, Rooney PA, Trowbridge JO, Rose JP. Coronary thrombosis and platelet/fibrin microemboli in death associated with acute myocardial infarction. Br Heart J 1988;59: 196–200.

43. Falk E. Unstable angina with fatal outcome: dynamic coronary thrombosis leading to infarction and/or sudden death. Autopsy evidence of recurrent mural thrombosis with peripheral embolization culminating in total vascular occlusion. Circulation 1985;71:699–708.

44. Mehta P, Mehta J. Platelet function studies in coronary artery disease. V. Evidence for enhanced platelet microthrombus formation activity in acute myocardial infarction. Am J Cardiol 1979;43:757–760.

45. El-Maraghi N, Genton E. The relevance of platelet and fibrin thromboembolism of the coronary microcirculation, with special reference to sudden cardiac death. Circulation 1980;62: 936–944.

46. Kowey PR, Verrier RL, Lown B, Handin RI. Influence of intracoronary platelet aggregation on ventricular electrical properties during partial coronary artery stenosis. Am J Cardiol 1983; 51:596–602.

47. Roe MT, Harrington RA, Prosper DM, Pieper KS, Bhatt DL, Lincoff AM, Simoons ML, Akkerhuis M, Ohman EM, Kitt MM, Vahanian A, Ruzyllo W, Karsch K, Califf RM, Topol EJ. Clinical and therapeutic profile of patients presenting with acute coronary syndromes who do not have significant coronary artery disease. Circulation 2000;102:1101–1106.

48. Eguchi H, Ikeda H, Murohara T, Yasukawa H, Haramaki N, Sakisaka S, Imaizumi T. Endothelial injuries of coronary arteries distal to thrombotic sites: role of adhesive interaction between endothelial P-selectin and leukocyte sialyl LewisX. Circ Res 1999;84:525–535.

49. Mutin M, Canavy I, Blann A, Bory M, Sampol J, Dignat-George F. Direct evidence of endothelial injury in acute myocardial infarction and unstable angina by demonstration of circulating endothelial cells. Blood 1999;93:2951–2958.

50. Combes V, Simon AC, Grau GE, Arnoux D, Camoin L, Sabatier F, Mutin M, Sanmarco M, Sampol J, Dignat-George F. In vitro generation of endothelial microparticles and possible prothrombotic activity in patients with lupus anticoagulant. J Clin Invest 1999;104:93–102.

51. Henn V, Slupsky JR, Grafe M, Anagnostopoulos I, Forster R, Muller-Berghaus G, Kroczek RA. CD40 ligand on activated platelets triggers an inflammatory reaction of endothelial cells. Nature 1998;391:591–594.

52. Aukrust P, Muller F, Ueland T, Berget T, Aaser E, Brunsvig A, Solum NO, Forfang K, Froland SS, Gullestad L. Enhanced levels of soluble and membrane-bound CD40 ligand in patients with unstable angina : possible reflection of T lymphocyte and platelet involvement in the pathogenesis of acute coronary syndromes. Circulation 1999;100:614–620.

53. Hermann A, Weber AA, Schror K. Clopidogrel inhibits platelet adhesion and platelet-dependent mitogenesis in vascular smooth muscle cells. Thromb Res 2002;105:173–175.

54. Heeschen C, Dimmeler S, Hamm CW, van den Brand MJ, Boersma E, Zeiher AM, Simoons ML. Soluble CD40 ligand in acute coronary syndromes. N Engl J Med 2003;348:1104–1111.

55. Slupsky JR, Kalbas M, Willuweit A, Henn V, Kroczek RA, Muller-Berghaus G. Activated platelets induce tissue factor expression on human umbilical vein endothelial cells by ligation of CD40. Thromb Haemost 1998;80:1008–1014.

56. Ikeda H, Ueyama T, Murohara T, Yasukawa H, Haramaki N, Eguchi H, Katoh A, Takajo Y, Onitsuka I, Ueno T, Tojo SJ, Imaizumi T. Adhesive interaction between P-selectin and sialyl Lewis(x) plays an important role in recurrent coronary arterial thrombosis in dogs. Arterioscler Thromb Vasc Biol 1999;19:1083–1090.

57. Lefer AM, Campbell B, Scalia R, Lefer DJ. Synergism between platelets and neutrophils in provoking cardiac dysfunction after ischemia and reperfusion: role of selectins. Circulation 1998;98:1322–1328.

58. Katopodis JN, Kolodny L, Jy W, Horstman LL, De Marchena EJ, Tao JG, Haynes DH, Ahn YS. Platelet microparticles and calcium homeostasis in acute coronary ischemias. Am J Hematol 1997;54:95–101.

59. Neumann FJ, Marx N, Gawaz M, Brand K, Ott I, Rokitta C, Sticherling C, Meinl C, May A, Schomig A. Induction of cytokine expression in leukocytes by binding of thrombin-stimulated platelets. Circulation 1997;95:2387–2394.

60. Bhatt DL, Topol EJ. Scientific and therapeutic advances in antiplatelet therapy. Nat Rev Drug Discov 2003;2:15–28.

61. Simon DI, Xu H, Ortlepp S, Rogers C, Rao NK. 7E3 monoclonal antibody directed against the platelet GPIIb/IIIa cross-reacts with the leukocyte integrin Mac-1 and blocks adhesion to fibrinogen and ICAM-1. Arterioscler Thromb Vasc Biol 1997;17:528–535.

62. Reverter JC, Beguin S, Kessels H, Kumar R, Hemker HC, Coller BS. Inhibition of platelet-mediated, tissue factor-induced thrombin generation by the mouse/human chimeric 7E3 antibody. Potential implications for the effect of c7E3 Fab treatment on acute thrombosis and ''clinical restenosis''. J Clin Invest 1996;98:863–874.

63. Coleman KR, Braden GA, Willingham MC, Sane DC. Vitaxin, a Humanized Monoclonal Antibody to the Vitronectin Receptor, Reduces Neointimal Hyperplasia and Total Vessel Area After Balloon Injury in Hypercholesterolemic Rabbits. Circ Res 1999;84:1268–1276.

64. Gawaz M, Neumann FJ, Dickfeld T, Reininger A, Adelsberger H, Gebhardt A, Schomig A. Vitronectin receptor (alpha(v)beta3) mediates platelet adhesion to the luminal aspect of endothelial cells: implications for reperfusion in acute myocardial infarction. Circulation 1997;96:1809–1818.

65. Lincoff AM, Kereiakes DJ, Mascelli MA, Deckelbaum LI, Barnathan ES, Patel KK, Frederick B, Nakada MT, Topol EJ. Abciximab suppresses the rise in levels of circulating inflammatory markers after percutaneous coronary revascularization. Circulation 2001;104:163–167.

66. Lenderink T, Boersma E, Heeschen C, Vahanian A, de Boer MJ, Umans V, van den Brand MJ, Hamm CW, Simoons ML. Elevated troponin T and C-reactive protein predict impaired outcome for 4 years in patients with refractory unstable angina, and troponin T predicts benefit of treatment with abciximab in combination with PTCA. Eur Heart J 2003;24:77–85.

67. Aronow HD, Shishehor MH, Davis DA, et al. White blood cell count predicts microembolic Doppler signals during carotid stenting: a link between inflammation and embolization. Circulation 2002;106:2–577.

68. Willerson JT, Golino P, Eidt J, Campbell WB, Buja LM. Specific platelet mediators and unstable coronary artery lesions. Experimental evidence and potential clinical implications. Circulation 1989;80:198–205.

69. Eidt JF, Ashton J, Golino P, McNatt J, Buja LM, Willerson JT. Thromboxane A2 and serotonin mediate coronary blood flow reductions in unsedated dogs. Am J Physiol 1989;257: H873–H882.

70. Yao SK, Ober JC, Krishnaswami A, Ferguson JJ, Anderson HV, Golino P, Buja LM, Willerson JT. Endogenous nitric oxide protects against platelet aggregation and cyclic flow variations in stenosed and endothelium-injured arteries. Circulation 1992;86:1302–1309.

71. Eidt JF, Allison P, Noble S, Ashton J, Golino P, McNatt J, Buja LM, Willerson JT. Thrombin is an important mediator of platelet aggregation in stenosed canine coronary arteries with endothelial injury. J Clin Invest 1989;84:18–27.

72. Yao SK, Ober JC, McNatt J, Benedict CR, Rosolowsky M, Anderson HV, Cui K, Maffrand JP, Campbell WB, Buja LM, et al. ADP plays an important role in mediating platelet aggregation and cyclic flow variations in vivo in stenosed and endothelium-injured canine coronary arteries. Circ Res 1992;70:39–48.

73. Wilson RF, Laxson DD, Lesser JR, White CW. Intense microvascular constriction after angioplasty of acute thrombotic coronary arterial lesions. Lancet 1989;1:807–811.

74. Hirsh PD, Hillis LD, Campbell WB, Firth BG, Willerson JT. Release of prostaglandins and thromboxane into the coronary circulation in patients with ischemic heart disease. N Engl J Med 1981;304:685–691.

75. Ostrovsky L, King AJ, Bond S, Mitchell D, Lorant DE, Zimmerman GA, Larsen R, Niu XF, Kubes P. A juxtacrine mechanism for neutrophil adhesion on platelets involves platelet-activating factor and a selectin-dependent activation process. Blood 1998;91:3028–3036.

76. Huang Q, Wu M, Meininger C, Kelly K, Yuan Y. Neutrophil-dependent augmentation of PAF-induced vasoconstriction and albumin flux in coronary arterioles. Am J Physiol 1998; 275:H1138–H1147.

77. Moliterno DJ. Anticoagulants and their use in acute coronary syndromes. In: Topol EJ, Ed. Textbook of Interventional Cardiology. 3rd ed.. Philadelphia: W.B. Saunders Company, 1999: 25–51.

78. Taniyama Y, Ito H, Iwakura K, Masuyama T, Hori M, Takiuchi S, Nishikawa N, Higashino Y, Fujii K, Minamino T. Beneficial effect of intracoronary verapamil on microvascular and myocardial salvage in patients with acute myocardial infarction. J Am Coll Cardiol 1997; 30:1193–1199.

79. Ito H, Taniyama Y, Iwakura K, Nishikawa N, Masuyama T, Kuzuya T, Hori M, Higashino Y, Fujii K, Minamino T. Intravenous nicorandil can preserve microvascular integrity and myocardial viability in patients with reperfused anterior wall myocardial infarction. J Am Coll Cardiol 1999;33:654–660.

80. Gibson CM, Cannon CP, Daley WL, Dodge JT, Alexander B, Marble SJ, McCabe CH, Raymond L, Fortin T, Poole WK, Braunwald E. TIMI frame count: a quantitative method of assessing coronary artery flow. Circulation 1996;93:879–888.

81. Gibson CM, Ryan KA, Murphy SA, Mesley R, Marble SJ, Giugliano RP, Cannon CP, Antman EM, Braunwald E. Impaired coronary blood flow in nonculprit arteries in the setting of acute myocardial infarction. The TIMI Study Group. Thrombolysis in myocardial infarction. J Am Coll Cardiol 1999;34:974–982.

82. Gowda MS, Vacek JL, Hallas D. One-year outcomes of diabetic versus nondiabetic patients with non-Q-wave acute myocardial infarction treated with percutaneous transluminal coronary angioplasty. Am J Cardiol 1998;81:1067–1071.

83. Aronson D, Rayfield EJ, Chesebro JH. Mechanisms determining course and outcome of diabetic patients who have had acute myocardial infarction. Ann Intern Med 1997;126: 296–306.

84. Barsness GW, Peterson ED, Ohman EM, Nelson CL, DeLong ER, Reves JG, Smith PK, Anderson RD, Jones RH, Mark DB, Califf RM. Relationship between diabetes mellitus and long-term survival after coronary bypass and angioplasty. Circulation 1997;96:2551–2556.

85. Mak KH, Moliterno DJ, Granger CB, Miller DP, White HD, Wilcox RG, Califf RM, Topol EJ. Influence of diabetes mellitus on clinical outcome in the thrombolytic era of acute myocardial infarction. GUSTO-I Investigators. Global Utilization of Streptokinase and Tissue Plasminogen Activator for Occluded Coronary Arteries. J Am Coll Cardiol 1997;30:171–179.

86. Gu K, Cowie CC, Harris MI. Diabetes and decline in heart disease mortality in US adults. JAMA 1999;281:1291–1297.

87. Tschoepe D, Roesen P. Heart disease in diabetes mellitus: a challenge for early diagnosis and intervention. Exp Clin Endocrinol Diabetes 1998;106:16–24.

88. Knobler H, Savion N, Shenkman B, Kotev-Emeth S, Varon D. Shear-induced platelet adhesion and aggregation on subendothelium are increased in diabetic patients. Thromb Res 1998;90: 181–190.

89. Iwase E, Tawata M, Aida K, Ozaki Y, Kume S, Satoh K, Qi R, Onaya T. A cross-sectional evaluation of spontaneous platelet aggregation in relation to complications in patients with type II diabetes mellitus. Metabolism 1998;47:699–705.

90. Tschoepe D, Driesch E, Schwippert B, Lampeter EF. Activated platelets in subjects at increased risk of IDDM. DENIS Study Group. Deutsche Nikotinamid Interventionsstudie. Diabetologia 1997;40:573–577.

91. Silva JA, Escobar A, Collins TJ, Ramee SR, White CJ. Unstable angina. A comparison of angioscopic findings between diabetic and nondiabetic patients. Circulation 1995;92: 1731–1736.

92. Akasaka T, Yoshida K, Hozumi T, Takagi T, Kaji S, Kawamoto T, Morioka S, Yoshikawa J. Retinopathy identifies marked restriction of coronary flow reserve in patients with diabetes mellitus. J Am Coll Cardiol 1997;30:935–941.

93. Yokayama I, Momomura SI, Ohtake T, Yonekura K, Nishikawa J, Sasaki YMO. Reduced Myocardial Flow Reserve in Non-Insulin Dependent Diabetes Mellitus. J Am Coll Cardiol 1997;30:1472–1477.

94. Tschoepe D, Rauch U, Schwippert B. Platelet-leukocyte-cross-talk in diabetes mellitus. Horm Metab Res 1997;29:631–635.

95. Bhatt DL, Marso SP, Lincoff AM, Wolski KE, Ellis SG, Topol EJ. Abciximab reduces mortality in diabetics following percutaneous coronary intervention. J Am Coll Cardiol 2000; 35:922–928.

96. Antman EM, Grudzien C, Sacks DB. Evaluation of a rapid bedside assay for detection of serum cardiac troponin T. JAMA 1995;273:1279–1282.

97. Antman EM, Tanasijevic MJ, Thompson B, Schactman M, McCabe CH, Cannon CP, Fischer GA, Fung AY, Thompson C, Wybenga D, Braunwald E. Cardiac-specific troponin I levels to predict the risk of mortality in patients with acute coronary syndromes. N Engl J Med 1996;335:1342–1349.

98. Hamm CW, Goldmann BU, Heeschen C, Kreymann G, Berger J, Meinertz T. Emergency room triage of patients with acute chest pain by means of rapid testing for cardiac troponin T or troponin I. N Engl J Med 1997;337:1648–1653.

99. Newby LK, Christenson RH, Ohman EM, Armstrong PW, Thompson TD, Lee KL, Hamm CW, Katus HA, Cianciolo C, Granger CB, Topol EJ, Califf RM. Value of serial troponin T measures for early and late risk stratification in patients with acute coronary syndromes. The GUSTO-IIa Investigators. Circulation 1998;98:1853–1859.

100. Hamm CW, Heeschen C, Goldmann B, Vahanian A, Adgey J, Miguel CM, Rutsch W, Berger J, Kootstra J, Simoons ML. Benefit of abciximab in patients with refractory unstable angina in relation to serum troponin T levels. c7E3 Fab Antiplatelet Therapy in Unstable Refractory Angina (CAPTURE) Study Investigators. N Engl J Med 1999;340:1623–1629.

101. Heeschen C, van Den Brand MJ, Hamm CW, Simoons ML. Angiographic findings in patients with refractory unstable angina according to troponin T status. Circulation 1999;100: 1509–1514.

102. Hamm CW, Heeschen C, Goldmann BU, White HD. Benefit of Tirofiban in High-Risk Patients with Unstable Angina Identified by Troponins in the PRISM Trial. Circulation 1999; 100:1–775.

103. Heeschen C, Hamm CW, Goldmann B, Deu A, Langenbrink L, White HD. Troponin concentrations for stratification of patients with acute coronary syndromes in relation to therapeutic efficacy of tirofiban. PRISM Study Investigators. Platelet Receptor Inhibition in Ischemic Syndrome Management. Lancet 1999;354:1757–1762.

104.  Lindahl B, Toss H, Siegbahn A, Venge P, Wallentin L. Long-term mortality in unstable coronary artery disease in relation to markers of myocardial damage and inflammation. Circulation 1999;100:1–372.

105.  Lindahl B, Diderholm E, Kontny F, Lagerqvist B, Husted S, Stahle E, Swahn E, Wallentin L. Long term treatment with low molecular weight heparin (dalteparin) reduces cardiac events in unstable coronary artery disease with troponin-T elevation: A FRISCII substudy. Circulation 1999;100:1–498.

106.  Ito H, Okamura A, Iwakura K, Masuyama T, Hori M, Takiuchi S, Negoro S, Nakatsuchi Y, Taniyama Y, Higashino Y, Fujii K, Minamino T. Myocardial perfusion patterns related to thrombolysis in myocardial infarction perfusion grades after coronary angioplasty in patients with acute anterior wall myocardial infarction. Circulation 1996;93:1993–1999.

107.  Ito H, Maruyama A, Iwakura K, Takiuchi S, Masuyama T, Hori M, Higashino Y, Fujii K, Minamino T. Clinical implications of the 'no reflow' phenomenon. A predictor of complications and left ventricular remodeling in reperfused anterior wall myocardial infarction. Circulation 1996;93:223–228.

108.  Porter TR, Li S, Oster R, Deligonul U. The clinical implications of no reflow demonstrated with intravenous perfluorocarbon containing microbubbles following restoration of Thrombolysis In Myocardial Infarction (TIMI) 3 flow in patients with acute myocardial infarction. Am J Cardiol 1998;82:1173–1177.

109.  Sakuma T, Hayashi Y, Sumii K, Imazu M, Yamakido M. Prediction of short- and intermediate-term prognoses of patients with acute myocardial infarction using myocardial contrast echocardiography one day after recanalization. J Am Coll Cardiol 1998;32:890–897.

110.  Wu KC, Kim RJ, Bluemke DA, Rochitte CE, Zerhouni EA, Becker LC, Lima JA. Quantification and time course of microvascular obstruction by contrast- enhanced echocardiography and magnetic resonance imaging following acute myocardial infarction and reperfusion. J Am Coll Cardiol 1998;32:1756–1764.

111.  Rochitte CE, Lima JA, Bluemke DA, Reeder SB, McVeigh ER, Furuta T, Becker LC, Melin JA. Magnitude and time course of microvascular obstruction and tissue injury after acute myocardial infarction. Circulation 1998;98:1006–1014.

112.  Wu KC, Zerhouni EA, Judd RM, Lugo-Olivieri CH, Barouch LA, Schulman SP, Blumenthal RS, Lima JA. Prognostic significance of microvascular obstruction by magnetic resonance imaging in patients with acute myocardial infarction. Circulation 1998;97:765–772.

113.  Fernandez AR, Sequeira RF, Chakko S, Correa LF, de Marchena EJ, Chahine RA, Franceour DA, Myerburg RJ. ST segment tracking for rapid determination of patency of the infarct-related artery in acute myocardial infarction. J Am Coll Cardiol 1995;26:675–683.

114.  Schroder R, Dissmann R, Bruggemann T, Wegscheider K, Linderer T, Tebbe U, Neuhaus KL. Extent of early ST segment elevation resolution: a simple but strong predictor of outcome in patients with acute myocardial infarction. J Am Coll Cardiol 1994;24:384–391.

115.  Schroder R, Wegscheider K, Schroder K, Dissmann R, Meyer-Sabellek W. Extent of early ST segment elevation resolution: a strong predictor of outcome in patients with acute myocardial infarction and a sensitive measure to compare thrombolytic regimens. A substudy of the International Joint Efficacy Comparison of Thrombolytics (INJECT) trial. J Am Coll Cardiol 1995;26:1657–1664.

116.  Dissmann R, Schroder R, Busse U, Appel M, Bruggemann T, Jereczek M, Linderer T. Early assessment of outcome by ST-segment analysis after thrombolytic therapy in acute myocardial infarction. Am Heart J 1994;128:851–857.

117.  Krucoff MW, Croll MA, Pope JE, Granger CB, O'Connor CM, Sigmon KN, Wagner BL, Ryan JA, Lee KL, Kereiakes DJ, et al. Continuous 12-lead ST-segment recovery analysis in the TAMI 7 study. Performance of a noninvasive method for real-time detection of failed myocardial reperfusion. Circulation 1993;88:437–446.

118.  Krucoff MW, Croll MA, Pope JE, Pieper KS, Kanani PM, Granger CB, Veldkamp RF, Wagner BL, Sawchak ST, Califf RM. Continuously updated 12-lead ST-segment recovery analysis for myocardial infarct artery patency assessment and its correlation with multiple simultaneous early angiographic observations. Am J Cardiol 1993;71:145–151.

119. Langer A, Krucoff MW, Klootwijk P, Veldkamp R, Simoons ML, Granger C, Califf RM, Armstrong PW. Noninvasive assessment of speed and stability of infarct-related artery reperfusion: results of the GUSTO ST segment monitoring study. Global Utilization of Streptokinase and Tissue Plasminogen Activator for Occluded Coronary Arteries. J Am Coll Cardiol 1995;25:1552–1557.
120. Veldkamp RF, Green CL, Wilkins ML, Pope JE, Sawchak ST, Ryan JA, Califf RM, Wagner GS, Krucoff MW. Comparison of continuous ST-segment recovery analysis with methods using static electrocardiograms for noninvasive patency assessment during acute myocardial infarction. Thrombolysis and Angioplasty in Myocardial Infarction (TAMI) 7 Study Group. Am J Cardiol 1994;73:1069–1074.
121. Santoro GM, Valenti R, Buonamici P, Bolognese L, Cerisano G, Moschi G, Trapani M, Antoniucci D, Fazzini PF. Relation between ST-segment changes and myocardial perfusion evaluated by myocardial contrast echocardiography in patients with acute myocardial infarction treated with direct angioplasty. Am J Cardiol 1998;82:932–937.
122. van 't Hof AW, Liem A, de Boer MJ, Zijlstra F. Clinical value of 12-lead electrocardiogram after successful reperfusion therapy for acute myocardial infarction. Zwolle Myocardial Infarction Study Group. Lancet 1997;350:615–619.
123. de Lemos JA, Antman EM, Gibson M, McCabe CH, Giugliano RP, Murphy SA, Frey MJ, Van der Wieken R, Van de Werf F, Braunwald E. Abciximab improves both epicardial flow and myocardial reperfusion in ST elevation myocardial infarction: A TIMI 14 analysis. Circulation 1999;100:1–649.
124. Neumann FJ, Blasini R, Schmitt C, Alt E, Dirschinger J, Gawaz M, Kastrati A, Schomig A. Effect of GPIIb/IIIa receptor blockade on recovery of coronary flow and left ventricular function after the placement of coronary-artery stents in acute myocardial infarction. Circulation 1998;98:2695–2701.
125. Agati L, Voci P, Hickle P, Vizza DC, Autore C, Fedele F, Feinstein SB, Dagianti A. Tissue-type plasminogen activator therapy versus primary coronary angioplasty: impact on myocardial tissue perfusion and regional function 1 month after uncomplicated myocardial infarction. J Am Coll Cardiol 1998;31:338–343.
126. Assmus B, Schachinger V, Teupe C, Britten M, Lehmann R, Dobert N, Grunwald F, Aicher A, Urbich C, Martin H, Hoelzer D, Dimmeler S, Zeiher AM. Transplantation of Progenitor Cells and Regeneration Enhancement in Acute Myocardial Infarction (TOPCARE-AMI). Circulation 2002;106:3009–3017.
127. Britten MB, Abolmaali ND, Assmus B, Lehmann R, Honold J, Schmitt J, Vogl TJ, Martin H, Schachinger V, Dimmeler S, Zeiher AM. Infarct remodeling after intracoronary progenitor cell treatment in patients with acute myocardial infarction (TOPCARE-AMI): mechanistic insights from serial contrast-enhanced magnetic resonance imaging. Circulation 2003;108:2212–2218.

# 5

# Plaque Vulnerability (Insights from Intravascular Ultrasound, Optical Coherence Tomography, and Thermography)

**Samir R. Kapadia, Murat E. Tuzcu, and Steven E. Nissen**
*The Cleveland Clinic Foundation*
*Cleveland, Ohio, U.S.A.*

## INTRODUCTION

In recent years, many potential methods for determining the likelihood for disruption of a coronary atherosclerotic plaque have emerged. The promising diagnostic tools include imaging techniques that characterize plaque morphology and composition, as well as other techniques that focus on quantifying plaque inflammation to identify vulnerable plaques [1]. Imaging techniques are based on ultrasounds, light (infrared or X-rays), or magnetic resonance. Thermography and the biochemical markers can detect inflammation. This chapter will focus on the development of intravascular ultrasound based imaging techniques, optical coherence tomography and thermography in detecting vulnerable plaques.

## VULNERABLE PLAQUE

When a patient presents with acute coronary syndrome (ACS), the atherosclerotic plaque responsible for the event is defined as a culprit plaque. In other words, a culprit plaque or lesion in the coronary artery is a retrospective diagnosis. Several studies have attempted to characterize culprit plaques from victims of sudden cardiac death. The histopathology of these lesions is summarized in Table 1 [2,3].

The concept of ''vulnerable plaque'' is to prospectively identify a rupture prone plaque. Therefore, the term should be carefully employed when a study is prospectively designed to identify plaque that will become a culprit plaque in the near future. The precise histological characteristics of vulnerable plaques are not known. One attempt to define major and minor criteria for the diagnosis of a vulnerable plaque is presented in Table 2 [2,3]. Since the plaque characteristics are dynamic and the risk of thrombosis is a continuum, the precise distinction of a stable from unstable plaque is difficult. Further, it is important to note that many ruptured plaques do not necessarily lead to clinical symptoms

**Table 1**  Underlying Pathologies of "Culprit" Coronary Lesions

Ruptured plaques (70%)
   Stenotic (20%)
   Nonstenotic (50%)
Nonruptured plaques (30%)
   Erosion
   Calcified nodule
   Others/Unknown

but may only lead to asymptomatic progression of a lesion. This adds to the complexity in defining a vulnerable plaque because a vulnerable plaque may not present a culprit lesion for ACS but may progress to a more stenotic lesion that may or may not become symptomatic.

## IMAGING TECHNIQUES: PRINCIPLES AND EQUIPMENT

### Ultrasound Imaging

*"Standard" Intravascular Ultrasound Imaging*

Unlike conventional angiographic imaging, which generates shadows based on the atomic density of the tissues, ultrasound images are based on reflections from interfaces between tissues having different acoustic properties. Therefore, the strength and signal quality of the ultrasound beam returning to the transducer (backscatter) determines whether the ultrasound scanner visualizes a particular structure. The acoustic impedance of tissue determines the amplitude of the backscatter and the intensity of image. Acoustic properties of the tissues are determined by specific gravity, compressibility, and viscosity. Of these, the first two are of greatest importance in clinical imaging, and most of the differences in soft tissue are probably due to differences in specific gravity. In normal coronary arteries,

**Table 2**  Criteria for Defining Vulnerable Plaque, Based on the Study of Culprit Plaques

**Major criteria**
   Active inflammation (monocyte/macrophage and sometimes T-cell infiltration)
   Thin cap with large lipid core
   Endothelial denudation with superficial platelet aggregation
   Fissured plaque
   Stenosis 90%
**Minor criteria**
   Superficial calcified nodule
   Glistening yellow
   Intraplaque hemorrhage
   Endothelial dysfunction
   Outward (positive) remodeling

collagen creates the strongest backscatter of the signal; thus, adventitia, with its high collagen content, strongly reflects ultrasound. On the other hand, the media of coronary arteries consists predominantly of smooth muscle cells and very little collagen; thus, this layer reflects little of the ultrasound signal. The inner elastic membrane reflects ultrasound well due to its dense elastic tissue. The blood within the vessel lumen exhibits a characteristic pattern in intravascular ultrasound (IVUS) examinations. At frequencies greater than 25 MHz, the lumen is characterized by blood flow seen as subtle, finely textured echoes moving in a characteristic swirling pattern. In many clinical situations, the presence of blood ''speckle'' can assist image interpretation by confirming communication between dissection planes and the lumen. The pattern of blood speckle is dependent upon the velocity of flow, exhibiting increased intensity and a more coarse texture when flow is reduced. This latter property can represent a confounding variable if examination is performed during a slow flow condition because the increased echogenicity of blood may interfere with delineation of the blood tissue interface. Increasing the frequency of the ultrasound to greater than 40 MHz also increases blood contrast dramatically due to Rayleigh scattering [4].

In a normal coronary artery, the discrete echodense layer at the lumen–wall interface is caused by the reflections of the internal elastic lamina, which is often referred to as intima. The tunica media is visualized as a distinct subintimal sonolucent layer, which is limited by an outer echodense media–adventitia interface. The outer or trailing edge of the adventitia is indistinct, as it merges into the surrounding perivascular connective tissue. The echodense intima and adventitia with the sonolucent medial layer in between give the arterial wall a trilaminar appearance. In the younger population, the internal elastic membrane is not dense enough to reflect ultrasound signal giving a typical monolayer appearance [5] (Figure 1).

The equipment required to perform intracoronary ultrasound consists of two major components, a catheter incorporating a miniaturized transducer and a console containing the electronics necessary to reconstruct the image. Since the transducer is placed in close proximity to the vessel wall, high ultrasound frequencies (30–50 MHz) can be employed for high-resolution coronary imaging. At 30 MHz, the wavelength is approximately 50 $\mu$m, which permits axial resolution of approximately 100 $\mu$m. Determinants of lateral resolution are more complicated and dependent on imaging depth and beam shape. Typically, lateral resolution for a 30 MHz device will average approximately 250 $\mu$m at typical distances in coronary imaging [6]. Two different transducer designs have emerged— mechanically rotated devices and multielement electronic arrays. Although, initially, the mechanically rotated catheters tended to have better images, especially in the near field, artifacts are more likely with this type of catheter. However, the difference in image quality has diminished significantly with recent advances. Both of these catheter systems are now commercially available in the United States.

IVUS imaging has provided insights into the severity of lesions, remodeling of the vessels and, to some extent, the morphology of the lesions responsible for ACS. The tissue characterization has been improved using some improvisations of this ''standard'' technology.

*Virtual Histology*

Gray scale IVUS images are generated by incorporating intensity and timing of the reflected ultrasound. Although videodensitometric analysis is the most straightforward technique for quantifying IVUS data, these data are at the end of a long processing chain, including many nonlinear stages. The purpose of such transformations is to provide a

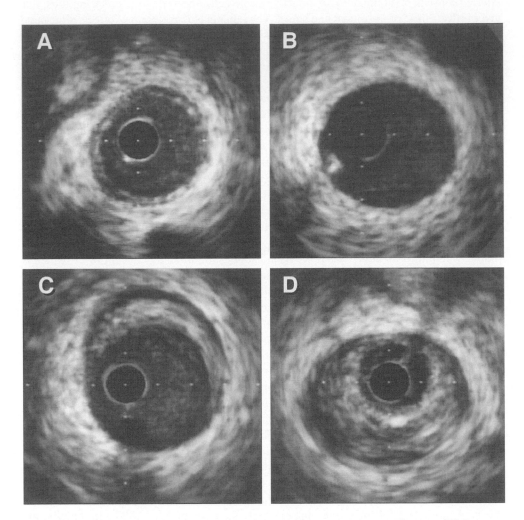

**Figure 1** Intravascular ultrasound images from stable coronary artery disease. (**A**) Appearance of a coronary artery with minimal intimal thickening. In the center of the lumen is the intravascular ultrasound catheter. Lumen of the artery shows blood speckles, which are more apparent on the real-time images. The lumen is separated from the sonolucent media by the minimally thickened intima. The media is separated from adventitia by the external elastic lamina (EEM). Adventitia merges with the surrounding connective tissue without clear demarcation. The scale superimposed on the image represents 1 mm between each marker. Intimal thickness is measured from lumen to EEM and therefore includes the media. The area subtended by the EEM is also referred to as the vessel area. Lumen area plus intimal area equals the vessel area. (**B**) In the younger population, the internal elastic membrane does not reflect ultrasound signal and therefore is not visualized. This gives a typical monolayer appearance with lumen area equal to EEM area. (**C**) A typical eccentric, noncircumferential plaque. (**D**) A typical advanced atherosclerotic plaque with 2 × 2-mm residual lumen.

pleasing image on the screen. The problem with using such data for tissue structure analysis is that their relation with the original acoustic signal is highly distorted and can even be altered by display controls such as brightness and gain. The spectral analysis of the backscatter signal prior to processing provides significantly more information regarding the tissue structure.

Various different parameters can be used to characterize backscatter information. Integrated backscatter is one of the commonly used parameters. Integrated backscatter is calculated by integrating the power spectrum of the received signal over the meaningful bandwidth of the transducer. Therefore, it is a measure of the mean reflected ultrasonic energy from a particular region of tissue [7].

Extensive clinical evaluation of the properties of integrated backscatter has demonstrated that changes in its magnitude, cycle dependent variation, and timing of peak and trough levels can all be influenced by a variety of disease processes [8,9]. However, due to the lack of standardization in the acquisition and processing of the raw radio frequency (RF) data sets, it is hard to compare results from different studies. One such protocol using multiple different characteristics of the backscatter including the integrated backscatter has advanced to clinical testing [10,11]. In this protocol, average spectrum from region of interest was identified and a normalized spectrum is calculated using a spectrum from

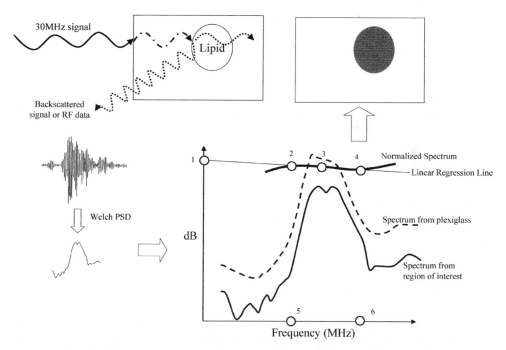

**Figure 2** Schematic representation of methodology for virtual histology. The backscatter from the plaque is processed with Welch Power Spectral Density (PSD) to derive averaged spectrum from region of interest. Averaged spectrum from region of interest (*solid line*) is normalized using spectrum from plexiglass (*dotted line*) as baseline. Parameters are identified from the normalized spectrum and then used to compute classification tree for plaque characterization. There are, (a) Y intercept; (b) maximum power; (c) mid-band fit; (d) minimum power; (e) and (f) frequencies at maximum and minimum powers. The other two parameters used but not shown in this figure were slope of regression line and integrated backscatter.

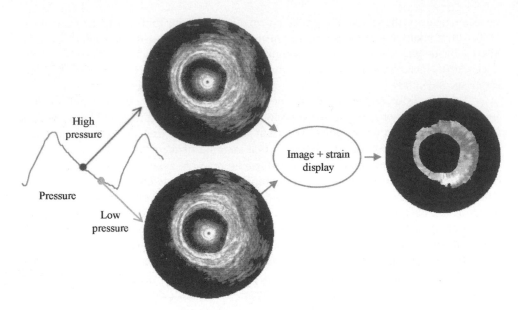

**Figure 3**  Principle of intravascular elastography. The intravascular ultrasound (IVUS) image is acquired at high and low intraluminal pressure. Radial strain in the tissue is determined by cross-correlation of IVUS image with pressure data. The data are then displayed on gray scale (or color) in the same orientation as an IVUS image.

imaging plexiglass (Figure 2). A database of parameters was then generated using accurate matching with the histology information. Once the system was trained, it was tested in human ex vivo coronary arteries with good success. This methodology accurately identified plaque content by classifying them in fibrous, fibrolipid, calcium, and calcified necrosis. The data can be displayed as an IVUS image, with specific color-coding for different tissues.

## Intravascular Elastography

Elastography is an imaging technique based on tissue deformation [12]. The rate of deformation (strain) of the tissue is directly related to the mechanical properties. In the blood vessel, the change in the lumen is determined using IVUS, and continuous blood pressure measurements are made using a guide catheter connected to a transducer. Using this information, the elastogram (image of the radial strain) is plotted complementary to the IVUS image. Since the acting force is applied on the lumen boundaries, a surface based assessment of the mechanical properties has been developed and is called palpography. This technique assesses the local mechanical properties of tissue using its deformation caused by the intraluminal pressure (Figure 3).

## OPTICAL COHERENCE TOMOGRAPHY

Optical Coherence Tomography (OCT) is analogous to ultrasound imaging, except that infrared light waves are used rather than acoustic waves [13]. An optical beam is focused into the tissue, and the echo time delay of light reflected from internal microstructure at different depths is measured by interferometry. In ultrasound, the time the ultrasound pulse takes to travel to a surface and be reflected back can be measured by an electronic clock. However, this is not possible with optical techniques because of the high speed of light. This limitation is overcome with the use of a reference light path and interferometry. Light is generated from either an infrared low-coherence diode (similar to compact disc players) or a femtosecond laser source. The beam is split evenly, half to the sample and half to a reference mirror. The reflected light intensity from structures within the tissue is measured by recombining its signal with that returning from the moving reference mirror (the distance to which is accurately known). Interference occurs only when the two paths are matched within the coherence length of the source, allowing micron scale ranging.

Image information is obtained by performing repeated axial measurements at different transverse positions as the optical beam is scanned across the tissue. The resulting data constitute a two-dimensional map of the backscattering or reflectance from internal architectural morphology and cellular structures in the tissue. This technique is commonly used in ophthalmology, where transparent tissues are interrogated. However, the application of OCT for intravascular imaging involves imaging of tissues that are nontransparent. Although vascular and other tissues strongly absorb visible wavelengths of light, most tissues are relatively nonabsorbent at infrared wavelengths. Thus, imaging depth is limited by light scattering rather than absorption. By performing OCT imaging at longer infrared wavelengths (1300 nm vs. 800 nm conventionally used in ophthalmic OCT), the imaging depth in vascular tissues can be increased to permit full thickness imaging of the vessel. The axial resolution of images achieved using OCT can be greater than 20 μm, which is much better than other available methods for imaging (Figure 4). Current limitations of OCT remain significant and are related predominantly to the features of a light-based energy source, including poor tissue penetration and interference from blood. The latter necessitates techniques similar to angioscopy that displace blood, such as saline injection

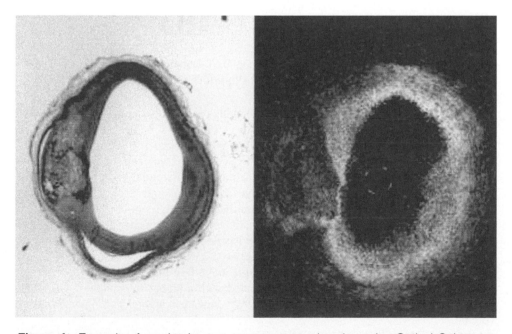

**Figure 4** Example of ex vivo human coronary artery imaging using Optical Coherence Tomography (OCT). Remarkable details of the plaque architecture can be appreciated with this imaging technique.

with or without a proximal occlusion balloon. These maneuvers limit prolonged image acquisition and preclude screening long arterial segments.

## THERMOGRAPHY

Inflammation of the atherosclerotic plaque has been increasingly implicated in the plaque rupture. The inflammatory reaction is manifested by the local invasion of macrophages and lymphocytes, and the deposition of matrix metalloproteinases that degrade the supporting collagen and promote plaque fragility. One of the hallmarks of inflammation is the increase in the temperature of the inflamed tissue. Various investigators have tried to measure temperature of atherosclerotic plaque in carotid and coronary arteries with a catheter-based thermistor with a temperature differentiation of 0.05°C and a spatial resolution of 0.5 mm [14]. It is possible that the blood flow in the vessel cools down the surface of the plaque and that accurate measurement of temperature may be a transient interruption of the blood flow.

## CLINICAL DATA IN ACUTE CORONARY SYNDROMES FROM VARIOUS IMAGING TECHNIQUES

### "Standard" Intravascular Ultrasound

The important clinical information derived from the standard IVUS interrogation can be divided into information on plaque morphology, lesion severity, and remodeling.

*Plaque Morphology*

Intravascular ultrasound studies have shown that, in patients with angiographically severe coronary disease, clinical symptoms correlate primarily with plaque characteristics rather than with the severity of stenosis [15,16]. Ruptured plaques identified by IVUS correlate with clinical presentation of ACS [16] (Figure 5 and 6). Ruptured plaques are characterized by an echolucent zone within a plaque, with a thin ulcerated fibrous cap (type I), or by deep ulceration in the plaque (type II).

Morphological characteristics of a "vulnerable plaque" on IVUS examination have not been prospectively tested. However, various studies have described morphology of culprit lesions in patients with unstable angina and compared it to the morphology of lesions in patients with stable angina. Kearney et al. reported the presence of a demarcated inner layer in unstable lesions, delimited by a fine circumferential line (Figure 7). This pattern was noted in 77% (14 out of 18) of unstable lesions and in 7% (1 out of 15) of stable lesions.[17] Rasheed et al. performed a multivariate analysis to identify independent predictors of plaque morphology and found stable angina, age greater than 60 years, and location of a lesion in distal segments to be independent predictors an echodense plaque [18]. Gyongyosi et al. studied the correlation between coronary atherosclerosis risk factors and plaque morphology in patients with unstable angina. In this study, hypercholesterolemia, smoking, and male gender were associated with a higher frequency of thrombus. Diabetes mellitus and hypercholesterolemia were independent predictors for greater plaque volume.[19]

Ge et al. identified ruptured plaques (Figure 8) with intravascular ultrasound examination and compared the characteristics of these plaques with those without evidence of rupture. The area of the emptied plaque cavity ($4.1 \pm 3.2$ mm$^2$) with rupture was larger

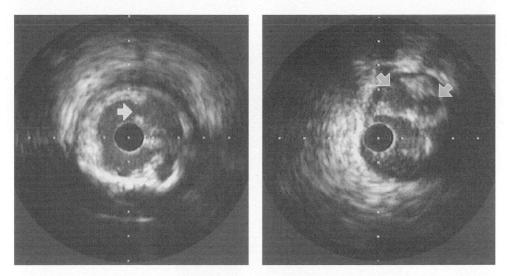

**Figure 5** In the image on the left plaque rupture is demonstrated (*arrow*) involving lateral aspect of the plaque. The irregular margins of the ulcerated fibrous cap are well visualized. The panel on the right shows the same artery just distal to the site seen in the left panel. Intraplaque dissection with "excavation" of the plaque core is seen (*arrows*). Contrast injection proved communication of this echolucent area with the lumen.

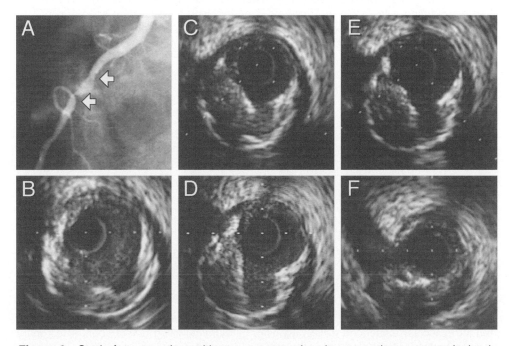

**Figure 6** Study from a patient with new onset angina demonstrating a severe lesion in the right coronary artery on angiography. Ultrasound revealed an extensive spontaneous plaque rupture with a large residual ulcer. Panels B through F indicate sequential ultrasound images obtained from the points indicated by the arrows. In panels B and F small defects in the fibrous cap are visible. In the images from the center of the plaque (**C**, **D**, **E**), a deep ulcer is evident.

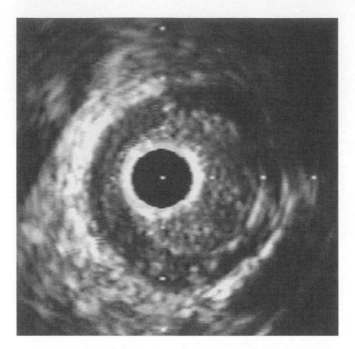

**Figure 7**   This IVUS image shows lumen filled with material that has echogenicity greater than surrounding plaque that, on real-time images, gives a scintillating appearance. The "line of demarcation" between this structure and atheromatous plaque is seen distinctly between 9 o'clock and 2 o'clock. This is consistent with thrombus as suggested by Kearney and her colleagues.

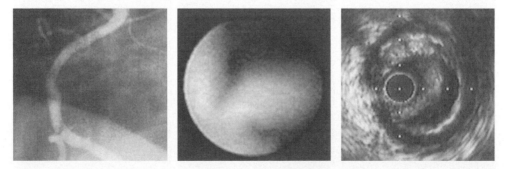

**Figure 8**   This is an example of acute plaque rupture seen with angiography, angioscopy, and intravascular ultrasound (IVUS) imaging. Intraluminal filling defect seen on coronary angiography could be interpreted as thrombus or ruptured plaque with dissection. The shape of the intraluminal structure on IVUS image helps to identify it as a ruptured plaque rather than a thrombus. This was verified to be the case as demonstrated by angioscopy in the middle panel.

than the echolucent zone in the plaques without rupture ($1.32 \pm 0.79$ mm$^2$; $p = 0.001$). The authors suggested that a lipid core greater than 1 mm$^2$ or a lipid core to plaque ratio greater than 20% and a fibrous cap thinner than 0.7 mm characterized a vulnerable plaque. This study also identified the site of plaque rupture and showed that shoulder region of the plaque is the most likely (55% in this study) site for rupture. Plaque erosion, where the underlying lipid core is not exposed to the lumen, is a recognized mechanism for ACS. However, in the study be Ge et al., only 10% of the plaques had superficial ulceration. This may be due to the limited resolution of current IVUS equipment.

Because thrombus formation is the hallmark of unstable lesion, attempts have been made to characterize thrombus with IVUS examination (Figure 9). Despite the high-frequency imaging provided by IVUS, it is still unreliable in differentiating acute thrombi from echolucent plaques, probably due to the similar echodensity of lipid and loose connective tissue within the plaque and stagnant blood forming the thrombus. In vitro comparison of ultrasound imaging to angioscopy revealed that it is less reliable for the diagnosis of thrombi. The sensitivity of ultrasound was low (57%), although the specificity remained high (91%), but both were lower than angioscopy (sensitivity and specificity of 100%) [20]. Several small observational studies attempted to define the IVUS appearance of a coronary thrombus. A thrombus was defined as low echogenic material within the lumen demonstrating slight synchronic pulsation and significantly different acoustic impedance at the interface between it and the more echogenic plaque [17,21,22]. Suspicion of thrombus according to ultrasound criteria was based on visualization of a structure with low signal intensity and very soft echoes, clearly separated from the adjacent vessel wall. Chemarin-Alibelli et al. studied ultrasound characteristics of thrombus in acute myocardial infarction (MI) patients undergoing directional atherectomy after thrombolytic therapy and confirmed the presence of thrombus with histology [23]. The sensitivity of IVUS detection of thrombus compared to histology was 84%, and specificity was 71%. All patients studied within

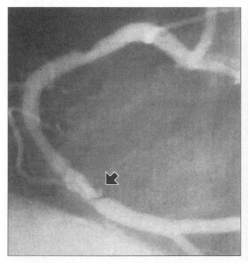 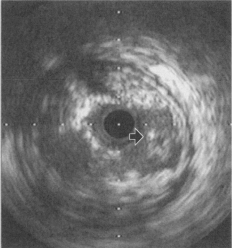

**Figure 9**   This angiogram and intravascular ultrasound (IVUS) images were obtained from patient presenting with acute inferior wall myocardial infarction (MI) after successful reperfusion with thrombolytic therapy. Angiogram suggests a flap-like intraluminal filling defect. IVUS imaging uncovers a complex ruptured plaque with irregular borders and evidence of thrombus (*arrow*) in the ulcer.

the first 5 days of acute MI (n = 12) had a thrombus protruding in the lumen that was characterized by bright, speckled, echogenic material that scintillated with movement. On the other hand, in patients undergoing IVUS examination after 5 days of acute MI (n = 18), echogenic thrombus protruding in the lumen was rarely found. The older thrombus was more difficult to identify, as the speckled appearance was replaced with a more echogenic linear pattern.

Bocksch et al. performed IVUS imaging in 50 patients with acute MI within 6 hours after the onset of chest pain before percutaneous coronary angioplasty [22]. Following angiographic documentation of a proximal occlusion, a 3.5 mechanical ultrasound catheter (30 MHz) was advanced successfully through the lesion in 42 of 50 patients (84%). Only 75 ± 22 seconds were added to the total time of procedure, which was 42 minutes. In 37 (88%) patients, ultrasound differentiated between a thrombus characterized by a pulsatile, low echogenic, intraluminal material with a negative imprint of the IVUS catheter and a highly echogenic atherosclerotic plaque. The plaque was eccentric in 32 (76%) patients with area stenosis of 48 ± 14%. Interestingly, contrary to other literature, the majority (76%) of the plaques were described as eccentric hard plaques with evidence of calcification in 83%.

Calcium is often considered a hallmark of "old" atherosclerotic lesions. Hodgson et al. found that patients with unstable angina had more soft echolucent regions and fewer calcified plaques than patients with stable angina [24]. De Servi et al. [25] suggested that ultrasound images consistent with focal calcification are actually common in plaques that cause ACS. In 43 patients with unstable angina, 54% had either mild or heavily calcific deposits at the suspected culprit lesion site. Interestingly, patients in the Braunwald class IB were more likely to have focal calcific deposits than patients in class II or IIIB, in whom soft, noncalcified lesions were most common. In a much larger series (n = 1442), the independent predictors of the arc of target lesion calcium included patient age, stable angina and lesion site, and reference segment plaque burden [26]. However, the vast majority of patients with ACS and at least moderate angiographic disease have identifiable coronary calcium by ultra-fast computed tomography (CT). Patients with no calcium are younger and tend to be active cigarette smokers [27]. In patients with ACS but no angiographically critical stenoses, the number of segments with calcified plaques increases linearly with an increase in number of diseased segments [28].

*Multifocal disease*

IVUS imaging studies in patients presenting with ACS have demonstrated lesions with characteristics of plaque rupture at multiple sites other than the culprit lesion [29–33]. Schoenhagen et al. reported from Controlled Abciximab and Device Investigation to Lower Late Angioplasty Complications (CADILLAC) trial that 19% of the patients with acute MI had evidence of plaque ulceration proximal to culprit lesion site [33]. This has also been observed in the histological studies [34]. The histologic studies also demonstrate that episodes of plaque rupture are frequent and only occasionally result in ACS [35].

*Culprit Lesion Severity*

Angiographic studies have demonstrated that the severity of coronary stenosis alone is inadequate to accurately predict the time or location of a subsequent coronary occlusion that will produce a myocardial infarction. Little and colleagues found that 66% of the patients had less than 50% maximal narrowing in the infarct vessel prior to infarction and that 17% had less than 50% stenosis, yet all had at least luminal irregularities [36]. Further, patients with uncomplicated stable angina have more severe and extensive atherosclerosis compared with those with unheralded acute MI, also underscoring the absence of correlation between angiographic severity of disease and clinical presentation. It has been postulated that progression of a lesion occurs with repeated plaque rupture and plaque stabilization cycles with few or no symptomatic episodes until the stenosis reaches a significant level [37–39]. This theory provides one explanation for greater severity of stenosis in patients with stable plaques compared with the stenosis in patients with unstable plaques. Ge et al. reported intravascular imaging data from 139 studies in 144 consecutive patients with angina [16]. Ruptured plaques, characterized by a plaque cavity and a tear on the thin fibrous cap, were identified in 31 patients. Culprit lesion stenosis in patients with evident plaque rupture (n = 31) was more than in patients without IVUS evidence of plaque rupture (n = 108) (56 ± 16% vs. 68 ± 13%; p = 0.001). Of note, the plaque area was not significantly different between the groups. Some other studies have reported a larger plaque burden in patients with unstable coronary artery disease compared to those with stable coronary syndrome. However, almost uniformly the area stenosis of ruptured plaques is less than the stable plaques [15,40]. These findings underscore the importance of remodeling in unstable atherosclerotic plaques (vide infra).

Infrequently, patients with ACS have angiographically normal coronary arteries. It has been hypothesized that the mechanism of acute MI in these patients is temporary occlusion of the infarct related vessel by spasm or thrombus or a combination of both. In these patients, IVUS examination may help to uncover the mechanism for MI. Mild disease with large thrombus, spontaneous dissection, posttraumatic dissections, and, at times, moderate or even severe disease can be unraveled by IVUS examination (Figure 10) [41–43].

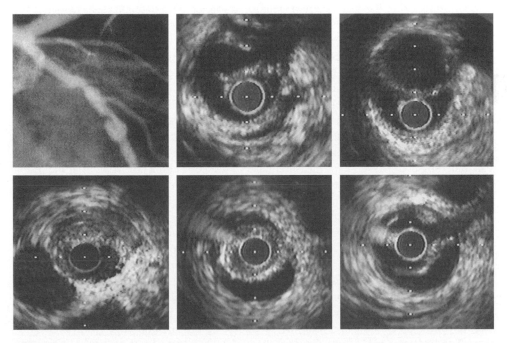

**Figure 10** Occasionally a focal plaque rupture extends longitudinally along the vessel and results in spontaneous dissection of the coronary artery. In this example, the angiogram displayed a complex series of "focal" lesions extending over a 30-mm length of the vessel. However, ultrasound revealed diffuse disease with extensive dissection involving approximately 40 mm of the vessel.

Myocardial bridging is usually asymptomatic, but has been associated with acute MI in patients in the absence of risk factors for coronary artery disease. Although a common postmortem finding, myocardial bridging is manifest in up to 5% of patients undergoing diagnostic angiography. As coronary arterial blood flow is primarily diastolic, the relevance of bridging in clinical practice has been debated. However, deep muscle bridges can twist the coronary artery and compromise diastolic blood flow, and this disturbance in flow at the site of the bridge might increase the propensity for intimal damage or platelet aggregation. De Winter et al. reported a case of recurrent acute MI caused by a soft atheromatous plaque within a myocardial bridge [44]. This plaque was invisible during coronary angiography and could only be imaged using IVUS. In symptomatic patients with myocardial bridging, IVUS examination may be useful to rule out a significant atherosclerotic lesion within the bridged segment. Myocardial bridging is characterized by a specific echolucent half moon phenomenon over the bridge segment, which exists throughout the cardiac cycle; systolic compression of the bridge segment; accelerated flow velocity in early diastole (fingertip phenomenon); no or reduced systolic antegrade flow; retrograde flow in the proximal segment, which is provoked and enhanced by nitroglycerin injection [45].

*Remodeling*

*Remodeling* refers to the changes in arterial dimensions associated with the development of disease. Initially, it was described as increase in arterial size that accommodates the deposition of atherosclerotic plaque material, frequently referred to as positive remodeling. In recent years, histopathologic and IVUS studies have demonstrated a new dimension to arterial remodeling, the negative remodeling, or arterial shrinkage. At diseased sites, the artery may actually shrink in size and contribute to, instead of compensate for, the degree of luminal stenosis.

Different methodologies have been utilized for investigating remodeling by IVUS. Positive correlation between the plaque area and external elastic lamina (EEM) area with no correlation between the plaque area and lumen area at the lesion site has been used as evidence for positive remodeling. This method helps to study the presence or absence of significant remodeling for a group lesions, but does not allow quantification of remodeling for each lesion. Further, the negative remodeling cannot be studied with this methodology. Remodeling ratio, a quantitative measure of extent and direction of remodeling, can be calculated by comparing IVUS measurements of the vessel area (EEM area) at the lesion site to the EEM area at the corresponding proximal and/or distal reference sites. Positive remodeling is typically defined as a remodeling ratio greater than 1.05, and negative remodeling as a remodeling ratio less than 0.95. A 5% difference in the lesion and reference site traditionally is considered insignificant and represents variability of measurement [46]. However, when this method is utilized for the quantification of remodeling, vessel tapering, obstruction of blood flow by IVUS catheter, and possible remodeling of the ''reference site'' can confound these measurements. Serial measurements of lumen, plaque, and vessel area at the lesion site can provide the most rigorous evidence for remodeling, but the logistics of this type of study and the practical difficulties in identifying the same exact site on follow-up examination limit the usefulness of this methodology [47].

Schoenhagen et al. studied culprit lesions in 76 patients with unstable angina and acute infarction and compared them to lesions in 40 patients presenting with stable angina. Positive and negative remodeling at the lesion sites were defined as remodeling ratio greater than 1.05 and less than 0.95, respectively. In the unstable patients, EEM area, plaque area, and remodeling ratio were significantly larger than the corresponding measurements in the stable patients. Positive remodeling was more prevalent in the unstable group (51% vs. 18%, p = 0.002) and negative remodeling was more prevalent in the stable group (58% vs. 33%, p = 0.002) [46]. Smits et al. reported identical results from a similarly designed study [48]. In another study, Gyongyosi et al. reported their data from 60 of 95 consecutively admitted patients with unstable angina where positive remodeling was more frequent compared to negative remodeling (37% vs. 23%). Patients with adaptive remodeling showed more thrombi and plaque disruption and larger plaque and vessel cross-sectional areas. Patients with constrictive remodeling were significantly older and had a higher angina score [49]. Nakamura et al. also reported more frequent positive remodeling of the culprit lesion in patients with ACS compared to patients with stable angina pectoris (74% vs. 37%) [50]. The extent of remodeling was also greater in patients with unstable symptoms (remodeling ratio of 1.13 ± 0.10 vs. 0.0.96 ± 0.13).

The direction and extent of remodeling also depends on the plaque composition and patient characteristics. Arc of calcium has been identified as an independent negative predictor of adequate remodeling, whereas hard plaques were defined as an independent predictor of negative remodeling [51–53]. Age has also been thought to play an important role in direction of remodeling in patients with unstable angina [19].

The relation of remodeling to unstable plaque may be pathophysiologically linked. Interestingly, histologic markers of plaque vulnerability have been correlated to positive remodeling in peripheral arteries [54]. In a study of 50 femoral arteries, 1521 sections were stained for the presence of macrophages (CD68), T-lymphocytes (CD45R), smooth muscle cells (alpha-actin), and collagen. Significantly more macrophages, more lymphocytes, less collagen, and less alpha actin staining were observed with larger plaque and vessel areas. These histologic markers of cellularity and inflammation, traditionally associated with vulnerable plaque, were more prevalent in larger and more remodeled plaques [54]. Further, human vascular cells can produce the matrix metalloproteinases (MMPs) that may play a crucial role in vascular remodeling during development, growth, and rupture of an atherosclerotic plaque [55,56]. These markers may provide an explanation for the positive remodeling seen in large, lipid-laden plaques with activated macrophages encountered in unstable angina. Further studies are needed to examine whether the extent and direction of remodeling can predict clinical outcome.

*Tissue Characterization with Standard Intravascular Ultrasound*

Tissue characterization with standard IVUS examination has been difficult, with limited success for an individual lesion. Typically, a "soft" plaque is defined as a plaque with at least 80% area containing material with less echo-reflectivity than the adventitia, and an arc of calcium less than 10 degrees. A fibrous plaque is defined as having echo-reflectivity as bright as or brighter than the adventitia of at least 80% of the plaque and mixed as plaque that contain both low and high echo-reflective areas. Fibrous and mixed plaques are categorized as hard plaques.

Earlier studies have demonstrated the reliability of ultrasound imaging in predicting the composition of the atherosclerotic plaque. Gussenhoven et al. compared the histology of the plaques in 1100 sections obtained from fresh human arteries to the corresponding ultrasound appearance [57]. Lipid-laden lesions appeared as hypoechoic areas, while "soft" echoes represented fibromuscular lesions. Dense fibrous or calcified tissues were recognized as bright echoes, the latter characterized by shadows obscuring the underlying internal elastic lamina (back shadow) (Figure 11). Lesions containing lipid, fibromuscular tissue, and areas of calcification were described as shadows of variable echodensity. In lipid-laden or fibromuscular lesions with prominent overlying fibrous "caps," a more

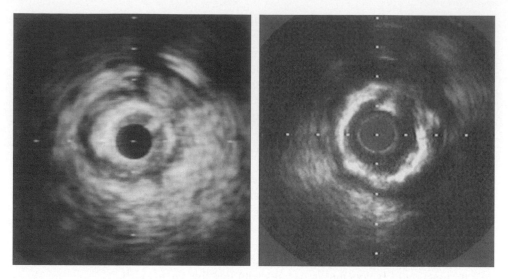

**Figure 11** On the left panel, the plaque has fibrous appearance between 7 o'clock and 2 o'clock with echodensity equal to or greater than the surrounding adventitia. Note that there is no acoustic shadowing. On the right side is an example of a superficially calcified plaque with overt shadowing.

reflective structure separating the soft echoes from the lumen was identified. In a study of human coronary arteries, the plaque composition was accurately predicted by visual assessment of ultrasound images in 96% of 112 quadrants of 21 arteries [58]. Fibrous and calcified plaque quadrants were correctly identified in almost all images (100 out of 103, 97%), but only 7 of 9 quadrants (78%) with predominantly lipid deposits were correctly diagnosed (Figure 12).

Ultrasound imaging has shown significant superiority over fluoroscopy or angiography in the detection of coronary calcification (Figure 13). The severity of calcification has been quantified according to the angle subtended by the calcified arc of the vessel wall [59]. In a clinical series of 110 patients undergoing transcatheter therapy, target lesion calcification was detected by ultrasound and fluoroscopy in 84 and 50 patients, respectively (76% vs. 14%, $p < 0.001$). There was a correlation between the severity of calcification by ultrasound and its detection by fluoroscopy; calcium in two or more quadrants ($\geq$ 180°) or greater than or equal to 5-mm long, which increased the fluoroscopic detection rates to 74% and 86%, respectively [60]. The depth of calcification, as determined by ultrasound, also influences the recognition of calcification on fluoroscopy [61]. In a retrospective analysis of the angiographic and ultrasound images of 183 consecutive interventional patients, calcification was detected in 138 patients by ultrasound and in 63 by fluoroscopy. The sensitivity and specificity of angiography was 46% and 82%, respectively. The assessment by the two techniques was concordant in 92 cases and discordant in 91 cases. The arc of calcium measured by ultrasound was greater in patients with angiographically visible calcification than in those without (175° $\pm$ 85° versus 108° $\pm$ 71°; $p = 0.0001$). When calcium was detected angiographically, the calcification detected by ultrasound was likely greater than 90 degrees and superficial in location, whereas if no calcification could be visualized on the angiogram, the chance of detecting a large superficial arc of calcium by ultrasound was low (12%). Additionally, when calcification

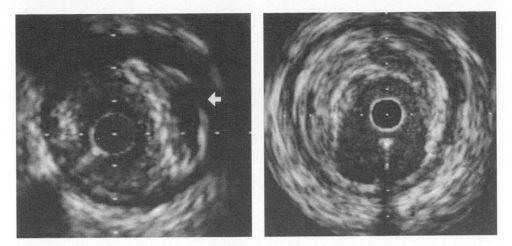

**Figure 12**   Image on the left shows echolucent area within the plaque (*arrow*) with intact, relatively thick fibrous cap. The image to the right shows thinning of the fibrous cap over the echolucent area (between 12 o'clock and 3 o'clock). A real-time image demonstrated independent movement of the thin fibrous cap suggestive of recent plaque rupture. Injection of the contrast was made to confirm communication of the echolucent area with the lumen.

was angiographically detectable at remote sites and not at the target lesion, the probability of detection of target lesion calcification by ultrasound was high.

However, the accuracy of conventional videodensitometric analysis in identifying different atherosclerotic plaque types is limited to differentiating only three basic types of plaque: highly echo-reflective regions with acoustic shadows often corresponding to calcified tissue; echo-dense areas representing fibrosis or microcalcification; and echo-lucent intimal thickening corresponding to fibrotic, thrombotic/haemorrhagic or lipid tissue, or a mixture of these elements. More objective, quantitative texture analysis of videodensitometric data has not led to significant improvements in the ability to discriminate detailed plaque composition [62,63].

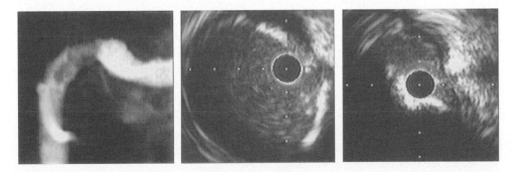

**Figure 13**   Some lesions with "classic" angiographic appearance of unstable plaque have unsuspected features by ultrasound. This patient presented with a non–Q wave infarction and only angiographic finding was a large intraluminal filling defect in the proximal right coronary artery suggestive of thrombus. Intravascular ultrasound (IVUS) examination showed extensive, heavily calcified plaque (*right panel*) with a relatively disease-free proximal segment (*middle panel*).

## Virtual Histology

Validation of the radiofrequency data has been performed using ex vivo analysis of the human coronary arteries [11]. Eighty-eight plaques from 51 left anterior descending coronary arteries were imaged ex vivo at physiological pressure with the use of 30-MHz IVUS transducers. After IVUS imaging, the arteries were pressure-fixed and corresponding histology was collected in matched images. Regions of interest, selected from histology, were 101 fibrous regions, 56 fibrolipidic regions, 50 calcified regions, and 70 calcified-necrotic regions. Classification schemes for model building were computed for autoregressive and classic Fourier spectra by using 75% of the data. The remaining data were used for validation. Autoregressive classification schemes performed better than those from classic Fourier spectra with accuracies of 90% for fibrous regions, 92.3% for fibrolipidic regions, 91% for calcified regions, and 90% for calcified-necrotic regions in the training data set and 80%, 81%, 93%, and 86% in the test data, respectively [11]. The automated real-time system is now available for clinical investigation, and meaningful data from in vivo studies are beginning to emerge.

## Intravascular Palpography

Elastographic experiments were performed in excised human coronary (n = 4) and femoral (n = 9) arteries [64]. Elastographic data and histology matching was performed using the IVUS images. The cross-sections were segmented in regions (n = 125) based on the strain value on the elastogram. The dominant plaque types in these regions (fibrous, fibrofatty, or fatty) were obtained from histology and correlated with the average strain and echo intensity. Mean strain values of 0.27%, 0.45%, and 0.60% were found for fibrous, fibrofatty and fatty plaque components, respectively. The strain for the three plaque types as determined by histology differed significantly (p = 0.0002). This difference was independent of the type of artery (coronary or femoral) and was mainly evident between fibrous and fatty tissue (p = 0.0004). The plaque types did not reveal echo-intensity differences in the IVUS echogram (p = 0.992). Conversion of the strain into Young's modulus values resulted in 493 kPa, 296 kPa, and 222 kPa for fibrous, fibrofatty, and fatty plaques, respectively. Although the individual values may change with different systems, the ratio between fibrous and fatty material remains similar [65]. Subsequently, the technique was validated in pig coronary arteries with atherosclerosis [66]. Ex vivo human coronary experiments have been performed to characterize "vulnerable plaque." In 24 diseased coronary arteries, 54 cross-sections were studied, with histology showing 26 vulnerable plaques and 28 nonvulnerable plaques. Higher strain correlated with vulnerability of the plaque. Linear regression showed high correlation between the strain in caps and the amount of macrophages (p < 0.006) and an inverse relation between the amount of smooth muscle cells and strain (p < 0.0001). Receiver-operator characteristic analysis revealed a maximum predictive power for a strain value threshold of 1.26% resulting in an area under the receiver-operator characteristic curve of 0.85. To detect vulnerable plaques, the sensitivity was 88% and the specificity was 89%. Plaques, which are declared vulnerable in elastography, had a thinner cap than nonvulnerable plaques (p < 0.0001) [67]. This promising technique is at the stage of collecting in vivo human data.

## Optical Coherence Tomography

OCT characteristics of various plaque components have been established by ex vivo histologic correlation [13]. In this study, OCT image criteria for three types of plaque were formulated by analysis of a subset (n = 50) of arterial segments. OCT images of fibrous plaques were characterized by homogeneous, signal-rich regions; fibrocalcific plaques by well-delineated, signal-poor regions with sharp borders; and lipid-rich plaques by signal-poor regions with diffuse borders. Independent validation of these criteria was accomplished by analyzing 307 segments, demonstrating a sensitivity and specificity in the range of 70–79% and 97–98% for fibrous plaques, 95–96% and 97% for fibrocalcific plaques, and 90–94% and 90–92% for lipid-rich plaques, respectively.

In a comparison with high-resolution IVUS, OCT has proven equivalent in detecting plaque and discerning fibrous and calcified plaque morphologies [68]. In terms of resolution, OCT was found to be superior, allowing identification of intimal hyperplasia, internal and external elastic laminas, and regions of lipid-rich plaque not detected by IVUS. Recently, the ability of OCT to detect and quantify macrophage infiltration was demonstrated in an autopsy study [69]. The presence of macrophages within the fibrous cap, identified by immunoperoxidase staining for CD68, was correlated with the optical signal such that a sensitivity and specificity of 100% was achieved for the detection of an arbitrary quantity of greater than 10% CD68-positive macrophages within that imaged region.

## Thermography

Casscells et al. measured intimal surface temperatures in carotid artery samples obtained by endarterectomy [70]. The samples were probed with a thermistor (24-gauge needle tip; accuracy 0.1°C; time contrast 0.15 s). Plaques showed several regions in which the surface temperatures varied reproducibly by 0.2–0.3°C, but 37% of plaques had substantially warmer regions (0.4–2.2°C). Points with substantially different temperatures could not be distinguished from one another by the naked eye and were sometimes very close to one another ($< 1$ mm apart). Temperature correlated positively with cell density ($r = 0.68$; $p = 0.0001$) and inversely with the distance of the cell clusters from the luminal surface ($r = -0.38$; $p = 0.0006$). Most cells were macrophages. In an in vivo setting, Verheye et al. examined temperature heterogeneity in the rabbit aorta [71]. The animals received either a normal or cholesterol-rich (0.3%) diet for 6 months before undergoing thermography of the surface of aortic arch and descending aorta. In the animals receiving a normal diet, plaque formation and temperature heterogeneity were absent. In hypercholesterolemic rabbits, plaque formation was prominent in the thoracic aorta and showed markedly elevated temperature heterogeneity that increased with plaque thickness. Importantly, after 3 months of cholesterol lowering, plaque thickness remained unchanged, but temperature heterogeneity was significantly decreased. Thus, in vivo temperature heterogeneity of rabbit atherosclerotic plaques were determined by plaque composition.

Clinically, coronary arterial temperature differentials are greater in patients who present with acute coronary events. Stefanadis et al. studied 90 patients; 45 with normal coronary arteries, 15 with stable angina, 15 with unstable angina, and 15 with acute MI [72]. Temperature was constant within the arteries of the control subjects, whereas most arteriosclerotic plaques showed higher temperature compared with healthy-appearing portions of the vessel wall. Temperature differences between arteriosclerotic plaques and healthy-appearing portions increased progressively from stable angina to acute MI patients (difference of plaque temperature from background temperature, $0.106 \pm 0.110$°C in stable angina, $0.683 \pm 0.347$°C in unstable angina, and $1.472 \pm 0.691$°C in acute MI). Heterogeneity within the plaque was shown in 20%, 40%, and 67% of the patients, respectively, whereas no heterogeneity was observed in the control subjects.

Stefanadis et al. prospectively investigated the relation between temperature difference between the atherosclerotic plaques and angiographically healthy vessel wall and event-free survival among 86 patients undergoing successful percutaneous intervention [73]. The study group consisted of patients with effort angina (34.5%), unstable angina

(34.5%), and acute MI (30%). Temperature difference increased progressively from effort angina to acute MI (0.132 ± 0.18°C in effort angina, 0.637 ± 0.26°C in unstable angina, and 0.942 ± 0.58°C in acute MI). The median clinical follow-up period was 18 months. Temperature difference was greater in patients with adverse cardiac events than in patients without events (temperature difference: 0.939 ± 0.49°C vs. 0.428 ± 0.42°C; p < 0.0001). Temperature difference was a strong predictor of adverse cardiac events during follow-up (odds ratio 2.14; p = 0.043). The threshold of temperature difference above which the risk of an adverse cardiac event was significantly increased was 0.5°C. The incidence of adverse cardiac events in patients with a temperature difference greater than or equal to 0.5°C was 41%, as compared to 7% in patients with a temperature difference less than 0.5°C (p < 0.001). The same group observed that coronary thermal heterogeneity was reduced by statin treatment [74]. They reported that, in 72 patients, 21 had effort angina, 32 had unstable angina, and 19 had acute MI. In the overall group of patients, 37 received statins for greater than 4 weeks and 35 did not receive statins. Temperature difference was higher in the group not treated with statins compared to the group treated with statins (0.56 ± 0.41°C vs. 0.29 ± 0.33°C; p < 0.01). A progressive increase in temperature difference by type of clinical syndrome was observed in both groups. Multivariate analysis showed that treatment with statins was an independent factor associated with temperature variation after correcting for the effect on temperature of the various clinical syndromes (p < 0.05).

The Pressure Wire™ (Radi Medical Systems, Inc. Wilmington, MA), a pressure sensing 0.014″ wire, can also measure the difference in temperature of blood when placed in the coronary arteries. Preliminary studies have shown that there may be a detectable temperature gradient in the coronary arteries. The blood near the inflamed plaque may have a greater temperature compared to blood near a relatively normal vessel wall. However, more rigorous studies are needed before determining the significance of such information.

The exact mechanism of temperature elevation remains unknown. Macrophages have a high metabolic turnover rate exceeding that of most other cells [75]. Oxygen consumption of lipid-laden foam cells is three times higher than that of smooth muscle cells [76]. Further, some macrophage subpopulations may express mitochondrial uncoupling proteins, which are homologs of thermogenin. Thermogenin produces heat in brown fat tissue [77]. Accordingly, it is plausible that areas of macrophage accumulation display enhanced heat production, which can be detected by intracoronary temperature recordings. Cell adhesion molecules, which mark the inflammatory process central to the pathogenesis of coronary artery disease, have been correlated with temperature differentials at culprit lesions in ACS. However, there appears to be a significant overlap between temperature differentials in stable and unstable presentations of coronary artery disease, and there is no clear evidence that temperature differentials are related to specific plaque vulnerability rather than a generalized marker of inflammation. Similarly, individual variations in temperature heterogeneity have been documented; it has been suggested that these variations have arisen from altered blood flow through a stenotic lesion or because of systemic inflammation or medication, all features that question thermography's capacity to assess individual plaque vulnerability.

## REFERENCES

1. Tuzcu EM, Schoenhagen P. Acute coronary syndromes, plaque vulnerability, and carotid artery disease: the changing role of atherosclerosis imaging. J Am Coll Cardiol; 2003;42:1033-6.

2. Naghavi M, Libby P, Falk E, Casscells SW, Litovsky S, Rumberger J, Badimon JJ, Stefanadis C, Moreno P, Pasterkamp G, Fayad Z, Stone PH, Waxman S, Raggi P, Madjid M, Zarrabi A, Burke A, Yuan C, Fitzgerald PJ, Siscovick DS, de Korte CL, Aikawa M, Airaksinen KE, Assmann G, Becker CR, Chesebro JH, Farb A, Galis ZS, Jackson C, Jang IK, Koenig W, Lodder RA, March K, Demirovic J, Navab M, Priori SG, Rekhter MD, Bahr R, Grundy SM, Mehran R, Colombo A, Boerwinkle E, Ballantyne C, Insull W, Jr, Schwartz RS, Vogel R, Serruys PW, Hansson GK, Faxon DP, Kaul S, Drexler H, Greenland P, Muller JE, Virmani R, Ridker PM, Zipes DP, Shah PK, Willerson JT. From vulnerable plaque to vulnerable patient: a call for new definitions and risk assessment strategies: Part II. Circulation; 2003; 108:1772-8.

3. Naghavi M, Libby P, Falk E, Casscells SW, Litovsky S, Rumberger J, Badimon JJ, Stefanadis C, Moreno P, Pasterkamp G, Fayad Z, Stone PH, Waxman S, Raggi P, Madjid M, Zarrabi A, Burke A, Yuan C, Fitzgerald PJ, Siscovick DS, de Korte CL, Aikawa M, Juhani Airaksinen KE, Assmann G, Becker CR, Chesebro JH, Farb A, Galis ZS, Jackson C, Jang IK, Koenig W, Lodder RA, March K, Demirovic J, Navab M, Priori SG, Rekhter MD, Bahr R, Grundy SM, Mehran R, Colombo A, Boerwinkle E, Ballantyne C, Insull W, Jr, Schwartz RS, Vogel R, Serruys PW, Hansson GK, Faxon DP, Kaul S, Drexler H, Greenland P, Muller JE, Virmani R, Ridker PM, Zipes DP, Shah PK, Willerson JT. From vulnerable plaque to vulnerable patient: a call for new definitions and risk assessment strategies: Part I. Circulation; 2003;108:1664-72.

4. Kuo IY, Shung KK. High frequency ultrasonic backscatter from erythrocyte suspension. IEEE Trans Biomed Eng; 1994;41:29-34.

5. Fitzgerald PJ, St.Goar FG, Connolly AJ, Pinto FJ, Billingham ME, Popp RL, Yock PG. Intravascular ultrasound imaging of coronary arteries. Is three layers the norm? Circulation; 1992; 86:154-158.

6. Nissen SE. Application of intravascular ultrasound to characterize coronary artery disease and assess the progression or regression of atherosclerosis. Am J Cardiol; 2002;89:24B-31B.

7. Wickline SA, Shepard RK, Daugherty A. Quantitative ultrasonic characterization of lesion composition and remodeling in atherosclerotic rabbit aorta. Arterioscler Thromb; 1993;13: 1543-50.

8. Barzilai B, Madaras EI, Sobel BE, Miller JG, Perez JE. Effects of myocardial contraction on ultrasonic backscatter before and after ischemia. Am J Physiol; 1984;247:H478-83.

9. Fitzgerald PJ, McDaniel MM, Rolett EL, James DH, Strohbehn JW. Two-dimensional ultrasonic variation in myocardium throughout the cardiac cycle. Ultrason Imaging; 1986;8:241-51.

10. Nair A, Kuban BD, Obuchowski N, Vince DG. Assessing spectral algorithms to predict atherosclerotic plaque composition with normalized and raw intravascular ultrasound data. Ultrasound Med Biol; 2001;27:1319-31.

11. Nair A, Kuban BD, Tuzcu EM, Schoenhagen P, Nissen SE, Vince DG. Coronary plaque classification with intravascular ultrasound radiofrequency data analysis. Circulation; 2002; 106:2200-6.

12. de Korte CL, Schaar JA, Mastik F, Serruys PW, van der Steen AF. Intravascular elastography: from bench to bedside. J Interv Cardiol; 2003;16:253-9.

13. Yabushita H, Bouma BE, Houser SL, Aretz HT, Jang IK, Schlendorf KH, Kauffman CR, Shishkov M, Kang DH, Halpern EF, Tearney GJ. Characterization of human atherosclerosis by optical coherence tomography. Circulation; 2002;106:1640-5.

14. Stefanadis C, Toutouzas K, Tsiamis E, Vavuranakis M, Kallikazaros I, Toutouzas P. Thermography of human arterial system by means of new thermography catheters. Catheter Cardiovasc Interv; 2001;54:51-8.

15. Erbel R, Ge J, Gorge G, Baumgart D, Haude M, Jeremias A, von Birgelen C, Jollet N, Schwedtmann J. Intravascular ultrasound classification of atherosclerotic lesions according to American Heart Association recommendation. Coron Artery Dis; 1999;10:489-99.

16. Ge J, Chirillo F, Schwedtmann J, G Gr, Haude M, Baumgart D, Shah V, von Birgelen C, Sack S, Boudoulas H, Erbel R. Screening of ruptured plaques in patients with coronary artery disease by intravascular ultrasound. Heart; 1999;81:621-627.

17. Kearney P, Erbel R, Rupprecht HJ, Ge J, Koch L, Voigtlander T, Stahr P, Gorge G, Meyer J. Differences in the morphology of unstable and stable coronary lesions and their impact on the mechanisms of angioplasty. An in vivo study with intravascular ultrasound. Eur Heart J; 1996;17:721-30.

18. Rasheed Q, Nair R, Sheehan H, Hodgson JM. Correlation of intracoronary ultrasound plaque characteristics in atherosclerotic coronary artery disease patients with clinical variables. Am J Cardiol; 1994;73:753-8.

19. Gyongyosi M, Yang P, Hassan A, Weidinger F, Domanovits H, Laggner A, Glogar D. Coronary risk factors influence plaque morphology in patients with unstable angina. Coron Artery Dis; 1999;10:211-9.

20. Siegel RJ, Ariani M, Fishbein MC, Chae JS, Park JC, Maurer G, Forrester JS. Histopathologic validation of angioscopy and intravascular ultrasound. Circulation; 1991;84:109-17.

21. Bocksch WG, Schartl M, Beckmann SH, Dreysse S, Paeprer H. Intravascular ultrasound imaging in patients with acute myocardial infarction: comparison with chronic stable angina pectoris. Coron Artery Dis; 1994;5:727-35.

22. Bocksch W, Schartl M, Beckmann S, Dreysse S, Fleck E. Intravascular ultrasound imaging in patients with acute myocardial infarction. Eur Heart J; 1995;16 Suppl J:46-52.

23. Chemarin-Alibelli MJ, Pieraggi MT, Elbaz M, Carrie D, Fourcade J, Puel J, Tobis J. Identification of coronary thrombus after myocardial infarction by intracoronary ultrasound compared with histology of tissues sampled by atherectomy. Am J Cardiol; 1996;77:344-9.

24. Hodgson JM, Reddy KG, Suneja R, Nair RN, Lesnefsky EJ, Sheehan HM. Intracoronary ultrasound imaging: correlation of plaque morphology with angiography, clinical syndrome and procedural results in patients undergoing coronary angioplasty. J Am Coll Cardiol; 1993; 21:35-44.

25. De Servi S, Arbustini E, Marsico F, Bramucci E, Angoli L, Porcu E, Costante AM, Kubica J, Boschetti E, Valentini P, Specchia G. Correlation between clinical and morphologic findings in unstable angina. Am J Cardiol; 1996;77:128-32.

26. Mintz GS, Pichard AD, Popma JJ, Kent KM, Satler LF, Bucher TA, Leon MB. Determinants and correlates of target lesion calcium in coronary artery disease: a clinical, angiographic and intravascular ultrasound study. J Am Coll Cardiol; 1997;29:268-74.

27. Schmermund A, Baumgart D, Gorge G, Seibel R, Gronemeyer D, Ge J, Haude M, Rumberger J, Erbel R. Coronary artery calcium in acute coronary syndromes: a comparative study of electron-beam computed tomography, coronary angiography, and intracoronary ultrasound in survivors of acute myocardial infarction and unstable angina. Circulation; 1997;96:1461-9.

28. Schmermund A, Baumgart D, Adamzik M, Ge J, Gronemeyer D, Seibel R, Sehnert C, Gorge G, Haude M, Erbel R. Comparison of electron-beam computed tomography and intracoronary ultrasound in detecting calcified and noncalcified plaques in patients with acute coronary syndromes and no or minimal to moderate angiographic coronary artery disease. American Journal of Cardiology; 1998;81:141-6.

29. Goldstein JA, Demetriou D, Grines CL, Pica M, Shoukfeh M, O'Neill WW. Multiple complex coronary plaques in patients with acute myocardial infarction. N Engl J Med; 2000;343:915-22.

30. Zairis MN, Papadaki OA, Manousakis SJ, Thoma MA, Beldekos DJ, Olympios CD, Festeridou CA, Argyrakis SK, Foussas SG. C-reactive protein and multiple complex coronary artery plaques in patients with primary unstable angina. Atherosclerosis; 2002;164:355-9.

31. Rioufol G, Finet G, Ginon I, Andre-Fouet X, Rossi R, Vialle E, Desjoyaux E, Convert G, Huret JF, Tabib A. Multiple atherosclerotic plaque rupture in acute coronary syndrome: a three-vessel intravascular ultrasound study. Circulation; 2002;106:804-8.

32. Maehara A, Mintz GS, Bui AB, Walter OR, Castagna MT, Canos D, Pichard AD, Satler LF, Waksman R, Suddath WO, Laird JR, Jr, Kent KM, Weissman NJ. Morphologic and angiographic features of coronary plaque rupture detected by intravascular ultrasound. J Am Coll Cardiol; 2002;40:904-10.

33. Schoenhagen P, Stone GW, Nissen SE, Grines CL, Griffin J, Clemson BS, Vince DG, Ziada K, Crowe T, Apperson-Hanson C, Kapadia SR, Tuzcu EM. Coronary plaque morphology

and frequency of ulceration distant from culprit lesions in patients with unstable and stable presentation. Arterioscler Thromb Vasc Biol; 2003;23:1895-900.

34. Burke AP, Kolodgie FD, Farb A, Weber DK, Malcom GT, Smialek J, Virmani R. Healed plaque ruptures and sudden coronary death: evidence that subclinical rupture has a role in plaque progression. Circulation; 2001;103:934-40.

35. Casscells W, Naghavi M, Willerson JT. Vulnerable atherosclerotic plaque: a multifocal disease. Circulation; 2003;107:2072-5.

36. Little WC, Constantinescu M, Applegate RJ, Kutcher MA, Burrows MT, Kahl FR, Santamore WP. Can coronary angiography predict the site of a subsequent myocardial infarction in patients with mild-to-moderate coronary artery disease? Circulation; 1988;78:1157-66.

37. Davies MJ. Stability and instability: two faces of coronary atherosclerosis. The Paul Dudley White Lecture 1995. Circulation; 1996;94:2013-20.

38. Mann J, Davies MJ. Mechanisms of progression in native coronary artery disease: role of healed plaque disruption. Heart; 1999;82:265-8.

39. Ge J, Haude M, Gorge G, Liu F, Erbel R. Silent healing of spontaneous plaque disruption demonstrated by intracoronary ultrasound. Eur Heart J; 1995;16:1149-51.

40. Weissman NJ, Sheris SJ, Chari R, Mendelsohn FO, Anderson WD, Breall JA, Tanguay JF, Diver DJ. Intravascular ultrasonic analysis of plaque characteristics associated with coronary artery remodeling. Am J Cardiol; 1999;84:37-40.

41. Williams MJ, Restieaux NJ, Low CJ. Myocardial infarction in young people with normal coronary arteries. Heart; 1998;79:191-4.

42. Morocutti G, Spedicato L, Vendrametto F, Bernardi G. [Intravascular echocardiography (ICUS) diagnosis of post-traumatic coronary dissection involving the common trunk. A case report and review of the literature]. G Ital Cardiol; 1999;29:1034-7.

43. Kearney P, Erbel R, Ge J, Zamorano J, Koch L, Gorge G, Meyer J. Assessment of spontaneous coronary artery dissection by intravascular ultrasound in a patient with unstable angina. Cathet Cardiovasc Diagn; 1994;32:58-61.

44. de Winter RJ, Kok WE, Piek JJ. Coronary atherosclerosis within a myocardial bridge, not a benign condition. Heart; 1998;80:91-3.

45. Ge J, Jeremias A, Rupp A, Abels M, Baumgart D, Liu F, Haude M, Görge G, Von Birgelen C, Sack S, Erbel R. New signs characteristic of myocardial bridging demonstrated by intracoronary ultrasound and Doppler. Eur Heart J; 1999;20:1707-1716.

46. Schoenhagen P, Ziada KM, Nissen SE, Tuzcu EM. Arterial remodeling in stable versus unstable coronary syndromes: an intravascular ultrasound study (abstract ). Circulation; 1998;98:I-368.

47. Ziada KM, Kapadia SR, Crowe TD, T BC, M RS, V O, E NS, M TE. Adaptive Coronary Remodeling is Evident in Later Stages of Transplant Vasculopathy: A Serial Intravascular Ultrasound Study. Journal of the American College of Cardiology; 1999;33:90A.

48. Smits PC, Pasterkamp G, Quarles van Ufford MA, Eefting FD, Stella PR, de Jaegere PP, Borst C. Coronary artery disease: arterial remodelling and clinical presentation. Heart; 1999; 82:461-4.

49. Gyongyosi M, Yang P, Hassan A, Weidinger F, Domanovits H, Laggner A, Glogar D. Arterial remodelling of native human coronary arteries in patients with unstable angina pectoris: a prospective intravascular ultrasound study. Heart; 1999;82:68-74.

50. Nakamura M, Nishikawa H, Mukai S, Setsuda M, Tamada H, Suzuki H, Ohnishi T, Kakuta Y, Lee DP, Yeung AC. Comparison of Coronary Remodeling in the Culprit Lesion in the Acute Coronary Syndrome and Stable Angina Pectoris. J Am Coll Cardiol; 1999;33 (suppl A):18A.

51. Tauth J, Pinnow E, Sullebarger JT, Basta L, Gursoy S, Lindsay J, Jr, Matar F. Predictors of coronary arterial remodeling patterns in patients with myocardial ischemia. Am J Cardiol; 1997;80:1352-5.

52. Mintz GS, Kent KM, Pichard AD, Satler LF, Popma JJ, Leon MB. Contribution of inadequate arterial remodeling to the development of focal coronary artery stenoses. An intravascular ultrasound study [see comments]. Circulation; 1997;95:1791-8.

53. Sabate M, Kay IP, de Feyter PJ, van Domburg RT, Deshpande NV, Ligthart JM, Gijzel AL, Wardeh AJ, Boersma E, Serruys PW. Remodeling of atherosclerotic coronary arteries varies in relation to location and composition of plaque. Am J Cardiol; 1999;84:135-40.

54. Pasterkamp G, Schoneveld AH, van der Wal AC, Haudenschild CC, Clarijs RJ, Becker AE, Hillen B, Borst C. Relation of arterial geometry to luminal narrowing and histologic markers for plaque vulnerability: the remodeling paradox [see comments]. J Am Coll Cardiol; 1998; 32:655-62.

55. Rajavashisth TB, Xu XP, Jovinge S, Meisel S, Xu XO, Chai NN, Fishbein MC, Kaul S, Cercek B, Sharifi B, Shah PK. Membrane type 1 matrix metalloproteinase expression in human atherosclerotic plaques: evidence for activation by proinflammatory mediators. Circulation; 1999;99:3103-9.

56. Galis ZS, Sukhova GK, Lark MW, Libby P. Increased expression of matrix metalloproteinases and matrix degrading activity in vulnerable regions of human atherosclerotic plaques. J Clin Invest; 1994;94:2493-503.

57. Gussenhoven EJ, Essed CE, Lancee CT, Mastik F, Frietman P, van Egmond FC, Reiber J, Bosch H, van Urk H, Roelandt J. Arterial wall characteristics determined by intravascular ultrasound imaging: an in vitro study. J Am Coll Cardiol; 1989;14:947-52.

58. Potkin BN, Bartorelli AL, Gessert JM, Neville RF, Almagor Y, Roberts WC, Leon MB. Coronary artery imaging with intravascular high-frequency ultrasound. Circulation; 1990;81: 1575-1585.

59. Honye J, Mahon DJ, Jain A, White CJ, Ramee SR, Wallis JB, al-Zarka A, Tobis JM. Morphological effects of coronary balloon angioplasty in vivo assessed by intravascular ultrasound imaging. Circulation; 1992;85:1012-25.

60. Mintz GS, Douek P, Pichard AD, Kent KM, Satler LF, Popma JJ, Leon MB. Target lesion calcification in coronary artery disease: an intravascular ultrasound study. J Am Coll Cardiol; 1992;20:1149-55.

61. Tuzcu EM, Berkalp B, De Franco AC, Ellis SG, Goormastic M, Whitlow PL, Franco I, Raymond RE, Nissen SE. The dilemma of diagnosing coronary calcification: angiography versus intravascular ultrasound. J Am Coll Cardiol; 1996;27:832-8.

62. Rasheed Q, Dhawale PJ, Anderson J, Hodgson JM. Intracoronary ultrasound-defined plaque composition: computer-aided plaque characterization and correlation with histologic samples obtained during directional coronary atherectomy. Am Heart J; 1995;129:631-7.

63. Peters RJ, Kok WE, Bot H, Visser CA. Characterization of plaque components with intracoronary ultrasound imaging: an in vitro quantitative study with videodensitometry. J Am Soc Echocardiogr; 1994;7:616-23.

64. de Korte CL, Pasterkamp G, van der Steen AF, Woutman HA, Bom N. Characterization of plaque components with intravascular ultrasound elastography in human femoral and coronary arteries in vitro. Circulation; 2000;102:617-23.

65. Varghese T, Techavipoo U, Liu W, Zagzebski JA, Chen Q, Frank G, Lee FT, Jr. Elastographic measurement of the area and volume of thermal lesions resulting from radiofrequency ablation: pathologic correlation. AJR Am J Roentgenol; 2003;181:701-7.

66. de Korte CL, Sierevogel MJ, Mastik F, Strijder C, Schaar JA, Velema E, Pasterkamp G, Serruys PW, van der Steen AF. Identification of atherosclerotic plaque components with intravascular ultrasound elastography in vivo: a Yucatan pig study. Circulation; 2002;105:1627-30.

67. Schaar JA, De Korte CL, Mastik F, Strijder C, Pasterkamp G, Boersma E, Serruys PW, Van Der Steen AF. Characterizing vulnerable plaque features with intravascular elastography. Circulation; 2003;108:2636-41.

68. Jang IK, Bouma BE, Kang DH, Park SJ, Park SW, Seung KB, Choi KB, Shishkov M, Schlendorf K, Pomerantsev E, Houser SL, Aretz HT, Tearney GJ. Visualization of coronary atherosclerotic plaques in patients using optical coherence tomography: comparison with intravascular ultrasound. J Am Coll Cardiol; 2002;39:604-9.

69. Tearney GJ, Yabushita H, Houser SL, Aretz HT, Jang IK, Schlendorf KH, Kauffman CR, Shishkov M, Halpern EF, Bouma BE. Quantification of macrophage content in atherosclerotic plaques by optical coherence tomography. Circulation; 2003;107:113-9.

70. Casscells W, Hathorn B, David M, Krabach T, Vaughn WK, McAllister HA, Bearman G, Willerson JT. Thermal detection of cellular infiltrates in living atherosclerotic plaques: possible implications for plaque rupture and thrombosis. Lancet; 1996;347:1447-51.

71. Verheye S, De Meyer GR, Van Langenhove G, Knaapen MW, Kockx MM. In vivo temperature heterogeneity of atherosclerotic plaques is determined by plaque composition. Circulation; 2002;105:1596-601.

72. Stefanadis C, Diamantopoulos L, Vlachopoulos C, Tsiamis E, Dernellis J, Toutouzas K, Stefanadi E, Toutouzas P. Thermal heterogeneity within human atherosclerotic coronary arteries detected in vivo: A new method of detection by application of a special thermography catheter. Circulation; 1999;99:1965-71.

73. Stefanadis C, Toutouzas K, Tsiamis E, Stratos C, Vavuranakis M, Kallikazaros I, Panagiotakos D, Toutouzas P. Increased local temperature in human coronary atherosclerotic plaques: an independent predictor of clinical outcome in patients undergoing a percutaneous coronary intervention. J Am Coll Cardiol; 2001;37:1277-83.

74. Stefanadis C, Toutouzas K, Vavuranakis M, Tsiamis E, Tousoulis D, Panagiotakos DB, Vaina S, Pitsavos C, Toutouzas P. Statin treatment is associated with reduced thermal heterogeneity in human atherosclerotic plaques. Eur Heart J; 2002;23:1664-9.

75. Newsholme P, Newsholme EA. Rates of utilization of glucose, glutamine and oleate and formation of end-products by mouse peritoneal macrophages in culture. Biochem J; 1989;261: 211-8.

76. Bjornheden T, Bondjers G. Oxygen consumption in aortic tissue from rabbits with diet-induced atherosclerosis. Arteriosclerosis; 1987;7:238-47.

77. Zarrabi A, Gul K, Willerson JT, Casscells W, Naghavi M. Intravascular thermography: a novel approach for detection of vulnerable plaque. Curr Opin Cardiol; 2002;17:656-62.

# 6

# Differences Between Unstable Angina and Acute Myocardial Infarction: Pathophysiological and Clinical Spectrum

**Jacqueline Saw**
*The Cleveland Clinic Foundation*
*Cleveland, Ohio, U.S.A.*

**David J. Moliterno**
*University of Kentucky*
*Lexington, Kentucky, U.S.A.*

## INTRODUCTION

The acute coronary syndromes (ACS) belong to a diagnostic and pathophysiological continuum of acute myocardial ischemia, with or without evidence of myonecrosis, and encompass unstable angina, non–ST-segment elevation myocardial infarction (NSTEMI), and ST-segment elevation myocardial infarction (STEMI) (Figure 1). At the interface between unstable angina and myocardial infarction (MI), these entities become nearly indistinct as most features are shared. Indeed, the phrase "unstable angina" was first used by Conti [1] and Fowler [2] in the early 1970s to specifically describe symptom complexes intermediate in severity between stable angina pectoris and MI. Other terms used to describe unstable angina also show its close apposition to MI: intermediate coronary syndrome and preinfarction angina [2–5]. On the other hand, a number of features distinguish unstable angina from acute MI. These differences are seen in the pathophysiologic as well as the clinical spectrum of ACS, and they affect the diagnosis, treatment, and outcome. This chapter will review the shared features and distinguishing characteristics of unstable angina and acute MI regarding etiology, pathology, and clinical course.

### Definitions

The first distinction between unstable angina and acute MI can be seen when considering their definitions or classifications. Unstable angina has a broad, less-distinct definition, whereas the definition of acute MI is specific. The diversity of clinical conditions that cause unstable angina, its varying intensity and frequency of pain, and its unpredictability have made classification challenging [6]. Nonetheless, a clinical classification based on symptom presentation has been widely adopted, specifically angina symptoms that are present at rest, new-onset, or increasing in severity (Table 1). Braunwald [7] suggested a more detailed classification scheme based upon angina severity, clinical circumstances,

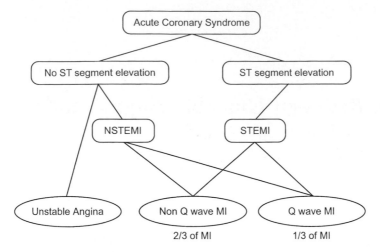

**Figure 1**  Schematic representation of the varied presentations of acute coronary syndromes. (Adapted from Ref. 9) About one-third of acute myocardial infarctions result in Q-waves, whereas approximately two-thirds are non–Q-wave myocardial infarctions (From Ref. 147).

presence of electrocardiographic changes, and intensity of antianginal therapy (Table 2). Patients in Class I have new or accelerated *exertional* angina, whereas those in Class II have subacute ($>$ 48 hours since last pain) or Class III acute ($\leq$ 48 hours since last pain) *rest* angina. Among approximately 3000 consecutive 1996 hospital admissions for unstable angina in the United States, the Global Unstable Angina Registry And Treatment Evaluation (GUARANTEE) study reported that one-third of patients had new or accelerated symptoms associated with exertion, whereas two-thirds presented with symptoms at rest [8]. The clinical circumstances associated with unstable angina are further categorized as type A (secondary [extrinsic to the coronary arterial bed, e.g., anemia, fever, hypoxia]), B (primary [due to coronary arterial narrowing]), or C (postinfarction [$<$ 2 weeks after infarction]). The intensity of antianginal therapy is subclassified as: 1 (no treatment), 2 (usual oral therapy), and 3 (intense therapy, such as intravenous nitroglycerin). A patient with atherosclerotic heart disease and acute chest pain during minimal activity or at rest while taking usual medical therapy would be categorized as Class IIIB$_2$. This is by far the most common presentation.

In contrast, acute MI is commonly separated into distinct categories by electrocardiographic criteria: NSTEMI and STEMI, and more traditionally, non–Q-wave MI and Q-

**Table 1**  Three Major Presentations of Unstable Angina

| | |
|---|---|
| Rest angina | Prolonged angina occurring at rest, usually lasting $>$20 minutes |
| New-onset angina | New-onset angina of at least Canadian Cardiovascular Society (CCS) class III severity |
| Increasing angina | Angina that is increasing in severity, frequency, duration, or lower threshold of precipitation (requires increase in CCS class $\geq$1 to at least class III severity) |

**Table 2**   Braunwald Classification of Unstable Angina

| | | |
|---|---|---|
| Severity | **I** | Symptoms with exertion |
| | **II** | Symptoms at rest: subacute (2–30 days prior) |
| | **III** | Symtoms at rest: acute (within prior 48 hours) |
| Precipitant | **A** | Secondary |
| | **B** | Primary |
| | **C** | Postinfarction |
| Therapy presents | | |
| During symptoms | **1** | No treatment |
| | **2** | Usual angina therapy |
| | **3** | Maximal therapy |

wave MI. It is accepted that MI represents loss of cardiomyocytes due to prolonged myocardial ischemia, and was previously defined by the World Health Organization (WHO) as the presence of 2 of the following 3 characteristics: (a) typical ischemic symptoms, (b) a rise and fall in serial cardiac enzymes, and (c) changes on serially obtained electrocardiograms. The joint consensus document by the European Society of Cardiology and the American College of Cardiology describes a redefinition of MI, which more precisely incorporated biochemical (including elevation in troponin level), electrocardiographic, pathologic and clinical presentations (Table 3) [9]. Several investigators have since compared the diagnostic capability of both criteria and concluded that the redefined criteria substantially increased the diagnosis of acute MI incidence (by at least $> 25\%$), as well as the diagnosis of patients with worse 6-month outcomes who were otherwise missed by the WHO criteria [10–13].

Acute STEMI is defined as new ST-segment elevation in two or more contiguous leads that is greater than or equal to 0.1 mV. The exceptions are posterior MI (defined by ST-segment depression $\geq$ 0.1 mV in V1 and V2) and new left-bundle branch block. Patients with STEMI have occlusion or impending occlusion of a major epicardial coronary artery, with potentially large myocardium in jeopardy, and require immediate myocardial reperfusion therapy (thrombolysis or percutaneous intervention). Progression to electrocar-

**Table 3**   Redefinition of Myocardial Infarction by the Joint European Society of Cardiology/American College of Cardiology Committee

**Criteria for acute, evolving or recent MI**
Either one of the following criteria satisfies the diagnosis for an acute, evolving or recent MI:
   (1) Typical rise and gradual fall (troponin) or more rapid rise and fall (CKMB) of biochemical markers of myocardial necrosis with at least one of the following:
     a. Ischemic symptoms
     b. Development of pathologic Q waves on ECG
     c. ECG changes indicative ischemia (ST segment elevation or depression)
     d. Coronary artery intervention
   (2) Pathologic findings of an acute MI
**Criteria for established MI**
Any one of the following criteria satisfies the diagnosis for established MI:
   (1) Development of new pathological Q waves on serial ECGs.
   (2) Pathological findings of a healed or healing MI.

From Ref. 9

diographic pathological Q waves (Q-wave MI) occurs in the absence of timely reperfusion, indicating an established MI. On the other hand, NSTEMI is defined as the presence of myonecrosis (elevated troponin or creatine kinase myocardial band (CKMB) levels to > 99th percentile of reference controls) in the absence of ST-segment elevation [9,14]. Patients with either STEMI or NSTEMI can subsequently progress to either Q-wave MI or non–Q-wave MI (Figure 1).

## PATHOPHYSIOLOGY

### Supply–Demand Mismatch

The myocardial ischemia of unstable angina and MI, like all causes of tissue ischemia, results from excessive demand or inadequate supply of oxygen and nutrients. *Excess demand* from increased myocardial workload (heart rate-systolic pressure product) is responsible for nearly all cases of stable angina, approximately one-third of unstable angina episodes, and very rare cases of MI. For example, in Braunwald class I unstable angina, stable symptoms accelerate and become more intense, frequent, or easily provoked, and this heightened demand forces outstripping of the myocardial blood supply. Conversely, *inadequate supply* alone is responsible for few cases of stable angina, two-thirds of unstable angina episodes, and almost all MI. The etiology of the supply–demand mismatch can be further classified as primary or secondary. Primary causes of ischemia are from obstructive coronary lesions. Secondary causes are varied, extrinsic to the coronary arterial bed, and are more often seen in unstable angina than acute infarction. These precipitants of myocardial ischemia usually increase myocardial demands in the presence of underlying noncritical coronary artery stenoses. Table 4 lists common examples of secondary disorders which increase myocardial oxygen demand (e.g., fever, thyrotoxicosis, cocaine) or decrease oxygen supply (e.g., hypoxemia, anemia) and can lead to the transient ischemia of unstable angina or, rarely, infarction.

**Table 4**   Secondary Cause of Myocardial Ischemia

Increase Myocardial Oxygen Demand
  Fever
  Tachyarrhythmias
  Malignant hypertension
  Thyrotoxicosis
  Pheochromocytoma
  Cocaine
  Amphetamines
  Aortic stenosis
  Supravalvular aortic stenosis
  Obstructive cardiomyopathy
  Aortovenous shunts
  High output states
  Congestive failure
Decreased oxygen supply
  Anemia
  Hypoxemia
  Polycythemia

*Source*: Adapted from Ref. 46.

## Plaque Disruption

Braunwald class II and III unstable angina and nearly all cases of myocardial infarction are the result of reduction in coronary arterial perfusion associated with atherosclerotic plaque disruption and thrombosis. Atherosclerotic plaques that are prone to rupture (i.e., vulnerable plaques) typically have large lipid cores, thin fibromuscular collagen cap, low smooth muscle cell density, abundant inflammatory infiltrate, high macrophage density, and high concentrations of matrix metalloproteinases and tissue factor (see Chapter 5). As the lipid-rich plaque grows, production of macrophage proteases [15] and neutrophil elastases [16] within the plaque cause thinning of the overlying fibromuscular cap. This, in combination with circumferential wall stress and blood flow shear stress, can lead to endothelial erosion, plaque fissuring, or plaque rupture, especially at the junction of the cap and the vessel wall (Chapter 3). The extent of plaque disruption occurs over a spectrum, with endothelial erosion and most minor fissuring being occult and moderate-to-large disruptions leading to acute infarction. Minor plaque ulceration with relatively small areas of exposed subendothelium explains some cases of unstable angina. Because the area of damage is limited, coronary flow remains brisk, accumulation of thrombus does not occur, and the lesion heals uneventfully (Figure 2). Falk and others have histologically [17] and angiographically [18] demonstrated that coronary stenoses of unstable angina are the result of repeated episodes of plaque ulceration and healing with a resultant gradual increase in plaque volume. During vessel wall repair, the lesion may increase its fibrous content (thrombus organization) thereby limiting the extent of future disruptions.

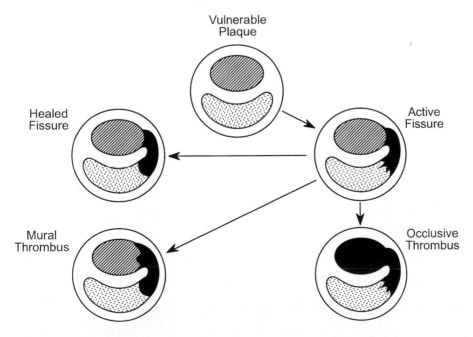

**Figure 2**  Schematic diagram of an atherosclerotic plaque rupture. Several outcomes follow plaque rupture including uneventful healing if the fissure is small and no clinically siginficant thrombus forms. If plaque rupture is extensive or the thromus formed is significant, partial or transient vessel occlusion may occur with resultant unstable angina or non–Q-wave myocardial infarction. If complete occlusion occurs and remains present, myocardial necrosis may occur leading to Q-wave myocardial infarction.

In contrast, in acute MI the extent of plaque disruption is larger, thrombus accumulation is occlusive, and tissue infarction results. In several reports of acute MI, the underlying plaque was found to be immature, i.e., a recently developed, soft underlying stenosis of only mild to moderate lumen diameter narrowing (approximately 70% of lesions had < 50% diameter stenosis prior to rupture) [19]. Unfortunately, these inflamed vulnerable atherosclerotic plaques that are prone to rupture causing clinical events, are not well distinguished by diagnostic angiography alone. For instance, coronary artery plaques prone to rupture tend to have positive remodeling, with larger lipid content and macrophage count [20], which would require intravascular ultrasound (IVUS) for detection during angiography. Whether or not vessel occlusion occurs depends on many factors, including the extent of vessel disruption, rheology of blood (vessel diameter, lesion geometry, and distal vasoconstriction), platelet aggregability, and the balance of endogenous hemostatic and thrombolytic factors.

*Inflammation*

Inflammation has recently been shown to play a pivotal role in the pathogenesis of atherosclerosis and ACS, having been linked to all stages of vulnerable plaque development, from lipid deposition to plaque rupture and thrombosis. Indeed, patients with ACS not only accumulate coronary arterial bed inflammatory infiltrates but also express systemic signs of inflammation, such as increased concentrations of acute phase reactants (e.g., C-reactive protein, serum amyloid A protein, fibrinogen) [21–23], proinflammatory cytokines (e.g., interleukin 1, 6 and 18, myeloperoxidase, tumor necrosis factor α) [24–27], adhesion molecules (e.g., intercellular adhesion molecule 1, P-selectin, E-selectin) [28–30], circulating matrix metalloproteinases [31,32], and circulating activated inflammatory cells (e.g., neutrophils, lymphocytes, monocytes). Patients with such high states of inflammatory stress have been shown to be at increased risk for future vascular events

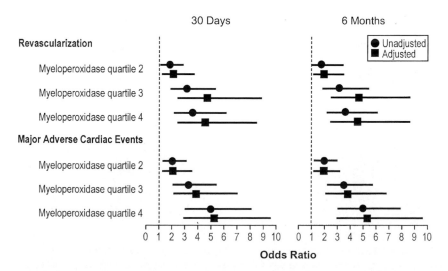

**Figure 3**   Odds ratio and 95% confidence interval of 30-days and 6-months revascularization and major adverse cardiac events (myocardial infarction, reinfarction, need for revascularization, or death) among patients with negative troponin T presenting with chest pain. (Adapted from Ref. 25)

[33]. For example, increased plasma levels of myeloperoxidase (secreted by activated leukocytes with inflammation) was recently shown to independently predict 30-day and 6-month major adverse cardiac events (MACE), irrespective of troponin levels, among 604 patients presenting with chest pain thought due to ACS [25]. Figure 3 shows the adjusted odds ratios of revascularization and MACE according to quartiles of myeloperoxidase levels in patients with persistently negative troponin T.

*Thrombosis*

The thrombotic process following plaque rupture is multistaged and begins with the exposure of subendothelial constituents such as collagen, von Willebrand factor (vWF), fibronectin, and vitronectin. These matrix components are recognized by platelet surface receptors (primarily glycoprotein [GP] Ib) and platelet attachment to the vessel wall (adhesion) occurs. As platelets adhere to the vessel wall, they become activated. During activation, platelets secrete a host of substances from their alpha-granules, which lead to vasoconstriction, chemotaxis, mitogenesis, and activation of neighboring platelets [34] (Figure 4). The released substances include thromboxane $A_2$, serotonin, fibrinogen, plaminogen activator

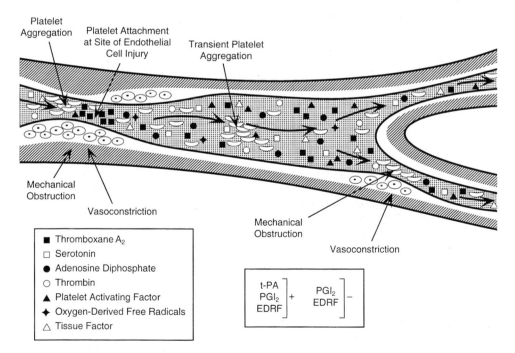

**Figure 4** Schematic diagram of mechanism underlying primary acute coronary syndromes. At the site of atherosclerotic plaque (anatomic obstruction) endothelial injury is present. This in combination with the release of vasoactive and platelet activating substances such as thromboxane A2, serotonin, thrombin, and adenosine diphosphate (ADP) causes a physiologic obstruction superimposed on the anatomic obstruction. Platelet activation and aggregation can occur as a result of these substances or in response to exposure of the subendothelial matrix following plaque fissuring or rupture. Platelets release additional vasoactive factors and fibrinogen which, in turn, leads to further vasoconstriction, platelet activation, thrombin formation, and potentially vessel obstruction. (From Ref. 44)

inhibitor (PAI-1), and growth factors. Platelet activation leads to the recruitment and "functionalization" of GPIIb/IIIa integrins or specialized surface receptors, which mediate aggregation (platelet–platelet binding). Aggregated platelets accelerate the production of thrombin by providing the surface for the binding of cofactors required for the conversion of prothrombin to thrombin. In a reciprocating fashion, thrombin is a potent agonist for further platelet activation and it stabilizes the thrombus by converting fibrinogen to fibrin. Sherman et al. [35] performed angioscopy in 10 patients with unstable angina. Distinctive intimal abnormalities were observed in all patients, 4 of whom had complex plaque morphology and 7 of whom had identifiable thrombus. Patients with accelerating symptoms had complex plaque morphology while those with rest angina consistently had intracoronary thrombus. In contrast to the nonocclusive thrombus of unstable angina, the thrombus associated with MI is transiently or persistently occlusive. Depending on the extent and duration of occlusion, the presence of collateral vessels, and the area of myocardium perfused, non–Q-wave or Q-wave infarction results. Infarction in the absence of atherothrombosis is rare and may be secondary to disorders such as those producing secondary unstable angina. In addition, unusual conditions such as nonthrombotic embolism, myocardial contusion, and aortic dissection, may lead to MI, as listed in Table 5.

   Since thrombus is believed to be responsible for the vast majority of ACS, several investigations have been performed to assess serologic factors associated with hemostasis and endogenous thrombolysis. For example, fibrinopeptide A (polypeptide fragment

**Table 5**   Causes of Myocardial Infarction Without Atherothrombosis

Nonatherosclerotic coronary arterial narrowing or compression
   Spasm (Prinzmetal's angina)
   Dissection of the aorta with coronary ostium compression
   Dissection of coronary artery
   Anomalous coronary artery origin
Emboli
   Endocarditis
   Atheroma or air associated with invasive coronary artery procedures
   Cardiac myxoma
   Thromboembolism from prosthetic valve
   Thromboembolism from left atrium or ventricle
Excessive myocardial oxygen demand
   Aortic stenosis
   Aortic insufficiency
   Hypertrophic cardiomyopathy
   Thyrotoxicosis
   Cocaine or amphetamines
Inadequate myocardial oxygen supply
   Carbon monoxide poisoning
   Hypoxemia
   Anemia
   Sustained hypotension
Miscellaneous
   Chest wall or myocardial trauma
   Radiation-induced coronary fibrosis
   Arteritis

cleaved from fibrinogen when thrombin converts it to fibrin), prothrombin fragment 1 + 2, D-dimer, and PAI-1 levels are substantially elevated in patients with unstable angina compared with patients without ACS [36–40].

*Vasoconstriction and Cyclic Flow Variation*

Continuous monitoring in patients with unstable angina at rest has revealed that many first display a decrease in coronary sinus blood flow. This is followed by typical electrocardiographic changes of ischemia and then chest discomfort. Heart rate and systolic arterial pressure also may rise in response to chest pain [41,42]. These episodes of ischemia, as well as those documented by Holter monitoring [43], resolve minutes later and may recur cyclically during disease instability. Episodic platelet aggregation at the site of coronary stenoses have been shown to be responsible for the cyclic flow reduction and transient myocardial ischemia in animal models [44]. In short, most subjects with rest angina have recurrent, transient reduction in coronary blood supply secondary to vasoconstriction and thrombus formation at the site of atherosclerotic plaque rupture. These events occur as a complex interaction among the vascular wall, leukocytes, platelets, and atherogenic lipoproteins. Among patients with MI, these events may also occur as prodromal angina or during early recanalization of the infarct-related artery.

## THE CLINICAL SPECTRUM

### Epidemiology

Acute coronary syndromes are the leading causes of hospitalizations for adults in the United States. The incidence of unstable angina is increasing, and approximately 800,000 hospitalizations each year are due to unstable angina. A similar number of unstable angina episodes likely occur outside the hospital and are unrecognized or managed in the outpatient setting. With heightened public awareness, improved survival following acute MI, and an increasing proportion of the population being of advanced age, this number should continue to rise despite primary and secondary prevention measures. The incidence of MI is currently estimated at 650,000 annually in the United States, and approximately 250,000 people die annually of coronary heart disease before hospitalization [45]. Several studies have suggested that the incidence of unstable angina has steadily increased to exceed that of acute MI [46].

### Demographics

The demographics of ACS mainly reflect the risk factors associated with atherosclerosis. Most patients hospitalized are between 50 and 70 years-old, with patients having unstable angina being slightly older. Because the Global Use of Stratgies to Open Occluded Coronary Arteries (GUSTO) IIb study [47] simultaneously enrolled patients across the spectrum of ACS, its data are particularly relevant to assess the underlying demographics. Of the 12,142 patients enrolled in this study, the median ages for those with STEMI and no ST-segment elevation (patients with unstable angina or NSTEMI) were 63 and 66 years, respectively (Figure 5). Perhaps because females represent a greater percentage of the elderly population, they have a relatively greater presence in the ACS patients without STEMI. While men more commonly have ACS than women, the ratio of men to women with no ST-segment elevation (2:1) is lower than for patients with STEMI (3:1). Coronary artery disease (CAD) risk factors—hypertension, hypercholesterolemia, and tobacco

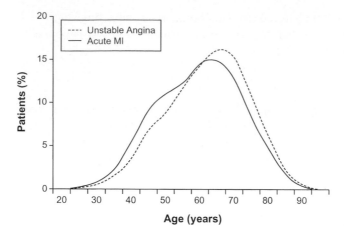

**Figure 5** Histogram of the age of patients enrolled in the Global Use of Strategies to Open Occluded Coronary Arteries (GUSTO) IIb study [47] separated by diagnosis of non–ST segment elevation (unstable angina and non–Q-wave myocardial infarction) or ST-segment elevation (Q-wave myocardial infarction). The median ages for those with acute myocardial infarction and unstable angina were 63 and 66 years, respectively.

use—are present in 30–40% of patients with an ACS, whereas diabetes is usually present in 15–20% (Table 6). Again, perhaps because of somewhat older age, those without STEMI are more likely to have diabetes, hypertension, and hypercholesterolemia compared to patients with STEMI. Finally, for several reasons, including more advanced age, more extensive CAD, and a higher representation of vessel reocclusion, patients without STEMI are more likely to have had a prior infarction or myocardial revacularization procedure.

## Physical and Laboratory Assessment

The key differentiations of unstable angina from NSTEMI and STEMI are based on electro-cardiographic and enzymatic evidence of myonecrosis. It is more difficult, often impossi-

**Table 6**  Baseline Characteristics of Patients with Acute Coronary Syndromes in GUSTO-IIb

| Characteristic | No ST-segment elevation (n = 8011) | ST-segment elevation (n = 4131) |
|---|---|---|
| Age (years) | 66 | 63 |
| Systolic blood pressure (mmHg) | 139 | 130 |
| Female gender (%) | 33 | 24 |
| Diabetes (%) | 19 | 16 |
| Hypertension (%) | 48 | 40 |
| Hypercholesterolemia (%) | 41 | 36 |
| Current smoker (%) | 27 | 41 |
| Prior myocardial infarction (%) | 32 | 17 |
| Prior CABG (%) | 12 | 5 |
| Prior PTCA (%) | 11 | 6 |

Data for continuous variables are median values. CABG=coronary artery bypasss grafting; PTCA=percutaneous transluminal coronary angioplasty.
From GUSTO-IIb: Ref. 29

ble, to differentiate these syndromes based on clinical presentations. Patients with unstable angina, by definition, present with new-onset chest pain, or chest pain that is more intense or more easily provoked compared to patients with stable angina (Table 1). Patients with acute MI may have pain or associated signs and symptoms (e.g. nausea, dyspnea, diaphoresis) of greater severity and longer duration than that of unstable angina, but they may be of similar hemodynamic stability. For example, in the GUSTO-IIb study, the proportion of patients in Killip class I, II, and III–IV (88%, 11%, and 1%, respectively) was identical for patients presenting with STEMI or no ST-segment elevation. Reasons for this lack of difference in Killip class may stem from the study's relatively homogeneous population shaped by the inclusion and exclusion criteria. Nonetheless, cardiogenic shock is infrequent among patients with unstable angina since substantial myonecrosis have not occurred, as opposed to patients with acute MI. The Killip classification is a well-established prognostic indicator for patients presenting with acute STEMI. A study by Khot et al. evaluated this classification in 26,090 patients with NSTEMI, and also found that higher Killip class was associated with higher mortality for NSTEMI patients at 30 days (2.8% class I, 8.8% class II, 14.4% class III/IV, $p < 0.001$) and 6 months (5.0% class I, 14.7% class II, 23.0% class III/IV, $p < 0.001$) [48].

Elevation of the ST-segment is interpreted as transmural myocardial ischemia, as opposed to subendocardial ischemia associated with ST-segment depression or T-wave inversion of unstable angina or NSTEMI. Interestingly, continuous electrocardiographic recordings by Holter monitoring in subjects with unstable angina reveal frequent episodes of ST-segment abnormalities without associated symptoms, (i.e., silent ischemia), and this may be related to cyclic flow variation in the culprit lesion. Gottlieb et al. [43] found that greater than 50% of unstable angina patients in the intensive care unit had silent ischemia during aggressive medical therapy, and this portended a worse prognosis. The recent development of more sensitive markers of myocardial-cell injury (Chapter 13), such as troponin I or T, has provided evidence of cell necrosis in some subjects with unstable angina [49,50]. Hamm et al. observed circulating cardiac troponin T, an intracellular contractile protein not normally found in blood, in 39% of subjects with acute angina at rest (Braunwald Class III). Among these subjects with detected troponin T, 30% manifested an MI (i.e., electrocardiographic changes and elevated levels of creatine kinase MB activity) days later. In contrast, no subject with accelerated (Class I) or subacute (Class II) unstable angina had detectable troponin T. These data nicely demonstrate the pathophysiological continuum of acute myocardial ischemia such that subjects with the most severe unstable angina have minimal but detectable myocardial-cell necrosis, thereby bordering the conventional definition of MI. The hallmark of unstable angina is unpredictability, but specific prognostic indicators, such as silent ischemia on Holter monitoring or detected circulating cardiac troponin, are helpful to stratify patients with unstable angina into groups who need early angiography and revascularization vs. conservative medical therapy.

Multiple studies have shown that troponin levels can be used to guide treatment strategies for unstable angina and NSTEMI, including both interventional (invasive or initially conservative) and antithrombotic (with low molecular-weight heparin and GPIIb/IIIa inhibitors) therapies. Table 7 describes the relative risks of clinical outcomes according to various treatment strategies, based on whether troponin levels are elevated or not. Six randomized trials showed that an early invasive treatment strategy reduces ischemic events compared to an initially conservative medical strategy [51–56], particularly among patients with positive troponin levels (see ''Antiplatelet'' section under ''Treatment and Outcomes''). This discrepancy in benefit was also demonstrated with the use of low molecular-

**Table 7**  Relative Risk of Clinical Outcomes According to Elevated or Nonelevated Troponin
Levels with Various Treatment Strategies

| Agent/Strategy | Comparisons | N | Endpoints | Troponin + ve | Troponin − ve | Relative Risk* | P value* |
|---|---|---|---|---|---|---|---|
| LMW heparin (59) | Enoxaparin | 359 | Death, MI, or UR at 14d | 21% | 9% | 0.53 | 0.007 |
|  | Heparin |  |  | 40% | 6% | 1.6 | NS |
| Glycoprotein IIb/IIa inhibitor (57,60,61) | Abciximab | 1265 | Death or MI at 6mth | 9.5% | 9.4% | 0.40 | 0.002 |
|  | Placebo |  |  | 23.9 | 7.5% | 1.3 | 0.47 |
|  | Tirofiban | 2222 | Death or MI at 30d | 4.3% | 5.7% | 0.33 | < 0.001 |
|  | Placebo |  |  | 13.0% | 4.9% | 1.2 | NS |
|  | Lamifiban | 1160 | Death, MI, or recurrent ischemia at 30d | 11.0% | 10.8% | 0.57 | 0.01 |
|  | Placebo |  |  | 19.4% | 11.2% | 0.96 | 0.86 |
| Invasive strategy (52) | Invasive | 2220 | Death, MI, or rehospitalization at 6mth | 14.8% | 16.7% | 0.61 | < 0.001 |
|  | Conservative |  |  | 24.2% | 14.8% | 1.12 | 0.46 |

* Relative risks and P values are given comparing enoxaparin vs. heparin, glycoprotein IIb/IIIa inhibtors
   vs. placebo, and invasive vs. conservative strategies. LMW, low molecular-weight; NS, nonsignificant; MI,
   myocardial infarction; UR, urgent revascularization.

weight heparin and GPIIb/IIIa inhibitors, whereby those with an elevated troponin level
benefited from these antithrombotic strategies, as opposed to no benefit when troponin
was not elevated [57–61].

## Coronary Anatomy

Angiographic studies in patients with unstable angina have differed greatly regarding the
observed presence and severity of coronary atherosclerosis, presence of thrombosis, and
lesion morphology. These inconsistencies are understandable when considering the diversity of patients falling under the definition of unstable angina, as well as when considering
the timing and limitations of angiography. Data from some series [62–64] suggest that
one, two, and three-vessel severe coronary stenoses occur in approximately 15, 35, and
50% of unstable angina patients, respectively. Compared to subjects with stable angina
or first MI, these data suggest more extensive CAD in patients with unstable angina.
Autopsy studies in patients with unstable angina support the finding from angiography
that these subjects have more extensive CAD [65] and eccentrically located stenoses [66]
compared to those with stable angina. In contrast, the Thrombolysis in Myocardial Infarction (TIMI) IIIA study [67] which evaluated the effects of thrombolytic therapy on culprit
lesions in subjects with ischemia at rest, found one-, two-, and three-vessel disease in
35%, 39%, and 26%, respectively. These data are more similar to those found in subjects
with chronic stable angina.

Thrombus has been frequently reported on coronary angiography among patients
with unstable angina. It is especially prevalent among those with rest angina within the
preceding 24 hours (> 50%) [68–70], but less so among those with remote chest pain
within the previous month (< 10%) [71]. The incidence of angiographic occlusive thrombus is more common in patients presenting with acute MI, both Q-wave [72] and non–
Q-wave [73] infarctions. DeWood et al. showed that total coronary occlusion was present
in 87% of patients within 4 hours of presentation of a Q-wave MI [72]. These and similar
studies have also shown the incidence of angiographically demonstrable thrombus to stead-

ily decrease in the hours to days following MI, remaining evident in 40–50% of subjects at 2 weeks. This is often due to spontaneous endogenous thrombolysis in some individuals, which, if occurring within minutes, can avoid myocardial-cell necrosis (unstable angina).

## Noninvasive Cardiac Assessment

In addition to routine 12-lead electrocardiography to discern the presence of previous infarction, ST-segment or T-wave abnormalities, the use of continuous electrocardiographic observation by Holter monitoring may also provide helpful information. Abnormal ST-segment shifts can be observed in roughly one-third of patients, depending on the criteria of ST-segment deviation, timing of monitoring relative to disease instability, and the intervening medical therapy. Exercise electrocardiographic testing is also helpful; among men, shorter exercise duration, lower maximal rate-pressure product, and exercise-induced angina or ST-segment depression have correlated with unfavorable outcome [74,75]. Table 8 describes the stress test parameters that have been shown to predict adverse outcomes and multivessel CAD [76]. In multivariable analysis, Wilcox et al. [77] found that predischarge exercise tests added independent prognostic information to known important clinical descriptors (e.g., recurrent rest pain and evolutionary T-wave changes). However, the positive predictive value for future ischemic events with routine exercise testing is low, even among patients with recent myocardial injury [78].

Nuclear scintigraphy, assessing regional myocardial perfusion using thallium$^{201}$, can be performed at rest, i.e., between anginal episodes, or in combination with physiologic or pharmacologic stress. Pooling data from several studies [79–83], the sensitivity of thallium$^{201}$ imaging at rest alone for the detection of severe coronary artery stenoses averages less than 60%. With the addition of dipyridamole, a pharmacologic "stress," thallium$^{201}$ imaging in patients with unstable angina increases sensitivity to 90% while maintaining a specificity of approximately 80% [84]. When present, perfusion defects can provide prognostic information; Wackers et al. [79] observed perfusion defects in 76% of subjects who had a complicated clinical course compared to 32% of those who had an uncomplicated outcome following an ACS. Assessing myocardial tissue metabolism with positron emission tomography (PET) using 5-fluordeoxyglucose in patients with unstable angina demonstrates increased glucose consumption at rest compared to subjects with stable angina. This occurs in the absence of symptoms or electrocardiographic evidence of myocardial ischemia and also suggests a state of prolonged or chronic hypoperfusion.

**Table 8** Exercise Stress Test Parameters Associated with Adverse Prognosis

1. Duration of symptom-limiting exercise $< 6$ METs
2. Failure to increase systolic blood pressure $\geq 120$ mm Hg, or a sustained decrease $\geq 10$ mm Hg, or below rest levels, during progressive exercise
3. ST segment depression $\geq 2$ mm, downsloping ST segment, starting at $< 6$ METs, involving $\geq 5$ leads, persisting $\geq 5$ min into recovery
4. Exercise-induced ST segment elevation (aV$_r$ excluded)
5. Angina pectoris at low exercise workloads
6. Reproducible sustained ($> 30$ sec) or symptomatic ventricular tachycardia

From: Ref. 76.

Thus, nuclear myocardial studies can detect and localize severe coronary stenoses with a moderate to high sensitivity; however, a substantial percentage of subjects who have an untoward outcome may not be prospectively identified.

## Invasive Assessment

Since numerous studies have demonstrated that greater than or equal to 80% of subjects with unstable angina have important atherosclerotic CAD and that this percent is higher postinfarction, some physicians feel it is prudent to directly define the extent and severity of disease in these patients during index hospitalization. Indeed, among 1,457 consecutive hospital admissions with unstable angina in the GUARANTEE study [8] who underwent angiography, 82% had significant CAD. Other reasons cited for early angiographic assessment include evidence that roughly half of these subjects have left main or three-vessel CAD and may benefit from prompt surgical revascularization. These points, combined with an overall moderate positive predictive value of noninvasive assessments, suggest that a significant percentage of important coronary lesions may be initially unappreciated without angiography. Finally, a small percentage of patients presenting with unstable angina will have angiographically normal coronary arteries. For these patients and for those with minimal coronary arterial lesions following MI, their prognosis is very good. In large-scale studies such as GUSTO-IIb, GUARANTEE, and PURSUIT (Platelet Glycoprotein IIb/IIIa in Unstable Angina Receptor Suppression Using Integrilin Therapy) [8,47,85], approximately 60–80% of patients undergo coronary angiography during the initial hospitalization. This percentage is similar for those with unstable angina and acute MI.

## TREATMENT AND OUTCOME

### Medical Therapy

Since there is significant overlap in the pathophysiology of unstable angina and acute MI, there are many similarities in treatment strategies. As mentioned, the pathophysiologic cornerstone of unstable angina and acute MI is the formation of thrombus, which involves platelets and a number of plasma and tissue factors. Treatment of this thrombotic process, therefore, can be directed at platelets, thrombin, fibrin and other coagulation factors. The respective categories of therapy are: (a) antiplatelet agents (Chapters 17–19), such as aspirin, ticlopidine, and potent platelet GPIIb/IIIa inhibitors, (b) antithrombins (Chapter 21), such as heparin and hirudin, (c) fibrinolytic agents or plasminogen activators (Chapters 9 and 10), and (d) inhibitors of vitamin K-dependent coagulation proteins, such as warfarin. Since inhibitors of the vitamin K-dependent factors usually take days to become effective, they are not clinically important in the unstable phase of ACS. Rather, most patients presenting with unstable angina or infarction will receive a combination of rapid-acting anticoagulant therapies, such as intravenous heparin and oral aspirin.

### Antiplatelets

The benefit of aspirin, thienopyridines, and platelet GPIIb/IIIa inhibitors alone or in combination with heparin in the treatment of unstable angina has been proven in many randomized trials. Such trials of antiplatelet therapies in ACS are detailed in Chapters 18–20. In general, several observations can be made when assessing the relative benefit of antiplatelet therapies in the spectrum of ACS. Pooling data from over 2,000 patients with unstable angina using aspirin [86–89], the occurrence of infarction or death in the early weeks was reduced from 11.8% (control) to 6.0% (aspirin).

In the setting of an acute STEMI, aspirin was shown to reduce mortality by 23% in the Second International Study of Infarct Survival (ISIS-2) [90]. More recently, aspirin's role in achieving infarct-artery patency is suggested by a smaller study indicating that, when chewed, aspirin alone is taken in the hyperacute phase of an MI, stable reperfusion can be achieved in nearly 50% of patients, compared with 25% in controls [91]. The ability of aspirin to reduce the risk of recurrent cardiovascular complications in patients who have survived an MI has been studied in 8 trials involving nearly 16,000 patients [92]. Collectively, these 8 studies demonstrate a one-third reduction in the risk of nonfatal MI and a one-fourth decrease in the occurrence of MI, stroke, or vascular death. In brief, because of the platelet-centric etiology of most ACS, aspirin plays a fundamental role in both the treatment of unstable angina and acute MI.

Ticlopidine and clopidogrel (thienopyridines) also reduce secondary ischemic events of ACS [93,94]. Most recently, the CURE (Clopidogrel in Unstable angina to prevent Recurrent Events) trial showed that combining clopidogrel with aspirin reduced the composite endpoints of cardiovascular death, nonfatal MI, and stroke by 20% in over 12,000 patients with non–ST-elevation ACS, compared to aspirin alone [95]. The newest and most potent antiplatelet agents are the GPIIb/IIIa receptor inhibitors. These agents have become standard therapy in patients undergoing percutaneous coronary interventions (PCI) and as empirical therapy for ACS patients without ST elevation. The 6 main trials are: GUSTO-IV ACS, PRISM, PRISM-PLUS (PRISM in Patients Limited by Unstable Signs and Symptoms), PURSUIT, PARAGON-A (Platelet IIb/IIIa Antagonism for the Reduction of Acute Coronary Syndrome Events in a Global Organization Network), and PARAGON-B [96–100]. In a meta-analysis of these 6 trials by Boersma et al., a small reduction in death or MI was observed with a GPIIb/IIIa antagonist (11.8% compared with 10.8% with placebo, $p = 0.015$) [101]. The relative treatment benefit was similar irrespective of baseline characteristics, except the female subgroup. Data from GPIIb/IIIa antagonists PCI trials also showed similar results with enhanced benefit in those presenting with ACS. Pooled data from the EPIC, EPILOG, and EPISTENT trials similarly showed reduction in 1 year death or MI rates in 3,478 ACS patients with abciximab (6.7% compared with 13.3% for placebo) [102]. Importantly, several posthoc analyses have shown that patients most likely to receive benefit are those with NSTEMI at presentation (elevated troponin levels) as compared to those with unstable angina (no evidence for myocardial necrosis at entry). For example, in PRISM there was no reduction in the 30-day death or MI composite by tirofiban among those who were troponin-I negative (heparin 4.9% vs. tirofiban 5.7%). In contrast, those who were troponin-I positive had a 67% reduction in 30-day events with tirofiban (13.0% vs. 4.3%, $p < 0.001$) (Figure 6 and Table 7) [60].

In the setting of STEMI, several phase II studies have been completed using adjunctive GPIIb/IIIa antagonists with fibrinolytic therapy (Thrombolysis and Angioplasty in Myocardial Infarction [TAMI] 8 103, Integrilin to manage platelet aggregation to prevent coronary thrombosis in acute myocardial infarction [IMPACT-AMI] 104, and platelet aggregation receptor antagonist dose investigation for reperfusion gain in myocardial infarction [PARADIGM] 105 studies), which showed the combination of GPIIb/IIIa antagonists to thrombolytic strategies to be feasible and safe. Each also showed promise for the improvement of myocardial reperfusion, but alone or in combination, there was no demonstration of a reduction in 30-day mortality. The strategies for patency enhancement in the emergency department (SPEED) [106] and thrombolysis in myocardial infarction (TIMI) 14A [107] studies randomized patients to abciximab alone, fibrinolytic alone, or the combination of abciximab with reduced-dose fibrinolytic therapy to assess 60 to 90-

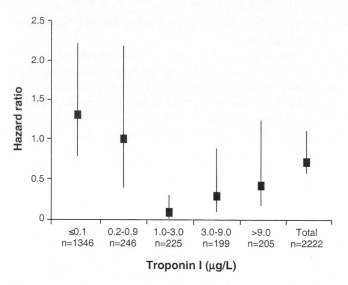

**Figure 6**  Adjusted hazard ratios (decrease 30-day death or MI) and 95% confidence intervals for treatment with tirofiban by troponin quartiles. Hazard ratios below 1.0 favor treatment with tirofiban. (From Ref. 60)

minute TIMI grade flow. The INTRO-AMI (Integrilin and low-dose Thrombolysis in Acute Myocardial Infarction) [108] was performed similarly using eptifibatide and reduced-dose t-PA. Collectively, these studies show an approximately 15% absolute increase in 60 to 90-minute TIMI-3 flow (55% in the fibrinolytic alone group vs. 70% in the abciximab plus *reduced-dose* fibrinolytic groups).

*Antithrombins*

Heparin is a mucopolysaccharide that inhibits thrombin via the heparin–antithrombin complex, which increases antithrombin activity several thousand fold. Clinically, many trials have been performed using heparin in unstable angina and in conjunction with thrombolytic therapy for acute MI. These trials are detailed in Chapter 21. Oler and colleagues performed a meta-analysis of 6 trials with over 1,300 patients who were treated with heparin activated partial thromboplastin time ([aPTT] 1.5–2x control) in addition to 75 to 650 mg aspirin per day for patients with unstable angina. With the addition of heparin, there was a trend (p = 0.06) for a lower rate of the composite of death or MI during inpatient therapy (relative risk = 0.67), though this was lost at follow-up weeks to months later (relative risk = 0.82) [109]. When more potent antiplatelet therapy is utilized, such as the GPIIb/IIIa inhibitors studied in PARAGON and PRISM, the modest benefit of heparin therapy is likely to be further attenuated.

      The antithrombin effect of heparin is lost when thrombin is bound to fibrin or the endothelium; as well, heparin can be inactivated by platelet factor 4 and heparinases. Low-molecular-weight heparins (LMWH) have more inhibitory activity against factor Xa and are less inactivated by platelet factor 4. New antithrombins, such as hirudin and hirulog (bivalirudin) differ from heparin in that they are effective against free, as well as bound thrombin and they do not require antithrombin as a cofactor. Both LMWH and hirudin have been studied in ACS and shown to be effective. Examples include the efficacy and safety of subcutaneous enoxaparin in non–Q-wave coronary events (ESSENCE) study [110], which randomized 3,171 patients with unstable angina or non–Q-wave MI to

LMWH (enoxaparin) or unfractionated heparin for 2 to 8 days. At 30-day follow-up, the rate of death, (re)infarction, and recurrent ischemia was reduced 15% (23.3% to 19.8%, p = 0.017) by enoxaparin. The rate of death or (re)infarction was reduced 20% (p = 0.081). Similar to the IIb/IIIa inhibitor studies of unstable angina, patients in these LMWH trials who were troponin positive appear to derive particular benefit (Table 7). At 40-day follow-up in the fragmin in unstable coronary artery disease (FRISC) study, dalteparin reduced the incidence of death or MI by 48% as compared with placebo among patients who were troponin positive. For patients who were troponin negative, no reduction in events was seen (4.7% placebo vs. 5.7% dalteparin) [111]. Similarly, when hirudin was compared to heparin for all ACS in the GUSTO-IIb study among 12,142 patients, the rate of death or (re)infarction was slightly reduced (9.8% to 8.9%, OR = 0.89, p = 0.058) [112]. In the organization to assess strategies for ischemic syndromes (OASIS) II trial, the use of recombinant hirudin (lepirudin) in patients with unstable angina and NSTEMI was associated with a trend to lower primary endpoint of death or MI at 7 days (3.6% hirudin vs. 4.2% heparin, p = 0.077) [113]. An upcoming trial, the ACUITY (Acute Catheterization and Urgent Intervention Triage StrategY) trial, will evaluate the use of bivalirudin in approximately 13,800 patients with ACS.

In summary, the similarly important benefit provided to the outcome of unstable angina, non–Q-wave, and Q-wave MI by antiplatelet and antithrombin therapies cements the common underlying pathophysiology and acute pharmacologic management. On the other hand, the spectrum of disease acuity and the importance of underlying thrombus are evidenced by those studies showing that most of the benefit of potent antiplatelet and antithrombin therapy is extended to patients who are troponin positive.

*Fibrinolytic Therapy*

Since coronary thrombus formation is known to be pathophysiologically responsible for unstable angina, as it is in MI, fibrinolysis for unstable angina seems intuitive. The earliest trials of fibrinolytic agents in unstable angina were without control populations and demonstrated little benefit. These were followed by angiographic trials of intracoronary thrombolysis in ACS and revealed angiographic improvement; however, without substantial clinical benefit. A number of placebo-controlled trials have been performed with intravenous thrombolytic agents used in conjunction with aspirin and heparin [114–127]. The results from these trials, assessing the incidence of nonfatal infarctions and death, vary substantially. Three of the four largest trials did observe a tendency for more nonfatal infarctions among subjects receiving thrombolytic therapy. While none of these differences was strongly powered, a formal meta-analysis [128] of nearly 2,500 patients demonstrated a paradoxically higher (p < 0.05) rate of nonfatal infarction or the combination of death and infarction (12.4% vs. 11.0%) among subjects receiving thrombolysis. The risk of major bleeding events was also higher among patients receiving thrombolytic therapy.

The worsened outcomes for unstable angina patients receiving thrombolysis are in striking contrast to patients with acute MI who gain unarguable survival benefit from thrombolytic therapy. These points are evidenced by data from the Fibrinolytic Therapy Trialists' Collaborative Group [129]. This study group combined nine large-scale international thrombolytic trials, reporting data from 58,600 patients treated with thrombolytic therapy, including 32,346 with ST-segment elevation and 4,237 with ST-segment depression. Whereas those with ST-segment elevation had a 19% higher survival rate if treated with thrombolytic therapy, there was a 10% lower survival rate among those with ST-segment depression receiving thrombolysis compared to placebo. This translated into 14 excess deaths per 1,000 ST-segment depression patients treated. Not surprisingly there was also an excess of serious bleeding events and stroke among those receiving thrombo-lytic therapy. In short, among the many areas of similar pharmacologic therapies for treatment of ACS, thrombolytic therapy is a clear exception and should be reserved for patients with ST-segment elevation or bundle-branch morphology.

*Antianginals*

The obvious goal of antianginal therapy is to reverse the oxygen supply–demand mismatch by minimizing requirements and maximizing delivery of tissue nutrients. Secondary pre-cipitants (such as anemia and hypoxemia) should be corrected. Nitrates, the century-old category of antianginals, remain a therapeutic mainstay for patients with ACS. A recent study of platelet function in whole blood found intravenous nitroglycerin to inhibit aggrega-tion, an effect that was substantial and rapidly reversible [130]. Other possible beneficial effects of nitroglycerin include an increase in coronary collateral blood flow [131] and a favorable redistribution of regional flow [132]. Important caveats to nitrate therapy include rapid (< 24 hour) development of drug tolerance with continuous therapy (i.e., without a nitrate-free interval) and reported induction of heparin resistance [133,134].

Beta-adrenergic blocking agents serve a number of important roles in the treatment of myocardial ischemia. Their main function, blocking adrenergic receptors, serves to blunt heart rate increases that occur in response to physical exertion, chest pain, or as a reflex to vasodilators. In addition, beta-blockers decrease blood pressure and myocardial contractility, each thereby lowering myocardial oxygen demands. Clinical trials of beta-adrenoreceptor blockers in the setting of stable and unstable angina have shown decreases in both ischemic symptoms and occurrence of MI [135]. Another potential benefit of beta-adrenergic blocking agents is inhibition of platelet aggregation, which has been observed in several in vitro studies [136,137]. Beta-blockers, alone or in combination with other agents, have been shown to reduce the relative risk of MI by 10–15% [138,139]. Infrequent situations of angina where beta-blocker therapy should be avoided include nonischemic exacerbation of heart failure, cocaine-induced coronary vasoconstriction [140], and vaso-spastic angina [141]. Beta-blockers should be used cautiously or avoided in those suscepti-ble to reactive (bronchospastic) airway disease. Cardioselective beta-blockers, such as metoprolol and atenolol, are preferred to the nonselective beta-blockers because they pro-duce fewer unwanted (noncardiac) effects.

Calcium channel antagonists are effective in lowering blood pressure and decreasing chest pain frequency among patients with stable angina. They are generally considered safe, provided there is no important systolic ventricular dysfunction or reflex tachycardia. The use of short-acting calcium channel antagonists in the treatment of unstable angina has produced mixed results and should be avoided as first-line agents. By partially blocking the flux of calcium ions into muscle cells, calcium channel blockers cause relaxation of vascular smooth muscle and the myocardium. Like other vasodilators, these effects intui-tively decrease myocardial oxygen consumption. The Holland interuniversity nifedipine/metoprolol trial (HINT) [135] was a double-blind, placebo-controlled, randomized study of medical therapies in 515 subjects with unstable angina. Among subjects receiving nifedipine without pretreatment or concomitant beta-blocker therapy, the event ratio of recurrent ischemia or infarction was 1.15 relative to placebo. When nifedipine was used in combination with metoprolol or initiated among patients already receiving beta-blockade, respective cardiac event ratios were 0.80 and 0.68 compared to placebo. Diltiazem, on the other hand, was shown to be equally effective to propranolol in reducing episodes of symptomatic ischemia and produced a similar long-term outcome regarding cardiovascular events [142]. The newest calcium channel antagonists, nicardipine and amlodipine, reportedly have minimal to no cardiodcprcssant or chronotropic effects, so that they can be used safely in combination with beta-blockers or used in patients with known chronic heart failure [143].

Because patients with acute MI often have more ischemia, they are more likely to receive a fuller or more aggressive antianginal regimen. For example, in the GUSTO-IIb study, nearly all patients were treated with beta-blockers, though patients with MI were more likely to receive them intravenously (25% vs. 13%) [112]. Patients suffering infarction are also more likely to receive angiotensin-converting enzyme inhibtors to reduce afterload and favorably affect ventricular remodeling. In summary, nitrates, beta-adrenergic antagonists, and calcium channel blockers are each able to lower myocardial oxygen demands, weakly inhibit platelet aggregation, and reduce the frequency of chest pain in stable and ACS. Although, nifedipine monotherapy should be avoided because it appears to increase the risk of nonfatal MI in the early hours of angina instability, likely due to reflex sympathetic stimulation.

## Invasive Procedures

The proportion of patients with unstable angina or MI who undergo cardiac catheterization is similar, approximately 40% undergo coronary revascularization in the days to weeks following presentation. However, patients with acute MI are more likely to undergo PCI, whereas those with unstable angina undergo PCI and surgical revascularization with a similar frequency. Nine randomized trials have compared an early invasive vs. an initially conservative medical strategy of managing ACS without STEMI, the most recent 6 trials demonstrated benefit with the routine invasive strategy [51–56], especially among patients with positive troponin levels (Table 7). In the Treat Angina with Aggrastat and determine Cost of Therapy with a Invasive or Conservative Strategy (TACTICS) TIMI-18 trial, 2,220 patients with unstable angina or NSTEMI who had ST-segment depression or T wave inversion, positive cardiac enzymes, or history of CAD, were randomized to an early invasive or a more conservative strategy [52]. All patients received aspirin, heparin, and tirofiban. At 6 months, the primary composite endpoint of death, MI, or rehospitalization for ACS was reduced significantly with the invasive group (15.9% vs. 19.4% conservative, odds ratio = 0.78, p = 0.025). However, this benefit was confined to those with troponin T greater than 0.01 ng/mL (14.8% invasive vs. 24.2% conservative, odds ratio = 0.55, p < 0.001), with no overt benefit when troponin T was less than or equal to 0.01 ng/mL (16.7% invasive vs. 14.8% conservative, odds ratio = 1.15; p = 0.46). Similarly, in the FRISC II trial, which randomized 2,457 patients with unstable coronary syndromes to invasive or conservative strategies, the reduction of death and MI was more significant among those with elevated troponin T levels (> 0.01 ng/mL) (risk ratio 0.7, 95% confidence interval 0.53 to 0.93) compared with nonelevated troponin T levels (risk ratio 0.77; 95% confidence interval 0.54 to 1.11) [51].

## OUTCOME

### Bleeding and Stroke Events

Severe bleeding, usually defined as greater than 5 g of hemoglobin loss or bleeding that results in hemodynamic compromise, occurs in a relatively low frequency (1–1.5%) in both patients with unstable angina and MI. Transfusions are required in 5–10% of hospitalized patients with ACS. Among patients with electrocardiographic evidence of ischemia at rest, either Braunwald class II–III unstable angina or acute MI, transfusions are consistently used in approximately 10% of patients [47]. The incidence of all strokes (hemorrhagic and nonhemorrhagic) is roughly similar among the acute coronary syndromes. Patients with acute infarction are more likely to receive thrombolytic therapy, which is associated with a higher risk of hemorrhagic stroke. On the other hand, patients with unstable angina are more likely to be elderly and have slightly higher systolic blood pressure, which are also known risk factors for intracranial hemorrhage. Thus, the incidence of all strokes is between 0.7 to 1.2%, with a slight preponderance among those with MI due to hemorrhagic events.

### Death and (Re)infarction

In the late 1980s, studies reported the incidence of MI in the early weeks following non–ST-elevation ACS to be approximately 10% and the incidence of death 4%. The TIMI-IIIB investigators in the early 1990s [126] reported a 6-week nonfatal MI incidence of 5.4% and death of 2.4%. Similarly, the overall rate of death or MI at 30 days in GUSTO-IIb was 9.4% and the rate of stroke was 1% [47]. More recent ACS studies (with strict guidelines for monitoring creatine-kinase (CK) elevations, definitions of MI, and blinded adjudication of events) report a 30-day composite of death or nonfatal MI of approximately 12% for medically treated patients [144]. With these important adverse cardiac events in mind, an assertive approach should be initially taken in all patients to ameliorate ongoing or recurrent myocardial ischemia. The outcome for unstable angina patients found to be troponin positive or with electrocardiographic ST-segment depression or T-wave inversion have an outcome similar to patients with acute infarction (Figure 7). Savonitto and colleagues [145] showed among the 12,142 GUSTO-IIb patients that the 30-day death or MI rate was 5.5% for those with T-wave inversion, 9.4% with ST-segment elevation, 10.5% with ST-segment depression, and 12.4% for those with ST-segment elevation and depression. Other predictors for long-term outcome for those with unstable angina include age, baseline hemodynamics, and underlying left ventricular systolic function. The most recent trial combining aggressive pharmacological and mechanical strategies for non–ST-elevation ACS, such as TACTICS-TIMI 18 [52], have halved the early rate of death or nonfatal

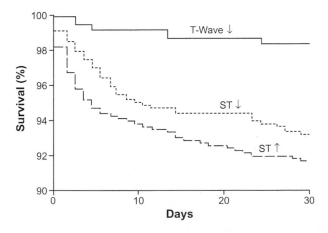

**Figure 7**  Correlation of 30-day mortality and electrocardiogram on presentation in the Global Use of Strategies to Open Occluded Coronary Arteries (GUSTO) IIa study. A dichotomous outcome for patients with unstable angina could be seen when separated according to the presenting electrocardiogram. Patients presenting with isolated T-wave inversion (T-wave↓) had a relatively low mortality. In contrast, patients with ST-segment depression (ST→) had a significantly worse outcome which paralleled that of patients with acute myocardial infarction (ST↓). (Data from Ref. 148)

**Table 9** Independent Predictors of 30-Day Adverse Ischemic Events* (Death or MI)

| Gusto-I | Gusto-IIb | Pursuit |
|---|---|---|
| Age | Age | Age |
| Systolic blood pressure | MI at enrollment | MI at enrollment |
| Killip class | Heart failure | Geographic region |
| Heart rate | ST-depression | ST-depression |
| MI location | Tachycardia | Female gender |
| Prior MI | Diabetes | Heart failure |

* 30-day outcome modeling from GUSTO-I (ST-elevation MI patients) are for independent predictors of death (data from Ref. 146); Outcome from both GUSTO-IIb and PURSUIT (non-ST-elevation patients) are independent predictors for death or (re)infarction at 30 days. These leading six predictors supply more than 90% of the independent predictive value for outcome. MI, myocardial infarction.
(Data from Ref. 47 and Ref. 85)

MI to approximately 6%. Likewise, for patients with acute STEMI, the 30-day mortality ranges from 4–8% depending on the initial strategy employed for perfusion restoration. The 30-day incidence of recurrent infarction is 5% and the risk of stroke is approximately 1%. Independent predictors of mortality and (re)infarction for patients with unstable angina and non–Q-wave MI, and predictors of mortality for patients with Q-wave MI [146], have been statistically determined and are compared in Table 9.

## CONCLUSION

In summary, the acute coronary syndromes (unstable angina, NSTEMI, and STEMI) belong to a continuum of myocardial ischemia with many similarities with respect to pathophysiology, diagnosis, and treatment. Among patients presenting with unstable angina and dynamic electrocardiographic changes, one-third will have subsequent evidence for myocardial necrosis, developing NSTEMI, and thus crossing the line into infarction. Despite many similarities, there are unique differences that distinguish unstable angina and MI. These include differences in response to thrombolytic therapy and clinical outcomes. Both electrocardiographic (the presence of ST elevation or depression, or T inversion) and biochemical findings help risk-stratify patients and guide the appropriate treatment strategy. Patients treated with a combined early approach of contemporary pharmacologic and mechanical reperfusion strategies have the best outcome. Novel research in inflammatory markers, genomics, antiplatelet, antithrombotic, and revascularization therapies are ongoing and will hopefully further improve the clinical outcomes of the spectrum of ACS.

## REFERENCES

1. Conti CR, Greene B, Pitt B et al. Coronary surgery in unstable angina pectoris. Circulation 1971;44(suppl II):II–154.
2. Fowler NO. ''Preinfarction angina: a need for an objective definition and for a controlled clinical trial of its management. Circulation 1971;44:755–758.
3. Wood P. Acute and subacute coronary insufficiency. Br Med J 1961(I):1779–1782.

4.  Vakil RJ. Preinfarction syndrome: Management and follow-up. Am J Cardiol 1964;14:55–63.
5.  Scanlon PJ, Ncmickas R, Moran JF, Talano JV, Amirparviz F, Pifarre R. Accelerated angina pectoris: Clinical hemodynamic, arteriographic, and therapeutic experience in 85 patients. Circulation 1973;47:19–26.
6.  Fuster V, Chesebro JH. Mechanisms of unstable angina. N Engl J Med 1986;315:1023–1024.
7.  Braunwald E. Unstable angina. A classification. Circulation 1989;80:410–414.
8.  Moliterno DJ, Aguirre FV, Cannon CP et al. The Global unstable angina registry and treatment evaluation. Circulation 1996;94:I.
9.  Myocardial infarction redefined—a consensus document of The Joint European Society of Cardiology/American College of Cardiology Committee for the redefinition of myocardial infarction. Eur Heart J 2000;21:1502–1513.
10. Ferguson JL, Beckett GJ, Stoddart M, Walker SW, Fox KA. Myocardial infarction redefined: the new ACC/ESC definition, based on cardiac troponin, increases the apparent incidence of infarction. Heart 2002;88:343–347.
11. Collinson PO, Rao AC, Canepa-Anson R, Joseph S. Impact of European Society of Cardiology/American College of Cardiology guidelines on diagnostic classification of patients with suspected acute coronary syndromes. Ann Clin Biochem 2003;40:156–160.
12. Meier MA, Al-Badr WH, Cooper JV et al. The new definition of myocardial infarction: diagnostic and prognostic implications in patients with acute coronary syndromes. Arch Intern Med 2002;162:1585–1589.
13. Trevelyan J, Needham EW, Smith SC, Mattu RK. Sources of diagnostic inaccuracy of conventional versus new diagnostic criteria for myocardial infarction in an unselected UK population with suspected cardiac chest pain, and investigation of independent prognostic variables. Heart 2003;89:1406–1410.
14. Braunwald E, Antman EM, Beasley JW et al. ACC/AHA guidelines for the management of patients with unstable angina and non-ST-segment elevation myocardial infarction. A report of the American College of Cardiology/American Heart Association Task Force on Practice Guidelines (Committee on the Management of Patients With Unstable Angina). J Am Coll Cardiol 2000;36:970–1062.
15. Aceti A, Taliani G, Bac C, Sebastiani A. Monocyte activation and increased procoagulant activity in unstable angina. Lancet 1990;336:1444–1446.
16. Dinerman JL, Mehta JL, Saldeen TGP et al. Increased neutrophil elastase release in unstable angina pectoris and acute myocardial infarction. J Am Coll Cardiol 1990;15:1559–1563.
17. Falk E. Unstable angina with fatal outcome: dynamic coronary thrombosis leading to infarction and/or sudden death. Circulation 1985;71:699–708.
18. Moise A, Théroux P, Taeymans Y et al. Unstable angina and progression of coronary atherosclerosis. N Engl J Med 1983;309:685–689.
19. Falk E, Shah P, Fuster V. Coronary plaque disruption. Circulation 1995;92:657–671.
20. Varnava AM, Mills PG, Davies MJ. Relationship between coronary artery remodeling and plaque vulnerability. Circulation 2002;105:939–943.
21. Haverkate F, Thompson SG, Pyke SD, Gallimore JR, Pepys MB. Production of C-reactive protein and risk of coronary events in stable and unstable angina. European Concerted Action on Thrombosis and Disabilities Angina Pectoris Study Group. Lancet 1997;349:462–466.
22. Ridker PM, Stampfer MJ, Rifai N. Novel risk factors for systemic atherosclerosis: a comparison of C-reactive protein, fibrinogen, homocysteine, lipoprotein(a), and standard cholesterol screening as predictors of peripheral arterial disease. Jama 2001;285:2481–2485.
23. Morrow DA, Rifai N, Antman EM et al. Serum amyloid A predicts early mortality in acute coronary syndromes: A TIMI 11A substudy. J Am Coll Cardiol 2000;35:358–362.
24. Biasucci LM, Liuzzo G, Fantuzzi G et al. Increasing levels of interleukin (IL)-1Ra and IL-6 during the first 2 days of hospitalization in unstable angina are associated with increased risk of in-hospital coronary events. Circulation 1999;99:2079–2084.
25. Brennan ML, Penn MS, Lente F et al. Prognostic value of myeloperoxidase in patients with chest pain. N Engl J Med 2003;349:1595–604.
26. Ridker P, Rifai N, Stampfer M et al. Plasma concentration of interleukin-6 and the risk of future myocardial infarction among apparently healthy men. Circulation 2000;101:1767–1772.

27. Blankenberg S, Luc G, Ducimetiere P et al. Interleukin-18 and the Risk of Coronary Heart Disease in European Men: The Prospective Epidemiological Study of Myocardial Infarction (PRIME). Circulation 2003;108:2453–2459.

28. Hwang S, Ballantyne C, Sharrett A et al. Circulating adhesion molecules VCAM-1, ICAM-1, and E-selectin in carotid atherosclerosis and incident coronary heart disease cases. The Atherosclerosis Risk Communities (ARIC) study. Circulation 1997;96:4219–4225.

29. Ridker PM, Hennekens CH, Roitman-Johnson B, Stampfer MJ, Allen J. Plasma concentration of soluble intercellular adhesion molecule 1 and risks of future myocardial infarction in apparently healthy men. Lancet 1998;351:88–92.

30. Ridker PM, Buring JE, Rifai N. Soluble P-selectin and the risk of future cardiovascular events. Circulation 2001;103:491–495.

31. Inokubo Y, Hanada H, Ishizaka H, Fukushi T, Kamada T, Okumura K. Plasma levels of matrix metalloproteinase-9 and tissue inhibitor of metalloproteinase-1 are increased in the coronary circulation in patients with acute coronary syndrome. Am Heart J 2001;141: 211–217.

32. Ikeda U, Shimada K. Matrix metalloproteinases and coronary artery diseases. Clin Cardiol 2003;26:55–59.

33. Libby P, Ridker PM, Maseri A. Inflammation and atherosclerosis. Circulation 2002;105: 1135–1143.

34. Coller BS. The role of platelets in arterial thrombosis and the rationale for blockade of platelet GP IIb/IIIa receptors as antithrombotic therapy. Eur Heart J 1995;16:11–15.

35. Sherman CT, Litvack F, Grundfest W et al. Coronary angioscopy in patients with unstable angina pectoris. N Engl J Med 1986;315:913–919.

36. Wilensky RL, Bourdillon P, Vix VA, Zeller JA. Intracoronary artery thrombus formation in unstable angina: a clinical, biochemical and angiographic correlation. J Am Coll Cardiol 1993;21:692–699.

37. Merlini PA, Bauer KA, Oltrona L et al. Persistent activation of coagulation mechanism in unstable angina and myocardial infarction. Circulation 1994;90:61–68.

38. Théroux P, Latour J, Leger-Gauthier C, DeLara J. Fibrinopeptide A and platelet factor levels in unstable angina pectoris. Circulation 1987;75:156–162.

39. Kruskal JB, Commerford PJ, Franks JJ, Kirsch RE. Fibrin and fibrinogen-related antigens in patients with stable and unstable coronary artery disease. N Engl J Med 1987;309:1361–1365.

40. Zalewski A, Shi Y, Nardone D et al. Evidence for reduced fibrinolytic activity in unstable angina at rest. Circulation 1991;83:1685–1691.

41. Chierchia S, Brunelli C, Simonetti I, Lazzari M, Maseri A. Sequence of events in angina at rest: primary reduction in coronary flow. Circulation 1980;61:759–768.

42. Davies GJ, Bencivelli W, Fragasso G et al. Sequence and magnitude of ventricular volume changes in painful and painless myocardial ischemia. Circulation 1988;78:310–319.

43. Gottlieb SO, Weisfeldt ML, Ouyang P, Mellits ED, Gerstenblith G. Silent ischemia as a marker for early unfavorable outcomes in patients with unstable angina. N Engl J Med 1986; 314:1214–1219.

44. Willerson JT, Golino P, Eidt J, Campbell WB, Buja LM. Specific platelet mediators and unstable coronary artery lesions experimental evidence and potential clinical implications. Circulation 1989;80:198–205.

45. American Heart Association. Heart Disease and Stroke Statistics—2003 Update. Dallas. Texas: American Heart Association, 2002.

46. Théroux P, Liddon R-M. Unstable angina: pathogenesis, diagnosis and treatment. Curr Prob Cardiol 1993;18:157–231.

47. The Global Use of Strategies to Open Occluded Coronary Arteries (GUSTO) IIb Investigators. A comparison of recombinant hirudin with heparin for the treatment of acute coronary syndromes. N Engl J Med 1996;335:775–782.

48. Khot UN, Jia G, Moliterno DJ et al. Prognostic importance of physical examination for heart failure in non-ST-elevation acute coronary syndromes: the enduring value of Killip classification. JAMA 2003;290:2174–2181.

49. Hamm C, Ravkilde J, Gerhardt W et al. The prognostic value of serum troponin T in unstable angina. N Engl J Med 1992;327:146–150.

50. Katus HA, Diederich KW, Hoberg E, Kubler W. Circulating cardiac myosin light chains in patients with angina at rest: identification of a high risk subgroup. J Am Coll Cardiol 1988; 11:487–493.

51. Wallentin L, Lagerqvist B, Husted S, Kontny F, Stahle E, Swahn E. Outcome at 1 year after an invasive compared with a non-invasive strategy in unstable coronary-artery disease: the FRISC II invasive randomised trial. FRISC II Investigators. Fast Revascularisation during Instability in Coronary artery disease. Lancet 2000;356:9–16.

52. Cannon CP, Weintraub WS, Demopoulos LA et al. Comparison of early invasive and conservative strategies in patients with unstable coronary syndromes treated with the glycoprotein IIb/IIIa inhibitor tirofiban. N Engl J Med 2001;344:1879–1887.

53. Michalis LK, Stroumbis CS, Pappas K et al. Treatment of refractory unstable angina in geographically isolated areas without cardiac surgery. Invasive versus conservative strategy (TRUCS study). Eur Heart J 2000;21:1954–1959.

54. Spacek R, Widimsky P, Straka Z et al. Value of first day angiography/angioplasty in evolving Non-ST segment elevation myocardial infarction: an open multicenter randomized trial. The VINO Study. Eur Heart J 2002;23:230–238.

55. Fox KA, Poole-Wilson PA, Henderson RA et al. Interventional versus conservative treatment for patients with unstable angina or non-ST-elevation myocardial infarction: the British Heart Foundation RITA 3 randomised trial. Randomized Intervention Trial of unstable Angina. Lancet 2002;360:743–751.

56. Neumann F. Intracoronary Stenting With Antithrombotic Regimen Cooling-Off ISAR-COOL) Study. Presented at the American Heart Association Scientific Sessions. Chicago, Nov 17–20, 2002.

57. Hamm CW, Heeschen C, Goldmann B et al. Benefit of abciximab in patients with refractory unstable angina in relation to serum troponin T levels. c7E3 Fab Antiplatelet Therapy in Unstable Refractory Angina (CAPTURE) Study Investigators. N Engl J Med 1999;340: 1623–1629.

58. Lindahl B, Venge P, Wallentin L. Troponin T identifies patients with unstable coronary artery disease who benefit from long-term antithrombotic protection. Fragmin in Unstable Coronary Artery Disease (FRISC) Study Group. J Am Coll Cardiol 1997;29:43–48.

59. Morrow DA, Antman EM, Tanasijevic M et al. Cardiac troponin I for stratification of early outcomes and the efficacy of enoxaparin in unstable angina: a TIMI-11B substudy. J Am Coll Cardiol 2000;36:1812–1817.

60. Heeschen C, Hamm CW, Goldmann B et al. Troponin concentrations for stratification of patients with acute coronary syndromes in relation to therapeutic efficacy of tirofiban. Lancet 1999;354:1757–1762.

61. Newby LK, Ohman EM, Christenson RH et al. Benefit of glycoprotein IIb/IIIa inhibition in patients with acute coronary syndromes and troponin t-positive status: the paragon-B troponin T substudy. Circulation 2001;103:2891–2896.

62. Luchi RJ, Scott SM, Deupree RH. and the Principal Investigators and Their Associates of Veterans Administration Cooperative Study No 28. Comparison of medical and surgical treatment for unstable angina pectoris. N Engl J Med 1987;316:977–984.

63. CASS Principal Investigators and their associates. Myocardial infarction and mortality in the Coronary Artery Surgery Study (CASS) randomized trial. N Engl J Med 1984;310:750–758.

64. Alison HW, Russell ROJ, Mantle JA, Kouchoukos NT, Moraski RE, Rackley CE. Coronary anatomy and arteriography in patients with unstable angina pectoris. Am J Cardiol 1978;41: 204–209.

65. Roberts W. Qualitative and quantitative comparison of amounts of narrowing by atherosclerotic plaques in the major epicardial coronary arteries at necropsy in sudden coronary death, transmural acute myocardial infarction, transmural healed myocardial infarction and unstable angina pectoris. Am J Cardiol 1989;64:324–328.

66. Saner GE, Gobel FL, Salomonowitz E et al. The disease-free wall in coronary atherosclerosis: Its relation to the degree of obstruction. J Am Coll Cardiol 1985;6:1096.

67. The TIMI IIIA Investigators. Early effects of tissue-type plasminogen activator added to conventional therapy on the culprit coronary lesion in patients presenting with ischemic cardiac pain at rest: results of the thrombolysis in myocardial ischemia (TIMI IIIA) Trial. Circulation 1993;87:38–52.

68. Freeman MR, Williams AE, Chisholm RJ, Armstrong PW. Intracoronary thrombus and complex morphology in unstable angina. Circulation 1989;80:17–23.

69. Capone G, Wolf NM, Meyer B, Meister SG. Frequency of intracoronary filling defects by angiography in angina pectoris at rest. Am J Cardiol 1985;56:403–406.

70. Gotoh K, Minamino T, Katoh O et al. The role of intracoronary thrombus in unstable angina: angiographic assessment and thrombolytic therapy during ongoing anginal attacks. Circulation 1988;77:526–534.

71. Vetrovec GW, Cowley MJ, Overton H, Richardson DW. Intracoronary thrombus in syndromes of unstable myocardial ischemia. Am Heart J 1981;102:1202.

72. De Wood MA, Spores J, Notske R et al. Prevalence of total coronary occlusion during the early hours of transmural myocardial infarction. N Engl J Med 1980;303:897–902.

73. DeWood MA, Stifter WF, Simpson CS et al. Coronary arteriographic findings soon after non-Q-wave myocardial infarction. N Engl J Med 1986;315:417–423.

74. Swahn E, Areskog M, Berglund U et al. Predictive importance of clinical findings and a predischarge exercise test in patients with suspected unstable coronary artery disease. Am J Cardiol 1987;59:208.

75. Butman SM, Olson HG, Butman LK. Early exercise testing after stabilization of unstable angina: correlation with coronary angiographic findings and subsequent cardiac events. Am Heart J 1986;111:11–18.

76. Chaitman B. Exercise Stress Testing In: Braunwald E, Ed. Heart Disease: A Textbook of Cardiovascular Medicine. 5th edition ed. Philadelphia: WB Saunders, 1997:162.

77. Wilcox I, Freedman B, Allman KC et al. Prognostic significance of a predischarge exercise test in risk stratification after unstable angina pectoris. J Am Coll Cardiol 1991;18:677–683.

78. Pitt B. Evaluation of the Postinfarct Patient. Circulation 1995;91:1855–1860.

79. Wackers FJT, Lie KI, Liem KL et al. Thallium-201 scintigraphy in unstable angina pectoris. Circulation 1978;57:738–741.

80. Brown KA, Okada RD, Boucher CA, Phillips HR, Strauss HW, Pohost GM. Serial thallium-201 imaging at rest in patients with unstable and stable angina pectoris: relationship of myocardial perfusion at rest to presenting clinical syndrome. Am Heart J 1983;106:70–77.

81. Berger BC, Watson DD, Burwell LR et al. Redistribution of thallium at rest in patients with stable and unstable angina and the effects of coronary artery bypass surgery. Circulation 1979;60:1114–1125.

82. Gerwitz H, Beller GA, Strauss HW ct al. Transient defects of resting thallium scans in patients with coronary artery disease. Circulation 1979;59:707–713.

83. Freeman MR, Chisholm RJ, Armstrong PW. Usefulness of exercise electrocardiography and thallium scintigraphy in unstable angina pectoris in predicting the extent and severity of coronary artery disease. Am J Cardiol 1988;62:1164–1170.

84. Zhu YY, Chung WS, Botvinick EH et al. Dipyridamole perfusion scintigraphy: the experience with its application in one hundred seventy patients with known or suspected unstable angina. Am Heart J 1991;121:33–43.

85. The PURSUIT Trial Investigators. Inhibition of platelet glycoprotein IIb/IIIa with eptifibatide in patients with acute coronary syndromes. N Engl J Med 1998;339:436–463.

86. Cairns JA, Gent M, Singer J et al. Aspirin, sulfinpyrazone, or both in unstable angina. N Engl J Med 1985;313:1369–1375.

87. Lewis HDJ, Davis JW, Archibald DG et al. Protective effects of aspirin against acute myocardial infarction and death in men with unstable angina. N Engl J Med 1983;309:396–403.

88. Théroux P, Ouimet H, McCans J et al. Aspirin, heparin, or both to treat acute unstable angina. N Engl J Med 1988;319:1105–1111.

89. Wallentin LC. the Research Group on Instability in Coronary Artery Disease in Southeast Sweden. Aspirin (75 mg/day) after an episode of unstable coronary artery disease: long-term

effects on the risk for myocardial infarction, occurrence of severe angina and the need for revascularization. J Am Coll Cardiol 1991;18:1587–1593.

90. ISIS-2 (Second International Study of Infarct Survival) Collaborative Group. Randomized trial of intravenous streptokinase, oral aspirin, both, or neither among 17,187 cases of suspected acute myocardial infarction; ISIS-2. Lancet 1988;II:349.

91. Freifeld A, Rabinowitz B, Kaplinsky E et al. Aspirin-induced reperfusion in acute myocardial infarction. J Am Coll Cardiol 1995:310A.

92. Antiplatelet Trialists' Collaboration. Collaborative overview of randomised trials of antiplatelet therapy - I. Prevention of death, myocardial infarction, and stroke by prolonged antiplatelet therapy in various categories of patients. Br Med J 1994;308:81–106.

93. Balsano F, Rizzon P, Violi F et al. Antiplatelet treatment with ticlopidine in unstable angina. A controlled multicenter clinical trial. Circulation 1990;82:17–26.

94. CAPRIE Steering Commitee. A randomised, blinded, trial of clopidogrel versus aspirin in patients at risk of ischaemic events (CAPRIE). Lancet 1996;348:1329–1339.

95. Yusuf S, Zhao F, Mehta S, Chrolavicius S, Tognoni G, Fox K. Effects of clopidogrel in addition to aspirin in patients with acute coronary syndrome without ST-segment elevation. N Engl J Med 2001;345:494–502.

96. The GUSTO-IV ACS Investigators. Effect of glycoprotein IIb/IIIa receptor blocker abciximab on outcome in patients with acute coronary syndromes without early coronary revascularisation: the GUSTO IV-ACS randomised trial. Lancet 2001;357:1915–1924.

97. The PRISM Investigators. A comparison of aspirin plus tirofiban with aspirin plus heparin for unstable angina. N Engl J Med 1998;338:1498–1505.

98. The PRISM-PLUS Investigators. Inhibition of the platelet glycoprotein IIb/IIIa receptor with tirofiban in unstable angina and non-Q-wave myocardial infarction. N Engl J Med 1998;338: 1488–1497.

99. The PURSUIT Investigators. Inhibition of platelet glycoprotein IIb/IIIa with eptifibitide in patients with acute coronary syndromes. N Engl J Med 1998;339:436–443.

100. The PARAGON Investigators. International, randomized, controlled trial of lamifiban (a platelet glycoprotein IIb/IIIa inhibitor), heparin, or both in unstable angina. Circulation 1998; 97:2386–2395.

101. Boersma E, Harrington R, Moliterno D et al. Platelet glycoprotein IIb/IIIa inhibitors in acute coronary syndromes: a meta-analysis of all major randomised clinical trials. Lancet 2002; 359:189–198.

102. Roe M, Gum P, Booth J et al. Consistent and durable reduction in death and myocardial infarction with abciximab during coronary intervention in acute coronary syndromes and stable angina. Circulation 1999;100:I–187.

103. Kleiman NS, Ohman EM, Califf RM et al. Profound inhibition of platelet aggregation with monoclonal antibody 7E3 Fab after thrombolytic therapy: Results of the Thrombolysis and Angioplasty in Myocardial Infarction (TAMI) 8 Pilot Study. J Am Coll Cardiol 1993;22: 381–389.

104. Ohman E, Kleinman N, Gacioch G et al. Combined accelerated tissue-plasminogen activator and glycoprotein IIb/IIIa integrin receptor blockade with Integrilin in acute myocardial infarction: results of a randomized, placebo-controlled, dose-ranging trial. Circulation 1997;95: 846–854.

105. Moliterno D, Harrington R, Califf R, Rapold H, Topol E. for the PARADIGM Investigators. Randomized, placebo-controlled study of Lamifiban with thrombolytic therapy for the treatment of acute myocardial infarction: rationale and design for the Platelet Aggregation Receptor Antagonist Dose Investigation and Reperfusion Gain in Myocardial Infarction (PARADIGM) study. J Thromb Thrombolysis 1996;2:165–169.

106. The Strategies for Patency Enhancement in the Emergency Department (SPEED) Group. Trial of abciximab with and without low-dose reteplase for acute myocardial infarction. Circulation 2000;101:2788–2794.

107. Antman EM, Giugliano RP, Gibson CM et al. Abciximab facilitates the rate and extent of thrombolysis: results of the thrombolysis in myocardial infarction (TIMI) 14 trial. Circulation 1999;99:2720–2732.

108. Brener SJ, Zeymer U, Adgey AA et al. Eptifibatide and low-dose tissue plasminogen activator in acute myocardial infarction: the integrilin and low-dose thrombolysis in acute myocardial infarction (INTRO AMI) trial. J Am Coll Cardiol 2002;39:377–386.

109. Oler A, Whooley MA, Oler J, Grady D. Adding heparin to aspirin reduces the incidence of myocardial infarction and death in patients with unstable angina: a meta-analysis. JAMA 1996;2276:811–815.

110. Cohen M, Demers C, Gurfinkel EP et al. A comparison of low-molecular-weight heparin with unfractionated heparin for unstable coronary artery disease. N Engl J Med 1997;337: 447–452.

111. Lindahl B, Venge P, Wallentin L. Troponin T identifies patients with unstable coronary artery disease who benefit from long-term antithrombotic protection. Fragmin in Unstable Coronary Artery Disease (FRISC) Study Group. J Am Coll Cardiol 1997;29:43–48.

112. Investigators GI. A comparison of recombinant hirudin with heparin for the treatment of acute coronary syndromes. The Global Use of Strategies to Open Occluded Coronary Arteries (GUSTO) IIb investigators. N Engl J Med 1996;335:775–782.

113. Effects of recombinant hirudin (lepirudin) compared with heparin on death, myocardial infarction, refractory angina, and revascularisation procedures in patients with acute myocardial ischaemia without ST elevation: a randomised trial. Organisation to Assess Strategies for Ischemic Syndromes (OASIS-2) Investigators. Lancet 1999;353:429–438.

114. Ardissino D, Barberis P, De Servi S et al. Recombinant tissue-type plasminogen activator followed by heparin compared with heparin alone for refractory unstable angina pectoris. Am J Cardiol 1990;66:910–914.

115. Bar F, Verheugt F, Materne P et al. Thrombolysis in patients with unstable angina improves the angiographic but not the clinical outcome: Results of UNASEM, a multicenter, randomized, placebo-controlled, clinical trial with anistreplase. Circulation 1992;86:131–137.

116. Charbonnier B, Bernadet P, Schiele F, Thery C, Bauters C. Intravenous thrombolysis by recombinant plasminogen activator (rt-PA) in unstable angina: a multicenter study versus placebo. Archives des Maladies du Couer des Vaisseaux 1992;85:1471–1477.

117. Freeman MR, Langer A, Wilson RF, Morgan CD, Armstrong PW. Thrombolysis in unstable angina. Randomized double-blind trial of t-PA and placebo. Circulation 1992;85:150–157.

118. Gold HK, Coller BS, Yasuda T et al. Rapid and sustained coronary artery recanalization with combined bolus injection of recombinant tissue-type plasminogen activator and monoclonal antiplatelet GP IIb/IIIa antibody in a canine preparation. Circulation 1988;77:670–677.

119. Karlsson J, Berglund U, Bjorkholm A et al. Thrombolysis with recombinant human tissue-type plasminogen activator during instability in coronary artery disease - effect on myocardial ischemia and need for coronary revascularization. Am Heart J 1992;124:1419–1426.

120. Neri Serneri G, Gensini GF, Poggesi L et al. Effect of heparin, aspirin, or alteplase in reduction of myocardial ischaemia in refractory unstable angina. Lancet 1990;335:615–618.

121. Nicklas J, Topol E, Kander N et al. Randomized, double-blind, placebo-controlled trial of tissue plasminogen activator in unstable angina. J Am Coll Cardiol 1989;13:434–441.

122. Roberts MJ, McNeil AJ, Dalzell GW et al. Double-blind randomized trial of alteplase versus placebo in patients with chest pain at rest. Eur Heart J 1993;14:1536–1542.

123. Saran RK, Bhandari K, Narain VS et al. Intravenous streptokinase in the management of a subset of patients with unstable angina: a randomized controlled trial. Int J Cardiol 1990;28: 209–213.

124. Schreiber T, Rizik D, White C et al. Randomized trial of thrombolysis versus heparin in unstable angina. Circulation 1992;86:1407–1414.

125. Scrutinio D, Biasco MG, Rizzon P. Thrombolysis in unstable angina: results of clinical studies. Am J Cardiol 1991;68:99B–104B.

126. The TIMI IIIB Investigators. Effects of tissue-type plasminogen activator and a comparison of early invasive and conservative strategies in unstable angina and non-Q-wave myocardial infarction: results of the TIMI IIIB trial. Circulation 1994;89:1545–1556.

127. Williams DO, Topol EJ, Califf RM et al. Intravenous recombinant tissue-type plasminogen activator in patients with unstable angina pectoris. Circulation 1990;82:376–383.

128. Moliterno D, Sapp S, Topol E. The paradoxical effect of thrombolytic therapy for unstable angina: meta-analysis. J Am Coll Cardiol 1994;23:288A.

129. Fibrinolytic Therapy Trialists' (FTT) Collaborative Group. Indications for fibrinolytic therapy in suspected acute myocardial infarction: collaborative overview of early mortality and major morbidity results from all randomised trials of more than 1000 patients. Lancet 1994;343: 311–322.

130. Diodati J, Theroux P, Latour JG, Lacoste L, Lam JYT, Waters D. Effects of nitroglycerin at therapeutic doses on platelet aggregation in unstable angina pectoris and acute myocardial infarction. Am J Cardiol 1990;66:683–688.

131. Cohen MV, Downey JM, Sonnenblick EH, Kirk ES. The effects of nitroglycerin on coronary collaterals and myocardial contractility. J Clin Investig 1973;52:2836–2847.

132. Bache RJ, Ball RM, Cobb FR, Rembert JC, Greenfield JC. Effects of nitroglycerin on transmural myocardial blood flow in the unanesthetized dog. J Clin Investig 1975;55:1219–1228.

133. Becker RC, Corrao JM, Bovill EG et al. Intravenous nitroglycerin-induced heparin resistance: a qualitative antithrombin III abnormality. Am Heart J 1990;119:1254–1261.

134. Habbab MA, Haft JI. Heparin resistance induced by intravenous nitroglycerin. Arch Intern Med 1987;147:857–860.

135. Lubsen J, Tijssen JGP. for the HINT Research Group. Efficacy of nifedipine and metoprolol in the treatment of unstable angina in the coronary care unit: findings from the Holland Interuniversity Nifedipine/Metoprolol Trial (HINT). Am J Cardiol 1987;60:18A–25A.

136. Gasser JA, Betterridge DJ. Comparison of the effects of carvedilol, propranolol, and verapamil on in vitro platelelt function in healthy volunteers. J Cardiovasc Pharmacol 1991;18(suppl 4):S29–S34.

137. Ondriasova E, Ondrias K, Stasko A, Nosal R, Csollei J. Comparison of the potency of five potential beta-adrenergic blocking drugs and eight calcium channel blockers to inhibit platelet aggregation and to perturb liposomal membranes prepared from platelet lipids. Physiol Res 1992;41:267–272.

138. Yusuf S, Wittes J, Friedman L. Overview of results of randomized trials in heart disease: II. Unstable angina, heart failure, primary prevention with aspirin, and risk factor modification. JAMA 1988;260:2259–2263.

139. Tijssen JG, Lubsen J. Early treatment of unstable angina with nifedipine and metoprolol—the HINT trial. J Cardiovasc Pharmacol 1988;12((Suppl 71)).

140. Lange RA, Cigarroa RG, Flores ED, Hillis LD. Potentiation of cocaine-induced coronary vasoconstriction by beta-adrenergic blockade. Ann Intern Med 1990;112:897–903.

141. Robertson RM, Wood AJJ, Vaughn WK et al. Exaccerbation of vasotonic angina pectoris by propranolol. Circulation 1982;65:281–285.

142. Théroux P, Taeymans Y, Morissette D, Bosch X, Pelletier GB, Waters DD. A randomized study comparing propranolol and diltiazem in the treatment of unstable angina. J Am Coll Cardiol 1985;5:717–722.

143. Packer M, O'Connor C, Ghali J et al. Effect of amlodipine on morbidity and mortality in severe chronic heart failure. N Engl J Med 1996;335:1107–1114.

144. Moliterno DJ, White HD. Unstable angina: PARAGON, PURSUIT, PRISM, and PRISM-PLUS. In: Lincoff AM, Topol EJ, Eds. Contemporary Cardiology: Platelet Glycoprotein IIb/IIIa Inhibitors in Cardiovascular Disease. Totowa. NJ: Humana Press, 1999:201–227.

145. Savonitto S, Ardissino D, Granger C et al. Prognostic value of the admission electrocardiogram in acute coronary syndromes. JAMA 1999;281:707–713.

146. Lee KL, Woddlief LH, Topol EJ et al. Predictors of 30-day mortality in the era of reperfusion for acute myocardial infarction. Results from an international trial of 41,021 patients. GUSTO-I Investigators. Circulation 1995;91:1659–1668.

147. Rogers WJ, Canto JG, Lambrew CT et al. Temporal trends in the treatment of over 1.5 million patients with myocardial infarction in the US from 1990 through 1999: the National Registry of Myocardial Infarction 1, 2 and 3. J Am Coll Cardiol 2000;36:2056–2063.

148. Moliterno D, Sgarbossa E, Armstrong P et al. A major dichotomy in unstable angina outcome: ST depression vs. T-wave inversion—GUSTO II results. J Am Coll Cardiol 1996;27:182A.

# 7

# Acute ST-Segment Elevation Myocardial Infarction: The Open Artery and Tissue Reperfusion

**Peter Sinnaeve and Frans Van de Werf**
*Gasthuisberg University Hospital*
*Leuven, Belgium*

## INTRODUCTION

Two considerations have had a tremendous impact on the modern management of ST-segment elevation acute myocardial infarction (STEMI). First, occlusive thrombosis superimposed on a ruptured plaque in an epicardial coronary artery was firmly established as the usual proximate cause of STEMI [1]. Coronary artery occlusion sets off a wave front of myocardial necrosis, spreading from endocardium to epicardium, with an inverse relation between the time to perfusion and the ultimate size and extent of transmurality of the infarct [2]. Transmural myocardial infarction, as opposed to subendocardial myocardial infarction, is characterized pathologically by necrosis involving not only the inner half but also significant amounts of the outer half of the ventricular wall, and electrocardiographically by the ST-segment elevation/Q-wave pattern. Secondly, restoration of coronary artery patency was found to correlate with survival. Recanalization can be achieved by pharmacologic dissolution of the coronary clot (fibrinolysis). Current fibrinolytic therapy consists of intravenous bolus administration of a plasminogen activator that dissolves the fibrin matrix of a thrombus. Alternatively, mechanical interventions within the occluded coronary artery may restore patency. Although the link between patency and survival is intuitively appealing and was firmly supported by laboratory animal experiments, only in the early 1990s did the Global Utilization of Streptokinase and TPA for Occluded Coronary Arteries (GUSTO) I study convincingly establish the "open-artery hypothesis" (Fig. 1).

## GUSTO-I AND THE OPEN ARTERY

The GUSTO-I trial enrolled 41,021 patients within 6 hours after the onset of STEMI to one of four different fibrinolytic regimens: streptokinase with either intravenous or subcutaneous heparin; front-loaded recombinant tissue-type plasminogen activator (rt-PA) with intravenous heparin; or a combination of streptokinase and rt-PA with intravenous heparin [3]. Before GUSTO-I, the open-artery hypothesis was challenged. Whereas earlier

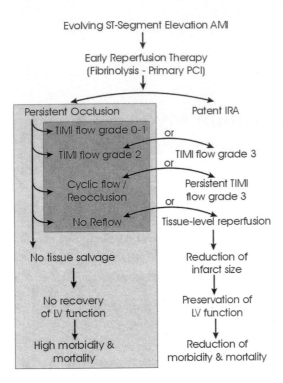

**Figure 1**  Reperfusion paradigm

patency studies demonstrated that rt-PA recanalized vessels more efficiently than streptokinase [4,5], no significant survival difference emerged from large-scale mortality trials,
such as the Gruppo Italiano per lo Studio della Streptochi-nasi nell'Infarto Miocardico
(GISSI) 2/International Study Group [6] and the Third International Study of Infarct Survival (ISIS-3) [7] trials, which compared rt-PA with streptokinase in patients with STEMI.

Two explanations for this apparent discrepancy were put forward: fibrinolytic agents
improve clinical outcome largely by mechanisms other than early coronary artery revascularization (implying that the open-artery hypothesis is not valid), or, alternatively, the
dosing of rt-PA in the GISSI-2/International Study Group [6] and ISIS-3 [7] trials was
suboptimal, thereby masking the superiority of this agent (implying that the open-artery
hypothesis still holds true). GUSTO-I was designed to solve this controversy. To explore
the relation between coronary artery patency status and clinical outcome, a subset of 2,431
patients was also evaluated angiographically [8]. Moreover, to optimize the frequency,
speed and durability or rt-PA-induced reperfusion, the administration of rt-PA was accelerated or "front-loaded," implying infusion of two-thirds of the dose over the first 30
minutes and of the total dose (maximally 100 mg) over 90 minutes instead of 3 hours [9],
and combined with immediate intravenous heparin [10].

As in most patency studies, angiographic characterization of coronary artery flow
in GUSTO-I relied on the scoring system introduced by the thrombolysis in myocardial
infarction (TIMI) study group (Table 1) [11]. The regimen inducing the greatest reperfusion
benefit at 90 minutes—i.e., accelerated or front-loaded rt-PA in conjunction with aspirin
and immediate intravenous heparin—also produced the greatest survival benefit: 30-day
mortality rates were 6.3% after accelerated rt-PA vs. 7.3% after streptokinase-only strategies (p = 0.001). The survival benefit with rt-PA was already apparent at 24 hours. TIMI

**Table 1**  TIMI Flow Grades

---

0  No penetration of contrast beyond point of obstruction
1  Contrast penetrates the point of obstruction but does not
   completely opacify the entire distal vessel
2  Complete contrast opacification of the infarct-related vessel
   but either contrast opacification or washout is delayed
3  Brisk, "normal" flow

---

flow grade 3 rates following accelerated rt-PA were significantly higher at 90 minutes than the streptokinase regimens (54% vs. 31%, $p < 0.001$), but not at 180 minutes (43% vs. 38%, $p = NS$) or later. The failure of this angiographic ''catch-up phenomenon'' by streptokinase to equalize survival rates indirectly underscores the relative importance of early reperfusion over late patency.

Figure 2 relates TIMI flow grades at 90 minutes to 30-day mortality in GUSTO-I. Mortality in patients with TIMI flow grade 2 at 90 minutes was not significantly different from the mortality with TIMI flow grades 0 or 1 at 90 minutes and approximately twice the mortality with TIMI flow grade 3. A meta-analysis of the GUSTO-I and four other angiographic studies elaborated these findings: the odds ratio for early mortality following TIMI flow grade 3 perfusion at 90 minutes 3 was 0.45 (95% Confidence Interval (CI) 0.34 to 0.61, $p < 0.0001$) vs. TIMI flow grade less than 3, and 0.54 (95% CI 0.37 to 0.78, $p = 0.001$) vs. TIMI flow grade 2 [12].

The 30-day mortality differences among the four fibrinolytic strategies compared in the main GUSTO-I trial (all 41,021 patients) could be predicted very accurately ($R^2$ = 0.92) from differences in 90-minute TIMI grade 3 flow rates in the angiographic substudy [13]. This close match between mortality differences predicted from early patency data and actual mortality supports the paradigm that early and complete coronary artery reperfusion is a critical mechanism underlying the life-saving potential of fibrinolytic therapy.

Patency of the infarct related artery (IRA) was also associated with longer-term benefits. Among the 12,864 patients enrolled in GUSTO-I who underwent coronary angi-

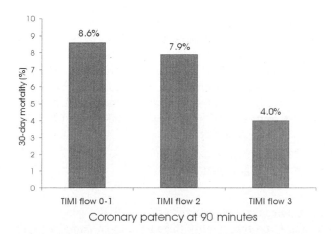

**Figure 2**  30-day mortality according to coronary patency at 90 minutes in GUSTO-I

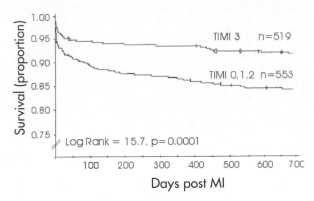

**Figure 3**  Two-year survival curves for patients with 90-minute thrombolysis in myocardial infarction (TIMI) flow. (Modified from Ref. 16)

ography and who had no previous mechanical or surgical intervention, one-year mortality was significantly lower in patients with patent IRA than patients with occluded IRA: 3.3% vs. 8.5% in medically treated patients; 2.5% vs. 8.5% in patients who underwent coronary artery bypass surgery [14]. The survival benefit of 1% of accelerated rt-PA over streptokinase observed after 30 days was unchanged at 1 year [15], and the survival benefit of early TIMI grade 3 flow, regardless of the lytic given, was amplified at 2 years (Figure 3) [16].

   Successful fibrinolysis also resulted in improved left ventricular function. Irrespective of treatment assignment, left ventricular ejection fraction at 90 minutes was significantly better in patients with than without TIMI grade 3 flow (62% vs. 55%, respectively, p < 0.001) [17]. The aforementioned meta-analysis confirmed the relation between early IRA patency and left ventricular (LV) function: acute and convalescent ejection fraction, regional wall motion, and risk of heart failure were each significantly better in patients achieving TIMI grade 3 flow than TIMI grade 2 or lower epicardial flow [12]. Although differences were small, patients treated with rt-PA in GUSTO-I had better preserved left ventricular function than patients given streptokinase [18]. Accordingly, cardiac complications associated with poor left ventricular function were less frequent in the rt-PA group, supporting previous observations in placebo-controlled trials of a lower cardiac morbidity in the fibrinolysis arm. Indeed, the incidence of major in-hospital events, including serious arrhythmias and congestive heart failure, is consistently lower with fibrinolytic regimens that result not only in better survival but also in less morbidity among survivors.

   Reocclusion eliminated the advantages of initially successful fibrinolysis. The 30-day mortality in patients with documented reocclusion in the angiographic substudy of GUSTO-I was 12%, compared with 1.1% in patients with early and persistently patent coronary arteries (p < 0.001) and 8.8% in those with initially occluded IRAs [19].

## PROMPT, COMPLETE, AND SUSTAINED CORONARY RECANALIZATION

GUSTO-I, thus, convincingly demonstrated that the potential of fibrinolytic agents to save myocardium and lives depends primarily on their ability to induce *early, complete,* and *sustained* coronary artery recanalization.

## Early Reperfusion

The benefits conferred by fibrinolytic therapy are clearly time-dependent. Even without fibrinolytic therapy, endogenous fibrinolysis assures high late-coronary artery patency rates (> 54% overall patency at 3 weeks) [20]. The rate by which infused plasminogen activators speed up this natural process determines their impact on morbidity and mortality. Although administering fibrinolytic agents up to 12 hours after the onset of symptoms may be beneficial in terms of outcome [21], every minute that reperfusion is postponed will inevitably entail more extensive necrosis. Early in the course of STEMI, the thrombus may be smaller and easier to lyse. In a meta-analysis, the proportional mortality reduction following fibrinolytic therapy was calculated to be 44% (95% CI 32%–53%) in patients treated within 2 hours vs. 20% (95% CI 15%–25%) in those treated later (p = 0.001) [22]. Also, treatment delay is associated with less successful ST-segment recovery and subsequent higher long-term mortality rates [23].

## Complete Reperfusion

Coronary reflow needs to be brisk to substantially improve prognosis. Conventionally, persistently occluded IRAs (comprising TIMI flow grades 0 and 1) were regarded as fibrinolytic failures, whereas patent IRAs (TIMI flow grades 2 and 3) denoted fibrinolytic successes. GUSTO-I and other studies demonstrated that TIMI grade 2 flow is associated with a clearly worse clinical outcome than TIMI grade 3 flow [13,24–27]. Irrespective of the question whether TIMI grade 2 flow is the cause or consequence of impaired tissue reperfusion, the immediate goal of coronary fibrinolysis should be the rapid and persistent restoration of TIMI grade 3 flow. Interestingly, 67% of patients in GUSTO-I with TIMI grade 2 flow at 90 minutes had improved to TIMI grade 3 flow at day 5 to 7. These patients had significantly better left ventricular function than patients with persistent TIMI grade 0, 1 or 2 flow [28].

Also, flow has been shown to be globally slower at 90 minutes after fibrinolysis, even in nonculprit coronary arteries [29,30]. A slower global flow is associated with adverse outcome [29]. Since flow recovery in nonculprit vessels is linked to that in the culprit artery [29], rapid and complete recanalization of the IRA and, hence, nonculprit vessels can have a global impact on preservation of LV function and ultimately improve outcome.

## Sustained Reperfusion

Angiographically documented acute coronary reocclusion occurs in 5 to 10% of patients, resulting in a significant deterioration of left ventricular function and a steep increase in in-hospital mortality [31]. Combined data from GUSTO-I and GUSTO-III indicate that patients with an in-hospital reinfarction have a three-fold higher risk of dying [32]. Although early reinfarction is also associated with higher long-term mortality rates, death seems to occur early [32,33], and can be, in part, prevented by instant reopening of the artery with refibrinolysis or mechanical revascularization [34]. Late reocclusions are also frequent, occurring in up to 20 to 30% of previously patent infarct-related vessels [35,36]. Rethrombosis may be mediated by the interaction of vasospasm, aggregating platelets, clot-bound thrombin, the thrombogenicity of partially lysed clot and ruptured atheroma, or the persistence of a flow-limiting stenosis and high shear stress. Paradoxical procoagulant and platelet-activating side effects of fibrinolytic agents might also trigger reocclusion, especially with fibrin-specific drugs [37]. Indeed, in a pooled analysis of 15 trials, accelerated rt-PA was associated with higher rates of reocclusion within 48 hours of administration compared to streptokinase (9.2% vs. 3.7% respectively) [38], underscoring the importance of antithrombotic cotherapy with fibrin-selective fibrinolytics.

## MARKERS FOR SUCCESSFUL REPERFUSION

### Epicardial Patency

The direct correlation between coronary artery patency and survival, derived from the open-artery theory, validates patency trials for assessing the clinical value of reperfusion strategies. Traditionally, TIMI flow at 60 or 90 minutes has been the primary end point of many trials. Yet, this evaluation carries possible flaws and some *caveats* must be considered [39,40]. Patency may have resulted from successful pharmacologic dissolution of the occlusive thrombus by the fibrinolytic drug, but may also have occurred spontaneously or may have been present before drug infusion. Recanalization (as opposed to patency) studies include a pretreatment angiogram to confirm baseline occlusion of the IRA. Forceful injection of contrast dye directly in the occluded IRA may mechanically promote recanalization in the absence of any pharmacologic dissolution of thrombus. Also, 60 or 90 minutes is an arbitrary time point and may be too late to appreciate the true efficacy of a fibrinolytic regimen in view of time-dependent benefits of fibrinolytic therapy.

As stated before, the angiographic definition of successful pharmacologic reperfusion has recently been narrowed: not overall patency (TIMI flow grades 2 and 3) but rather complete patency (TIMI flow grades 3) predicts improved clinical outcome. Moreover, the conventional categorical TIMI flow classification is hampered by high interobserver variability. TIMI frame counting has been advocated as a continuous, more reproducible, objective, and quantitative index of coronary reperfusion than conventional TIMI 3 flow grading [41]. TIMI frame count represents the number of cineframes needed for contrast dye to reach standardized distal coronary landmarks. The longer left anterior descending coronary artery TIMI frame counts are divided by 1.7 to correct for the disparities in vessel length between the left anterior descending artery and the circumflex or right coronary artery (corrected TIMI frame count). Only a third of patients with an open IRA (TIMI 2 or 3) at 90 minutes after fibrinolytic therapy were found to achieve flow truly within the normal range (corrected TIMI frame count < 28). TIMI frame counting has been validated and its relationship to major clinical end points after fibrinolysis has been established [39].

Studies suggest that IRA patency is a significant predictor of late survival independent of late ventricular function [42,43]. The finding that mortality benefits produced by fibrinolytics frequently exceeded their impact on systolic left ventricular function has evoked the postulation that even late recanalization may improve outcome by mechanisms other than myocardial salvage and infarct size reduction [44–46]. These mechanisms include enhanced provision of a conduit for augmentation of collateral flow [47,48], electrical stability [49–51], reduction of left ventricular wall stress and aneurysm formation, and attenuation of left ventricular remodeling and dilatation [52,53]. Acute reperfusion therapy has been shown to reduce ventricular volume, even beyond the time frame for myocardial salvage [54,55]. Also, in the late assessment of thrombolytic efficacy (LATE) study, patients treated between 6 and 12 hours after symptom onset had a significant 25% reduction in mortality [56]. Nevertheless, the relation between late opening, LV function, and outcome is less clear in randomized studies. In a Japanese study, late (> 24 hours) recanalization of the infarct-related artery was associated with improved LV function and long-term outcome [57]. In contrast, reopening an occluded left anterior descending coronary artery (LAD) three days to four weeks after a myocardial infarction was associated with a trend toward worsening LV function compared to conservative treatment in the open artery trial (TOAT) study [58]. Still, it is likely that late reopening of a proximal occlusion of a large coronary artery could be beneficial in selected patients, especially those with decreased LV function. This hypothesis is currently being tested in the Open Artery Trial (OAT) [59].

Furthermore, a single angiogram at 60 or 90 minutes only provides a snapshot, neglecting the dynamic process involved in the formation and dissolution of a coronary thrombus. Cyclic flow and frank reocclusion often follow initially successful recanalization. Angiographic trials sometimes incorporate an angiogram at 24 hours to assess (early) reocclusion. As mentioned earlier, late reocclusions occur frequently.

A final limitation concerns the invasive nature and the logistic challenge of the angiographic assessment of early coronary patency. Noninvasive and reliable reperfusion markers, readily available for routine use, have been validated. Despite these *caveats*, the frequency of inducing early and sustained coronary artery TIMI flow grade 3 remains a standard measure of reperfusion efficacy.

## Tissue Reperfusion

Patency of the large epicardial vessels does not equal reestablishment of tissue-level perfusion, the ultimate goal of any reperfusion strategy [40]. Studies on the coronary microcirculation with contrast echocardiography [60,61] and positron emission tomography (PET) [62,63] suggest that impaired myocardial tissue perfusion persists in over one-third of patients despite restoration of TIMI grade 3 perfusion. This "no-reflow" phenomenon may be a consequence of extensive cellular necrosis and microcirculatory damage, which has been shown to extend further over 48 hours after reperfusion [64,65]. Clot dislodgement with downstream migration of microemboli and "reperfusion injury" are also implicated, especially during primary PCI [66]. The new concepts of microcirculation damage and impaired tissue perfusion have introduced new important tools for evaluating the microcirculation and tissue perfusion [67]. On the basis of myocardial tissue flow measurements by PET within the first 24 hours of acute MI, patients with TIMI flow grade 3 of the IRA at 90 minutes could be divided in three groups. Patients with severely impaired regional myocardial flow ($< 50\%$ of normally perfused myocardium) despite successful fibrinolysis had no recovery of left ventricular function at 3 months. Patients with high flow ($> 75\%$ of normal) showed preserved regional contractile function at 3 months. Patients with intermediate flow (50–75% of normal) showed functional improvement only when a PET mismatch, indicative of viable but ischemically compromised myocardium, was present and an additional revascularization procedure was performed [62]. PET may, thus, be helpful in selecting patients for additional revascularization.

Success of reperfusion at tissue level can be assessed noninvasively using cardiac markers [68,69], resolution of ST-segment elevation [70,71], or the combination of both (Table 2) [72]. ST-segment resolution, reflecting myocardial reperfusion, has been shown to improve short-term and long-term mortality [73–75]. In the TIMI-14 trial, a combination of symptom and ST-elevation resolution and myoglobin washout was especially predictive of TIMI grade 3 flow [72]. Other noninvasive methods to detect reperfusion at tissue level include magnetic resonance imaging [76], positron emission tomography [62], contrast-enhanced echocardiography [77] and transthoracic Doppler ultrasound [78,79]. Myocardial reperfusion at tissue level can also be adequately assessed invasively using the TIMI myocardial perfusion (TMP) score, based on myocardial "blushing" after contrast injection. Low TMP grades have been shown to be related to increased mortality [80]. Moreover, even in patients with normal epicardial (TIMI 3) flow, a TMP grade of 3 (normal tissue

**Table 2**   Evaluation of Myocardial Tissue Reperfusion

| Noninvasive | Invasive |
| --- | --- |
| Resolution of ST-segment elevation (70,71) | TIMI myocardial perfusion grade (80) |
| Contrast echocardiography (77) | Intracoronary Doppler (81) |
| Cardiac markers (68,69) | |
| Transthoracic Doppler (78,79) | |
| Magnetic resonance imaging (76) | |
| Positron emission tomography (62) | |

perfusion) was associated with a much lower 30-day mortality rate (0.7% vs. 4.7% for TMP grade ≤ 2) (Figure 4) [80].

## REPERFUSION AND THE OPEN-ARTERY PARADIGM BEYOND GUSTO-I

### Fibrinolysis

The most effective fibrinolytic regimen in GUSTO-I (i.e., accelerated rt-PA combined with aspirin and immediate intravenous heparin) achieved TIMI flow 3 in the IRA at 90

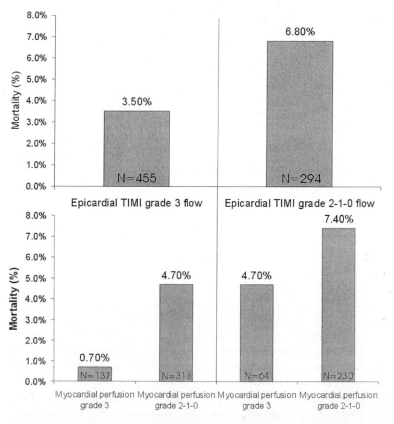

**Figure 4**   30-day mortality in relation to tissue perfusion with or without thrombolysis in myocardial infarction (TIMI) flow grade 3. (Modified from Ref. 80)

minutes only in just over half of patients, and streptokinase-based regimens in but one-third [8]. Failure of fibrinolysis may be related to clot composition: platelet-rich clots exhibit an intrinsic resistance to lysis with conventional agents. Hemorrhage within the plaque may mechanically prevent pharmacological coronary artery recanalization. Also, inhibitors may neutralize the exogenously administered plasminogen activators (e.g., pre-formed anti-streptokinase antibodies for streptokinase and anisoylated plasminogen-streptokinase activator complex (APSAC), and plasminogen activator inhibitor [PAI-1] for rt-PA).

On average, the onset of restoration of antegrade coronary blood flow is delayed for 30 to 45 minutes with intravenous infusions of conventional fibrinolytic agents. Frequent reocclusions undo the initial gain. This high incidence of primary and secondary treatment failures, together with the appreciation that even sustained TIMI 3 flow does not equal restoration of tissue perfusion, as discussed before, may account for modest mean salvage of left ventricular function following fibrinolysis in placebo-controlled trials [20,46]. The same mechanisms may explain why large patency differences do not consistently translate into equally large mortality and morbidity differences and why extra gain from fibrinolytic therapy after hospital discharge is usually absent [82]. Indeed, in GUSTO-I, a 65% increase in TIMI 3 patency with rt-PA relative to streptokinase accounted for only a 14% relative or 1% absolute mortality reduction [3]. In most trials, survival curves after hospital discharge did not diverge further, but ran parallel for 1 to 10 years [15,83–87]. The presumption that fibrinolytic therapy in patients with a very poor residual left ventricular function only postpones death by a few weeks to months, may contribute to this phenomenon. Likewise, the (very) low ejection fractions of these early reperfused patients may mask the gain obtained in other reperfused patients and, therefore, distort the comparison with surviving patients not treated with fibrinolytic agents or treated with less potent agents [46].

To improve on shortcomings of first-generation fibrinolytic agents, several new fibrinolytics have been developed in the past decade. Of these, reteplase and tenecteplase are the most extensively studied agents. Reteplase is a mutant of rt-PA in which the finger, the kringle-1 domain and epidermal growth factor domains were removed. This results in a decreased plasma clearance, which permits double-bolus administration. However, the removal of the finger domain diminishes fibrin specificity [37], while inactivation by PAI-1 remains similar, as with alteplase. Tenecteplase, also derived from rt-PA after mutations at three places, has increased plasma half-life allowing convenient single-bolus administration, increased fibrin binding and specificity, and higher resistance to PAI-1. As a consequence, tenecteplase leads to faster recanalization compared with alteplase [88]. Tenecteplase also has higher thrombolytic potency on platelet-rich clots than its parent molecule [89].

Reteplase was associated with superior patency rates compared with rt-PA in the Reteplase Angiographic Phase II International Dose-finding Study (RAPID) I and II trials [90,91]. However, higher TIMI-3 rates at 90 minutes with reteplase did not translate in lower mortality rates at 30 days or one year compared to rt-PA in the 15,059-patient GUSTO-III trial [86,92]. Likewise, using cardiac markers, tenecteplase was found to induce prompt recanalization (< 40 min) in significantly more patients than rt-PA (76% vs. 56%) [88], while patency rates with tenecteplase were similar to rt-PA in the TIMI 10A and 10B trials [93,94]. In the 16,949-patient assessment of the safety and efficacy of a new thrombolytic (ASSENT-2) trial [95], tenecteplase and alteplase were shown to be equivalent for 30-day mortality. One-year mortality rates also remained similar [83]. The two treatments did not differ significantly in any subgroup analysis, except for a lower 30-day mortality with tenecteplase in patients treated after 4 hours of symptom onset, suggesting that increased fibrin specificity of tenecteplase may induce a better outcome in late-treated patients. Thus, both ASSENT-2 and GUSTO-III studied fibrinolytics with features that promised to provide earlier, more complete, and sustained coronary patency, but in terms of outcome, at best, showed equivalency toward accelerated rt-PA. In retrospect, this should not be surprising in view of the much lower improvements in epicardial patency with reteplase and tenecteplase, compared to the 65% increase in the rate of TIMI 3 flow needed for a 1% absolute reduction in mortality with rt-PA.

## Antithrombotic Cotherapy

In GUSTO-I, aspirin and unfractionated heparin were added to rt-PA as antithrombotic cotherapy. In recent years, different antithrombotic strategies have been tested in combination with fibrinolytics, in order to improve patency rates, tissue reperfusion, and reduce ischemic complications such as death, reinfarction, and recurrent ischemia.

When combined with fibrinolysis, low-molecular-weight heparins (LMWH, Chapter 20) have been shown to induce and preserve higher patency rates compared to conventional unfractionated heparin. Studies have shown a reduction in reinfarction and reocclusion rates and enhanced late patency with the use of LMWH in ACS [96–98]. In the ASSENT-3 study, enoxaparin and full-dose tenecteplase significantly reduced the risk for ischemic complications (reinfarction and refractory ischemia). A significant improvement in the primary efficacy and safety end point was seen with tenecteplase and enoxaparin when compared to standard tenecteplase and unfractionated heparin (UFH). Nevertheless, no difference between enoxaparin and UFH in 30-day and one-year mortality was seen.

The addition of glycoprotein (GP) IIb/IIIa inhibitors such as abciximab, eptifibatide, and tirofiban (Chapter 17) to fibrinolytic regimens might also overcome some of the drawbacks of fibrinolysis, such as recurrent ischemia and reocclusion due to the prothrombotic side effects of fibrinolytic drugs [99,100]. This results in a reduction in angiographically evident thrombus, improving epicardial and tissue perfusion [101]. The TIMI-14, Strategies for Patency Enhancement in the Emergency Department (SPEED), and INTRO-AMI trials [102–104] all indicate that abciximab with half-dose fibrinolytic (rPA or rt-PA) not only enhances recanalization of the culprit epicardial vessel but also improves tissue reperfusion (as evaluated by the amount of ST-segment resolution) and facilitates coronary interventions if needed [105,106]. In the INTRO-AMI trial, the highest 60-minute reperfusion rates were seen in patients treated with half-dose rt-PA and double-bolus eptifibatide followed by a 48-hour infusion (60-minute TIMI grade 3 flow rate of 65% vs. 40% for full-dose alteplase alone) [102]. In the TIMI 14 study, reperfusion rates were evaluated after half-dose alteplase with standard-dose abciximab vs. standard dose alteplase alone in 888 patients. Abciximab with half-dose alteplase significantly enhanced reperfusion at 90 minutes in the TIMI-14 trial, with TIMI 3 flow in 72%, compared to 43% with alteplase alone [107]. The effect of low-dose reteplase with abciximab on early reperfusion was tested in 528 patients in the SPEED trial [103]. TIMI grade 3 flow rate was only 27% when abciximab was used in monotherapy, and 47% with full-dose reteplase alone; the highest TIMI 3 flow rate (61%) was observed in the group that received reduced double-bolus reteplase in combination with abciximab and heparin. The effect of improved epicardial patency rates on outcome with combination therapy using abciximab was tested in the GUSTO-V and ASSENT-3 trials [108,109]. In the GUSTO-V trial, an open-label noninferiority trial, 16,588 patients were randomized to either reteplase or half-dose reteplase with weight-adjusted abciximab [110]. Thirty-day mortality rates were 5.9% for reteplase and 5.6% for the combined reteplase-abciximab group. One-year follow-up mortality rates were identical: 8.4% [87]. Combination therapy with reteplase and abciximab resulted in a significant reduction of ischemic complications after acute MI. Similarly, in the ASSENT-3 study, a significant decrease in ischemic complications with abciximab plus half-dose tenecteplase was observed, without significant difference in 30-day and one-year mortality rates [108]. Taken together, trials with newer antithrombotic cotherapies indicate that modest improvements in coronary patency do not easily translate in lower short-term and long-term mortality rates, although most of these studies are only powered for combined end points. As stated earlier, differences in patency need to be fairly large to detect a mortality benefit. Alternatively, differences between treatment groups in the number of coronary interventions might obscure an existing benefit in outcome [111].

## Prehospital Fibrinolysis and Patency

Since GUSTO-I, it has been difficult to improve on treatment delays using conventional in-hospital strategies [112]. Time lost between symptom onset and hospitalization remains a crucial contributor to treatment delay in STEMI. In the National Registry of Myocardial Infarction (NRMI)-II registry, mean delay was 5.5 hours, with 1 in 3 patients presenting after 4 hours [113]. Since the introduction of bolus fibrinolytics, prehospital treatment of STEMI has gained momentum. Administering fibrinolysis before arrival in the hospital has been shown to reduce treatment delays [114,115], reduce the incidence of cardiogenic shock [116], and decrease mortality after MI [117,118]. Recent data from the prehospital Comparison of Angioplasty versus Prehospital Thrombolysis in Acute Myocardial Infarction (CAPTIM) trial also emphasizes the importance of initiation of reperfusion therapy very soon after symptom onset: patients treated in the prehospital setting within two hours of symptom onset had significantly lower mortality rates than those transferred to a hospital for primary PCI [120]. Prehospital treatment is discussed in further detail in Chapter 8.

## Reperfusion and Primary PCI

Pooled analysis of data from all randomized controlled trials including a total of 2,606 patients with STEMI indicates that 30-day mortality after primary angioplasty is significantly lower (4.4%) than after fibrinolytic therapy (6.5%, odds ratio (OR) 0.66, 95% CI 0.46–0.94, p = 0.02) [120]. A recent meta-analysis suggests that this benefit persists even if the patients need to be transported to another center with an interventional team [121]. Yet, when comparing fibrinolysis with relatively delayed primary PCI, there seems to be no mortality benefit [122–124]. Offering the opportunity of direct angioplasty represents a major logistical challenge in daily practice and requires permanent availability of experienced interventional cardiologists, technical and paramedic support, and skilled surgical backup. Still, in patients with a high risk for intracranial hemorrhage and in patients with cardiogenic shock, primary angioplasty is clearly the treatment of choice.

In primary PCI, time-to-treatment seems to be especially important in the first two hours. Although the rate of ischemic complications is lower in patients treated early (< 2 hours of symptom onset), the impact of later presentation (> 2 hours) on mortality is less clear compared with fibrinolysis [125]. Nevertheless, mortality increases when door-to-balloon times exceed 2 hours, but this might, in part, reflect poorer quality of care [126]. Similar to delayed administration of fibrinolytics, survival after primary PCI beyond the first few hours seems to rely less on recovery of LV function [127], although improved LV indices have been reported with ischemia times up to 12 hours [54]. Apparently, increasing time-to-angioplasty especially has an impact on patients with increased risk of ischemic complications [128]. Nevertheless, the open-artery paradigm, in general, seems to hold up in primary PCI. In the Abciximab before Direct angioplasty and stenting in Myocardial Infarction Regarding Acute and Long-term follow-up (ADMIRAL) study, adjunctive therapy with the glycoprotein (GP) IIb/IIIa inhibitor abciximab to primary stent implantation in patients with STEMI was associated with higher pre- and postprocedural

TIMI flow grade 3 rates and subsequently fewer ischemic complications at 30 days and 6 months [129].

Similar to fibrinolysis, significant numbers of patients also do not show signs of adequate tissue reperfusion after successful primary PCI [71,130]. As with fibrinolysis, inadequate myocardial tissue reperfusion after primary PCI predicts worse LV function and outcome [131]. This suggests that concomitant therapy to protect the microcirculation could also be beneficial with primary angioplasty and stenting. Indeed, the GPIIb/IIIa inhibitor abciximab improves microvascular perfusion and LV function after primary PCI [132]. Since this has been translated into improved outcome in randomized trials, abciximab has become standard in primary PCI [129,133]. Mechanical protection of the microcirculation against microembolization using distal filter devices also helps to improve tissue reperfusion during primary PCI [134].

## Pharmacoinvasive Strategies and Reperfusion

In primary PCI studies, 10 to 20% of patients with STEMI appear to have spontaneous epicardial reperfusion before the intervention [135–137]. Normal epicardial flow before the intervention is a predictor of outcome. In the four primary angioplasty in myocardial infarction (PAMI) trials, mortality was 0.5% with TIMI grade 3 flow before the intervention, compared with 2.8% or 4.4% with TIMI flow 2 or TIMI flow 0/1, respectively (Figure 5) [137]. Patients with reperfusion before the procedure also have better preserved left ventricular function and less progression to heart failure and cardiogenic shock [135,137]. Similarly, adequate tissue perfusion before a primary PCI is associated with improved outcome, irrespective of epicardial reperfusion [138]. These findings suggest that fibrinolysis during the interval between presentation and primary PCI might have an impact on outcome after STEMI [139]. Surprisingly, earlier trials comparing routine immediate angioplasty following fibrinolysis with more conservative treatment, in the absence of continued or recurrent ischemia, showed that the invasive approach was associated with a higher complication rate, including abrupt artery closure, reinfarction, and death [140–145]. Also, in patients undergoing primary PCI for STEMI, adjunctive therapy with streptokinase before and during the intervention was not associated with improved outcome in a small study [146]. One explanation for these unexpected findings is that traditional fibrinolytic strategies activate platelets and the coagulation system, promoting thrombotic complications in the setting of angioplasty. It is likely that the reduced dose of the fibrinolytic and the coadministration of more potent antiplatelet agents like the GPIIb/IIIa inhibitors may significantly reduce the risk of early interventions. The SPEED trial studied the effect of

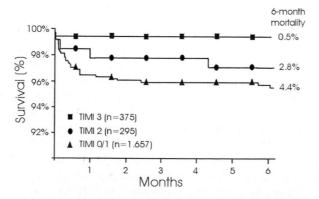

**Figure 5**   6-month mortality in patients with thrombolysis in myocardial infarction (TIMI) flow grade 3 before primary angioplasty in the four PAMI trials. (Modified from Ref. 137)

different doses of reteplase with abciximab on epicardial reperfusion in patients presenting with STEMI [103]. Of the 528 patients, 323 underwent a PCI within 60 to 90 minutes of presentation. The combined end point of death, reinfarction, and urgent revascularization was significantly lower than in patients who did not undergo early PCI (5.6% vs. 16.0%, p = 0.001) [105]. The discrepancy with earlier trials was contributed to the use of a GPIIb/IIIa inhibitor and stents. The plasminogen-activator angioplasty compatibility trial (PACT) has also shown that, even in the absence of a GPIIb/IIIa antagonist, coronary interventions can be safely performed immediately following a single bolus of 50 mg rt-PA [147]. Furthermore, this approach was associated with a better-preserved left ventricular function when compared with primary PCI alone. Other recent small trials have confirmed these promising findings [148,149]. The strategy of early pharmacological reperfusion followed by planned mechanical intervention is currently being studied in the ASSENT-4 PCI and Facilitated Intervention with Enhanced Reperfusion Speed to Stop Events (FINESSE) trials [150].

## CONCLUSION

Prompt, complete, and sustained recanalization of the IRA is a prerequisite for tissue reperfusion and is mandatory to reduce mortality and morbidity of patients with STEMI. In recent years we have witnessed a vast expansion of the ''coronary reperfusion arsenal.'' Different pharmacologic and mechanical revascularization strategies have been compared with reference to efficacy, safety, and cost, frequently evoking vigorous debate. Taken together, newer, often more expensive, approaches offer a benefit over older strategies that is only marginal, compared with the benefit of *any* timely reperfusion therapy over merely supportive therapy. In other words, rapid treatment aimed at reperfusion is more important than the actual choice of a treatment modality. In practice, the best choice will often depend on on-the-spot availability. If an important time-delay before hospital arrival is anticipated (e.g., transport time > 90 minutes), prehospital fibrinolysis must be considered. Undoubtedly, research will continue to refine and optimize methods to detect and to achieve myocardial tissue reperfusion and to reset the standards of care for STEMI. Also, in the future, prompt diagnosis and restoration of tissue flow will remain the cornerstone of successful therapy for STEMI.

## REFERENCES

1. DeWood MA, Spores J, Notske R, Mouser LT, Burroughs R, Golden MS, Lang HT. Prevalence of total coronary occlusion during the early hours of transmural myocardial infarction. N Engl J Med 1980;303:897–902.
2. Reimer KA, Lowe JE, Rasmussen MM, Jennings RB. The wavefront phenomenon of ischemic cell death. 1. Myocardial infarct size vs. duration of coronary occlusion in dogs. Circulation 1977;56:786–794.
3. An international randomized trial comparing four thrombolytic strategies for acute myocardial infarction. The GUSTO investigators. N Engl J Med 1993;329:673–682.
4. The Thrombolysis in Myocardial Infarction (TIMI) trial. Phase I findings. TIMI Study Group. N Engl J Med 1985;312:932 936.
5. Verstraete M, Bernard R, Bory M, Brower RW, Collen D, de Bono DP, Erbel R, Huhmann W, Lennane RJ, Lubsen J. Randomised trial of intravenous recombinant tissue-type plasminogen activator versus intravenous streptokinase in acute myocardial infarction. Report from the European Cooperative Study Group for Recombinant Tissue-type Plasminogen Activator. Lancet 1985;1:842–847.

6.  GISSI-2: a factorial randomised trial of alteplase versus streptokinase and heparin versus no heparin among 12,490 patients with acute myocardial infarction. Gruppo Italiano per lo Studio della Sopravvivenza nell'Infarto Miocardico. Lancet 1990;336:65–71.

7.  ISIS-3: a randomised comparison of streptokinase vs tissue plasminogen activator vs anistreplase and of aspirin plus heparin vs aspirin alone among 41,299 cases of suspected acute myocardial infarction. ISIS-3 (Third International Study of Infarct Survival) Collaborative Group. Lancet 1992;339:753–770.

8.  The effects of tissue plasminogen activator, streptokinase, or both on coronary-artery patency, ventricular function, and survival after acute myocardial infarction. The GUSTO Angiographic Investigators. N Engl J Med 1993;329:1615–1622.

9.  Neuhaus KL, Feuerer W, Jeep-Tebbe S, Niederer W, Vogt A, Tebbe U. Improved thrombolysis with a modified dose regimen of recombinant tissue-type plasminogen activator. J Am Coll Cardiol 1989;14:1566–1569.

10. Bleich SD, Nichols TC, Schumacher RR, Cooke DH, Tate DA, Teichman SL. Effect of heparin on coronary arterial patency after thrombolysis with tissue plasminogen activator in acute myocardial infarction. Am J Cardiol 1990;66:1412–1417.

11. Chesebro JH, Knatterud G, Roberts R, Borer J, Cohen LS, Dalen J, Dodge HT, Francis CK, Hillis D, Ludbrook P. Thrombolysis in Myocardial Infarction (TIMI) Trial, Phase I: A comparison between intravenous tissue plasminogen activator and intravenous streptokinase. Clinical findings through hospital discharge. Circulation 1987;76:142–154.

12. Anderson JL, Karagounis LA, Califf RM. Meta-analysis of five reported studies on the relation of early coronary patency grades with mortality and outcomes after acute myocardial infarction. Am J Cardiol 1996;78:1–8.

13. Simes RJ, Topol EJ, Holmes DR, White HD, Rutsch WR, Vahanian A, Simoons ML, Morris D, Betriu A, Califf RM. Link between the angiographic substudy and mortality outcomes in a large randomized trial of myocardial reperfusion. Importance of early and complete infarct artery reperfusion. GUSTO-I Investigators. Circulation 1995;91:1923–1928.

14. Puma JA, Sketch MH, Thompson TD, Simes RJ, Morris DC, White HD, Topol EJ, Califf RM. Support for the open-artery hypothesis in survivors of acute myocardial infarction: analysis of 11,228 patients treated with thrombolytic therapy. Am J Cardiol 1999;83:482–487.

15. Califf RM, White HD, Van de Werf FJ, Sadowski Z, Armstrong PW, Vahanian A, Simoons ML, Simes RJ, Lee KL, Topol EJ. One-year results from the Global Utilization of Streptokinase and TPA for Occluded Coronary Arteries (GUSTO-I) trial. GUSTO-I Investigators. Circulation 1996;94:1233–1238.

16. Ross AM, Coyne KS, Moreyra E, Reiner JS, Greenhouse SW, Walker PL, Simoons ML, Draoui YC, Califf RM, Topol EJ, Van De WF, Lundergan CF. Extended mortality benefit of early postinfarction reperfusion. GUSTO-I Angiographic Investigators. Global Utilization of Streptokinase and Tissue Plasminogen Activator for Occluded Coronary Arteries Trial. Circulation 1998;97:1549–1556.

17. Lundergan CF, Reiner JS, McCarthy WF, Coyne KS, Califf RM, Ross AM. Clinical predictors of early infarct-related artery patency following thrombolytic therapy: importance of body weight, smoking history, infarct-related artery and choice of thrombolytic regimen: the GUSTO-I experience. Global Utilization of Streptokinase and t-PA for Occluded Coronary Arteries. J Am Coll Cardiol 1998;32:641–647.

18. The effects of tissue plasminogen activator, streptokinase, or both on coronary-artery patency, ventricular function, and survival after acute myocardial infarction. The GUSTO Angiographic Investigators. N Engl J Med 1993;329:1615–1622.

19. Reiner JS, Lundergan CF, van den BM, Boland J, Thompson MA, Machecourt J, Py A, Pilcher GS, Fink CA, Burton JR. Early angiography cannot predict postthrombolytic coronary reocclusion: observations from the GUSTO angiographic study. Global Utilization of Streptokinase and t-PA for Occluded Coronary Arteries. J Am Coll Cardiol 1994;24:1439–1444.

20. Granger CB, White HD, Bates ER, Ohman EM, Califf RM. A pooled analysis of coronary arterial patency and left ventricular function after intravenous thrombolysis for acute myocardial infarction. Am J Cardiol 1994;74:1220–1228.

21. Indications for fibrinolytic therapy in suspected acute myocardial infarction: collaborative overview of early mortality and major morbidity results from all randomised trials of more than 1000 patients. Fibrinolytic Therapy Trialists' (FTT) Collaborative Group. Lancet 1994; 343:311–322.

22. Boersma E, Maas AC, Deckers JW, Simoons ML. Early thrombolytic treatment in acute myocardial infarction: reappraisal of the golden hour. Lancet 1996;348:771–775.

23. Fu Y, Goodman S, Chang WC, Van de Werf FJ, Granger CB, Armstrong PW. Time to treatment influences the impact of ST-segment resolution on one-year prognosis: insights from the assessment of the safety and efficacy of a new thrombolytic (ASSENT-2) trial. Circulation 2001;104:2653–2659.

24. Clemmensen P, Ohman EM, Sevilla DC, Wagner NB, Quigley PS, Grande P, Wagner GS. Importance of early and complete reperfusion to achieve myocardial salvage after thrombolysis in acute myocardial infarction. Am J Cardiol 1992;70:1391–1396.

25. Kennedy JW. Optimal management of acute myocardial infarction requires early and complete reperfusion. Circulation 1995;91:1905–1907.

26. Lenderink T, Simoons ML, van Es GA, Van de Werf F, Verstraete M, Arnold AE. Benefit of thrombolytic therapy is sustained throughout five years and is related to TIMI perfusion grade 3 but not grade 2 flow at discharge. The European Cooperative Study Group. Circulation 1995;92:1110–1116.

27. Vogt A, von Essen R, Tebbe U, Feuerer W, Appel KF, Neuhaus KL. Impact of early perfusion status of the infarct-related artery on short-term mortality after thrombolysis for acute myocardial infarction: retrospective analysis of four German multicenter studies. J Am Coll Cardiol 1993;21:1391–1395.

28. Reiner JS, Lundergan CF, Fung A, Coyne K, Cho S, Israel N, Kazmierski J, Pilcher G, Smith J, Rohrbeck S, Thompson M, Van De WF, Ross AM. Evolution of early TIMI 2 flow after thrombolysis for acute myocardial infarction. GUSTO-1 Angiographic Investigators. Circulation 1996;94:2441–2446.

29. Gibson CM, Ryan KA, Murphy SA, Mesley R, Marble SJ, Giugliano RP, Cannon CP, Antman EM, Braunwald E. Impaired coronary blood flow in nonculprit arteries in the setting of acute myocardial infarction. The TIMI Study Group. Thrombolysis in myocardial infarction. J Am Coll Cardiol 1999;34:974–982.

30. French JK, Straznicky IT, Webber BJ, Aylward PE, Frey MJ, Adgey AA, Williams BF, McLaughlin SC, White HD. Angiographic frame counts 90 minutes after streptokinase predict left ventricular function at 48 hours following myocardial infarction. Heart 1999;81:128–133.

31. Ohman EM, Califf RM, Topol EJ, Candela R, Abbottsmith C, Ellis S, Sigmon KN, Kereiakes D, George B, Stack R. Consequences of reocclusion after successful reperfusion therapy in acute myocardial infarction. TAMI Study Group. Circulation 1990;82:781–791.

32. Hudson MP, Granger CB, Topol EJ, Pieper KS, Armstrong PW, Barbash GI, Guerci AD, Vahanian A, Califf RM, Ohman EM. Early reinfarction after fibrinolysis: experience from the global utilization of streptokinase and tissue plasminogen activator (alteplase) for occluded coronary arteries (GUSTO I) and global use of strategies to open occluded coronary arteries (GUSTO III) trials. Circulation 2001;104:1229–1235.

33. Gibson CM, Karha J, Murphy SA, James D, Morrow DA, Cannon CP, Giugliano RP, Antman EM, Braunwald E. Early and long-term clinical outcomes associated with reinfarction following fibrinolytic administration in the Thrombolysis in Myocardial Infarction trials. J Am Coll Cardiol 2003;42:7–16.

34. Barbash GI, Birnbaum Y, Bogaerts K, Hudson M, Lesaffre E, Fu Y, Goodman S, Houbracken K, Munsters K, Granger CB, Pieper K, Califf RM, Topol EJ, Van de Werf FJ. Treatment of reinfarction after thrombolytic therapy for acute myocardial infarction: an analysis of outcome and treatment choices in the global utilization of streptokinase and tissue plasminogen activator for occluded coronary arteries (gusto I) and assessment of the safety of a new thrombolytic (assent 2) studies. Circulation 2001;20(103):954–960.

35. Brouwer MA, Bohncke JR, Veen G, Meijer A, van Eenige MJ, Verheugt FW. Adverse long-term effects of reocclusion after coronary thrombolysis. J Am Coll Cardiol 1995;26: 1440–1444.

36. White HD, French JK, Hamer AW, Brown MA, Williams BF, Ormiston JA, Cross DB. Frequent reocclusion of patent infarct-related arteries between 4 weeks and 1 year: effects of antiplatelet therapy. J Am Coll Cardiol 1995;25:218–223.

37. Hoffmeister HM, Kastner C, Szabo S, Beyer ME, Helber U, Kazmaier S, Baumbach A, Wendel HP, Heller W. Fibrin specificity and procoagulant effect related to the kallikrein-contact phase system and to plasmin generation with double-bolus reteplase and front-loaded alteplase thrombolysis in acute myocardial infarction. Am J Cardiol 2000;86:263–268.

38. Barbagelata NA, Granger CB, Oqueli E, Suarez LD, Borruel M, Topol EJ, Califf RM. TIMI grade 3 flow and reocclusion after intravenous thrombolytic therapy: a pooled analysis. Am Heart J 1997;133:273–282.

39. Gibson CM, Murphy SA, Rizzo MJ, Ryan KA, Marble SJ, McCabe CH, Cannon CP, Van De WF, Braunwald E. Relationship between TIMI frame count and clinical outcomes after thrombolytic administration. Thrombolysis In Myocardial Infarction (TIMI) Study Group. Circulation 1999;99:1945–1950.

40. Lincoff AM, Topol EJ. Illusion of reperfusion. Does anyone achieve optimal reperfusion during acute myocardial infarction? Circulation 1993;88:1361–1374.

41. Gibson CM, Cannon CP, Daley WL, Dodge JT, Alexander B, Marble SJ, McCabe CH, Raymond L, Fortin T, Poole WK, Braunwald E. TIMI frame count: a quantitative method of assessing coronary artery flow. Circulation 1996;93:879–888.

42. Lamas GA, Flaker GC, Mitchell G, Smith SC, Gersh BJ, Wun CC, Moye L, Rouleau JL, Rutherford JD, Pfeffer MA. Effect of infarct artery patency on prognosis after acute myocardial infarction. The Survival and Ventricular Enlargement Investigators. Circulation 1995; 92:1101–1109.

43. White HD, Cross DB, Elliott JM, Norris RM, Yee TW. Long-term prognostic importance of patency of the infarct-related coronary artery after thrombolytic therapy for acute myocardial infarction. Circulation 1994;89:61–67.

44. Kim CB, Braunwald E. Potential benefits of late reperfusion of infarcted myocardium. The open artery hypothesis. Circulation 1993;88:2426–2436.

45. Nash JA. The open infarct-related artery: theoretical and practical considerations. Coron Artery Dis 1995;6:739–749.

46. Van de Werf FJ. Discrepancies between the effects of coronary reperfusion on survival and left ventricular function. Lancet 1989;1:1367–1369.

47. Braunwald E. Myocardial reperfusion, limitation of infarct size, reduction of left ventricular dysfunction, and improved survival. Should the paradigm be expanded? Circulation 1989; 79:441–444.

48. Califf RM, Topol EJ, Gersh BJ. From myocardial salvage to patient salvage in acute myocardial infarction: the role of reperfusion therapy. J Am Coll Cardiol 1989;14:1382–1388.

49. Gang ES, Lew AS, Hong M, Wang FZ, Siebert CA, Peter T. Decreased incidence of ventricular late potentials after successful thrombolytic therapy for acute myocardial infarction. N Engl J Med 1989;321:712–716.

50. Newby KH, Thompson T, Stebbins A, Topol EJ, Califf RM, Natale A. Sustained ventricular arrhythmias in patients receiving thrombolytic therapy: incidence and outcomes. The GUSTO Investigators. Circulation 1998;98:2567–2573.

51. Sager PT, Perlmutter RA, Rosenfeld LE, McPherson CA, Wackers FJ, Batsford WP. Electrophysiologic effects of thrombolytic therapy in patients with a transmural anterior myocardial infarction complicated by left ventricular aneurysm formation. J Am Coll Cardiol 1988;12: 19–24.

52. Hochman JS, Choo H. Limitation of myocardial infarct expansion by reperfusion independent of myocardial salvage. Circulation 1987;75:299–306.

53. Lavie CJ, O'Keefe JH, Chesebro JH, Clements IP, Gibbons RJ. Prevention of late ventricular dilatation after acute myocardial infarction by successful thrombolytic reperfusion. Am J Cardiol 1990;66:31–36.

54. Miura H, Kiuchi K, Nejima J, Takano T. Limitation of infarct size and ventricular remodeling in patients with completely reperfused anterior acute myocardial infarction—the potential role of ischemia time. Clin Cardiol. 2002;25:566–571.

55. Pfeffer MA, Braunwald E. Ventricular remodeling after myocardial infarction. Experimental observations and clinical implications. Circulation 1990;81:1161–1172.

56. Late Assessment of Thrombolytic Efficacy (LATE) study with alteplase 6–24 hours after onset of acute myocardial infarction. Lancet 1993;342:759–766.

57. Horie H, Takahashi M, Minai K, Izumi M, Takaoka A, Nozawa M, Yokohama H, Fujita T, Sakamoto T, Kito O, Okamura H, Kinoshita M. Long-term beneficial effect of late reperfusion for acute anterior myocardial infarction with percutaneous transluminal coronary angioplasty. Circulation 1998;98:2377–2382.

58. Yousef ZR, Redwood SR, Bucknall CA, Sulke AN, Marber MS. Late intervention after anterior myocardial infarction: effects on left ventricular size, function, quality of life, and exercise tolerance: results of the Open Artery Trial (TOAT Study). J Am Coll Cardiol 2002; 40:869–876.

59. Sadanandan S, Buller C, Menon V, Dzavik V, Terrin M, Thompson B, Lamas G, Hochman JS. The late open artery hypothesis—a decade later. Am Heart J 2001;142:411–421.

60. Ito H, Tomooka T, Sakai N, Yu H, Higashino Y, Fujii K, Masuyama T, Kitabatake A, Minamino T. Lack of myocardial perfusion immediately after successful thrombolysis. A predictor of poor recovery of left ventricular function in anterior myocardial infarction. Circulation 1992;85:1699–1705.

61. Ito H, Maruyama A, Iwakura K, Takiuchi S, Masuyama T, Hori M, Higashino Y, Fujii K, Minamino T. Clinical implications of the ''no reflow'' phenomenon. A predictor of complications and left ventricular remodeling in reperfused anterior wall myocardial infarction. Circulation 1996;93:223–228.

62. Maes A, Van de Werf FJ, Nuyts J, Bormans G, Desmet W, Mortelmans L. Impaired myocardial tissue perfusion early after successful thrombolysis. Impact on myocardial flow, metabolism, and function at late follow-up. Circulation 1995;92:2072–2078.

63. Maes AF, Van de Werf FJ, Mesotten LV, Flamen PB, Kuzo RS, Nuyts JL, Mortelmans L. Early assessment of regional myocardial blood flow and metabolism in thrombolysis in myocardial infarction flow grade 3 reperfused myocardial infarction using carbon-11-acetate. J Am Coll Cardiol 2001;37:30–36.

64. Ambrosio G, Weisman HF, Mannisi JA, Becker LC. Progressive impairment of regional myocardial perfusion after initial restoration of postischemic blood flow. Circulation 1989; 80:1846–1861.

65. Rochitte CE, Lima JA, Bluemke DA, Reeder SB, McVeigh ER, Furuta T, Becker LC, Melin JA. Magnitude and time course of microvascular obstruction and tissue injury after acute myocardial infarction. Circulation 1998;98:1006–1014.

66. Falk E, Thuesen L. Pathology of coronary microembolisation and no reflow. Heart 2003;89: 983–985.

67. Eeckhout E, Kern MJ. The coronary no-reflow phenomenon: a review of mechanisms and therapies. Eur Heart J 2001;22:729–739.

68. Ellis AK, Little T, Masud AR, Liberman HA, Morris DC, Klocke FJ. Early noninvasive detection of successful reperfusion in patients with acute myocardial infarction. Circulation 1988;78:1352–1357.

69. Jurlander B, Clemmensen P, Ohman EM, Christenson R, Wagner GS, Grande P. Serum myoglobin for the early non-invasive detection of coronary reperfusion in patients with acute myocardial infarction. Eur Heart J 1996;17:399–406.

70. Schroder R, Wegscheider K, Schroder K, Dissmann R, Meyer-Sabellek W. Extent of early ST segment elevation resolution: a strong predictor of outcome in patients with acute myocardial infarction and a sensitive measure to compare thrombolytic regimens. A substudy of the International Joint Efficacy Comparison of Thrombolytics (INJECT) trial. J Am Coll Cardiol 1995;26:1657–1664.

71. van't Hof AW, Liem A, de Boer MJ, Zijlstra F. Clinical value of 12-lead electrocardiogram after successful reperfusion therapy for acute myocardial infarction. Zwolle Myocardial infarction Study Group. Lancet 1997;350:615–619.

72. de Lemos JA, Morrow DA, Gibson CM, Murphy SA, Rifai N, Tanasijevic M, Giugliano RP, Schuhwerk KC, McCabe CH, Cannon CP, Antman EM, Braunwald E. Early noninvasive

detection of failed epicardial reperfusion after fibrinolytic therapy. Am J Cardiol 2001;88: 353–358.

73. Anderson RD, White HD, Ohman EM, Wagner GS, Krucoff MW, Armstrong PW, Weaver WD, Gibler WB, Stebbins AL, Califf RM, Topol EJ. Predicting outcome after thrombolysis in acute myocardial infarction according to ST-segment resolution at 90 minutes: a substudy of the GUSTO-III trial. Global Use of Strategies To Open occluded coronary arteries. Am Heart J 2002;144:81–88.

74. French JK, Andrews J, Manda SO, Stewart RA, McTigue JJ, White HD. Early ST-segment recovery, infarct artery blood flow, and long-term outcome after acute myocardial infarction. Am Heart J 2002;143:265–271.

75. Johanson P, Jernberg T, Gunnarsson G, Lindahl B, Wallentin L, Dellborg M. Prognostic value of ST-segment resolution-when and what to measure. Eur Heart J 2003;24:337–345.

76. Wu KC, Zerhouni EA, Judd RM, Lugo-Olivieri CH, Barouch LA, Schulman SP, Blumenthal RS, Lima JA. Prognostic significance of microvascular obstruction by magnetic resonance imaging in patients with acute myocardial infarction. Circulation 1998;97:765–772.

77. Wu KC, Kim RJ, Bluemke DA, Rochitte CE, Zerhouni EA, Becker LC, Lima JA. Quantification and time course of microvascular obstruction by contrast-enhanced echocardiography and magnetic resonance imaging following acute myocardial infarction and reperfusion. J Am Coll Cardiol 1998;32:1756–1764.

78. Voci P, Mariano E, Pizzuto F, Puddu PE, Romeo F. Coronary recanalization in anterior myocardial infarction: the open perforator hypothesis. J Am Coll Cardiol 2002;40:1205–1213.

79. Lee S, Otsuji Y, Minagoe S, Hamasaki S, Toyonaga K, Negishi M, Tsurugida M, Toda H, Tei C. Noninvasive evaluation of coronary reperfusion by transthoracic Doppler echocardiography in patients with anterior acute myocardial infarction before coronary intervention. Circulation 2003;108:2763–2768.

80. Gibson CM, Cannon CP, Murphy SA, Ryan KA, Mesley R, Marble SJ, McCabe CH, Van de Werf FJ, Braunwald E. Relationship of TIMI myocardial perfusion grade to mortality after administration of thrombolytic drugs. Circulation 2000;101:125–130.

81. Kawamoto T, Yoshida K, Akasaka T, Hozumi T, Takagi T, Kaji S, Ueda Y. Can coronary blood flow velocity pattern after primary percutaneous transluminal coronary angioplasty [correction of angiography] predict recovery of regional left ventricular function in patients with acute myocardial infarction? Circulation 1999;100:339–345.

82. Van de Werf FJ. Thrombolysis for acute myocardial infarction. Why is there no extra benefit after hospital discharge? Circulation 1995;91:2862–2864.

83. Sinnaeve P, Alexander J, Belmans A, Bogaerts K, Langer A, Diaz R, Ardissino D, Vahanian A, Pehrsson K, Armstrong P, Van de Werf FJ. One-year follow-up of the ASSENT-2 trial: a double-blind, randomized comparison of single-bolus tenecteplase and front-loaded alteplase in 16,949 patients with ST-elevation acute myocardial infarction. Am Heart J 2003; 146:27–32.

84. Franzosi MG, Santoro E, De Vita C, Geraci E, Lotto A, Maggioni AP, Mauri F, Rovelli F, Santoro L, Tavazzi L, Tognoni G. Ten-year follow-up of the first megatrial testing thrombolytic therapy in patients with acute myocardial infarction: results of the Gruppo Italiano per lo Studio della Sopravvivenza nell'Infarto-1 study. The GISSI Investigators. Circulation 1998; 98:2659–2665.

85. Long-term effects of intravenous thrombolysis in acute myocardial infarction: final report of the GISSI study. Gruppo Italiano per lo Studio della Streptochi-nasi nell'Infarto Miocardico (GISSI). Lancet 1987;2:871–874.

86. Topol EJ, Ohman EM, Armstrong PW, Wilcox R, Skene AM, Aylward P, Simes J, Dalby A, Betriu A, Bode C, White HD, Hochman JS, Emanuelson H, Vahanian A, Sapp S, Stebbins A, Moliterno DJ, Califf RM. Survival outcomes 1 year after reperfusion therapy with either alteplase or reteplase for acute myocardial infarction: results from the Global Utilization of Streptokinase and t-PA for Occluded Coronary Arteries (GUSTO) III Trial. Circulation 2000; 102:1761–1765.

87. Lincoff AM, Califf RM, Van de Werf FJ, Willerson JT, White HD, Armstrong PW, Guetta V, Gibler WB, Hochman JS, Bode C, Vahanian A, Steg PG, Ardissino D, Savonitto S, Bar

F, Sadowski Z, Betriu A, Booth JE, Wolski K, Waller M, Topol EJ. Mortality at 1 year with combination platelet glycoprotein IIb/IIIa inhibition and reduced-dose fibrinolytic therapy vs conventional fibrinolytic therapy for acute myocardial infarction: GUSTO V randomized trial. JAMA 2002;288:2130–2135.

88. Binbrek A, Rao N, Absher PM, Van de Werf FJ, Sobel BE. The relative rapidity of recanalization induced by recombinant tissue-type plasminogen activator (r-tPA) and TNK-tPA, assessed with enzymatic methods. Coron Artery Dis 2000;11:429–435.

89. Collen D, Stassen JM, Yasuda T, Refino C, Paoni N, Keyt B, Roskams T, Guerrero JL, Lijnen HR, Gold HK. Comparative thrombolytic properties of tissue-type plasminogen activator and of a plasminogen activator inhibitor-1-resistant glycosylation variant, in a combined arterial and venous thrombosis model in the dog. Thromb Haemost 1994;72:98–104.

90. Smalling RW, Bode C, Kalbfleisch J, Sen S, Limbourg P, Forycki F, Habib G, Feldman R, Hohnloser S, Seals A. More rapid, complete, and stable coronary thrombolysis with bolus administration of reteplase compared with alteplase infusion in acute myocardial infarction. RAPID Investigators. Circulation 1995;91:2725–2732.

91. Bode C, Smalling RW, Berg G, Burnett C, Lorch G, Kalbfleisch JM, Chernoff R, Christie LG, Feldman RL, Seals AA, Weaver WD. Randomized comparison of coronary thrombolysis achieved with double-bolus reteplase (recombinant plasminogen activator) and front-loaded, accelerated alteplase (recombinant tissue plasminogen activator) in patients with acute myocardial infarction. The RAPID II Investigators. Circulation 1996;94:891–898.

92. A comparison of reteplase with alteplase for acute myocardial infarction. The Global Use of Strategies to Open Occluded Coronary Arteries (GUSTO III) Investigators. N Engl J Med 1997;337:1118–1123.

93. Cannon CP, McCabe CH, Gibson CM, Ghali M, Sequeira RF, McKendall GR, Breed J, Modi NB, Fox NL, Tracy RP, Love TW, Braunwald E. TNK-tissue plasminogen activator in acute myocardial infarction. Results of the Thrombolysis in Myocardial Infarction (TIMI) 10A dose-ranging trial. Circulation 1997;95:351–356.

94. Cannon CP, Gibson CM, McCabe CH, Adgey AA, Schweiger MJ, Sequeira RF, Grollier G, Giugliano RP, Frey M, Mueller HS, Steingart RM, Weaver WD, Van de Werf FJ, Braunwald E. TNK-tissue plasminogen activator compared with front-loaded alteplase in acute myocardial infarction: results of the TIMI 10B trial. Thrombolysis in Myocardial Infarction (TIMI) 10B Investigators. Circulation 1998;98:2805–2814.

95. Single-bolus tenecteplase compared with front-loaded alteplase in acute myocardial infarction: the ASSENT-2 double-blind randomised trial. Assessment of the Safety and Efficacy of a New Thrombolytic Investigators. Lancet 1999;354:716–722.

96. Turpie AG, Antman EM. Low-molecular-weight heparins in the treatment of acute coronary syndromes. Arch Intern Med 2001;161:1484–1490.

97. Wallentin L, Dellborg DM, Lindahl B, Nilsson T, Pehrsson K, Swahn E. The low-molecular-weight heparin dalteparin as adjuvant therapy in acute myocardial infarction: the ASSENT PLUS study. Clin Cardiol 2001;24:I12–I14.

98. Ross AM, Molhoek P, Lundergan C, Knudtson M, Draoui Y, Regalado L, Le LV, Bigonzi F, Schwartz W, de Jong E, Coyne K. Randomized comparison of enoxaparin, a low-molecular-weight heparin, with unfractionated heparin adjunctive to recombinant tissue plasminogen activator thrombolysis and aspirin: second trial of Heparin and Aspirin Reperfusion Therapy (HART II). Circulation 2001;104:648–652.

99. Bertram U, Moser M, Peter K, Kuecherer HF, Bekeredjian R, Straub A, Nordt TK, Bode C, Ruef J. Effects of Different Thrombolytic Treatment Regimen with Abciximab and Tirofiban on Platelet Aggregation and Platelet-Leukocyte Interactions: A Subgroup Analysis from the GUSTO V and FASTER Trials. J Thromb Thrombolysis 2002;14:197–203.

100. Coulter SA, Cannon CP, Ault KA, Antman EM, Van de Werf FJ, Adgey AA, Gibson CM, Giugliano RP, Mascelli MA, Scherer J, Barnathan ES, Braunwald E, Kleiman NS. High levels of platelet inhibition with abciximab despite heightened platelet activation and aggregation during thrombolysis for acute myocardial infarction: results from TIMI (thrombolysis in myocardial infarction) 14. Circulation 2000;101:2690–2695.

101. Gibson CM, de Lemos JA, Murphy SA, Marble SJ, McCabe CH, Cannon CP, Antman EM, Braunwald E. Combination therapy with abciximab reduces angiographically evident thrombus in acute myocardial infarction: a TIMI 14 substudy. Circulation 2001;103: 2550–2554.

102. Brener SJ, Zeymer U, Adgey AA, Vrobel TR, Ellis SG, Neuhaus KL, Juran N, Ivanc TB, Ohman EM, Strony J, Kitt M, Topol EJ. Eptifibatide and low-dose tissue plasminogen activator in acute myocardial infarction: the integrilin and low-dose thrombolysis in acute myocardial infarction (INTRO AMI) trial. J Am Coll Cardiol 2002;39:377–386.

103. Trial of abciximab with and without low-dose reteplase for acute myocardial infarction. Strategies for Patency Enhancement in the Emergency Department (SPEED) Group. Circulation 2000;20(101):2788–2794.

104. Antman EM, Gibson CM, de Lemos JA, Giugliano RP, McCabe CH, Coussement P, Menown I, Nienaber CA, Rehders TC, Frey MJ, Van Der WR, Andresen D, Scherer J, Anderson K, Van de Werf FJ, Braunwald E. Combination reperfusion therapy with abciximab and reduced dose reteplase: results from TIMI 14. The Thrombolysis in Myocardial Infarction (TIMI) 14 Investigators. Eur Heart J 2000;21:1944–1953.

105. Herrmann HC, Moliterno DJ, Ohman EM, Stebbins AL, Bode C, Betriu A, Forycki F, Miklin JS, Bachinsky WB, Lincoff AM, Califf RM, Topol EJ. Facilitation of early percutaneous coronary intervention after reteplase with or without abciximab in acute myocardial infarction: results from the SPEED (GUSTO-4 Pilot) Trial. J Am Coll Cardiol 2000;36:1489–1496.

106. de Lemos JA, Antman EM, Gibson CM, McCabe CH, Giugliano RP, Murphy SA, Coulter SA, Anderson K, Scherer J, Frey MJ, Van Der Wieken R, Van de Werf FJ, Braunwald E. Abciximab improves both epicardial flow and myocardial reperfusion in ST-elevation myocardial infarction. Observations from the TIMI 14 trial. Circulation 2000;101:239–243.

107. Antman EM, Giugliano RP, Gibson CM, McCabe CH, Coussement P, Kleiman NS, Vahanian A, Adgey AA, Menown I, Rupprecht HJ, Van Der Wieken R, Ducas J, Scherer J, Anderson K, Van de Werf FJ, Braunwald E. Abciximab facilitates the rate and extent of thrombolysis: results of the thrombolysis in myocardial infarction (TIMI) 14 trial. The TIMI 14 Investigators. Circulation 1999;99:2720–2732.

108. Efficacy and safety of tenecteplase in combination with enoxaparin, abciximab, or unfractionated heparin: the ASSENT-3 randomised trial in acute myocardial infarction. Lancet 2001; 358:605–613.

109. Topol EJ. Reperfusion therapy for acute myocardial infarction with fibrinolytic therapy or combination reduced fibrinolytic therapy and platelet glycoprotein IIb/IIIa inhibition: the GUSTO V randomised trial. Lancet 2001;357:1905–1914.

110. Topol EJ, Moliterno DJ, Herrmann HC, Powers ER, Grines CL, Cohen DJ, Cohen EA, Bertrand M, Neumann FJ, Stone GW, DiBattiste PM, Demopoulos L. Comparison of two platelet glycoprotein IIb/IIIa inhibitors, tirofiban and abciximab, for the prevention of ischemic events with percutaneous coronary revascularization. N Engl J Med 2001;344: 1888–1894.

111. Dubois CL, Belmans A, Granger CB, Armstrong PW, Wallentin L, Fioretti PM, Lopez-Sendon JL, Verheugt FW, Meyer J, Van de Werf F. Outcome of urgent and elective percutaneous coronary interventions after pharmacologic reperfusion with tenecteplase combined with unfractionated heparin, enoxaparin, or abciximab. J Am Coll Cardiol 2003;42:1178–1185.

112. Gibler WB, Armstrong PW, Ohman EM, Weaver WD, Stebbins AL, Gore JM, Newby LK, Califf RM, Topol EJ. Persistence of delays in presentation and treatment for patients with acute myocardial infarction: The GUSTO-I and GUSTO-III experience. Ann Emerg Med 2002;39:123–130.

113. Goldberg RJ, Gurwitz JH, Gore JM. Duration of, and temporal trends (1994–1997) in, prehospital delay in patients with acute myocardial infarction: the second National Registry of Myocardial Infarction. Arch Intern Med 1999;159:2141–2147.

114. Wallentin L, Goldstein P, Armstrong PW, Granger CB, Adgey AA, Arntz HR, Bogaerts K, Danays T, Lindahl B, Makijarvi M, Verheugt F, Van de Werf FJ. Efficacy and safety of tenecteplase in combination with the low-molecular-weight heparin enoxaparin or unfraction-

ated heparin in the prehospital setting: the Assessment of the Safety and Efficacy of a New Thrombolytic Regimen (ASSENT)-3 PLUS randomized trial in acute myocardial infarction. Circulation 2003;108:135–142.

115.  Morrow DA, Antman EM, Sayah A, Schuhwerk KC, Giugliano RP, deLemos JA, Waller M, Cohen SA, Rosenberg DG, Cutler SS, McCabe CH, Walls RM, Braunwald E. Evaluation of the time saved by prehospital initiation of reteplase for ST-elevation myocardial infarction: results of The Early Retavase-Thrombolysis in Myocardial Infarction (ER-TIMI) 19 trial. J Am Coll Cardiol 2002;40:71–77.

116.  Bonnefoy E, Lapostolle F, Leizorovicz A, Steg G, McFadden EP, Dubien PY, Cattan S, Boullenger E, Machecourt J, Lacroute JM, Cassagnes J, Dissait F, Touboul P. Primary angioplasty versus prehospital fibrinolysis in acute myocardial infarction: a randomised study. Lancet 2002;360:825–829.

117.  Morrison LJ, Verbeek PR, McDonald AC, Sawadsky BV, Cook DJ. Mortality and prehospital thrombolysis for acute myocardial infarction: A meta-analysis. JAMA 2000;283:2686–2692.

118.  Mathew TP, Menown IB, McCarty D, Gracey H, Hill L, Adgey AA. Impact of pre-hospital care in patients with acute myocardial infarction compared with those first managed in-hospital. Eur Heart J 2003;24:161–171.

119.  Steg G, Bonnefoy E, Chabaud S, Lapostolle F, Dubien P, Cristofini P, Leizorovicz A, Touboul P. Impact of time to treatment on mortality after prehospital fibrinolysis or primary angioplasty—Data from the CAPTIM randomized clinical trial. Circulation 2003;108:2851–2856.

120.  Weaver WD, Simes RJ, Betriu A, Grines CL, Zijlstra F, Garcia E, Grinfeld L, Gibbons RJ, Ribeiro EE, DeWood MA, Ribichini F. Comparison of primary coronary angioplasty and intravenous thrombolytic therapy for acute myocardial infarction: a quantitative review. JAMA 1997;278:2093–2098.

121.  Dalby M, Bouzamondo A, Lechat P, Montalescot G. Transfer for primary angioplasty versus immediate thrombolysis in acute myocardial infarction: a meta-analysis. Circulation 2003; 108:1809–1814.

122.  Every NR, Parsons LS, Hlatky M, Martin JS, Weaver WD. A comparison of thrombolytic therapy with primary coronary angioplasty for acute myocardial infarction. Myocardial Infarction Triage and Intervention Investigators. N Engl J Med 1996;335:1253–1260.

123.  Rogers WJ, Dean LS, Moore PB, Wool KJ, Burgard SL, Bradley EL. Comparison of primary angioplasty versus thrombolytic therapy for acute myocardial infarction. Alabama Registry of Myocardial Ischemia Investigators. Am J Cardiol 1994;74:111–118.

124.  Danchin N, Vaur L, Genes N, Etienne S, Angioi M, Ferrieres J, Cambou JP. Treatment of acute myocardial infarction by primary coronary angioplasty or intravenous thrombolysis in the ''real world'': one-year results from a nationwide French survey. Circulation 1999;99: 2639–2644.

125.  Zijlstra F, Patel A, Jones M, Grines CL, Ellis S, Garcia E, Grinfeld L, Gibbons RJ, Ribeiro EE, Ribichini F, Granger C, Akhras F, Weaver WD, Simes RJ. Clinical characteristics and outcome of patients with early ($<$ 2 h), intermediate (2–4 h) and late ($>$ 4 h) presentation treated by primary coronary angioplasty or thrombolytic therapy for acute myocardial infarction. Eur Heart J 2002;23:550–557.

126.  Cannon CP, Gibson CM, Lambrew CT, Shoultz DA, Levy D, French WJ, Gore JM, Weaver WD, Rogers WJ, Tiefenbrunn AJ. Relationship of symptom-onset-to-balloon time and door-to-balloon time with mortality in patients undergoing angioplasty for acute myocardial infarction. JAMA 2000;283:2941–2947.

127.  Brodie BR, Stuckey TD, Wall TC, Kissling G, Hansen CJ, Muncy DB, Weintraub RA, Kelly TA. Importance of time to reperfusion for 30-day and late survival and recovery of left ventricular function after primary angioplasty for acute myocardial infarction. J Am Coll Cardiol 1998;32:1312–1319.

128.  Antoniucci D, Valenti R, Migliorini A, Moschi G, Trapani M, Buonamici P, Cerisano G, Bolognese L, Santoro GM. Relation of time to treatment and mortality in patients with acute myocardial infarction undergoing primary coronary angioplasty. Am J Cardiol 2002; 89:1248–1252.

129. Montalescot G, Barragan P, Wittenberg O, Ecollan P, Elhadad S, Villain P, Boulenc JM, Morice MC, Maillard L, Pansieri M, Choussat R, Pinton P. Platelet glycoprotein IIb/IIIa inhibition with coronary stenting for acute myocardial infarction. N Engl J Med 2001;344: 1895–1903.

130. Claeys MJ, Bosmans J, Veenstra L, Jorens P, De Raedt H, Vrints CJ. Determinants and prognostic implications of persistent ST-segment elevation after primary angioplasty for acute myocardial infarction: importance of microvascular reperfusion injury on clinical outcome. Circulation 1999;99:1972–1977.

131. Lepper W, Sieswerda GT, Vanoverschelde JL, Franke A, de Cock CC, Kamp O, Kuhl HP, Pasquet A, Voci P, Visser CA, Hanrath P, Hoffmann R. Predictive value of markers of myocardial reperfusion in acute myocardial infarction for follow-up left ventricular function. Am J Cardiol 2001;88:1358–1363.

132. Petronio AS, Rovai D, Musumeci G, Baglini R, Nardi C, Limbruno U, Palagi C, Volterrani D, Mariani M. Effects of abciximab on microvascular integrity and left ventricular functional recovery in patients with acute infarction treated by primary coronary angioplasty. Eur Heart J 2003;24:67–76.

133. Tcheng JE, Kandzari DE, Grines CL, Cox DA, Effron MB, Garcia E, Griffin JJ, Guagliumi G, Stuckey T, Turco M, Fahy M, Lansky AJ, Mehran R, Stone GW. Benefits and Risks of Abciximab Use in Primary Angioplasty for Acute Myocardial Infarction. The Controlled Abciximab and Device Investigation to Lower Late Angioplasty Complications (CADILLAC) Trial. Circulation 2003;108:1316–1323.

134. Limbruno U, Micheli A, De Carlo M, Amoroso G, Rossini R, Palagi C, Di BV, Petronio AS, Fontanini G, Mariani M. Mechanical prevention of distal embolization during primary angioplasty: safety, feasibility, and impact on myocardial reperfusion. Circulation 2003;108: 171–176.

135. Brodie BR, Stuckey TD, Hansen C, Muncy D. Benefit of coronary reperfusion before intervention on outcomes after primary angioplasty for acute myocardial infarction. Am J Cardiol 2000;85:13–18.

136. Stone GW, Brodie BR, Griffin JJ, Morice MC, Costantini C, St Goar FG, Overlie PA, Popma JJ, McDonnell J, Jones D, O'Neill WW, Grines CL. Prospective, multicenter study of the safety and feasibility of primary stenting in acute myocardial infarction: in-hospital and 30-day results of the PAMI stent pilot trial. Primary Angioplasty in Myocardial Infarction Stent Pilot Trial Investigators. J Am Coll Cardiol 1998;31:23–30.

137. Stone GW, Cox D, Garcia E, Brodie BR, Morice MC, Griffin J, Mattos L, Lansky AJ, O'Neill WW, Grines CL. Normal flow (TIMI-3) before mechanical reperfusion therapy is an independent determinant of survival in acute myocardial infarction: analysis from the primary angioplasty in myocardial infarction trials. Circulation 2001;104:636–641.

138. Gibson CM, Cannon CP, Murphy SA, Marble SJ, Barron HV, Braunwald E. Relationship of the TIMI myocardial perfusion grades, flow grades, frame count, and percutaneous coronary intervention to long-term outcomes after thrombolytic administration in acute myocardial infarction. Circulation 2002;105:1909–1913.

139. Cannon CP. Multimodality reperfusion therapy for acute myocardial infarction. Am Heart J 2000;140:707–716.

140. Immediate vs delayed catheterization and angioplasty following thrombolytic therapy for acute myocardial infarction. TIMI II A results. The TIMI Research Group. JAMA 1988;260: 2849–2858.

141. Comparison of invasive and conservative strategies after treatment with intravenous tissue plasminogen activator in acute myocardial infarction. Results of the thrombolysis in myocardial infarction (TIMI) phase II trial. The TIMI Study Group. N Engl J Med 1989;320:618–627.

142. SWIFT trial of delayed elective intervention v conservative treatment after thrombolysis with anistreplase in acute myocardial infarction. SWIFT (Should We Intervene Following Thrombolysis?) Trial Study Group. BMJ 1991;302:555–560.

143. Califf RM, Topol EJ, Stack RS, Ellis SG, George BS, Kereiakes DJ, Samaha JK, Worley SJ, Anderson JL, Harrelson-Woodlief L. Evaluation of combination thrombolytic therapy

and timing of cardiac catheterization in acute myocardial infarction. Results of thrombolysis and angioplasty in myocardial infarction--phase 5 randomized trial. TAMI Study Group. Circulation 1991;83:1543–1556.

144. Simoons ML, Arnold AE, Betriu A, de Bono DP, Col J, Dougherty FC, von Essen R, Lambertz H, Lubsen J, Meier B. Thrombolysis with tissue plasminogen activator in acute myocardial infarction: no additional benefit from immediate percutaneous coronary angioplasty. Lancet 1988;1:197–203.

145. Topol EJ, Califf RM, George BS, Kereiakes DJ, Abbottsmith CW, Candela RJ, Lee KL, Pitt B, Stack RS, O'Neill WW. A randomized trial of immediate versus delayed elective angioplasty after intravenous tissue plasminogen activator in acute myocardial infarction. N Engl J Med 1987;317:581–588.

146. O'Neill WW, Weintraub R, Grines CL, Meany TB, Brodie BR, Friedman HZ, Ramos RG, Gangadharan V, Levin RN, Choksi N. A prospective, placebo-controlled, randomized trial of intravenous streptokinase and angioplasty versus lone angioplasty therapy of acute myocardial infarction. Circulation 1992;86:1710–1717.

147. Ross AM, Coyne KS, Reiner JS, Greenhouse SW, Fink C, Frey A, Moreyra E, Traboulsi M, Racine N, Riba AL, Thompson MA, Rohrbeck S, Lundergan CF. A randomized trial comparing primary angioplasty with a strategy of short-acting thrombolysis and immediate planned rescue angioplasty in acute myocardial infarction: the PACT trial. PACT investigators. Plasminogen-activator Angioplasty Compatibility Trial. J Am Coll Cardiol 1999;34:1954–1962.

148. Fernandez-Aviles F, Alonso J, Castro-Beiras A, Vazquez N, Blanco J, Alonso J, Lopez-Mesa J, Fernandez-Vazquez F. Randomized trial comparing stenting within 24 hours of thrombolysis versus conservative ischaemia-guided approach to thrombolysed ST-elevated acute myocardial infarction. Final results of the GRACIA trial (abstract). Eur Heart J 2003; 24:704.

149. Scheller B, Hennen B, Hammer B, Walle J, Hofer C, Hilpert V, Winter H, Nickenig G, Bohm M. Beneficial effects of immediate stenting after thrombolysis in acute myocardial infarction. J Am Coll Cardiol 2003;42:634–641.

150. Herrmann HC, Kelley MP, Ellis SG. Facilitated PCI: rationale and design of the FINESSE trial. J Invasive Cardiol 2001;13(suppl A):10A–15A.

# 8

# Prehospital Treatment of Acute Myocardial Infarction

**Kevin J. Beatt and Farzin Fath-Ordoubadi**
*Hammersmith Hospital*
*London, England*

## INTRODUCTION

The concept of prehospital management of myocardial infarction was introduced in the mid-1960s in recognition of the very substantial loss of life occurring before patients could be admitted to the hospital. At a time when there was no effective treatment for the majority of patients with this condition, 60% of patients died within the first hour and many failed to reach a hospital within the first 12 hours [1]. At present, each year around 800,000 people in the United States suffer an acute myocardial infarction (MI) and at least 213,000 will die as a result. Surveys show more than 50% of these deaths are still within the first hour, with the percentage rising to 80% within the first 24 hours [2,3]. Despite the recognized improvement in mortality of those reaching the hospital, this has not been matched by the same improvement in prehospital mortality.

The importance of ventricular fibrillation as an early cause of death and the ability of resuscitation and cardioversion to have an impact on mortality were the factors that initially drove the development of prehospital programs for treatment of acute MI. The logistic difficulties of providing the service were such that any benefits were confined to a relatively small proportion of the overall MI population, bringing into question the value of this type of care. However, the value of early vessel patency achieved either by thrombolysis or primary angioplasty has prompted the development of strategies to facilitate rapid triage and treatment of the patient with an evolving myocardial infarction. The London Ambulance Service is both the busiest and largest in the world, receiving over 1 million calls per year and transporting around 700,000 patients to hospital. Annually, they respond to over 38,000 emergency calls for adults with chest pain. Currently, 77% of patients with chest pain due to acute MI are attended to in less than 8 minutes from the time of call for help. This compares with a figure approaching 50% only 2 years ago.

It is now clear that the initiation of very early treatment, before 90% of patients are seen in the hospital, is more beneficial than previously thought. This has led to a renewed emphasis on prehospital management of MI.

## PREHOSPITAL RECOGNITION OF ACUTE MYOCARDIAL INFARCTION

Since the diagnosis of MI and the decision to give thrombolysis depends on electrocardiograph (ECG) findings, emergency personnel should be able to perform and correctly interpret the ECG findings. In the study by Gemmill et al [3], primary care physicians were equipped with an ECG machine and asked to undertake a home recording in 69 patients with suspected MI. Only 75% of ECGs were successfully completed; of these, the recording was satisfactory in only 60%. In McCrea and Saltissi's study [4], primary care physicians were asked to interpret a series of different ECGs. Although 82% of primary care physicians were able to recognize a normal ECG, recognition of an acute abnormality was less reliable. Between 33% and 66% correctly identified acute transmural ischemia or infarction depending on the specific trace presented. Accurate localization of the site of the infarct was achieved by 8% to 30% of participants, while only 22% to 25% correctly interpreted nonacute abnormalities.

Another potentially important technology, as used in the myocardial infarction triage and intervention (MITI) trial, is the ability to transmit ECG information by cellular telephone, which was demonstrated to be a feasible and reliable method of screening, especially when reperfusion therapy is being considered. In this study, ECGs equipped with a computer algorithm were particularly useful with a high sensitivity (about 80%) and specificity (about 98%) for identifying patients with acute MI and ST-segment elevation [5].

## CARDIOPULMONARY RESUSCITATION

For almost 40 years, it has been recognized that prehospital resuscitation and prompt treatment of life-threatening arrhythmias can be effective at reducing mortality [6]. Ventricular fibrillation is the only important cause of death in patients who die in the first hour following the onset of MI and may be 25 times more common in this early period than the in-hospital occurrence [2]. In the majority of cases, provided treatment is immediate, direct current (DC) cardioversion will successfully terminate the arrhythmia. Many studies have shown that trained nonmedical personnel are able to deliver effective treatment [7]. The principal limitation of prehospital resuscitation as a treatment strategy is the inability to provide trained personnel to cover every event, a situation made particularly difficult as patients may not seek medical help or consider asking for it until the moment of collapse, despite having the pain of an evolving MI.

### Targeting Levels of Expertise

Initial attempts to resuscitate patients in the community relied primarily on the expertise of trained ambulance staff. However, it soon became clear that even a prompt ambulance response was unable to arrive soon enough in many cases, and there was a need to have a larger, more responsive body of personnel trained in cardiopulmonary resuscitation (CPR). Observations in Seattle prior to the introduction of thrombolytic therapy showed that 28% of those found in a state of cardiac arrest were eventually discharged from the hospital. If cardioversion was performed by the first responder to a call for help, the survival was 38%; if performed by someone witnessing the arrest, survival was 70%. The ability of a witness to perform resuscitation rather than having to wait the extra time for a paramedic team to arrive was estimated to result in an additional 100 lives saved per 1,000 patients treated. These observations led to the concept and subsequent development of a two-tier system; the first, early response tier system, consisting of personnel more likely to be in the vicinity, trained in resuscitation, and, if possible, equipped with defibrillators. Groups targeted for training include firemen, police officers, railway personnel, selected individuals in large establishments, and relatives of patients who are at risk for MI.

In Seattle, this approach has achieved a response time of 3.1 minutes for the first tier (generally without defibrillators) and 6.2 minutes for the more experienced, highly trained second tier [8].

The impact of such services is difficult to evaluate. Randomized trials are clearly not possible within the same community, and sequential outcomes analyses are of limited value because of the changing rate of cardiac mortality in most communities. A 62% reduction in prehospital mortality in patients more than 70 years old was observed after the introduction of a prehospital CPR program [9]. Just over one-third of the patients with acute MI to whom the unit attended had experienced a cardiac arrest. One-third of these died despite resuscitative measures, 18% during ambulance transport. These observations, which are free from the influence of thrombolytic agents, were used to crudely estimate a benefit of 15 lives saved per 100,000 population each year. Data from Belfast, comparing two similar communities in the same city, one with a mobile coronary care unit and one without, supported these findings. Community mortality was 63% where there was no specific prehospital service and 50% where there was, the difference being most apparent in younger patients [10]. The median delay from onset of symptoms to hospital admission was 135 minutes with the prehospital service and 256 minutes without. Although these results are not impressive by today's standards, they do indicate that with concerted efforts, resources, and dedication, it is possible to develop services that provide an effective means of resuscitating a significant number of patients. A degree of benefit can be achieved by concentrating resources for training and the provision of equipment, particularly portable defibrillators, on paramedical staff. However, a far more substantial benefit can be achieved by having a more widespread body of expertise, with potential first responders able to perform cardiopulmonary resuscitation and cardioversion. In contrast, the focusing of resources on individuals who will be called upon to resuscitate infrequently may be unrewarding. A survey among 200 primary care physicians who were supplied portable defibrillators as part of a British Heart Foundation initiative showed that over a 1-year period, 53 attempts at resuscitation were made. However, only 19 arrests occurred in the near vicinity of a physician, with 13 patients being successfully cardioverted and nine surviving to hospital discharge. On average, a primary physician will use the defibrillator only once every 4 years in this setting.

Automated external defibrillators (AEDs) are now more portable and simpler to use. The latest device measures $6 \times 22 \times 20$ cm and weighs 2 kg. This device is designed to make possible the use of defibrillation by individuals other than paramedics and hospital staff. In fact, it has been demonstrated that during mock cardiac arrest, the speed of AED use by untrained children was only slightly slower than that of professionals [11]. Ease of use and widespread availability will allow many more patients to be treated effectively by cardioversion.

## PREHOSPITAL THROMBOLYSIS

The benefit of thrombolytic therapy is greatest when it is given early after the onset of symptoms. Early animal studies have demonstrated a temporal relationship between the extent of myocardial damage and duration of coronary artery occlusion [9]. In the dog model, 64% of involved myocardium is salvageable after 40 minutes of coronary artery occlusion, whereas after 3 hours, only 11% is salvageable [12]. In determining the optimal use of thrombolysis, it is crucial to establish whether *substantial* additional benefit can be achieved by administering thrombolysis in the first 1 or 2 hours after the onset of pain. Mortality reduction in those treated within 1 hour of symptom onset in the Second

International Study of Infarct Survivals (ISIS-2) [13] was 56%, and, in the First Gruppo Italiano per lo Studio della Streptochinasi nell'Infarcto miocardico (GISSI-1) [14], was 46%, whereas the mortality reduction in those treated between 3 and 6 hours was 17% in the latter study. In the First Global Utilization of Streptokinase and Tissue Plasminogen Activator for Occluded Coronary Arteries (GUSTO-1) study [15], the 30-day mortality rate in patients treated within 2 hours of onset of symptoms was 5.5%, and 9.0% in those treated after 4 hours. In the MITI prehospital thrombolytic trial [5], the mortality rate in those treated within 70 minutes of symptom onset was as low as 1.2%, compared with 8.7% in those who were treated after that time. There was no detectable evidence of myocardial damage in 40% of cases who were treated early using quantitative thallium tomography. Close examination of the effect of time to thrombolysis on outcome following an acute MI has shown that in the first 1 to 2 hours after the onset of chest pain, the relationship between time of treatment and survival is exponential [16,17] (Fig. 1). However, the relationship becomes more linear after this period. This analysis suggests that the benefit of thrombolytic therapy was 65, 37, 26, and 29 lives saved per 1,000 treated patients in the 0–1, 1–2, 2–3, and 3–6-hour interval, respectively. Proportional mortality reduction was significantly higher in patients treated within 2 hours than in those treated later (44% vs. 20%; p = 0.001).

   Although the importance of time to treatment may be influenced by factors such as the presence or absence of collaterals, myocardial workload, preconditioning, and episodes of flow and no flow, which may occur during a stuttering infarct, studies have now confirmed that early, complete, and sustained reperfusion of the infarct-related artery remains the most crucial factor in preventing death and impairment of cardiac function following MI in most patients. A major confounding factor limiting the benefit of thrombolytic therapy is the failure to initiate treatment in the first 1 to 1.5 hour after symptom onset. The different components in the delay to administration of thrombolytic therapy have been documented [18]:

1.   Failure of most patients to react rapidly and appropriately to symptoms.
2.   Long time delays from summoning help to hospital arrival, the median time from onset of chest pain and hospital admission in most hospitals being between 81 to 160 minutes.
3.   Delays from hospital arrival to treatment, with a median delay time of 31 to 80 minutes [19].

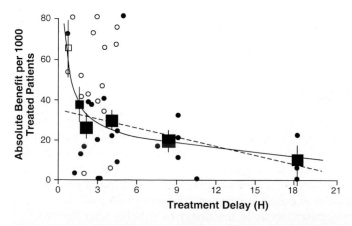

**Figure 1**   Absolute 35-day mortality reduction vs. treatment. (From Ref. 16)

A logical step to reducing the prehospital delay is for thrombolytic therapy to be brought and administered to the patient whether in his or her home or out in the community.

## Clinical Trials of Prehospital vs. In-Hospital Thrombolysis

The first study of prehospital thrombolysis was published by Koren et al. in 1985 [20]. In this study, nine patients received prehospital streptokinase at home given by a physician attached to a mobile coronary care unit (MCCU), and 44 received hospital treatment. Patients treated less than 1.5 hours after the onset of pain had a significantly higher global ejection fraction (56% $\pm$ 15 vs. 47% $\pm$ 14; $p < 0.05$) and a lower QRS score (5.6 $\pm$ 4.9 vs. 8.6 $\pm$ 5.5; $P < 0.01$) compared with patients receiving treatment between 1.5 and 4 hours after the onset of chest pain. Patients treated earlier by the MCCU also had better left ventricular function than patients treated in the hospital. There are now several trials confirming the feasibility and safety of prehospital thrombolysis in widely varying circumstances and settings [21–26].

Having established the feasibility and safety of prehospital thrombolysis, randomized studies comparing prehospital with hospital thrombolysis were required to determine if a reduction in mortality could be achieved. There are now eight such studies published [27–34]. Design characteristics of these studies are shown in Table 1. The number of patients recruited ranged from 57 to 5,469. Six studies [27–31,33] required presence of diagnostic ST-segment elevation whereas two studies [32,34] recruited all patients with a suspected infarct. The time saved by giving prehospital thrombolysis varied from 34 to 130 minutes depending on the setting in which the trial was carried out, with the greatest saving achieved in patients living in rural areas (Table 2).

The European Myocardial Infarction Project (EMIP) study [34] has been the largest of the randomized studies. (n = 5,469) In this multicenter study, enrollment was carried out by MCCU staff from 163 centers in 15 European countries and Canada. There was a nonsignificant trend toward a lower mortality in the prehospital treated group (9.7% vs. 11.1%; p = 0.08).

Partly because of the small number of patients involved, these studies individually did not show a significant reduction in in-hospital or 30-day mortality in the prehospital-treated group [35]. However, analysis of pooled data from these studies shows a significantly lower mortality in favor of the prehospital-treated group [36,37] (Fig. 2). In this overview, the mortality was 9% in the prehospital- and 10.8% in hospital-treated group (p = 0.01). This represents a reduction in mortality of 16.7%, translating into 18 extra

**Table 1**  Design Characteristics of Randomized Trials of Prehospital Thrombolysis

| Author | Design | Thrombolyte | Setting | Treating Physician | Delay (Hours) | Age Limit (years) |
|---|---|---|---|---|---|---|
| McNeil | DB | t-PA | Urban | Dr | <4 | <75 |
| Castaigne | Open | APSAC | Urban | Dr | <3 | <75 |
| Barbash | Open | t-PA | Urban | Dr | <4 | <72 |
| Schofer | DB | Urokinase | Urban | Dr | <4 | <70 |
| GREAT | DB | APSAC | Rural | GP | <4 | No limit |
| McAleer | Open | SK | Rural | Dr | <6 | No limit |
| EMIP | DB | APSAC | MC | Dr | <6 | No limit |
| MITI | Open | t-PA | MC | Remote Dr | <6 | <75 |

DB, double blind; MC, multicenter; GP, general practitioner; Dr, hospital physician

**Table 2**   Time Saving on Prehospital Thrombolysis

| Study | Median time to prehospital Rx (min) | Median time to hospital Rx (min) | Time saving (min) |
|---|---|---|---|
| McNeil | 119 | 187 | 68 |
| Castaigne | 131 | 180 | 60 |
| Barbash | 96 | 132 | 40 |
| Schofer | 85 | 137 | 43 |
| GREAT | 101 | 240 | 130 |
| McAleer | 138 | 172 | 34 |
| EMIP | 130 | 190 | 55 |
| MITI | 77 | 110 | 33 |

lives saved per 1,000 patients treated in the community (Table 3). In addition, it has been shown that early diagnosis of MI at home reduces the time to administration of thrombolytic therapy in the hospital by mobilization of the hospital team for immediate evaluation and treatment on the patient's arrival [27].

## Optimal Setting for Prehospital Thrombolysis

As discussed earlier, the greatest benefit of thrombolytic therapy is achieved when it is given within 1 to 1.5 hours after onset of chest pain. Prehospital thrombolysis should therefore, be considered in locations where achieving this goal would not otherwise be

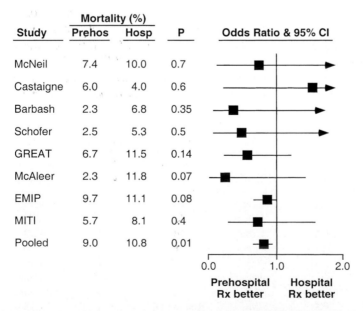

**Figure 2**   Overview of randomized trials prehospital vs. hospital thrombolysis. Mortality rates, odds ratio, and 95% CL for the individual studies and the pooled data are shown.

**Table 3**  Overview of Mortality Data from Randomized Trials of Prehospital Thrombolysis

| Study | No. of deaths/total no. | | |
|-------|---------|---------|---------|
| | Prehosp | Hosp | *p* value |
| McNeil | 2/27 | 3/30 | .7 |
| Castaigne | 3/50 | 2/50 | .6 |
| Barbash | 1/43 | 3/44 | .35 |
| Schofer | 1/40 | 2/38 | .5 |
| GREAT | 11/163 | 17/148 | .14 |
| McAleer | 1/43 | 12/102 | .07 |
| EMIP | 266/2750 | 303/2719 | .08 |
| MITI | 10/175 | 15/185 | .4 |
| Pooled | 295/3291 | 357/3316 | .01 |

possible. In particular, it should be considered in places where the transfer time from home to hospital is greater than 90 minutes. In the Grampian Region Early Anistreplase Trial (GREAT) study, there was a 42% reduction in 3-month mortality in the prehospital-treated group (p = 0.04), where the time saved by giving prehospital thrombolysis was greater than 90 minutes [32]. Similarly, in the EMIP study [34], there was a significant 42% (p = 0.05) reduction in mortality in the prehospital subgroup who received treatment greater than 90 minutes sooner than the hospital group. Settings that would, therefore, be most suited for prehospital thrombolysis are those where the distance between home and hospital is greater than 10 km, such as rural areas and regions where MCCUs with a fast response rate have already been established, in particular in cities where traffic jams may be a major problem.

## Adverse Events

In the prehospital-treated group of the EMIP study [34], there was a small but significantly greater rate of ventricular fibrillation (2.5% vs. 1.6%; p = 0.02) and shock (including cardiogenic and allergic shock and those with symptomatic hypotension [6.3% vs. 3.9%; p < 0.001]) in the period between the arrival of the emergency medical team and hospital admission. However, a greater rate of ventricular fibrillation and shock following admission in the hospital-treated group meant that the overall rates of these two complications were similar in the two groups. There were no significant differences in the incidence of other major complications, including cardiac arrest, acute pulmonary edema, and stroke, up until the time of hospital discharge.

## Choice of Thrombolytic Agent

Several agents have been used in the prehospital trials. Thrombolytics differ in fibrin specificity, potency and resistance to inactivation by plasminogen activation inhibitor 1. These differences translate clinically to variations in the frequency of administration. For example, anistreplase is given as a bolus injection over 5 minutes making it the most commonly used thrombolytic in the community. However, it must be kept at 2 to 8°C and not frozen. It is rendered ineffective by exposure to normal temperature for more than 2 or 3 hours and has a relatively short shelf life. In the GUSTO-1 study [15], irrespective of the thrombolytic therapy used, patients with a fully patent artery (referred to as TIMI grade 3) 90 minutes after commencement of treatment had the lowest mortality rate (4.4%), compared with 8.9% in those with an occluded artery at 90 minutes. In an overview of 4,687 patients with MI who underwent coronary angiography 90 minutes following thrombolysis, the mortality rate was lowest in patients with TIMI grade 3 flow (3.7%) and significantly lower than in those with TIMI 2 (6.6%; $p = 0.0003$), or TIMI 0/1 (9.2%; $p < 0.0001$) flow [38]. In view of the importance of very early reperfusion, it makes sense to optimize the benefit of prehospital treatment by giving an agent that achieves the highest early patency rate.

Accelerated t-PA has been shown to be associated with a better 90-minutes TIMI 3 flow compared with both streptokinase [39] and APSAC [40]. However, it has the disadvantage of requiring a more complicated infusion regimen. Although this agent could be given as bolus injections, this may be associated with an increased risk of hemorrhagic complications [41]. A recombinant form of t-PA called reteplase has been shown to be at least as effective as accelerated t-PA without compromising safety [41,42]. In addition, this drug has the advantage of ease of administration. The usual regimen for this drug is two bolus injections of 10 units, given 30 minutes apart. This enables the first injection to be given in the community and the second in the hospital following reassessment of the patient. In this way, should the diagnosis be wrong or side effects develop, the second dose could be withheld.

Tenecteplase is a recombinant homologue of t-PA that differs in structure by the substitution of 3 amino acids resulting in a greater specificity for fibrin and a longer plasma half-life. The Assessment of the Safety and Efficacy of a New Thrombolytic (ASSENT) 2 investigators compared tenecteplase with alteplase and found the same 30-day mortality (6.2%) in both groups and similar rates of in-hospital coronary revascularisation. The 30-day mortality rate was the same (6.2%) in both groups, and the rates of in-hospital procedures (e.g., percutaneous transluminal coronary angioplasty, stent placement, coronary artery bypass graft surgery) were similar.

## Logistic Problems

The principal arguments against the widespread use of prehospital thrombolysis are concerned with the logistics of implementing this service in a comprehensive manner, and the emerging evidence for the benefit of primary angioplasty. Chest pain is common, and whereas many patients may seek medical attention, the number with acute MI who are eligible for thrombolysis is relatively small. In any prehospital thrombolysis program, the service will be called upon to screen a large number of patients, where only a few will benefit. In the MITI study [5], during a 3-year period, 8,863 patients with chest pain were examined by five paramedic units operating in the city of Seattle. Of these, 1,973 (22%) met the criteria for a history of acute MI, and only 483 had ST-segment elevation on ECG while 360 (4%) were eligible for thrombolysis according to the trial's inclusion criteria.

On average, each paramedic unit administered prehospital thrombolytics only 24 times a year. The involvement of individual paramedics was even less, as each unit was manned by several paramedics covering a 24-hour rotation. In a similar study combining the prehospital experience of units in Nashville and Cincinnati [44], only 27 (4.8%) of 562 people screened for chest pain were candidates for thrombolytic therapy. In that study, a decline in paramedic skills was noted because of lack of experience resulting from the infrequent administration of a thrombolytic agent. The majority of patients with MI who did not receive thrombolysis were more than 75 years old, which was considered an exclusion criterion. Eliminating the age limit may increase the proportion of patients receiving prehospital thrombolysis to 32% [34], but the number of patients treated per individual paramedic per year will remain relatively small. The situation is worse when a primary care physician is involved in giving prehospital thrombolysis. In the United Kingdom, a primary care physician has, on average, about 1,000 patients in his or her practice, and, although many patients with chest pain will be seen each year, only two to eight of them will have MIs [45]. Similarly, only 5% of cardiac arrest events are witnessed by a primary care physician. This underlines a central problem in any thrombolysis or resuscitation program in the community, something that is not properly addressed in the randomized trials, as only the relatively few patients suitable for prehospital treatment are included in the analysis. Interpretation of the randomized trials should be performed with a full understanding of how limited and selected the sample populations may be.

The cost/benefit analysis of prehospital thrombolysis is difficult and controversial, as any individual assessment can only apply to the region surveyed and may vary dramatically with differing regions. For example, in regions where there is a longer time to transport to the hospital, the benefits will be greater [33,34]. Prehospital thrombolysis is cheaper where there is already an established and well-trained paramedic system.

## Prehospital Thrombolysis vs Primary Angioplasty

Primary angioplasty is emerging as the prefered treatment of acute ST segment elevation myocardial infarction[46]. Data from the DANish trial in Acute Myocardial Infarction-2 (DANAMI 2), Primary Angioplasty in patients transferred from General community hospitals to specialized percutaneous coronary intervention Units with or without Emergency thrombolysis (PRAGUE), and Air Primary Angioplasty in Myocardial Infarction (AIR PAMI) study have shown that delays of up to 3 hours can be incurred in transporting patients to PCI centers while still maintaining a benefit of primary Percutaneous Coronary Intervention (PCI) over thrombolysis administered in the local center [47–49]. Can the very early administration of prehospital thrombolysis match the advantages of primary angioplasty in terms of improved outcome and reduced complications? The Comparison of Angioplasty and Prehospital Thrombolysis in acute Myocardial infarction (CAPTIM) trial [50] attempted to answer this question by randomizing patients who presented within 6 hours of an acute ST-elevation MI to prehospital thrombolyisis or transfer for primary angioplasty by a mobile emergency care unit. This study planned to recruit 2,400 patients initially, but, due to lack of finances and slow recruitment, only 840 patients were recruited. Despite this, there was a trend towards a 24% relative reduction of the composite endpoint of 30-day death, reinfarction, or disabling stroke in favor of primary Percutaneous Transluminal Coronary Angioplasty (PTCA). Subgroup analysis of patients randomised within the first 2 hours of symptom onset showed no significant difference between prehospital lysis and primary PCI in patients reaching the primary endpoint (7.4% vs. 6.6 respectively). However there was significantly cardiogenic shock (1.3% vs. 5.3% $p = 0.032$ and a trend towards lower 30 day mortality in the thrombolytic group (2.2% vs. 5.7% $p = 0.058$). This trend was reversed in patients randomized outside the 2 hours window.

## Prehospital Treatment of Myocardial Infarction in the Primary Angioplasty Era: The Role of Facilitated Primary PCI

While the mainstay of prehospital treatment is still stabilization of rhythm and hemodynamics, it is important to determine whether the early administration of antiplatelet, antithrombin, or thrombolytic agents at this time may facilitate the success of primary angioplasty.

The burden of thrombus frequently seen at the time of urgent angioplasty, particularly where there is a delay in treatment, compromises sustained and complete reperfusion. In particular, the use of stents in this setting is associated with the release of plaque material/thrombus into the distal vascular bed [51–54], which may significantly compromise microvascular flow.

Adjunctive agents given early enough may lead to more complete epicardial and microvascular flow (TIMI 3 flow) with a subsequent improvement in outcome [55] A pooled analysis of the 4 PAMI trials has shown that those patients who, at the time of primary PCI, are found to have TIMI 3 flow prior to intervention are less likely to develop complications related to left ventricular failure and have both improved early and late survival rates [56].

Therapies that reduce the burden of thrombus, facilitate early arterial patency and can be given in the prehospital period are worthy of further investigation.

## Use of Thrombolytics with Primary Angioplasty

Early randomized trials found full dose thrombolysis prior to angioplasty to be associated with increased abrupt closure and bleeding complication [57–59]. More recently, the Primary Angioplasty/Alteplase Compatibility Trial (PACT) study found administration of half-dose alteplase followed by immediate angiography and angioplasty to be safe with no increased bleeding risk when compared to primary PCI on its own [60]. The improvement may be due to increased operator experience, the use of stents, or the availability of antiplatelet agents.

The Grupo de Análisis de la Cardiopatia Isquémica Agunda (GRACIA) 2 trial provides further evidence that adjunctive thrombolysis is safe. It compared optimal PCI within 180 minutes to immediate tenecteplase administration followed by PCI within 3 to 12 hours of symptom onset. The risk of bleeding complications was low in both groups and clinical outcomes were similar despite more complete ST resolution in patients having facilited PCI. Although a number of studies have suggested an improvement in perfusion by surrogate endpoints, there is no convincing evidence demonstrating an improvement in outcome.

Further studies are being conducted to determine the role of adjunctive thrombolysis. This is the subject of the ASSENT 4 and Facilitated Intervention with Enhanced Reperfusion Speed to Stop Events (FINESSE) trials, which are currently recruiting.

## The Use of Glycoprotein IIb/IIIa Inhibitors with Primary Angioplasty

One of the first trials to explore this area assessed the use of abciximab (bolus 0.25 mg/kg plus infusion 0.125 microgram/kg/min) given immediately to ST-segment elevation MIs referred for urgent primary angioplasty [61]. Compared to placebo, patients treated with abciximab had a 59% reduction in the primary end point (death, reinfarction, or urgent target vessel revascularization [TVR]) at 30 days. At 6 months, the combination of early abciximab and revascularization produced a 50% reduction in the incidence of death alone (3.3% with abciximab vs 7.3% with placebo), but this did not reach statistical significance (p = 0.19). These improvements in outcome were reflected in the higher rate of TIMI 3 flow both prior to and following revascularisation. (TIMI 3 flow prior to revascularisation was 16.8% in the abciximab group and 4.8% in the placebo group, p = 0.01, and, immediately following revascularization, 95.1% in the abciximab group as apposed to 86.7% in the placebo group, p = 0.04).

In the Controlled Abciximab and Device Investigation to Lower Late Angioplasty Complications (CADILLAC) trial [62], abciximab was given later, at the time of the acute intervention. Included were patients with acute coronary syndromes with and without ST-

segment elevation. Treatment consisted of abciximab or placebo in conjunction with balloon angioplasty alone or the elective use of stents in a two-by-two design. The two stent
groups were associated with the most favorable outcome in terms of composite of death,
stroke, reinfarction, and target vessel revascularisation, with little further benefit with the
use of abciximab.

The very low mortality rates prevent meaningful comparison of this endpoint, in
part, because of the enrollment of patients without ST-segment elevation.

Administering Tirofiban to patients prior to transfer for PCI in the Ongoing Tirofiban
in Myocardial infarction Evaluation (ON-TIME) trial showed lower rates of TIMI-0, 1,
and 2 flow, but there was no benefit in terms of event rates when compared to placebo.

## USE OF THROMBOLYTIC AND IIB/IIIA COMBINATION THERAPY WITH PRIMARY ANGIOPLASTY

The TIMI-14 investigators demonstrated that combination therapy with abciximab and reduced dose t-PA had a 59% rate of complete ST segment resolution at 90 minutes compared
with 37% in those treated with t-PA alone. Furthermore of all patients found to have TIMI
3 flow at 90 minutes patients treated with combination therapy remained significantly more
likely to achieve complete ST segment resolution than those receiving t-PA alone (69% versus 44%) These findings suggest that abciximab not only improves TIMI 3 coronary arterial
patency but has a beneficial effect on the coronary microvasclature. The TIMI 14 investigators did not encourage coronary intervention in the first 90 minutes.

Retrospective subgroup analysis of the small number of patients undergoing PCI in
the Strategies for Patency Enhancement in the Emergency Department (SPEED) trial
showed that PCI performed after combination therapy increased the rates of TIMI 3 flow
from 47% to 87% and decreased corrected TIMI frame counts, an indication of improved
microvascular flow.

These studies indicate that combination therapy appears to have a synergistic effect in
achieving not only epicardial vessel patency but improving coronary microcirculation. It is
unclear what impact this will have on clinical outcome. The role of adjunctive pharmacotherapy prior to mechanical intervention remains unclear and further studies are addressing this.

## OTHER ADJUVANT THERAPY

### Aspirin

Aspirin has been shown to be beneficial in patients with unstable angina or acute MI
[13,64] In the second international study of infarct survivals (ISIS-2) study, 5-week vascular mortality was reduced by 23% when aspirin was given alone and by 42% when it was
given together with streptokinase within 24 hours of the onset of chest pain [13]. There
is no study that examines the role of early prehospital aspirin on mortality, but subgroup
analysis from ISIS-2 study [13] showed that there was a nonsignificant trend of 16%
reduction in mortality in patients who received aspirin within 2 hours of the onset of chest
pain compared with patients who received treatment within 5 to 12 hours. Furthermore,
experimental studies have shown that effective inhibition of platelet activity can be
achieved within 1 hour of administration of aspirin [65].

### Beta-Blockers

The only study that has examined the use of β-blockers in a prehospital setting is the
Thrombolysis Early in Acute Heart Attack Trial (TEAHAT) [66]. In this study, 352 patients

with acute MI were randomized to receive placebo or t-PA. All patients with no contraindications also received intravenous metoprolol. In 29% of patients, intravenous metoprolol was started prior to hospital admission, and only patients with chest pain lasting less than 2 hours 45 minutes were recruited. Thirty-seven percent of patients had contraindications to β-blockers, the most frequent of which were a heart rate of less than 60 beats per minute or hypotension. No side effects of metoprolol, either alone or in combination with t-PA, was observed during the prehospital phase. Patients treated with metoprolol had lower incidence of Q-wave infarction, congestive cardiac failure, and ventricular fibrillation. There was also a reduction in infarct size, as assessed by cardiac enzymes, in patients who had a β-blocker in addition to t-PA. The TIMI IIB trial [67] compared immediate intravenous metoprolol within 6 hours of onset of chest pain (a mean of 42 minutes after initiation of t-PA administration) to delayed oral metoprolol (on day 6). Subgroup analysis showed that very early treatment was associated with significant benefit compared with delayed treatment with a reduction in 6-week mortality or reinfarction of 61% (p = 0.01) when metoprolol was given within 2 hours of onset of symptoms. A similar marked benefit was also observed in patients treated with intravenous β-blockers within the first 2 hours in the ISIS-1 study [68]. Despite the evidence, the use of intravenous (IV) β-blockers is small.

## Antiarrhythmics

Patients with acute MI are at risk of ventricular fibrillation, cardiac arrest, and sudden death within the first hours after the onset of chest pain. These findings prompted several trials of prophylactic antiarrhythmic drug administration following acute MI, with disappointing results. A meta-analysis of trials of prophylactic lidocaine has shown a significant (35%) reduction in ventricular fibrillation but a nonsignificant (38%) increase in mortality [69]. The increased mortality could be a result of an increased risk of bradyarrhythmias, atrioventricular block, and asystole with the use of lidocaine. Similarly, class Ia and Ic drugs may lead to increased mortality following acute MI [70]. Trials with amiodarone, a class III agent, have been more promising [71]. However, its effect very early after the onset of infarction has not been assessed. The routine use of antiarrhythmic drugs following acute MI is, therefore, not recommended.

## SUMMARY

There have been highly significant advances in prehospital treatment of acute MI over the past few years. The importance of rapid response to the patient presenting in the community with chest pain is now well recognized. Those healthcare professionals responding to emergency calls should be able to reliably diagnose acute MI, initiate early management and manage the early complications of rhythm disturbance, the principle cause of death at this time. Additionally, prehospital diagnosis of MI allows for rapid transfer to selected specialist hospitals for the appropriate administration of definitive treatments including revascularization.

Primary angioplasty has been shown to be associated with improved outcome and decreased complication rate compared to thrombolysis, even when there are delays in transfer of up to 3 hours to the interventional center. The role of adjunctive therapy prior to mechanical reperfusion is still under evaluation with most recent studies demonstrating no increase in bleeding complications, improved indices of perfusion but no clear improvement in clinical outcomes. Where primary angioplasty is available with little delay, there may be no need to consider adjunctive therapy. On the other hand, where there is likely to be a delay of more than one hour, it seems likely that some form of adjunctive therapy will be shown to be useful.

Prehospital thrombolysis is the preferred treatment where primary angioplasty is not available or where the patient presents within the golden hours and there will be a considerable delay before mechanical reperfusion can be instituted. Further investigations are necessary to define these issues more precisely. For patients suffering an MI, the early attendance of trained personnel and successful resuscitation is still the measure that will save most lives. Primary angioplasty, or the early prehospital administration of thrombolysis where an interventional center is not readily available will lead to further significant improvements in outcome.

## REFERENCES

1. Bainton CR, Peterson DR. Deaths from coronary heart disease in persons fifty years of age and younger. A community-wide study. N Engl J Med 1963;268:569–575.
2. Tunstall-Pedoe H, Kuulasmaa K, Amouyel P, Arveiler D, Rajakangas AM, Pajak A. Myocardial infarction and coronary deaths in the World Health Organization MONICA Project. Registration procedures, event rates, and case-fatality rates in 38 populations from 21 countries in four continents. Circulation 1994;90:583–612.
3. Gemmill JD, Lifson WK, Rae AP, Hillis WS, Dunn FG. Assessment by general practitioners of suitability of thrombolysis in patients with suspected acute myocardial infarction. Br Heart J 1993;70:503–506.
4. McCrea WA, Saltissi S. Electrocardiogram interpretation in general practice: relevance to prehospital thrombolysis. Br Heart J 1993;70:219–225.
5. Kudenchuk PJ, Ho MT, Weaver WD, Litwin PE, Martin JS, Eisenberg MS, Hallstrom AP, Cobb LA, Kennedy JW. Accuracy of computer-interpreted electrocardiography in selecting patients for thrombolytic therapy. MITI Project Investigators. J Am Coll Cardiol 1991;17: 1486–1491.
6. Pantridge JF, Geddes JS. A mobile intensive-care unit in the management of myocardial infarction. Lancet 1967;2:271–273.
7. National Heart, Lung and Blood Institutes of Health. Patient/bystander recognition and action : rapid identification and treatment of acute myocardial infarction, National Heart Attach Program (NHAAP). National Institues of Health NIH Publication 1993:93–3303. 2004.
8. Weaver WD, Cobb LA, Hallstrom AP, Fahrenbruch C, Copass MK, Ray R. Factors influencing survival after out-of-hospital cardiac arrest. J Am Coll Cardiol 1986;7:752–757.
9. Crampton RS, Aldrich RF, Gascho JA, Miles JR, Stillerman R. Reduction of prehospital, ambulance and community coronary death rates by the community-wide emergency cardiac care system. Am J Med. 1975;58:151–165.
10. Mathewson ZM, McCloskey BG, Evans AE, Russell CJ, Wilson C. Mobile coronary care and community mortality from myocardial infarction. Lancet 1985;1:441–444.
11. Gundry JW, Comess KA, DeRook FA, Jorgenson D, Bardy GH. Comparison of naive sixth-grade children with trained professionals in the use of an automated external defibrillator. Circulation 1999;100:1703–1707.
12. Reimer KA, Lowe JE, Rasmussen MM, Jennings RB. The wavefront phenomenon of ischemic cell death. 1. Myocardial infarct size vs duration of coronary occlusion in dogs. Circulation 1977;56:786–794.
13. Randomised trial of intravenous streptokinase, oral aspirin, both, or neither among 17,187 cases of suspected acute myocardial infarction: ISIS-2. ISIS-2 (Second International Study of Infarct Survival) Collaborative Group. Lancet 1988;2:349–360.
14. Effectiveness of intravenous thrombolytic treatment in acute myocardial infarction. Gruppo Italiano per lo Studio della Streptochinasi nell'Infarto Miocardico (GISSI). Lancet 1986;1: 397–402.
15. An international randomized trial comparing four thrombolytic strategies for acute myocardial infarction. The GUSTO investigators. N Engl J Med 1993;329:673–682.
16. Boersma E, Maas AC, Deckers JW, Simoons ML. Early thrombolytic treatment in acute myocardial infarction: reappraisal of the golden hour. Lancet 1996;348:771–775.

17. Fath-Ordoubadi F, Beatt KJ. Fibrinolytic therapy in suspected acute myocardial infarction. Lancet 1994;343:912.

18. Weaver WD. Time to thrombolytic treatment: factors affecting delay and their influence on outcome. J Am Coll Cardiol 1995;25:3S–9S.

19. Birkhead JS. Time delays in provision of thrombolytic treatment in six district hospitals. Joint Audit Committee of the British Cardiac Society and a Cardiology Committee of Royal College of Physicians of London. BMJ 1992;305:445–448.

20. Koren G, Weiss AT, Hasin Y, Appelbaum D, Welber S, Rozenman Y, Lotan C, Mosseri M, Sapoznikov D, Luria M. Prevention of myocardial damage in acute myocardial ischemia by early treatment with intravenous streptokinase. N Engl J Med 1985;313:1384–1389.

21. Kereiakes DJ, Weaver WD, Anderson JL, Feldman T, Gibler B, Aufderheide T, Williams DO, Martin LH, Anderson LC, Martin JS. Time delays in the diagnosis and treatment of acute myocardial infarction: a tale of eight cities. Report from the Pre-hospital Study Group and the Cincinnati Heart Project. Am Heart J 1990;120:773–780.

22. Weaver WD, Eisenberg MS, Martin JS, Litwin PE, Shaeffer SM, Ho MT, Kudenchuk P, Hallstrom AP, Cerqueria MD, Copass MK. Myocardial Infarction Triage and Intervention Project—phase I: patient characteristics and feasibility of prehospital initiation of thrombolytic therapy. J Am Coll Cardiol 1990;15:925–931.

23. Very early thrombolytic therapy in suspected acute myocardial infarction. The Thrombolysis Early in Acute Heart Attack Trial Study Group. Am J Cardiol 1990;65:401–407.

24. Roth A, Barbash GI, Hod H, Miller HI, Rath S, Modan M, Har-Zahav Y, Keren G, Bassan S, Kaplinsky E. Should thrombolytic therapy be administered in the mobile intensive care unit in patients with evolving myocardial infarction? A pilot study. J Am Coll Cardiol 1990; 15:932–936.

25. The Belgian Eminase Prehospital Study (BEPS). BEPS Collaborative Group. Prehospital thrombolysis in acute myocardial infarction. Eur Heart J 1991;12:965–967.

26. Bouten MJ, Simoons ML, Hartman JA, van Miltenburg AJ, van der DE, Pool J. Prehospital thrombolysis with alteplase (rt-PA) in acute myocardial infarction. Eur Heart J 1992;13: 925–931.

27. Weaver WD, Cerqueira M, Hallstrom AP, Litwin PE, Martin JS, Kudenchuk PJ, Eisenberg M. Prehospital-initiated vs hospital-initiated thrombolytic therapy. The Myocardial Infarction Triage and Intervention Trial. JAMA 1993;270:1211–1216.

28. McNeill AJ, Cunningham SR, Flannery DJ, Dalzell GW, Wilson CM, Campbell NP, Khan MM, Patterson GC, Webb SW, Adgey AA. A double blind placebo controlled study of early and late administration of recombinant tissue plasminogen activator in acute myocardial infarction. Br Heart J 1989;61:316–321.

29. Castaigne ADHCD-MA. Prehospital use of APSAC: results of a placebo-controlled study. Am J Cardiol 1989;64(suppl A):30–33.

30. Barbash GI, Roth A, Hod H, Miller HI, Modan M, Rath S, Zahav YH, Shachar A, Basen S, Battler A. Improved survival but not left ventricular function with early and prehospital treatment with tissue plasminogen activator in acute myocardial infarction. Am J Cardiol 1990;66:261–266.

31. Schofer J, Buttner J, Geng G, Gutschmidt K, Herden HN, Mathey DG, Moecke HP, Polster P, Raftopoulo A, Sheehan FH. Prehospital thrombolysis in acute myocardial infarction. Am J Cardiol 1990;66:1429–1433.

32. Grampian Region Early Anistreplase Trial (GREAT) Investigators. Feasibility, safety, and efficacy of domiciliary thrombolysis by general practitioners: Grampian region early anistreplase trial. BMJ 1992;305:548–553.

33. McAleer B, Ruane B, Burke E, Cathcart M, Costello A, Dalton G, Williams JR, Varma MP. Pre hospital Thrombolysis in rural community:short and long term survival. Cardiovasc Drugs Ther 1992;6:369–372.

34. Prehospital thrombolytic therapy in patients with suspected acute myocardial infarction. The European Myocardial Infarction Project Group. N Engl J Med 1993;329:383–389.

35. Fath-Ordoubadi F, Al-Mohammad A, Huehns TY, Beatt KJ. Meta-analysis of randomised trials of prehospital thrombolysis. Circulation 1994;90:I–325.

36. Fibrinolytic Therapy Trialists' (FTT) Collaborative Group. Indications for fibrinolytic therapy in suspected acute myocardial infarction: collaborative overview of early mortality and major morbidity results from all randomised trials of more than 1000 patients. Lancet 1994;343: 311–322.

37. Morrison LJ, Verbeek PR, McDonald AC, Sawadsky BV, Cook DJ. Mortality and prehospital thrombolysis for acute myocardial infarction: A meta-analysis. JAMA 2000;283:2686–2692.

38. The effects of tissue plasminogen activator, streptokinase, or both on coronary-artery patency, ventricular function, and survival after acute myocardial infarction. The GUSTO Angiographic Investigators. N Engl J Med 1993;329:1615–1622.

39. Neuhaus KL, von Essen R, Tebbe U, Vogt A, Roth M, Riess M, Niederer W, Forycki F, Wirtzfeld A, Maeurer W. Improved thrombolysis in acute myocardial infarction with front-loaded administration of alteplase: results of the rt-PA-APSAC patency study (TAPS). J Am Coll Cardiol 1992;19:885–891.

40. A comparison of continuous infusion of alteplase with double-bolus administration for acute myocardial infarction. The Continuous Infusion versus Double-Bolus Administration of Alteplase (COBALT) Investigators. N Engl J Med 1997;337:1124–1130.

41. Bode C, Smalling RW, Berg G, Burnett C, Lorch G, Kalbfleisch JM, Chernoff R, Christie LG, Feldman RL, Seals AA, Weaver WD. Randomized comparison of coronary thrombolysis achieved with double-bolus reteplase (recombinant plasminogen activator) and front-loaded, accelerated alteplase (recombinant tissue plasminogen activator) in patients with acute myocardial infarction. The RAPID II Investigators. Circulation 1996;94:891–898.

42. Randomised, double-blind comparison of reteplase double-bolus administration with streptokinase in acute myocardial infarction (INJECT): trial to investigate equivalence. International Joint Efficacy Comparison of Thrombolytics. Lancet 1995;346:329–336.

43. Single-bolus tenecteplase compared with front-loaded alteplase in acute myocardial infarction: the ASSENT-2 double-blind randomised trial. Assessment of the Safety and Efficacy of a New Thrombolytic Investigators. Lancet 1999;354:716–722.

44. Gibler WB, Kereiakes DJ, Dean EN, Martin L, Anderson L, Abbottsmith CW, Blanton J, Blanton D, Morris JA Jr, Gibler CD. Prehospital diagnosis and treatment of acute myocardial infarction: a north-south perspective. The Cincinnati Heart Project and the Nashville Prehospital TPA Trial. Am Heart J 1991;121:1–11.

45. Fath-Ordoubadi F, Dana A, Tork A, Huehns TY, Beatt KJ. Prehospital Thrombolysis: a survey of UK's General Practitioners' Views and skills in two different settings (urban vs rural) (abstract). Eur Heart J 1996;17:569.

46. Keeley EC, Boura JA, Grines CL. Primary angioplasty versus intravenous thrombolytic therapy for acute myocardial infarction: a quantitative review of 23 randomised trials. Lancet 2003;361:13–20.

47. Andersen HR, Nielsen TT, Rasmussen K, Thuesen L, Kelbaek H, Thayssen P, Abildgaard U, Pedersen F, Madsen JK, Grande P, Villadsen AB, Krusell LR, Haghfelt T, Lomholt P, Husted SE, Vigholt E, Kjaergard HK, Mortensen LS; DANAMI-2 Investigators. A comparison of coronary angioplasty with fibrinolytic therapy in acute myocardial infarction. N Engl J Med 2003;349:733–742.

48. Widimsky P, Groch L, Zelizko M, Aschermann M, Bednar F, Suryapranata H. Multicentre randomized trial comparing transport to primary angioplasty vs immediate thrombolysis vs combined strategy for patients with acute myocardial infarction presenting to a community hospital without a catheterization laboratory. The PRAGUE study. Eur Heart J 2000;21: 823–831.

49. Stone GW, Grines CL, Cox DA, Garcia E, Tcheng JE, Griffin JJ, Guagliumi G, Stuckey T, Turco M, Carroll JD, Rutherford BD, Lansky AJ; Controlled Abciximab and Device Investigation to Lower Late Angioplasty Complications (CADILLAC) Investigators. Comparison of angioplasty with stenting, with or without abciximab, in acute myocardial infarction. N Engl J Med 2002;346:957–966.

50. Bonnefoy E, Lapostolle F, Leizorovicz A, Steg G, McFadden EP, Dubien PY, Cattan S, Boullenger E, Machecourt J, Lacroute JM, Cassagnes J, Dissait F, Touboul P; Comparison

of Angioplasty and Prehospital Thrombolysis in Acute Myocardial Infarction Study group. Primary angioplasty versus prehospital fibrinolysis in acute myocardial infarction: a randomised study. Lancet 2002;360:825–829.

51. Schatz RA, Baim DS, Leon M, Ellis SG, Goldberg S, Hirshfeld JW, Cleman MW, Cabin HS, Walker C, Stagg J. Clinical experience with the Palmaz-Schatz coronary stent. Initial results of a multicenter study. Circulation 1991;83:148–161.

51a. de Lemos JA, Antman EM, Gibson CM, McCabe CH, Giugliano RP, Murphy SA, Coulter SA, Anderson K, Schere J, Frey MJ, Van der Wieken R, Van de Werf F, Braunwald E. Abciximab improves both epicardial flow and myocardial reperfusion in ST-elevation myocardial infarction. Observation from the TIMI 14 trial. Circulation 2000;101:239–243.

52. Agrawal SK, Ho DS, Liu MW, Iyer S, Hearn JA, Cannon AD, Macander PJ, Dean LS, Baxley WA, Roubin GS. Predictors of thrombotic complications after placement of the flexible coil stent. Am J Cardiol 1994;73:1216–1219.

53. Mak KH, Belli G, Ellis SG, Moliterno DJ. Subacute stent thrombosis: evolving issues and current concepts. J Am Coll Cardiol 1996;27:494–503.

54. Alfonso F, Rodriguez P, Phillips P, Goicolea J, Hernandez R, Perez-Vizcayno MJ, Fernandez-Ortiz A, Segovia J, Banuelos C, Aragoneillo P, Macaya C. Clinical and angiographic implications of coronary stenting in thrombus-containing lesions. J Am Coll Cardiol 1997;29: 725–733.

55. Neumann FJ, Blasini R, Schmitt C, Alt E, Dirschinger J, Gawaz M, Kastrati A, Schomig A. Effect of glycoprotein IIb/IIIa receptor blockade on recovery of coronary flow and left ventricular function after the placement of coronary-artery stents in acute myocardial infarction. Circulation 1998;98:2695–2701.

56. DeGeare VS, Stone GW, Grines L, Brodie BR, Cox DA, Garcia E, Wharton TP, Boura JA, O'Neill WW, Grines CL. Angiographic and clinical characteristics associated with increased in-hospital mortality in elderly patients with acute myocardial infarction undergoing percutaneous intervention (a pooled analysis of the primary angioplasty in myocardial infarction trials). Am J Cardiol 2000;86:30–34.

57. Topol EJ, Califf RM, George BS, Kereiakes DJ, Abbottsmith CW, Candela RJ, Lee KL, Pitt B, Stack RS, O'Neill WW. A randomized trial of immediate versus delayed elective angioplasty after intravenous tissue plasminogen activator in acute myocardial infarction. N Engl J Med 1987;317:581–588.

58. Immediate vs delayed catheterization and angioplasty following thrombolytic therapy for acute myocardial infarction. TIMI II A results. The TIMI Research Group. JAMA 1988;260: 2849–2858.

59. SWIFT trial of delayed elective intervention v conservative treatment after thrombolysis with anistreplase in acute myocardial infarction. SWIFT (Should We Intervene Following Thrombolysis?) Trial Study Group. BMJ 1991;302:555–560.

60. Ross AM, Coyne KS, Reiner JS, Greenhouse SW, Fink C, Frey A, Moreyra E, Traboulsi M, Racine N, Riba AL, Thompson MA, Rohrbeck S, Lundergan CF. A randomized trial comparing primary angioplasty with a strategy of short-acting thrombolysis and immediate planned rescue angioplasty in acute myocardial infarction: the PACT trial. PACT investigators. Plasminogen-activator Angioplasty Compatibility Trial. J Am Coll Cardiol 1999;34:1954–1962.

61. Montalescot G, Barragan P, Wittenberg O, Ecollan P, Elhadad S, Villain P, Boulenc JM, Morice MC, Maillard L, Pansieri M, Choussat R, Pinton P; ADMIRAL Investigators, Abciximab before Direct Angioplasty and Stenting in Myocardial Infarction Regarding Acute and Long-term Follow-up. Platelet glycoprotein IIb/IIIa inhibition with coronary stenting for acute myocardial infarction. N Engl J Med 2001;344:1895–1903.

62. Stone GW, Grines CL, Cox DA, Garcia E, Tcheng JE, Griffin JJ, Guagliumi G, Stuckey T, Turco M, Carroll JD, Rutherford BD, Lansky AJ; Controlled Abciximab and Device Investigations to Lower Late Angioplasty Complication (CADILLAC) Investigators. Comparison of angioplasty with stenting, with or without abciximab, in acute myocardial infarction. N Engl J Med 2002;346:957–966.

63. Trial of abciximab with and without low-dose reteplase for acute myocardial infarction. Strategies for Patency Enhancement in the Emergency Department (SPEED) Group. Circulation 2000;101:2788–2794.

64. Hirsh J, Dalen JE, Fuster V, Harker LB, Salzman EW. Asprin and other platelet-active drugs: the relationship between dose, effectiveness, and side effects (abstract). Chest 1992;102: 327s–336s.

65. Round A, Marshall AJ. Survey of general practitioners' prehospital management of suspected acute myocardial infarction. BMJ 1994;309:375–376.

66. Risenfors M, Herlitz J, Berg CH, Dellborg M, Gustavsson G, Gottfridsson C, Lomsky M, Swedberg K, Hjalmarsson A. Early Treatment with Thrombolysis and beta-blocked in suspected acute Myocardial Infarction: results from the TEAHAT study. (abstract). J Int Med 1991;229:35–42.

67. Roberts R, Rogers WJ, Mueller HS, Lambrew CT, Diver DJ, Smith HC, et al. Immediate versus deferred beta-blockade following thrombolytic therapy in patients with acute myocardial infarction. Results of the Thrombolysis in Myocardial Infarction (TIMI) II-B Study. Circulation 1991;83:422–437.

68. Randomised trial of intravenous atenolol among 16,027 cases of suspected acute myocardial infarction: ISIS-1. First International Study of Infarct Survival Collaborative Group. Lancet 1986;2:57–66.

69. MacMahon S, Collins R, Peto R, Koster RW, Yusuf S. Effects of prophylactic lidocaine in suspected acute myocardial infarction. An overview of results from the randomized, controlled trials. JAMA 1988;260:1910–1916.

70. Effect of the antiarrhythmic agent moricizine on survival after myocardial infarction. The Cardiac Arrhythmia Suppression Trial II Investigators. N Engl J Med 1992;327:227–233.

71. Kudenchuk PJ, Cobb LA, Copass MK, Cummins RO, Doherty AM, Fahrenbruch CE, Hallstrom AP, Murray WA, Olsufka M, Walsh T. Amiodarone for resuscitation after out-of-hospital cardiac arrest due to ventricular fibrillation. N Engl J Med 1999;341:871–878.

# 9

# Fibrinolysis for ST-Elevation Myocardial Infarction: First and Second Generation Agents

**Eric R. Bates**
*Division of Cardiovascular Diseases*
*Department of Internal Medicine*
*University of Michigan*
*Ann Arbor, MI, U.S.A.*

## INTRODUCTION

The development of fibrinolytic therapy for ST-elevation myocardial infarction (STEMI) stands as a paradigm for cooperation between basic science, clinical research, and industry. The result has been the elucidation of the pathogenesis of STEMI, the development of an important new class of pharmacological agents, and the legitimization of multicenter randomized trials as the standard for proving clinical utility. Most importantly, fibrinolytic therapy has been shown to restore infarct artery patency, reduce infarct size, preserve left ventricular function, and decrease mortality in patients with STEMI.

Three seminal events ushered in the "fibrinolytic era." First, DeWood and colleagues [1] performed coronary angiography in patients with STEMI and showed that as many as 85% had thrombotic coronary artery occlusion in the early hours of transmural myocardial infarction (MI). Second, Rentrop and coworkers [2] demonstrated acute reperfusion of occluded infarct arteries with streptokinase. Third, Reimer et al. [3] demonstrated in a dog model that myocardial necrosis, after coronary artery occlusion spread from the endocardial surface to the epicardial surface over a period of hours, restoration of arterial patency before three hours preserved an epicardial rim of viable muscle.

The Western Washington randomized trial of intracoronary streptokinase [4] and the Netherlands Interuniversity Cardiology Institute trial [5] stimulated intense interest in the potential of fibrinolytic therapy, which resulted in an unprecedented explosion in clinical research activity. It is beyond the scope of this review to accurately document the many invaluable accomplishments and observations made by the efforts of so many talented investigators. Nevertheless, the cumulative work of the Thrombolysis and Angioplasty in Myocardial Infarction (TAMI) investigators [6–15] (Table 1), the Thrombolysis in Myocardial Infarction (TIMI) investigators [16–28] (Table 2), the European Cooperative Study Group (ECSG) investigators [29–34] (Table 3), the Gruppo Italiano per lo Studio Della Sopravvivenza nell'Infarto Miocardico (GISSI) investigators [35–37] (Table 4), the International Study of Infarct Survival (ISIS) investigators [38–41] (Table 5), and the

**Table 1**  The Thrombolysis and Angioplasty in Myocardial Infarction (TAMI) Trials

| Trial | Syndrome | Comparison | No. of Patients | Major Findings |
|-------|----------|------------|-----------------|----------------|
| TAMI-1 (6) | STEMI <4–6h | t-PA plus immediate vs. delayed PTCA. | 386 | No advantage for immediate PTCA |
| TAMI-2 (7) | STEMI <4–6h | Combination thrombolysis with t-PA and UK | 146 | Safe and may reduce reocclusion after rescue PTCA |
| TAMI-3 (8) | STEMI <4–6h | t-PA plus immediate vs. 90" delayed IV heparin | 134 | No difference |
| TAMI-4 (9) | STEMI <6h | t-PA ± prostacyclin | 50 | Negative pharmacokinetic interaction |
| TAMI-UK (10) | STEMI <6h | High dose UK | 102 | Safe and effective mono-therapy |
| TAMI-5 (11) | STEMI <6h | 1. t-PA vs. UK vs. combination<br>2. Immediate vs. delayed cardiac catheterization | 575 | 1. Combination reduced in-hospital events<br>2. Early catheterization may benefit |
| TAMI-6 (12) | STEMI 6–24h | Late t-PA vs. placebo | 197 | t-PA improves patency and prevents LV cavity dilation |
| TAMI-7(13) | STEMI <6h | Accelerated t-PA regimes ± UK | 232 | No regimen better than Neuhaus front-loading (58) |
| TAMI-8 (14) | STEMI <6h | t-PA plus platelet GP IIb/IIIa inhibition. | 70 | ↑ patency with potent platelet inhibition |
| TAMI-9 (15) | STEMI <6h | t-PA plus fluosol vs. placebo | 430 | No difference |

GP, glycoprotein; IV, intravenous; LV, left ventricular; PTCA, percutaneous transluminal coronary angioplasty; STEMI, ST elevation myocardial infarction; t-PA, tissue plasminogen activator; UK, urokinase.

Global Utilization of Strategies to Open Occluded Coronary Arteries (GUSTO) investigators [42–46] are noteworthy.

This review will summarize information on the first- and second-generation fibrinolytic agents including streptokinase, alteplase, duteplase, anistreplase, urokinase, and saruplase. Characteristics of the two drugs available in the United States are shown in Table 6.

## STREPTOKINASE

Tillet and Garner [47] discovered in 1933 that a filtrate of b-hemolytic strains of Streptococcus could dissolve human thrombus. Streptokinase is a single chain nonenzyme protein which forms a 1:1 stoichiometric complex with plasminogen. The streptokinase-plasminogen activator complex then converts plasminogen to plasmin, which initiates fibrinolysis. Intravenous streptokinase was initially used in the late 1950s for STEMI [48]

**Table 2**   The Thrombolysis in Myocardial Infarction (TIMI) Streptokinase and Alteplase Trials

| Trial | Syndrome | Comparison | No. of Patients | Major Findings |
|---|---|---|---|---|
| TIMI-I (16) | STEMI <7h | t-PA vs. SK | 290 | ↑ reperfusion with t-PA |
| TIMI-IIA (17) | STEMI <4h | t-PA plus immediate PTCA vs. delayed PTCA | 586 | No benefit from immediate PTCA |
| TIMI-IIB (18) | STEMI <4h | 1. t-PA plus routine PTCA vs. PTCA for recurrent ischemia. 2. Intravenous vs. delayed beta blockade | 3,262 | 1. No benefit from routine PTCA. 2. ↓ reinfarction, ischemia with early B-blocker. |
| TIMI-IIIA (19) | UA/NSTEMI | t-PA vs. placebo | 306 | Small benefit for t-PA in stenosis severity. |
| TIMI-IIIB (20) | UA/NSTEMI | 1. t-PA vs. placebo  2. Early invasive vs. conservative strategy | 1,473 | 1. No benefit t-PA, possible harm  2. Minimal benefit early PTCA; no difference death or MI |
| TIMI-4 (21) | STEMI <6h | Accelerated t-PA vs. APSAC vs. Combination | 382 | Better 60" patency with t-PA, ↓ 6 week mortality. |
| TIMI-5 (22) | STEMI <6h | Hirudin vs. heparin with t-PA | 246 | ↑ Patency with hirudin 18–36 hr, ↓ death and recurrent MI. |
| TIMI-6 (23) | STEMI <6h | Hirudin vs. heparin with SK | 193 | Trend for ↓ recurrent MI, ↓ CHF, ↑ EF with hirudin. |
| TIMI-9A (24) | STEMI <12h | Hirudin vs. heparin with thrombolytics | 757 | Excessive bleeding. |
| TIMI-9B (25) | STEMI <12h | Hirudin vs. heparin with thrombolytics | 3,002 | No difference. |
| TIMI-10B (26) | STEMI <12h | Accel t-PA vs. TNK | 886 | Equivalent patency. |
| TIMI-14 (27) | STEMI <12h | Full dose lytic vs. Abciximab plus reduced dose SK, t-PA, r-PA | 888 | Higher patency with abciximab plus reduced dose lytic. |
| TIMI-17 (In-TIME-II) (28) | STEMI <6h | Accel rt-PA vs. lanoteplase. | 15,078 | No difference. |

APSAC, anisoylated plasminogen streptokinase activator complex; CHF, congestive heart failure; EF, ejection fraction; MI, myocardial infarction; STEMI, non-ST elevation myocardial infarction; PTCA, percutaneous transluminal coronary angioplasty; r-PA, recombinant plasminogen activator; SK, streptokinase; STEMI, ST elevation myocardial infarction; TNK, tenecteplase; t-PA, tissue plasminogen activator.

**Table 3**   The European Cooperative Study Group (ECSG) Trials

| Trial | Syndrome | Comparison | No. of Patients | Major Findings |
|---|---|---|---|---|
| ECSG-1 (29) | STEMI <6h | t-PA vs. SK | 129 | ↑ patency with t-PA. |
| ECSG-2 (30) | STEMI <6h | t-PA vs. placebo | 129 | ↑ patency with t-PA. |
| ECSG-3 (31) | STEMI <4h | 6h t-PA infusion vs. placebo in patent infarct artery | 123 | No difference in late reocclusion. |
| ECSG-4 (32) | STEMI <5h | t-PA ± PTCA at 2h | 367 | PTCA detrimental. |
| ECSG-5 (33) | STEMI <5h | t-PA vs. placebo. | 721 | ↓ infarct size, trend ↓ mortality |
| ECSG-6 (34) | STEMI <6h | t-PA± heparin. | 652 | Better patency with heparin. |

PTCA, percutaneous transluminal coronary angioplasty; STEMI, ST elevation myocardial infarction; t-PA, tissue plasminogen activator.

and was tested in several multicenter trials in the 1960s and 1970s [49]. Unfortunately, improvement in left ventricular function and mortality were inconsistently found because of inadequate doses and late implementation of therapy. Immediate arteriographic recanalization following intracoronary injection of streptokinase during STEMI was first reported by Chazov [50] and later in the English literature by Rentrop, et al [2]. These observations legitimized fibrinolytic therapy for STEMI and initiated the angiographic evaluation of mechanisms and clinical benefit.

## Coronary Patency, Infarct Size, and Left Ventricular Function

The conventional dose of 1.5 million units over 60 minutes for intravenous streptokinase was derived empirically by Schroeder and colleagues [51]. Sixty and 90 minute patency rates are approximately 50% and 2–3 hour patency rates are 70% [52] (Table 7).

Enzymatic estimation of infarct size in the Netherlands Interuniversity Cardiology Institute study [53] of intracoronary streptokinase demonstrated a 51% decrease in infarct size in patients treated within one hour of onset of symptoms, of 31% treated, between one and two hours, and of 13% treated, between two and four hours. The Intravenous

**Table 4**   The Gruppo Italiano per lo Studio della Sopravvivenza nell'Infarto Miocardico (GISSI) Trials

| Trial | Syndrome | Comparison | No. of Patients | Major Findings |
|---|---|---|---|---|
| GISSI-1 (35) | STEMI <12h | SK vs. placebo | 11,806 | ↓ mortality with SK. |
| GISSI-2 (36) | STEMI <6h | 1. t-PA vs. SK<br>2. SQ heparin vs. placebo | 12,490 | 1. No mortality difference.<br>2. No mortality difference. |
| GISSI-3 (37) | STEMI <24h | 1. Nitrate vs. placebo<br>2. Lisinopril vs. placebo | 19,394 | 1. No mortality difference.<br>2. Mild mortality benefit. |

SK, streptokinase; STEMI, ST elevation myocardial infarction; SQ, subcutaneous.

**Table 5** The International Study of Infarct Survival (ISIS) Trials

| Trial | Syndrome | Comparison | No. of Patients | Major Findings |
|---|---|---|---|---|
| ISIS-1 (38) | Suspected MI <12h | Atenolol vs. placebo | 16,027 | ↓ mortality with atenolol. |
| ISIS-2 (39) | Suspected MI <24h | SK vs. placebo ± ASA | 17,187 | ↓ mortality with SK, ASA; lowest with both. |
| ISIS-3 (40) | Suspected MI <24h | 1. Duteplase vs. SK vs. APSAC<br>2. SQ heparin vs. placebo | 39,713 | 1. No mortality difference.<br>2. No mortality difference. |
| ISIS-4 (41) | Suspected MI <24h | 1. Magnesium vs. placebo<br>2. Nitrate vs. placebo<br>3. Captopril vs. placebo | 58,050 | 1. No mortality difference.<br>2. No mortality difference.<br>3. Mild mortality benefit. |

APSAC, anisoylated plasminogen streptokinase activator complex; ASA, aspirin; MI, myocardial infarction; SK, streptokinase; SQ, subcutaneous.

**Table 6** Characteristics of Thrombolytic Drugs

| | Streptokinase | Alteplase |
|---|---|---|
| Plasma clearance time (min) | 15–25 | 4–8 |
| Fibrin specificity | Minimal | Moderate |
| Plasminogen binding | Indirect | Direct |
| Potential allergic reaction | Yes | No |
| Typical dose | $1.5 \times 10^6$ units | 100 mg |
| Administration (min) | 60 | 90 |
| Cost ($) | 568 | 2750 |

**Table 7** Infarct Artery Patency Results*

| Time | Control | Streptokinase | Alteplase (3h) | Alteplase (90 min) | Anistreplase | Urokinase |
|---|---|---|---|---|---|---|
| 60 min | 15 (6–24) | 48 (41–56) | 57 (52–61) | 74 (70–77) | 61 (55–67) | – |
| 90 min | 21 (11–31) | 51 (48–55) | 70 (68–72) | 84 (82–87) | 70 (66–74) | 60 (55–64) |
| 2–3 hr | 24 (14–35) | 70 (65–75) | 73 (65–80) | | 74 (68–80) | 58 (48–68) |
| 1 day | 21 (9–32) | 86 (82–89) | 84 (82–86) | 86 (82–90) | 80 (77–83) | – |
| 3–21 days | 61 (57–64) | 73 (70–78) | 80 (78–81) | 89 (85–94) | 85 (81–89) | 72 (63–81) |

* percent (95% confidence interval)
Adapted from Ref. 52

Streptokinase in Acute Myocardial infarction (ISAM) trial [54] measured a lower enzymatic infarct size in patients treated within three hours after onset of pain, but no difference in patients treated later.

Likewise, early treatment is associated with preservation of approximately six ejection fraction points [55,56]. End-systolic volume measurements are smaller in treated patients [55,57].

## Mortality Trials

The Western Washington intracoronary streptokinase trial [4] randomized 134 patients to streptokinase and 116 patients to control. Recanalization was achieved in 68% of the streptokinase-treated group and 30-day mortality was significantly reduced (3.7 vs 11.2%).

The Netherlands Interuniversity Cardiology Institute trial [5] allocated 264 patients to conventional treatment and 269 to intracoronary streptokinase, the last 117 of which were first treated with 500,000 units of intravenous streptokinase. Time to treatment was 80 minutes faster than in the Western Washington trial and the recanalization rate was higher (79%). Mortality rates at 28 days were significantly reduced with streptokinase (5.9 vs 11.7%).

The ISAM trial [54] randomized 1,741 patients to intravenous streptokinase or control within six hours of symptom onset. Mortality at 21 days was lower than expected in the control group, rendering the trial underpowered to detect a treatment difference. However, the insignificant relative reduction in mortality associated with streptokinase therapy (6.3 vs. 7.1%) was similar to that seen in the GISSI-1 trial [35].

The GISSI-1 trial [35] randomized 11,806 patients to either intravenous streptokinase or control within 12 hours of symptom onset. Mortality at 21 days was 10.7% in the streptokinase group vs. 13% in the control group, an 18% reduction. The largest reduction (47%) was seen when treatment was initiated within one hour of symptom onset.

The ISIS-2 trial [39] randomized 17,187 patients within 24 hours of the onset of symptoms of suspected MI to streptokinase, aspirin, both, or neither. Streptokinase alone reduced five-week vascular mortality (9.2% vs. 12%) and the combination of aspirin plus streptokinase additionally reduced mortality (8% vs. 13.2%).

The Estudio Multicentrico Estreptoquinasa Republicas de America del Sur (EMERAS) trial [58] found an insignificant 14% reduction (11.7% vs. 13.2%) in hospital mortality in 2,080 patients randomized to streptokinase or placebo 6–12 hours after symptom onset, but no benefit in patients presenting after 12–24 hours.

## ALTEPLASE

Tissue plasminogen activator (t-PA) is a naturally occurring single chain serine protease normally secreted by vascular endothelium. It was first obtained from the Bowes melanoma cell line and is now produced by recombinant DNA techniques. Native t-PA and alteplase (rt-PA) have a binding site for fibrin, which causes a great affinity for attaching to thrombus and preferentially lysing it, although systemic plasminogen activation occurs at clinical doses.

## Coronary Patency, Infarct Size, and Left Ventricular Function

The TIMI-I [16] and ECSG-1 [29] studies established higher 90-minute patency rates for rt-PA than streptokinase. The TIMI-II trial [18] began with a dose of 150 mg over six hours, but this was reduced to 100 mg over three hours because of an unacceptable rate of intracerebral hemorrhage. Numerous studies established a 90-minute patency rate of 70% with this dose [52], a success rate equal to that achieved with streptokinase 2–3 hours after initiation of therapy (Table 7). Neuhaus and colleagues [59] accelerated the dosing, infusing the total dose of 100 mg before the 90-minute angiogram and achieved a 90-minute patency rate of 91%. Purvis and coworkers [60] tested double bolus (two 50 mg injections 30 minutes apart) alteplase and demonstrated 93% patency rates at 90 minutes. Subsequent testing has established that a weight-adjusted accelerated or front-loaded dose (15 mg bolus, 0.75 mg/kg over 30 minutes, 0.5 mg/kg over 60 minutes) is superior to double bolus dosing and achieves 90-minute patency rates of approximately 82% [43,52].

The ECSG-5 trial [33] was a double-blind, placebo-controlled trial in 721 patients treated within five hours of symptom onset. The cumulative myocardial enzyme release over 72 hours was 20% lower in patients treated with alteplase. Three small trials [61–63] had previously revealed a 6–7% higher ejection fraction in patients treated with alteplase. The ECSG-5 [33] trial measured a 2.2% higher ejection fraction and lower end-diastolic and end-systolic volumes in patients randomized to alteplase.

## Mortality Trials

The Anglo-Scandinavian Study of Early Thrombolysis (ASSET) [64] randomized 5,011 patients with less than five hours of symptoms to alteplase or placebo. Although patients received intravenous heparin, aspirin was not given. At one month, mortality was reduced by 26% with alteplase (7.2% vs. 9.8%).

The Late Assessment of Thrombolytic Efficacy (LATE) study [65] randomized 5,711 patients with symptoms between 6 and 24 hours from onset to alteplase or placebo. A significant 26% reduction in 35-day mortality (8.9 vs. 12%) was found in the 6–12 hour group, but no difference was seen between 12–24 hours.

The ECSG-5 trial [33] randomized 721 patients with less than 5 hours of symptoms to alteplase or placebo. Despite only small differences in ejection fraction, the 14–day mortality was reduced with alteplase (2.8 vs. 5.7%).

There have been two comparative trials of alteplase vs. streptokinase (Table 8). The GISSI-2 trial [36] tested a 3-hour alteplase infusion and found no treatment advantage. The 12,490 patients from GISSI-2 were added to 8,401 recruited elsewhere to form the International Study [66], with no mortality difference between alteplase and streptokinase (8.9% vs. 8.5%). In contrast, the GUSTO-I trial [42] tested the accelerated dose combined with intravenous heparin and found a significant mortality reduction (6.3 vs. 7.3%).

Finally, the Continuous Infusion vs. Double Bolus Administration of Alteplase (CO-BALT) trial [67], comparing double bolus dosing with the accelerated dose in 7,169

**Table 8**  Study Design of Thrombolytic Megatrials

| | International (65)* | ISIS-3 (40) | GUSTO-1 (42) |
|---|---|---|---|
| Sample size | 20,891 | 41,299 | 41,021 |
| Thrombolytic regimen | 1. Streptokinase | 1. Streptokinase | 1. Streptokinase |
| | 2. Alteplase (3 hr) | 2. Duteplase (4 hr) | 2. Alteplase (90 min) |
| | | 3. Anistreplase | 3. Streptokinase/Alteplase |
| Heparin regimen | 12,500 IU SQ BID | 12,500 IU SQ BID | 12,500 IU SQ BID or |
| | or placebo | or placebo | 1,000–1,200 IU/hr |
| Delay in heparin Rx | 12 hr | 4 hr | 4 hr SQ 0 hr IV |

* Includes 12,490 patients from GISSI-2 trial.

patients, was prematurely stopped when no mortality benefit (8.0% vs. 7.5%) was seen during an interim analysis.

## The TAMI Trials

The TAMI Study Group (Table 1) completed 10 studies [6–15] of various alteplase and urokinase, therapeutic regimens in STEMI focusing on dosing and adjunctive therapies. Angiography was used to assess infarct artery patency and left ventricular function. Ten different doses of alteplase were given, with an accelerated dose similar to the dose used by Neuhaus et al. [59] having the highest patency rate [13]. Treating patients 6–24 hours after symptom onset improved early patency (65% vs. 27%) and preserved end-diastolic volume (TAMI-6) [12]. The strategy of immediate Percutaneous Transluminal Coronary Angioplasty (PTCA) after successful fibrinolysis offered no clinical benefit (TAMI-1) [6], but acute angiography and rescue PTCA as necessary was feasible and potentially useful (TAMI-1 [6], TAMI-5 [11]). Immediate heparin administration did not facilitate fibrinolysis (TAMI-3) [8], as suggested in animal studies, but more potent platelet inhibition with a monoclonal antibody directed against the platelet glycoprotein (GP) IIb/IIIa receptor did improve patency (TAMI-8) [14]. Preclinical studies suggesting that prostacyclin and fluosol decreased reperfusion injury by inhibiting free radicals and neutrophil activity, and improved left ventricular function were not confirmed in the TAMI-4 [9] and TAMI-9 [15] studies, respectively. Furthermore, the TAMI dataset was analyzed in a number of publications to examine patient selection, clinical outcomes, and prognosis [68].

## The TIMI Trials

In parallel with the TAMI investigators, the TIMI investigators were also studying fibrinolysis with streptokinase and alteplase [16–28] (Table 2). After demonstrating superior recanalization rates for rt-PA compared with streptokinase in TIMI-1 [16], the TIMI-II [17,18] trial showed no advantage for PTCA immediately or 18–48 hours after thrombolysis vs. a selective strategy of treating postinfarction ischemia. The TIMI-III trial [19,20] examined patients with unstable angina and NSTEMI. Patients treated with alteplase instead of placebo had a higher rate of MI (8.3% vs. 4.6%) and a 0.55% risk of intracerebral hemorrhage. An early invasive strategy with angiography, rather than an early conservative strategy with routine medical care and risk stratification, was associated with no difference in death or MI, but fewer patients were rehospitalized or taking antianginal medications at 6 weeks. In TIMI-4 [21], accelerated alteplase had higher patency rates and improved clinical benefit, compared with anistreplase or combination thrombolytic therapy. Hirudin, a direct thrombin inhibitor, achieved a more consistent level of anticoagulation than heparin when tested with alteplase in TIMI-5 [22] and streptokinase in TIMI-6 [23]. Clinical endpoints were also improved. However, a high dose was associated with an unacceptable rate of intracerebral hemorrhage in TIMI-9 [24] and a lower dose had no survival advantage [25].

The TIMI-10B trial showed equivalent patency rates with accelerated alteplase and tenecteplase [26]. Coadministration of abciximab with reduced dose alteplase or reteplase increased patency rates in TIMI-14 [27]. There was no mortality difference between accelerated alteplase and laneteplase in TIMI-17, but intracerebral hemorrhage rates were higher with lanoteplase [28]. The TIMI dataset has also produced a number of important publications [69].

## DUTEPLASE

Duteplase is a nearly pure two-chain form of rt-PA. It differs from alteplase, only in the substitution of methionine for valine at position 245 in the amino acid sequence in the kringle 2 region. Duteplase produced a 90-minute patency rate of 69% in 488 patients when given over four hours, with 0.4 megaunits/kg given in the first hour (including a 10% bolus) and 0.2 megaunits/kg given over the subsequent three hours [70]. As with the conventional alteplase dose of 100 mg over three hours used in the GISSI-2 trial [36], two-thirds the dose was administered by 90 minutes. This dose was used in the ISIS-3 trial [40] where no mortality difference was seen between streptokinase (10.6%), duteplase (10.3%), and anistreplase (10.5%). Patency results and the mortality data from GISSI-2 and ISIS-3 suggest that duteplase and alteplase are clinically equivalent. Duteplase was withdrawn from further development after loss of a patent infringement legal suit to the manufacturer of alteplase.

## ANISTREPLASE

Anistreplase (anisoylated plasminogen streptokinase activator complex, APSAC) is a stoichiometric combination of streptokinase and human lys-plasminogen. An anisoyl group reversibly bound to the catalytic center of the plasminogen moiety slowly undergoes deacylation prior to direct plasminogen activation. The delayed onset of action permits the agent to be administered over a few minutes.

### Coronary Patency, Infarct Size, and Left Ventricular Function

A dose of 30 mg injected over five minutes contains approximately one million units of streptokinase. Patency rates are equivalent to those seen with the three-hour alteplase dose, with a 70% 90-minute patency rate [52].

The APSAC Multicenter Trial Group [71] found no difference in peak creatine kinase activity, although the time to peak activity was shorter with anistreplase vs. placebo. In contrast, Bassand et al. [72] demonstrated a 31% decrease in infarct size measured by single photon emission computed tomography. Similarly, the former trial [71] showed no difference in left ventricular function, whereas the latter trial [72] found a 6% higher mean left ventricular ejection fraction with anistreplase.

### Mortality Trials

The APSAC Intervention Mortality Study (AIMS) [73] randomized 1,258 patients to anistreplase or placebo within six hours from symptom onset. The trial was stopped prematurely due to the 47% mortality reduction seen with anistreplase (6.4% vs. 12.1%).

There have been five comparative trials involving anistreplase, streptokinase, and rt-PA. The Second Thrombolytic Trial of Eminase in Acute Myocardial Infarction (TEAM-2) [74] compared anistreplase and streptokinase, showing comparable patency and mortality (5.9% vs. 7.1%) results in 370 patients. The TEAM-3 trial [75] documented equivalent patency rates and mortality (6.2% vs. 7.9%) between anistreplase and standard alteplase in 325 patients. The ISIS-3 study [40] showed no difference in mortality between streptokinase, duteplase and anistreplase. The rt-PA-APSAC Patency Study (TAPS) [76] showed higher patency and lower mortality (2.4% vs. 8.1%) for accelerated alteplase vs. anistreplase in 435 patients. Similarly, TIMI-4 [21] showed the same mortality advantage

(2.2% vs. 8.8%) for accelerated alteplase compared with anistreplase in 382 patients. Anistreplase was withdrawn from the U.S. market in 2000.

## UROKINASE

Urokinase is a double chain serine protease derived initially from urine and subsequently, from neonatal renal parenchymal cell cultures. It directly activates plasminogen without forming an activator complex, like alteplase, but like streptokinase, it is not specific for fibrin-bound thrombus.

Urokinase can be given as a bolus, like alteplase, or infused over 60 to 90 minutes. Mathey and coworkers [77] injected a bolus of 2 million units and documented a 60% patency rate at 60 minutes in 50 patients. Four other trials had similar patency rates at 90 minutes with 3 million unit infusion protocols [10,11,78,79]. Mortality trials have not been performed, and intravenous urokinase (unlike intracoronary urokinase) is not formally approved by the Food and Drug Administration for use in STEMI.

Urokinase has been used in combination with alteplase [7,11,13,80], producing an improved 90-minute patency rate of 72% and low reocclusion rates. However, other trials [21,42] of combination thrombolytic therapy have not demonstrated clinical benefit and there may be an increased risk of intracerebral hemorrhage.

## SARUPLASE

Saruplase is a recombinant unglycosylated form of single chain urokinase (pro-urokinase). It exhibits relative fibrin specificity, a short half-life, and concomitant need for adjunctive heparin infusion. Saruplase has generally been administered as a 20 mg bolus and a 60 mg infusion over 60 minutes. In the Pro-Urokinase in Myocardial Infarction (PRIMI) trial [81], saruplase patency rates were superior to streptokinase and equivalent to those seen with standard alteplase and anistreplase. The Comparative Trial of Saruplase vs. Streptokinase (COMPASS) trial [82] showed that 30-day mortality rates were at least as low with saruplase as streptokinase (5.7 vs. 6.7%). The Study in Europe of Saruplase and Alteplase in Myocardial Infarction (SESAM) trial [83] found equivalent patency, reocclusion, and complication rates, compared with standard alteplase.

## COMPLICATIONS

The major complication of fibrinolytic therapy is bleeding. Although fibrin-specific agents were expected to result in fewer bleeding complications, the large comparative trials found no difference in bleeding or transfusion rates [35,38,42]. The true incidence of bleeding has been difficult to determine because of underreporting in larger trials of streptokinase, the subjective nature of the events, and the variable use of invasive procedures. In GUSTO-I [42], the transfusion rate was 10%. Concomitant use of heparin increases bleeding risk, particularly when the activated partial thrombin time (aPTT) exceeds 100 seconds [84]. Therefore, therapeutic heparin is not recommended with the longer acting agents streptokinase and anistreplase, although it is given with alteplase and saruplase to prevent infarct artery reocclusion. Many patients have conditions that increase the risk of serious bleeding and are absolute contraindications for fibrinolytic therapy [85]. These include aortic dissection, acute pericarditis, active bleeding, previous cerebral hemorrhage, intracerebral vascular or neoplastic disease, and major surgery, organ biopsy, or trauma in the preceding two weeks. Relative contraindications include blood pressure greater than 180/110 mm Hg, history of stroke, prolonged or traumatic cardiopulmonary resuscitation, puncture of a noncompressible vessel, and major surgery or trauma in the preceding 2–4 weeks. When life-threatening bleeding occurs, heparin should be discontinued. Therapeutic interventions include protamine to normalize the aPTT, cryoprecipitate to increase fibrinogen levels, fresh frozen plasma to replace clotting factors, platelet transfusions if the bleeding time is prolonged, and packed red blood cells to restore hemoglobin mass [86]. A computerized tomographic scan of the head should be performed to document suspected intracranial hemorrhage.

The most devastating complication of thrombolytic therapy is intracerebral hemorrhage. Data from clinical trials and unselected populations suggest that the risk is 0.5–1% [87]. At least half the patients die and severe disability occurs in an additional 25%. Increased risk is associated with age greater than 65 years, hypertension, and low body-weight [88]. More potent fibrinolytic agents increase risk. In GUSTO-I [42], an excess of two intracerebral hemorrhages per 1,000 patients was seen with alteplase compared with streptokinase. It is important to note, however, that fibrinolytic therapy decreases late, presumably thrombotic, stroke, so there is no overall excess in stroke.

Streptokinase and anistreplase are antigenic. Because of antibody formation, re-treatment should not be given after four days of the initial exposure to avoid neutralization of streptokinase activity [89]. Moreover, mild allergic reactions (fever, rash, rigor, broncho-spasm) occur in 5%, including anaphylactic shock in 0.2%, and release of bradykinin produces hypotension in 5–10% [39].

Early reports suggested that reocclusion rates were higher with alteplase (14%) than with streptokinase, anistreplase, or urokinase (8%) [87]. However, no differences were seen in GUSTO-I [42], perhaps due to the use of monitored intravenous heparin with alteplase. Additionally, there does not appear to be any difference between agents in rates of recurrent ischemia (20%) or reinfarction (4%).

The incidence of atrial and ventricular arrhythmias, congestive heart failure, and cardiogenic shock were each reduced by an absolute 1% with alteplase versus streptokinase in GUSTO-1 [42].

## CONCLUSION

First generation fibrinolytics, including streptokinase, anistreplase, and urokinase, are not fibrin specific and activate plasminogen systemically. Second-generation fibrinolytics, including alteplase, duteplase, and saruplase, preferentially activate plasminogen at the fibrin clot. Accelerated or front-loaded alteplase, administered with intravenous heparin for 24–48 hours, has proven to be the best fibrinolytic strategy tested to date. Its superior ability to restore early normal blood flow to the infarct artery has been associated with improved left ventricular function and lower mortality and morbidity rates than the other agents. Bolus administration of alteplase, or combination therapy with alteplase and strep-tokinase, anistreplase, or urokinase, have not proven to be superior strategies. The standard three-hour infusion of alteplase appears to produce clinical outcomes similar to streptoki-nase, anistreplase, and saruplase. Anistreplase is the easiest to administer and streptokinase is the least expensive agent. Long-term follow-up demonstrates that the short-term reduc-tion in mortality is maintained for at least one year [90–93].

The link between normal infarct artery blood flow, preserved left ventricular function and mortality reduction documented in GUSTO-I [42,43] has stimulated new efforts to develop superior lytic agents (Chapter 10) and new adjunctive strategies. The wealth of information provided by the studies summarized in this review has clearly established the benchmarks against which new strategies will be tested.

## REFERENCES

1. DeWood MA, Spores J, Notske R, Mouser LT, Burroughs R, Golden MS, Lang HT. Prevalence of total coronary occlusion during the early hours of transmural infarction. N Engl J Med 1980;303:897–902.
2. Rentrop KT, Blanke H, Karsch KR, Weigand V, Kostering H. Acute myocardial infarction: Intracoronary application of nitroglycerine and streptokinase. Clin Cardiol 1979;2:354–363.
3. Reimer KA, Lowe JE, Rasmussen MM, Jennings RB. The wave-front phenomenon of ischemic death. I. Myocardial infarct size vs duration of coronary occlusion in dogs. Circulation 1977; 56:786–794.
4. Kennedy JW, Ritchie JL, Davis KB, Fritz JK. Western Washington randomized trial of intracoronary streptokinase in acute myocardial infarction. N Engl J Med 1983;309:1477–1482.
5. Simoons M, Van den Brand M, De Zwaan C, Verheugt FWA, Remme WJ, Serruys PW, Bär F, Res J, Krauss XH, Vermeer F, Lubsen J. Improved survival after early thrombolysis in acute myocardial infarction: A randomized trial of the Interuniversity Cardiology Institute in the Netherlands. Lancet 1985;2:578–582.
6. Topol EJ, Califf RM, George BS, Kereiakes DJ, Abbottsmith CW, Candela RJ, Lee KL, Pitt B, Stack RS, O'Neill WW. A randomized trial of immediate versus delayed elective angioplasty after intravenous tissue plasminogen activator in acute myocardial infarction. N Engl J Med 1987;317:581–588.
7. Topol EJ, Califf RM, George BS, Kereiakes DJ, Rothbaum D, Candela RJ, Abbottsmith CW, Pinkerton CA, Stump DC, Collen D, Lee KL, Pitt B, Kline EM, Boswick JM, O'Neill WW, Stack RS. Coronary arterial thrombolysis with combined infusion of recombinant tissue-type plasminogen activator and urokinase in patients with acute myocardial infarction. Circulation 1988;77:1100–1107.
8. Topol EJ, George BS, Kereiakes DJ, Stump DC, Candela RJ, Abbottsmith CW, Aronson L, Pickel A, Boswick JM, Lee KL, Ellis SG, Califf RM. A randomized controlled trial of intravenous tissue plasminogen activator and early intravenous heparin in acute myocardial infarction. Circulation 1989;79:281–286.
9. Topol EJ, Ellis SG, Califf RM, George BS, Stump DC, Bates ER, Nabel EG, Walton JA, Candela RJ, Lee KL, Kline EM, Pitt B. Combined tissue-type plasminogen activator and prostacyclin therapy for acute myocardial infarction. J Am Coll Cardiol 1989;14:877–884.
10. Wall TC, Phillips HR, Stack RS, Mantell S, Aronson L, Boswick J, Sigmon K, DiMeo M, Chaplin D, Whitcomb D, Pasi D, Zawodniak M, Hajisheik M, Hegde S, Barker W, Tenney R, Califf RM. Results of high dose intravenous urokinase for acute myocardial infarction. Am J Cardiol 1990;65:124–131.
11. Califf RM, Topol EJ, Stack RS, Ellis SG, George BS, Kereiakes DJ, Samaha JK, Worley SJ, Anderson JL, Harrelson-Woodlief L, Wall TC, Phillips HR, Abbottsmith CW, Candela RJ, Flanagan WH, Sasahara AA, Mantell SJ, Lee KL. Evaluation of combination thrombolytic therapy and timing of cardiac catheterization in acute myocardial infarction. Results of Thrombolysis and Angioplasty in Myocardial Infarction - Phase 5 randomized trial. Circulation 1991; 83:1543–1556.
12. Topol EJ, Califf RM, Vandormael M, Grines CL, George BS, Sanz ML, Wall T, O'Brien M, Schwaiger M, Aguirre FV, Young S, Popma JJ, Sigmon KN, Lee KL, Ellis SG. A randomized trial of late reperfusion therapy for acute myocardial infarction. Circulation 1992;85: 2090–2099.
13. Wall TC, Califf RM, George BS, Ellis SG, Samaha JK, Kereiakes DJ, Worley SJ, Sigmon K, Topol EJ. Accelerated plasminogen activator dose regimens for coronary thrombolysis. J Am Coll Cardiol 1992;19:482–489.
14. Kleiman NS, Ohman EM, Califf RM, George BS, Kereiakes D, Aguirre FV, Weisman H, Schaible T, Topol EJ. Profound inhibition of platelet aggregation with monoclonal antibody 7E3 fab after thrombolytic therapy: Results of the Thrombolysis and Angioplasty in Myocardial Infarction (TAMI) 8 pilot study. J Am Coll Cardiol 1993;22:381–389.
15. Wall TC, Califf RM, Blankenship J, Talley JD, Tannenbaum M, Schwaiger M, Gacioch G, Cohen MD, Sanz M, Leimberger JD, Topol EJ. Intravenous fluosol in the treatment of acute

myocardial infarction: Results of the Thrombolysis and Angioplasty in Myocardial Infarction 9 trial. Circulation 1994;90:114–120.

16. The TIMI Study Group. The Thrombolysis in Myocardial Infarction (TIMI) Trial. Phase 1 findings. N Engl J Med 1985;312:932–936.

17. Rogers WJ, Baim DS, Gore JM, Brown BG, Roberts R, Williams DO, Chesebro JH, Babb JD, Sheehan FH, Wackers FJT, Zaret BL, Robertson TL, Passamani ER, Ross R, Knatterud GL, Braunwald E. for the TIMI II-A Investigators. Comparison of immediate invasive, delayed invasive, and conservative strategies after tissue-type plasminogen activator. Results of the Thrombolysis in Myocardial Infarction (TIMI) Phase II-A Trial. Circulation 1990;81: 1457–1476.

18. TIMI Study Group. Comparison of invasive and conservative strategies after treatment with intravenous tissue plasminogen activator in acute myocardial infarction. Results of the Thrombolysis in Myocardial Infarction (TIMI) Phase II Trial. N Engl J Med 1989;320:618–627.

19. The TIMI IIIA Investigators. Early effects of tissue-type plasminogen activator added to conventional therapy on the culprit lesion in patients presenting with ischemic cardiac pain at rest. Results of the Thrombolysis in Myocardial Ischemia (TIMI-IIIA) Trial. Circulation 1993; 87:38–52.

20. The TIMI-IIIB Investigators. Effects of tissue plasminogen activator and a comparison of early invasive and conservative strategies in unstable angina and non–Q-wave myocardial infarction: Results of the TIMI IIIB Trial. Circulation 1994;89:1545–1556.

21. Cannon CP, McCabe CH, Diver DJ, Herson S, Greene RM, Shah PK, Sequeira RF, Leya F, Kirshenbaum JM, Magorien RD, Palmeri ST, Davis V, Gibson CM, Poole WK, Braunwald E. Comparison of front-loaded recombinant tissue-type plasminogen activator, anistreplase and combination thrombolytic therapy for acute myocardial infarction: Results of the Thrombolysis in Myocardial Infarction (TIMI) 4 trial. J Am Coll Cardiol 1994;24:1602–1610.

22. Cannon CP, McCabe CH, Henry TD, Schweiger M, Gibson RS, Mueller HS, Becker RC, Kleiman NS, Haugland JM, Anderson JL, Sharaf BL, Edwards S, Rogers W, Williams DO, Braunwald E. A pilot trial of recombinant desulfatohirudin compared with tissue-type plasminogen activator and aspirin for acute myocardial infarction: Results of the Thrombolysis in Myocardial Infarction (TIMI) 5 trial. J Am Coll Cardiol 1994;23:993–1003.

23. Lee LV. Initial experience with hirudin and streptokinase in acute myocardial infarction: Results of the Thrombolysis in Myocardial Infarction (TIMI) 6 trial. Am J Cardiol 1995;75: 7–13.

24. Antman EM. Hirudin in acute myocardial infarction: Safety report from the Thrombolysis and Thrombin Inhibition in Myocardial Infarction (TIMI) 9A trial. Circulation 1994;90:1624–1630.

25. Antman EM. Hirudin in acute myocardial infarction. Thrombolysis and Thrombin Inhibition in Myocardial Infarction (TIMI) 9B Trial. Circulation 1996;94:911–921.

26. Cannon CP, Gibson CM, McCabe CH, Adgey AAJ, Schweiger MJ, Sequeira RF, Grollier G, Giugliano RP, Frey M, Meuller HS, Steingart RM, Weaver WD, Van de Werf F, Braunwald E. for the Thrombolysis in Myocardial Infarction (TIMI) 10B Investigators. TNK-tissue plasminogen activator compared with front-loaded alteplase in acute myocardial infarction: Results of the TIMI 10B trial. Circulation 1998;98:2805–2814.

27. Antman EM, Giugliano RP, Gibson CM, McCabe CH, Coussement P, Kleiman NS, Vahanian A, Adgey AAJ, Menown I, Rupprecht H-J, Van der Wieken R, Ducas J, Scherer J, Anderson K, Van de Werf F, Braunwald E. for the TIMI 14 investigators. Abciximab facilitates the rate and extent of thrombolysis: Results of the thrombolysis in myocardial infarction (TIMI) 14 trial. Circulation 1999;99:2720–2732.

28. In-TIME-II Investigators. Intravenous NPA for the treatment of myocardium infracting; IN-TIME-II, a double-blind comparison of single-bolus lanteplase vs accelerated alteplase for the treatment of patients with acute myocardial infarction. Eur Heart J 2000;21:2005–2013.

29. Verstraete M, Bernard R, Bory M, Brower RW, Collen D, de Bono DP, Erbel R, Huhmann W, Lennane RJ, Lubsen J, Mathey D, Meyer J, Michels HR, Rutsch W, Schartl M, Schmidt W, Uebis R, von Essen R. Randomised trial of intravenous recombinant tissue-type plasminogen activator versus intravenous streptokinase in acute myocardial infarction. Lancet 1985;1: 842–847.

30. Verstraete M, Bleifeld W, Brower RW, Charbonnier B, Collen D, de Bono DP, Dunning AJ, Lennane RJ, Lubsen J, Mathey DG, Michel PL, Raynaud PH, Schofer J, Vahanian A, Vanheke J, van de Kley GA, Van de Werf F, von Essen R. Double-blind randomised trial of intravenous tissue-type plasminogen activator versus placebo in acute myocardial infarction. Lancet 1985; 2:965–969.

31. Verstraete M, Arnold AER, Brower RW, Collen D, de Bono DP, De Zwaan C, Erbel R, Hillis WS, Lennane RJ, Lubsen J, Mathey D, Reid DS, Rutsch W, Schartl M, Schofer J, Serruys PW, Simoons ML, Uebis R, Vahanian A, Verheugt FWA, von Essen R. Acute coronary thrombolysis with recombinant human tissue-type plasminogen activator: Initial patency and influence of maintained infusion on reocclusion rate. Am J Cardiol 1987;60:231–237.

32. Simoons ML, Betriu A, Col J, von Essen R, Lubsen J, Michel PL, Rutsch W, Schmidt W, Thery C, Vahanian A, Willems GM, Arnold AER, DeBono DP, Dougherty PC, Lambertz H, Meier B, Raynaud P, Sanz GA, Uebis R, Van de Werf F, Wood D, Verstraete M. Thrombolysis with tissue plasminogen activator in acute myocardial infarction: No additional benefit from immediate percutaneous coronary angioplasty. Lancet 1988;1:197–202.

33. Van de Werf F, Arnold AER. Intravenous tissue plasminogen activator and size of infarct, left ventricular function, and survival in acute myocardial infarction. Br Med J 1988;297: 1374–1379.

34. de Bono DP, Simoons ML, Tijssen J, Arnold AE, Betriu A, Burgersdijk C, Lopez Bescos L, Mueller E, Pfisterer M, Zijlstra F, Verstraete M, Van de Werf F. Effect of early intravenous heparin on coronary patency, infarct size, and bleeding complications after alteplase thrombolysis: Results of a randomised double blind European Cooperative Study Group trial. Br Heart J 1992;67:122–128.

35. Gruppo Italiano per lo Studio della Streptochinasi nell'infarto Miocardico (GISSI). Effectiveness of intravenous thrombolytic treatment in acute myocardial infarction. Lancet 1986;1: 397–401.

36. Gruppo Italiano per lo Studio Della Sopravvivenza nell'infarto Miocardico. GISSI-2: a factorial randomised trial of alteplase versus streptokinase and heparin versus no heparin among 12,490 patients with acute myocardial infarction. Lancet 1990;336:65–71.

37. Gruppo Italiano per lo Studio della Sopravvivenza nell'Infarto Miocardico. GISSI-3: effects of lisinopril and transdermal glyceryl trinitrate singly and together on 6-week mortality and ventricular function after acute myocardial infarction. Lancet 1994;343:1115–1122.

38. ISIS-1 (First International Study of Infarct Survival) Collaborative Group. Randomised trial of intravenous atenolol among 16,027 cases of suspected acute myocardial infarction: ISIS-1. Lancet 1986;2:57–66.

39. ISIS-2 (Second International Study of Infarct Survival) Collaborative Group. Randomised trial of intravenous streptokinase, oral aspirin, both, or neither among 17,187 cases of suspected acute myocardial infarction: ISIS-2. Lancet 1988;2:349–360.

40. ISIS-3 (Third International Study of Infarct Survival) Collaborative Group. ISIS-3: A randomized comparison of streptokinase vs tissue plasminogen activator vs anistreplase and of aspirin plus heparin vs aspirin alone among 41,299 cases of suspected acute myocardial infarction. Lancet 1992;339:753–770.

41. ISIS-4 (Fourth International Study of Infarct Survival) Collaborative Group. ISIS-4: A randomized factorial trial assessing early oral captopril, oral mononitrate, and intravenous magnesium sulphate in 58,050 patients with suspected acute myocardial infarction. Lancet 1995;345: 669–685.

42. The GUSTO Investigators: An international randomized trial comparing four thrombolytic strategies for acute myocardial infarction. N Engl J Med 1993;329:673–682.

43. The GUSTO Angiographic Investigators. The effects of tissue plasminogen activator, streptokinase, or both on coronary-artery patency, ventricular function, and survival after acute myocardial infarction. N Eng J Med 1993;329:1615–1622.

44. GUSTO IIa Investigators. Randomized trial of intravenous heparin versus recombinant hirudin for acute coronary syndromes. Circulation 1994;90:1631–1637.

45. GUSTO-IIb Investigators. A comparison of recombinant hirudin versus heparin for the treatment of acute coronary syndromes. N Engl J Med 1996;335:775–782.

46. GUSTO-III Investigators. An international, multicenter, randomized comparison of reteplase with alteplase for acute myocardial infarction. N Engl J Med 1997;337:1118–1123.

47. Tillet WS, Garner RI. The fibrinolytic activity of hemolytic streptococci. J Experimental Med 1933;58:485–502.

48. Fletcher AP, Alkjaersig N, Smyrniotis FE, Sherry S. The treatment of patients suffering from early myocardial infarction with massive and prolonged streptokinase therapy. Trans Assoc Am Physicians 1958;71:287–296.

49. Yusuf S, Collins R, Peto R, Furberg C, Stampfer MJ, Goldhaber SZ, Hennekens CH. Intravenous and intracoronary fibrinolytic therapy in acute myocardial infarction: Overview of results on mortality, reinfarction, and side-effects from 33 randomized controlled trials. Eur Heart J 1985;6:556–585.

50. Chazov EI, Mateeva LS, Mazaev AV, Sargin KE, Sadovskaia GV. Intracoronary administration of fibrinolysis in acute myocardial infarction. Ter Arkh 1976;48:8–19.

51. Schröder GV, Biamino G, von Leitner ER, Linderer T, Brueggeman T, Heitz J, Vohringer HF, Wegscheider K. Intravenous short-term infusion of streptokinase in acute myocardial infarction. Circulation 1983;67:536–548.

52. Granger CB, White H, Bates ER, Ohman EM, Califf RM. Patency profiles and left ventricular function after intravenous thrombolysis: A pooled analysis. Am J Cardiol 1994;74:1220–1228.

53. Simoons ML, Serruys PW, van den Brand M, Res J, Verheugt FWA, Krauss XH, Remme WJ, Bär F, de Zwaan C, van der Laarse A, Vermeer F, Lubsen J. Early thrombolysis in acute myocardial infarction: Limitation of infarct size and improved survival. J Am Coll Cardiol 1986;7:717–728.

54. ISAM Study Group: A prospective trial of intravenous streptokinase in acute myocardial infarction (I.S.A.M.). Mortality, morbidity and infarct size at 21 days. N Engl J Med 1986; 314:1465–1471.

55. Serruys PW, Simoons ML, Suryapranata H, Vermeer F, Wijns W, van den Brand M, Bär F, de Zwaan C, Krauss XH, Remme WJ, Res J, Verheugt FWA, Van Domburg R, Lubsen J, Hugenholtz PG. Preservation of global and regional left ventricular function after early thrombolysis in acute myocardial infarction. J Am Coll Cardiol 1986;7:729–742.

56. White HD, Norris RM, Brown MA, Takayama M, Maslowski A, Bass NM, Ormiston JA, Whitlock T. Effect of intravenous streptokinase on left ventricular function and early survival after acute myocardial infarction. N Engl J Med 1987;317:850–855.

57. White HD, Norris RM, Brown MA, Brandt P, Whitlock R, Wild CJ. Left ventricular end-systolic volume as the major determinant of survival after recovery from myocardial infarction. Circulation 1987;76:41–51.

58. EMERAS (Estudio Multicentrico Estreptoquinasa Republica de America de Sur) Collaborative Group. Randomised trial of late thrombolysis in patients with suspected acute myocardial infarction. Lancet 1993;342:767–772.

59. Neuhaus K-L, Feuerer W, Jeep-Tebbe S, Niederer W, Vogt A, Tebbe U. Improved thrombolysis with a modified dose regimen of recombinant tissue-type plasminogen activator. J Am Coll Cardiol 1989;14:1556–1559.

60. Purvis JA, McNeill AJ, Rizwan A, Siddiqui RA, Roberts MJD, McClements BM, McEnearney D, Campbell NPS, Kahn MM, Webb SW, Wilson CM, Adgey AAJ. Efficacy of 100 mg of double-bolus alteplase in achieving complete perfusion in the treatment of acute myocardial infarction. J Am Coll Cardiol 1994;23:6–10.

61. Guerci AD, Gerstenblith G, Brinker JA, Chandra NC, Gottlieb SO, Bahr RD, Weiss JL, Shapiro EP, Flaherty JT, Bush DE, Chew PH, Gottlieb SH, Halperin HR, Ouyang P, Walford GD, Bell WR, Fatterpaker AK, Llewellyn M, Topol EJ, Healy B, Siu CO, Becker LC, Weisfeldt ML. A randomized trial of intravenous tissue plasminogen activator for acute myocardial infarction with subsequent randomization to elective coronary angioplasty. N Engl J Med 1987;317:1613–1618.

62. O'Rourke M, Baron D, Keogh A, Kelly R, Nelson G, Barnes C, Raftos J, Rivers J, Graham K, Hillman K, Newman H, Healey J, Woolridge J, Rivers J, White H, Whitlock R, Norris R. Limitation of myocardial infarction by early infusion of recombinant tissue-type plasminogen activator. Circulation 1988;77:1311–1315.

63. National Heart Foundation of Australia Coronary Thrombolysis Group: Coronary thrombolysis and myocardial salvage by tissue plasminogen activator given up to 4 hours after onset of myocardial infarction. Lancet 1988;1:203–207.

64. Wilcox RG, von der Lippe G, Olsson CG, Jensen G, Skene AM, Hampton JR. Trial of tissue plasminogen activator for mortality reduction in acute myocardial infarction: The Anglo-Scandinavian Study of Early Thrombolysis (ASSET). Lancet 1988;2:525–530.

65. LATE Study Group. Late assessment of thrombolytic efficacy (LATE) study with alteplase 6–12 hours after onset of acute myocardial infarction. Lancet 1993;342:759–766.

66. International Study Group. In-hospital mortality and clinical course of 20,891 patients with suspected acute myocardial infarction randomized between alteplase and streptokinase with or without heparin. Lancet 1990;336:71–75.

67. The COBALT Investigators. A comparison of continuous infusion of alteplase with double-bolus administration for acute myocardial infarction. The continuous infusion versus double bolus administration of alteplase (rt-PA): The COBALT trial. N Engl J Med 1997;337:1124–1130.

68. Barseness GW, Ohman EM, Califf RM, Kereiakes DJ, George BS, Topol EJ. The Thrombolysis and Angioplasty in Myocardial Infarction (TAMI) trials: A decade of reperfusion strategies. J Intervent Card 1996;9:89–115.

69. Cannon CP, Braunwald E, McCabe CH, Antman EM. The Thrombolysis in Myocardial Infarction (TIMI) trials: The first decade. J Intervent Cardiol 1995;8:117–135.

70. Kalbfleisch JM, Kurnik PB, Thadani U, DeWood MA, Kent R, Magorien RD, Jain AC, Spaccavento LJ, Morris DL, Taylor GJ, Perry JM, Kutcher MA, Gorfinkel HJ, Littlejohn JK. Myocardial infarct artery patency and reocclusion rates after treatment with duteplase at the dose used in the International Study of Infarct Survival-3. Am J Cardiol 1993;71:386–392.

71. Meinertz T, Kasper W, Schumacher M, Just H. The German multicenter trial of anisoylated plasminogen streptokinase activator complex versus heparin for acute myocardial infarction. Am J Cardiol 1988;62:347–351.

72. Bassand JP, Machecourt J, Cassagnes J, Anguenot T, Lusson R, Borel E, Peycelow P, Wolf E, Ducellier D. Multicenter trial of intravenous anisoylated plasminogen streptokinase activator complex (APSAC) in acute myocardial infarction: Effects on infarct size and left ventricular function. J Am Coll Cardiol 1989;13:988–997.

73. AIMS Trial Study Group: Effect of intravenous APSAC on mortality after acute myocardial infarction: Preliminary report of a placebo-controlled clinical trial. Lancet 1988;1:545–549.

74. Anderson JL, Sorenson S, Moreno F, Hackworthy R, Browne K, Dale HT, Leya F, Dangoisse V, Eckerson H, Marder V. Multicenter patency trial of intravenous APSAC compared with streptokinase in acute myocardial infarction. Circulation 1991;88:126–140.

75. Anderson JL, Becker LC, Sorenson SG, Karagounis LA, Browne KF, Shah PK, Morris DC, Fintel DJ, Mueller HS, Ross AM, Hall SM, Askins JK, Doorey AJ, Grines CL, Moreno FL, Marder VJ. APSAC versus alteplase in acute myocardial infarction: Comparative effects on left ventricular function, morbidity and 1-day coronary artery patency. J Am Coll Cardiol 1992;20:753–766.

76. Neuhaus K-L, Von Essen R, Tebbe U, Vogt A, Roth M, Riess M, Niederer W, Forycki F, Wirtzfeld A, Maeurer W, Limbourg P, Merx W, Haerten K. Improved thrombolysis in acute myocardial infarction with front-loaded administration of alteplase: Results of the rt-PA-APSAC Patency Study (TAPS). J Am Coll Cardiol 1992;19:885–891.

77. Mathey DG, Schofer J, Sheehan FH, Becher H, Tilsner V, Dodge HT. Intravenous urokinase in acute myocardial infarction. Am J Cardiol 1985;55:878–882.

78. Neuhaus KL, Tebbe U, Gotwik M, Weber M, Feurer W, Niederer W, Haerer W, Praetorius F, Grosser KD, Huhmann W, Hoepp HW, Alber G, Sheikhzadeh A, Schneider B. Intravenous recombinant tissue plasminogen activator (rt-PA) and urokinase in acute myocardial infarction: Results of the German Activator Urokinase Study (GAUS). J Am Coll Cardiol 1988;12:581–587.

79. Whitlow PL, Bashore TM. Catheterization/Rescue Angioplasty Following Thrombolysis (CRAFT) study: Acute myocardial infarction treated with recombinant tissue plasminogen activator versus urokinase (abstr). J Am Coll Cardiol 1991;17:276A.

80. Urokinase and Alteplase in Myocardial Infarction Collaborative Group (URALMI). Combination of urokinase and alteplase in the treatment of myocardial infarction. Coron Art Dis 1991; 2:225–235.

81. PRIMI Trial Study Group: Randomized double-blind trial of recombinant prourokinase against streptokinase in acute myocardial infarction. Lancet 1989;1:863–868.

82. Tebbe U, Michels R, Adgey J, Boland J, Caspi AVI, Charbonnier B, Windeler J, Barth H, Groves R, Hopkins GR, Fennell W, Betriu A, Ruda M, Milczoch J. Randomized, double-blind study comparing saruplase with streptokinase therapy in acute myocardial infarction: the COMPASS equivalence trial. J Am Coll Cardiol 1998;31:487–493.

83. Bär FW, Meyer J, Vermeer F, Michels R, Charbonnier B, Haerten K, Spiecker M, Macaya C, Hanssen M, Heras M, Boland JP, Morice M-C, Dunn FG, Uebis R, Hamm C, Ayzenberg O, Strupp G, Withagen AJ, Klein W, Windeler J, Hopkins G, Barth H, von Fisenne MJM. for the SESAM Study Group. Comparison of saruplase and alteplase in acute myocardial infarction. Am J Cardiol 1997;79:727–732.

84. Granger CB, Hirsh J, Califf RM, Col J, White HD, Betriu A, Woodlief LH, Lee KL, Bovill EG, Simes RJ, Topol EJ. Activated partial thromboplastin time and outcome after thrombolytic therapy for acute myocardial infarction. Results from the GUSTO-I trial. Circulation 1996; 93:870–878.

85. Ryan TJ, Antman EM, Brooks NH, Califf RM, Hillis LD, Hiratzka LF, Rapaport E, Riegel BJ, Russell RO, EE III, Weaver WD. 1999 update: ACC/AHA guidelines for the management of patients with acute myocardial infarction: A report of the American College of Cardiology/ American Heart Association Task Force on Practice Guidelines (Committee on Management of Acute Myocardial Infarction). J Am Coll Cardiol 1999;34:890–911.

86. Sane DC, Califf RM, Topol EJ, Stump DC, Mark DB, Greenberg CS. Bleeding during thrombolytic therapy for acute myocardial infarction: Mechanisms and management. Ann Intern Med 1989;111:1010–1022.

87. Granger CB, Califf RM, Topol EJ. Thrombolytic therapy for acute myocardial infarction. Drugs 1992;44:293–325.

88. Simoons ML, Maggioni AP, Knatterud G, Leimberger JD, de Jaegere P, van Domburg R, Boersma E, Franzosi MG, Califf R, Schroeder R, Braunwald E. Individual risk assessment for intracranial hemorrhage during thrombolytic therapy. Lancet 1993;342:1523–1528.

89. White HD. Thrombolytic treatment for recurrent myocardial infarction. Avoid repeating streptokinase or anistreplase. Br Med J 1991;302:429–430.

90. Gruppo Italiano per lo Studio della streptochinasi nell 'Infarto Miocardico (GISSI): Long-term effects of intravenous thrombolysis in acute myocardial infarction. Final report of the GISSI study. Lancet 1987;2:871–877.

91. AIMS Trial Study Group: Long-term effects of intravenous anistreplase in acute myocardial infarction: Final report of the AIMS study. Lancet 1990;335:427–431.

92. Wilcox RG, von der Lippe C, Olsson CG, Jensen G, Skene AM, Hampton JR. Effects of Alteplase in acute myocardial infarction: 6-month results from the ASSET study. Lancet 1990; 335:1175–1178.

93. Califf RM, White HD, van de Werf F, Sadowski Z, Armstrong PW, Vahanian A, Simoons ML, Simes RJ, Lee KL, Topol EJ. One-year results from the Global Utilization of Streptokinase and TPA for Occluded Coronary Arteries (GUSTO-1) Trial. Circulation 1996;94:1233–1238.

# 10

# Third-Generation Fibrinolytic Agents and Combined Fibrinoplatelet Lysis for Acute Myocardial Infarction

**Sorin J. Brener**
*The Cleveland Clinic Foundation*
*Cleveland, Ohio, U.S.A.*

## INTRODUCTION

Acute ST-elevation myocardial infarction (STEMI) affects 30–50% of patients presenting with an acute coronary syndrome (ACS) and requires immediate reperfusion therapy. The benefits of such an intervention have been amply documented [1,2]. Beyond extending survival, it improves myocardial salvage, preserves an open artery as a source of collateral flow, and limits the danger of malignant arrhythmias. Fibrinolytic therapy has been studied extensively over the last two decades and has remained the mainstay of reperfusion therapy because of its universal and rapid availability. Chapter 9 reviews in detail the significant contributions to these goals of the first two generations of lytic agents, as well as their important limitations.

Since the last update of this monograph, the main developments in the field of fibrinolysis with third-generation agents have been more in the refinement of the administration regimen and adjunctive treatment, rather than in the synthesis of new compounds. The ideal fibrinolytic agent remains elusive. The latest compounds continue to achieve arterial patency in approximately 60% of patients at 60 minutes from administration and be hampered by a rate of intracranial hemorrhage of 0.6%–1.0%, not significantly different from the performance of the accelerated regimen of tissue plasminogen activator (t-PA). We will review in this chapter the newest evidence from trials utilizing reteplase (r-PA), tenecteplase (TNK-t-PA) and staphylokinase, with or without adjunctive platelet inhibition, as well as other aspects of adjunctive therapy. Lanoteplase (n-PA) has not become commercially available and will not be reviewed [3].

The impetus for the addition of potent platelet inhibition (beyond aspirin) to lysis stems from a number of small-scale Phase II trials, which demonstrated that a regimen of reduced-dose fibrinolysis and full-dose intravenous glycoprotein (GP) IIb/IIIa inhibition has the potential to enhance arterial patency [4,5] and improve markers of epicardial and myocardial reperfusion [6] (discussed in detail in Chapter 12). The ability of oral platelet inhibitors, such as thienopyridines, to promote fibrinolysis is currently under investigation.

Restoration of myocardial perfusion, beyond the achievement of epicardial patency, has been at the forefront of research in the last few years because of its tremendous impact on survival and myocardial salvage. In a study involving 886 patients with acute myocardial infarction (MI), restoration of normal myocardial perfusion (''blush score'' or tissue myocardial perfusion grade III) has been associated with a 30-day mortality of 2.0%, while lesser degrees of successful reperfusion had higher rates of death (4.4% and 6.0%, p = 0.05). Importantly, even in patients with normal epicardial flow, normalized myocardial perfusion conferred a marked survival advantage, 0.73% vs. 2.9% vs. 5.0%, p = 0.03 [7]. In multivariate analysis, the blush score maintained its independent predictive value, while more classical parameters of reperfusion, epicardial flow grade and frame counts, became insignificantly associated with mortality.

## Reteplase

Recombinant plasminogen activator (reteplase, r-PA, Figure 1) is a nonglycosylated deletion mutant of wild-type t-PA, expressed in *Escherichia coli*. It maintains the kringle-2 and protease domains, but lacks the kringle 1, finger, and epidermal growth factor domains. It becomes active after in vitro refolding. In comparison with t-PA, these modifications result in preferential activation of fibrin bound plasminogen, a longer half-life in animals, healthy volunteers and patients [8], enhanced fibrinolytic potency, and lower affinity for endothelial cells [9]. The profile of plasma reteplase activity is monophasic ($t_{1/2}$ = 11.2 minutes), while the reteplase antigen activity displays a biphasic curve with an initial $t_{1/2}$ of 13.9 minutes and a terminal $t_{1/2}$ of almost 3 hours. These observations, made in healthy volunteers [10], suggested that there is dissociation between the antigenic and lytic activity of reteplase. Reteplase-specific antibodies were not detected in 2,400 patients treated initially with this drug.

Reteplase was tested in numerous clinical trials and compared with streptokinase [11] and t-PA [12–14]. In the pivotal Global Utilization of Strategies To open Occluded arteries (GUSTO) III Trial [14], reteplase and t-PA were compared with respect to 30-day mortality in nearly 15,000 patients. Despite initial evidence that reteplase improves rate of Thrombolysis in Myocardial Infarction (TIMI) grade III flow at 90 minutes[12], the mortality was 7.47% for reteplase and 7.24% for t-PA (P = 0.61). This near identity persisted at 1 year [15].

t-PA

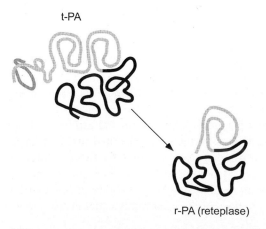

r-PA (reteplase)

**Figure 1**   Transformation from t-PA to reteplase.

The latest and largest trial utilizing reteplase in acute MI was the Global Utilization of Strategies To open Occluded arteries (GUSTO) V study [16] The 16,588 patients, enrolled at 820 hospitals in 20 countries, were randomized 1:1 to double-bolus reteplase (10 U each, 30 min apart) or half-dose double-bolus reteplase (5 U each, 30 min apart) and full dose abciximab. Some important features of these patients are presented in Table 1. The primary end-point was all cause mortality by 30 days. Sixteen prespecified ischemic complications were also tabulated. Notable is the fact that time from symptom onset to administration of therapy has remained stable at approximately 3 hours. Patients scheduled for immediate primary mechanical revascularization, those with even one markedly abnormal blood pressure measurement (systolic $> 180$ mmHg or diastolic $> 110$ mmHg), or those with prior stroke or weighing more than 120 Kg, were excluded.

The statistical considerations of the GUSTO V trial included both the capability to detect superiority of the combination therapy (80% power for 15% reduction in 30-day mortality, assuming a rate of 7.4% with reteplase alone) and the ability to declare the combination therapy noninferior to the monotherapy arm, as long as the excess in mortality observed in the experimental arm did not surpass 10% of the control (reteplase alone) arm rate.

At 30 days, the mortality in the combination arm was 5.62% vs. 5.91% in the reteplase alone arm, or 0.95 (0.83–1.08), $p = 0.45$, satisfying the criteria for noninferiority. (Figure 2) Prespecified subgroup analyses of death by age, gender, presence of diabetes, infarct location, or time from symptom onset to lysis did not reveal any important interactions with treatment arm, as far as ischemic events were concerned. Reinfarction (2.3% vs. 3.5%, $p < 0.001$) and need for rescue urgent percutaneous coronary intervention (5.6% vs. 8.6%, $p < 0.001$) were significantly reduced by the combination therapy. When urgent percutaneous coronary intervention (PCI) was needed up to day 7, the pre-PCI incidence of TIMI flow III was 35% vs. 29% in the combination and monotherapy arms, respectively ($p < 0.001$), while post-PCI the rate of TIMI III flow in both groups was 75%. Paradoxically, it is possible that more frequent need for urgent rescue PCI in the monotherapy arm may have improved outcome in that group, thus reducing the advantage of combination therapy [17]. All but two of post-MI ischemic and arrhythmic complications (pulmonary embolism and pericarditis) were insignificantly less frequent in the combination arm.

**Table 1**  Baseline characteristics of patients enrolled in GUSTO V

|  | Reteplase (n = 8260) | Reteplase+Abciximab (n = 8328) |
|---|---|---|
| Age, y | 61±12 | 62±12 |
| Female gender, % | 25 | 25 |
| Caucasian race, % | 96 | 96 |
| Weight <75 Kg, % | 44 | 45 |
| Hypertension, % | 33 | 35 |
| Hyperlipidemia, % | 16 | 18 |
| Diabetes mellitus, % | 16 | 16 |
| Smoking, % | 46 | 45 |
| Prior MI, % | 15 | 16 |
| Prior heart failure, % | 3 | 3 |
| Prior revascularization, % | 10 | 10 |
| Qualifying anterior MI, % | 37 | 38 |
| Time from symptom onset, h | 2.9±1.6 | 3.1±2.2 |

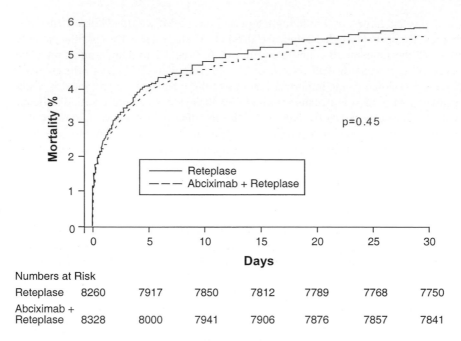

**Figure 2**  Mortality at 30 days in GUSTO V. (From Ref. 16)

The safety of the combination therapy was inferior to that of reteplase alone. There was twice as much severe bleeding (1.1% vs. 0.5%, p < 0.001) and twice as much moderate bleeding (3.5% vs. 1.8%, p < 0.001). Transfusion of blood products was increased by 50% in recipients of combination therapy (5.7% vs. 4.0%, respectively, p < 0.001). Intracranial hemorrhage (ICH) occurred in 0.6% of both groups (p = 0.80). Nevertheless, ICH was nearly twice as common in patients older than 75 years receiving combination therapy, compared with monotherapy (2.1% vs. 1.1%, p = 0.07, Figure 3). In younger patients, the incidence of ICH was lower in the combination arm than in the monotherapy group, such that there was a significant interaction between ICH and treatment, p = 0.032 [18]. It is notable that the reteplase monotherapy arm in GUSTO V had a significantly lower rate of ICH than a similarly treated group of patients in GUSTO III (0.6% vs. 0.9%, p = 0.015). The same magnitude of difference in 30-day mortality was also observed, 5.9% vs. 7.4%, p < 0.001, suggesting a possibly lower risk population and improved adjunctive care. Indeed, median age was 2 years younger in GUSTO V and anterior MI was significantly less frequent, 37% vs. 48% (p < 0.001).

Although the combination therapy was not superior to reteplase monotherapy, it was expected that the significant difference in in-hospital re-MI would translate into a survival benefit by 1 year, particularly when the mortality rate at 30 days was the lowest recorded in any fibrinolytic trial at that time. With nearly complete follow-up (99.4%), the 1-year mortality rate was identical in the two groups, at 8.4%, p = 1.0 [19]. Again, there were no significant interactions with treatment in the prespecified subgroups mentioned earlier. (Figure 4) Even in the patients with anterior MI younger than 75 years, the mortality at 1 year was 7.1% vs. 8.0%, for combination and monotherapy, respectively, p = 0.21.

## Tenecteplase

The need to improve the pharmacokinetics of t-PA and to reduce its susceptibility to circulating inhibitors led to a systematic approach to submolecular modifications of t-PA

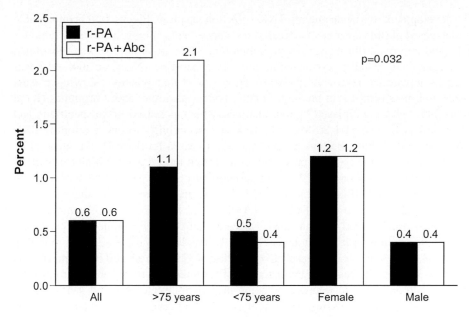

**Figure 3**  Incidence of ICH in Gusto V (From Ref. 16 and Ref. 18).

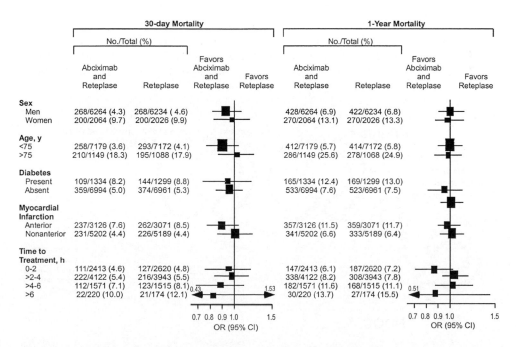

**Figure 4**  Subgroup analysis for treatment interaction in GUSTO V for 30-day and 1-year mortality. (From Ref. 19)

and the development of a triple mutant, TNK-t-PA (tenecteplase, Figure 5). It is remarkable for its decreased plasma clearance, increased resistance to plasminogen activator inhibitor (PAI-1), and improved fibrin specificity. A threonine (T) at position 103 was substituted by asparagine and added a glycosylation site. An asparagine (N) at position 117 was replaced by glutamine, removing a glycosylation site at that position, slowing plasma clearance and increasing fibrin binding. Finally, lysine, histidine, and 2 arginines (K) at positions 296–299 were replaced by four alanines, which increased fibrin specificity and enhanced resistance to PAI-1 80-fold. The lack of susceptibility to inactivation by PAI-1 is an important attribute, because it combats the increased levels of PAI-1 secreted by platelets activated by the lytic agent. Collen et al. tested tenecteplase initially in various experimental thrombosis models [20], and subsequently it was compared with t-PA in numerous Phase II and III clinical studies [21–24]. In the Assessment of the Safety and Efficacy of a New Thrombolytic Regimen (ASSENT-2) trial [24], 16,949 patients with acute MI were randomized to front-loaded accelerated t-PA or weight-adjusted tenecteplase, in conjunction with aspirin and heparin. Thirty-day covariate adjusted mortality was identical, 6.15% and 6.18%, respectively, while ICH occurred in 0.94% and 0.93%, respectively. Besides the ease of administration of tenecteplase, it caused fewer episodes of bleeding and appeared to improve outcome in patients treated beyond 4 hours from symptom onset, 7% vs. 9.2%, respectively, p = 0.018. Of even greater interest was the effect of weight-adjustment of tenecteplase dose in elderly women (> 75 years) of low weight (< 67 Kg). ICH occurred in 1.14% of tenecteplase- and 3.02% of t-PA-treated patients with these characteristics.

The latest clinical trial of tenecteplase in acute ST-elevation MI is the Assessment of the Safety and Efficacy of a New Thrombolytic Regimen (ASSENT-3) [25]. Over 6,000 patients within 6 hours of symptom onset were randomized to one of three arms in a 1:1:1 scheme: Full-dose, weight-adjusted tenecteplase with weigh-adjusted unfractionated heparin (UFH, 60 u/Kg, max 4,000 u bolus and 12 u/h, max. 1,000 u/h infusions) for up to 48 hours (control arm), or full-dose, weight-adjusted tenecteplase with fixed IV bolus and twice-daily weight-adjusted enoxaparin SQ low-molecular weight heparin (LMWH) for up to 7 days or until discharge or revascularization, or half-dose weight-adjusted tenecteplase with IV abciximab for 12 hours and lower dose weight-adjusted (40 u/Kg, max 3,000 u bolus

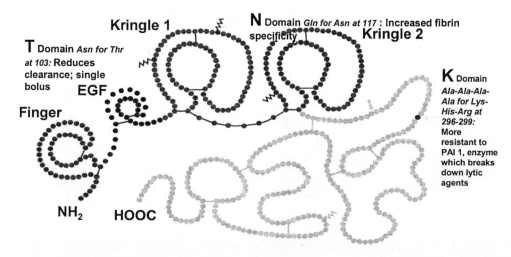

**Figure 5**   Transformation from t-PA to tenecteplase

**Table 2** Baseline characteristics of patients enrolled in ASSENT-3

| | TNK+UFH (n=2038) | TNK+ENOX (n=2040) | TNK+Abciximab (n=2017) |
|---|---|---|---|
| Age, y | 61±13 | 61±12 | 61±12 |
| Female gender, % | 23 | 23 | 24 |
| Weight, Kg | 79±15 | 79±15 | 79±16 |
| Hypertension, % | 41 | 41 | 41 |
| Diabetes mellitus, % | 18 | 19 | 18 |
| Smoking, % | 47 | 44 | 47 |
| Prior MI, % | 14 | 14 | 13 |
| Prior revascularization, % | 9 | 10 | 9 |
| Qualifying anterior MI, % | 38 | 39 | 39 |
| Time from symptom onset, h | 3.1±1.6 | 3.0±1.7 | 3.1±1.4 |

and 7 u/h, max. 800 u/h infusion) UFH for up to 48 hours. The activated partial prothrombin time (aPTT) in the unfractionated heparin (UFH) arms was measured 3 hours after initiation of therapy and maintained at 50–70 seconds. Angiography and revascularization, as in GUSTO V, was left at the discretion of the investigator. The primary efficacy endpoint was the composite of 30-day death and in-hospital reinfarction or refractory ischemia, while the combined efficacy and safety endpoint included the above and ICH or major bleeding. The study was powered (80%) to exclude with 95% confidence a higher than 1% absolute difference between the control arm and each of the experimental combinations. The important baseline characteristics of the three groups are shown in Table 2.

At 30 days, the primary efficacy endpoint was achieved in 15.4%, 11.4% and 11.1%, respectively, $p < 0.001$. (Figure 6) The primary efficacy and safety endpoint was attained in 17.0%, 13.8% and 14.1%, respectively, $p = 0.008$. The major adverse events in each arm are detailed in Table 3. Urgent PCI was needed in 14.4%, 11.9% and 9.1%, respectively,

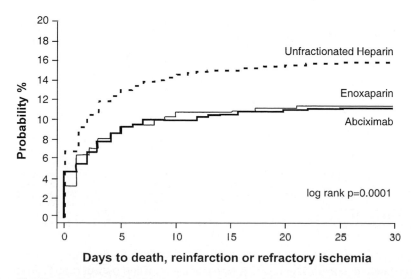

**Figure 6** The combined primary endpoint of death, re-MI or refractory ischemia in AS-SENT-3. (From Ref. 25)

**Table 3**   Major Adverse Events in ASSENT-3

|                        | TNK+UFH (n = 2038) | TNK+ENOX (n = 2040) | TNK+Abciximab (n = 2017) | p value |
|------------------------|--------------------|---------------------|--------------------------|---------|
| Death, 30 d, %         | 6.0                | 5.4                 | 6.6                      | 0.25    |
| In-hospital re-MI, %   | 4.2                | 2.7                 | 2.2                      | 0.0009  |
| In-hospital ischemia, %| 6.5                | 4.6                 | 3.2                      | < 0.0001|
| In-hospital ICH, %     | 0.9                | 0.9                 | 0.9                      | 0.98    |
| Major bleeding. %      | 2.2                | 3.0                 | 4.3                      | 0.0005  |
| Urgent PCI, %          | 14.4               | 11.9                | 9.1                      | < 0.0001|

ASSENT, Assessment of the safety and efficacy of a New Thrombolytic; TNK, tenecteplase; UFH, unfractionated heparin; ENOX, Enoxaparin; MI, myocardial infarction; ICH, intracranial hemorrhage; PCI, percutaneous coronary intervention years

$p < 0.001$. Overall ICH rates were 0.9% in each arm. There was a statistically significant interaction between treatment arm and outcome (combined efficacy and safety) in patients over age 75 years and in diabetics, disfavoring the abciximab arm. (Figure 7) The latter interaction was particularly surprising in view of previously observed benefit of abciximab in diabetics and remains unexplained. Nevertheless, like in GUSTO V, patients older than 75 years had worse outcome with combination fibrin and platelet lysis than with conventional fibrinolysis.

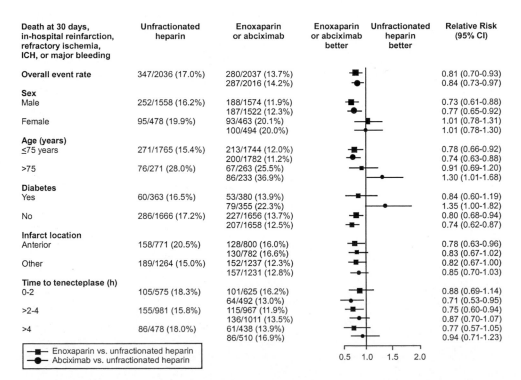

**Figure 7**   Subgroup analysis for treatment interaction in ASSENT-3 for the combined primary efficacy and safety endpoint. There was a significant interaction between abciximab therapy and age (p = 0.001) and between abciximab therapy and diabetes (p = 0.0007). (From Ref. 25)

Beyond the comparison of tenecteplase-based monotherapy and combination therapy, the ASSENT-3 trial refocused our attention on the importance of anti-thrombin therapy in the management of acute MI, as discussed later.

## Recombinant Staphylokinase

Renewed interest in staphylokinase [26]emerged after the successful cloning of its gene in 1980, followed by its expression in *E. Coli* [27]. Elucidation of its molecular interactions revealed a most interesting mechanism of fibrin selectivity, with great potential for clinical application. Like streptokinase, staphylokinase binds in a 1:1 stoichiometric complex with plasminogen. In contrast to streptokinase, the staphylokinase–plasminogen complex is inactive, requiring the transformation to staphylokinase-plasmin to expose its active site and become an effective plasminogen activator. In the absence of fibrin, this latter complex is quickly inactivated by $\alpha_2$-antiplasmin (a process greatly retarded by fibrin), while its predecessor is not. Furthermore, staphylokinase is released for recycling to other plasminogen molecules after the inactivation occurs. The interactions described above confer staphylokinase a unique mechanism for fibrin selectivity. First, the agent is not activated in the absence of fibrin. In contrast, where fibrin is present, small amounts of plasmin on the fibrin surface form an active staphylokinase–plasmin complex, bound to fibrin via the lysine binding sites of plasmin, and protected from rapid inhibition by $\alpha_2$-antiplasmin. Later on, after the thrombus undergoes dissolution, the staphylokinase-plasmin complex is released and inactivated, effectively interrupting further plasminogen activation.

After initial testing in humans [28] and comparison with t-PA [29], staphylokinase, as the modified SAK 42D, was used in the Collaborative Angiographic Patency Trial of Recombinant Staphylokinase (CAPTORS) [30]. Using doses between 15 and 45 mg given as a continuous 30-minute infusion (20% of the dose as bolus) in 82 patients, Armstrong et al. demonstrated a rate of TIMI III flow at 60 minutes of 62%, irrespective of dose. The same investigators refined the molecule using a pegulated SAK 42D staphylokinase variant and compared various doses of PEG-SAK to t-PA in a total of 500 patients [31]. Only at the highest dose, 0.05 mg/Kg did PEG-SAK achieve similar rates of TIMI III flow as t-PA (43% vs. 41%), while lower doses had inferior efficacy. The safety of the compound was also comparable to t-PA.

## Adjunctive Antithrombin Therapy

The prototypical antithrombin agent used with fibrinolysis has been UFH. Its many deficiencies include unpredictable volume of distribution and binding to plasma proteins, unpredictable anticoagulation despite weight-adjusted regimens, inhibition by platelet-derived platelet factor 4, and rebound thrombosis after discontinuation. The latter was observed in the GUSTO I trial and has prompted renewed interest in more sustained and slowly weaning anticoagulation [32,33]. LMWH, and particularly enoxaparin, has been studied extensively in ACS without persistent ST-segment elevation [34–36] and became the logical candidate for evaluation in ST-segment elevation MI. Most of the studies were performed with second-generation lytics, such as t-PA. Because of more predictable anticoagulant effect, reduced bleeding incidence [24]· and lack of need for monitoring, enoxaparin promised to facilitate fibrinolysis and maintain patency of the infarct artery beyond the initial few days after MI. The latter point is particularly important as symptomatic or silent reocclusion is frequent and occurs in 12% of patients with demonstrated patency at 90 minutes after lysis by 7 days [37]. The consequence of reocclusion is a three-fold higher mortality before hospital discharge, 11% vs. 4.5%, p = 0.01 [38]. Some of the predictors of reocclusion, such as the presence of residual thrombus, are particularly amenable to treatment with antithrombin therapy. Indeed, encouraging results were obtained in the Heparin and Aspirin Reperfusion Therapy (HART II) trial [39]. Among 400 patients treated with accelerated t-PA and randomized to enoxaparin or UFH, 90-minute TIMI II or III flow was obtained in 80% and 75%, respectively. It is likely that more effective anticoagulation achieved with enoxaparin was responsible for this trend [40]. Importantly, at 5–7 days, reocclusion in patients with initial TIMI III flow was significantly less frequent in enoxaparin treated patients, 3.1% vs. 9.1%, p < 0.01.

Similar results were observed in the Enoxaparin as Adjunctive Antithrombin Therapy for ST-Elevation Myocardial Infarction (ENTIRE-TIMI) 23 trial [41]. In a $2 \times 2$ factorial design, 483 patients received either full-dose tenecteplase with UFH or enoxaparin (IV bolus and SQ injections), or half-dose tenecteplase and abciximab with UFH or enoxaparin. Although 60-minute patency was not improved overall by enoxaparin-based regimens, compared with UFH, the incidence of re-MI was 1.8% in patients receiving enoxaparin vs. 8.2% for UFH, p = 0.01. Even in patients receiving abciximab, reinfarction was 1.8% for enoxaparin and 3.9% for UFH, suggesting a significantly lower rate of reocclusion. This difference in reinfarction was present both in patients who did (n = 224, 2.8% vs. 8.8%) and in those who did not (n = 259, 1.1% vs. 7.6%) undergo PCI.

Even when combined with a less potent lytic agent, enoxaparin improves outcome. In the acute myocardial infarction-streptokinase (AMI-SK) trial, 496 patients received streptokinase and were randomized to UFH or enoxaparin (IV bolus and SQ injections) for 3–8 days. Partial or complete ST-segment resolution at 180 minutes was more frequent with enoxaparin, 80% vs. 67%, p = 0.004. The primary endpoint, TIMI III flow at predischarge angiography (day 5–10) was achieved in 70% vs. 58%, p = 0.01. This was associated with a reduction in 30-day death, re-MI or recurrent angina from 21% to 13%, p = 0.03 [42].

If one adds the data from the ASSENT-3 PLUS trial of prehospital lytic administration (discussed in Chapter 8) [43] and from the Enoxaparin vs. Unfractionated Heparin After Thrombolytic therapy for Acute Myocardial Infarction [44], all these 5 trials have consistently demonstrated a reduction in reinfarction when enoxaparin is used as the antithrombin agent, regardless of the lytic agent used. Safety concerns, particularly the use in patients older than 75 years [43] and the combination with GPIIa/IIIb, require additional intensive research.

Another approach to adjunctive antithrombin therapy is the use of a direct thrombin inhibitor, such as bivalirudin. White et al. reported in the Hirulog and Early Reperfusion or Occlusion (HERO-2) trial on 17,073 patients treated with streptokinase and randomized to bivalirudin or UFH. While the 30-day mortality was similar (10.8% vs. 10.9%, respectively), adjudicated re-MI within 96 hours was reduced by 30% with bivalirudin (adjusted hazard ratio 0.70 [0.56–0.87], p = 0.001) [45]. Intracranial hemorrhage (ICH) (p = 0.09) and major bleeding (p = 0.07) tended to be more common in the bivalirudin group.

A synthetic factor Xa inhibitor, Pentalyse, was compared with UFH, as an adjunct to t-PA, in 333 patients with acute MI. As with LMWH, the patency of the infarct-artery at 90 minutes was similar among the various dosing groups. At follow-up angiogram (5–7 days), patients treated with Pentalyse demonstrated less reocclusion than those receiving UFH [46].

## Other Adjunctive Therapy to Fibrinolysis

In addition to antithrombin and antiplatelet therapy, other modalities to enhance the fibrinolytic effect of available preparations have been tested, mostly with second- rather than third-generation lytics.

Mahaffey et al. tested the utility of a 3-hour infusion of adenosine or placebo in conjunction with t-PA or streptokinase in 236 patients. There was a significant 67% reduction in scintigraphic infarct size in patients with anterior MI treated with adenosine (15% vs. 45%, p = 0.014), while clinical events did not differ between the groups [47].

The Limitation of Myocardial Infarction Following Thrombolysis in Acute Myocardial Infarction (LIMIT AMI) Study compared anti-CD18 with placebo as adjunct to t-PA in 394 patients with acute MI. Compared with placebo, inhibition of leucocyte aggregation did not result in a reduction in infarct size, persistence of ST-segment elevation or in an improvement in rate of TIMI 3 flow [48].

In a related attempt to investigate the role of complement activation in reperfusion injury, Mahaffey et al. compared Pexelizumab, a C5 inhibitor, to placebo in patients treated with lytic therapy. Among 943 patients receiving placebo, bolus only or bolus and infusion of Pexelizumab, there was no difference in clinical events at 90 days, or in enzymatic infarct size [49].

## Summary and Personal Perspective

Fibrinolytic therapy will continue to be the cornerstone of reperfusion therapy in the majority of patients with acute ST-segment elevation MI. Inherent limitations of these agents, resulting from their insufficient ability to penetrate aging thrombus and the pro-thrombotic state they engender, make the search for the ideal adjunctive therapy ever so more critical. It does not appear, at this time, that a new, more potent lytic is emerging. Instead, utilization of single- or double-bolus compounds and effective thrombin and platelet inhibition promise to deliver early arterial patency in 60–70% of patients. Appropriate and timely adjustment of the adjunctive therapy, based on age, weight, gender and renal function, may limit bleeding complications. The growing population older than 75 years poses an important challenge because of high mortality rate and susceptibility to bleeding complications, including ICH. Prompt and judicious use of early mechanical intervention can bridge the reperfusion gap in the remainder of patients and solidify the early benefits of pharmacotherapy in the majority of acute MI subjects.

## REFERENCES

1. The GUSTO Angiographic Investigators. The effects of tissue plasminogen activator, streptokinase, or both on coronary-artery patency, ventricular function, and survival after acute myocardial infarction. N Engl J Med 1993;329:1615–1621.
2. Fibrinolytic Therapy Trialists' (FTT) Collaborative Group. Indications for fibrinolytic therapy in suspected acute myocardial infarction: collaborative overview of early mortality and major morbidity results from all randomised trials of more than 1000 patients. Lancet 1994;343: 311–322.
3. den Heijer P, Vermeer F, Ambrosioni E, Sadowski Z, Lopez-Seendon JL, von Essen R, Beaufils P, Thadani U, Adgey J, Pierard L, Brinker J, Davies RF, Smalling RW, Wallentin L, Caspi A, Pangerl A, Trickett L, Hauck C, Henry D, Chew P. Evaluation of a weight-adjusted single-bolus plasminogen activator in patients with myocardial infarction: a double-blind, randomized angiographic trial of lanoteplase versus alteplase. Circulation 1998;98:2117–2125.
4. Antman EM, Giugliano RP, Gibson CM, McCabe CH, Coussement P, Kleiman NS, Vahanian A, Adgey AA, Menown I, Rupprecht HJ, Van der Wieken R, Ducas J, Scherer J, Anderson K, Van de Werf F, Braunwald E. Abciximab facilitates the rate and extent of thrombolysis: results of the thrombolysis in myocardial infarction (TIMI) 14 trial. The TIMI 14 Investigators. Circulation 1999;99:2720–2732.

5.  Brener SJ, Zeymer U, Adgey AA, Vrobel TR, Ellis SG, Neuhaus KL, Juran N, Ivanc TB, Ohman EM, Strony J, Kitt M, Topol EJ. Eptifibatide and low-dose tissue plasminogen activator in acute myocardial infarction: the integrilin and low-dose thrombolysis in acute myocardial infarction (INTRO-AMI) trial. J Am Coll Cardiol 2002;39:377–386.

6.  de Lemos JA, Antman EM, Gibson CM, McCabe CH, Giugliano RP, Murphy SA, Coulter SA, Anderson K, Scherer J, Frey MJ, Van Der Wieken R, Van De Werf F, Braunwald E. Abciximab improves both epicardial flow and myocardial reperfusion in ST-elevation myocardial infarction. Observations from the TIMI 14 trial. Circulation 2000;101:239–243.

7.  Gibson CM, Cannon CP, Murphy SA, Ryan KA, Mesley R, Marble SJ, McCabe CH, Van De Werf F, Braunwald E. Relationship of TIMI myocardial perfusion grade to mortality after administration of thrombolytic drugs. Circulation 2000;101:125–130.

8.  Martin U, Sponer G, Strein K. Evaluation of thrombolytic and systemic effects of the novel recombinant plasminogen activator BM 06.022 compared with alteplase, anistreplase, streptokinase and urokinase in a canine model of coronary artery thrombosis. J Am Coll Cardiol 1992;19:433–440.

9.  Hu CK, Kohnert U, Wilhelm O, Fischer S, Llinas M. Tissue-type plasminogen activator domain-deletion mutant BM 06.022: modular stability, inhibitor binding, and activation cleavage. Biochemistry 1994;33:11760–11766.

10. Martin U, van Mollendorf E, Akpan W, Kientsch-Engel R, Kaufmann B, Neugebauer G. Pharmacokinetic and hemostatic properties of the recombinant plasminogen activator BM 06.022 in healthy volunteers. Thromb Haemost 1991;66:569–574.

11. International Joint Efficacy Comparison of Thrombolytics Investigators. Randomised, double-blind comparison of reteplase double-bolus administration with streptokinase in acute myocardial infarction (INJECT): trial to investigate equivalence. Lancet 1995;346:329–336.

12. Bode C, Smalling RW, Berg G, Burnett C, Lorch G, Kalbfleisch JM, Chernoff R, Christie LG, Feldman RL, Seals AA, Weaver WD. Randomized comparison of coronary thrombolysis achieved with double-bolus reteplase (recombinant plasminogen activator) and front-loaded, accelerated alteplase (recombinant tissue plasminogen activator) in patients with acute myocardial infarction. The RAPID II Investigators. Circulation 1996;94:891–898.

13. Smalling RW, Bode C, Kalbfleisch J, Sen S, Limbourg P, Forycki F, Habib G, Feldman R, Hohnloser S, Seals A. More rapid, complete, and stable coronary thrombolysis with bolus administration of reteplase compared with alteplase infusion in acute myocardial infarction. RAPID Investigators. Circulation 1995;91:2725–2732.

14. The Global Use of Strategies to Open Occluded Coronary Arteries (GUSTO III) Investigators. A comparison of reteplase with alteplase for acute myocardial infarction. N Engl J Med 1997; 337:1118–1123.

15. Topol EJ, Ohman EM, Armstrong PW, Wilcox R, Skene AM, Aylward P, Simes J, Dalby A, Betriu A, Bode C, White HD, Hochman JS, Emanuelson H, Vahanian A, Sapp S, Stebbins A, Moliterno DJ, Califf RM. Survival outcomes 1 year after reperfusion therapy with either alteplase or reteplase for acute myocardial infarction: results from the Global Utilization of Streptokinase and t-PA for Occluded Coronary Arteries (GUSTO) III Trial. Circulation 2000; 102:1761–1765.

16. Topol EJ. Reperfusion therapy for acute myocardial infarction with fibrinolytic therapy or combination reduced fibrinolytic therapy and platelet glycoprotein IIb/IIIa inhibition: the GUSTO V randomised trial. Lancet 2001;357:1905–1914.

17. Gibson CM, Karha J, Murphy SA, James D, Morrow DA, Cannon CP, Giugliano RP, Antman EM, Braunwald E. Early and long-term clinical outcomes associated with reinfarction following fibrinolytic administration in the thrombolysis in myocardial infarction trials. J Am Coll Cardiol 2003;42:7–16.

18. Savonitto S, Armstrong PW, Lincoff AM, Jia G, Sila CA, Booth J, Terrosu P, Cavallini C, White HD, Ardissino D, Califf RM, Topol EJ. Risk of intracranial haemorrhage with combined fibrinolytic and glycoprotein IIb/IIIa inhibitor therapy in acute myocardial infarction. Dichotomous response as a function of age in the GUSTO V trial. Eur Heart J 2003;24:1807–1814.

19. Lincoff AM, Califf RM, Van De Werf F, Willerson JT, White HD, Armstrong PW, Guetta V, Gibler WB, Hochman JS, Bode C, Vahanian A, Steg PG, Ardissino D, Savonitto S, Bar

F, Sadowski Z, Betriu A, Booth JE, Wolski K, Waller M, Topol EJ. Mortality at 1 year with combination platelet glycoprotein IIb/IIIa inhibition and reduced-dose fibrinolytic therapy vs conventional fibrinolytic therapy for acute myocardial infarction: GUSTO V Randomized Trial. JAMA 2002;288:2130–2135.

20. Collen D, Stassen JM, Yasuda T, Refino C, Paoni N, Keyt B, Roskams T, Guerrero JL, Lijnen HR, Gold HKet al. Comparative thrombolytic properties of tissue-type plasminogen activator and of a plasminogen activator inhibitor-1-resistant glycosylation variant, in a combined arterial and venous thrombosis model in the dog. Thrombosis & Haemostasis 1994;72:98–104.

21. Cannon C, McCabe C, Gibson M, Ghali M, Sequeira R, McKendall G, Breed J, Modi N, Fox N, Tracy R, Lowe T, Braunwald E. Investigators ftTA. TNK-tissue pasminogen activator in acute myocardial infarction. Results of the Thrombolysis in Myocardial Infarction (TIMI) 10A dose-ranging study. Circulation 1997;95:351–356.

22. Cannon CP, Gibson CM, McCabe CH, Adgey AA, Schweiger MJ, Sequeira RF, Grollier G, Giugliano RP, Frey M, Mueller HS, Steigart RM, Weaver WD, Van de Werf F, Braunwald E. TNK-tissue plasminogen activator compared with front-loaded alteplase in acute myocardial infarction: results from the TIMI 10B trial. Circulation 1998;98:2805–2814.

23. Van de Werf F, Cannon CP, Luyten A, Houbracken K, McCabe CH, Berioli S, Bluhmki E, Sarelin H, Wang-Clow F, Fox NL, Braunwald E. Safety assessment of single-bolus administration of TNK tissue plasminogen activator in acute myocardial infarction: the ASSENT-1 trial. Am Heart J 1999;137:786–791.

24. Assessment of the Safety and Efficacy of a New Thrombolytic Investigators. Single-bolus tenecteplase compared with front-loaded alteplase in acute myocardial infarction: the ASSENT-2 double-blind randomised trial. Lancet 1999;354:716–722.

25. The ASSENT-3 Investigators. Efficacy and safety of tenecteplase in combination with enoxaparin, abciximab, or unfractionated heparin: the ASSENT-3 randomised trial in acute myocardial infarction. Lancet 2001;358:605–613.

26. Collen D, Lijnen HR. Staphylokinase, a fibrin-specific plasminogen activator with therapeutic potential? Blood 1994;84:680–686.

27. Schlott B, Hartmann M, Guhrs KH, Birch-Hirschfeid E, Pohl HD, Vanderschueren S, Van de Werf F, Michoel A, Collen D, Behnke D. High yield production and purification of recombinant staphylokinase for thrombolytic therapy. Bio/Technology. 1994;12:185–9.

28. Collen D, Van de Werf F. Coronary thrombolysis with recombinant staphylokinase in patients with evolving myocardial infarction. Circulation 1993;87:1850–1853.

29. Vanderschueren S, Barrios L, Kerdsinchai P, Van den Heuvel P, Hermans L, Vrolix M, De Man F, Benit E, Muyldermans L, Collen Det al. A randomized trial of recombinant staphylokinase versus alteplase for coronary artery patency in acute myocardial infarction. The STAR Trial Group. Circulation 1995;92:2044–9.

30. Armstrong PW, Burton JR, Palisaitis D, Thompson CR, Van de Werf F, Rose B, Collen D, Teo KK. Collaborative angiographic patency trial of recombinant staphylokinase (CAPTORS). Am Heart J 2000;139:820–823.

31. Armstrong PW, Burton J, Pakola S, Molhoek PG, Betriu A, Tendera M, Bode C, Adgey AA, Bar F, Vahanian A, Van de Werf F. Collaborative Angiographic Patency Trial Of Recombinant Staphylokinase (CAPTORS II). Am Heart J 2003;146:484–488.

32. Granger CB, Hirsch J, Califf RM, Col J, White HD, Betriu A, Woodlief LH, Lee KL, Bovill EG, Simes RJ, Topol EJ. Activated partial thromboplastin time and outcome after thrombolytic therapy for acute myocardial infarction: results from the GUSTO-I trial. Circulation 1996;93:870–878.

33. Granger CB, Becker R, Tracy RP, Califf RM, Topol EJ, Pieper KS, Ross AM, Roth S, Lambrew C, Bovill EG. Thrombin generation, inhibition and clinical outcomes in patients with acute myocardial infarction treated with thrombolytic therapy and heparin: results from the GUSTO-I Trial. GUSTO-I Hemostasis Substudy Group. Global Utilization of Streptokinase and TPA for Occluded Coronary Arteries. J Am Coll Cardiol 1998;31:497–505.

34. Antman EM, McCabe CH, Gurfinkel EP, Turpie AG, Bernink PJ, Salein D, Bayes De Luna A, Fox K, Lablanche JM, Radley D, Premmereur J, Braunwald E. Enoxaparin prevents death

and cardiac ischemic events in unstable angina/non-Q-wave myocardial infarction. Results of the thrombolysis in myocardial infarction (TIMI) 11B trial. Circulation 1999;100:1593–1601.

35. Cohen M, Demers C, Gurfinkel EP, Turpie AG, Fromell GJ, Goodman S, Langer A, Califf RM, Fox KA, Premmereur J, Bigonzi F. A comparison of low-molecular-weight heparin with unfractionated heparin for unstable coronary artery disease. Efficacy and Safety of Subcutaneous Enoxaparin in Non-Q-Wave Coronary Events Study Group. N Engl J Med 1997;337: 447–452.

36. Antman EM, Cohen M, McCabe C, Goodman SG, Murphy SA, Braunwald E. Enoxaparin is superior to unfractionated heparin for preventing clinical events at 1-year follow-up of TIMI 11B and ESSENCE. Eur Heart J 2002;23:308–314.

37. Gibson CM, Cannon CP, Piana RN, Breall JA, Sharaf B, Flatley M, Alexander B, Diver DJ, McCabe CH, Flaker GCet al. Angiographic predictors of reocclusion after thrombolysis: results from the Thrombolysis in Myocardial Infarction (TIMI) 4 trial. J Am Coll Cardiol 1995;25: 582–589.

38. Ohman EM, Califf RM, Topol EJ, Candela R, Abbottsmith C, Ellis S, Sigmon KN, Kereiakes D, George B, Stack R. Consequences of reocclusion after successful reperfusion therapy in acute myocardial infarction. TAMI Study Group. Circulation 1990;82:781–791.

39. Ross AM, Molhoek P, Lundergan C, Knudtson M, Draoui Y, Regalado L, Le Louer V, Bigonzi F, Schwartz W, de Jong E, Coyne K. Randomized comparison of enoxaparin, a low-molecular-weight heparin, with unfractionated heparin adjunctive to recombinant tissue plasminogen activator thrombolysis and aspirin: second trial of Heparin and Aspirin Reperfusion Therapy (HART II). Circulation 2001;104:648–652.

40. Hsia J, Kleiman N, Aguirre F, Chaitman BR, Roberts R, Ross AM. Heparin-induced prolongation of partial thromboplastin time after thrombolysis: relation to coronary artery patency. HART Investigators. J Am Coll Cardiol 1992;20:31–35.

41. Antman EM, Louwerenburg HW, Baars HF, Wesdorp JCL, Hamer B, Bassand J-P, Bigonzi F, Pisapia G, Gibson CM, Heidbuchel H, Braunwald E, Van de Werf F. for the ENTIRE-TIMI 23 Investigators. Enoxaparin as Adjunctive Antithrombin Therapy for ST-Elevation Myocardial Infarction: Results of the ENTIRE-Thrombolysis in Myocardial Infarction (TIMI) 23 Trial. Circulation 2002;105:1642–1649.

42. Simoons M, Krzeminska-Pakula M, Alonso A, Goodman S, Kali A, Loos U, Gosset F, Louer V, Bigonzi F. Improved reperfusion and clinical outcome with enoxaparin as an adjunct to streptokinase thrombolysis in acute myocardial infarction. The AMI-SK study. Eur Heart J 2002;23:1282–1290.

43. Wallentin L, Goldstein P, Armstrong PW, Granger CB, Adgey AA, Arntz HR, Bogaerts K, Danays T, Lindahl B, Makijarvi M, Verheugt F, Van de Werf F. Efficacy and safety of tenecteplase in combination with the low-molecular-weight heparin enoxaparin or unfractionated heparin in the prehospital setting: the Assessment of the Safety and Efficacy of a New Thrombolytic Regimen (ASSENT)-3 PLUS randomized trial in acute myocardial infarction. Circulation 2003;108:135–142.

44. Baird SH, Menown IB, McBride SJ, Trouton TG, Wilson C. Randomized comparison of enoxaparin with unfractionated heparin following fibrinolytic therapy for acute myocardial infarction. Eur Heart J 2002;23:627–632.

45. White H. Thrombin-specific anticoagulation with bivalirudin versus heparin in patients receiving fibrinolytic therapy for acute myocardial infarction: the HERO-2 randomised trial. Lancet 2001;358:1855–1863.

46. Coussement PK, Bassand JP, Convens C, Vrolix M, Boland J, Grollier G, Michels R, Vahanian A, Vanderheyden M, Rupprecht HJ, Van de Werf F. A synthetic factor-Xa inhibitor (ORG31540/SR9017A) as an adjunct to fibrinolysis in acute myocardial infarction. The PENTALYSE study. Eur Heart J 2001;22:1716–1724.

47. Mahaffey KW, Puma JA, Barbagelata NA, DiCarli MF, Leesar MA, Browne KF, Eisenberg PR, Bolli R, Casas AC, Molina-Viamonte V, Orlandi C, Blevins R, Gibbons RJ, Califf RM, Granger CB. Adenosine as an adjunct to thrombolytic therapy for acute myocardial infarction: results of a multicenter, randomized, placebo-controlled trial: the Acute Myocardial Infarction STudy of ADenosine (AMISTAD) trial. J Am Coll Cardiol 1999;34:1711–1720.

48. Baran KW, Nguyen M, McKendall GR, Lambrew CT, Dykstra G, Palmeri ST, Gibbons RJ, Borzak S, Sobel BE, Gourlay SG, Rundle AC, Gibson CM, Barron HV. Double-blind, randomized trial of an anti-CD18 antibody in conjunction with recombinant tissue plasminogen activator for acute myocardial infarction: limitation of myocardial infarction following thrombolysis in acute myocardial infarction (LIMIT AMI) study. Circulation 2001;104:2778–2783.

49. Mahaffey KW, Granger CB, Nicolau JC, Ruzyllo W, Weaver WD, Theroux P, Hochman JS, Filloon TG, Mojcik CF, Todaro TG, Armstrong PW. Effect of pexelizumab, an anti-C5 complement antibody, as adjunctive therapy to fibrinolysis in acute myocardial infarction: the COMPlement inhibition in myocardial infarction treated with thromboLYtics (COMPLY) trial. Circulation 2003;108:1176–1183.

# 11

# Diagnosis of Acute Coronary Syndromes in the Emergency Department: Evolution of Chest Pain Centers

**Andra L. Blomkalns and Brian W. Gibler**
*University of Cincinnati College of Medicine*
*Cincinnati, Ohio, U.S.A.*

## INTRODUCTION

Each year in the United States, it is estimated that nearly 8 million patients present to the emergency departments (ED) with complaints of chest discomfort or other symptoms consistent with potential acute manifestations of acute coronary syndrome (ACS). Typically, over half of these patients are admitted for further diagnostic evaluation, yet fewer than 20% are ultimately diagnosed with ACS. Hospital beds and inpatient resources are scarce in the current environment. These admissions could potentially be avoided by evaluating low to moderate risk patients in a chest pain center (CPC) [1–4] in the emergency setting.

Patients with chest discomfort and possible ACS represent a high-risk group requiring a protocol-driven approach and specific ED resources. During this protocol, patients must be evaluated for myocardial necrosis, rest ischemia, and exercise-induced ischemia. This evaluation is needed to appropriately determine if a patient is safe to be discharged home from the ED with outpatient follow-up, or to identify ACS requiring treatment and hospitalization.

The concept of rapid diagnostic and treatment protocols in the ED for specific disease processes is not new. Similar evaluations for trauma patients have been widely accepted for many years. These same tenants of early evaluation, appropriate risk stratification and rapid intervention, are also most appropriate for the patient presenting with possible ACS to the emergency setting. Just as trauma centers have certification procedures and adopted regulations, CPCs should individually adopt basic principles of evaluation and set minimum standards for quality assurance/improvement. This crucial evaluation and risk stratification period in the ED is the chief rationale for a CPC.

## IMPLEMENTATION

Implementation of a CPC can be challenging. Several components are required to appropriately, efficiently, and cost-effectively evaluate this patient group. These include:

1.  Sufficient and dedicated space to evaluate and observe the patients
2.  Nursing staff and other emergency personnel that are knowledgeable and dedicated to this evaluation
3.  Emergency physician staff that can be nearby and capable of caring for these patients
4.  Collaboration of Cardiologist colleagues to develop protocols, provide testing, patient follow-up, and admission to the hospital if necessary
5.  Availability of Nuclear Cardiology and Radiology colleagues for the emergent performance and reading of nuclear imaging studies if required in a given hospital's CPC protocol
6.  Laboratory personnel to run serial cardiac biomarker measurements
7.  Primary care physicians that understand the scope and limitations of a CPC evaluation and a willingness to provide long term follow-up, particularly for patients without ACS.

A variety of physical models exist for CPCs. Several of these models are illustrated in Table 1 and Figures 1 and 2. References for each center's protocol are provided. Each model takes into account the specific patient population, cardiologist collaboration, nuclear imaging availability, and ED resources necessary to design the optimal CPC for that hospital's environment. In most CPC protocols, collaborative discussions between emergency physicians and cardiologists at a given institution will determine the optimal protocol, which reflects the skills and resources for the individual hospital.

Most CPCs provide care for patients in an area adjacent, but separate from, the general emergency patient population, often in conjunction with other observation unit (OU) protocols. As these patients are frequently in the ED for 6 hours or more, it is desirable to provide many of the in-hospital comforts not generally available in a traditional ED. These may include comfortable hospital beds, meals, television sets, and telephones to maximize patient convenience and satisfaction. Such space allocation and additional resources may be difficult to obtain for those emergency physicians considering starting a new CPC, therefore, some of these protocols may have to be performed within the regular ED, utilizing available resources.

A successful CPC also requires a nursing staff dedicated to the care of these patients with special needs. These patients will require frequent assessment, close monitoring, noninvasive testing, serial cardiac marker testing and ECG acquisition. These tasks are generally in excess of those expected for a typical ED patient and may require additional personnel training and staffing in the CPC as appropriate for the individual institution and ED. The overall success of the unit depends on adherence to the systematic evaluation protocol and substantial nursing independence.

**Table 1**  Medical College of Virginia CPC Protocol

| Level | AMI Risk | ACS Risk | Strategy | Disposition |
|-------|----------|----------|----------|-------------|
| 1 | Very high | Very high | Fibrinolysis/PCI | CCU |
| 2 | High | High | ASA, Heparin, NTG, IIb/IIIa | CCU |
| 3 | Moderate | Moderate | Markers + nuclear imaging | 9h observation |
| 4 | Low | Mod or low | Nuclear Imaging | Home and OI stress test |
| 5 | Very Low | Very low | As needed | Home |

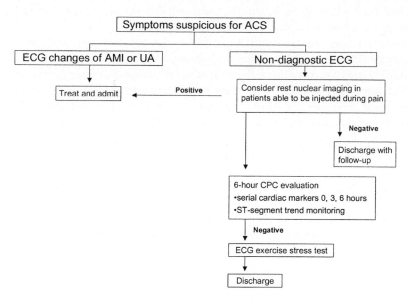

**Figure 1** University of Cincinnati "Heart ER" strategy. (From Ref. 63)

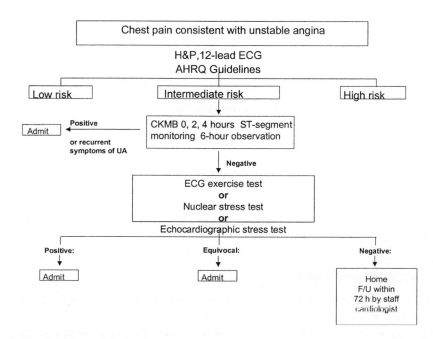

**Figure 2** Mayo Clinic strategy.

While most of these patients are placed on CPC protocols that require little emergency physician interaction, these patients must be continually reevaluated and reassessed. ACS is a dynamic process and can easily progress over the course of the patient's evaluation. Symptom changes, cardiac marker positivity, and ECG changes should prompt immediate therapy and potential cardiac catheterization laboratory intervention. The emergency physician must stay integrally involved with the patient's care to provide this intervention. A successful CPC requires the cooperation of many health care professionals, both in the ED and around the participating institution. An absolutely critical component of successful CPC operation is the collaboration and cooperation of cardiologists and radiologists. Cardiology involvement in CPC protocols is intuitive, for many reasons. For one, formulation, knowledge, and acceptance of CPC protocols, in particular, for each institution is mandatory. Secondly, many CPC protocols successfully employ the use of provocative testing or echocardiography and these tests generally require the expert interpretation of a cardiologist [5–10].

While collaboration between Emergency Medicine and Cardiology is intuitive, integration with nuclear cardiologists and radiologists is pivotally important to the success of any CPC as well. Radionuclide perfusion imaging has emerged as an important tool in many centers for assessing patients with and without known cardiovascular disease, and also in evaluating the patient presenting to the ED with possible ACS. Technitium-99 sestamibi tomographic imaging is the most common agent currently being used in patients presenting to the ED with suspected ACS and can be available 24 hours per day, seven days a week [11,12]. Studies have shown that positive rest perfusion imaging accurately identifies patients at high risk for adverse cardiac events at rest [13]. Perfusion imaging has thus become a cornerstone of evaluation for many units [14,15].

The diagnostic sensitivity of myocardial perfusion imaging is dependent on the timing of injection in relation to chest pain. The major obstacles for radionuclide studies have traditionally included cost and accessibility. The perfusion agents have a 6- to 12-hour shelf life, and thus, have to be prepared several times a day to be available for acute imaging in an emergency environment. Collaboration with Nuclear Cardiology and Radiology colleagues is paramount for this reason. Timely evaluation of these patients requires immediate access to these studies, and timely reading and reporting of the results to the emergency physician.

In addition, the laboratory must be supportive of a CPC. Ideally, bedside point-of-care testing for cardiac biomarkers provides rapid data collection for these patients as Creative Kinase (CK)-MB and in particular, the troponins I and T, allow risk stratification to be performed expeditiously [16]. A collaborative relationship between emergency physicians, radiologists, and laboratorians can insure a consistent and effective evaluation of patients in the CPC. Finally, primary care physicians need to be supportive of the CPC and willing to have patients evaluated in this protocol-driven process. Communication between emergency physicians and the patient's primary care physician can assure careful follow-up and compliance after evaluation.

## RISK STRATIFICATION IN THE ED

The protocols developed for CPCs must provide testing to evaluate every patient for three different possibilities: myocardial necrosis, rest ischemia, and exercise induced ischemia. Numerous studies in several different hospital environments have proved the utility of the CPC. Even early CPCs, without the benefits of cardiac troponins and immediate nuclear imaging, were successful in safely evaluating patients at low probability for acute myocardial infarction [17].

Early myocardial necrosis "rule-out" protocols challenged the traditional notion of a 24-hour period required to detect acute myocardial infarction. Lee and colleagues' multicenter trial validated a 12-hour algorithm using Creative kinase (CK); Creative kinase-MB fraction and CK-MB in patients identified as "low-risk" through assessment of clinical characteristics in the ED. "Low-risk" was defined as the probability of acute myocardial infarction (AMI) less than 7%. Patients with CK-MB levels lower than 5% of the total CK without recurrent chest pain after 12 hours had a 0.5% missed AMI rate while identifying 94% of AMI patients [18]. Farkouh et al. demonstrated the utility of a CPC protocol and CK-MB measurements for patients identified as intermediate risk for adverse cardiac events. In this study, patients underwent 6 hours of observation, followed by provocative testing. In a higher-risk patient population than typical for CPCs, this protocol identified all patients with short- and long-term cardiac events while using fewer resources over a six-month time period [19]. Symptom onset to patient presentation is a crucial factor in the interpretation of cardiac marker protocols. Marker release kinetics vary with time. As time to ED presentation may be as short as 90 minutes or as long as several days, no single cardiac biomarker determination is suitable for adequately "ruling-out" myocardial necrosis [5,20,21]. In one of the first studies with a CPC protocol, Gibler et al. used a nine-hour protocol with serial CK-MB at 0, 3, 6, and 9 hours along with continuous electrocardiographic (ECG) monitoring, echocardiography, and real-time exercise testing in the ED. They found that serial markers alone had a sensitivity and specificity for AMI of 100% and 98%, respectively [5]. The American Heart Association currently recommends serial cardiac biomarker determinations to increase sensitivity for detecting necrosis, rather than a single determination on ED presentation.

Several other studies have examined the value of cardiac markers in the risk stratification of heterogenous patients with chest pain presenting to the ED. In a multicenter study of over 5,000 patients in 53 EDs, the relative risk of ischemic complications and death for emergency patients with positive CK-MB at 0 or 2 hours was 16.1 and 25.4, respectively [22]. Serial CK-MB results have also proved to be sensitive for myocardial necrosis detection when collected at 0 and 3 hours after ED presentation. Young et al. found a 93% and 95% sensitivity and specificity when combining zero, three, and net change in CK-MB level to make this determination. As expected, this sensitivity improved with increased time from symptom onset [23]. Serial marker measurements and comparison of marker elevation over 3 to 6 hours also improved sensitivity for MI [24–26]. Even minor elevations of CK-MB, as small as twice the upper limit of normal, are associated with an increased 6-month mortality when compared with those with normal levels [27].

Serial CK/CK-MB protocols have largely become the diagnostic standard for AMI in the CPC setting. Most all studied protocols use a specific threshold, above which is diagnostic for AMI or ACS. Fesmire et al. studied a promising approach of change in CK-MB levels within the normal range over the course of ED evaluation. In his population of 710 CPC patients, a CK-MB increase or delta of 1.6 ng/mL over 2 hours was more sensitive for AMI than a second CK-MB drawn 2 hours after patient arrival (93.8% vs. 75.2%) [26]. Validation of these new approaches in protocols will add to the further utility of markers in the CPC setting.

The beneficial attributes of myoglobin have made it a commonly used cardiac biomarker in the CPC setting. The diagnostic strength of myoglobin lies in its early release kinetics and sensitivity, while its primary weakness is that myoglobin lacks specificity. Davis et al. showed that serial myoglobin levels were 93% sensitive and 79% specific in detecting MI in patients within 2 hours of arrival [28]. Similarly, Tucker at al. showed a myoglobin sensitivity of 89% in patients with nondiagnostic ECGs within 2 hours of ED presentation [29]. Myoglobin appears to achieve maximal diagnostic accuracy within 5 hours after symptom onset [30].

Therefore, it is reasonable and recommended that the early cardiac biomarker of myocardial necrosis, myoglobin, should be combined with other more specific cardiac markers when used in CPC protocols. Brogan et al. found that a combination of carbonic anhydrase III and serum myoglobin was more sensitive and equally specific as CK-MB in patients presenting early within 3 hours of symptom onset [31]. In contrast, Kontos et al. reported less encouraging results from a study of 2,093 patients combining CK, CK-MB, and myoglobin obtained at 0, 3, 6, and 8 hours. A CK-MB level greater than 8.0 ng/mL at 3 hours was 93% sensitive and 98% specific for AMI, adding myoglobin decreased the specificity to 86% with no significant increase in sensitivity [3].

Much like the other cardiac biomarkers, myoglobin levels become increasingly useful when drawn in a serial fashion. In a study of 133 consecutive admitted chest-pain patients, myoglobin levels were obtained at 2, 3, 4, and 6 hours after symptom onset. This regimen was found to be 86% sensitive for AMI at 6 hours. The negative predictive value (NPV) in patients with negative myoglobin levels during 6 hours of evaluation and without doubling over any 2-hour period was 97% for AMI [29]. As CPCs continue to evolve, aggressive and innovative marker strategies have been developed. McCord et al. [32] found that acute myocardial infarction can be excluded 90 minutes after patient presentation using point-of-care myoglobin and cardiac troponin I.

Data from protocols using myoglobin measurements in patients with lower risk for AMI can be conflicting. In a study of 3075 low-risk CPC patients with AMI prevalence of 1.4%, a 4-hour serial myoglobin protocol was reported as 100% sensitive for AMI [9]. Conversely, in a study of 368 patients whose MI prevalence was 11%, the sensitivity and specificity of myoglobin at zero and 2 to 3 hours was only 61% and 68%. A myoglobin change or increase did not improve diagnostic performance [25].

Myoglobin in the CPC setting is best used in a serial fashion, along with another more specific cardiac biomarker of necrosis, particularly one of the troponins. It is most valuable when used in patients presenting very early in the time course of symptoms and less so for remote events.

Troponins I and T have revolutionized the risk stratification of chest pain patients in CPC protocols and are now considered essential to the emergency management of ACS. They have been proved extremely valuable and sensitive in the diagnosis of myocardial necrosis [33,34]. In addition to diagnosis of myocardial necrosis in ACS, the troponins are valuable for risk stratification of both low- and high-risk patient populations. Troponin-release kinetics mimic CK-MB due to an initial cytosolic release, but remain elevated for days to weeks after AMI due to the breakdown of the contractile apparatus over this period.

The main issues surrounding the cardiac troponins include: (a) cutoff values for troponin I, and (b) appropriately defining the time of chest pain onset in the context of the ED presentation. While significant effort has been made to determine the "superior" troponin, most large studies and analyses have determined that cTnI and cTnT can both identify patients at risk for adverse cardiac events.[33–36]

Cardiac TnT is detected at slightly lower serum levels than most cTnI assays and has proved valuable in the emergency setting for early identification of myocardial necrosis. The GUSTO-II investigators compared cTnI and cTnT in short-term risk stratification of ACS patients. This model compared troponins collected within 3.5 hours of ischemic symptom onset. Ohman and colleagues found that cTnT showed a greater association with 30-day mortality ($Chi^2 = 18.0$, $p < 0.0001$) than cTnI ($Chi^2 = 12.5$, $p = 0.0002$) [37]. These authors concluded that cTnT is a strong, independent predictor of short-term outcome in ACS patients, and serial levels useful in determining the risk of adverse cardiac events [38,39].

As with all new cardiac markers, initial studies on troponin risk stratification were initially performed on patients with known ACS. Studies using cTnI in ACS patients showed a statistically significant increase in mortality among those patients with levels greater than 0.4 ng/mL [40]. Stubbs and colleagues [41] showed that patients with elevated baseline cTnT levels have up to four times higher mortality than ACS patients with normal values.

While the increased risk for troponin positive patients is now well established, the degree of risk varies greatly between studies and patient populations. Meta-analyses have helped to identify clinically useful parameters when using troponins for the evaluation of patients. One such analysis in high risk patients performed by Wu and colleagues demonstrated a cumulative odds ratio of a positive cTnT for the development of AMI or death from hospital discharge to 34 months was 4.3 (2.8–6.8 95% CI) [42]. The cumulative odds ratio of a positive cTnT for predicting need for cardiac revascularization within the same period was 4.4 (3.0–6.5 95% CI). Another analysis involving greater than 18,000 patients in 21 ACS studies found that troponin positive patients had an odds ratio of 3.44 for death or MI at 30 days. Troponin positive patients without ST-segment elevation and patients with unstable angina carried odds ratios of 4.93 and 9.39 for adverse cardiac outcomes [36].

Benamer et al. compared the prognostic value of cTnI combined with C-reactive protein (CRP) in patients with unstable angina. They found that while 23% of patients with elevated cTnI had major in-hospital cardiac events; there was no such prognostic significance associated with CRP [43]. Currently, CRP is not routinely used in the emergency setting to risk stratify patients.

Troponin applications in low- to moderate-risk patients presenting to EDs have shown similar encouraging results. Tucker et al. used a comprehensive marker strategy including myoglobin, CK-MB, troponin I, and troponin T in ED patients over 24 hours after arrival. As would be expected within the first 2 hours of presentation, CK-MB and myoglobin maintained better sensitivity. The troponins were useful only when measured 6 or more hours after arrival. Sensitivities and specificities of 82% and 97% for troponin I and 89% and 84% for troponin T were obtained [44]. Troponin use seems to be more beneficial in later or delayed patient presentations. In a study of 425 patients using serial troponin I and CK-MB over 16 hours, Brogan et al. showed no increase in sensitivity or specificity between troponin and CK-MB in patients with symptoms <24 hours. However, in patients presenting greater than 24 hours of symptoms after symptom onset, troponin I had a sensitivity of 100% compared with 56.5% for CK-MB [45].

Sayre et al. showed that patients with a troponin T level of 0.2 ng/L or greater were 3.5 times more likely to have a cardiac complication within 60 days of ED presentation [46]. In a CPC population, Newby et al. determined that cTnT positive patients had angiographically significant lesions (89% vs. 49%) and positive stress testing (46% vs. 14%) more frequently than cTnT negative patients. Long-term mortality was also shown to be higher in cTnT positive patients (27% vs. 7%) [47]. Johnson et al. studied a heterogeneous patient population admitted from an urban teaching hospital and found that cTnT was elevated in 31% of patients without MI who had major short-term complications, as compared to CK-MB activity and mass [34].

Other authors have found that while patients with troponin positivity are at higher risk for adverse cardiac events, the test in isolation lacks sensitivity. Kontos et al. found that while cTnI positive patients were more likely to have significant complications (43% vs 12%), the sensitivity for these end points was low (14%) [48]. Similarly, Polanczyk et al. demonstrated that peak cTnI greater than 0.4 ng/mL was associated with only a 47% sensitivity and 80% specificity for a major cardiac event within 72 hours of presentation [49].

The recent publication of standards redefining acute myocardial infarction has brought troponin to the forefront of both diagnosis and risk stratification in this patient population [50]. In a reanalysis of the data from The Second Platelet IIb/IIIa Antagonism for the Reduction of Acute Coronary Syndrome Events in Global Organization Network (PARAGON B), Global Utilization of Streptokinase and Tissue Plasminogen Activator for Occluded Coronary Artery (GUSTO IIa), and The chest pain evaluation by creative kinase-MB, myoglobin, and troponin I (CHECKMATE) studies, patients with baseline troponin elevation without CK-MB elevation were found to be at increased risk for early and short-term adverse outcomes [39,51–54]. McCord et al. found that troponin, and myoglobin measurement over a nine hour period was most predictive of adverse events in their CPC population [55].

In the future, it is likely that CPCs will incorporate a multimarker approach of cardiac bio-markers that includes some combination of myoglobin, CK-MB, and troponin, as well as an inflammatory marker, such as C-reactive protein (CRP) [43,56]. Additional markers, such as brain matriuretic peptide (BNP), myeloperoxidase and albumin cobalt binding assays, have been investigated and show promising results as well [56–61].

Rapid perfusion imaging has been a major diagnostic improvement for the evaluation of ACS in CPCs. Perfusion imaging has been used in a variety of settings with great success. Tatum and colleagues found that patients with normal imaging findings had a one-year event rate of 3% no MI or death, compared to 42% with 11% experiencing MI and 8% cardiac death [14].

The opportunity exists to educate patients about the risk factors for coronary artery disease during their stay in the CPC. For many patients, coming to the ED represents a key interventional moment where education risk factor modification may be particularly effective [62].

## SPECIFIC INSTITUTIONAL PROTOCOLS

Over the years, several manifestations of CPCs have evolved. Each of these models has been successfully adapted to specific institutions and patient populations. An individual institution should carefully evaluate their patient population, physician expertise, physical structure, staffing model, and hospital environment to most adequately determine their optimal CPC protocol.

The University of Cincinnati Center for Emergency Care "Heart ER" was one of the first ED-based CPCs, having been established in October 1991 (Figure 1). Since then, over 2,600 patients have been admitted to the Heart ER program and are considered to be a low- to moderate-risk cohort for ACS. Serial cardiac biomarkers, including CK-MB, myoglobin, and cTnT levels, are drawn at 0, 3, and 6 hours. The original protocol utilized continuous ST-segment trend monitoring, which has since been discontinued, as it was found not be helpful with this low-prevalence/low-risk population. Graded exercise testing, or Tc-99m sestamibi radionuclide scanning, is now performed, depending on patient's functional status and test availability. Patients having negative evaluations in the Heart ER are released to home with careful follow-up as an outpatient [5].

In the first 2,131 consecutive patients evaluated over a six-year period, 309 (14.5%) required admission and 1,822 (85.5%) were released to home from the ED. Of admitted patients, 94 (30%) were found to have a cardiac cause for their chest pain. Follow-up of 1,696 patients discharged from the Heart ER to home yielded nine cardiac events (0.53%, CI 0.24%–1.01%; 7 Percutaneous Coronary Angiography (PTCA), 1 Coronary artery bypass grafting (CABG), 1 death) [63].

These data suggest that the Heart ER program at the University of Cincinnati provides a safe and effective means for evaluating low- to moderate-risk patients with possible ACS presenting to the ED.

Other institutions have also developed effective chest pain center strategies. The Medical College of Virginia has an elegant protocol, which risk stratifies chest pain patients into five distinct levels on ED presentation (Table 1) [14,64]. Level 1 patients have ST-segment elevation acute myocardial infarction while level 5 patients have a clearly noncardiac cause for their chest discomfort. Triage level severity dictates treatment and further diagnostic studies. Intermediate level patients (levels 2 and 3) include individuals with variable probability of unstable angina, or non–ST-segment elevation AMI. These patients are admitted to the CCU for the diagnosis of ACS while less acute patients (level 4) undergo serial biomarker determination and Tc-99m sestamibi radionuclide imaging from the ED, then released to home after a negative evaluation.

The University of California at Davis protocol employs a novel use of immediate exercise treadmill testing without serial cardiac biomarker determination. In a recent study of 1,000 patients, 13% were positive and 64% negative for ischemia. The remaining 23% of the patients had nondiagnostic tests. There were no adverse events due to exercise testing and no mortality in each of the patient evaluation groups on 30-day follow-up. These authors concluded that immediate exercise testing of low-risk patients is safe and accurate for the determination of which patients can be safely discharged from the ED [6].

Mayo Clinic separates patients into low-, intermediate-, and high-risk categories according to Agency for Health Care Policy Research (AHCPR) guidelines (Figure 2). Intermediate risk patients are evaluated with CK-MB levels at 0, 2, and 4 hours while undergoing continuous ST-segment trend monitoring and six hour observation. If this evaluation in negative, an ECG exercise test, a nuclear stress test, or an echocardiographic stress test is performed. Patients with positive or equivocal evaluations are admitted while patients with negative evaluations are discharged to home with a 72-hour follow-up [19].

Lastly, Brigham and Women's Hospital divides patients into three groups: UA or AMI, possible ischemia, and nonischemia. Patients with unstable angina or AMI are admitted while nonischemic chest pain patients are discharged from the CPC. The intermediate, or "possible ischemia," group either undergoes exercise treadmill testing with a 6-hour period of observation or a 12-hour period of observation. At the end of the observation period, stable patients are discharged to home. Nichol et al. evaluated the impact of this pathway approach in a retrospective cohort of 4,585 patients and found that a 17% reduction in admissions and an 11% reduction in length of stay would occur if even fewer than 50% of eligible patients for observation and exercise testing had participated [65].

From these protocols, it is apparent that physicians from each institution must tailor their CPC protocols to their patient population, expertise, and resource availability to properly identify patients with ACS. Each hospital and patient population represents a unique environment with specific needs and resources that must be reflected in the ultimate CPC design and implementation.

Of important note, once the patient "clears" the CPC protocol and does not appear to have ACS, the individual can safely be discharged to home with appropriate follow-up arranged. Adequate attention must be given to the cause of the patient's discomfort, even if it is determined not likely to be cardiac in nature. Further evaluation for gastrointestinal, psychiatric, or musculoskeletal causes of chest pain must be explored. Patients require outpatient provocative testing, if not received in the CPC protocol, to further delineate their cardiac risk. These tests must be followed and acted upon by a cardiologist or primary care physician. Closure of this evaluation loop is essential to provide appropriate patient care.

## COST EFFECTIVENESS

Continued economic constraints and scarce inpatient resources discourage unnecessary inpatient admissions, making CPC protocols more relevant in today's emergency environments than in the past. "Rule-out MI" is no longer an acceptable diagnosis to assign low- and moderate-risk patients with chest pain on admission. Increased financial pressures exerted by federal and private insurers on physicians and hospitals have stressed the necessity for more CPCs. Emergency physicians, in particular, have been challenged to develop more efficient and cost-effective strategies to evaluate these patients [66,67].

Admissions for ultimately diagnosed "noncardiac" chest pain cost our society billions of dollars annually [68]. The CPC has allowed physicians to condense a hospital admission into a 6- to 12-hour evaluation, risk stratification, and observation period which has proved most cost-effective. Even CPCs of a decade ago proved to have significant economic advantages over hospital admission [9,69,70]. Roberts et al. determined that accelerated diagnostic protocols for low-risk patients with chest pain saved total hospital costs while reducing hospitalization rates and patient length of stay [71]. Ultimately each CPC must be formulated and evaluated based on the target patient population, hospital occupancy and resources, and reimbursement patterns. The use of CPCs offers the opportunity for a continuous evolution towards optimal patient care and cost savings.

In general, protocol and guideline driven medicine is effective for the evaluation of multiple disease processes in the ED, chest discomfort included. Continuous quality improvement should be an integral part of the continued assessment of any CPC [72]. The 2002 ACC/AHA guidelines for unstable angina/non–ST-segment elevation myocardial infarction must be reflected in any CPC protocol. This would include diagnostic and treatment strategies for patients in these units [73].

It is important to stress that CPCs are optimally used for the evaluation of low- to moderate-risk patients, and not "no-risk" patients presenting to the ED. Evaluating all patients presenting with chest discomfort in a CPC protocol would indeed be an inefficient use of ED and hospital resources. Vigorous quality assurance/improvement analysis should be used to ensure that appropriate patients are being admitted for evaluation to a CPC. A committee consisting of cardiologists and emergency physicians should meet frequently to assess all aspects of their CPC protocol. Continuous assessment of alternative, more effective, and possibly less expensive programs will improve care standards for these units over time. The Society for Chest Pain Centers and Providers has already begun a process where certification of a hospital's CPC can be obtained. Already, the last decade has seen a remarkable evolution of cardiac biomarker regimens and diagnostic and prognostic testing for the evaluation of patients with possible ACS. Future advances must be integrated into a CPC protocol to optimize diagnostic and therapeutic outcomes.

As more and more reports of successful CPCs are published and evidence expands for cost-effectiveness, it will be an expectation, rather than an exception, that EDs and hospitals have such units. Further success and improved patient outcomes will fuel the demand for these innovative protocols.

## REFERENCES

1. Pope JH, Aufderheide TP, Ruthazer R, Woolard RH, Feldman JA, Beshansky JR, Griffith JL, Selker HP. Missed diagnoses of acute cardiac ischemia in the emergency department. N Engl J Med 2000;342(16):1163–1170.
2. Nourjah P. National hospital ambulatory medical care survey: 1997 emergency department summary. Advance data from vital and health statistics. 0. 0: National Center for Health Statistics, 2001. Report No. 304.

3. Kontos MC, Anderson FP, Schmidt KA, Ornato JP, Tatum JL, Jesse RL. Early diagnosis of acute myocardial infarction in patients without ST- segment elevation. Am J Cardiol 1999; 83(2):155–158.

4. Graff LG, Dallara J, Ross MA, et al. Impact on the care of the emergency department chest pain patient from the chest pain evaluation registry (CHEPER) study. Am J Cardiol 1997; 80(5):563–568.

5. Gibler WB, Runyon JP, Levy RC, et al. A rapid diagnostic and treatment center for patients with chest pain in the emergency department. Ann Emerg Med 1995;25(1):1–8.

6. Amsterdam EA, Kirk JD, Diercks DB, Lewis WR, Turnipseed SD. Immediate exercise testing to evaluate low-risk patients presenting to the emergency department with chest pain. J Am Coll Cardiol 2002;40(2):251–256.

7. Amsterdam EA, Lewis WR, Kirk JD, Diercks DB, Turnipseed S. Acute ischemic syndromes. Chest pain center concept. Cardiol Clin 2002;20(1):117–136.

8. Zalenski RJ, McCarren M, Roberts R, et al. An evaluation of a chest pain diagnostic protocol to exclude acute cardiac ischemia in the emergency department. Arch Intern Med 1997;157(10): 1085–1091.

9. Mikhail MG, Smith FA, Gray M, Britton C, Frederiksen SM. Cost-effectiveness of mandatory stress testing in chest pain center patients. Ann Emerg Med 1997;29(1):88–98.

10. Levitt MA, Promes SB, Bullock S, et al. Combined cardiac marker approach with adjunct two-dimensional echocardiography to diagnose acute myocardial infarction in the emergency department [see comments]. Ann Emerg Med 1996;27(1):1–7.

11. Hilton TC, Thompson RC, Williams HJ, Saylors R, Fulmer H, Stowers SA. Technetium-99m sestamibi myocardial perfusion imaging in the emergency room evaluation of chest pain. J Am Coll Cardiol 1994;23(5):1016–1022.

12. Gersh BJ. Noninvasive imaging in acute coronary disease. A clinical perspective. Circulation 1991;84(3 Suppl):I140–147.

13. Kontos MC, Anderson FP, Hanbury CM, Roberts CS, Miller WG, Jesse RL. Use of the combination of myoglobin and CK-MB mass for the rapid diagnosis of acute myocardial infarction. Am J Emerg Med 1997;15(1):14–19.

14. Tatum JL, Jesse RL, Kontos MC, et al. Comprehensive strategy for the evaluation and triage of the chest pain patient. Ann Emerg Med 1997;29(1):116–125.

15. Abbott BG, Wackers FJ. Emergency department chest pain units and the role of radionuclide imaging. J Nucl Cardiol 1998;5(1):73–79.

16. Lee-Lewandrowski E, Corboy D, Lewandrowski K, Sinclair J, McDermot S, Benzer TI. Implementation of a point-of-care satellite laboratory in the emergency department of an academic medical center. Impact on test turnaround time and patient emergency department length of stay. Arch Pathol Lab Med 2003;127(4):456–460.

17. Gaspoz JM, Lee TH, Cook EF, Weisberg MC, Goldman L. Outcome of patients who were admitted to a new short-stay unit to "rule-out" myocardial infarction. Am J Cardiol 1991; 68(2):145–149.

18. Lee TH, Juarez G, Cook EF, et al. Ruling out acute myocardial infarction. A prospective multicenter validation of a 12-hour strategy for patients at low risk. N Engl J Med 1991; 324(18):1239–1246.

19. Farkouh ME, Smars PA, Reeder GS, et al. A clinical trial of a chest-pain observation unit for patients with unstable angina. Chest Pain Evaluation in the Emergency Room (CHEER) Investigators. N Engl J Med 1998;339(26):1882–1888.

20. Lambrew CT, Bowlby LJ, Rogers WJ, Chandra NC, Weaver WD. Factors influencing the time to thrombolysis in acute myocardial infarction. Time to Thrombolysis Substudy of the National Registry of Myocardial Infarction-1. Arch Intern Med 1997;157(22):2577–2782.

21. Newby LK, Rutsch WR, Califf RM, et al. Time from symptom onset to treatment and outcomes after thrombolytic therapy. GUSTO-1 Investigators. J Am Coll Cardiol 1996;27(7):1646–1655.

22. Hoekstra JW, Hedges JR, Gibler WB, Rubison RM, Christensen RA. Emergency department CK-MB: a predictor of ischemic complications. National cooperative CK-MB project group. Acad Emerg Med 1994;1(1):17–27.

23. Young GP, Gibler WB, Hedges JR, et al. Serial creatine kinase-MB results are a sensitive indicator of acute myocardial infarction in chest pain patients with nondiagnostic electrocardiograms: the second Emergency Medicine Cardiac Research Group Study. Acad Emerg Med 1997;4(9):869–877.

24. Gibler WB, Young GP, Hedges JR, et al. Acute myocardial infarction in chest pain patients with nondiagnostic ECGs: serial CK-MB sampling in the emergency department. The Emergency Medicine Cardiac Research Group. Ann Emerg Med 1992;21(5):504–512.

25. Polanczyk CA, Lee TH, Cook EF, Walls R, Wybenga D, Johnson PA. Value of additional two-hour myoglobin for the diagnosis of myocardial infarction in the emergency department. Am J Cardiol 1999;83(4):525–529.

26. Fesmire FM, Percy RF, Bardoner JB, Wharton DR, Calhoun FB. Serial creatinine kinase (CK) MB testing during the emergency department evaluation of chest pain: utility of a 2-hour deltaCK-MB of + 1.6ng/ml. Am Heart J 1998;136(2):237–244.

27. Alexander JH, Sparapani RA, Mahaffey KW, et al. Association between minor elevations of creatine kinase-MB level and mortality in patients with acute coronary syndromes without ST-segment elevation. PURSUIT Steering Committee. Platelet glycoprotein IIb/IIIa in unstable angina: receptor suppression using integrilin therapy. JAMA 2000;283(3):347–353.

28. Davis CP, Barrett K, Torre P, Wacasey K. Serial myoglobin levels for patients with possible myocardial infarction. Acad Emerg Med 1996;3(6):590–597.

29. Tucker JF, Collins RA, Anderson AJ, et al. Value of serial myoglobin levels in the early diagnosis of patients admitted for acute myocardial infarction. Ann Emerg Med 1994;24(4):704–708.

30. de Winter RJ, Lijmer JG, Koster RW, Hoek FJ, Sanders GT. Diagnostic accuracy of myoglobin concentration for the early diagnosis of acute myocardial infarction. Ann Emerg Med 2000;35(2):113–120.

31. Brogan GX, Vuori J, Friedman S, et al. Improved specificity of myoglobin plus carbonic anhydrase assay versus that of creatine kinase-MB for early diagnosis of acute myocardial infarction. Ann Emerg Med 1996;27(1):22–28.

32. McCord J, Nowak RM, McCullough PA, et al. Ninety-minute exclusion of acute myocardial infarction by use of quantitative point-of-care testing of myoglobin and troponin I. Circulation 2001;104(13):1483–1488.

33. Falahati A, Sharkey SW, Christensen D, et al. Implementation of serum cardiac troponin I as marker for detection of acute myocardial infarction. Am Heart J 1999;137(2):332–337.

34. Johnson PA, Goldman L, Sacks DB, et al. Cardiac troponin T as a marker for myocardial ischemia in patients seen at the emergency department for acute chest pain. Am Heart J 1999;137(6):1137–1144.

35. Ottani F, Galvani M, Ferrini D, et al. Direct comparison of early elevations of cardiac troponin T and I in patients with clinical unstable angina. Am Heart J 1999;137(2):284–291.

36. Ottani F, Galvani M, Nicolini FA, et al. Elevated cardiac troponin levels predict the risk of adverse outcome in patients with acute coronary syndromes. Am Heart J 2000;140(6):917–927.

37. Christenson RH, Duh SH, Newby LK, et al. Cardiac troponin T and cardiac troponin I: relative values in short- term risk stratification of patients with acute coronary syndromes. GUSTO-IIa Investigators. Clin Chem 1998;44(3):494–501.

38. Newby LK, Christenson RH, Ohman EM, et al. Value of serial troponin T measures for early and late risk stratification in patients with acute coronary syndromes. The GUSTO-IIa Investigators. Circulation 1998;98(18):1853–1859.

39. Ohman EM, Armstrong PW, Christenson RH, et al. Cardiac troponin T levels for risk stratification in acute myocardial ischemia. GUSTO IIA Investigators. N Engl J Med 1996;335(18):1333–1341.

40. Antman EM, Tanasijevic MJ, Thompson B, et al. Cardiac-specific troponin I levels to predict the risk of mortality in patients with acute coronary syndromes. N Engl J Med 1996;335(18):1342–1349.

41. Stubbs P, Collinson P, Moseley D, Greenwood T, Noble M. Prognostic significance of admission troponin T concentrations in patients with myocardial infarction. Circulation 1996;94(6):1291–1297.

42. Wu AH, Lane PL. Metaanalysis in clinical chemistry: validation of cardiac troponin T as a marker for ischemic heart diseases. Clin Chem 1995;41(8 Pt 2):1228–1233.

43. Benamer H, Steg PG, Benessiano J, et al. Comparison of the prognostic value of C-reactive protein and troponin I in patients with unstable angina pectoris. Am J Cardiol 1998;82(7): 845–850.

44. Tucker JF, Collins RA, Anderson AJ, Hauser J, Kalas J, Apple FS. Early diagnostic efficiency of cardiac troponin I and Troponin T for acute myocardial infarction. Acad Emerg Med 1997; 4(1):13–21.

45. Brogan GX, Hollander JE, McCuskey CF, et al. Evaluation of a new assay for cardiac troponin I vs creatine kinase-MB for the diagnosis of acute myocardial infarction. Biochemical Markers for Acute Myocardial Ischemia (BAMI) Study Group. Acad Emerg Med 1997;4(1):6–12.

46. Sayre MR, Kaufmann KH, Chen IW, et al. Measurement of cardiac troponin T is an effective method for predicting complications among emergency department patients with chest pain. Ann Emerg Med 1998;31(5):539–549.

47. Newby LK, Kaplan AL, Granger BB, Sedor F, Califf RM, Ohman EM. Comparison of cardiac troponin T versus creatine kinase-MB for risk stratification in a chest pain evaluation unit. Am J Cardiol 2000;85(7):801–805.

48. Kontos MC, Anderson FP, Alimard R, Ornato JP, Tatum JL, Jesse RL. Ability of troponin I to predict cardiac events in patients admitted from the emergency department. J Am Coll Cardiol 2000;36(6):1818–1823.

49. Polanczyk CA, Lee TH, Cook EF, et al. Cardiac troponin I as a predictor of major cardiac events in emergency department patients with acute chest pain. J Am Coll Cardiol 1998;32(1): 8–14.

50. Myocardial infarction redefined–a consensus document of The Joint European Society of Cardiology/American College of Cardiology Committee for the redefinition of myocardial infarction. J Am Coll Cardiol 2000;36(3):959–969.

51. Rao SV, Ohman EM, Granger CB, et al. Prognostic value of isolated troponin elevation across the spectrum of chest pain syndromes. Am J Cardiol 2003;91(8):936–940.

52. Newby LK, Storrow AB, Gibler WB, et al. Bedside multimarker testing for risk stratification in chest pain units: The chest pain evaluation by creatine kinase-MB, myoglobin, and troponin I (CHECKMATE) study. Circulation 2001;103(14):1832–1837.

53. Newby LK, Ohman EM, Christenson RH, et al. Benefit of glycoprotein IIb/IIIa inhibition in patients with acute coronary syndromes and troponin t-positive status: the paragon-B troponin T substudy. Circulation 2001;103(24):2891–2896.

54. Apple FS, Wu AH, Jaffe AS. European Society of Cardiology and American College of Cardiology guidelines for redefinition of myocardial infarction: how to use existing assays clinically and for clinical trials. Am Heart J 2002;144(6):981–986.

55. McCord J, Nowak RM, Hudson MP, et al. The prognostic significance of serial myoglobin, troponin I, and creatine kinase-MB measurements in patients evaluated in the emergency department for acute coronary syndrome. Ann Emerg Med 2003;42(3):343–350.

56. Sabatine MS, Morrow DA, de Lemos JA, et al. Multimarker approach to risk stratification in non-ST elevation acute coronary syndromes: simultaneous assessment of troponin I, C-reactive protein, and B-type natriuretic peptide. Circulation 2002;105(15):1760–1763.

57. Gibler WB, Blomkalns AL, Collins SP. Evaluation of chest pain and heart failure in the emergency department: impact of multimarker strategies and B-type natriuretic Peptide. Rev Cardiovasc Med 2003;4(Suppl 4):S47–S55.

58. Brennan ML, Penn MS, Van Lente F, et al. Prognostic value of myeloperoxidase in patients with chest pain. N Engl J Med 2003;349(17):1595–1604.

59. Russell CJ, Exley AR, Ritchie AJ. Widespread coronary inflammation in unstable angina. N Engl J Med 2003;348(19):1931.

60. Baldus S, Heeschen C, Meinertz T, et al. Myeloperoxidase serum levels predict risk in patients with acute coronary syndromes. Circulation 2003;108(12):1440–1445.

61. Bhagavan NV, Lai EM, Rios PA, et al. Evaluation of human serum albumin cobalt binding assay for the assessment of myocardial ischemia and myocardial infarction. Clin Chem 2003; 49(4):581–585.

62. Bahr RD. The changing paradigm of acute heart attack prevention in the emergency department: a futuristic viewpoint?. Ann Emerg Med 1995;25(1):95–96.

63. Storrow AB, Gibler WB, Walsh RA. An emergency department chest pain rapid diagnosis and treatment unit: results from a six year experience. Circulation 1999;98:I–425.

64. Jesse RL, Kontos MC. Evaluation of chest pain in the emergency department. Curr Probl Cardiol 1997;22(4):149–236.

65. Nichol G, Walls R, Goldman L, et al. A critical pathway for management of patients with acute chest pain who are at low risk for myocardial ischemia: recommendations and potential impact. Ann Intern Med 1997;127(11):996–1005.

66. National Heart Attack Alert Program issues report on how to shorten intervention time. Am Fam Physician 1994;50(7: 1569):73–74, 76.

67. Emergency department: rapid identification and treatment of patients with acute myocardial infarction. National Heart Attack Alert Program Coordinating Committee, 60 Minutes to Treatment Working Group. Ann Emerg Med 1994;23(2):311–329.

68. Weingarten SR, Ermann B, Riedinger MS, Shah PK, Ellrodt AG. Selecting the best triage rule for patients hospitalized with chest pain. Am J Med 1989;87(5):494–500.

69. Gomez MA, Anderson JL, Karagounis LA, Muhlestein JB, Mooers FB. An emergency department-based protocol for rapidly ruling out myocardial ischemia reduces hospital time and expense: results of a randomized study (ROMIO). J Am Coll Cardiol 1996;28(1):25–33.

70. Lee TH. Emergency Department Observation Units: Has the Time Come?. J Thromb Thrombolysis 1996;3(3):257–261.

71. Roberts RR, Zalenski RJ, Mensah EK, et al. Costs of an emergency department-based accelerated diagnostic protocol vs hospitalization in patients with chest pain: a randomized controlled trial. JAMA 1997;278(20):1670–1676.

72. Group NHAAPNCCCPW. Critical pathways for managment of patients with acute coronary syndromes: An assessment by the National Heart Attack Alert Program. Am Heart J 2002; 143:777–789.

73. Braunwald E, Antman EM, Beasley JW, Califf RM, Cheitlin MD, Hochman JS. ACC/AHA 2002 Guideline Update for the Management of Patients With Unstable Angina and Non–ST-Segment Elevation Myocardial Infarction. A report of the American College of Cardiology, American Heart Association Task Force on Practice Guidelines (Commitee on the management of patients with unstable angina). Circulation 2002;106(14):1893–1900.

# 12

# Facilitated Percutaneous Coronary Intervention for Acute Myocardial Infarction

**Sorin J. Brener**
*The Cleveland Clinic Foundation*
*Cleveland, Ohio, U.S.A.*

## INTRODUCTION

Timely administration of reperfusion therapy has been the focus of our efforts to improve outcome in patients with acute ST-elevation myocardial infarction (MI). For two decades, the debate between proponents of pharmacologically mediated lytic therapy and the supporters of mechanical revascularization (percutaneous coronary intervention [PCI]) has generated a wealth of information from randomized clinical trials (RCT) [1]. They showed that, in selected patients and clinical environments, PCI is superior to fibrinolysis with respect to death, reinfarction, need for repeat revascularization, and major bleeding complications, particularly intracranial hemorrhage (Figure 1). Two additional modifiers have added fuel to the controversy. On one hand, recent trials comparing on-site administration of lytics to patient transfer to a PCI center have shown again that transfer is better than fibrinolysis, particularly with respect to prevention of reinfarction and to patients presenting beyond 2–3 hours from symptom onset. These trials were performed in Europe and were remarkable for a very short (< 60 min) and uneventful transport (Figure 2) [2]. On the other hand, prehospital administration of fibrinolysis has reemerged as an appealing option, particularly when supported by physician-manned emergency medical services, rapid transfer to a facility with PCI capabilities, and aggressive treatment of lytic failure [3,4].

In the United States, recent data from the National Registry of Myocardial Infarction (NRMI 4) reveal a less encouraging reality (French W., XIXth George Washington Reperfusion Symposium, 2003). As of 2003, only 39% of patients are treated with PCI within 90 minutes [5] of hospital arrival (door-to-balloon), but only 4% of hospitals managed to treat at least 75% of their myocardial infarction (MI) patients. The median door-to-balloon time is 105 min for men and 115 min for women. Transfer for primary PCI takes more than 2 hours, bringing the total time from arrival at first hospital to balloon inflation to 171 minutes (Figure 3). Because of these delays and the overall improvement in general medical therapy, the in-hospital mortality of patients treated with lytics and PCI is nearly identical, 4.3% vs. 4.4%, respectively.

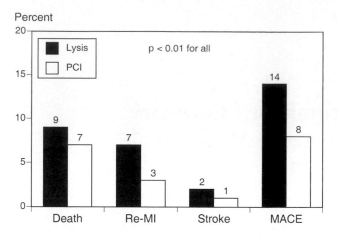

**Figure 1** Meta-analysis of 23 trials (7,739 patients) comparing short-term outcome of primary PCI with fibrinolysis. (Adapted from Ref. 1)

In this chapter, we review the emerging data supporting the concept of combination of pharmacological and mechanical reperfusion, the so-called ''pharmacoinvsive recanalization strategy'' (Fig. 4) [6].

## Rationale for Facilitated PCI

Early attempts to routinely perform PCI after lysis have been disappointing [7–9]. Inadequate PCI equipment, the prothrombotic state engendered by lytics with concomitant platelet activation, the inability to seal the dissections invariably created by balloon angioplasty, and the lack of protection of the microcirculation from embolization were all factors in creating the adage that lysis and immediate PCI cannot be complementary. Stents, glyco-

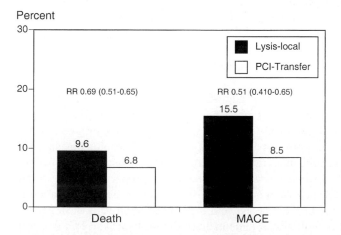

**Figure 2** Meta-analysis of 5 trials (2,466 patients) comparing the short-term outcome (death, re-MI or stroke) of primary PCI after hospital transfer with on-site fibrinolysis. (Adapted from Ref. 2).

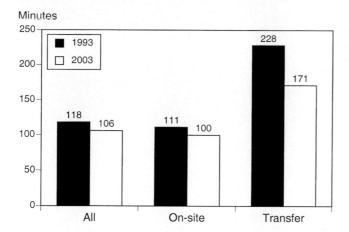

**Figure 3**  Secular trends in door-to balloon times in the National Registry of Myocardial Infarction (NRMI)-4. (French W, preliminary data.)

protein (GP) IIb/IIIa inhibitors, emboli protection devices (EPD), inflammatory modulation and metabolic interventions have made great strides in eliminating those concerns.

The critical concept at the basis for the quest for the most effective strategy of facilitating PCI in acute MI is that myocardial survival is a time-dependent phenomenon. While the quality of reperfusion obtained with PCI is superior to that of lytics, one has to try to apply it as soon as possible in order to prevent irreversible myocardial loss. Many analyses have addressed the issue of delay to reperfusion with somewhat contradictory conclusions [10–14]. Although the total time from symptom onset to restoration of normal flow would appear to be the logical parameter to correlate with outcome, difficulties in assessing it may explain some of the conflicting results. Fluctuating arterial patency, collateral flow, pain threshold and other factors can render that determination imprecise. The delay from hospital arrival to PCI is easier to measure, but is really important only if it reflects total ischemic time. Recent studies, including adjustment for baseline characteristics suggest that delay in performing PCI are associated with worse outcome [14], although the slope of the "penalty" is milder than for lysis [15], consistent with the fact that PCI achieves more consistently reperfusion than lytics, particularly in aging thrombi.

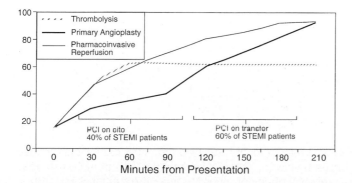

**Figure 4**  Theoretical model of facilitated PCI. (From Ref. 6)

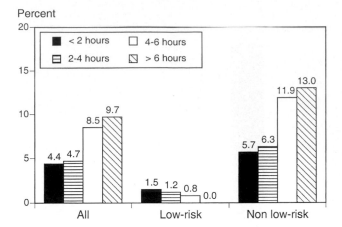

**Figure 5** One-year mortality according to door-to-balloon time in 1,791 patients treated with primary PCI and categorized by low (n = 545) or nonlow (n = 1,246) pre-PCI risk. Risk assessment is based on the presence of any of: prior MI, age > 70, anterior MI, SBp < 100 mmHg, HR > 100 bpm, atrial arrhythmias, Killip class > 1 [9]. (Adapted from Ref. 14)

The best explanation for the disparity in time dependency of the strategies can be gleaned from the examination of pre-PCI risk, i.e., patients at low-risk have little deterioration of benefit with more delayed PCI, while those at high(er) risk pay a steep penalty for each additional hour that passes before reperfusion (Figure 5 and 6) [13,14].

One can also relate delays in reperfusion and their link to outcome with the presence or absence of flow in the infarct artery at initial angiogram. Brodie et al. [16] and Stone et al. [17] have shown that patients arriving to angiography with a patent artery have a better angiographic and clinical outcome than those without flow (Figure 7). These data

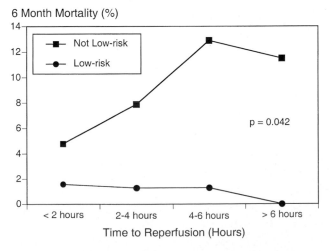

**Figure 6** Six-month mortality according to door-to-balloon time in 1,362 patients treated with primary PCI and categorized by low (n = 394) or nonlow (n = 942) pre-PCI risk. Risk assessment is based on the presence of any of: prior MI, age > 70, anterior MI, SBp < 100 mmHg, HR > 100 bpm, atrial arrhythmias, Killip class > 1 [9]. (From Ref. 13)

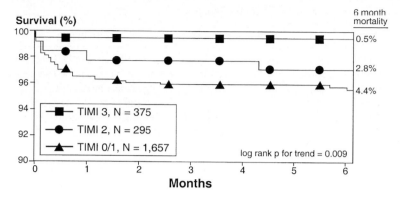

**Figure 7** Impact of pre-PCI flow in the infarct-related artery on 6-month survival. (From Ref. 17)

are intuitively expected and pose the challenge of implementing a pharmacological strategy that has the best efficacy in restoring flow before PCI without a prohibitive bleeding risk. Such an approach will also limit the incidence of malignant ventricular arrhythmia, prevent the development of cardiogenic shock [3] and lessen the probability of reperfusion injury.

Three approaches to facilitation of PCI have been tried and will be reviewed in the following sections. We do not distinguish between PCI performed only in response to clinically evident or angiographically proven failed pharmacological lysis or that, which follows routinely, and in proximity to pharmacological pre-treatment. The former has been insufficiently studied in RCT [18], except in one old study [19], while the latter more closely mirrors our practice.

## Fibrinolysis before PCI

After the unfavorable experience with immediate PCI in the late 1980s [7–9], 4 contemporary trials of varying designs and size examined the role of fibrinolysis before PCI (Table 1). In general, all patients received aspirin and an antithrombin agent and were randomized to lytic or placebo before undergoing angiography and PCI or coronary artery bypass grafting (CABG), as appropriate. The studies were too small to detect important differences in clinical outcome. Some notable findings, though, were:

1. Pre-PCI infarct artery patency was higher in pretreated patients (Figure 8).
2. PCI success was not affected by pretreatment and was high in both groups, with rates of thrombolysis in myocardial infarction (TIMI 3) flow greater than 85%, in general.
3. Subtle measures of reperfusion, such as regional wall motion, and even global ejection fraction (EF) were improved in patients with a patent artery before PCI, regardless of whether they were pretreated. For example, in the plasminogen-activator angioplasty compatibility trial (PACT) [20], convalescent EF was 62.4% in patients with patent infarct related artery (IRA) on arrival to angiography vs. 57.3% in those with delays greater than 1 hour to reperfusion ($p < 0.05$).
4. With the exception of Streptokinase or angioplasty in myocardial Infarction (SAMI) [21], there was no important excess bleeding in those treated with lytics before PCI.

**Table 1**   Recent Trials of Facilitation of PCI with Fibrinolysis

| Trial | Year | N | Lytic | Antithrombin | Comments |
|-------|------|-----|-------|--------------|----------|
| SAMI (21) | 1992 | 122 | SK | UFH | No difference in PCI success |
| PACT (20) | 1999 | 606 | t-PA | UFH | No difference in PCI success |
| PRAGUE-1 (45)* | 2000 | 201 | SK | UFH | Transport median time 106 min |
| GRACIA-2** | 2003 | 212 | TNK | LMWH | PCI in 3–12 hours |

* Excluding patients treated on-site with SK
** Preliminary data

The largest, albeit nonrandomized, experience with PCI after lysis comes from the analysis of large trials of fibrinolytic agents. In TIMI 10B, patients undergoing rescue PCI for failed lysis showed improved survival at 2 years, compared with those not treated (log-rank p = 0.03) [22]. In a combined analysis of over 20,000 patients enrolled in four fibrinolysis trials, the same investigators demonstrated again that adjunctive or rescue PCI after lysis is associated with improved outcome (Figure 9) [23]. The recently published Arbeitsgemeinschaft Leitende Kardiologische Krankenhausarzte (ALKK) registry also showed that, in stable patients 8–42 days after lysis, PCI confers a substantial advantage in long-term (4.5 years) survival, compared with medical therapy alone, 96% vs. 89%, p = 0.02 [24]. Similarly, the Southwest German Interventional Study in Acute Myocardial Infarction (SIAM III) trial compared the utility of stenting the IRA within 6 hours of fibrinolysis vs. later stenting at 2 weeks. Among 163 patients, the 6-month incidence of death, re-MI, or revascularization was 25.6% vs. 50.6%, p = 0.001, respectively [25].

The recurring observation from these randomized and nonrandomized series is that early PCI after fibrinolysis reduces the risk of re-MI, related to an unstable IRA plaque, residual thrombus, and significant platelet activation. Indeed, early PCI was associated with a 66% reduction in re-MI (1.6% vs. 4.5%, p < 0.001) among 20,101 patients enrolled in fibrinolysis trials [23]. The significance of this reduction is critical because re-MI is associated with a 3-fold increase in 30-day mortality (16.4% vs. 6.2%, p < 0.001). Ob-

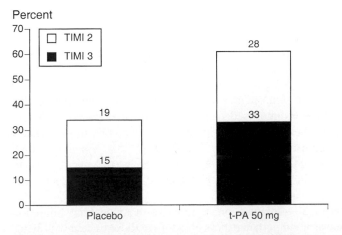

**Figure 8**   Impact of pre-PCI fibrinolysis on infarct-artery flow. (Adapted from Ref. 20)

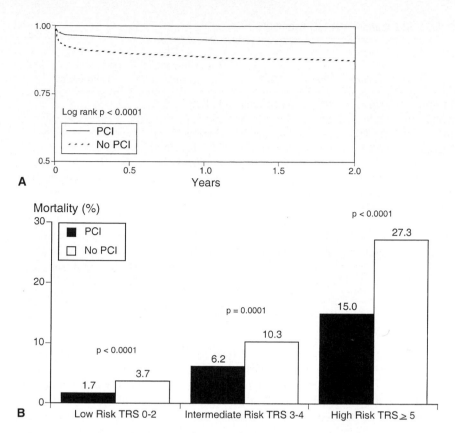

**Figure 9** In-hospital PCI after fibrinolysis improves 2-year survival, regardless of pre-PCI risk. (From Ref. 23)

viously, as the risk for re-MI increases as time from lysis passes, earlier PCI is likely to have a greater benefit than more delayed intervention.

## Glycoprotein Inhibitor (GPI) before Percutaneous Coronary Intervention

Eight trials have addressed specifically, in various designs, the utility of GPI alone, mostly abciximab, before primary PCI. (Table 2) The important lessons from these trials were:

1. The effect of GPI on arterial patency is time-dependent, such that earlier administration (in ambulance/ED) has a better chance to result in a patent artery before PCI than infusion just before balloon inflation (Figure 10).
2. GPI cannot reproduce the patency rates of fibrin-specific lytics. Only about 30% of pretreated patients, at most, achieve TIMI 3 flow before PCI.
3. GPI reduces 30-day ischemic events, mostly by preventing reinfarction and need for urgent target vessel revascularization. (Figure 11) This effect is durable for at least 6 months.
4. When PCI is performed with GPI pretreatment, other measures of reperfusion are improved, such as coronary flow characteristics [26], speed of reperfusion [27], and myocardial perfusion.

**Table 2**  Trials of Facilitation of PCI with GPI

| Trial | Year | N | GPI | Time (or difference in time) to angiogram | Comments |
|---|---|---|---|---|---|
| RAPPORT (46) | 1998 | 483 | Abciximab | In Lab | |
| Neumann (26) | 1998 | 200 | Abciximab | In Lab | Flow velocity |
| GRAPE (47) | 1999 | 60 | Abciximab | Average 45 min | |
| ADMIRAL (28) | 2001 | 300 | Abciximab | 25% in ambulance (60 min) | |
| CADILLAC (29) | 2002 | 1800 | Abciximab | In Lab | After angiogram |
| TIGER-PA (48) | 2003 | 100 | Tirofiban | 33 min | Early vs. late tirofiban |
| INTAMI* | 2003 | | | | |
| | | 74 | Eptifibatide | N/A | Early vs. late eptifibatide |
| On-TIME* | 2003 | 507 | Tirofiban | 59 min | Early vs. late tirofiban |

* Preliminary data

It is notable that in the Abciximab before Direct stenting in Myocardial Infarction Regarding Acute and Long-term follow-up (ADMIRAL) trial [28], the reduction in ischemic events with abciximab was most pronounced in the subset (approximately 25%) of patients receiving the drug in the ambulance—2.5% vs 21.1%, p < 0.05—while those randomized in the angiography suite derived a nonsignificant benefit, 8.3% vs. 12.4%, respectively. Furthermore, although in the Controlled Abciximab and Device Investigation to Lower Late Angioplasty Complications [29] trial, there was no difference among stented patients between those randomized to placebo or abciximab in the primary 6-month endpoint, at 30 days patients treated with abciximab had a significantly lower rate of ischemic events 5.0% vs. 7.1%, p = 0.04, predominantly related to prevention of subacute stent thrombosis.

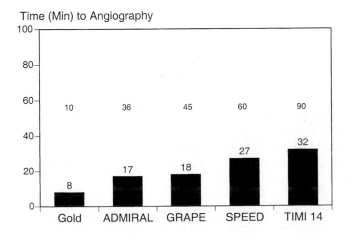

**Figure 10**  Impact of time from administration of abciximab prior to primary PCI on pre-PCI arterial patency (%, TIMI 3 flow). (Adapted from Ref. 52, Ref. 28, Ref. 47, Ref. 38, Ref. 49)

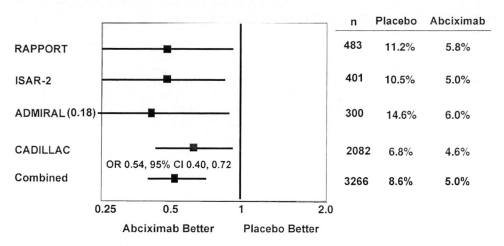

| | n | Placebo | Abciximab |
|---|---|---|---|
| RAPPORT | 483 | 11.2% | 5.8% |
| ISAR-2 | 401 | 10.5% | 5.0% |
| ADMIRAL (0.18) | 300 | 14.6% | 6.0% |
| CADILLAC | 2082 | 6.8% | 4.6% |
| Combined | 3266 | 8.6% | 5.0% |

OR 0.54, 95% CI 0.40, 0.72

0.25    0.5    1    2.0

Abciximab Better    Placebo Better

**Figure 11** Incidence of major adverse ischemic events at 30 days after primary PCI with or without abciximab. (From Ref. 53)

## COMBINATION LYTICS AND GPI BEFORE PCI

Two large clinical trials without mandatory immediate angiography, powered to detect differences in mortality at 30 days, have failed to show that combination half-dose lytic and full-dose GPI therapy was superior to lytic monotherapy in absence of systematic revascularization [30,31]. Despite a reduction in re-MI [30,32] and its complications [30] with combination therapy, there was no difference in survival at 1 year [33]. Combination therapy with abciximab and fibrinolysis (tissue plasminogen activator (t-PA) or tenecteplase (TNK) in reduced dose) decreased the need for urgent PCI [30,32]. Similar results were noted when fibrinolysis was combined with enoxaparin [32]. When needed, though, urgent PCI in patients treated with combination therapy resulted in inferior results than in those treated with conventional fibrinolysis, probably reflecting a significant bias in patient selection [32]. A worrisome increased incidence of intracranial hemorrhage was consistently observed in patients older than 75 years of age receiving combination therapy [34].

Smaller trials, utilizing combination therapy and mandating immediate angiography and revascularization when feasible, have aimed both at documenting improved arterial patency at initial angiography, as well as examining the facilitation of immediate PCI. (Table 3) They contributed the following to the concept of facilitated PCI:

1. Arterial patency was higher in patients receiving combination therapy at 60–90 minutes from drug administration than in patients receiving either monotherapy (Figure 12). The magnitude of the increased patency was smaller than expected (approximately 10–15%) and did not translate in improved clinical events.
2. Markers of reperfusion before PCI, such as ST-segment resolution, myocardial blush scores, or absence of thrombus were improved in the combination arm [35–37].
3. PCI results were not influenced by type of pretreatment and were more dependent on the patency of the IRA before procedure [38].
4. Bleeding complications tended to occur more commonly in patients receiving combination therapy than in those treated with monotherapy. For example, in integrilin and tenecteplase in acute myocardial infarction (INTEGRITI), major bleeding occurred in 8% of combination therapy and in 3% of TNK-alone pa-

**Table 3**   Trials of Facilitation of PCI with Combination Fibrinolysis and GPI

| Trial | Year | N | Lytic | GPI |
|-------|------|---|-------|-----|
| TIMI 14 (49) | 1999 | 888 | t-PA | Abciximab |
| SPEED (38) | 2000 | 485 | r-PA | Abciximab |
| INTRO-AMI (37) | 2002 | 649 | t-PA | Eptifibatide |
| ENTIRE TIMI 23 (50) | 2002 | 483 | TNK | Abciximab |
| INTEGRITI (51) | 2003 | 438 | TNK | Eptifibatide |
| BRAVE* | 2003 | 253 | r-PA | Abciximab |

* Presented at the American Heart Association Annual Meeting, Orlando, 2003

tients, while in the integrilin and low-dose thrombolysis therapy in acute myocardial infarction (INTRO-AMI) the rates were 11% and 6%, respectively. An augmentation of the risk of major bleeding was observed in Enoxaparin as Adjunctive Antithrombin Therapy for ST-Elevation Myocardial Infarction (ENTIRE)-TIMI 23 for patients receiving enoxaparin instead of unfractionated heparin and combination therapy, 8.5% vs. 5.2%, respectively. In the TNK monotherapy arm, the respective rates were 1.9% vs. 2.4%.

Interestingly, in the latest trial of facilitated PCI, Bavarian Reperfusion Alternatives Evaluation (BRAVE) [38a], infarct size was not different between patients treated with r-PA and abciximab or abciximab alone prior to angiography and primary PCI (13% vs. 11.5%, p = 0.81) (Kastrati A., American Heart Association Annual Meeting, Orlando, 2003). As expected, those treated with combination therapy had a higher rate of TIMI 3 flow at initial angiogram, 40% vs. 18%, p < 0.01, while both groups had 87% TIMI 3 flow at the completion of PCI. The incidence of clinical events was also similar, while major bleeding occurred, predictably, more often in the combination arm, 5.6% vs. 1.6%, p < 0.05.

Two large clinical trials are currently underway to investigate the utility of fibrinolysis with or without GPI prior to PCI. The Facilitated Intervention with Enhanced Reperfusion Speed to Stop Events (FINESSE) trial will enroll approximately 3,000 patients with

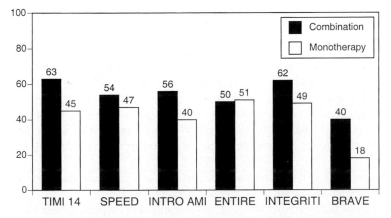

**Figure 12**   Incidence of TIMI 3 (%) flow at 60–90 min in patients treated with combination GPI and reduced-dose fibrinolysis therapy vs. monotherapy (lysis or GPI). All monotherapy groups consisted of fibrinolysis, except for BRAVE (Abciximab).

high-risk acute MI and an expected door-to-balloon time of 1–4 hours to one of three arms: half-dose r-PA with abciximab, abciximab alone, or abciximab administered only after arrival to angiography suite. The Assessment of the Safety and Efficacy of a New Thrombolytic (ASSENT)-4 trial will enroll approximately 4,000 patients with high-risk acute MI into one of two arms: TNK and enoxaparin or enoxaparin alone as pretreatment before PCI (GPI optional). It is hoped that by 2005, results from both trials will be available.

## Other facilitating strategies

Acute MI constitutes a profound inflammatory stimulus. Leukocyte accumulation in the infarcting myocardium may be responsible for reperfusion injury. The Hu23F2G Anti-Adhesion to Limit Cytotoxic Injury Following AMI (HALT-MI) study tested the role of CD11/CD18 integrin receptor blockade prior to primary PCI, performed within 6 hours of symptom onset [39]. Among 420 patients randomized to one of two doses of the antibody or placebo, the final scintigraphic infarct size was 16% for placebo, 17.2% for low-dose and 16.6% for high-dose antibody (p = NS). There was no particular benefit in patients with anterior MI or those treated within 2 hours of symptom onset.

Eniporide, an inhibitor of the Na/H proton exchange mechanism was studied because of its potential to reduce calcium overload and reperfusion injury. In the Evaluation of the Safety and Cardioprotective Effects of Eniporide in Acute Myocardial Infarction (ESCAMI) trial, 1,389 patients with acute MI were randomized to placebo or escalating doses of Eniporide before reperfusion therapy [40]. In the dose-finding phase, there appeared to be a reduction in infarct size in the subset treated with PCI and high-dose Eniporide. Nevertheless, in the confirmation phase of the trial, these findings could not be replicated among recipients of placebo, 100 mg or 150 mg of Eniporide undergoing PCI. Death rates were nonsignificantly higher in the active treatment arm.

An agent similar to Eniporide, Cariporide, was studied in a small study of 100 patients with anterior MI treated with primary PCI [41]. Compared with placebo, Cariporide reduced the area under the curve for creatine Kinase (CK) release (p = 0.047) and showed a trend towards improved restoration of segmental function in the infarct territory.

Recently, Pexelizumab, a complement fragment C5 inhibitor, was shown to be beneficial in acute MI patients undergoing primary PCI. In the complement inhibition in myocardial infarction treated with angioplasty (COMMA) trial, 960 patients were randomized to placebo or two doses of Pexelizumab before primary PCI. The CK area under the curve was not different among the groups and the composite 90-day event rate was similar [42]. Unexpectedly, the mortality at 90 days was significantly lower in the bolus and infusion group than in the bolus alone or placebo groups (1.8% vs. 4.2% vs. 5.9%, respectively, p = 0.014). This hypothesis-generating observation will be tested in approximately 3,000-patient trial, sufficiently powered to detect differences in mortality.

A different approach to metabolic manipulations has been investigated in studies of glucose-insulin-potassium (GIK) supplementation before reperfusion therapy, which attempt to reduce the oxidative stress associated with reperfusion injury. In a recent trial of 940 patients scheduled for primary PCI, open-label administration of the GIK solution for 8–12 hours resulted in a nonsignificant reduction in 30-day mortality (4.8% vs. 5.8% for placebo) [43]. In a posthoc analysis, the patients presenting in Killip Class I had a significant reduction in mortality (1.2% vs. 4.2%, p = 0.01).

Finally, the outcome of primary PCI could be further improved by mechanical means. Recently, the utilization of an emboli-protection device, the FilterX (Genentech, San Francisco, CA) wire was assessed in acute MI [44]. In 53 consecutive patients, the filter retrieved debris in 100% of analyzed specimens. The rate of blush score 3 was 66%, compared with 36% in a matched cohort not treated with the filter. There was a lower peak of CK-MB and greater improvement in regional wall motion in the experimental group, as well. A large trial, entitled Enhanced Myocardial Efficacy and Removal by Asperation (EMERALD), is currently evaluating this strategy in a large population.

## Summary and personal perspective

Secular trends in the presentation features of acute coronary syndromes (ACS) indicate that fewer patients will be presenting with ST-segment elevation MI, and more will have the non–ST-elevation ACS. Slowly, the distinctions between the two syndromes will fade in favor of a unified reperfusion strategy that encompasses effective upstream pharmacological intervention followed by timely and efficient mechanical reperfusion. The challenge for the next few years is to identify the optimal upstream pharmacology that will facilitate PCI without increasing the hazard of bleeding.

Based on the data reviewed in this chapter, certain potential strategies can be envisioned. It is clear that antithrombotic therapy will retain its importance. Potent dual antiplatelet therapy (probably aspirin and clopidogrel), as well as an effective antithrombin agent, such as enoxaparin or a direct-thrombin inhibitor, will constitute the platform to which fibrinolysis and/or GPI will be added. Eventually, the concept of facilitated PCI will incorporate effective modification of the metabolic milieu to preserve the myocardium prior to, and prevent injury after reperfusion. Anti-inflammatory interventions, such as those achieved by certain antithrombotic medications, are likely to contribute to lowering the incidence of recurring events. These adjunctive therapies will enhance the benefit obtained from immediate revascularization, performed with optimal protection of the microcirculation and antiproliferative agents deployed locally for prevention of restenosis. All these interventions need to be considered in the context of an ageing population, in whom the effects of multiple medications tend to results in more side effects, particularly bleeding.

Meanwhile, additional research is needed to identify the correct ingredients and recipe for this cocktail and, potentially, develop genetically based markers for customization of therapy.

## REFERENCES

1.  Keeley EC, Boura JA, Grines CL. Primary angioplasty versus intravenous thrombolytic therapy for acute myocardial infarction: a quantitative review of 23 randomized trials. Lancet 2003;361:13–20.
2.  Zijlstra F. Angioplasty vs thrombolysis for acute myocardial infarction: a quantitative overview of the effects of interhospital transportation. Eur Heart J 2003;24:21–3.
3.  Bonnefoy E, Lapostolle F, Leizorovicz A, Steg G, McFadden EP, Dubien PY, Cattan S, Boullenger E, Machecourt J, Lacroute JM, Cassagnes J, Dissait F, Touboul P. Primary angioplasty versus prehospital fibrinolysis in acute myocardial infarction: a randomized study. Lancet 2002;360:825–829.
4.  Wallentin L, Goldstein P, Armstrong PW, Granger CB, Adgey AA, Arntz HR, Bogaerts K, Danays T, Lindahl B, Makijarvi M, Verheugt F, Van de Werf F. Efficacy and safety of tenecteplase in combination with the low-molecular-weight heparin enoxaparin or unfractionated heparin in the prehospital setting: the Assessment of the Safety and Efficacy of a New Thrombolytic Regimen (ASSENT)-3 PLUS randomized trial in acute myocardial infarction. Circulation 2003;108:135–142.
5.  Force AAT. ACC/AHA guidelines for percutaneous coronary intervention. J Am Coll Cardiol 2001;37:2215–2238.
6.  Dauerman HL, Sobel BE. Synergistic treatment of ST-segment elevation myocardial infarction with pharmacoinvasive recanalization. J Am Coll Cardiol 2003;42:646–51.

7. Simoons M, Betriu A, Col J, von Essen R, Lubsen J, Michel P, Rutsch W, Schmidt W, Thery C, Vahanian A, Willems G, Arnold A, De Bono D, Dougherty F, Lambertz H, Meier B, Raynaud P, Sanz G, Serruys P, Uebis R, Van De Werf F, Wood D. Thrombolysis with tissue plasminogen activator in acute myocardial infarcton: No additional benefit from immediate percutaneous coronary angioplasty. Lancet 1988:197–202.

8. Topol E, aliff R, George B, Kereiakes D, Abbottsmith C, Candela R, Lee K, Pitt B, Stack R, O'Neill W. A randomized trial of immediate versus delayed elective angioplasty after intravenous tissue plasminogen activator in acute myocardial infarction. N Engl J Med 1987; 317:581–588.

9. Comparison of invasive and conservative strategies after treatment with intravenous tissue plasminogen activator in acute myocardial infarction. Results of the thrombolysis in myocardial infarction (TIMI) phase II trial. The TIMI Study Group. N Engl J Med 1989;320:618–27.

10. Berger PB, Ellis SG, Holmes DR, Granger CB, Criger DA, Betriu A, Topol EJ, Califf RM. Relationship between delay in performing direct coronary angioplasty and early clinical outcome in patients with acute myocardial infarction: results from the global use of strategies to open occluded arteries in Acute Coronary Syndromes (GUSTO-IIb) trial. Circulation 1999; 100:14–20.

11. Cannon CP, Gibson CM, Lambrew CT, Shoultz DA, Levy D, French WJ, Gore JM, Weaver WD, Rogers WJ, Tiefenbrunn AJ. Relationship of symptom-onset-to-balloon time and door-to-balloon time with mortality in patients undergoing angioplasty for acute myocardial infarction. JAMA 2000;283:2941–7.

12. Brener SJ, Ellis SG, Sapp SK, Betriu A, Granger CB, Burchenal JE, Moliterno DJ, Califf RM, Topol EJ. Predictors of death and reinfarction at 30 days after primary angioplasty: the GUSTO IIb and RAPPORT trials. Am Heart J 2000;139:476–81.

13. Antoniucci D, Valenti R, Migliorini A, Moschi G, Trapani M, Buonamici P, Cerisano G, Bolognese L, Santoro GM. Relation of time to treatment and mortality in patients with acute myocardial infarction undergoing primary coronary angioplasty. Am J Cardiol 2002; 89:1248–1252.

14. De Luca G, Suryapranata H, Zijlstra F, van't Hof AW, Hoorntje JC, Gosselink AT, Dambrink JH, de Boer MJ. Symptom-onset-to-balloon time and mortality in patients with acute myocardial infarction treated by primary angioplasty. J Am Coll Cardiol 2003;42:991–997.

15. Zijlstra F, Patel A, Jones M, Grines CL, Ellis S, Garcia E, Grinfeld L, Gibbons RJ, Ribeiro EE, Ribichini F, Granger C, Akhras F, Weaver WD, Simes RJ. Clinical characteristics and outcome of patients with early (<2 h), intermediate (2–4 h) and late (>4 h) presentation treated by primary coronary angioplasty or thrombolytic therapy for acute myocardial infarction. Eur Heart J 2002;23:550–7.

16. Brodie BR, Stuckey TD, Hansen C, Muncy D. Benefit of coronary reperfusion before intervention on outcomes after primary angioplasty for acute myocardial infarction. Am J Cardiol 2000;85:13–8.

17. Stone GWMD, Cox DMD, Garcia EMD, Brodie BRMD, Morice M-CMD, Griffin JMD, Mattos LMD, Lansky AJMD, O'Neill WWMD, Grines CLMD. Normal Flow (TIMI-3) Before mechanical reperfusion therapy is an independent determinant of survival in acute myocardial infarction: analysis from the Primary Angioplasty in Myocardial Infarction Trials. Circulation 2001;104:636–641.

18. Ellis SG, Da Silva ER, Spaulding CM, Nobuyoshi M, Weiner B, Talley JD. Review of immediate angioplasty after fibrinolytic therapy for acute myocardial infarction: insights from the RESCUE I, RESCUE II, and other contemporary clinical experiences. Am Heart J 2000; 139:1046–1053.

19. Ellis SG, da Silva ER, Heyndrickx G, Talley JD, Cernigliaro C, Steg G, Spaulding C, Nobuyoshi M, Erbel R, Vassanelli C, et al. Randomized comparison of rescue angioplasty with conservative management of patients with early failure of thrombolysis for acute anterior myocardial infarction. Circulation 1994;90:2280–2284.

20. Ross AM, Coyne KS, Reiner JS, Greenhouse SW, Fink C, Frey A, Moreyra E, Traboulsi M, Racine N, Riba AL, Thompson MA, Rohrbeck S, Lundergan CF. A randomized trial compar-

ing primary angioplasty with a strategy of short-acting thrombolysis and immediate planned rescue angioplasty in acute myocardial infarction: the PACT trial. PACT investigators. Plasminogen-activator Angioplasty Compatibility Trial. [In Process Citation.]. J Am Coll Cardiol 1999;34:1954–1962.

21. O'Neill WW, Weintraub R, Grines CL, Meany TB, Brodie BR, Friedman HZ, Ramos RG, Gangadharan V, Levin RN, Choksi N, et al. A prospective, placebo-controlled, randomized trial of intravenous streptokinase and angioplasty versus lone angioplasty therapy of acute myocardial infarction. Circulation 1992;86:1710–1717.

22. Gibson CM, Cannon CP, Murphy SA, Marble SJ, Barron HV, Braunwald E. Relationship of the TIMI myocardial perfusion grades, flow grades, frame count, and percutaneous coronary intervention to long-term outcomes after thrombolytic administration in acute myocardial infarction. Circulation 2002;105:1909–1913.

23. Gibson CM, Karha J, Murphy SA, James D, Morrow DA, Cannon CP, Giugliano RP, Antman EM, Braunwald E. Early and long-term clinical outcomes associated with reinfarction following fibrinolytic administration in the thrombolysis in myocardial infarction trials. J Am Coll Cardiol 2003;42:7–16.

24. Zeymer U, Uebis R, Vogt A, Glunz HG, Vohringer HF, Harmjanz D, Neuhaus KL. Randomized comparison of percutaneous transluminal coronary angioplasty and medical therapy in stable survivors of acute myocardial infarction with single vessel disease: a study of the Arbeitsgemeinschaft Leitende Kardiologische Krankenhausarzte. Circulation 2003;108: 1324–1328.

25. Scheller B, Hennen B, Hammer B, Walle J, Hofer C, Hilpert V, Winter H, Nickenig G, Bohm M. Beneficial effects of immediate stenting after thrombolysis in acute myocardial infarction. J Am Coll Cardiol 2003;42:634–641.

26. Neumann FJ, Blasini R, Schmitt C, Alt E, Dirschinger J, Gawaz M, Kastrati A, Schomig A. Effect of glycoprotein IIb/IIIa receptor blockade on recovery of coronary flow and left ventricular function after the placement of coronary-artery stents in acute myocardial infarction. Circulation 1998;98:2695–2701.

27. Brener SJ, Barr LA, Burchenal JE, Wolski KE, Effron MB, Topol EJ. Effect of abciximab on the pattern of reperfusion in patients with acute myocardial infarction treated with primary angioplasty. RAPPORT investigators. ReoPro And Primary PTCA Organization and Randomized Trial. Am J Cardiol 1999;84:728–730, A8.

28. Montalescot G, Barragan P, Wittenberg O, Ecollan P, Elhadad S, Villain P, Boulenc JM, Morice MC, Maillard L, Pansieri M, Choussat R, Pinton P. Platelet glycoprotein IIb/IIIa inhibition with coronary stenting for acute myocardial infarction. N Engl J Med 2001;344: 1895–1903.

29. Stone GW, Grines CL, Cox DA, Garcia E, Tcheng JE, Griffin JJ, Guagliumi G, Stuckey T, Turco M, Carroll JD, Rutherford BD, Lansky AJ. the Controlled Abciximab and Device Investigation to Lower Late Angioplasty Complications (CADILLAC) Investigators. Comparison of Angioplasty with Stenting, with or without Abciximab, in Acute Myocardial Infarction. N Engl J Med 2002;346:957–966.

30. Topol EJ. Reperfusion therapy for acute myocardial infarction with fibrinolytic therapy or combination reduced fibrinolytic therapy and platelet glycoprotein IIb/IIIa inhibition: the GUSTO V randomised trial. Lancet 2001;357:1905–1914.

31. Efficacy and safety of tenecteplase in combination with enoxaparin, abciximab, or unfractionated heparin: the ASSENT-3 randomised trial in acute myocardial infarction. Lancet 2001; 358:605–613.

32. Dubois CL, Belmans A, Granger CB, Armstrong PW, Wallentin L, Fioretti PM, Lopez-Sendon JL, Verheugt FW, Meyer J, Van de Werf F. Outcome of urgent and elective percutaneous coronary interventions after pharmacologic reperfusion with tenecteplase combined with unfractionated heparin, enoxaparin, or abciximab. J Am Coll Cardiol 2003;42:1178–1185.

33. Lincoff AM, Califf RM, Van De Werf F, Willerson JT, White HD, Armstrong PW, Guetta V, Gibler WB, Hochman JS, Bode C, Vahanian A, Steg PG, Ardissino D, Savonitto S, Bar F, Sadowski Z, Betriu A, Booth JE, Wolski K, Waller M, Topol EJ. Mortality at 1 year with combination platelet glycoprotein IIb/IIIa inhibition and reduced-dose fibrinolytic therapy

vs. conventional fibrinolytic therapy for acute myocardial infarction: GUSTO V randomized trial. JAMA 2002;288:2130–2135.

34. Savonitto S, Armstrong PW, incoff AM, Jia G, Sila CA, Booth J, Terrosu P, Cavallini C, White HD, Ardissino D, Califf RM, Topol EJ. Risk of intracranial haemorrhage with combined fibrinolytic and glycoprotein IIb/IIIa inhibitor therapy in acute myocardial infarction. Dichotomous response as a function of age in the GUSTO V trial. Eur Heart J 2003;24:1807–1814.

35. de Lemos JA, Antman EM, Gibson CM, McCabe CH, Giugliano RP, Murphy SA, Coulter SA, Anderson K, Scherer J, Frey MJ, Van Der Wieken R, Van De Werf F, Braunwald E. Abciximab improves both epicardial flow and myocardial reperfusion in ST-elevation myocardial infarction. Observations from the TIMI 14 trial. Circulation 2000;101:239–243.

36. Gibson CM, de Lemos JA, Murphy SA, Marble SJ, McCabe CH, Cannon CP, Antman EM, Braunwald E. Combination therapy with abciximab reduces angiographically evident thrombus in acute myocardial infarction: a TIMI 14 substudy. Circulation 2001;103: 2550–2554.

37. Brener SJ, Zeymer U, Adgey AA, Vrobel TR, Ellis SG, Neuhaus KL, Juran N, Ivanc TB, Ohman EM, Strony J, Kitt M, Topol EJ. Eptifibatide and low-dose tissue plasminogen activator in acute myocardial infarction: the integrilin and low-dose thrombolysis in acute myocardial infarction (INTRO AMI) trial. J Am Coll Cardiol 2002;39:377–386.

38. Herrmann HC, Moliterno DJ, Ohman EM, Stebbins AL, Bode C, Betriu A, Forycki F, Miklin JS, Bachinsky WB, Lincoff AM, Califf RM, Topol EJ. Facilitation of early percutaneous coronary intervention after reteplase with or without abciximab in acute myocardial infarction: results from the SPEED (GUSTO-4 Pilot) Trial. J Am Coll Cardiol 2000;36:1489–1496.

38a. Kastrati A, Mehilli J, Schlotterbeck K, Dotzer F, Dirschinger J, Schmitt C, Nekolla SG, Seyfarth M, Martinoff S, Markwadt C, Clermont G, Gerbig HW, Leiss J, Schwarger M, Schomig A. Early administration of reteplase plus abciximab vs. abciximab alone in patients with acute myocardial infarction referred for percutaneous coronary intervention: a randomized controlled trial. JAMA 2004;291:947–54.

39. Faxon DP, Gibbons RJ, Chronos NA, Gurbel PA, Sheehan F. The effect of blockade of the CD11/CD18 integrin receptor on infarct size in patients with acute myocardial infarction treated with direct angioplasty: the results of the HALT-MI study. J Am Coll Cardiol 2002; 40:1199–1204.

40. Zeymer U, Suryapranata H, Monassier JP, Opolski G, Davies J, Rasmanis G, Linssen G, Tebbe U, Schroder R, Tiemann R, Machnig T, Neuhaus KL. The Na($+$)/H($+$) exchange inhibitor eniporide as an adjunct to early reperfusion therapy for acute myocardial infarction. Results of the evaluation of the safety and cardioprotective effects of eniporide in acute myocardial infarction (ESCAMI) trial. J Am Coll Cardiol 2001;38:1644–1650.

41. Rupprecht HJ, vom Dahl J, Terres W, Seyfarth KM, Richardt G, Schultheibeta HP, Buerke M, Sheehan FH, Drexler H. Cardioprotective effects of the Na($+$)/H($+$) exchange inhibitor cariporide in patients with acute anterior myocardial infarction undergoing direct PTCA [see comments]. Circulation 2000;101:2902–2908.

42. Granger CB, Mahaffey KW, Weaver WD, Theroux P, Hochman JS, Filloon TG, Rollins S, Todaro TG, Nicolau JC, Ruzyllo W, Armstrong PW. Pexelizumab, an Anti-C5 Complement Antibody, as Adjunctive Therapy to Primary Percutaneous Coronary Intervention in Acute Myocardial Infarction: The COMplement inhibition in Myocardial infarction treated with Angioplasty (COMMA) Trial. Circulation 2003;108:1184–1190.

43. van der Horst IC, Zijlstra F, van't Hof AW, Doggen CJ, de Boer MJ, Suryapranata H, Hoorntje JC, Dambrink JH, Gans RO, Bilo HJ. Glucose-insulin-potassium infusion inpatients treated with primary angioplasty for acute myocardial infarction: the glucose-insulin-potassium study: a randomized trial. J Am Coll Cardiol 2003;42:784–791.

44. Limbruno U, Micheli A, De Carlo M, Amoroso G, Rossini R, Palagi C, Di Bello V, Petronio AS, Fontanini G, Mariani M. Mechanical Prevention of Distal Embolization During Primary Angioplasty: Safety, Feasibility, and Impact on Myocardial Reperfusion. Circulation 2003; 108:171–176.

45. Widimsky P, Groch L, Zelizko M, Aschermann M, Bednar F, Suryapranata H. Multicentre randomized trial comparing transport to primary angioplasty vs immediate thrombolysis vs

combined strategy for patients with acute myocardial infarction presenting to a community hospital without a catheterization laboratory. The PRAGUE study [see comments]. Eur Heart J 2000;21:823–831.

46. Brener SJ, Barr LA, Burchenal JE, Katz S, George BS, Jones AA, Cohen ED, Gainey PC, White HJ, Cheek HB, Moses JW, Moliterno DJ, Effron MB, Topol EJ. Randomized, placebo-controlled trial of platelet glycoprotein IIb/IIIa blockade with primary angioplasty for acute myocardial infarction. ReoPro and Primary PTCA Organization and Randomized Trial (RAP-PORT) Investigators. Circulation 1998;98:734–741.

47. van den Merkhof LF, Zijlstra F, Olsson H, Grip L, Veen G, Bar FW, van den Brand MJ, Simoons ML, Verheugt FW. Abciximab in the treatment of acute myocardial infarction eligible for primary percutaneous transluminal coronary angioplasty. Results of the Glycoprotein Receptor Antagonist Patency Evaluation (GRAPE) pilot study. J Am Coll Cardiol 1999; 33:1528–1532.

48. Lee DP, Herity NA, Hiatt BL, Fearon WF, Rezaee M, Carter AJ, Huston M, Schreiber D, DiBattiste PM, Yeung AC. Adjunctive platelet glycoprotein IIb/IIIa receptor inhibition with tirofiban before primary angioplasty improves angiographic outcomes: results of the TIrofiban Given in the Emergency Room before Primary Angioplasty (TIGER-PA) pilot trial. Circulation 2003;107:1497–1501.

49. Antman EM, Giugliano RP, Gibson CM, McCabe CH, Coussement P, Kleiman NS, Vahanian A, Adgey AA, Menown I, Rupprecht HJ, Van der Wieken R, Ducas J, Scherer J, Anderson K, Van de Werf F, Braunwald E. Abciximab facilitates the rate and extent of thrombolysis: results of the thrombolysis in myocardial infarction (TIMI) 14 trial. The TIMI 14 Investigators. Circulation 1999;99:2720–2732.

50. Antman EM, Louwerenburg HW, Baars HF, Wesdorp JCL, Hamer B, Bassand J-P, Bigonzi F, Pisapia G, Gibson CM, Heidbuchel H, Braunwald E, Van de Werf F. for the ENTIRE-TIMI 23 Investigators. Enoxaparin as Adjunctive Antithrombin Therapy for ST-Elevation Myocardial Infarction: Results of the ENTIRE-Thrombolysis in Myocardial Infarction (TIMI) 23 Trial. Circulation 2002;105:1642–1649.

51. Giugliano RP, Roe MT, Harrington RA, Gibson CM, Zeymer U, Van de Werf F, Baran KW, Hobbach HP, Woodlief LH, Hannan KL, Greenberg S, Miller J, Kitt MM, Strony J, McCabe CH, Braunwald E, Califf RM. ombination reperfusion therapy with eptifibatide and reduced-dose tenecteplase for ST-elevation myocardial infarction: results of the integrilin and tenecteplase in acute myocardial infarction (INTEGRITI) Phase II Angiographic Trial. J Am Coll Cardiol 2003;41:1251–1260.

52. Gold HK, Garabedian HD, Dinsmore RE, Guerrero LJ, Cigarroa JE, Palacios IF, Leinbach RC. Restoration of coronary flow in myocardial infarction by intravenous chimeric 7E3 antibody without exogenous plasminogen activators. Observations in animals and humans. Circulation 1997;95:1755–1759.

53. Kandzari DE, Hasselbad V, Tcheng JE, Stone GW, Califf RM, Kastrati A, Neumann FJ, Brener SJ, Montalescot G, Kong DF, Harrington RA. Improved clinical outcomes with abciximab therapy in acute myocardial infarction: a systemic overview of randomized clinical trials. Am Heart J 2004;147:457–462.

# 13

# Regional Centers of Excellence for the Care of Patients with Acute Coronary Syndromes

**Dean J. Kereiakes**
*The Carl and Edyth Lindner Center for Research and Education*
*Ohio State University*
*Cincinnati, Ohio, U.S.A.*

The past decade has witnessed a remarkable evolution in our understanding of the pathogenesis of acute coronary syndromes (ACS), which, in turn, has prompted a similar evolution in pharmacologic and catheter-based therapies. Concomitantly, great strides have been made in our ability to accurately risk-stratify patients who present with ACS. Spontaneous plaque rupture, often precipitated by a generalized multicentric inflammatory arteritis [1–3], results in endothelial denudation with exposure of collagen, atherosclerotic debris, and other subintimal thrombogenic vessel wall components. Platelet adherence, activation, and aggregation follows with fibrin incorporation leading to thrombus propagation [4–6]. The severity of the resultant clinical syndrome is manifest in direct proportion to the degree of restriction in coronary blood flow, ranging from asymptomatic (insignificant restriction) to non–ST-segment elevation ACS (NSTACS), which includes both unstable angina and non–ST segment elevation myocardial infarction (NSTEMI), that is associated with severe coronary flow restriction, and, finally, ST-segment elevation myocardial infarction (STEMI), which is usually secondary to complete coronary occlusion [4,7,8]. As the pathogenesis of coronary flow restriction is multifactorial (platelets, organized thrombus, vasomotion, and mechanical obstruction), it is best addressed by a multimodal approach to therapy (antiplatelet, anticoagulant, fibrinolytic, and percutaneous catheter-based intervention) implemented in a timely manner. Indeed, the rapid restoration of normal coronary blood flow via pharmacological and/or mechanical recanalization of an occluded coronary artery limits the extent of myocardial necrosis and reduces mortality. A concerted, integrated approach to therapy of ACS is complicated by the diversity and extent of resources required for comprehensive treatment of this disease spectrum. Furthermore, any analysis of therapeutic strategies for ACS must consider resource (both technical facility and manpower) availability, logistic as well as economic concerns.

## SCOPE OF THE PROBLEM

The number of deaths from myocardial infarction (MI) in the United States alone exceeds (seven-fold) that for all-cause trauma in the general population, and is twenty-fold higher for persons more than 65 years of age [9]. The approach of creating specialized centers of care for treating victims of trauma has been validated for improving clinical outcomes [10,11]. The lack of specialized centers of care for patients with acute ischemic heart disease is not commensurate with the magnitude of this public health problem. In addition, the facts that the vast majority of hospitals lack tertiary invasive facilities for coronary revascularization and that much of the United States (and other countries) include large, sparsely populated areas with long travel distances required to reach a more populous area where a "regional center of excellence" may exist, mandate a more "global" integrated approach to the treatment of ACS [12–16] Indeed, the reality that only a minority of patients who experience an acute MI will receive any specific therapy directed at coronary reperfusion has prompted some thought-leaders to view the scope of this problem in perspective: "The opportunity to provide reperfusion to a larger proportion of patients worldwide represents a far greater health issue than attempts to tease out the small differences that may exist among populations treated with percutaneous coronary intervention vs. drug therapy" [17]. Conversely, in industrialized nations, the "optimal" strategy for reperfusion (pharmacologic vs. mechanical) has become a point of contention, confounded by economic and reimbursement considerations. This divergence of interest and opinion bridges a broach spectrum from those who contend, "the real issue is not whether the creation of specialized centers for care of those (ACS) patients would provide an important advance, but rather how to create them" [15] to those who suggest "clear compelling evidence of the benefits of ACS regionalization within the United States and a better understanding of its potential consequences are needed before implementing a national policy of regionalized ACS care". Recent data supporting the relative safety and efficacy of percutaneous coronary intervention (PCI) vs. thrombolytic reperfusion for MI [19–21] have been largely extrapolated out of context to rationalize the proliferation of PCI programs into community hospitals without cardiac surgical facilities [22–24]. This proliferation of PCI and cardiac surgical programs comes at a time when resource pools for both subspecialized nursing staff and cardiovascular physician providers are taxed to "crisis" proportions [25–27]. In addition, the proliferation of small volume interventional programs poses yet another challenge to "the continuous cycle of quality" [28]. Multiple national initiatives, such as Get with the Guidelines™ [29], the Cardiac Hospitalization Atherosclerosis Management program (CHAMPS) [30], the Guidelines Applied to Practice (GAP) project [31], the National Registry of myocardial infarction (NRMI) [32], and the Can Rapid Risk Stratification of Unstable Angina Patients Suppress Adverse outcomes with early implementation of the ACC/AHA guidelines (CRUSADE) project [33] have emphasized a focus on system quality by systematically measuring processes and outcomes. In general, patients have better clinical outcomes when treated in centers that commonly encounter the clinical problem with which the patient is afflicted ("practice makes perfect").

Patients with more complex cardiovascular illnesses (MI, congestive heart failure) appear to fare better with subspecialty cardiology compared with generalist's care [34–37]. Both compliance with clinical practice guidelines and the ability to monitor or audit guideline adherence are greater in higher volume, regional programs [38,39]. Current financial considerations present a complicating and constraining effect on efforts to regionalize care for ACS to specialized centers of excellence. Not only is coronary heart disease the preeminent cause of death and disability, it is also a critical determinant of financial success for many hospitals in the United States. Cardiovascular service lines are traditionally profitable, and profitability from cardiovascular procedures are often used to offset deficits from other services. One proviso to this scenario is that profitability is usually volume-driven and this relationship provides a link (volume) for quality outcome measures.

## ST-SEGMENT ELEVATION MYOCARDIAL INFARCTION

The rapidity, extent, and durability of coronary reperfusion are important determinants of prognosis in acute myocardial infarction. Primary PCI results in higher infarct-related coronary artery reperfusion rates and has been demonstrated to be superior to fibrinolytic therapy in reducing mortality, recurrent ischemia and stroke [19–21]. Nevertheless, the vast majority of hospitals lack tertiary invasive revascularization facilities and, thus, most therapeutic strategies have focused on pharmacologic reperfusion with intravenous fibrinolytics as either monotherapy or to facilitate (precede) planned catheter-based intervention. Most randomized comparative trials of fibrinolytic vs. PCI therapy for acute MI have involved tertiary high-volume enrollment centers [19–21]. More recently, several studies have evaluated the strategy of transfer to a tertiary center for PCI vs. on-site fibrinolytic therapy in a community hospital setting [40–46]. From this cumulative experience, several observations can be made.

First, the relative advantage of PCI vs. fibrinolytic therapy is dependent on the case volume experience of both the interventional cardiologist and the hospital facility providing the service [47–53]. The best clinical outcomes and, hence, the greatest relative advantage for PCI, are obtained by the highest-volume operators and institutions. Indeed, no advantage in favor of PCI may be evident in "low volume" institutions. Secondly, the advantage for PCI (vs. fibrinolytics) may depend on the time course of implementation [55]. Only recently have the time dependent efficacies for both mechanical and pharmacologic reperfusion been scrutinized and relative differences between these strategies become evident. For example, the time from infarct symptom onset to initiation of fibrinolytic reperfusion is a critical determinant for both successful coronary recanalization and survival. Conversely, the relationship between infarct duration, prior to PCI recanalization, with either procedural success or survival, is less direct [56–61]. Although PCI consistently yields higher coronary patency rates at 60 and 90 minutes following initiation of therapy, with less residual coronary stenosis and lower reocclusion rates, this strategy usually entails an obligate additional time delay for implementation [62–64]. A recent analysis suggests that the survival benefit associated with PCI (vs. fibrinolytics) may be lost if the delay-to-initiation (door-to-balloon time) exceeds more than 1 hour, compared with the time delay (door-to-needle time) for initiating fibrinolysis [55]. Interestingly, door-to-balloon times vary significantly with the time of hospital arrival (24-hour clock) [65] and are inversely proportional to hospital volumes of primary PCI procedures [65–69]. Although door-to-balloon times of less than 120 minutes have been associated with improvement in hospital survival [66], recent data from the NRMI 2,3 registries demonstrates that door-to-balloon times of less than 2.2 hours were observed only between the hours of 8 am and 5 pm [65]. Third, transport to a regional center for PCI yields superior clinical outcomes when compared with onsite (community hospital) fibrinolytic therapy, despite time delays incurred during the transport process (Figure 1) [45,46].

Recent meta-analyses of multiple randomized clinical trials have demonstrated a reduction in mortality, recurrent ischemia and stroke for patients transported to a regional center for PCI, as compared with those patients randomly assigned to receive immediate (on-site) fibrinolysis (Figure 2), despite the additional 70–103 minutes required for transport [45,46]. The explanation for this finding is likely multifactorial and may include the fact that clinical outcomes after PCI are less dependent on time delay from infarct symptom onset to therapy. Furthermore, regional interventional centers treat larger numbers of patients and, thus, may provide incremental benefit based on volume credentialing and access to adjunctive technologies [66]. Importantly, no adverse clinical outcomes have been observed as a consequence of transport in thousands of patients included in these analyses.

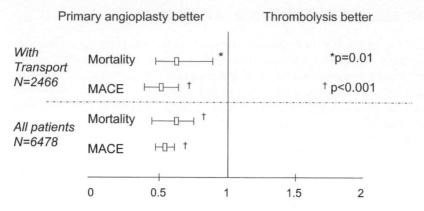

**Figure 1** Meta-analysis of multiple randomized trials demonstrating relative benefit of primary angioplasty (vs. thrombolysis) for all studies (all patients) as well as studies which involve transport to a regional center for primary angioplasty vs. "on-site" thrombolytic therapy (with transport). (From Ref. 45)

Lastly, based largely on data favoring PCI (vs. fibrinolysis) derived in regional centers, many community hospitals in the United States have sought to implement PCI reperfusion programs in the absence of elective provisions for percutaneous coronary intervention. Few prospective studies have evaluated the outcomes of PCI at centers without on-site cardiac surgical facilities. Most data in support of this practice are derived from observational series [70–77] and one prematurely terminated, randomized clinical trial [78]. The rates of surgical coronary revascularization during the index hospitalization in these studies have been between 5.3 and 7.0%. Although the requirement for emergency surgical coronary revascularization following primary PCI for acute MI is uncommon in the era of

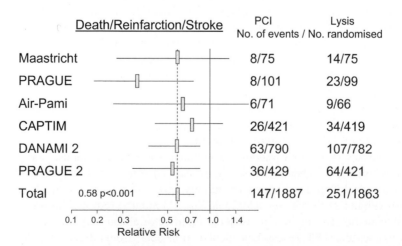

**Figure 2** Meta-analysis of multiple randomized trials which compared on-site fibrinolysis vs. transfer to a regional center for primary PCI in the treatment of acute ST segment elevation myocardial infarction. A reduction in the composite occurrence of death, reinfarction or stroke was observed in favor of transfer for primary angioplasty. (From Ref. 46)

coronary stenting and optimized pharmacotherapy (platelet glycoprotein [GP] IIb/IIIa inhibition and thienopyridine therapy), recent data suggest that clinical outcomes of surgery in these patients are guarded, patient acuity is high and morbidity/mortality is substantial [79]. These sobering results reflect current practice, despite existing American College of Cardiology/American Hospital Association (ACC/AHA) guideline recommendations that call for "formalized written protocols in place for immediate (within 1 hour) and efficient transfer of patients to the nearest cardiac surgical facility which are reviewed/tested on a regular (quarterly) basis" [80]. Whether or not current guidelines are being strictly implemented in facilities without on-site cardiac surgical backup, or if further guideline modifications should be made, remains to be determined. Finally, a single randomized trial directly evaluated whether on-site fibrinolysis or PCI provides the optimal therapeutic strategy for hospitals without cardiac surgical facilities. The Atlantic Cardiovascular Patient Outcomes Research Team (C-PORT) [78] trial involved participating community hospitals in Maryland and Massachusetts and randomly assigned 451 patients presenting with STEMI to receive either PCI or fibrinolysis "on-site." Extensive in-service training of hospital staff, consignment inventory of angioplasty supplies and performance of PCI procedures by relatively high-volume operators from neighboring communities were notable features. This trial was prematurely stopped due to lack of funding when less than 20% of the projected study volume had been enrolled. Patients randomly assigned to PCI had a lower incidence (p = 0.03) of the composite endpoint of death, reinfarction, or stroke at both 30 days and 6 months following treatment. (Table 1). Of note was the rather high rate of stroke (3.5%) in the fibrinolytic-treated patients in comparison with patients randomly assigned to primary PCI (1.3%). The incidence of stroke observed in fibrinolytic-treated patients in the C-PORT trial appears to be several-fold higher than observed in prior trials of fibrinolytic therapy for MI (0.5–1.1%) (Figure 3). Although many community hospitals in the United States have implemented PCI programs without on-site cardiac surgical facilities on the basis of C-PORT data, several pertinent questions remain. Should the results of a single, randomized trial in 451 patients become the standard of care for general practice? What is the statistical validity for a p value of 0.03 in favor of PCI benefit (vs. fibrinolysis) when less than 20% of the projected study volume has been enrolled? Why were not prespecified, more rigorous statistical requirements (i.e., p < 0.01 required for statistical significance) applied following premature study termination? Finally, in retrospect, the inclusion of a third randomized arm for transport to a regional

**Table 1**   C-PORT Primary Outcomes

|  | Fibrinolytic % (n=211) | Primary PCI % (n=171) | p value |
|---|---|---|---|
| *6 Weeks* | | | |
| Death | 7.1 | 5.3 | 0.44 |
| Reinfarction | 8.8 | 4.9 | 0.09 |
| Stroke | 3.5 | 1.3 | 0.13 |
| Composite | 17.7 | 10.7 | 0.03 |
| *6 Months* | | | |
| Death | 7.1 | 6.2 | 0.72 |
| Reinfarction | 10.6 | 5.3 | 0.04 |
| Stroke | 4.0 | 2.2 | 0.28 |
| Composite | 19.9 | 12.4 | 0.03 |

Adapted from Ref. 78

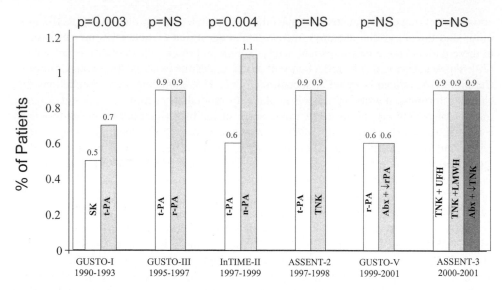

**Figure 3** Incidence of intracranial hemorrhage as reported in major trials of fibrinolytic therapy for the treatment of acute myocardial infarction. (AMI, acute myocardial infarction; SK, streptokinase; Abx, abciximab; LMWH, low-molecular-weight heparin; UFH, unfractionated heparin). Data abstracted from GUSTO 1-(Global Utilization of Streptokinase and Tissue Plasminogen Activator for Occluded Coronary Arteries); GUSTO 3 (Global Use of Strategies to Open occluded coronary arteries); ASSENT 2 (Assessment of the Safety and Efficacy of a New Thrombolytic agent); GUSTO-V (Global Utilization of Streptokinase and Tissue-plasminogen activator of Occluded arteries); and ASSENT 3 (Assessment of the Safety & Efficacy of New Thrombolytic Regimens) trials.

center for PCI would have been a useful comparator (vs. on-site community hospital PCI), particularly in the context of both logistic considerations for PCI program proliferation in community hospitals, as well as the previously cited benefis of immediate transport to a regional center for PCI (vs. on-site fibrinolysis). Beyond the intricacies of which reperfusion strategy employed in which clinical scenario is "best" is the growing realization that reperfusion therapy is not being provided to many victims of STEMI worldwide. As logistical considerations limit the performance of PCI within 2 hours of presentation (door-to-balloon time) in most patients, the timely administration of fibrinolytic therapy (door-to-needle time ≤ 30 minutes) should be applied (in the absence of specific contraindications) to most patients. Immediate patient transfer to a regional center following initiation of fibrinolysis is appropriate to facilitate angiography and PCI (if feasible) for fibrinolytic failure (rescue) and for recurrent ischemia/infarction.

Of note, reinfarction following successful fibrinolysis usually occurs early during the index hospitalization, is often unpredictable and is associated with increased mortality in long-term follow-up [81,82]. Successful coronary revascularization with PCI following fibrinolytic therapy during the index hospitalization is associated with a lower risk of recurrent myocardial infarction and mortality regardless of patient Thrombolysis In Myocardial Infarction (TIMI) risk stratification [81–83]. (Figure 4A,B). Surgical coronary revascularization appears to be associated with a similar degree of benefit for patients in both intermediate- and high-TIMI risk score strata. (Figure 5A,B) Clearly, definitive revascularization plays an integral role both as primary therapy for STEMI or following initial therapy with fibrinolysis [81–84]. Therefore, strategies for direct, immediate, or at least early transport

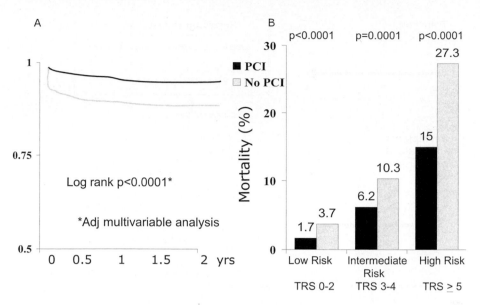

**Figure 4** (**A**) Kaplan Meier curves for mortality over time in patients either treated with percutaneous coronary intervention (PCI) or not (no PCI) during their index hospitalization following thrombolytic therapy for acute myocardial infarction. (**B**) Mortality during follow-up by thrombolysis in myocardial infarction (TIMI) risk score (TRS) strata for patients treated with PCI vs. no PCI following thrombolytic therapy for acute myocardial infarction. (From Ref. 81)

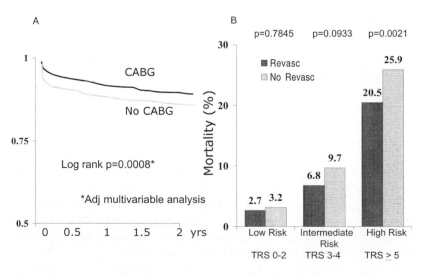

**Figure 5** (**A**) Kaplan Meier curves for mortality over time in patients treated with coronary artery bypass graft surgery (CABG) or not (no CABG) during their index hospitalization following thrombolytic therapy for acute myocardial infarction. (**B**) Mortality by thrombolysis in myocardial infarction (TIMI) risk score (TRS) strata for patients treated with CABG or no CABG following thrombolytic therapy for acute myocardial infarction. (From Ref. 81)

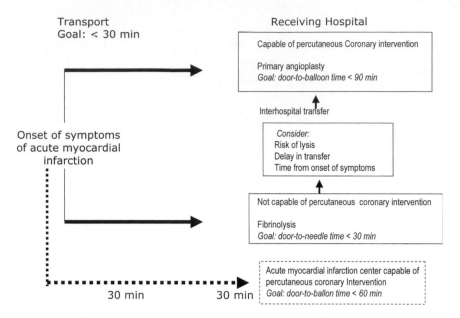

**Figure 6**  Suggested triage of patients with myocardial infarction and ST-segment elevation. (From Ref. 14)

of patients with STEMI to regional centers for interventional care would appear to assure optimal clinical outcomes (Figure 6). As recently suggested, "now is the time to discard the practice of transporting patients with acute myocardial infarction to the nearest hospital and to transport preferentially to centers of excellence for primary percutaneous coronary intervention" [14]. Such "regional centers of excellence" should be equipped with high quality digital radiographic imaging, hemodynamic monitoring systems, and a broad inventory of PCI supplies [12,13]. Intra-aortic balloon pump counterpulsation (IABP) devices and staff adequately trained to operate them are mandatory. Indeed, among STEMI patients with cardiogenic shock who have IABP placement, mortality has been inversely correlated with the number of IABP procedures performed at the facility where treatment is being provided [85]. Mortality is lowest at those institutions where IABP use is most frequent. Regional centers should have access to new technologies designed to limit myocardial injury and enhance functional recovery including adjunctive pharmacotherapies [86,87], as well as devices for distal embolic protection and/or thrombus removal [88]. Ideally, innovative therapies such as hypothermia to limit infarct size would be investigated [89,90]. These "state-of-the-art" technologies are not likely to be employed by low-volume operators at small community hospitals. Furthermore, regional centers must implement "the continuous cycle of quality" for evidence-based quality improvement [28]. Accurate, audited performance and acuity measures must be tracked. Such efforts will enhance and integrate care for patients with STEMI and is consistent with the model for care, which currently exists in the regional emergency system for trauma.

## NON–ST-SEGMENT ELEVATION ACUTE CORONARY SYNDROME

The prognosis for patients with NSTACS is guarded, even following treatment with aspirin, unfractionated heparin, nitrates, and beta-blockers. Despite these therapies, patients with

NSTACS are still at appreciable risk for death (approximately 6%), recurrent myocardial infarction (approximately 11%), or need for coronary revascularization (PCI approximately 30%, surgery approximately 27%) for up to one year after initial presentation [91–95]. In the era before coronary stenting and advances in adjunctive pharmacotherapy, guidelines for the treatment of NSTACS promoted ''conservatism'' to avoid the ''hazard'' of early coronary revascularization [96]. Both early randomized clinical trials [91,97] and retro-spective clinical series [98], which compared a routine ''invasive'' approach using early angiography to routine medical stabilization with revascularization performed only for spontaneous or provoked (stress test) ischemia (''conservative'' therapy), suggested that early PCI (within 1 week of presentation) was associated with a high incidence of proce-dural failure and major adverse cardiovascular events. However, advances in catheter-based technology, adjunctive pharmacology and the ability to accurately assign relative risk to patients who present with NSTACS have prompted multiple revisions in guideline recommendations [7,8] and a rapid evolution in treatment strategies. For example, both coronary stenting [99] and adjunctive platelet GPIIb/IIIa blockade [100] therapy have significantly improved outcomes (reduced the incidence of death, recurrent myocardial infarction/ischemia, or the requirement for urgent repeat revascularization) in patients with NSTACS. Adjunctive therapy with GPIIb/IIIa inhibition improves outcomes in patients who subsequently undergo coronary revascularization (both PCI and surgical) [101,102], particularly those patients who have an elevated serum troponin level [103]. Indeed, the relative benefit for both GPIIb/IIIa inhibitor therapy (vs. placebo) [104] or a routine early invasive/revascularization treatment strategy (vs. routine medical therapy only) is greatest for those patients in the highest risk strata [105]. Patients who present with an elevated serum troponin or TIMI risk score 3 or higher manifest greater improvement in clini-cal outcomes following early coronary revascularization [106] (Figure 7, Figure 8). In addition, the presence, magnitude, and cumulative ''burden'' (number of electrocardio-graphic (ECG) leads with ST-segment change) of ST-segment depression predict benefit from an early invasive treatment strategy [107]. More recently, levels of pro-inflammatory cytokines (IL-6)(108) and markers of inflammation (sCD 40L) [109] have been directly

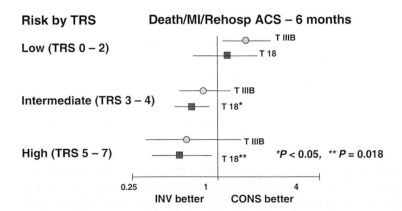

**Figure 7** Analysis of the Thrombolysis in Myocardial Infarction (TIMI) IIIB and the TACTICS 18 (Treat Angina with Aggrastat and Determine Cost of Therapy with an Invasive or Conserv-ative Strategy 18) trials with comparison of invasive (INV) treatment strategy vs. conservative (CONS) treatment strategy with respect to the occurrence of death, myocardial infarction (MI), or rehospitalization for acute coronary syndromes (rehosp ACS) to 6 months following enrollment by TIMI risk score (TRS) strata. (From Ref. 105)

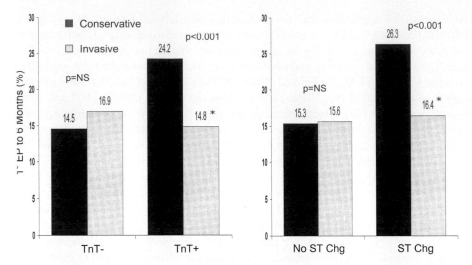

**Figure 8**   Predictive value of troponin (TNT) status and electrocardiographic ST-segment change (chg) on the primary endpoint (composite occurrence of death, myocardial infarction or requirement for rehospitalization for acute coronary syndromes) to 6 months following enrollment with either an invasive or conservative treatment strategy in the Treat Angina with Aggrastat and determine Cost of Therapy with an Invasive or Conservation Strategy—Thrombolysis in Myocardial Infarction 18 (TACTICS-TIMI 18) trial. Both positive troponin status and the presence of electrocardiographic ST segment change predicted the benefit of an invasive (vs. conservative) treatment strategy. (From Ref. 106)

correlated with subsequent mortality, as well as the magnitude of clinical benefit derived from adjunctive abciximab platelet GPIIb/IIIa inhibition (sCD 40L) or an invasive treatment strategy (IL-6). Similarly, the relative benefit (reduction in death, myocardial infarction, recurrent ischemia, or revascularization) attributable to the low-molecular-weight heparin enoxaparin (vs. unfractionated heparin) is most evident in those patients at highest risk as reflected by either TIMI risk score [110] or elevation in serum troponin [111]. Thus, the ability to accurately assign risk facilitates the appropriate triage of patients to an interventional center. Indeed, the "weight" of clinical trial data strongly supports the performance of early coronary angiography with revascularization, as indicated, and feasible for selected patients who present with NSTACS [112] (Figure 9).

Current guideline recommendations for early ($<$ 48 hours) coronary angiography in patients with NSTACS include those patients who have high-risk indicators [8]. Remarkably, recent reports from ongoing registries of ACS care show that early angiography ($<$ 48 hours) is being performed in less than half of NSTACS patients who present with an elevated serum troponin. Furthermore, the percentage of patients undergoing catheterization in-hospital does not appear to be influenced by either the presence or magnitude of serum troponin elevation (Figure 10A,B). Data have recently become available demonstrating that hospital adherence to ACC/AHA guideline recommended therapies and early ($<$ 48 hours) catheterization in high-risk patients is inversely correlated with in-hospital mortality [114,115]. Thus, a performance measure (hospital composite guideline adherence quartile) directly relates the process of care to mortality (Figure 11). Hospitals with the highest degree of guideline compliance ($>$ 80%) have a significantly lower in-hospital mortality for ACS when compared with hospitals in lower quartiles for guideline adherence.

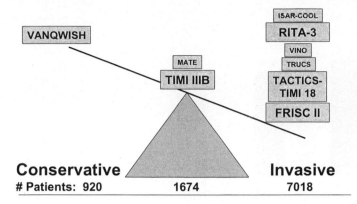

Conservative　　　　　　　　　　　　Invasive
# Patients: 920　　　　　1674　　　　　7018

**Figure 9** The cumulative weight of evidence from multiple randomized trials favors the invasive (vs. conservative) treatment strategy for unstable angina, non–ST-segment myocardial infarction (UA-NSTEMI). VANQWISH, Veterans Affair Non–Q-Wave Infarction Strategies in Hospital study; MATE, Medicine vs. Angioplasty for Thrombolytic Exclusions; TIMI IIIB, Thrombolysis in Myocardial Infarction IIIB; ISAR-COOL, Intracoronary Stenting With Antithrombotic Regimen Cooling-Off Trial; RITA-3, 3rd Randomized Interventional Treatment of Angina trial; VINO, Value of Intermediate angioplasty in Non–Q-wave infarction-Open randomized trial; TRUCS, Treatment of Refractory Unstable angina in geographically isolated areas without Cardiac Surgery. Invasive versus conservative strategy; TACTICS-TIMI 18, Treat Angina with Aggrastat and determine Cost of Therapy with an Invasive or Conservation Strategy—Thrombolysis in Myocardial Infarction 18; FRISC II, Fragmin and/or early Revascularization during InStability in Coronary artery disease. (From Ref. 106)

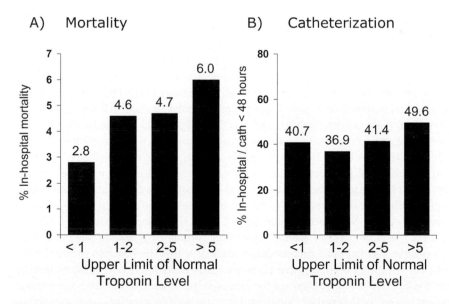

A)　Mortality　　　　　　　B)　Catheterization

**Figure 10** (A) In-hospital mortality by troponin level for patients with non–ST-segment elevation acute coronary syndrome enrolled into the **C**an **R**apid Risk Stratification of **U**nstable Angina Patients **S**uppress **AD**verse Outcomes with **E**arly Implementation of the ACC/AHA Guidelines (CRUSADE) registry. (B) The percentage of patients having cardiac catheterization during their index hospitalization by troponin level in the CRUSADE registry. (Adapted by Roe et al. Arch Int Med, in press).

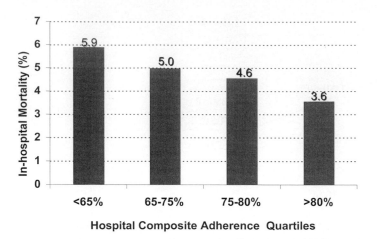

**Figure 11**   Relationship between process of care (hospital composite adherence to ACC/AHA recommended acute therapies and early catheterization) and mortality. (From Ref. 35)

Adjunctive therapy with clopidogrel has demonstrated early ($\leq$ 24 hours) benefit for reduction in death, myocardial infarction, stroke, or severe ischemia in patients presenting with NSTACS [116,117]. The clinical benefit provided by clopidogrel is not proportional to risk as reflected by the patient's TIMI risk score, but is symmetric across low-, intermediate- and high-risk patient cohorts [118]. Although early initiation of oral clopidogrel, particularly with a loading dose ($\geq$ 300 mg) improves outcomes for patients with NSTACS [119], it has been associated with an increased transfusion requirement and reoperation for bleeding in patients who, subsequently, require surgical coronary revascularization [120]. Coronary bypass surgery during the initial hospitalization for NSTACS may be required in 20% or more of patients and may be predictable based on clinical variables [121]. A multivariable analysis of the Treat Angina with Aggrastat® and Determine Cost of Therapy with Invasive or Conservative Strategy (TACTICS) TIMI-18 trial identified 8 variables (positive troponin, peripheral vascular disease, ST-segment deviation, prior angina, male gender, diabetes mellitus, hyperlipidemia, and prior aspirin therapy) as being independently associated with surgical coronary revascularization during the index hospitalization (Table 2). Using a simple scoring system to describe risk (1 point assigned to each variable if present, except troponin = 3 points), 41% of those patients with a cumulative score greater than 6 had surgical coronary revascularization during their index hospitalization [121]. When this same scoring system was applied retrospectively to the Thrombolysis In Myocardial Infarction (TIMI) 3B trial patient cohort, 37% of patients with a risk score greater than 6 points had coronary bypass surgery. Although further prospective validation of this model is needed, it may be possible to predict the relative risk for requirement of surgical coronary revascularization and, thus, to modify clopidogrel therapy accordingly. Concern for excessive perioperative bleeding has prompted recommendations for deferral of clopidogrel therapy until the time of coronary angiography, definition of coronary anatomy, and triage of the patient to either medical therapy or PCI (nonsurgical) coronary revascularization [116,122]. These recommendations place the pivotal triage point for initiation of clopidogrel therapy at the time of coronary angiography and, thus, emphasize the role of even earlier (< 24 hours) cardiac catheterization, particularly in higher risk patient subsets.

**Table 2** Eight variables independently associated with CABG—TACTICS TIMI 18

| Variable | Odds Ratio | 95% Confidence Interval | p value | Risk Score |
|---|---|---|---|---|
| (+) Troponin | 4.3 | 2.9–6.3 | < 0.0001 | 3 |
| Hx PVD | 2.0 | 1.2–3.4 | 0.009 | 1 |
| Standard deviation | 1.8 | 1.3–2.4 | < 0.0001 | 1 |
| Prior angina | 1.7 | 1.1–2.5 | 0.012 | 1 |
| Male gender | 1.6 | 1.2–2.2 | 0.002 | 1 |
| Diabetes | 1.5 | 1.1–2.0 | 0.011 | 1 |
| Prior aspirin | 1.4 | 1.1–1.9 | 0.026 | 1 |
| Hyperlipidemia | 1.4 | 1.1–1.9 | 0.017 | 1 |

Adapted from Ref. 121

## RECOMMENDATIONS

Several strategies have been proposed to make emergent angiography and PCI more readily available to patients who present with STEMI. One strategy has been to implement PCI reperfusion programs in community hospitals without provision for elective PCI procedures or cardiac surgical backup. The proliferation of low-volume PCI programs has been deemed "terribly unwise, impractical and expensive" [16] and will no doubt progressively tax severely limited resource pools of specially trained nurses and physicians. Furthermore, when annual primary PCI volumes are 36/year or less, outcomes are worse than following fibrinolysis [66]. In addition, the assimilation of new adjunctive therapies into practice will be less efficient and tracking compliance will be more complex in multiple small-volume programs than in regional high-volume centers.

Another strategy for which considerable rationale and support exists, is to develop regionalized centers of excellence for care in a manner similar to that which has been developed for trauma [12–16]. The focus of this strategy would be rapid diagnosis and risk stratification, implementation of protocol driven algorithms for guideline adherent care followed by efficient transport of appropriate patients to a regional care center. In patients who present with NSTACS and high-risk predictors (TIMI risk score ≥ 3; positive troponin; elevated myeloperoxidase 123 /inflammatory [IL-6 [108], sCD40L [109], NT-pro BNP [124], B-type Natriuretic Protein (BNP) [125], hsCRP [125]] markers) immediate or early (< 24 hours) transport to a regional center for coronary angiography and revascularization is recommended. Based on initial risk stratification, guideline adherent medical therapy should be implemented prior to transfer. Recent data suggest that our current system of nonregionalized care is suboptimal in dispensing guideline adherent care event to high-risk NSTACS patients [113]. For example, only 33.8 percent and 43 percent of patients with elevated serum troponin levels in the CRUSADE registry received early (< 24 hours) GPIIb/IIIa inhibitor therapy or early (< 48 hours) cardiac catheterization, respectively [113]. In patients with STEMI, emergent transfer to a tertiary care facility has been demonstrated to be safe and well tolerated with total transport time delays of < 2 hours. Despite the time delays incurred by transport, improved clinical outcomes have been observed following primary PCI compared with on-site (community hospital) fibrinolysis [45,46]. It should be noted, however, that the vast majority of patients who underwent primary PCI in these randomized trials, which compare transport for PCI versus on-site lysis, had their procedures at established tertiary PCI centers. It cannot be assumed that primary PCI in low volume centers, by low volume operators, will achieve the degree of benefit favoring PCI (vs. fibrinolysis) demonstrated in these comparative trials. In addition, emergency surgical revascularization, which may complicate 2% of primary PCI cases, will likely be more efficiently and safely implemented at a tertiary regional center. For NSTACS patients, early coronary angiography facilitates appropriate patient triage and definitive revascularization with safely expedited hospital discharge. Finally, in rural hospitals with prolonged (> 2 hours) transport times to tertiary regional centers, fibrinolytic monotherapy or combination reduced dose fibrinolytic plus abciximab therapy [127,128] in patients less than 75 years of age, should be initiated with implementation of transfer for failure to reperfuse and/or reocclusion recurrent ischemia. This specific benefit of facilitated PCI remains to be defined and is the subject of ongoing investigation [129,130].

## REFERENCES

1. Rioufol G, Finet G, Ginon I, Andre-Fouet X, Rossi R, Vialle E, Desjoyaux E, Convert G, Huret JF, Tabib A. Multiple atherosclerotic plaque rupture in acute coronary syndrome: a three-vessel intravascular ultrasound study. Circulation 2002;106:804–808.
2. Buffon A, Biasucci LM, Liuzzo G, D'Onofrio G, Crea F, Maseri A. Widespread coronary inflammation in unstable angina. N Engl J Med 2002;347:5–12.
3. Moreno PR, Falk E, Palacios IF, Newell JB, Fuster V, Fallon JT. Macrophage infiltration in acute coronary syndromes. Implications for plaque rupture. Circulation 1994;90:775–778.
4. Fuster V, Badimon L, Badimon JJ, Chesebro JH. The pathogenesis of coronary artery disease and the acute coronary syndromes. N Engl J Med 1992;326:242–250.
5. Waller BF, Gorfinkel HJ, Rogers FJ, Kent FM, Roberts WC. Early and late morphologic changes in major epicardial coronary arteries after percutaneous transluminal coronary angioplasty. Am J Cardiol 1984;53:42C–47C.
6. Waller BF, Pinkerton CA, Orr CM, Slack JD, VanTassel JW, Peters JW. Morphological observations late (greater than 30 days) after clinically successful coronary balloon angioplasty. Circulation 1991;83:128–141.
7. Braunwald E, Antman EM, Beasley JW, Califf RM, Cheitlin MD, Hochman JS, Jones RH, Kereiakes D, Kupersmith J, Levin TN, Pepine CJ, Schaeffer JW, Smith EE, Steward DE, Theroux P, Alpert JS, Eagle KA, Faxon DP, Fuster V, Gardner TJ, Gregoratos G, Russell RO, Smith SC. ACC/AHA guidelines for the management of patients with unstable angina and non–ST-segment elevation myocardial infarction. A report of the American College of Cardiology/American Heart Association Task Force on Practice Guidelines (Committee on the Management of Patients with Unstable Angina). J Am Coll Cardiol 2000;36:970–1062.
8. Braunwald E, Antman EM, Beasley JW, Califf RM, Cheitlin MD, Hochman JS, Jones RH, Kereiakes D, Kupersmith J, Levin TN, Pepine CJ, Schaeffer JW, Smith EE, Steward DE, Theroux P, Gibbons RJ, Alpert JS, Faxon DP, Fuster V, Gregoratos G, Hiratzka LF, Jacobs AK, Smith SC. American College of Cardiology/American Heart Association Task Force on Practice Guidelines (Committee on the Management of Patients With Unstable Angina). ACC/AHA guideline update for the management of patients with unstable angina and non–ST-segment elevation myocardial infarction-2002: summary article: a report of the American College of Cardiology/American Heart Association Task Force on Practice Guidelines (Committee on the Management of Patients With Unstable Angina). Circulation 2002; 106:1893–1900.
9. Anderson RN. Deaths: leading causes for 1999. National Vital Statistics Report. Vol. 49. Hyattsville. MD: National Center for Health Statistics, October 12, 2001.
10. Mullins RJ, Mann NC. Population-based research assessing the effectiveness of trauma systems. J Trauma 1999;47:S59–S66.
11. Nathens A, Jurkovich GJ, Rivar FP, Maier RV. Effectiveness of state trauma systems in reducing injury-related mortality: a national evaluation. J Trauma 2000;48:25–30.
12. Topol EJ, Kereiakes DK. Regionalization of care for acute ischemic heart disease: a call for specialized centers. Circulation 2003;107:1463–1466.

13. Califf RM, Faxon DP. Need for centers to care for patients with acute coronary syndromes. Circulation 2003;107:1467–1470.

14. Jacobs AK. Primary angioplasty for acute myocardial infarction—is it worth the wait? N Engl J Med 2003;349:798–800.

15. Willerson JT. Centers of Excellence. Circulation 2003;107:1471–1472.

16. Weaver WD. All hospitals are not equal for treatment of patients with acute myocardial infarction. Circulation 2003;108:1768–1771.

17. Eagle K, Goldman S, Avezum I, Budaj A, Sullivan CM, pez-Send n JL. and for the GRACE Investigators. Practice variation and missed opportunities for reperfusion in ST-segment elevation myocardial infarction: findings from the Global Registry of Acute Coronary Events (GRACE). Lancet 2002;359:373–377.

18. Deleted in proof.

19. Weaver WD, Simes RJ, Betriu A, Grines CL, Zijlstra F, Garcia E, Grinfeld L, Gibbons RJ, Ribeiro E, DeWood MA, Ribichini F. Comparison of primary coronary angioplasty and intravenous thrombolytic therapy for acute myocardial infarction. J Am Coll Cardiol 1997; 278:2093–2098.

20. Keeley EC, Boura JA, Grines CL. Primary angioplasty versus intravenous thrombolytic therapy for acute myocardial infarction: a quantitative review of 23 randomised trials. Lancet 2003;361:13–20.

21. Cannon CP. Primary percutaneous coronary intervention for all? J Am Med Assn 2002;287: 1987–1989.

22. Dzavik V, Rouleau J-L. Should all patients with an acute myocardial infarction present to a hospital with revascularization capabilities? J Am Coll Cardiol 2002;40:1041–1043.

23. Cannon CP, Baim DS. Expanding the reach of primary percutaneous coronary intervention for the treatment of acute myocardial infarction. J Am Coll Cardiol 2002;39:1720–1722.

24. McKay RG. Evolving strategies in the treatment of acute myocardial infarction in the community hospital setting. J Am Coll Cardiol 2003;42:642–645.

25. Fye WB. Cardiology workforce: there's already a shortage, and it's getting worse! J Am Coll Cardiol 2002;39:2077–2079.

26. Cooper RA. There's a shortage of specialists: is anyone listening? Acad Med 2002;77: 761–766.

27. Fye WB. Cardiology's workforce shortage: implication for patient care and research. Circulation 2004;109:813–816.

28. Califf RM, Peterson E, Gibbons RM, Brindis RG, Beller GA, Smith SC. American College of Cardiology; American Heart Association. Integrating quality into the cycle of therapeutic development. J Am Coll Cardiol 2002;40:1895–1901.

29. American Heart Association. Get With the Guidelines. Available at: http://www.americanheart.org/presenter.jhtml?identifier=1165 Accessed November 2003.

30. Fonarow GC, Gawlinski A, Moughrabi S, Tillisch JH. Improved treatment of coronary heart disease by implementation of a cardiac hospitalization atherosclerosis management program (CHAMP). Am J Cardiol 2001;87:819–822.

31. American College of Cardiology. Guidelines applied in practice. Available at http://www.acc.org/gap/gap.hun Accessed November 2003.

32. National registry of myocardial infarction. Home page. Available at: http://www.nrmi.org/index.html Accessed on November 2003.

33. Millenium Pharmaceuticals, Inc. CRUSADE Index. Available at http://www.millenium.com/clinicians/cardiovascular/crusade/index.asp Accessed November 2003.

34. Greenfield S, Kaplan SH, Kahn R, Ninomiya J, Griffith JL. Profiling care provided by different groups of physicians: effects of patient case-mix (bias) and physician-level clustering on quality assessment results. Ann Intern Med 2002;136:111 121.

35. Peterson ED, Roe MT, Li Y, Harrington RA, Brindis RG, Smith S, Gibler WB, Ohman EM. Influence of physician speciality on care and outcomes of acute coronary syndrome patients: results from CRUSADE. J Am Coll Cardiol 2003;41:534A (abstract).

36. Kim DH, Hunt SA. Heart failure management: caregiver versus care plan. Circulation 2003; 108:129–131.

37. Jong P, Gong Y, Liu PP, Austin PC, Lee DS, Tu JV. Care and outcomes of patients newly hospitalized for heart failure in the community treated by cardiologists compared with other specialists. Circulation 2003;108:184–191.

38. Allison JJ, Kiefe CI, Weissman NW, Person SD, Rousculp M, Canto JG, Bae S, Williams OD, Farmer R, Centor RM. Relationship of hospital teaching status with quality of care and mortality for medicare patients with acute MI. J Am Med Assn 2000;284:1256–1262.

39. Ayanian JZ, Weissman JS. Teaching hospitals and quality of care: a review of the literature. The Milbank Quarterly 2002;80:569–592.

40. Grines CL, Westerhausen DR, Grines LL, Hanlon JT, Logemann TL, Niemela M, Weaver WD, Graham M, Boura J, O'Neill WW, Balestrini C. for the Air PAMI Study Group. A randomized trial of transfer for primary angioplasty versus on-site thrombolysis in patients with high-risk myocardial infarction. The Air Primary Angioplasty in Infarction Study. J Am Coll Cardiol 2002;39:1713–1719.

41. Widimsky P, Groch L, Zelizko M, Aschermann M, Bednar F, Suryapranata H. Multicentre randomized trial comparing transport to primary angioplasty vs immediate thrombolysis vs combined strategy for patients with acute myocardial infarction presenting to a community hospital without a catheterization laboratory. The PRAGUE study. Eur Heart J 2000;21: 823–831.

42. Widimsky P, Budesinsky T, Vorac D, Groch L, Zelizko M, Aschermann M, Branny M, Staaasek J, Formanek P. on behalf of the PRAGUE study group investigators. Long distance transport for primary angioplasty vs. immediate thrombolysis in acute myocardial infarction. Eur Heart J 2003;24:94–104.

43. Andersen HR, Nielsen TT, Rasmussen K, Thuesen L, Kelbaek H, Thayssen P, Abildgaard U, Pedersen F, Madsen JK, Grande P, Villadsen ABCIXIMAB, Krusell LR, Haghfelt T, Lomholt P, Husted SE, Vigholt E, Kjaergard HK, Mortensen LS. for the DANAMI-2 investigators. A comparison of coronary angioplasty with fibrinolytic therapy in acute myocardial infarction. N Engl J Med 2003;349:733–742.

44. Vermeer F, Oude Ophuis AJM, Berg EJ, Brunninkuis LG, Wertner CJ, Goehmer AG, Lousberg AH, Dassen WR, Bar FW. Prospective randomized comparison between thrombolysis, rescue PTCA, and primary PTCA in patients with extensive myocardial infarction admitted to a hospital without PTCA facilities; a safety and feasibility study. Heart 1999;82:426–431.

45. Zijlstra F. Angioplasty vs. thrombolysis for acute myocardial infarction: a quantitative overview of the effects of interhospital transportation. Eur Heart J 2003;24:21–23.

46. Dalby M, Bouzamondo A, Lechat P, Montalescrot G. Transfer for primary angioplasty versus immediate thrombolysis in acute myocardial infarction—a meta-analysis. Circulation 2003; 108:1809–1814.

47. Thiemann DR, Coresh J, Oetgen WJ, Powe NR. The association between hospital volume and survival after acute myocardial infarction in elderly patients. New Engl J Med 1999;340: 1640–1648.

48. Magid DJ, Calonge BN, Rumsfeld JS, Cnto JG, Frederick PD, Every NR, Barron HV. for the National Registry of Myocardial infarction 2 and 3 investigators. Relation between hospital primary angioplasty volume and mortality for patients with acute MI treated with primary angioplasty vs. thrombolytic therapy. J Am Med Assn 2000;284:3131–3138.

49. Jollis JG, Romano PS. Volume-outcome relationship in acute myocardial infarction. J Am Med Assn 2000;284:3169–3171.

50. McGrath PD, Wennberg DE, Dickens JD, Siewers AE, Lucas FL, Malenka DJ, Kellett MA, Ryan TJ. Relation between operator and hospital volume and outcomes following percutaneous coronary interventions in the era of the coronary stent. J Am Med Assn 2000;284: 3139–3144.

51. Jollis JG, Peterson ED, DeLong ER, Mark DB, Collins SR, Muhlbaier LH, Pryor DB. The relation between the volume of coronary angioplasty procedures at hospitals treating Medicare beneficiaries and short-term mortality. N Engl J Med 1994;331:1625–1629.

52. Kimmel SE, Sauer WH, Brensinger C, Hirshfeld J, Haber HL, Localio AR. Relationship between coronary angioplasty laboratory volume and outcomes after hospital discharge. Am Heart J 2002;143:833–840.

53. Vaughan-Sarrazin MS, Hannan EL, Gormley CJ, Rosenthal GE. Mortality in medicare beneficiaries following coronary artery bypass graft surgery in states with and without certificate of need regulation. J Am Med Assn 2002;288:1859–1866.

54. Vakili BA, Brown DL. Relationship of total annual coronary angioplasty volume of physicians and hospitals on outcomes of primary angioplasty for acute myocardial infarciton (data from the 1995 Coronary Angiplasty Reporting system of the New York State Department of Health). Am J Cardiol 2003;91:726–728.

55. Nallamothu BK, Bates RK. Percutaneous coronary intervention versus fibrinolytic therapy in acute myocardial infarction: is timing (almost) everything? Am J Cardiol 2003;92:824–826.

56. Zijlstra F, Patel A, Jones M, Grines CL, Ellis S, Garcia E, Grinfeld L, Gibbons RJ, Ribeiro EE, Ribichini F, Granger C, Akhras F, Weaver WD, Simes RJ. for the PCAT collaboration. Clinical characteristics and outcome of patients with early (<2 h), intermediate (2–4 h), intermediate (2–4 h) and late (>4 h) presentation treated by primary coronary angioplasty or thrombolytic therapy for acute myocardial infarction. Eur Heart J 2002;23:550–557.

57. Brodie BR, Stone GW, Morice M-C, Cox DA, Garcia E, Mattos LA, Boura J, O'Neill WW, Stuckey TD, Milks S, Lansky AJ, Grines CL. for the Stent Primary Angioplasty in Myocardial Infarction Study Group. Am J Cardiol 2001;88:1085–1090.

58. Brodie BR, Stuckey TD, Muncy DB, Hansen CJ, Wall TC, Pulsipher M, Gupta N. Importance of time-to-reperfusion in patients with acute myocardial infarction with and without cardiogenic shock treated with primary percutaneous coronary intervention. Am Heart J 2003;145: 708–715.

59. Brodie BR, Cox DA, Stuckey TD, Turco M, Garcia E, Griffin JJ, Fahy M, Tcheng JE, Grines CL, Mehran R, Stone GW. How important is time to treatment with primary percutaneous coronary intervention for acute myocardial infarction? Results from the CADILLAC trial. J Am Coll Cardiol 2003;41:368A (abstract).

60. Santoro GM, Carrabba N, Barchielli A, Margheri M, Balzi D, Landini MC, Santoro G, Torri M, Lazzeri V, Buiatti E. Outcome of patients with acute myocardial infarction admitted to hospitals with and without facilities for primary percutaneous coronary intervention: data from the AMI-Florence registry. J Am Coll Cardiol 2003;41:358A (abstract).

61. De Luca G, Suryapranata H, van t' Hof AW, Hoormtje JC, de Boer M, Dambrink J, Zijlstra F. Relationship between time-to-reperfusionand 30-day mortality in patients with ST-segment elevation myocardial infarction treated with primary angioplasty. J Am Coll Cardiol 2003; 41:368A (abstract).

62. Singh M, Ting HH, Berger PB, Garratt KN, Holmes DR, Gersh BJ. Rationale for on-site cardiac surgery for primary angioplasty: a time for reappraisal. J Am Coll Cardiol 2002;39: 1881–1889.

63. Grines CL, Browne KF, Marco J, Rothbaum D, Stone GW, O'Keefe J, Overlie P, Donohue B, Chelliah N, Timmis GC, Vlietstra RE, Strzelecki M, Puchrowicz-Ochocki S, O'Neill WW. for the Primary Angioplasty in Myocardial Infarction Study Group. The primary angioplasty in myocardial infarction study group. A comparison of immediate angioplasty with thrombolytic therapy for acute myocardial infarction. N Engl J Med 1993;328:673–679.

64. Zijlstra F, de Boer MJ, Hoorntje JC, Reiffers S, Reiber JH, Suryapranata H. A comparison of immediate coronary angioplasty with intravenous streptokinase in acute myocardial infarction. N Engl J Med 1993;328:680–684.

65. Angeja BG, Gibson CM, Chin R, Frederick PD, Every NR, Ross AM, Stone GW, Barron HV. for the Participants in the National Registry of Myocardial Infarction 2–3. Predictors of door-to-balloon delay in primary angioplasty. Am J Cardiol 2002;89:1156–1161.

66. Cannon CP, Gibson CM, Lambrew CT, Shoultz DA, Levy D, French WJ, Gore JM, Weaver WD, Rogers WJ, Tiefenbrunn AJ. Relationship of symptom-onset-to-balloon time and door-to-balloon time with mortality in patients undergoing angioplasty for acute myocardial infarction. JAMA 2000;283:2941–2947.

67. Berger PB, Ellis SG, Holmes DR, Granger CB, Criger DA, Betriu A, Topol EJ, Califf RM. for the GUSTO-II Investigators. Relationship between delay in performing direct coronary angioplasty and early clinical outcome in patients with acute myocardial infarction: results

from the global use of strategies to open occluded arteries in acute coronary syndromes (GUSTO IIb) trial. Circulation 1999;100:14–20.

68. Serrano CV, Giraldez R, Nicolau JC, Venturinell M, Ramires JA, Zweier J. Differences between unstable angina and coronary angioplasty in platelet and leukocyte activation. J Am Coll Cardiol 2000;35:406A (abstract).

69. Cannon CP, Lambrew CT, Tiefenbrunn AJ, French WJ, Gore JM, Weaver D, Rogers WJ. for the NRMI-2 Investigators. Influence of door-to-balloon time on mortality in primary angioplasty results in 3,648 patients in the second national registry of myocardial infarction (NRMI-2). J Am Coll Cardiol 1996;27:61A (abstract).

70. Iannone LA, Anderson SM, Phillips SJ. Coronary angioplasty for acute myocardial infarction in a hospital without cardiac surgery. Tex Heart Inst J 1993;20:99–104.

71. Johnston JD, O'Neill WW, Slota P, Wharton TP, Turco MA, Stone GW, Brodie BR, Barsamian M, Graham M, Grines LL, Grines CL. Primary PTCA at community hospitals without surgical backup is performed as effectively and with less delay compared to tertiary care centers. Circulation 1998;98(Suppl I):I-770 (abstract).

72. Wharton TP, McNamara NS, Fedele FA, Jacobs MI, Gladstone AR, Funk EJ. Primary angioplasty for the treatment of acute myocardial infarction: experience at two community hospitals without cardiac surgery. J Am Coll Cardiol 1999;33:1257–1265.

73. Weaver WD, Litwin PE, Martin JS. the Myocardial Infarction Triage and Intervention Project Investigators. Use of direct angioplasty for treatment of patients with acute myocardial infarction in hospitals with and without on-site cardiac surgery. Circulation 1993;88:2067–2075.

74. Ting HH, Garratt KN, Tiede DJ. Percutaneous coronary intervention at two community hospitals without on-site cardiac surgical services supported with telemedicine. Circulation 2000;102(Suppl II):II735 (abstract).

75. Smyth DW, Richards AM, Elliott JM. Direct angioplasty for myocardial infarction: one-year experience in a center with surgical back-up 220 miles away. J Invasive Cardiol 1997;9: 324–332.

76. Brush JE, Thompson S, Ciuffo AA, Parker J, Stine RA, Mansfield CL, Hagerman P. Retrospective comparison of a strategy of primary coronary angioplasty versus intravenous thrombolytic therapy for acute myocardial infarction in a community hospital without surgical backup. J Invasive Cardiol 1996;8:91–98.

77. Ayres M. Coronary angioplasty for acute myocardial infarction in hospitals without cardiac surgery. J Invasive Cardiol 1995;7(Suppl F):40F–46F.

78. Aversano T, Aversano LT, Passamani E, Knatterud GL, Terrin ML, Williams DO, Forman SA. for the Atlantic Cardiovascular Patient Outcomes Research Team (C-PORT). Thrombolytic therapy vs. primary percutaneous coronary intervention for myocardial infarction in patients presenting to hospitals without on-site cardiac surgery: a randomized controlled trial. JAMA 2002;287:1943–1951.

79. Moscucci M, O'Donnell M, Share D, Maxwell-Eward A, Kline-Rogers E, De Franco AC, Meengs WL, Clark VL, McGinnity JG, De Gregorio M, Patel K, Eagle KA. Frequency and prognosis of emergency coronary artery bypass grafting after percutaneous coronary intervention for acute myocardial infarction. Am J Cardiol 2003;92:967–969.

80. Antman EM, Anbe DT, Armstrong PW, Bates ER, Green LA, Hand M, Hochman JS, Drumholz HM, Kushner FG, Lamas GA, Mullany CJ, Ornato JP, Pearle DL, Sloan MA, Smith SC. ACC/AHA guidelines for management of patients with ST-elevation myocardial infarction. Circulation. www.americanheart.org/downloadable/heart/1088697575586STEMIgood. pdf. Accessed online 07/06/04.

81. Gibson CM, Karha J, Murphy SA, James D, Morrow DA, Cannon CP, Giugliano RP, Antman EM, Braunwald E. for the TIMI study group. Early and long-term clinical outcomes associated with reinfarction following fibrinolytic administration in the thrombolysis in myocardial infarction trials. J Am Coll Cardiol 2003;42:7–16.

82. Dauerman HL. The early days after ST-segment elevation acute myocardial infarction: reconsidering the delayed invasive approach. J Am Coll Cardiol 2003;42:420–423.

83. Scheller B, Hennen B, Hammer B, Walle J, Hofer C, Hilpert V, Winter H, Nickenig G, Bohm M. for the SIAM III study group. Beneficial effects of immediate stenting after thrombolysis in acute myocardial infarction. J Am Coll Cardiol 2003;42:634–641.

84. Kernis SJ, Harjai KJ, Stone GW, Grines LL, Boura JA, Yerkey MW, O'Neill W, Grines CL. The incidence, predictors and outcomes of early reinfarction after primary angioplasty for acute myocardial infarction. J Am Coll Cardiol 2003;42:1173–1177.

85. Chen EW, Canto JG, Parsons LS, Peterson ED, Littrell KA, Every NR, Gibson CM, Hochman JS, Ohman M, Cheeks M, Barron HV. for the investigators in the National Registry of Myocardial Infarction (NRMI) 2. Relation between hospital intra-aortic balloon counterpulsation volume and mortality in acute myocardial infarction complicated by cardiogenic shock. Circulation 2003;108:951–957.

86. Tcheng JE, Kandzari DE, Grines CL, Cox DA, Effron M, Garcia E, Griffin JJ, Guagliumi G, Stuckey T, Turco M, Fahy M, Lansky AJ, Mehran R, Stone GW. for the CADILLAC investigators. Benefits and risks of abciximab use in primary angioplasty for acute myocardial infarction: the controlled abciximab and device investigation to lower late angioplasty complications (CADILLAC) trial. Circulation 2003;108:1316–1323.

87. Kandzari DE, Tcheng JE, Cohen DJ, Bakhai A, Grines CL, Cox DA, Effron M, Stuckey T, Griffin JJ, Turco M, Carroll JD, Fahy M, Mehran R, Stone GW. for the CADILLAC investigators. Feasibility and implications of an early discharge strategy after percutaneous intervention with abciximab in acute myocardial infarction (the CADILLAC trial). Am J Cardiol 2003; 92:779–784.

88. Limbruno U, Micheli A, De Carlo M, Amoroso G, Rossini R, Palagi C, Bello V, Petronio AS, Fontanini G, Mariani M. Mechanical prevention of distal embolization during primary angioplasty: safety, feasibility and impact of myocardial reperfusion. Circulation 2003;108: 171–176.

89. Herrmann HC. Optimizing outcomes in ST-segment elevation myocardial infarction. J Am Coll Cardiol 2003;42:1357–1359.

90. Dixon SR, Whitbourn RJ, Dae MW, Grube E, Sherman W, Schaer GL, Jenkins JS, Baim DS, Gibbons RJ, Kuntz RE, Popma JJ, Nguyen TT, O'Neill WW. Induction of mild systemic hypothermia with endovascular cooling during primary percutaneous coronary intervention for acute myocardial infarction. J Am Coll Cardiol 2002;40:1928–1934.

91. Boden WE, O'Rourke RA, Crawford MH, Blaustein AS, Deedwania PC, Zoble RG, Wexler LF, Kleiger RE, Pepine CJ, Ferry DR, Chow BK, Lavori PW. Outcomes in patients with acute non–Q-wave myocardial infarction randomly assigned to an invasive as compared with a conservative management strategy. Veterans Affairs Non–Q-Wave Infarction Strategies in Hospital (VANQWISH) Trial Investigators. N Engl J Med 1998;338:1785–1792.

92. Cohen M, Demers C, Garfinkel EP, Turpie AG, Fromell GJ, Goodman S, Langer A, Califf RM, Fox KA, Premmereur J, Bigonzi F. A Comparison of low-molecular weight heparin with unfractionated heparin for unstable coronary artery disease. N Engl J Med 1997;337: 447–452.

93. The Platelet Receptor Inhibition in Ischemic Syndrome Management in Patients Limited by Unstable Signs and Symptoms (PRISM-PLUS) Study Investigators. Inhibition of the platelet glycoprotein IIb/IIIa receptor with tirofiban in unstable angina and non–Q-wave myocardial infarction. N Engl J Med 1998;338:1488–1497.

94. The PURSUIT Trial investigators. Inhibition of platelet glycoprotein IIb/IIIa with eptifibatide in patients with acute coronary syndromes. N Engl J Med 1998;339:436–443.

95. The PARAGON investigators. International, randomized, controlled trial of lamfiban (a platelet glycoprotein IIb/IIIa inhibitor), heparin, or both in unstable angina. Circulation 1998;97: 2386–2395.

96. Braunwald E, Mark DB, Jones RH, Cheitlin MD, Fuster V, McCauley KM, Edwards C, Green LA, Mushlin AI, Swain JA, Smith EE, Cowan M, Rose GC, Concannon CA, Grines CL, Brown L, Lytle BW, Goldman L, Topol EJ, Willerson JT, Brown J, Archibald N. Unstable angina: diagnosis and management, Agency for health care policy and research and the National Heart, Lung and Blood Institute, Public Health Service. U.S. Department of Health and Human Services, Rockville, MD, National Center for Health Statistics, 1994.

97. Anderson HV, Cannon CP, Stone PH, Williams DO, McCabe CH, Knatterud GL, Thompson B, Willerson JT, Braunwald E. One-year results of the Thrombolysis in Myocardial Infarction

(TIMI) IIIB clinical trial. A randomized comparison of tissue-type plasminogen activator versus placebo and early invasive versus early conservative strategies in unstable angina and non–Q wave myocardial infarction. J Am Coll Cardiol 1995;26:1643–1650.

98. Myler RK, Shaw RE, Stertzer SH, Bashour TT, Ryan C, Hecht HS, Cumberland DC. Unstable angina and coronary angioplasty. Circulation 1990;82(3 Suppl):II88–95.

99. Singh M, Rihal CS, Berger PB, Bell MR, Grill DE, Garratt KN, Barseness GW, Holmes DR. Improving outcome over time of percutaneous coronary interventions in unstable angina. J Am Coll Cardiol 2000;36:674–678.

100. Chew DP, Moliterno DJ. A critical appraisal of platelet glycoprotein IIb/IIIa inhibition. J Am Coll Cardiol 2000;36:2028–2035.

101. Boersma E, Harrington RA, Moliterno DJ, White H, Theroux P, Van de Werf F, de Torbal A, Armstrong PW, Wallentin LC, Wilcox RG, Simes J, Califf RM, Topol EJ, Simoons ML. Platelet glycoprotein IIb/IIIa inhibitors in acute coronary syndromes: a meta-analysis of all major randomised clinical trials. Lancet 2002;359:189–198.

102. Roffi M, Moliterno DJ, Lauer MS, Reginelli J, Jia G, Topol EJ. Platelet glycoprotein IIb/IIIa antagonists are beneficial in patients with acute coronary syndromes who undergo in-hospital coronary artery bypass surgery. J Am Coll Cardiol 2003;41:351A (abstract).

103. Newby LK, Ohman EM, Christenson RH, Moliterno DJ, Harrington RA, White HD, Armstrong PW, Van de Werf F, Pfisterer M, Hasselblad V, Califf RM, Topol EJ. Circulation 2001;103:2891–2896.

104. Morrow DA, Sabatine MS, Cannon CP, Theroux P. Benefit of tirofiban among patients treated with coronary intervention: application of the TIMI risk score for unstable angina/non-ST. Circulation 2001;104:II–782 (abstract).

105. Sabatine MS, Morrow DA, Giugliano RP, Murphy SA, Demopoulos LA, Dibattiste PM, Weintraub WS, McCabe CH, Antman EM, Cannon CP, Braunwald E. Implicatons of upstream GP IIb/IIIa inhibition and stenting in the invasive management of UA/NSTEMI: a comparison of TIMI IIIb and TACTICS-TIMI 18. Circulation 2001;104:II549 (abstract).

106. Cannon C. Improving acute coronary syndrome care: the ACC/AHA guidelines and critical pathways. J Invasive Cardiol 2003;15:22B–27B.

107. Holmvang L, Clemmensen P, Lindahl B, Lagerqvist B, Venge P, Wagner G, Wallentin L, Grande P. Quantitative analysis of the admission electrocardiogram identifies patients with unstable coronary artery disease who benefit the most from early invasive treatment. J Am Coll Cardiol 2003;41:905–915.

108. Heeschen C, Dimmeler S, Hamm CW, Brand MJ, Boersma E, Zeiher AM, Simoons ML. CAPTURE Study Investigators. Soluble CD40 ligand in acute coronary syndromes. N Engl J Med. 2003;348:1104–1111.

109. Lindmark E, Diderholm E, Wallentin L, Siegbahn A. Relationship between interleukin 6 and mortality in patients with unstable coronary artery disease: effects of an early invasive or noninvasive strategy. JAMA 2001;286:2107–2113.

110. Antman EM, Cohen M, McCabe C, Goodman SG, Murphy SA, Braunwald E. TIMI 11B and ESSENCE Investigators. Enoxaparin is superior to unfractionated heparin for preventing clinical events at 1-year follow-up of TIMI 11B and ESSENCE. Eur Heart J 2002;23:308–314.

111. Bertrand ME, Simoons ML, Fox KA, Wallentin LC, Hamm CW, McFadden E, de Feyter PJ, Specchia G, Ruzyllo W. Management of acute coronary syndromes: acute coronary syndromes without persistent ST segment elevation; recommendations of the Task Force of the European Society of Cardiology. Eur Heart J 2000;21:1406–1432.

112. Cannon CP, Turpie AG. Unstable angina and non-ST-elevation myocardial infarction: initial antithrombotic therapy and early invasive strategy. Circulation 2003;107:2640–2645.

113. Roe MT, Peterson ED, Li Y, Harrington RA, Pollack CV, Brindis RG, Christenson RH, Smith SC, Gibler WB, Ohman M. Suboptimal adherence to the ACC/AHA non-ST elevation acute coronary syndrome practice guidelines for patients with positive troponin levels. J Am Coll Cardiol 2003;41:390A (abstract).

114. Roe MT, Parsons L, Pollack C, Canto JG, Barron HV, Every N, Rogers W, Peterson ED. Disparities in the treatment of acute myocardial infarction: underutilization of evidence-based

therapies for patients with non–ST-segment myocardial infarction. J Am Coll Cardiol 2003; 41:540A (abstract).

115. Roe MT, Peterson ED, Li Y, Pollack CV, Christenson RH, Peacock WF, Fesmire FM, Newby LK, Jesse RL, Hoekstra JW, Gibler WB, Ohman EM. for the CRUSADE investigators. Dissociation between risk stratification with cardiac troponin levels and adherence to the ACC/AHA guidelines for non-ST-elevation acute coronary syndromes. Arch Intern Med:In press.

116. Berger PB, Steinhubl S. Clinical implications of percutaneous coronary intervention-clopido-grel in unstable angina to prevent recurrent events (PCI-CURE) study: a US perspective. Circulation 2002;106:2284–2287.

117. Yusuf S, Mehta SR, Zhao F, Gersh BJ, Commerford PJ, Blumenthal M, Budaj A, Wittlinger T, Fox KA. Clopidogrel in Unstable angina to prevent Recurrent Events Trial Investigators. Early and late effects of clopidogrel in patients with acute coronary syndromes. Circulation 2003;107:966–972.

118. Budaj A, Yusuf S, Mehta SR, Fox KA, Tognoni G, Zhao F, Chrolavicius S, Hunt D, Keltai M, Franzosi MG. Clopidogrel in Unstable angina to prevent Recurrent Events (CURE) Trial Investigators. Benefit of clopidogrel in patients with acute coronary syndromes without ST-segment elevation in various risk groups. Circulation 2002;106:1622–1626.

119. Yusuf S, Zhao F, Mehta SR, Chrolavicius S, Tognoni G, Fox KK. Clopidogrel in Unstable Angina to Prevent Recurrent Events Trial Investigators. Effects of clopidogrel in addition to aspirin in patients with acute coronary syndromes without ST-segment elevation. New Engl J Med 2001;345:494–502.

120. Hongo RH, Ley J, Dick SE, Yee RR. The effect of clopidogrel in combination with aspirin when given before coronary artery bypass grafting. J Am Coll Cardiol 2002;40:231–237.

121. Sadanandan S, Cannon CP, Gibson CM, Desai R, Murphy SA, DiBattiste PM, Braunwald E. for the TACTICS TIMI-18 investigators. A risk score for predicting coronary artery bypass surgery in patients with non-ST elevation acute coronary syndromes. J Am Coll Cardiol 2003;41:391A (abstract).

122. Tcheng JE, Campbell ME. Platelet inhibition strategies in percutaneous coronary intervention: competition or coopetition? J Am Coll Cardiol 2003;42:1196–1198.

123. Brennan ML, Penn MS, Van Lente F, Nambi V, Shishehbor MH, Aviles RJ, Goormastic M, Pepoy ML, McErlean ES, Topol EJ, Nissen SE, Hazen SL. Prognostic value of myeloperoxi-dase in patients with chest pain. New Engl J Med 2003;349:1595.

124. Jernberg T, Stridsberg M, Venge P, Lindahl B. N-terminal pro brain natriuretic peptide on admission for early risk stratification of patients with chest pain and no ST-segment elevation. J Am Coll Cardiol 2002;40:437–445.

125. James S, Armstrong PW, Califf RM, Venge P, Simoons M, Wallentin L. A combination of Pro-BNP Och troponin T at baseline provide the best prediction of risk of death and myocardial infarction early after acute coronary syndrome. J Am Coll Cardiol 2003;41:353A (abstract).

126. de Lemos JA, Morrow DA, Bentley JH, Omland T, Sabatine MS, McCabe CH, Hall C, Cannon CP, Braunwald E. The prognostic value of B-type natriuretic peptide in patients with acute coronary syndromes. N Engl J Med 2001;345:1014–1021.

127. de Werf F, Baim DS. Reperfusion for ST-segment elevation myocardial infarction – an overview of current treatment options. Circulation 2002;105:2813–2816.

128. Hermann HC, Moliterno DJ, Ohman EM, Stebbins AL, Bode C, Betriu A, Forycki F, Miklin JS, Bachinsky WB, Lincoff AM, Califf RM, Topol EJ. Facilitation of early percutaneous coronary intervention after reteplase with or without abciximab in acute myocardial infarction – Results from the SPEED (GUSTO-4 Pilot) Trial. J Am Coll Cardiol 2000;36:1489–1496.

129. Dauerman HL, Sobel BE. Synergistic treatment of ST-segment elevation myocardial infarc-tion with pharmacoinvasive recanalization. J Am Coll Cardiol 2003;42:646–651.

130. Choo JK, Young JJ, Kereiakes DJ. Facilitated percutaneous coronary intervention: pharmaco-logic and mechanical synergy in reperfusion for ST elevation myocardial infarction. Acute Coronary Syndromes 2003;5:107–115.

# 14

# The Role of Troponin in Risk Stratification

**L. Kristin Newby**
*Duke University Medical Center*
*Durham, North Carolina, U.S.A.*

## INTRODUCTION

The acute coronary syndromes (ACS) represent a pathological, diagnostic, and risk contin-uum from unstable angina through myocardial infarction (MI) with or without ST-segment elevation. The management strategies and outcomes of patients who present with symp-toms of acute coronary ischemia depend upon where they fall within this spectrum. The ability to accurately diagnose and risk-stratify this group of patients at presentation and to provide continuous risk evaluation thereafter is critical, not only for patient outcome but also for efficiency of care. As the health care environment has evolved, our focus has also evolved from traditional categorical diagnosis to baseline and long-term risk stratification, and to methods that allow continuous risk assessment. Unfortunately, as shown by Lee and colleagues in 1986, the ability of physicians to accurately risk-stratify patients based on clinical factors alone is limited and subject to wide variability among physicians [1]. Neither experience nor practice setting of the physician significantly affects predictions of outcome [2].

The past two decades have seen extensive investigations into the use of various cardiac markers in addition to clinical factors and the electrocardiogram (ECG) to establish diagnosis and prognosis in ACS. The evolution of cardiac marker testing, particularly troponin testing, beyond simply documentation of myocardial necrosis to use for risk stratification and to guide treatment decisions has been a major contribution to the manage-ment of patients with ACS. This chapter will examine this evolution in cardiac marker testing with a focus on the use of troponin for risk stratification.

## TROPONIN AND EVOLUTION IN THE DEFINITION OF MYOCARDIAL INFARCTION

### The Ideal Marker

To be useful for diagnosis in the clinical setting, a serum marker of myocardial necrosis should be rapidly released early after the onset of ischemic symptoms and remain elevated for 12 to 24 hours in the serum, but not so long as to preclude detection of recurrent myocardial injury after an index event. It should be released in proportion to the degree of myocardial injury and should be very specific for myocardial cell damage vs. skeletal muscle or other tissue damage (that is, found in cardiac muscle but not in other tissues). To have a very sensitive, rapid quantitative assay for the marker would be ideal, but semiquantitative or qualitative whole-blood bedside assays are particularly useful in emergency departments, where on-line decisions can facilitate rapid identification and triage of ACS patients. Finally, for use in short- and long-term risk stratification, there should be a correlation between outcome and the presence or absence of a marker in the serum or the degree of elevation of the marker above "normal."

## Troponin and Redefinition of Myocardial Infarction

At the foundation of the assessment of a patient who presents with symptoms of suspected ACS are the directed history and physical examination and the 12-lead ECG. Yet, in most patients these components alone are insufficient to classify patients along the spectrum of ACS. Thus, measurement of serum cardiac markers of myocardial necrosis is a fundamental component of the evaluation. Until recently, the cardiac-specific isoenzyme of creatine kinase (CK), CK-MB, was the "gold standard" for biomarker diagnosis of MI and served as one diagnostic component of the World Health Organization—Monitoring trends and determinants in Cardiovascular disease (WHO-MONICA) study criteria for MI [3]. However, from autopsy series and myocardial biopsies performed during bypass surgery, it has been demonstrated that CK-MB does not detect all myocardial necrosis in patients with ACS [4,5].

### Cardiac Troponin T

The troponins comprise a group of three proteins (C, I, and T), which interact with tropomyosin to form the troponin–tropomyosin complex. This complex is part of the regulatory and structural backbone of the contractile apparatus of striated muscle (Figure 1). Troponin T is the 33-kDa structural component of the troponin complex that binds it to tropomyosin. Troponin T exists in three isoforms, skeletal (slow- and fast-twitch) muscle, and cardiac muscle. During fetal development, the cardiac and skeletal forms are coexpressed in both skeletal and cardiac tissues. In the adult, the cardiac isoform is expressed only in cardiac muscle and the skeletal form only in skeletal muscle [6]. With available monoclonal antibody techniques, cardiac troponin T (cTnT) is not detectable in serum from normal volunteers. Although, there is evidence, in the stressed human heart and in animal models, that the skeletal muscle isoform may be re-expressed [7,8], the current assay for cTnT does not appear to react with this isoform [9].

The majority of troponin T in the myocyte exists bound in the troponin–tropomyosin complex, however, there is a small cytoplasmic pool of about 6% of the total. Cardiac

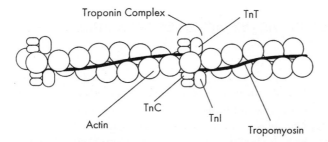

**Figure 1**   The troponin-tropomyosin complex. TnT, troponin T; TnC, troponin C ; TnI, troponin I.

troponin T is detectable in the serum above the reference range as early as 4 to 6 hours after onset of symptoms of ischemia, probably reflecting early release of the cytoplasmic pool, and remains elevated for 10 days to 2 weeks as a result of slower and sustained release of cTnT bound in the troponin-tropomyosin complex.

*Cardiac Troponin I*

Troponin I is a 23.5-kDa component of the troponin complex that inhibits the interaction of myosin and cross-bridges with the actin/tropomyosin complex and, thus, regulates striated muscle contraction. Like troponin T, troponin I exists in three isoforms, cardiac and skeletal (slow- and fast-twitch), that are specific to the given tissue. Also, similar to troponin T, troponin I exists predominantly bound within the troponin–tropomyosin complex, but it also has a small cytoplasmic pool of about 2.5% of the total. Unlike cTnT, the cardiac form of troponin I, cTnI, is never expressed in skeletal muscle, even during fetal development [6]. Cardiac troponin I is detectable in the serum slightly later than cTnT, about 6 hours after the onset of ischemia, and remains elevated for 7 to 10 days. Because of their long serum half-lives, neither cTnT nor cTnI is suitable for detection of reinfarction using currently available assays. However, because they do remain elevated for days, they may be able to reveal an MI that occurred in days past (when presentation of the patient to medical attention is delayed, for example), when other markers of MI have returned to normal.

*Redefinition of Myocardial Infarction*

The high sensitivity and specificity of assays for cardiac troponins T and I have led to the establishment of cardiac troponins and the new ''gold standard'' for the diagnosis of MI. This fundamental change is reflected in a 2000 consensus document from the European Society of Cardiology/American College of Cardiology (ESC/ACC) Joint Committee for the Redefinition of Myocardial Infarction, in which it is recommended that the definition of MI be changed to emphasize the use of cardiac troponins as the preferred marker of myocardial necrosis in the setting of ischemic symptoms [10]. The recommendations of this international committee of experts in clinical and laboratory medicine, pathology and epidemiology are summarized in Table 1.

*Other Markers of Myocardial Necrosis*

Although the cardiac troponins are now considered the ''gold standard'' for the definition of MI, other serum biomarkers may also be useful for diagnosis in patients presenting to

**Table 1**   Recommended Criteria for Myocardial Infarction Redefinition

Either one of:
1. Typical rise and gradual fall (troponin) or more rapid rise and fall (creatine kinase [CK]-MB) of biomarkers of myocardial necrosis with at least one of:
   A. ischemic symptoms
   B. development of pathologic q waves on 12-lead electrocardiogram
   C. ST-segment elevation or depression consistent with ischemia
   D. percutaneous coronary intervention
2. Pathological findings of acute myocardial infarction

Adapted from Ref. 10

the emergency room with ischemic symptoms. All markers are limited somewhat by their release and clearance kinetics in their ability to detect myocardial necrosis at a given time in a patient's clinical course. Figure 2 summarizes the time course of several commonly used markers of necrosis compared with troponins I and T.

The effect of these differing time courses of markers of myocardial necrosis on sensitivity for the diagnosis of MI over time was demonstrated in the Diagnostic Marker Cooperative Study and the Biochemical Markers of Acute Coronary Syndromes (BIOMACS) Study [11,12]. Because of these intrinsic characteristics of marker release and clearance and the inherent variability in timing of patient presentation after symptom onset, serial sampling of cardiac markers of necrosis at baseline, 6–9 hours and 12–24 hours, is recommended in the ESC/ACC document on redefinition of MI [10]. Support for these recommendations is provided by data from the Global Use of Strategies to Open Occluded Arteries in Acute Coronary Syndromes (GUSTO-IIa) troponin substudy, which showed incremental diagnostic yield and prognostic information by the addition of serial measures of troponin at 8 and 16 hours after baseline [13]. In this study, of 734 ACS patients, only 45% of cTnT-positive patients were identified by the baseline measure. Patients with positive baseline values had higher 30-day mortality (10%) compared with those who were identified as positive on later samples (5%), but among patients (n = 151) who remained negative on serial testing, mortality was 0% at 30 days.

As an alternative to serial sampling, the use of combinations of markers of myocardial necrosis with different release and clearance time courses has also been shown useful in both diagnosis and risk stratification among patients with suspected ACS. Newby and colleagues investigated the use of a multimarker strategy combining an early but non-specific necrosis marker (myoglobin) with later but more specific cardiac markers (cTnI and CK-MB) at the point of care in the Chest Pain Evaluation by CK-MB, Myoglobin, and Troponin I (CHECKMATE) study [14]. In this study of 1,005 chest-pain evaluation patients at 6 hospitals, not only did a multimarker strategy consisting of myoglobin, CK-MB, and cTnI measured simultaneously at the point of care, detect more marker-positive patients (18.9%) than single-marker testing in the hospital's local laboratory (5.2%), it did so approximately 1 hour earlier (2.5 hours vs. 3.4 hours, respectively). In this study, 228 patients had positive markers on serial testing with the multimarker strategy over

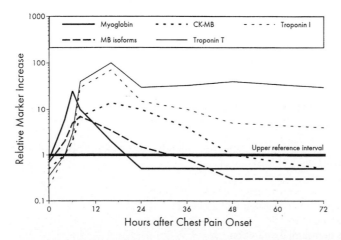

**Figure 2** Time course after symptom onset for various biochemical markers of myocardial necrosis. CK-MB = creatine kinase-MB isoenzyme.

9 12 hours. Of these, 137 were positive by only a single marker, and were negative by the other 2 markers. In addition, risk stratification for 30-day mortality using multimarker testing was superior to single-marker testing, and the multimarker testing result added independently to clinical characteristics and the ECG in multivariable modeling.

## ROLE OF TROPONIN IN ST-SEGMENT ELEVATION MYOCARDIAL INFARCTION

### Diagnosis and Prognosis in ST-segment Elevation Myocardial Infarction

When patients present with symptoms of acute myocardial ischemia and the ECG reveals ST-segment elevation, the diagnosis of acute MI is confirmed in over 90% of cases by serial CK-MB sampling [15,16]. The major decisions about acute treatment (thrombolytic therapy, direct angioplasty) and initial management (Cardiac Care Unit [CCU]-level care) in this group are made in response to the clinical and electrocardiographic diagnosis. Serum cardiac markers have largely played either a confirmatory role been used to document the extent of the infarct, or, in the case of thrombolytic therapy, assist in showing that reperfusion had occurred.

In the GUSTO-IIa troponin T substudy, Ohman and colleagues showed that a single cTnT measurement at baseline was able to risk-stratify patients presenting with acute coronary ischemia into those at high- or low-risk of in-hospital complications. Further, it added significant information, despite the presence of ST-segment elevation, in predicting short-term mortality in these patients [17]. Patients with ST-segment elevation who had cTnT more than 0.1 ng/mL had 13% mortality, compared with 4.7% in those with normal cTnT on admission. These findings have been confirmed by Stubbs and colleagues, who examined 240 patients with ST-segment elevation admitted to a general hospital [18]. Mortality was significantly higher (32% vs. 13% at 3 years) in patients with cTnT greater than 0.2 ng/mL.

The ability to risk-stratify patients with acute ST-segment elevation MI into high- and low-risk groups at admission could have important implications for both short- and long-term management decisions and for in-hospital resource use, length of stay, and costs. Lee and colleagues identified clinical characteristics at presentation that predicted mortality at 30 days in patients who underwent thrombolysis for ST-segment elevation MI [19]. Conversely, several other groups have described clinical features at day 3 or 4 that identify a low-risk population who could be discharged earlier after MI [20–22]. In the GUSTO-III troponin T substudy, Ohman and colleagues demonstrated in 12,666 patients with ST-segment elevation treated with either alteplase or reteplase, that a bedside whole-blood, qualitative cTnT result at presentation stratified risk for mortality and nonfatal postinfarction complications [23]. Patients who were cTnT-positive had significantly higher 30-day mortality than cTnT-negative patients (15.7% vs. 6.2%, p = 0.001). Further, the cTnT result provided independent prognostic information ($\chi^2$ 46, p = 0.001) when added to the clinical risk model developed by Lee.

Use of other myocardial necrosis markers may also improve risk stratification in ST-segment elevation MI, particularly for identifying low-risk patients. Srinivas and colleagues showed that using a myoglobin decision level of 239 ng/mL at 12 hours could separate patients with ST-segment elevation MI into groups, those with values 239 ng/mL or less who are at low risk for 30-day mortality (1.4%), and those with levels greater than 239 ng/mL who are at higher 30-day mortality risk (9.1%) [24]. In a multivariable model including age, sex, infarct artery location, and 90-minute Thrombolysis in Myocardial Infarction (TIMI) flow grade of CK-MB, cTnI, and myoglobin measured at various time points, only the 12-hour myoglobin added significantly in identifying low-risk patients. Similar to the use of markers to identify high-risk patients, identification of low-risk groups after ST-segment elevation MI could aid clinical management and discharge decisions.

Thus, the use of cardiac markers such as cardiac troponins in conjunction with clinical risk predictors and other necrosis markers in this population might be used prospectively to improve triage decisions and management strategies, including timing of discharge. Prospective validation of the utility of such measures remains to be undertaken, however.

## ROLE OF TROPONIN IN NON–ST-SEGMENT ELEVATION MYOCARDIAL INFARCTION

### Diagnosis of Non–ST-segment Elevation Myocardial Infarction

While the diagnosis of acute MI is relatively accurate in patients who present with ST-segment elevation, this group accounts for only a minority (about 5%) of the patients who ultimately are diagnosed with acute MI [15,25]. Beyond ST-segment elevation acute MI exists a diagnostic and risk continuum of ACS, including non–Q-wave or non–ST-segment elevation MI and unstable angina. The baseline ECG can help confirm a clinical suspicion of unstable angina but cannot differentiate non–ST-segment elevation MI from unstable angina [26,27]. If a patient with a history of symptoms suggestive of unstable angina is symptom-free upon examination, a baseline ECG with evidence of coronary artery disease (significant Q waves, deep symmetrical T-wave inversions, and resting ST-segment depression) supports the diagnosis. A normal ECG at baseline in the presence of symptoms does not exclude the diagnosis of unstable angina or non-ST-segment elevation MI, but it makes it less likely. Dynamic electrocardiographic changes with symptoms and symptom resolution strongly support the diagnosis, however.

Differentiation of non–ST-segment elevation MI from unstable angina is largely made, in retrospect, based on serial cardiac marker sampling over 24 hours. Even small amounts of myocardial necrosis, as measured by CK-MB or cardiac troponin sampling, portend a worse outcome [17,28,29], and because the best outcomes are likely obtained when specific therapy is started early, it is important to differentiate these two groups early and effectively. In addition, early risk assessment may improve triage decisions and facilitate development of diagnostic and management strategies. As described previously, a troponin ''gold standard'' has now been established for diagnosis of MI [10].

### Risk Stratification in Non–ST-segment Elevation Acute Coronary Syndromes

*Clinical Risk Stratification*

Just as the diagnostic boundaries between non–ST-segment elevation MI and unstable angina are blurred, so, too, is there a gradation of risk within ACS. Defining risk within the group is important for both patient management decisions and patient counseling. Clinical characteristics at presentation and diagnostic tools including the ECG and serum cardiac marker data can be used to help establish risk. The cardiac history and examination are often nonspecific, but prolonged pain at rest and the development of a transient S3 gallop, rales or other signs of congestive heart failure, hypotension, or new or more severe mitral regurgitation during symptoms suggest left ventricular dysfunction with ischemia and a higher short- and long-term risk of mortality [27,30].

Other baseline characteristics may also be important in risk stratification. Calvin and colleagues identified previous infarction, lack of β-blocker or calcium-channel blocker treatment, baseline ST-segment depression, and diabetes mellitus as predictors of death or acute MI in 393 patients presenting with unstable angina [31]. In a regression model developed in 1384 GUSTO-IIa patients with acute coronary ischemia, age, Killip class, systolic blood pressure, and previous hypertension were identified as significant predictors of 30-day mortality [32].

## The Electrocardiogram and Risk

Within the spectrum of non-ST-segment elevation ACS, the ECG remains an important prognostic tool. In particular, dynamic ST-segment elevation or depression and T-wave changes predict a higher risk of death or MI in unstable angina patients compared with normal tracings or nonspecific changes (26,27,33–35). In GUSTO-IIa, which included the spectrum of patients with ACS, the presenting electrocardiographic category (ST-segment elevation, ST-segment depression, T-wave inversion/normal, or confounding factors present) was an important predictor of short-term mortality in a multivariate survival model that also contained CK-MB and cTnT [17]. In comparing the categories, patients with confounding electrocardiographic factors (such as left bundle branch block, left ventricular hypertrophy, or paced rhythms) had the highest short-term mortality (11.6%), followed by those with ST-segment depression (8.0%), and ST-segment elevation (7.4%). Short-term mortality was the lowest (1.2%) in the group with T-wave inversion or a normal tracing.

## Risk Stratification with Troponin

As early as 1992, it was clearly demonstrated that elevation of cardiac troponins was associated with increased rates of major cardiac events in patients with unstable angina [36]. Since that time, numerous studies including landmark papers from the GUSTO-IIa troponin substudy with cTnT and the Thrombolysis in Myocardial Infarction (TIMI) IIIb troponin study with cTnI have confirmed the relationship of troponin elevation with mortality among patients with ACS (17,24,29,36–41). In each of these studies it was also demonstrated that the relationship of the magnitude of troponin elevation with mortality was nearly linear. Several meta-analyses have now solidified these relationships.

In a meta-analysis by Wu and colleagues in 1995, the odds ratio (OR) for death or MI in cTnT-positive unstable angina patients was 4.3 (95% confidence interval [CI], 2.8–6.8) [42]. A subsequent 1998 meta-analysis of both cTnT and cTnI studies by Olatidoye showed substantially increased risk in patients positive for either marker (cTnT: RR 2.7, 95% CI, 2.1–3.4; cTnI: RR 4.2, 95% CI, 2.7–6.4) [43]. More recently, two large meta-analyses have summarized the importance of troponin as a risk marker across the spectrum of ACS.

In a cohort of 18,982 patients from 21 studies, Ottani and colleagues demonstrated that relative to troponin-negative patients, the odds ratio for 30-day death or MI was 2.86 (95% CI, 2.35–3.47) among patients with ST-segment elevation MI, 4.93 (95% CI, 3.77–6.45) among patients with non–ST-segment elevation MI by traditional CK-MB diagnosis and importantly in the era of the troponin "gold standard," 9.39 (95% CI, 6.46–13.67) among patients with unstable angina [44]. Similarly, in a meta-analysis of 7 clinical trials and 19 cohort studies including 11,963 non–ST-segment elevation ACS patients, both short-term mortality (OR 3.1 [95% CI, 2.3–4.1]) and death or myocardial infarction (2.5 [95% CI, 2.0–3.1]) were significantly increased among troponin-positive patients [45]. Previous studies with older assays had suggested that cTnT might be superior to cTnI [46], but similar relationships were observed for both cTnT and cTnI in this meta-analysis [45].

Importantly, in these studies, cardiac troponins were shown to contribute information for risk stratification that was incremental to that provided by clinical and ECG characteristics obtained at patient presentation. In the Fragmin during instability in coronary artery disease (FRISC) trial, 976 patients with unstable angina were randomized to low-molecular-weight heparin or placebo. Cardiac troponin T was measured within 12 hours of presentation, and patients were followed for cardiac death or MI for 5 months [47]. The risk of events increased with increasing levels of cTnT ($<$ 0.06 ng/mL, 4.3%; 0.06–0.18 ng/mL, 10.5%; $>$ 0.18 ng/mL, 16.1%). In multivariable analysis, cTnT and the clinical variables, age, hypertension, number of antianginal drugs, and electrocardiographic changes, were identified as independent predictors of cardiac death or MI. Furthermore, Stubbs and colleagues have found similar results in a general unstable angina population [41].

Cardiac troponin I was a predictor of 42-day mortality in a retrospective analysis of 1404 patients with non–Q-wave MI or unstable angina randomized in the TIMI-IIIb trial [31]. The cutoff value used in this analysis was 0.4 ng/mL using the Dade Stratus II assay, below the cutoff of 1.5 ng/mL for the diagnosis of acute MI with this test. Troponin I was positive in 41% of patients; 32% had elevated CK-MB. Mortality was 3.7% in cTnI-positive patients, compared with 1.0% in cTnI-negative patients. The risk of mortality increased with increasing concentration of cTnI. In multivariable analysis, ST-segment depression (p $<$ 0.001), age greater than 65 years (p $=$ 0.026), and cTnI status on admission, (p $=$ 0.03) were independent predictors of 42-day mortality.

The GUSTO-IIa troponin T substudy, prospectively evaluated the prognostic significance of a single baseline measurement of cTnT in 855 patients across the spectrum of ACS [17]. In all, 755 patients had complete cTnT, CK-MB, and electrocardiographic information; 36% were cTnT-positive and 32% had elevated CK-MB. Mortality was highest in patients with electrocardiographic confounding factors (11.6%), and lowest in patients with normal tracings or only minor changes (1.2%). In cTnT-positive patients, 30-day mortality was 11.8%, compared with 3.9% in cTnT-negative patients. As shown in Figure 3, mortality increased with increasing concentrations of cTnT. The same mortality

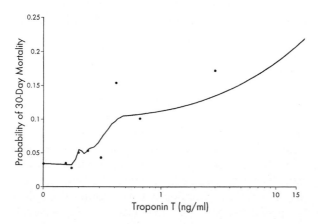

**Figure 3** Nonparametric estimates of the probability of 30-day mortality vs. admission troponin T level. Troponin T is plotted along a cube-root scale. Data density is shown at the top of the plot; each mark represents one patient. The solid circles represent simple mortality estimates from intervals of troponin T levels that were derived to contain at least 70 patients. (Reprinted from Ref. 17)

relationship in cTnT-positive vs. -negative patients held across all electrocardiographic categories (ST-segment elevation, ST-segment depression, confounders, and T-wave inversion/normal) (Table 2). In-hospital complications were likewise increased in the cTnT-positive patients. When the electrocardiographic category, CK-MB results, and cTnT value were considered in a mortality model, electrocardiographic findings followed by cTnT value and CK-MB were all predictors of 30-day mortality. The models were then adjusted for the presence of the other two variables; once the electrocardiographic findings and cTnT value were known, CK-MB contributed no further prognostic information. Cardiac troponin T added significantly even after the other two variables were known.

*Troponins for Risk Stratification in Patients with Renal Insufficiency*

Subsequent analyses from the GUSTO-IIa database confirmed the importance of troponin status in addition to clinical and electrocardiographic variables in both short- and long-term risk stratification among patients with ACS [13]. More recently, risk scores incorporating cardiac marker status at presentation with clinical variables have capitalized on the independent contributions of disparate types of information in risk stratification among patients with non-ST-segment elevation ACS [48,49].

While little doubt remains regarding the prognostic ability of troponin measures in discriminating high-risk patients with ACS, lingering concerns remain about their utility in patients with chronic renal insufficiency. Although cardiac troponins are clearly useful for both the diagnosis of myocardial necrosis and in assessing prognosis, they are cleared renally, and pathophysiology other than acute ischemia may lead to cardiac troponin release in patients with chronic renal insufficiency or end-stage renal disease.

Using data from 7,033 patients who presented with ischemic symptoms and signs and were enrolled in the GUSTO-IV trial, Aviles and colleagues examined the association between cTnT elevation, renal dysfunction and 30-day death or MI [50]. Twenty percent of patients with estimated creatinine clearance less than 58.4 mL/min had troponin levels of more than 0.1 ng/mL, the upper limit of normal for the cTnT assay studied. Figure 4 shows the relationship of cTnT elevation with 30-day death or MI in this cohort. Among patients with elevated cTnT there was a significantly increased risk of 30-day death or MI regardless of renal function; a risk which persisted after adjustment for potential confounders. Thus, among patients with signs and symptoms of ACS, troponin elevation is predictive of short-term adverse events regardless of renal function.

*Importance of Discordant Troponin and CK-MB Results*

Often in ACS patients CK-MB and a cardiac troponin are measured concurrently, and, in many cases, the results are discordant. Uncertainty remains about the appropriate management of these patients, particularly when clinical risk is otherwise low. Rao and colleagues investigated the association between isolated troponin elevation and 30-day outcomes in both ACS patients and in patients with low-risk chest pain [51]. Using combined data from the GUSTO IIa and Platelet IIb/IIIa Antagonism for the Reduction of Acute Coronary Syndrome Events in a Global Organization Network (PARAGON B) troponin substudies (high-risk), and data from the CHECKMATE study (low-risk) patients were grouped according to baseline marker status (troponin + /CK-MB + ; troponin + /CK-MB − ; troponin − /CK MB + ; troponin − /CK MB − ). As shown in Figure 5, troponin elevation at baseline without concurrent CK-MB elevation was associated with a significantly higher odds ratio for 30-day death or MI in both the high- and low-risk ACS patients. Risk for 30-day death or MI was similar among patients with isolated CK-MB elevation and patients with both markers negative.

**Table 2** Complications and 30-Day Outcomes in the GUSTO-IIa Troponin T Substudy by Electrocardiographic Category and Troponin T and Creatine Kinase-MB

|  | ST-segment Elevation | | | | ST-segment Depression | | | |
|---|---|---|---|---|---|---|---|---|
| 30-Day Outcomes | cTnT (+)[†] (n = 138) | cTnT (−) (n = 297) | CK-MB (+) (n = 143) | CK-MB (−) (n = 292) | cTnT (+) (n = 43) | cTnT (−) (n = 45) | CK-MB (+) (n = 30) | CK-MB (−) (n = 58) |
| Death | 18 (13.0) | 14 (4.7) | 15 (10.5) | 17 (5.8) | 5 (11.6) | 2 (4.4) | 4 (13.3) | 3 (5.2) |
| Myocardial infarction | 125 (90.6) | 241 (81.1) | 137 (95.8) | 229 (78.4) | 33 (76.8) | 17 (37.8) | 29 (96.7) | 21 (36.2) |
| Bypass surgery | 22 (15.9) | 41 (13.8) | 18 (12.6) | 45 (15.4) | 12 (27.9) | 11 (24.4) | 8 (26.7) | 15 (25.9) |
| Angioplasty | 35 (25.4) | 107 (36.0) | 43 (30.1) | 99 (33.9) | 9 (20.9) | 11 (24.4) | 8 (26.7) | 12 (20.7) |

|  | T-wave Inversion, Normal | | | | Confounding Electrocardiographic Factors[‡] | | | |
|---|---|---|---|---|---|---|---|---|
| 30-Day outcomes | cTnT (+) (n = 49) | cTnT (−) (n = 114) | CK-MB (+) (n = 44) | CK-MB (−) (n = 119) | cTnT (+) (n = 39) | cTnT (−) (n = 30) | CK-MB (+) (n = 28) | CK-MB (−) (n = 41) |
| Death | 2 (4.1) | 0 | 1 (2.3) | 1 (0.8) | 6 (15.4) | 2 (6.7) | 5 (17.9) | 3 (7.3) |
| Myocardial infarction | 43 (87.8) | 40 (35.1) | 43 (97.7) | 40 (33.6) | 31 (79.5) | 15 (50.7) | 27 (96.4) | 19 (46.3) |
| Bypass surgery | 10 (20.4) | 22 (19.3) | 8 (18.2) | 24 (20.2) | 3 (7.7) | 4 (13.3) | 0 | 7 (17.1) |
| Angioplasty | 18 (36.7) | 35 (30.7) | 16 (36.4) | 37 (31.1) | 11 (28.2) | 10 (33.3) | 10 (35.7) | 11 (26.9) |

Values are medians (25th, 75th percentiles) or frequencies (percentages). [†]Troponin T (cTnT) (+) = >0.1 ng/mL, (−) = ≤0.1 ng/mL, by core laboratory determination. [‡]Left bundle branch block, left ventricular hypertrophy, or paced rhythms. Adapted from Ref. 17.

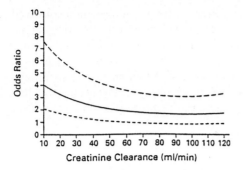

**Figure 4**  Adjusted odds ratio (solid line) with 95% confidence limits (dashed lines) for death or myocardial infarction by estimated creatinine clearance among patients with elevated troponin levels. (Reprinted from Ref. 50)

In a similar analysis from the CRUSADE Quality Improvement Registry, among 29,357 high-risk ACS patients, 28% had discordant troponin and CK-MB results within 36 hours of presentation (10% CK-MB + /troponin − ; 18% CK-MB − /troponin + ) [52]. In-hospital mortality was increased among groups with elevated troponin regardless of CK-MB status (4.45% for CK-MB − /troponin +  and 5.87% for CK-MB + /troponin + ), but CK-MB elevation in the absence of troponin elevation did not predict increased mortality. These studies highlight the importance of troponin as both an early and short-term marker of risk even when the results are discordant with traditional CK-MB measurement.

## Troponin to Guide Treatment in Patients with Acute Coronary Syndromes

That the cardiac markers have diagnostic and prognostic utility across the spectrum of chest pain patients has now, essentially, been proven beyond doubt. The evolution of

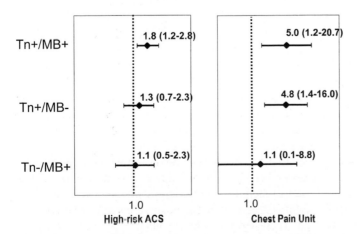

**Figure 5**  Adjusted odds ratio with 95% confidence intervals for death or myocardial infarction among high-risk acute coronary syndrome patients (left panel) and lower-risk chest pain unit patients (right panel) by troponin (Tn) and creatine kinase-MB (MB) status. (Adapted from Ref. 51)

cardiac marker testing has now taken us one step further, using the information conveyed by the results of cardiac marker testing to most appropriately and cost-effectively apply the rapidly growing therapeutic options available for ACS patients. Several studies have now shown that knowledge of troponin status in addition to clinical variables may be used to define high-risk populations who stand to gain the most from treatment with aggressive management strategies after an ACS or from the use of newer treatments such as the low molecular weight heparins or intravenous glycoprotein (GP) IIb/IIIa receptor antagonists.

*Low Molecular Weight Heparins*

The relationship of cardiac marker status with outcome by treatment strategy was extensively studied in 976 patients in the FRISC study. Among cTnT-positive patients, the risk of death or MI at 5–7 days was significantly reduced for patients receiving dalteparin compared with placebo (6.0% vs. 2.4%), such that the risk for cTnT-positive dalteparin-treated patients approached that of cTnT-negative patients receiving standard therapy (2.4%) [53]. Further, this treatment benefit was maintained for long-term follow-up. In contrast, among cTnT-negative patients at lower initial risk, the reduction in death or MI between treatment groups at 5 to 7 days was not statistically significant and was not present in long-term follow-up.

Similar results were observed with enoxaparin in a substudy of the TIMI 11b trial of enoxaparin vs. unfractionated heparin in patients with non–ST-segment elevation ACS [54]. Among baseline cTnI-positive patients at 14-day composite endpoint of death, MI or urgent revascularization was reduced by 47% among enoxaparin-treated patients, but among cTnI-negative patients no difference in outcomes by treatment was observed.

*Glyocoprotein IIb/IIIa Antagonists*

Studies of platelet glycoprotein IIb/IIIa receptor antagonists administered intravenously in the settings of percutaneous coronary intervention and ACS have shown a consistent and durable reduction in death or MI [55]. As with low-molecular weight heparins, data suggest that the results of cardiac marker testing along with clinical variables may identify subgroups of patients who benefit preferentially from the use of platelet GPIIb/IIIa antagonists.

Januzzi and colleagues showed that for the intravenous GPIIb/IIIa antagonist tirofiban in combination with heparin in patients with non–ST-segment elevation ACS, peak cTnI levels were significantly lower among patients who received tirofiban compared with standard heparin therapy alone suggesting a potential link between better outcomes in tirofiban-treated patients and troponin status [56]. Further, in conjunction with the Platelet-Receptor Inhibition for ischemic syndrome management (PRISM) study of 2,222 patients randomized to tirofiban or placebo, Heeschen and colleagues showed that among the 28% of patients with elevated cTnI (diagnostic threshold 1.0 ug/L) and the 29% of patients with elevated cTnT (diagnostic threshold 0.1 ug/L) measurements there was a significantly higher risk of 30-day rates of death or MI [57]. More importantly, they showed that troponin-positive status could be used to identify a subgroup of patients with ACS that benefited from the use of tirofiban. Among both the cTnI-positive patients who received tirofiban the hazard ratio for mortality (adjusted for other predictors) was 0.25 (95 % CI, 0.09–0.68). For MI, the adjusted hazard ratio was 0.37 (95% CI, 0.16–0.84). Table 3 reviews the event rates for these and other endpoints by cTnI status and treatment group in the PRISM study. Results were similar for cTnT. These marked reductions in 30-day death and MI occurred regardless of the overall management strategy (medical or

**Table 3** Event Rates Over Time by Troponin I Status

| | Troponin I-positive | | Troponin I-negative | |
|---|---|---|---|---|
| | Heparin (n = 324) | Tirofiban (n = 305) | Heparin (n = 801) | Tirofiban (n = 792) |
| **48 hours** | | | | |
| Refractory ischemia | 30 (9.3) | 10 (3.3) | 24 (3.05) | 17 (2.1) |
| Death or myocardial infarction | 11 (3.4) | 1 (0.3) | 5 (0.6) | 7 (0.9) |
| Death | 2 (0.6) | 0 | 0 | 3 (0.4) |
| Myocardial infarction | 9 (2.8) | 1 (0.3) | 5 (0.6) | 4 (0.5) |
| **7 days** | | | | |
| Refractory ischemia | 47 (14.5) | 26 (8.5) | 53 (6.6) | 59 (7.4) |
| Death or myocardial infarction | 30 (9.3) | 6 (2.0) | 18 (2.2) | 24 (3.0) |
| Death | 12 (3.7) | 2 (0.7) | 3 (0.4) | 7 (0.9) |
| Myocardial infarction | 18 (5.6) | 4 (1.3) | 14 (1.8) | 17 (2.1) |
| **30 days** | | | | |
| Refractory ischemia | 48 (14.8) | 31 (10.2) | 60 (7.5) | 72 (9.1) |
| Death or myocardial infarction | 42 (13.0) | 13 (4.3) | 39 (4.9) | 45 (5.7) |
| Death | 20 (6.2) | 5 (1.6) | 18 (2.3) | 18 (2.3) |
| Myocardial infarction | 22 (6.8) | 8 (2.6) | 21 (2.6) | 27 (3.6) |

Values are n (percent).
*Source*: Adapted from Ref. 57.

revascularization). There was no treatment benefit in the troponin-negative patients. Thus, troponin-positive status could be used to guide the use of tirofiban, reserving it for patients with the greatest benefit.

These results were extended by the results of a troponin T substudy from the Chimeric 7E3 Antiplatelet Therapy Unstable Angina Refractory to Standard Treatment (CAPTURE) trial. In CAPTURE, patients with refractory unstable angina were randomized to treatment with abciximab or placebo for 12 to 24 hours prior to, during and 12 hours following percutaneous intervention [58]. At all stages—before intervention, post-procedure and in follow-up, rates of MI were significantly lower in the abciximab-treated patients. The results of a cTnT substudy suggested that the observed treatment benefits were largely confined to patients who were cTnT-positive [59]. The relative risk (RR) of death or MI for abciximab treatment vs. placebo in patients with cTnT greater than 0.1 ng/mL was 0.32 (95% CI, 0.12–0.49), but, in patients with cTnT 0.1 ng/mL or less, there was no significant difference for treatment with abciximab vs. placebo, RR 1.26 (95% CI, 0.74–2.31). In this study, in addition to showing that the most benefit was gained by treating troponin-positive patients, it was also demonstrated that the potential mechanism for this benefit was related to the resolution of coronary thrombus [60]. Among cTnT-positive patients, visible thrombus was present at baseline angiography in 14.6% of cases compared with only 4.2% of cTnT-negative cases. Use of abciximab was highly associated with the resolution of thrombus and with greater improvement in TIMI flow among cTnT-positive patients (Table 4) suggesting the potential mechanism of the greater benefit of its use in cTnT-positive patients.

In the PARAGON B Troponin T Substudy, Newby and colleagues found a similar differential treatment effect by cTnT status [61]. The 30-day rate of death or MI was 19% among cTnT-positive patients who received placebo, but only 11% among those who received lamifiban. Among cTnT-negative patients, the corresponding 30-day rates of death or MI were 10.3% among patients receiving placebo and 9.6% among those random-

**Table 4**   TIMI flow after 18 to 24 hours of allocated treatment according to cTnT status

| cTnT-positive (n = 263) | | | | cTnT-negative (n = 589) | | | |
|---|---|---|---|---|---|---|---|
| TIMI flow at baseline | Abciximab | Placebo | P | TIMI flow at baseline | Abciximab | Placebo | P |
| TIMI 0 (n = 19) | − 1 | + 2 | 0.64 | TIMI 0 (n = 10) | + 1 | − 1 | 0.59 |
| TIMI 1 (n = 22) | − 5 | + 1 | 0.13 | TIMI 1 (n = 20) | − 1 | Equal | 0.87 |
| TIMI 2 (n = 65) | − 3 | + 1 | 0.16 | TIMI 2 (n = 119) | + 2 | − 1 | 0.43 |
| TIMI 3 (n = 157) | + 9 | − 4 | <0.001 | TIMI 3 (n = 440) | − 2 | + 2 | 0.06 |

*Source*: Adapted from Ref. 60

ized to lamifiban. In a meta-analysis of the CAPTURE, PRISM and PARAGON B troponin substudies shown in Figure 6, this interaction between troponin status and treatment effect was investigated further [61]. Among troponin-positive patients the pooled OR for 30-day death or MI was 0.34 (95% CI, 0.19–0.58); among troponin-negative patients no treatment benefit was observed (OR 1.06 [95% CI, 0.78–1.43]). The OR for the troponin status by treatment interaction was 0.33 (95% CI, 0.19–0.57).

In a subsequent meta-analysis that included results from all trials of small-molecule GPIIb/IIIa inhibitors in ACS patients, Boersma and colleagues observed a similar differential in treatment effect between troponin-positive and troponin-negative patients. The 30-day rate of death or MI was reduced significantly in patients with elevated baseline troponins, but this benefit did not extend to patients with normal baseline troponins [62].

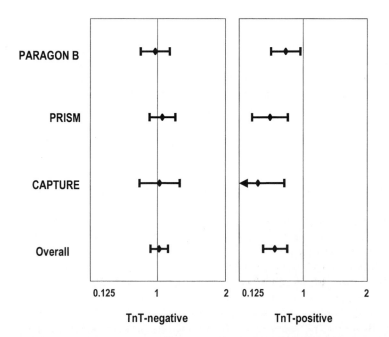

**Figure 6**   Odds ratio with 95% confidence intervals for treatment effect by troponin status (positive, *right panel*; negative, *left panel*) in various trials of glycoprotein IIb/IIIa inhibitors and overall. (Adapted from Ref. 61)

*Aggressive Interventional Strategies*

A recent study (FRISC II) of early invasive evaluation and revascularization if indicated vs. an early conservative strategy, reserving such evaluation and treatment for patients with recurrent symptoms or severe ischemia on treadmill testing showed a benefit favoring an early invasive strategy that was confined to cTnT-positive patients [63]. At 1 year, both death or MI were lower among cTnT-positive patients who underwent early revascularization for ACS (OR 0.70 [95% CI, 0.53–0.93]); for death alone the 1-year OR was 0.51 (95% CI, 0.28–0.94), but no benefit was observed among cTnT-negative patients.

Further, in a substudy of FRISC II, Diderholm and colleagues demonstrated the importance of ECG findings in conjunction with cTnT results to define high-risk patients who benefited most from an early invasive strategy [64]. In patients with both ST-segment depression and a cTnT greater than 0.03 ng/mL the early invasive strategy was associated with a reduction in 1-year death or MI from 22.1% to 13.2% (relative risk 0.60 [95% CI, 0.43–0.82]). Among patients with either one or the other of ST-segment depression or cTnT greater than 0.03 the risk reductions were smaller, and among those with neither finding, treatment effects were nonsignificant.

Among patients randomized to early invasive vs. a conservative strategy in the Treat Angina with Aggrastat and Determine Cost of Therapy with an Invasive or Conservative Strategy (TACTICS)-TIMI 18 trial, patients with elevated baseline cTnI levels (greater than 0.1 ng/mL) had significantly higher 30-day (11.7% vs. 5.5%, p < 0.001) and 6-month (20.1% vs. 14.2%, p < 0.001) rates of death or recurrent ischemia than cTnI-negative patients [65]. As in the FRISC II study, among cTnI-positive patients randomized to the early invasive strategy, there was a significant reduction in death, MI or rehospitalization at 6 months compared with the conservative strategy, but no treatment effect was observed among cTnI-negative patients.

Despite demonstration of the relationship between troponin elevation, risk and preferential treatment benefit, application of treatment based on troponin status has not been widely adopted even though these concepts have been incorporated into the American College of Cardiology/American Heart Association Guidelines for the Management of Patients with Unstable Angina and non–ST-segment Elevation Myocardial Infarction [66]. As shown by data from the CRUSADE Quality Improvement Initiative, among over 29,000 patients with high-risk ACS, in those with discordant CK-MB and troponin results, use of GPIIb/IIIa inhibitors was biased by the CK-MB result, despite the preponderance of evidence for use of these agents based on troponin-positivity [52]. Further, in a separate analysis from the CRUSADE registry, Roe and colleagues demonstrated that until troponin levels were greater than 5 times the upper limit of normal, neither troponin status (positive or negative) or the degree of elevation influenced the use of glycoprotein IIb/IIIa inhibitors or an early invasive catheterization strategy [67].

## Troponin and Other Markers of Risk

Two recent studies have addressed the use of combinations of biomarker, including the troponins, to enhance risk stratification in ACS patients. The Orbofibanin Patients with Unstable Coronary Syndromes (OPUS)-TIMI 16 investigators performed a nested case-control study to evaluate the utility of simultaneous measurements of serum C-reactive protein (CRP), cTnI and brain natriuretic peptide (BNP) in 450 patients within 72 hours of presentation with ACS [68]. They found that all three markers were independent predictors of 30-day and 10-month endpoints of death, MI, or congestive heart failure. Further, the number of markers that were elevated was directly correlated with outcome; for each additional elevated biomarker, there was a near-doubling of mortality risk. These results were validated in TACTICS-TIMI 18 patients in which, compared with patients with no elevated biomarkers, the 6-month risk of death, MI, or congestive heart failure was increased 2.1-fold among patients with one elevated marker, 3.1-fold with 2 elevated markers, and 3.6-fold with 3 elevated markers [68].

The utility of measuring markers of multiple processes (troponin, C-reactive protein, and N-terminal pro-brain natriuretic peptide) in determining risk in patients with ACS was also explored by the GUSTO-IV investigators [69]. In their analyses, the prognostic utility of an individual biomarker depended on the endpoint (mortality or MI) being assessed. Elevated levels of N-terminal pro-BNP, cTnT, and CRP, in addition to heart rate, creatinine clearance, and ST-segment depression, were all independently associated with 1-year mortality. Only cTnT, creatinine clearance, and ST-segment depression predicted risk for future MI. Additionally, the GUSTO-IV investigators demonstrated that the prognostic utility of cTnT and CRP differed over time, with cTnT providing more information for mortality risk-stratification at 30-days and CRP better for longer-term risk assessment [70].

### Troponin in the Chest Pain Unit

Each year in the United States, about 6 million people arrive at emergency departments with complaints of chest pain or other symptoms of possible cardiac ischemia. As described in detail in Chapter 11, accurate diagnosis and triage of this diverse group of patients can be difficult, but have important clinical, legal and economic implications. Graff and colleagues have shown that implementation of Chest Pain Units can cut the historical "miss" rate of MIs by 10-fold, from 4.3% to 0.4% [71].

Many strategies to improve diagnostic accuracy in these patients have been devised. Investigators have developed neural networks, diagnostic algorithms, and decision models to calculate the likelihood of acute MI (33,34,72–74), but the utility of these methods is generally limited by the available input. In part, because they are cumbersome and the use of these algorithms has not become widespread, despite testing and validation in multiple populations. Serial serum cardiac marker testing within short-stay observation units, sometimes called Chest Pain Units, has become widespread to evaluate the diverse group of chest pain patients who are not at high risk for myocardial ischemia, but in whom the diagnosis cannot be excluded.

Cardiac troponin T testing has shown promise for use in the low-risk chest pain unit population. In a meta-analysis of published reports of cTnT in chest pain patients, the odds ratio for coronary revascularization was 4.4 (95% CI, 3.0–6.5) with a positive cTnT result (24,38,41,43,75). Further, in an analysis of 383 consecutive patients in the Duke Chest Pain Unit, the rate of significant angiographic disease ($> 75\%$ stenosis) in cTnT-positive ($\geq 0.1$ ng/mL) patients was 89% compared with 49% in the cTnT-negative group ($p = 0.002$); the rate of multivessel disease among the cTnT-positive patients was also significantly higher (67% vs. 29%, $p = 0.003$) [75]. de Fillippi and colleagues have reported a similar association between troponin status and the presence of significant coronary artery disease at angiography in their chest pain cohort [76]. Both of these studies point out the high prevalence of underlying coronary artery disease among even troponin-negative patients considered low-to-moderate risk by clinical features alone. Therefore, the importance of stress testing or other means of risk stratification in troponin-negative patients prior to release from Chest Pain Units probably cannot be overemphasized. In support of this consideration, Lindahl and colleagues showed that, in the FRISC study, among 963 patients at all levels of cTnT values, including those with negative values, the stress test provided further risk stratification [77].

The prognostic value of troponin testing in the Chest Pain Unit setting has also been demonstrated. In the longest follow-up of a Chest Pain Unit population, the results from our study suggest that cTnT-positive status identifies a population at higher risk for total mortality (27% vs. 7%, p = 0.0001) and among those, cardiac mortality, than cTnT-negative patients [75]. As the clinical interpretation and application of such findings in the Chest Pain Unit population evolves and as new markers that detect ischemia rather than myocardial necrosis are developed, management strategies for otherwise low-risk chest pain patients will likely change—perhaps more aggressive in the positive patients, both early and in secondary prevention.

## Bedside Cardiac Marker Testing

Laboratory assays for most cardiac markers can now be done within 10 to 30 minutes of specimen receipt. Lost time in specimen ordering, collection, transport and result reporting add substantially to this time, however. In some institutions, this process may take as long as 2 to 3 hours [78], greatly diminishing the value of a test for which there is a rapid laboratory assay. Point-of-care testing could circumvent many of these problems by putting not only the results, but also the testing in the hands of the ordering physician. For example, real-time testing of blood glucose by a bedside device allows rapid and precise adjustments to insulin regimens in diabetic patients, which could not be achieved with laboratory assessments. Further, rapid point-of-care testing of the activated partial thromboplastin time (aPTT) in GUSTO-I resulted in fewer bleeding complications compared with usual laboratory-based testing and had a substantially shorter turnaround time [79].

As suggested by the work of Downie and colleagues [80], bedside assessment of serum markers of myocardial necrosis in real time may offer physicians the greatest ability to make rapid decisions about diagnosis and patient management approaches. Particularly in a Chest Pain Unit or to determine perfusion status after thrombolytic therapy, the availability of rapid bedside testing for cardiac markers would be important. This approach could offer not only the potential to improve the quality and effectiveness of critical management decisions but also the potential to advance the efficiency of patient care and reduce costs. In the CHECKMATE study, time to detection of patients with positive markers was reduced by 0.9 hours using point-of-care testing of a multimarker panel of necrosis markers. Further, in a single institution study of 939 marker tests, Christenson and colleagues demonstrated that the time from draw to reporting of results was a mean of 128 minutes (SD 47 minutes) using the local laboratory. Using point-of-care testing, the mean time from draw to result report was reduced to 15 minutes [81].

The prognostic utility of rapid bedside assays for cTnT and cTnI testing have also been demonstrated in clinical practice. In a GUSTO-III substudy, Ohman and colleagues demonstrated the ability of a rapid, bedside assay for cTnT to risk-stratify patients rapidly at presentation with acute MI, alone and combined with known clinical predictors of risk [23]. In addition, Hamm and colleagues showed that both cTnI and cTnT bedside qualitative assays were able to risk stratify patients across the full spectrum of chest pain presentations in the Emergency Department [82]. In their study the results for either marker sampled at presentation then 4 hours later was a strong independent predictor of 30-day mortality or MI in this broad chest pain population.

As health care systems evolve to emphasize and reward more efficient patient care, and as rapid advances in technology provide improved early treatment options, it will be increasingly important to determine the benefits to patient care and costs of point-of-care testing and to establish what role, if any, this method of assessment should play for patients with acute coronary syndromes or in the evaluation of chest pain patients with less clear diagnoses. A concerted multidisciplinary effort involving basic researchers, clinicians, and clinical laboratory personnel will be required to develop and study new assays, devices, and testing strategies and to define the optimal approach.

## CONCLUSIONS

Cardiac troponins have assumed the role of "gold standard" for detection of myocardial necrosis and the diagnosis of MI in patients with suspected ACS. The use of newer, more sensitive and specific markers and innovative testing strategies could greatly facilitate the process of care across the spectrum of diagnostic indications. The more recently documented prognostic importance of the troponins (cTnI and cTnT) alone and in combination with other biomarkers of risk will ultimately change the way we counsel ACS patients. Further, the growing evidence that identification of high-risk patients by troponin testing can identify patients who preferentially benefit from aggressive interventional strategies and potent and expensive antithrombotic therapy has the potential to improve clinical outcomes and improve resource use. The greatest challenge currently facing those who care for ACS patients is to apply this readily available information from troponin testing in clinical practice.

## REFERENCES

1.  Lee KL, Pryor DB, Harrell FE, Califf RM, Behar VS, Floyd WL, Morris JJ, Waugh RA, Whalen RE, Rosati R. Predicting outcome in coronary disease. Statistical models vs. expert clinicians. Am J Med 1986;80:553–560.
2.  Kong DF, Lee KL, Harrell FE, Boswick JM, Mark DB, Hlatky MA, Califf RM, Pryor D. Clinical experience and predicting survival in coronary disease. Arch Intern Med 1989;149: 1177–1181.
3.  Tunstall-Pedoe H, Kuulasmaa K, Amouyel P, Arveiler D, Rajakangas AM, Pajak A. Myocardial infarction and coronary deaths in the World Health Organization MONICA project: registration procedures, event rates, and case-fatality rates in 39 populations from 21 countries in four continents. Circulation 1994;90:583–612.
4.  Falk E. Unstable angina with fatal outcome: dynamic coronary thrombosis leading to infarction and/or sudden death. Autopsy evidence of recurrent mural thrombosis with peripheral embolization culminating in total vascular occlusion. Circulation 1985;71:699–708.
5.  Gotlieb AI, Freeman MR, Salerno TA, Lichtenstein SV, Armstrong P. Ultrastructural studies of unstable angina in living man. Mod Pathol 1991;4:75–80.
6.  Adams JE, Abendschein DR, Jaffe A. Biochemical markers of myocardial injury. Is MB creatine kinase the choice for the 1990s?. Circulation 1993;88:750–763.
7.  Anderson PAW, Malouf NN, Oakeley AE, Pagani ED, Allen P. Troponin T isoform expression in humans. Circ Res 1991;69:1226–1233.
8.  Saggin L, Gorza L, Ausoni S, Schiaffino S. Cardiac troponin T in developing, regenerating and denervated rat skeletal muscle. Development 1990;110:547–554.
9.  Ricchiuti V, Voss EM, Ney A, Odland M, Anderson PAW, Apple F. Cardiac troponin T isoforms expressed in renal diseased skeletal muscle will not cause false-positive results by the second generation cardiac troponin T assay by Boehringer Mannheim. Clin Chem 1998; 44:1919–1924.
10. The Joint European Society of Cardiology/American College of Cardiology Committee. Myocardial infarction redefined—a consensus statement of the joint ECS/ACC committee for the redefinition of myocardial infarction. J Am Coll Cardiol 2000;36:959–969.
11. Zimmerman J, Fromm R, Meyer D, et al. Diagnostic Marker Cooperative Study for the diagnosis of myocardial infarction. Circulation 1999;99:1671–1677.

12. Lindahl B, Venge P, Wallentin L. on behalf of the BIOMACS Study Group. Early diagnosis and exclusion of acute myocardial infarction using biochemical monitoring. Coron Artery Dis 1995;6:321–328.

13. Newby LK, Christenson RH, Ohman EM, Armstrong PW, Peck SL, Lee KL, Hamm CW, Katus HA, Cianciolo C, Granger CB, Topol EJ, Califf RM. for the GUSTO-IIa Investigators. Value of serial troponin T measures for early and late risk stratification in patients with acute coronary syndromes. Circulation 1998;98:1853–1859.

14. Newby LK, Storrow AB, Gibler WB, Garvey JL, Tucker JF, Kaplan AL, Schreiber DH, Tuttle RH, McNulty SE, Ohman E. Bedside multimarker testing for risk stratification in chest pain units: the CHECKMATE study. Circulation 2001;103:1832–1837.

15. Rude RE, Poole WK, Muller JE, Turi Z, Rutherford J, Parker C, Roberts R, Raabe DS, Gold HK, Stone P. Electrocardiographic and clinical criteria for the recognition of acute myocardial infarction based on analysis of 3,697 patients. Am J Cardiol 1983;52:936–942.

16. Yusuf S, Pearson M, Sterry H, Parish S, Ramsdale D, Rossi P, Sleight P. The entry ECG in the early diagnosis and prognostic stratification of patients with suspected acute myocardial infarction. Eur Heart J 1984;5:690–696.

17. Ohman EM, Armstrong PW, Christenson RH, Granger CB, Katus HA, Hamm CW, O'Hanesian MA, Wagner GS, Kleiman NS, Harrell FE, Califf RM, Topol EJ. for the GUSTO-IIa Investigators. Cardiac troponin T levels for risk stratification in acute myocardial ischemia. N Engl J Med 1996;335:1333–1341.

18. Stubbs P, Collinson P, Moseley D, Greenwood T, Noble M. Prognostic significance of admission troponin T concentrations in patients with myocardial infarction. Circulation 1996;94:1291–1297.

19. Lee KL, Woodlief LH, Topol EJ, Weaver WD, Betriu A, Col J, Simoons M, Aylward P, Van de Werf F, Califf RM. for the GUSTO-I Investigators. Predictors of 30-day mortality in the era of reperfusion for acute myocardial infarction. Results from an international trial of 14,021 patients. Circulation 1995;91:1659–1668.

20. Topol EJ, Burek K, O'Neill WW, Kewman DG, Kander NH, Shea MJ, Schork MA, Kirscht J, Juni JE, Pitt B. A randomized controlled trial of hospital discharge three days after myocardial infarction in the era of reperfusion. N Engl J Med 1988;318:1083–1088.

21. Mark DB, Sigmon K, Topol EJ, Kereiakes DJ, Pryor DB, Candela RJ, Califf R. Identification of acute myocardial infarction patients suitable for early hospital discharge after aggressive interventional therapy: results from the Thrombolysis and Angioplasty in Acute Myocardial Infarction registry. Circulation 1991;83:1186–1191.

22. Newby LK, Califf RM, Guerci A, Weaver WD, Col J, Horgan JH, Mark DB, Stebbins A, Van de Werf F, Gore JM, Topol EJ. for the GUSTO-I Investigators. Early discharge in the thrombolytic era: an analysis of criteria for uncomplicated infarction from the Global Utilization of Streptokinase and t-PA for Occluded Coronary Arteries (GUSTO) Trial. Am Coll Cardiol 1996;27:625–632.

23. Ohman EM, Armstrong PW, White HD, Granger CB, Wilcox RG, Weaver WD, Gibler WB, Stebbins AL, Cianciolo C, Califf RM, Topol E. Risk stratification with a point-of-care troponin T test in acute myocardial infarction. Am J Cardiol 1999;84:1281–1286.

24. Wu AH, Abbas SA, Green S, Pearsall L, Dhakam S, Azar R, Onoroski M, Senaie A, Mckay RG, Waters D. Prognostic value of cardiac troponin T in unstable angina pectoris. Am J Cardiol 1995;76:970–972.

25. Califf RM, Ohman E. The diagnosis of acute myocardial infarction. Chest 1992;101:106S–115S.

26. Karlson BW, Herlitz J, Pettersson P, Hallgren P, Strombom U, Hjalmarson A. One-year prognosis in patients hospitalized with a history of unstable angina pectoris. Clin Cardiol 1993;16:397–402.

27. Califf RM, Mark DB, Harrell FE, Hlatky MA, Lee KL, Rosati RA, Pryor D. Importance of clinical measures of ischemia in the prognosis of patients with documented coronary artery disease. J Am Coll Cardiol 1988;11:20–26.

28. Tardiff BE, Califf RM, Tcheng JE, Lincoff AM, Sigmon KN, Harrington RA, Mahaffey KW, Ohman EM, Teirstein PS, Blankenship JC, Kitt MM, Topol EJ. for the Integrilin (eptifibatide)

to Minimize Platelet Aggregation and Coronary Thrombosis-II (IMPACT-II) Investigators. Clinical outcomes after detection of elevated cardiac enzymes in patients undergoing percutaneous intervention. J Am Coll Cardiol 1999;33:88–96.

29. Antman EM, Tanasijevic MJ, Thompson B, Schactman M, McCabe CH, Cannon CP, Fischer GA, Fung AY, Thompson C, Wybenga D, Braunwald E. Cardiac-specific troponin I levels to predict the risk of mortality in patients with acute coronary syndromes. N Engl J Med 1996; 335:1342–1349.

30. Betriu A, Heras M, Cohen M, Fuster V. Unstable angina: outcome according to clinical presentation. J Am Coll Cardiol 1992;19:1659–1663.

31. Calvin JE, Klein LW, Van den Berg BJ, Meyer P, Condon JV, Snell RJ, Ramirez-Morgen LM, Parrillo J. Risk stratification in unstable angina: prospective validation of the Braunwald classification. JAMA 1995;273:136–141.

32. Woodlief LH, Lee KL, Califf RM. for the GUSTO IIa Investigators. Validation of a mortality model in 1384 patients with acute myocardial infarction. Circulation 1995;92(suppl I):I–776.

33. Selker HP, Griffith JL, D'Agostino R. A tool for judging coronary care unit admission appropriateness, valid for both real-time and retrospective use. A time-insensitive predictive instrument (TIPI) for acute cardiac ischemia: a multicenter study. Med Care 1991;29:610–627.

34. Goldman L, Cook EF, Brand DA, Lee TH, Rouan GW, Weisberg MC, Acampora D, Stasiulewicz C, Walshon J, Terranova G. A computer protocol to predict myocardial infarction in emergency department patients with chest pain. N Engl J Med 1988;318:797–803.

35. Rouan GW, Lee TH, Cook EF, Brand DA, Weisberg MC, Goldman L. Clinical characteristics and outcome of acute myocardial infarction in patients with initially normal or nonspecific electrocardiograms. A report from the Multicenter Chest Pain Study. Am J Cardiol 1989;64: 1087–1092.

36. Hamm CW, Ravkilde J, Gerhardt W, Jorgensen P, Peheim E, Ljungdahl L, Goldmann B, Katus H. The prognostic value of serum troponin T in unstable angina. N Engl J Med 1992; 327:146–150.

37. Ravkilde J, Horder M, Gerhardt W, Ljungdahl L, Pettersson T, Tryding N, Moller BH, Hamfelt A, Graven T, Asberg A. Diagnostic performance and prognostic value of serum troponin T in suspected acute myocardial infarction. Scand J Clin Lab Invest 1993;53:677–685.

38. Seino Y, Tomita Y, Takano T, Hayakawa H. Early identification of cardiac events with serum troponin T in patients with unstable angina. Lancet 1993;342:1236–1237.

39. Burlina A, Zaninotto M, Secchiero S, Rubin D, Accorsi F. Troponin T as a marker of ischemic myocardial injury. Clin Biochem 1994;27:113–121.

40. Ravkilde J, Nissen H, Horder M, Thygesen K. Independent prognostic value of serum creatine kinase isoenzyme MB mass, cardiac troponin T and myosin light chain levels in suspected acute myocardial infarction. Analysis of 28 months of follow-up in 196 patients. J Am Coll Cardiol 1995;25:574–581.

41. Stubbs P, Collinson P, Moseley D, Greenwood T, Noble M. Prospective study of the role of cardiac troponin T in patients admitted with unstable angina. Br Med J 1996;313:262–264.

42. Wu AHB, Lane P. Metaanalysis in clinical chemistry: validation of cardiac troponin T as a marker for ischemic heart diseases. Clin Chem 1995;41:1228–1233.

43. Olatidoye AG, Wu AH, Feng YJ, Waters D. Prognostic role of troponin T vs. troponin I in unstable angina pectoris for cardiac events with meta-analysis comparing published studies. Am J Cardiol 1998;81:1405–1410.

44. Ottani F, Galvani M, Nicolini FA, Ferrini D, Pozzati A, Di Pasquale G, Jaffe A. Elevated cardiac troponin levels predict the risk of adverse outcome in patients with acute coronary syndromes. Am Heart J 2000;140:917–927.

45. Heidenreich PA, Alloggiamento T, Melsop K, McDonald KM, Go AS, Hlatky M. The prognostic value of troponin in patients with non-ST elevation acute coronary syndromes: a meta-analysis. J Am Coll Cardiol 2001;38:478–485.

46. Christenson RH, Duh SH, Newby LK, Ohman EM, Califf RM, Granger CB, Peck S, Pieper KS, Armstrong PW, Katus HA, Topol EJ. for the GUSTO-IIa Investigators. Cardiac troponin T and cardiac troponin I: relative values in short-term risk stratification of patients with acute coronary syndromes. Clin Chem 1998;44:494–501.

47. Lindahl B, Venge P, Wallcntin L. for the FRISC Study Group. Relation between troponin T and the risk of subsequent cardiac events in unstable coronary artery disease. Circulation 1996; 93:1651–1657.

48. Antman EM, Cohen M, Bernink PJLM, McCabe CH, Horacek T, Papuchis G, Mautner B, Corbalan R, Radley D, Braunwald E. The TIMI risk score for unstable angina/non-ST elevation MI: a method for prognostication and therapeutic decision making. JAMA 2000;284:835–842.

49. Boersma E, Pieper KS, Steyerberg EW, Wilcox RG, Chang W-C, Lee KL, Akkerhuis M, Harrington RA, Deckers JW, Armstrong PW, Lincoff AM, Califf RM, Topol EJ, Simoons ML. for the PURSUIT Investigators. Circulation 2000;101:2557–2567.

50. Aviles RJ, Askari AT, Lindahl B, Wallentin L, Jia G, Ohman EM, Mahaffey KW, Newby LK, Califf RM, Topol EJ, Simoons ML, Lauer M. Troponin T levels in patients with acute coronary syndromes, with or without renal dysfunction. N Engl J Med 2002;346:2047–2052.

51. Rao SV, Ohman EM, Granger CB, Armstrong PW, Gibler WB, Christenson RH, McNulty SE, Stebbins A, Hasselblad V, Newby L. Prognostic value of isolated troponin elevation across the spectrum of chest pain syndromes. Am J Cardiol 2003;91:936–940.

52. Newby LK, Peterson ED, Chen A, Harrington RA, Pollack CV, Hoekstra JW, Christenson RH, Jesse RL, Gibler WB, Ohman EM, Roe M. Clinical implications of discordant creatine kinase-MB and troponin results in patients with acute coronary syndromes. J Am Coll Cardiol 2004;43:306A.

53. Lindahl B, Venge P, Wallentin L. for the Fragmin in Unstable Coronary Artery Disease (FRISC) Study Group. Troponin T identifies patients with unstable coronary artery disease who benefit from long-term anti-thrombotic protection. J Am Coll Cardiol 1997;29:43–48.

54. Morrow DA, Antman EM, Tanasijevic M, Rifai N, de Lemos JA, McCabe CH, Cannon CP, Braunwald E. Cardiac troponin I for the stratification for early outcomes and the efficacy of enoxaparin in unstable angina: a TIMI-11B substudy. J Am Coll Cardiol 2000;36:1812–1817.

55. Kong DF, Califf RM, Miller DP, Moliterno DJ, White HD, Harrington RA, Tcheng JE, Lincoff AM, Hasselblad V, Topol E. Clinical outcomes of therapeutic agents that block the platelet glycoprotein IIb/IIIa integrin in ischemic heart disease. Circulation 1998;98:2829–2835.

56. Januzzi JL, Hahn SS, Chae CU, Giugliano R, Lewandrowski K, Theroux P, Jang I. Effects of tirofiban plus heparin vs. heparin alone on troponin I levels in patients with acute coronary syndromes. Am JCardiol 2000;86:713–717.

57. Heeschen C, Hamm CW, Goldmann B, Deu A, Langenbrink L, White HD. for the PRISM Study Investigators. Troponin concentrations for stratification of patients with acute coronary syndromes in relation to therapeutic efficacy of tirofiban. Lancet 1999;354:1757–1762.

58. The CAPTURE Investigators. Randomised placebo-controlled trial of abciximab before and during coronary intervention in refractory unstable angina: the CAPTURE study. Lancet 1997; 349:1429–1435.

59. Hamm CW, Heeschen C, Goldmann B, Vahanian A, Adgey J, Miguel CM, Rutsch W, Berger J, Kootstra J, Simoons M. Benefit of abciximab in patients with refractory unstable angina in relation to serum troponin T levels. N Engl J Med 1999;340:1623–1629.

60. Heeschen C, van den brand MJ, Hamm CW, Simoons ML. for the CAPTURE Investigators. Angiographic findings in patients with refractory unstable angina according to troponin T status. Circulation 1999;104:1509–1514.

61. Newby LK, Ohman EM, Christenson RH, Moliterno DJ, Harrington RA, White HD, Armstrong PW, Van de Werf F, Pfisterer M, Hasselblad V, Califf RM, Topol E. Benefit of glycoprotein IIb/IIIa inhibition in patients with acute coronary syndromes and troponin T-positive status: the PARAGON-B troponin T substudy. Circulation 2001;103:2891–2896.

62. Boersma E, Harrington RA, Moliterno DJ, White H, Theroux P, Van de Werf F, de Torbal A, Armstrong PW, Wallentin LC, Wilcox RG, Simes J, Califf RM, Topol EJ, Simoons M. Platelet glycoprotein IIb/IIIa inhibitors in acute coronary syndromes: a meta-analysis of all major randomised clinical trials. Lancet 2002;359:189–198.

63. Wallentin L, Lagerqvist B, Husted S, Kontny F, Stahle E, Swahn E. Outcome at 1 year after an invasive compared with a non-invasive strategy in unstable coronary-artery disease: the FRISC II invasive randomised trial. Lancet 2000;356:9–16.

64. Diderholm E, Andren B, Frostfeldt G, Genberg M, Jernberg T, Lagerqvist B, Lindahl B, Venge P, Wallentin L. for the Fast Revascularisation during InStability in Coronary artery disease (FRISC II) Investigators. The prognostic and therapeutic implications of increased troponin T levels and ST depression in unstable coronary artery disease: the FRISC II invasive troponin T electrocardiogram substudy. Am Heart J 2002;143:760–767.

65. Morrow DA, Cannon CP, Rifai N, Frey MJ, Vicari R, Lakkis N, Robertson DH, Hille DA, DeLucca PT, DiBattiste PM, Demopoulos LA, Weintraub WS, Braunwald E. for the TACTICS-TIMI 18 Investigators. Ability of minor elevations of troponins I and T to predict benefit from an early invasive strategy in patients with unstable angina and non-ST elevation myocardial infarction: results from a randomized trial. JAMA 2001;286:2405–2412.

66. Braunwald E, Antman EM, Beasley JW, Califf RM, Cheitlin MD, Hochman JS, Jones RH, Kereiakes D, Kupersmith J, Levin TN, Pepine CJ, Schaeffer JW, Smith EE, Steward DE, Theroux P. ACC/AHA 2002 Guideline update for the management of patients with unstable angina and non-ST-segment elevation myocardial infarction—summary article: A report of the American College of Cardiology/American Heart Association Task Force on Practice Guidelines (Committee on Management of Patients with Unstable Angina). J Am Coll Cardiol 2002;40:1366–1374.

67. Roe MT, Peterson ED, Li Y, Harrington RA, Pollack CV, Brindis RG, Christenson RH, Smith SC, Gibler WB, Ohman E. Suboptimal adherence to the ACC.AHA non-ST elevation acute coronary syndrome practice guidelines for patients with positive troponin levels. J Am Coll Cardiol 2003;41:390A. Abstract.

68. Sabatine MS, Morrow DA, de Lemos JA, Gibson CM, Murphy SA, Rifai N, McCabe C, Antman EM, Cannon CP, Braunwald E. Multimarker approach to risk stratification in non-ST elevation acute coronary syndromes. Simultaneous assessment of troponin I, C-reactive protein, and B-type natriuretic peptide. Circulation 2002;105:1760–1763.

69. James SK, Lindahl B, Siegbahn A, Stridsberg M, Venge P, Armstrong P, Barnathan ES, Califf R, Topol EJ, Simoons ML, Wallentin L. N-terminal pro-brain natriuretic peptide and other risk markers for the separate prediction of mortality and subsequent myocardial infarction in patients with unstable coronary artery disease. A Global Utilization of Strategies to Open occluded arteries (GUSTO)-IV Substudy. Circulation 2003;108:275–281.

70. James SK, Armstrong P, Barnathan E, Califf R, Lindahl B, Siegbahn A, Simoons ML, Topol EJ, Venge P, Wallentin L. for the GUSTO-IV-ACS Investigators. Troponin and C-reactive protein have different relations to subsequent mortality and myocardial infarction after acute coronary syndrome: a GUSTO-IV substudy. J Am Coll Cardiol 2003;41:916–924.

71. Graff LG, Dallara J, Ross MA, Joseph AJ, Itzcovitz J, Andelman RP, Emerman C, Turbiner S, Espinosa JA, Severance H. Impact on the care of the emergency department chest pain patient from the Chest Pain Evaluation Registry (CHEPER) study. Am J Cardiol 1997;80: 563–568.

72. Mair J, Smidt J, Lechleitner P, Deinstl F, Puschendorf B. A decision tree for the early diagnosis of acute myocardial infarction in nontraumatic chest pain patients at hospital admission. Chest 1995;108:1502–1509.

73. Selker HP, Griffith JL, Patil S, Long WJ, D'Agostino R. A comparison of performance of mathematical predictive methods for medical diagnosis: identifying acute cardiac ischemia among emergency department patients. J Investig Med 1995;43:468–476.

74. Baxt WG, Skora J. Prospective validation of artificial neural network trained to identify acute myocardial infarction. Lancet 1996;347:12–15.

75. Newby LK, Kaplan AL, Granger BB, Sedor F, Califf RM, Ohman E. Comparison of cardiac troponin T vs. creatine kinase-MB for risk stratification in a Chest Pain Evaluation Unit. Am J Cardiol 2000;85:801–805.

76. de Fillippi CR, Parmar RJ, Potter MA, Tocchi M. Diagnostic accuracy, angiographic correlates and long-term risk stratification with the troponin T ultra sensitive rapid assay in chest pain patients at low risk for acute myocardial infarction. Eur Heart J 1998;19:N42–47.

77. Lindahl B, Andren B, Ohlsson J, Venge P, Wallentin L. for the FRISC Study Group. Risk stratification in unstable coronary artery disease. Additive value of troponin T determinations and pre-discharge exercise tests. Eur Heart J 1997;18:762–770.

78. Zolaga G. Evaluation of bedside testing options for the critical care unit. Chest 1990;97: 185S–190S.

79. Zabel KM, Granger CB, Becker RC, Bovill EG, Hirsh J, Aylward PE, Topol EJ, Califf RM. for the GUSTO Investigators. Use of bedside activated partial thromboplastin time monitor to adjust heparin dosing after thrombolysis for acute myocardial infarction: results of GUSTO-I. GlobalUtilization of Streptokinase and TPA for Occluded Coronary Arteries. Am Heart J 1998;136:868–76.

80. Downie AC, Frost PG, Fielden P, Joshi D, Dancy C. Bedside measurement of creatine kinase to guide thrombolysis on the coronary care unit. Lancet 1993;341:452–454.

81. Christenson R. Biochemical markers and the era of troponin. Maryland Medicine 2001(Suppl): 98–103.

82. Hamm CW, Goldmann BU, Heeschen C, Kreymann G, Berger J, Meinertz T. Emergency room triage of patients with acute chest pain by means of rapid testing for cardiac troponin T or troponin I. New Engl J Med 1997;337:1648–1653.

# 15

# B-Type Natriuretic Peptides in Acute Coronary Syndromes

**W. H. Wilson Tang and Gary S. Francis**
*The Cleveland Clinic Foundation*
*Cleveland, Ohio, U.S.A.*

## INTRODUCTION

The development of heart failure or left ventricular (LV) systolic dysfunction following acute coronary syndromes (ACS) remains prevalent despite major advances in the acute management of ACS. Many patients develop transient pulmonary congestion after ACS and have it resolve quickly, only to emerge years later as chronic heart failure. Patients may develop signs and symptoms of heart failure on admission ranging from mild-to-moderate symptoms to cardiogenic shock, or they may develop clinical heart failure later, sometimes years after the index event [1]. Data from several large-scale clinical trials have suggested that up to one-third of patients developed some degree of mild-to-moderate heart failure within 30 days following an acute ST-segment elevation myocardial infarction (STEMI) [2]. In the Second National Registry of Myocardial Infarction (NRMI-2), 19% of patients with acute STEMI had signs and symptoms of heart failure on admission [3]. More recently, the Global Registry of Acute Coronary Events (GRACE) registry extended these findings to the entire spectrum of ACS and demonstrated that new heart failure presentation occurred in 15% of patients with STEMI, 16% of patients with non-STEMI, and 9% of patients with unstable angina [4]. The latest data from the Valsartan in Acute Myocardial Infarction (VALIANT) Registry reported a much higher 24% incidence of postinfarction clinical heart failure and a 42% incidence of heart failure/LV systolic dysfunction in the 5,567 patients presenting with acute myocardial infarction [5]. What is more startling is that 18% patients with postinfarction LV systolic dysfunction had no overt signs and symptoms of heart failure. Recent data from the Cholesterol And Recurrent Events (CARE) trial further points out that postinfarction heart failure may occur in a time-dependent and linear pattern at a rate of 1.3% per year, with a direct consequence of a detectable interim myocardial infarction occurring in less than a quarter of postinfarction patients who subsequently develop heart failure [1]. These observations highlight the importance of a clinically silent reduction in LV function and its potential to associate with late heart failure from progressive LV remodeling at a time quite remote from the infarction. Recognition of such patients at an early point in time, prior to development of heart failure, would be a most attractive strategy to prevent heart failure. This is particularly

**309**

important now that we have therapies that reduce the progression from LV systolic dysfunction to chronic heart failure.

The majority of patients who develop postinfarction heart failure/LV systolic dysfunction continue to carry a substantially higher mortality risk. Despite improvements in the management of early in-hospital postinfarction heart failure (mortality 46% in 1975–1978 vs. 18% in 1993–1995), there remains a lack of improvement in the long-term prognosis of patients discharged with postinfarction heart failure (one-year mortality rate at 21%) [3]. However, aggressive medical strategies designed to prevent or reverse infarct-related LV remodeling require early detection. This has spurred enthusiasm for the search for biomarkers such as B-type natriuretic peptide (BNP) and N-terminal pro-BNP (NT-proBNP) in the setting of ACS to better identify patients at risk for poor outcomes, including heart failure and progressive LV remodeling.

### Brief Overview of B-Type Natriuretic Peptides

B-type natriuretic peptide and NT-proBNP belong to a family of naturally occurring hormones known as natriuretic peptides that are synthesized in cardiac myocytes. These peptides serve as the primary counter-regulatory hormones that are released in response to heightened ventricular wall stress (Figure 1). They are ''counter-regulatory'' because they promote vasodilation and, in some cases, a modest diuresis and natriuresis via activation of cyclic guanosine monophosphate (cGMP). They may also inhibit the sympathetic nervous system, aldosterone secretion, and myocardial interstitial matrix synthesis. The exact mechanism(s) responsible for regulating synthesis, release, and clearance of the 32-amino-acid peptide BNP is still unclear. The BNP gene has been located on the distal short arm of chromosome 1 [6]. The BNP mRNA is synthesized in bursts and is then transcribed into a 108-amino-acid precursor protein, proBNP, which coexists with the atrial natriuretic peptide (ANP) in the same secretory granules of myocites [7]. ProBNP is then cleaved at the time of its secretion to form BNP and its biologically inactive by-product, NT-proBNP. Unlike ANP, a long-term stimulus is general required to increase

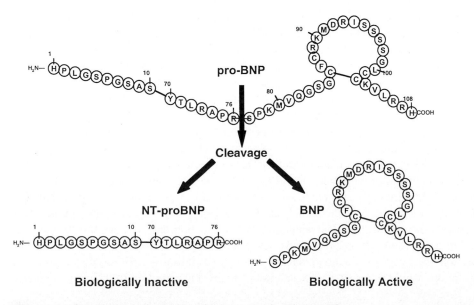

**Figure 1**    Synthesis and release of B-type natriuretic peptide.

plasma BNP concentration [8]. Upon release, BNP (but not NT-proBNP) exerts its biological effects via the A-type and B-type cGMP-mediated receptors. It is cleared by C-type receptors and neutral endopeptidases, particularly along the brush border of the kidney. It is too large a molecule to be filtered by the kidney or by dialysis, though its plasma concentrations are affected by reduced renal function.

Although BNP was discovered over 15 years ago, measurement of natriuretic hormones in the clinical setting has only recently been popularized with the availability of several commercially laboratory-based, point-of-care kits. The diagnostic utility of plasma BNP in patients with symptomatic heart failure is based on observations by several investigators [9–11], and has recently been confirmed by a large multicenter clinical trial (the Breathing-Not-Properly study) [12]. Plasma BNP or NT-proBNP in the normal range virtually exclude the diagnosis of heart failure as the cause of dyspnea. In contrast, high plasma-BNP levels are associated with the syndrome of heart failure and consistently relate to a poor prognosis [13].

As plasma BNP testing has become a routine laboratory test in the clinical setting, we are beginning to recognize the heterogeneity of plasma BNP and NT-proBNP levels as they relate to noncardiac factors such as age, gender, renal function, obesity, clinical setting, and even genetic predisposition [14–17]. Patterns of plasma BNP and NT-proBNP expression in the setting of myocardial ischemia are likely to be equally complex, and plasma levels will be influenced by multiple noncardiac factors.

## PATHOPHYSIOLOGY OF B-TYPE NATRIURETIC PEPTIDES IN MYOCARDIAL ISCHEMIA

The concept that myocardial ischemia may stimulate BNP release is supported by a number of experimental observations. In a rat coronary artery ligation model, tissue BNP concentration in both the infarcted and noninfarcted regions of the LV increased rapidly following experimental infarction. This occurred as early as 4 hours post-coronary occlusion. Myocardial tissue BNP was increased up to 5-fold by 1 day postinfarction compared with sham-operated rats [18]. The mechanism behind the increase in tissue BNP and subsequent plasma BNP or NT-proBNP are likely to be complex, but could involve the combination of hypoxia, intracellular acidosis, activation of the tissue renin-angiotensin-aldosterone system, and heightened sympathetic nervous activity [19–22]. Within the myocardium, BNP may decrease collagen synthesis (as well as diminished degradation of type I collagen) and increase matrix metalloproteinases via cGMP-protein kinase G signaling pathways, thereby inhibiting postinfarction LV remodeling [23,24].

In humans, one of the earliest manifestations of myocardial ischemia is a transient increase in LV wall tension [25]. In patients with chest pain syndromes, both plasma BNP and NT-proBNP levels are found to be significantly higher in the unstable angina group than in the atypical or stable angina groups, although it is worth noting that these concentrations are well below the conventional cutoff ranges for heart failure [26,27]. Furthermore, when plasma BNP levels are measured in patients with coronary disease during exercise-induced myocardial ischemia, patients have a significant but transient increase in plasma BNP levels. Interestingly, peak plasma BNP levels correlate well with both the size and degree of myocardial ischemia detected by thallium radionuclide imaging [28]. Direct demonstration of ischemia-related transient increase in plasma BNP levels has also been made during balloon inflation in the setting of uncomplicated percutaneous coronary intervention (PCI), even when there is unchanged intracardiac filling pressure [29,30]. Plasma BNP increases more than plasma ANP during percutaneous coronary angioplasty [30].

Are there any advantages or disadvantages between measuring plasma BNP or NT-proBNP in the ACS setting? Although several theoretical advantages have favored the use of plasma NT-proBNP measurements, including a more vigorous response to ischemia (corresponding to a greater rise in plasma levels) [31,32] and longer stability at room temperature [3,33], the two peptides appear to perform in a similar manner in several comparative postinfarction studies. Richards and colleagues studied 124 consecutive patients and sampled plasma BNP and NT-proBNP between 2–4 days postinfarction. They correlated radionuclide LV ejection fraction and plasma NT-proBNP at 2 to 4 days (r = −0.63, p < 0.0001) and 3 to 5 months (r = −0.58, p < 0.0001) after infarction and found the diagnostic performance of NT-proBNP to be comparable to that for plasma BNP. The optimal "cut-off" for detecting an LV ejection fraction of 40% or less during the first few days of admission was 145 pmol/L (equivalent to 1208 pg/mL) for NT-proBNP and 30 pmol/L (equivalent to 103 pg/mL) for BNP, with a sensitivity of 68–71% and specificity of 69%. Furthermore, both plasma BNP and NT-proBNP independently predicted LV ejection fraction and 2-year survival in a similar fashion [34]. In general, these two markers, plasma BNP and plasma NT-proBNP, behave rather similarly, even though a direct conversion has proven to be somewhat difficult.

## B-TYPE NATRIURETIC PEPTIDES IN ST-ELEVATION MYOCARDIAL INFARCTION

Several early studies have established that plasma BNP concentration increases after acute STEMI, although the pattern of elevation may differ depending on the size and extent of the infarct [35–37]. Interestingly, as with coronary angioplasty, plasma BNP concentrations do not correlate well with central filling pressures in the acute phase, but there is close correlation much later (at 4 weeks) [25]. In fact, the time course of the plasma BNP levels could be divided into two patterns: a monophasic pattern with one peak at about 16 hours after admission and a biphasic pattern with two peaks, one at 16 hours and one at 5 days after admission [25,38,39] (Figure 2). A similar biphasic profile has been observed with plasma NT-proBNP levels which peaks at 14–48 hours and again at 4–8 days postinfarction [40], There were significantly more patients with anterior infarction, symptomatic

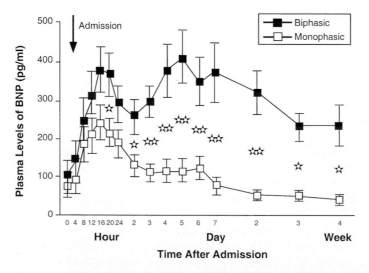

**Figure 2**  Time course of plasma BNP levels according to biphasic and monophasic patterns. *Statistically significant difference (p < 0.05). (Adapted from Ref. 25)

heart failure, higher levels of maximal creatine kinase isoenzyme (CK-MB), and lower LV ejection fraction in the biphasic group than in the monophasic group. Furthermore, several small studies have shown that higher plasma BNP or NT-proBNP correlates with both the LV ejection fraction measured during the acute phase of infarction and at 6 months, as well as predicting poorer long-term survival independent of the LV ejection fraction [36,37,40,41]. Most of the utility in measuring natriuretic peptides in ACS is in predicting the prognosis and not in aiding in the diagnosis, but changes in plasma BNP or NT-proBNP levels correspond to the time course of LV remodeling (Figure 3).

Since acute elevation of plasma BNP levels have been observed as early as 4 hours postangioplasty [29], it has been suggested that plasma BNP levels may rise even before conventional biomarkers of myocyte necrosis (cardiac troponin or CK-MB) can be detected. However, Gill and colleagues recently reported on a small cohort of patients where plasma NT-proBNP levels exhibited a greater absolute and proportional rise after acute myocardial infarction than ANP or BNP, achieving peak levels at 24 hours and remaining elevated on average for 12 weeks [32]. Since neither NT-proBNP nor BNP demonstrated significant advantages over traditional biomarkers in detecting the early phase of myocardial infarction (within the first 24 hours of admission), it is unlikely that plasma BNP will emerge as a conventional biomarker to detect myocardial necrosis at its onset. Moreover, since it rises both with angioplasty (ischemia in the absence of any measurable myocardial necrosis) and with acute myocardial infarction, it seems unlikely that a rise in plasma BNP or NT-proBNP will distinguish between myocardial necrosis and myocardial ischemia. This can explain its low predictive value in patients suffering from ACS in some reports [42].

Despite the general correlation between the degree of plasma BNP elevation and infarct size, the ability of plasma BNP to identify patients with significant myocardial damage early following acute myocardial infarction has been somewhat inconsistent. Two early small studies used a plasma BNP cut-off of 10 and 15 pmol/L (equivalent to 34 and 52 pg/mL, respectively) obtained on day 2 postinfarction and were able to distinguish between patients with impaired (LV ejection fraction < 40%) and those with preserved LV function [43,44]. However, in the Cooperative New Scandinavian Enalapril Survival Study II (CONSENSUS II) neurohormonal substudy, plasma natriuretic peptide was measured on the third day following acute myocardial infarction in 131 patients. Although there was a weak correlation between plasma BNP concentration and LV ejection fraction,

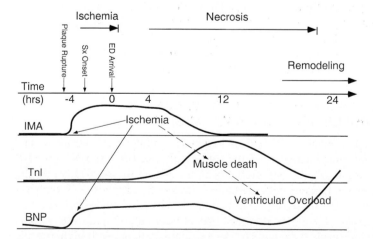

**Figure 3** Temporal relationship among markers of ischemia, necrosis, and B-type natriuretic peptide. (Adapted from Ref. 42a)

there was no clear distinction between baseline plasma BNP levels in those with LV ejection fraction of 45% or less and those with LV ejection fraction greater than 45% [41]. This limitation was also seen in long-term stable survivors of myocardial infarction as demonstrated in a West Glasgow cohort of 134 patients [45]. Plasma BNP, whether in the acute setting or in patients with chronic heart failure, provides only a very crude estimate of myocardial dysfunction. Rather, it better provides an additional prognostic factor that is associated with cardiac function. In ambiguous cases, it can help facilitate the diagnosis of heart failure, but this diagnosis remains primarily clinical. Like echocardiography, it can identify LV systolic and diastolic dysfunction, but provides no information regarding LV geometry, valvular insufficiency, or intracardiac shunts.

Bettencourt and colleagues evaluated 101 patients with acute myocardial infarction and no antecedent history of heart failure. Transthoracic echocardiography and plasma BNP measurements were performed on days 4–5 postinfarction, and there was good diagnostic accuracy of plasma BNP in detecting LV systolic and diastolic dysfunction. There was also excellent accuracy using plasma BNP for the prediction of death or the development of clinical heart failure over 12 months of follow-up [46]. These data were supported by observations from single-center studies whereby the observation was made that sustained elevation of plasma BNP and NT-proBNP levels following first transmural infarction up to 90 days is associated with evidence of progressive postinfarction LV remodeling and poorer prognosis (38,39,47–49). Using the Shionogi BNP assay at day 7 postinfarction, Nagaya and colleagues suggested that plasma BNP of 110 pg/mL or greater postinfarction identified patients who later developed myocardial remodeling (defined by an increase in indeped end-diastoluc volume (EDVI) $\geq$ 5 mL/m$^2$) with a sensitivity of 89% and a specificity of 75%; while plasma BNP less than 31 pmol/L (equivalent to 106 pg/mL) identified patients without subsequent myocardial remodeling, with a sensitivity of 75% and specificity of 78% [47]. Furthermore, a less than 25% decrease in plasma BNP from day 30 to day 90 identifies patients at risk for LV remodeling with a sensitivity of 100% and specificity of 83%. Persistence of elevated plasma BNP following acute myocardial infarction likely implies ongoing remodeling and risk for developing progressive heart failure.

In a recent analysis of the Optimal Therapy in Myocardial Infarction with the Angiotensin II Antagonist Losantan (OPTIMAAL) neurohormonal substudy, 235 patients with evidence of heart failure and/or LV systolic dysfunction following acute myocardial infarction were randomly allocated to losartan or captopril. Plasma NT-proBNP levels obtained at 3 days, 1 month and 1 year postinfarction were significantly higher in patients who died, not unexpectedly. Interestingly, follow-up (1-month or 1-year) but not baseline plasma NT-proBNP levels correlated with the total number of subsequent hospitalization days [50], reflecting the predictive power of persistently elevated plasma NT-proBNP levels in predicting clinical endpoints, such as death or heart failure progression.

## B-TYPE NATRIURETIC PEPTIDES IN NON–ST-ELEVATION MYOCARDIAL INFARCTION AND UNSTABLE ANGINA

The availability of blood samples in several multicenter, randomized controlled trials has provided valuable information regarding the role of plasma BNP and NT-proBNP measurements in predicting morbidity and mortality in the setting of non-STEMI. In the OPUS-TIMI 16 (Orbofiban in Patients with Unstable Coronary Syndromes—Thrombolysis In Myocardial Infarction 16) substudy, 2,525 patients hospitalized for ACS had blood samples obtained at a median of 40 hours after the onset of ischemic symptoms for plasma BNP assessment using the Biosite Triage assay. As expected, patients with higher levels of plasma BNP were more likely to develop congestive symptoms, had more ominous electrocardiographic changes, higher levels of CK-MB or other cardiac biomarkers, and

more renal insufficiency. Plasma BNP levels were also significantly and positively correlated with the extent of coronary atherosclerosis, and were significantly higher in patients
who ultimately died acute at 1 month and at 10 months. In particular, the 10-month
mortality increased in a stepwise fashion independent of other factors. Those patients with
plasma BNP levels greater than 80 pg/mL were more likely to die or progress to heart
failure, but did not have more recurrent nonfatal myocardial infarction (see Figure 4) [51].
These findings were validated by a case-controlled study of 681 patients enrolled in the
TIMI-11B (Thrombolysis In Myocardial Infarction 11B) study where blood samples were
obtained within 24 hours of admission for non-STEMI. Elevated plasma NT-proBNP
levels correlated with a higher risk of death 6 weeks following non-STEMI, but not with
recurrent infarction [52]. Additional data from Sahlgrenska and Uppsala Universities confirmed the association between elevated plasma NT-proBNP levels drawn at least 3 days
after hospitalization and poorer long-term prognosis for both non-STEMI and unstable

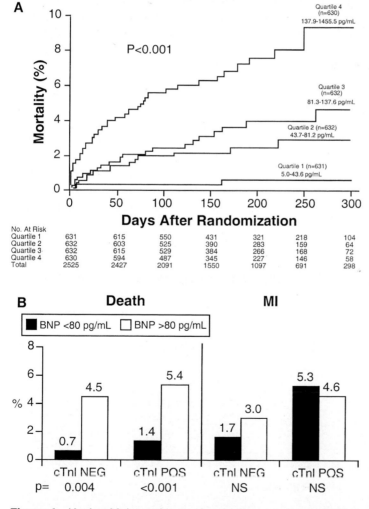

**Figure 4**   Kaplan-Meier estimate of mortality according to BNP quartiles in OPUS TIMI-16
(**A**), and risk of recurrent clinical events at 30 days stratified by baseline BNP and cardiac
troponin I levels (**B**) (Adapted from Ref. 55)

angina [53,54]. Compared with the lowest NT-proBNP quartile, patients in the second, third, and fourth quartiles had a relative risk of subsequent death over 40 months of 4.2, 10.7 and 26.6, respectively [54]. As expected, elevated plasma NT-proBNP levels remained an independent predictor of long-term mortality even when accounting for both the incidence of clinical heart failure during hospitalization and the degree of LV systolic dysfunction.

In a recent analysis of the TACTICS-TIMI 18 (Treat Angina with Aggrastat and determine Cost of Therapy with an Invasive or Conservative Strategy—Thrombolysis in Myocardial Infarction 18) trial, Morrow and colleagues measured plasma BNP levels prospectively in 1,676 patients with non-STEMI and unstable angina who were randomized to an early invasive strategy versus conservative management approach. Patients with baseline levels greater than 80 pg/mL were at higher mortality risks from as early as 7 days through 6 months of follow-up [55]. It is not unexpected that the higher the ''positive'' biomarkers, the greater the short- and long-term risks [56]. However, unlike cardiac troponin I, plasma BNP levels did not identify those patients who would more likely benefit from an early invasive strategy. Plasma BNP levels did add incremental benefit to cardiac troponin I levels in predicting morbidity and mortality postinfarction.

When the 2,019 patients with unstable coronary artery disease in the FRISC II (Fragmin and fast revascularization during instability in coronary artery disease) trial were classified into tertiles based on their NT-proBNP levels at admission, the risk ratios for two-year mortality in the upper tertile (NT-proBNP levels of > 905 ng/L in men and > 1,345 ng/L in women) were 4.1 (95% confidence interval [CI] 2.4 to 7.2) in the conservative treatment limb and 3.5 (95% CI 1.8 to 6.8) in the invasive treatment limb, as compared with patients in the lowest tertile [57]. Invasive treatment resulted in absolute mortality reductions of 3.6% (risk ratio 0.67, 95% CI 0.41 to 1.10) in the upper tertile and 0.6% (risk ratio 0.78, 95% CI 0.39 to 1.57) in the lowest and middle NT-proBNP tertiles. This association was independent of other prognostic markers such as interleukin-6 and troponin T levels. The largest mortality reduction achieved by invasive treatment (7.3% absolute) was in patients who were in the upper NT-proBNP tertile and who also had interleukin-6 levels of 5 mg/L or more. The fact that cardiac troponin T levels were not an independent

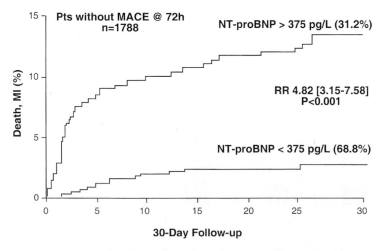

**Figure 5** Plasma NT-proBNP Levels at 72 Hours Predict Risk of 30-Day Death and Myocardial Infarction: PRISM (Adapted from Ref. 58. Presented at AHA Annual Scientific Sessions, 2002)

predictor of mortality, and that NT-proBNP and interleukin 6 were not predictors of future myocardial infarction, suggested that these biomarkers may represent different pathophysiologic processes. Recently, preliminary results from the PRISM (Platelet Receptor Inhibition in Ischemic Syndrome Management) substudy expanded this multimarker investigation to patients with unstable angina and no troponin elevation in the absence of myocardial necrosis. The PRISM investigators demonstrated that plasma levels of NT-proBNP had important prognostic predictive value. Furthermore, clinical stabilization is associated with rapid and significant reduction in plasma NT-proBNP levels, particularly when baseline plasma NT-proBNP levels are less than 400 ng/L at 72 hours. A relatively low plasma NT-proBNP may indicate a significantly better outcome at 30 days follow-up in the setting of non-STEMI (Figure 5) [58].

The largest published clinical series to date is the 6,809-patient substudy of the GUSTO-IV ACS (Global Use of Strategies To Open Occluded Coronary Arteries IV—Acute Coronary Syndrome) study, where plasma NT-proBNP levels correlated independently with age, female gender, low body weight, diabetes, renal dysfunction, history of myocardial infarction, heart failure, heart rate, ongoing myocardial damage, and time since onset of ischemia [59]. Increasing quartiles of NT-proBNP were related to increasing mortality rates of 1.8%, 3.9%, 7.7%, and 19.2% respectively. The combination of NT-proBNP and creatinine clearance provided the best prediction, with a 1-year mortality of

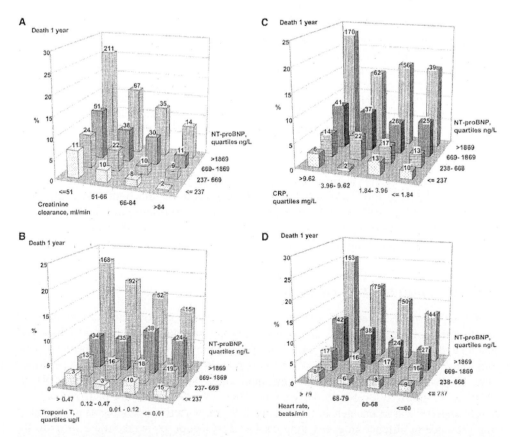

**Figure 6** Multimarker Risk Stratification in Acute Coronary Syndrome: GUSTO IV ACS Substudy. (From Ref. 59)

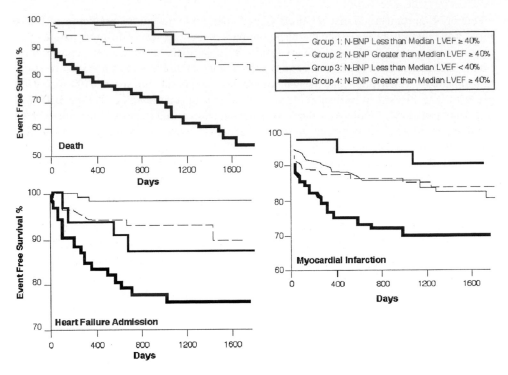

**Figure 7** Event-free survival in 666 patients with acute myocardial infarction for death (*top*), admission with heart failure (*middle*), and new myocardial infarction (*bottom*) according to combinations of plasma N-BNP above or below median levels and Lv ejection fraction < 40% or ≥ 40%. Group 1 (*fine line*): N-BNP less than median; Lv ejection fraction ≥ 40%. Group 2 (*dashed line*): N-BNP greater than median; Lv ejection fraction ≥ 40%. Group 3 (*medium line*): N-BNP less than median; Lv ejection fraction < 40%. Group 4 (*heavy line*): N-BNP greater than median; Lv ejection fraction < 40%. (Adapted from Ref. 60)

25.7% when both markers were in the top quartile (NT-proBNP > 1869 ng/L and creatinine clearance ≤ 51 mL/min) versus 0.3% with both markers in the bottom quartile (NT-proBNP ≤ 237 ng/L and creatinine clearance > 84 mL/min) (Figure 6). The combination of plasma NT-proBNP levels and LV ejection fraction at the time of admission has also been shown to predict long-term outcomes in a synergistic manner (Figure 7) [60].

## CAVEATS AND EXPERT OPINION

Although plasma BNP and NT-proBNP levels are specific for detecting compromise of cardiac performance, the added value of using baseline or sequential plasma BNP measurements to detect ischemia-specific cardiac dysfunction in the ACS setting (especially without knowledge of prior plasma BNP levels) is not proved. The majority of the published data are posthoc analyses from large-scale multicenter clinical trials using baseline plasma BNP or NT-proBNP levels to stratify patients into cohorts to compare their outcomes in a retrospective cohort manner. In these many trials, no objective assessments to determine the presence or absence of preexisting cardiac dysfunction or heart failure *prior* to the index ACS event were performed. Therefore elevated plasma BNP or NT-proBNP levels may simply reflect patients at high mortality risks irrespective of the ACS setting. Furthermore, as more and more BNP testing is performed in the clinical setting, we are also beginning to observe the very dynamic nature of plasma BNP and NT-proBNP synthesis, release, and clearance as it relates to thrombolysis and angioplasty, reperfusion, myocardial stunning, and cardiogenic shock. At present, the role of BNP in the pathophysiology of ACS remains largely unknown [61]. It may be largely epiphenomenon, a "bystander" that is associated with LV systolic dysfunction and thus prognosis. Unlike cardiac troponin, knowledge of plasma BNP or NT-proBNP values has not lead to important changes in management strategies or therapeutic choices in patients with ACS.

## CONCLUSION

We now have sufficient data regarding plasma BNP and NT-proBNP to say that these peptides are increased in patients with acute coronary syndromes, and that they have some prognostic power beyond cardiac troponin and other measures of clinical status. Nevertheless, BNP measurement is not routine but is rather more commonly used in a research setting. Most large databases are retrospectively reported on, and large prospective studies with natriuretic peptides in ACS would be a helpful step forward. As with heart failure, the regulation of synthesis, release, and activity of plasma BNP is not well understood. One should be mindful that numerous noncardiac factors, including age, gender, body weight, and renal function could influence plasma BNP and non-BNP levels. Additional studies to understand whether there is incremental value in knowing plasma BNP or NT-proBNP levels specific to the ACS setting will be necessary.

## REFERENCES

1. Lewis EF, Moye LA, Rouleau JL, Sacks FM, Arnold JM, Warnica JW, Flaker GC, Braunwald E, Pfeffer MA. Predictors of late development of heart failure in stable survivors of myocardial infarction: the CARE study. J Am Coll Cardiol; 2003;42:1446-1453.
2. Hasdai D, Topol EJ, Kilaru R, Battler A, Harrington RA, Vahanian A, Ohman EM, Granger CB, Van de Werf F, Simoons ML, O'Connor CM. Frequency, patient characteristics, and outcomes of mild-to-moderate heart failure complicating ST-segment elevation acute myocardial infarction: lessons from 4 international fibrinolytic therapy. Am Heart J; 2003;145:73-9.
3. Wu AH, Parsons L, Every NR, Bates ER. Hospital outcomes in patients presenting with congestive heart failure complicating acute myocardial infarction: A report from the Second National Registry of Myocardial Infarction (NRMI-2). J Am Coll Cardiol; 2002;40:1389-94.
4. Steg PG, Dabbous OH, Feldman LJ, Cohen-Solal A, Aumont MC, Lopez-Sendon J, Budaj A, Goldberg RJ, Klein W, Anderson FA Jr. Global Registry of Acute Coronary Events Investigators. Determinants and prognostic impact of heart failure complicating acute coronary syndromes: observations from the Global Registry of Acute Coronary Events (GRACE). Circulation; 2004;109(4):494-9.
5. Valazquez EJ, Weaver WD, Armstrong PW, Kilaru R, Diaz R, White HD, van Gilst WH, Spac J, O'Connor CM, Francis GS, Drexler H, Mareev VY, Maggioni AP, Leimberger JD, Myers M, Henis M, Califf RM. Heart failure and/or left ventricular systolic dysfunction complicating myocardial infarction is common and accounts for the majority of in-hospital myocardial infarction mortality: Results of the VALIANT Registry [Abstract 1038-71]. J Am Coll Cardiol; 2003;41;148A.
6. Cheung BMY, Kumana CR. Natriuretic peptides - relevance in cardiovascular disease. JAMA; 1998;280:1983-1984.
7. Nakamura S, Naruse M, Naruse K, Kawana M, Nishikawa T, Hosoda S, Tanaka I, Yoshimi T, Yoshihara I, Inagami T. Atrial natriuretic peptide and brain natriuretic peptide coexist in the secretory granules of human cardiac myocytes. Am J Hypertens; 1991;4:909-912.

8.   de Bold AJ, Buruneau BG, de Bold MLK. Mechanical and neuroendocrine regulation of the endocrine heart. Cardiovasc Res; 1996;31:7-18.

9.   Yamamoto K, Burnett JCJ, Jougasaki M, Nishimura RA, Bailey KR, Saito Y, Nakao K, Redfield MM. Superiority of brain natriuretic peptide as a hormonal marker of ventricular systolic and diastolic dysfunction and ventricular hypertrophy. Hypertension; 1996;28:988-994.

10.  Cheng V, Kazanagra R, Garcia A, Lenert L, Krishnaswamy P, Gardetto N, Clopton P, Maisel A. A rapid bedside test for B-type peptide predicts treatment outcomes in patients admitted for decompensated heart failure: a pilot study. J Am Coll Cardiol; 2001;37:386-391.

11.  Dao Q, Krishnaswamy P, Kazanegra R, Harrison A, Amirnovin R, Lenert L, Clopton P, Alberto J, Hlavin P, Maisel AS. Utility of B-type natriuretic peptide in the diagnosis of congestive heart failure in an urgent-care setting. J Am Coll Cardiol; 2001;37:379-85.

12.  Maisel AS, Krishnaswamy P, Nowak RM, McCord J, Hollander JE, Duc P, Omland T, Storrow AB, Abraham WT, Wu AH, Clopton P, Steg PG, Westheim A, Knudsen CW, Perez A, Kazane-gra R, Herrmann HC, McCullough PA. Rapid measurement of B-type natriuretic peptide in the emergency diagnosis of heart failure. N Engl J Med; 2002;347:161-167.

13.  Harrison A, Morrison LK, Krishnaswamy P, Kazanegra R, Clopton P, Dao Q, Hlavin P, Maisel AS. B-type natriuretic peptide predicts future cardiac events in patients presenting to the emergency department with dyspnea. Ann Emerg Med; 2002;39:131-8.

14.  Tang WH, Girod JP, Lee MJ, Starling RC, Young JB, Van Lente F, Francis GS. Plasma B-type natriuretic peptide levels in ambulatory patients with established chronic symptomatic systolic heart failure. Circulation; 2003;108:2964-7.

15.  Wang TJ, Larson MG, Levy D, Benjamin EJ, Corey D, Leip EP, Vasan RS. Heritability and genetic linkage of plasma natriuretic peptide levels. Circulation; 2003;108:13-16.

16.  Redfield MM, Rodeheffer RJ, Jacobsen SJ, Mahoney DW, Bailey KR, Burnett JCJ. Plasma brain natriuretic peptide concentration: impact of age and gender. J Am Coll Cardiol; 2002; 40:976-82.

17.  Raymond I, Groenning BA, Hildebrandt PR, Nilsson JC, Baumann M, Trawinski J, Pedersen F. The influence of age, sex and other variables on the plasma level of N-terminal pro brain natriuretic peptide in a large sample of the general population. Heart; 2003;89:745-751.

18.  Hama N, Itoh H, Shirakami G, Nakagawa O, Suga S, Ogawa Y, Masuda I, Nakanishi K, Yoshimasa T, Hashimoto Y, Yamaguchi M, Hori R, Yasue H, Nakao K. Rapid ventricular induction of brain natriuretic peptide gene expression in experimental acute myocardial infarc-tion. Circulation; 1995;92:1558-64.

19.  Toth M, Vuorinen KH, Vuolteenaho O, Hassinen IE, Uusimaa PA, Leppaluoto J, Ruskoaho H. Hypoxia stimulates release of ANP and BNP from perfused rat ventricular myocardium. Am J Physiol; 1994;266:H1572-80.

20.  Tunney TJ, Bachmann AW, Gordon RD. Response of atrial natriuretic peptide to adrenaline and noradrenaline infusion in man. Clin Exper Pharmacol Physiol; 1988;15:299-303.

21.  Tavi P, Laine M, Voutilainen S, Lehenkari P, Vuolteenaho O, Ruskoaho H, Weckstrom M. Potentiation of stretch-induced atrial natriuretic peptide secretion by intracellular acidosis. Am J Physiol; 1999;277:H405-H412.

22.  Focaccio A, Volpe M, Ambrosio G, Lembo G, Pannain S, Rubattu S, Enea I, Pignalosa S, Chiariello M. Angiotensin II directly stimulates release of atrial natriuretic factor in isolated rabbit hearts. Circulation; 1993;87:192-198.

23.  Tsuruda T, Boerrigter G, Huntley BK, Noser JA, Cataliotti A, Costello-Boerrigter LC, Chen HH, Burnett JCJ. Brain natriuretic peptide is produced in cardiac fibroblasts and induces matrix metalloproteinases. Circ Res; 2002;91:1127-34.

24.  Magga J, Puhakka M, Hietakorpi S, Punnonen K, Uusimaa P, Risteli J, Vuolteenaho O, Ruskoaho H, Peuhkurinen K. Atrial natriuretic peptide, B-type natriuretic peptide and serum collagen markers after acute myocardial infarction. J Appl Physiol; 2004; 96:1306-11.

25.  Morita E, Yasue H, Yoshimura M, Ogawa H, Jougasaki M, Matsumura T, Mukoyama M, Nakao K. Increased plasma levels of brain natriuretic peptide in patients with acute myocardial infarction. Circulation; 1993;88:82-91.

26. Kikuta K, Yasue H, Yoshimura M, Morita E, Sumida H, Kato H, Kugiyama K, Ogawa H, Okumura K, Ogawa Y, Nakao K. Increased plasma levels of B-type natriuretic peptide in patients with unstable angina. Am Heart J; 1996;132:101-7.

27. Talwar S, Squire IB, Downie PF, Davies JE, Ng LL. Plasma N terminal pro-brain natriuretic peptide and cardiotrophin 1 are raised in unstable angina. Heart; 2000;84:421-4.

28. Morimoto A, Nishikimi T, Takaki H, Okano Y, Matsuoka H, Takishita S, Kitamura K, Miyata A, Kangawa K, Matsuo H. Effect of exercise on plasma adrenomedullin and natriuretic peptide levels in myocardial infarction. Clin Exp Pharmacol Physiol; 1997;24:315-20.

29. Tateishi J, Masutani M, Ohyanagi M, Iwasaki T. Transient increase in plasma brain (B-type) natriuretic peptide after percutaneous transluminal coronary angioplasty. Clin Cardiol; 2000; 23:776-80.

30. Kyriakides ZS, Markianos M, Michalis L, Antoniadis A, Nikolaou NI, Kremastinos DT. Brain natriuretic peptide increases acutely and much more prominently than atrial natriuretic peptide during coronary angioplasty. Clin Cardiol; 2000;23:285-8.

31. Hunt PJ, Yandle TG, Nicholls MG, Richards AM, Espiner EA. The amino-terminal portion of pro-brain natriuretic peptide (Pro-BNP) circulates in human plasma. Biochem Biophys Res Commun; 1995;214:1175-1183.

32. Gill D, Seidler T, Troughton RW, Yandle TG, Frampton CM, Richards M, Lainchbury JG, Nicholls G. The vigorous response in plasma NT-BNP to acute myocardial infarction. Clin Sci (Lond); 2003; 106(2):135-9.

33. Wijbenga JAM, Balk AH, Boomsma F, Man in 't Veld AJ, Hall C. Cardiac peptides differ in their response to exercise: implications for patients with heart failure in clinical practice. Eur Heart J; 1999;20:1424-1248.

34. Richards AM, Nicholls MG, Yandle TG, Frampton C, Espiner EA, Turner JG, Buttimore RC, Lainchbury JG, Elliott JM, Ikram H, Crozier IG, Smyth DW. Plasma N-terminal pro-brain natriuretic peptide and adrenomedullin: new neurohormonal predictors of left ventricular function and prognosis after myocardial infarction. Circulation; 1998;97:1921-9.

35. Arakawa N, Nakawura M, Aoki H, Hiramori K. Relationship between plasma level of brain natriuretic peptide and myocardial infarct size. Cardiology; 1994;85:334-340.

36. Horio T, Shimada K, Kohno M, Yoshimura T, Kawarabayashi T, Yasunari K, Murakawa K, Yokokawa K, Ikeda M, Fukui T. Serial changes in atrial and brain natriuretic peptides in patients with acute myocardial infarction treated with early coronary angioplasty. Am Heart J; 1993;126:293-299.

37. Uusimaa P, Ruskoaho H, Vuolteenaho O, Niemela M, Lumme J, Ikaheimo M, Jounela A, Peuhkurinen K. Plasma vasoactive peptides after acute myocardial infarction in relation to left ventricular dysfunction. Int J Cardiol; 1999;69:5-14.

38. Nagaya N, Nishikimi T, Goto Y, Miyao Y, Kobayashi Y, Morii I, Daikoku S, Matsumoto T, Miyazaki S, Matsuoka H, Takishita S, Kangawa K, Matsuo H, Nonogi H. Plasma brain natriuretic peptide is a biochemical marker for the prediction of progressive ventricular remodeling after acute myocardial infarction. Am Heart J; 1998;135:21-8.

39. Crilley JG, Farrer M. Left ventricular remodelling and brain natriuretic peptide after first myocardial infarction. Heart; 2001;86:638-42.

40. Talwar S, Squire IB, Downie PF, McCullough AM, Campton MC, Davies JE, Barnett DB, Ng LL. Profile of plasma N-terminal proBNP following acute myocardial infarction. Correlation with left ventricular systolic dysfunction. Eur Heart J; 2000;21:1514-21.

41. Omland T, Aakvaag A, Bonarjee VV, Caidahl K, Lie RT, Nilsen DW, Sundsfjord JA, Dickstein K. Plasma brain natriuretic peptide as an indicator of left ventricular systolic function and long-term survival after acute myocardial infarction. Comparison with plasma atrial natriuretic peptide and N- terminal proatrial natriuretic peptide. Circulation; 1996;93:1963-9.

42. Panteghini M, Cuccia C, Bonetti G, Pagani F, Giubbini R, Bonini E. Rapid determination of brain natriuretic peptide in patients with acute myocardial infarction. Clin Chem Lab Med; 2003;41:164-168.

42a. Jesse RL. Neurohormonal regulation and the overlapping pathology between heart failure and acute coronary syndrome. Rev Cardiovasc Med 2003;4(Suppl.4):529–36.

43. Motwani JG, McAlpine H, Kennedy N, Struthers AD. Plasma brain natriuretic peptide as an indicator for angiotensin- converting-enzyme inhibition after myocardial infarction. Lancet; 1993;341:1109-13.

44. Choy AM, Darbar D, Lang CC, Pringle TH, McNeill GP, Kennedy NS, Struthers AD. Detection of left ventricular dysfunction after acute myocardial infarction: comparison of clinical, echocardiographic, and neurohormonal methods. Br Heart J; 1994;72:16-22.

45. McClure SJ, Caruana L, Davie AP, Goldthorp S, McMurray JJ. Cohort study of plasma natriuretic peptides for identifying left ventricular systolic dysfunction in primary care. BMJ; 1998; 317:516-519.

46. Bettencourt P, Ferreira A, Pardal-Oliveira N, Pereira M, Queiros C, Araujo V, Cerqueira-Gomes M, Maciel MJ. Clinical significance of brain natriuretic peptide in patients with postmyocardial infarction. Clin Cardiol; 2000;23:921-7.

47. Nagaya N, Goto Y, Nishikimi T, Uematsu M, Miyao Y, Kobayashi Y, Miyazaki S, Hamada S, Kuribayashi S, Takamiya M, Matsuo H, Kangawa K, Nonogi H. Sustained elevation of plasma brain natriuretic peptide levels associated with progressive ventricular remodelling after acute myocardial infarction. Clin Sci (Lond); 1999;96:129-36.

48. Nilsson JC, Groenning BA, Nielsen G, Fritz-Hansen T, Trawinski J, Hildebrandt PR, Jensen GB, Larsson HB, Sondergaard L. Left ventricular remodeling in the first year after acute myocardial infarction and the predictive value of N-terminal pro brain natriuretic peptide. Am Heart J; 2002;143:696-702.

49. Yoshitomi Y, Nishikimi T, Kojima S, Kuramochi M, Takishita S, Kangawa K, Matsuo H. Plasma natriuretic peptides as indicators of left ventricular remodeling after myocardial infarction. Int J Cardiol; 1998;64:153-160.

50. Orn S, Manhenke C, Squire IB, Aarsland T, Kristianson K, Dickstein K. Subacute elevated N-BNP consistently predicts increased mortality and morbidity following complicated acute myocardial infarction, an OPTIMAAL substudy [Abstract 486]. Eur J Heart Fail Suppl; 2003; 2:97.

51. de Lemos JA, Morrow DA, Bentley JH, Omland T, Sabatine MS, McCabe CH, Hall C, Cannon CP, Braunwald E. The prognostic value of B-type natriuretic peptide in patients with acute coronary syndromes. N Engl J Med; 2001;345:1014-21.

52. Omland T, de Lemos JA, Morrow DA, Antman EM, Cannon CP, Hall C, Braunwald E. Prognostic value of N-terminal pro-atrial and pro-brain natriuretic peptide in patients with acute coronary syndromes. Am J Cardiol; 2002;89:463-465.

53. Omland T, Persson A, Ng L, O'Brien R, Karlsson T, Herlitz J, Hartford M, Caidahl K. N-terminal pro-B-type natriuretic peptide and long-term mortality in acute coronary syndromes. Circulation; 2002;106:2913-8.

54. Jernberg T, Stridsberg M, Venge P, Lindahl B. N-terminal pro brain natriuretic peptide on admission for early risk stratification of patients with chest pain and no ST-segment elevation. J Am Coll Cardiol; 2002;40:437-445.

55. Morrow DA, de Lemos JA, Sabatine MS, Murphy SA, Demopoulos LA, DiBattiste PM, McCabe CH, Gibson CM, Cannon CP, Braunwald E. Evaluation of B-type natriuretic peptide for risk assessment in unstable angina/non-ST-elevation myocardial infarction: B-type natriuretic peptide and prognosis in TACTICS-TIMI 18. J Am Coll Cardiol; 2003;41:1264-72.

56. Sabatine MS, Morrow DA, de Lemos JA, Gibson CM, Murphy SA, Rifai N, McCabe CH, Antman EM, Cannon CP, Braunwald E. Multimarker approach to risk stratification in non-ST elevation acute coronary syndromes. Simultaneous assessment of troponin I, C-reactive protein, and B-type natriuretic peptide. Circulation; 2002;105:1760-3.

57. Jernberg T, Lindahl B, Siegbahn A, Andren B, Frostfeldt G, Lagerqvist B, Stridsberg M, Venge P, Wallentin L. N-terminal pro-brain natriuretic peptide in relation to inflammation, myocardial necrosis, and the effect of an invasive strategy in unstable coronary artery disease. J Am Coll Cardiol; 2003;42:1909-1916.

58. Heeschen C, Hamm CW, Mitrovic V, White HD. Prognostic value of B-type natriuretic peptide in patients with acute coronary syndromes [Abstract #2036]. Eur Heart J; 2002;:Abstr Suppl.

59. James SK, Lindahl B, Siegbahn A, Stridsberg M, Venge P, Armstrong P, Barnathan ES, Califf R, Topol EJ, Simoons ML, Wallentin L. N-terminal pro-brain natriuretic peptide and other risk markers for the separate prediction of mortality and subsequent myocardial infarction in

patients with unstable coronary artery disease: a Global Utilization of Strategies To Open occluded arteries (GUSTO)-IV substudy. Circulation; 2003;108:275-281.

60.  Richards AM, Nicholls MG, Espiner EA, Lainchbury JG, Troughton RW, Elliott J, Frampton C, Turner J, Crozier IG, Yandle TG. B-type natriuretic peptides and ejection fraction for prognosis after myocardial infarction. Circulation; 2003;107:2786-92.

61.  D'Souza SP, Baxter GFB Type natriuretic peptide: a good omen in myocardial ischaemia?. Heart; 2003;89:707-709.

# 16
## Inflammatory Markers in Acute Coronary Syndromes

**Mehdi H. Shishehbor and Stanley L. Hazen**
*The Cleveland Clinic Foundation*
*Cleveland, Ohio, U.S.A.*

## INTRODUCTION

Inflammation is a critical participant in all aspects of the cardiovascular disease process, spanning from generation of the first foam cell and atherosclerotic lesion, to development of the vulnerable plaque and consequent fissuring, rupture, and thrombosis [1,2]. The assumption that high-grade coronary artery stenoses are the cause of most acute coronary events has now been challenged from pathologic, invasive, and noninvasive techniques showing that most coronary events occur in lesions that obstruct less than 50% of the coronary lumen [3–6]. It is now clear that patients presenting with unstable angina have diffuse coronary inflammation regardless of the site of culprit lesion, indicating that patients with acute coronary syndromes have a heightened degree of systemic inflammation [7]. With the recognition that adverse coronary events predominantly arise from inflamed vulnerable plaque, and not flow-limiting stenoses, research has shifted focus to the role of inflammatory processes and molecular markers that serve to monitor these pathways. Biomarkers such as the acute phase reactant C-reactive protein (CRP), and more recently soluble CD40 ligand (sCD40L) and myeloperoxidase (MPO), are gaining in recognition as potential prognostic and diagnostic tools to detect "vulnerable patients" with "vulnerable plaques." The prognostic and diagnostic role of these and other novel inflammatory markers in acute coronary syndromes, and atherosclerotic risks, will be reviewed in this chapter.

## CRITICAL ROLE OF INFLAMMATION IN ATHEROSCLEROTIC DISEASE: FROM FATTY STREAK TO COMPLEX ATHEROSCLEROTIC PLAQUE

The initial step in atherosclerosis involves the formation of fatty streak. Modification of low-density lipoprotein (LDL) by chemical and oxidative processes, such as via enzymatic catalysts for initiation of lipid peroxidation like myeloperoxidase (MPO) and lipoxygenases, are believed to play a critical enabling role in the setting of hyperlipidemia [8–11]. Bioactive lipid oxidation products initiate and amplify the inflammatory milieu, inducing upregulation of endothelial and vascular cell adhesion molecules, chemotactic proteins, and other proinflammatory cytokines and chemokines [12,13]. Monocyte recruitment and diapedesis into arterial subendothelial space further fuels the inflammatory atherosclerotic process, including through differentiation into scavenger receptor-bearing macrophages, capable of taking up modified LDL leading to foam cell and lipid-laden atherosclerotic plaque formation [14]. Concomitant smooth muscle cell migration, proliferation, and elaboration of further inflammatory signaling molecules occurs, along with fibrous cap formation through synthesis of extracellular matrix proteins such as collagen and elastin [15].

A number of other inflammatory cells play a role in plaque progression. Lymphocytes, like monocytes, adhere to endothelial adhesion molecules and enter the subendothelial space. Once in the subendothelial space, they interact with monocytes/macrophages through sCD40L and its receptor, CD40. This interaction leads to production of mediators such as tissue factor and matrix metalloproteinases (MMPs), which play a significant role in plaque remodeling, thinning, rupture, and thrombosis [16,17]. Further, T cell lymphocytes in the subendothelial space encounter a number of antigens such as heat shock proteins, bacterial and viral antigens, and neoantigens on oxidized lipids and lipoproteins. These interactions can lead to further release of cytokines such as interferon-$\gamma$ (IFN-$\gamma$), which may play a significant role in plaque progression and rupture [18–21]. Thus, a constellation of inflammatory cell types, signaling molecules and oxidation/inflammatory pathways contribute to the genesis and evolution of the complex atherosclerotic plaque.

## INFLAMMATION AND VULNERABLE PLAQUE

The most widely studied, and mechanistically proven hypothesis for vulnerable plaque is rupture of fibrous cap and exposure of tissue factor to coagulation factors. The vulnerable plaque is a biologically active environment where inflammatory, immune, and smooth muscle cells interact with each other to generate a number of inflammatory cytokines and chemokines [22]. In addition to the generation of matrix proteins, smooth muscle cells and macrophages elaborate proteases such as collagense, gelatinases, and MMPs, which can break down collagen and elastin leading to weakening of fibrous cap [22,23]. This process is further propagated by other inflammatory elements such as MPO-generated oxidants that activate latent MMPs and other protease cascades [24–26]. Eventually, this process leads to thinning, fissuring, and instability of the fibrous cap, rendering it susceptible to rupture.

## INFLAMMATORY MARKERS AND ACUTE CORONARY SYNDROMES

### C-Reactive Protein

*Background*

C-reactive protein (CRP) is an acute phase reactant. First recognized during the acute phase of pneumococcal pneumonia [27], it is released from hepatocytes in response to acute and chronic inflammation [28]. Cytokines like IL-6 produced in response to inflammation lead to hepatic production of acute phase proteins such as CRP, serum amyloid A (SAA), ceruloplasmin, and fibrinogen. In addition to its function in innate host defense, CRP may worsen tissue damage by inducing release of inflammatory cytokines and tissue factor from monocytes [29 31]. Paradoxically, CRP may also attenuate inflammatory responses by diminishing accumulation of neutrophils at sites of inflammation and by reducing neutrophil adhesion to the endothelium [32]. CRP may also be involved in clearance of apoptotic cells by enhancing their uptake by macrophages [33]. Thus, CRP has both apparent pro- and anti-inflammatory actions.

While CRP clearly serves as a measure of inflammation [34], its role as a potential participant in atherothrombosis is less clear [35,36]. Some of the functions of CRP in innate host defenses have potential proatherogenic properties. In vitro studies demonstrate CRP can activate complement [37], enhance T-cell-mediated endothelial cell destruction [38,39], induce expression of adhesion molecules [38], stimulate macrophages to produce tissue factor [40], attenuate nitric oxide production [41,42], increases plasminogen activator inhibitor-1 expression and activity in human endothelial cells [43], upregulate angiotensin 1 receptor in vascular smooth muscle, inhibit angiogenesis, and promote intima-medial thickening in children [44]. Whether CRP functions to modulate processes within the atherosclerotic process remains unknown.

## CRP and Acute Coronary Syndromes

A substantial body of evidence supports the role of CRP as a risk factor for cardiovascular disease. Its clinical utility in acute cardiovascular risks, however, is less extensively studied. Increased serum levels of CRP herald worse short- and long-term prognosis in patients with unstable angina (Table 1). This association remains significant in most studies even after adjusting for traditional cardiac risk factors. For example, individuals with severe unstable angina in whom baseline CRP levels were 3 mg/L or more were at increased risk of recurrent ischemia, acute myocardial infarction, and need for revascularization procedures when compared to those with low serum CRP Levels [45]. In the thrombolysis in myocardial infarction (TIMI) 11A trial, highest mortality rates were seen in those with positive troponin and elevated CRP levels at baseline ($\geq$ 1.55 mg/dL), compared to those individuals with negative troponin and CRP less than 1.55 [46]. In the Fragmin and Fast Revascularization during Instability in Coronary Artery Disease (FRISC) trial, the prognostic value of CRP levels was analyzed by dividing the cohort into tertiles ($<$ 0.2, 0.2 to 1, and $>$ 1.0 mg/dL). The prevalence of death or nonfatal myocardial infarction at 5 months was 2.2, 3.6, and 7.5% for CRP tertiles 1, 2, and 3, respectively. After a mean follow-up of 37 months, cardiac death occurred in 16.5 percent of those with baseline third tertile CRP levels compared to only 5.7% in the first tertile [47].

In another large study of 2, 121 patients with angina (1,030 unstable, 743 stable, and 348 atypical angina), CRP levels were associated with coronary events in both stable and unstable angina [48]. In this study, a CRP value of greater than 3.0 mg/L was associated with two-fold increase in coronary events [48]. Toss et al. evaluated the prognostic value of CRP and fibrinogen in 965 patients with unstable angina or non–Q-wave myocardial infarction (MI). After 5 months, the probability of death was 7.5% in patients possessing the highest tertile for each marker compared to 2.2% in subjects with first tertile levels. After adjusting for multiple confounders, CRP levels were still predictive of death at 5 months (p = 0.012) [49]. Biasucci et al. evaluated CRP levels in 53 consecutive patients admitted to the acute coronary care unit with Braunwald class IIIB unstable angina. Blood samples were collected at baseline and after 3 months. An elevated CRP level at 3 months ($>$ 3 mg/L) was associated with 69% readmission rate for coronary instability or new MI, compared with 15% in those individuals with CRP levels less than 3 mg/L. In the same study, the prognostic value of SAA protein was similar to CRP; however, levels of fibrino-

**Table 1** Selected Studies of CRP C-Reactive Protein and Other Markers in Patients With Acute Coronary Syndromes

| Author | Patients | End Point(s) | Follow-up | Markers Examined | Results |
|---|---|---|---|---|---|
| Brennan et al., 2003 (85) | 604 patients with chest pain | MI, revascularization, or death | 30 days and 6 months | CRP, troponin T, and MPO | All markers were predictive of 30 days and 6 months major adverse cardiac events. |
| Baldus et al., 2003 (112) | 1090 patients with ACS | Death and MI | 6 months | CRP, MPO, troponin T, and sCD40L | All markers were independent predictor of risk at 6 months. |
| James et al., 2003 (53) | 6809 patients with ACS from GUSTO-IV substudy | Death and MI | 1 year | CRP, troponin T, and NT-proBNP | All markers were independently associated with 1-year mortality. |
| Sabatine et al., 2002 (54) | 450 patients with NSTEMI from OPUS-TIMI 16 and 1635 patients with NSTEMI from TACTICS-TIMI 18 | Composite of death, MI, or CHF | 30 days and 10 months | CRP, troponin I, and BNP | Additive predictive value for all markers. |
| Mueller et al., 2002 (51) | 1042 patients with non-ST-elevation acute coronary syndromes | Mortality | In hospital and 20 months | CRP | High in hospital mortality with CRP > 10mg/L. In addition, those with CRP > 10 mg/L had 4 times the risk of death at 20 months. |
| Heeschen et al., 2000 (52) | 447 patients with unstable angina | Death and MI | 6 months | CRP and troponin T | Both CRP and Troponin T were additive in predicting risk at 6 months. |
| Lindahl et al., 2000 (47) | 917 patients with unstable Coronary disease | CHD death | 37 months | CRP, fibrinogen, and troponin T | In multivariate analysis only CRP and troponin were independent predictors of risk. A CRP level > 10mg/L was additive to positive troponin in predicting outcome. |
| Biasucci et al., 1999 (50) | 53 patients with Braunwald class IIIB unstable angina | Death, MI, and Recurrent unstable angina | 1 year | CRP, SAA, Fibrinogen, | A CRP > 3mg/L was associated with recurrence of instability or new myocardial infarction. SAA had similar prognostic value as CRP. No association for fibrinogen |

| Study | Patients | Endpoint | Follow-up | Markers | Findings |
|---|---|---|---|---|---|
| Montalescot et al., 1998 (56) | 68 patients with unstable angina or non–Q-wave MI | Death, MI, revascularization, and recurrent angina | 14 days and 30 days | CRP, fibrinogen, von Willebrand factor antigen, endothelin-1, and troponin | No association between CRP and outcomes. von Willebrand factor was the only predictor of outcome. |
| Morrow et al., 1998 (46) | 437 patients with unstable angina or non–Q-wave MI | Death | 14 days | CRP and troponin T | Patients with CRP $\geq$ 1.55 and positive troponin T had the highest mortality. |
| Toss et al., 1997 (49) | 965 patients with unstable angina or non–Q-wave MI | Death and/or MI | 5 months | CRP and fibrinogen | Both CRP and fibrinogen were associated with death, however, no significant differences in the combined and point of death and/or myocardial infarction for CRP. |
| Haverkate et al., 1997 (48) | 2,121 outpatients (1,030 unstable, 743 stable, 287 atypical angina) | CHD events | 2 years | CRP and SAA | CRP > 3.6 mg/L was associated with greater than two-fold increase in outcome. No association with SAA. |
| Oltrona et al., 1997 (55) | 140 patient with unstable angina (Braunwald class IIIB) | Cardiac death MI, and revascularization | In hospital | CRP | No significant association between baseline CRP and in hospital events. |
| Liuzzo et al., 1994 (<5) | 32 patients with stable angina, 31 with severe unstable angina, and 29 with acute myocardial infarction | Cardiac death, MI, or urgent revascularization | In hospital | CRP, SAA, CK, Troponin T | A CRP level $\geq$ 0.3mg/dL and elevated SAA were associated with significant risk of in-hospital events. |

gen were not associated with clinical outcome [50]. More recently, Muller et al. evaluated the long-term prognostic value of CRP in 1,042 patients with non–ST-elevation acute coronary syndromes. After a mean follow up of 20 months, a CRP-level greater than 10 mg/L was significantly associated with long-term mortality (odds ratio = 3.8; 95% confidence level (CI) 2.3 to 6.2; <0.001) [51].

C-reactive protein also has additive predictive value to troponin and other risk factors in acute coronary syndromes. Numerous small studies (Table 1) have shown that the addition of CRP to troponin or other markers of myocardial damage, or functional impairment (e.g., brain natriuretic peptide, [BNP]) can have additive value for short- and long-term outcome. Heeschen and colleagues examined the additive predictive value of CRP and troponin in 447 patients with Braunwald class IIIB unstable angina in the Chimeric 7E3 Antiplatelet therapy in Unstable Refractory Angina (CAPTURE) trial [52]. After 6 months of follow-up, patients with negative troponin and a CRP level 10 mg/L or less had no coronary events while individuals with positive troponin and a CRP greater than 10 mg/L had a 5.3% mortality. In another study, Lindahl et al. measured CRP and troponin levels in 917 patients with unstable coronary disease in the FRISC trial [47]. These investigators also found an additive predictive value when CRP was combined with troponin.

Two recent large studies examined the additive predictive value of baseline BNP, troponin, and CRP in patients with unstable angina that were enrolled in Global Utilization of Streptokinase and Tissue Plasminogen Activator for Occluded Coronary Arteries (GUSTO-IV), Optimum Percutaneous Transluminal Coronary Angioplasty Compared with Routine Stent Strategy-Thrombolysis in Myocardial Infarction (OPUS-TIMI) 16, and Treat Angina with Aggrastat and Determine Cost of Therapy with an Invasive or Conservative Strategy-Thrombolysis in Myocardial Infarction (TACTICS-TIMI) 18 trials [53,54]. In the GUSTO-IV study of 6,809 patients, the authors showed that the addition of each marker into the logistic regression model improved prognostic value of the model for 1-year mortality. Sabatine et al. showed similar results in the OPUS-TIMI 16 trial of 450 patients, and TACTICS-TIMI 18 trial of 1,635 patients. In the TACTICS-TIMI 18 study, patients with one, two, or three elevated biomarkers had significantly higher risk of death, MI, or congestive heart failure (CHF) by 6 months (Odds ratio 2.1, 3.1, and 3.7, respectively).

Although most published studies provide evidence for an association between CRP levels and clinical outcome, it should be noted that several studies failed to show this association. Oltrono et al. studied the prognostic value of CRP in patients with Braunwald class IIIB angina using a cutoff value for CRP of 10 mg/L. No significant difference in cardiac events during hospitalization, or the incidence of ischemia at holter monitoring during the first 72 hours after hospitalization, were noted [55]. In another study, baseline and 48-hour CRP levels were measured in patients with unstable angina or non–Q-wave myocardial infarction. At 14 days there was no significant association between CRP levels (cutoff 5 mg/L) and clinical outcome [56].

*CRP and Revascularization*

C-reactive protein has also been shown to have prognostic value in patients undergoing percutaneous coronary interventions (PCI) or coronary bypass surgery. In a study by Chew et al., baseline CRP levels before PCI were predictive of death or MI at 30 days [57]. Similarly, Muller et al. showed that CRP was predictive of short- and long-term mortality in patients with acute coronary syndromes who underwent an invasive approach with coronary intervention. A CRP level greater than 10 mg/L posed a four-fold increase risk of long-term mortality [51]. Other studies have shown similar results [52,58–64]. More interesting, a number of studies have shown that patients with elevated CRP precoronary intervention get the most benefit from certain medications such as statins and clopidogrel [62,64].

*CRP and Primary Prevention*

A number of prospective epidemiological studies in individuals without known coronary artery disease (CAD) have demonstrated that CRP levels predict future cardiovascular events (Table 2) [65–81]. Interestingly, the association between CRP levels and future cardiovascular events has been independent of age, smoking, cholesterol levels, diabetes, and other major cardiac risk factors. Furthermore, CRP levels may also identify individuals at elevated global risk in whom LDL cholesterols levels are not elevated [71]. In this seminal study, CRP levels of more than 27,000 healthy American women were measured at baseline with follow-up for over a mean of eight years. CRP levels were predictive of cardiovascular events even after adjusting for Framingham risk score. In addition, CRP levels were a better predictor of cardiovascular outcome than LDL cholesterol. Lastly, the prognostic information obtained from CRP was additive to LDL cholesterol levels, strongly supporting the notion that CRP levels serve as a surrogate of a pathologically distinct mechanism from cholesterol, such as inflammation (Figure 1)

*Limitations of CRP as an Inflammatory Marker for ACS*

Many investigators have cautioned against the use of CRP as primary or secondary prevention marker [82,83]. They argue that CRP does not meet the criteria proposed by the Guide to Clinical Preventive Services and its accuracy, reliability, and likelihood of altering intervention has not been established. Furthermore, the minimal rise seen in CRP in patients with cardiovascular risk occurs readily secondary to multiple other conditions such as stress, high protein diet, minor inflammatory stimuli, and trauma. It has, thus, been argued that the predictive value seen in large observational population studies may not translate to the individual patient on a single date.

Another limitation of CRP is that it appears to fail to predict new cardiovascular events in patients that present initially with negative troponin [84]. For example, in a recent study of 604 consecutive patients presenting with chest pain, CRP was not predictive of 30-day and 6-month major cardiovascular events in patients who had negative troponin levels at presentation or were persistently troponin negative [85].

## CD40/CD40L

*Background*

Recent studies highlight a potential role of CD40 and its soluble ligand (sCD40L), in atherogenesis [86]. CD40 ligand is a trimeric, transmembrane protein that apparently participates in plaque formation [86]. Originally it was believed that CD40 and sCD40L were only expressed on the B-lymphocytes and $CD4^+$ T lymphocytes, and mediated the T cell-dependent B-cell activation and differentiation [87,88]. However, more recent studies indicate CD40 and sCD40L are present on a number of cells including vascular endothelial cells, smooth muscle cells, platelets, and other cell types. A number of pathophysiologically important events occur as the result of CD40/CD40L interaction and potentially participate in all stages of acute coronary syndromes. For example, sCD40L plays a significant role as a mediator between platelets and other cells such as endothelial cells and monocytes. This interaction leads to release of chemokines and adhesion molecules, which can further promote leukocyte recruitment to sites of vascular injury [16]. Furthermore, CD40 signaling can lead to expression of a number of proatherogenic mediators such as matrix metalloproteinases and caspase-1 [89,90].

**Table 2** Selected Studies of CRP C-Reactive Protein in Apparently Healthy Populations

| Author | Patients/Study Type | Primary End point (s) | Follow up | Results |
|---|---|---|---|---|
| Luc et al., 2003 (76) | Nested case-control study of healthy men Cases = 3178 Controls = 609 | MI | 5 yrs | After adjusting for interlukin-6, and fibrinogen, only interlukin-6 was associated with fatal CHD. |
| Ridker et al., 2002 (71) | Prospective study of 27,939 apparently healthy women | MI, ischemic stroke, coronary revascularization, or death from cardiovascular causes | 8 years | CRP was a stronger predictor of cardiovascular events than the LDL cholesterol level and it added prognostic information to Framingham risk score |
| Albert et al., 2002 (74) | Prospective, nested Case-Control study of men Cases = 97 Control = 192 | Sudden cardiac death | 17 yrs. | RR = 2.78 (1.35–5.72) for upper versus lower quartile. |
| Lowe G et al., 2001 (80) | 1,690 men in Speedwell Prospective Study | IHD | 75 months | Unadjusted 2.49 (1.44–4.30) upper versus lower tertile, however, after multivariate adjustment, it no longer was significant. |
| Pradhan et al., 2001 (79) | Nested case-control study of post menopausal women (WHI), Cases = 304 Controls = 304 | MI or death from CHD | 2.9 yrs | RR = 2.1 (1.1–4.1) upper versus lower quartile. |
| Ridker et al., 2001 (73) | Nested case-control Cases = 140 Controls = 140 | Symptomatic peripheral arterial disease | 9 yrs. | RR = 2.8 (1.3–5.9) for upper versus lower quartile. |
| Ridker et al., 2001 (72) | Prospective 5,742 participants (AFCAPS/Tex-CAPs) and West of Scotland Coronary Prevention Study | Coronary events | 5 yrs | RR = 1.7 (P = 0.01) for upper versus lower quartile. |
| Danesh et al., 2000 (66) | Nested case-control healthy men Case = 506 Control = 1025 | Fatal and nonfatal CHD | 12 yrs | RR = 2.13 (1.38–3.28) for upper third versus lower third. |
| Roivainen et al., 2000 (78) | Nested case-control study Cases = 241 Controls = 241 | MI or coronary death | 8.5 yrs | RR = 3.66 (1.97–6.81) upper versus lower quartile. |
| Packard et al., 2000 (81) | Nested case-control study Cases = 580 Control = 1160 | non-fatal MI, death from CHD, or revascularization | 6 yrs | CRP was no longer predictive of outcome after multivariate adjustment. |

| Study | Population | Endpoint | Follow-up | Result |
|---|---|---|---|---|
| Ridker et al., 2000 (70) | Prospective, nested case-control study among healthy post-menopausal women. Cases = 122 Controls = 244 | Death from CHD, nonfatal, MI, stroke, or need for coronary revascularization | 3 yrs | RR = 1.5 (1.1–2.1) for upper versus lower quartile. |
| Koenig et al., 1999 (75) | 936 men 45 to 64 years of age randomly selected | CHD | 8 yrs | RR = 1.60 (1.23–2.08) for 1 standard deviation increase in log-CRP level |
| Tracy et al., 1997 (65) | Nested case-control healthy elderly men and women, Cases = 146 Controls = 146 | Angina, MI, Death | 2.4 yrs. | RR = 2.67 (1.04–6.81) for upper quartile versus lower three for MI. |
| Ridker et al., 1997 (127) | Nested case-control study from physician's health study Cases = 543 Controls = 543 | MI, Ischemic stroke, and venous thrombosis | 8 yrs. | RR for MI = 2.9 ([?040] < 0.001) and for ischemic stroke = 1.9 (??? = 0.02) for upper versus lower quartile. |
| Kuller et al., 1996 (77) | Nested case-control study-MRFIT Cases = 246 Controls = 491 | Death, MI | 6–7 yrs MI 17 yrs death | RR (Death) = 4.3 (1.74–10.8) upper versus lower quartile. |

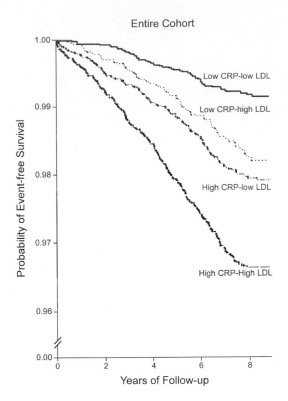

Entire Cohort

**Figure 1** Event-free survival among women with C-Reactive Protein (CRP) and LDL cholesterol levels above or below the median for the study population (From Ref. 71)

Platelets play a central role in atherothrombosis. Interestingly, 90% of the sCD40L found in plasma is thought to originate from activation of the platelets [91]. Upon activation, sCD40L is shed from the platelets and interacts with its receptor on a number of different cells. These interactions lead to release of a number of cytokines and chemokines, as shown in Figure 2. In addition, the interaction between platelets and endothelial cells through CD40–sCD40L interaction leads to increased expression of tissue factor, a potent procoagulant [92]. Hence, CD40 and its ligand are potential participants in atherothrombosis, and its serum level may have potential clinical implication.

*sCD40L and Acute Coronary Syndromes*

CD40L is a cell-associated 39-kDa protein; however, a soluble biologically active form exists (sCD40L). Aukrust et al. were first to show an association between sCD40L levels and unstable angina [93]. They analyzed soluble and membrane-bound CD40L in 29 patients with stable angina, 26 with unstable angina, and 19 controls. Patients with unstable angina had significantly higher levels of sCD40L compared to those with stable angina or controls. These studies also showed that platelets could release significant amounts of sCD40L once activated ex vivo, and that patients with unstable angina had significantly higher percentage of degranulated platelets compared to controls. In another study of 221 patients with acute coronary syndromes, sCD40L was associated with an increase risk of cardiovascular events. Compared to those with sCD40L of 5.0 μg or less per liter, individuals with sCD40L of 5.0 μg or more per liter had an adjusted hazard ratio of 2.71; 95%

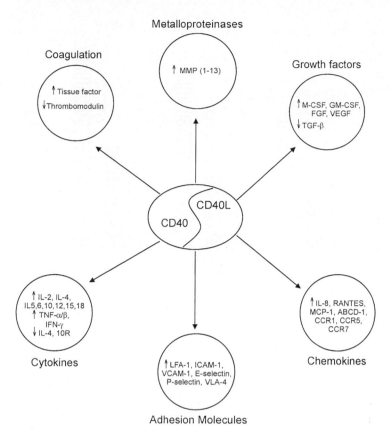

Metalloproteinases

Coagulation

Growth factors

↑ MMP (1-13)

↑ Tissue factor

↓ Thrombomodulin

↑ M-CSF, GM-CSF, FGF, VEGF

↓ TGF-β

CD40L

CD40

↑ IL-2, IL-4, IL5,6,10,12,15,18
↑ TNF-α/β, IFN-γ
↓ IL-4, 10R

Cytokines

↑ IL-8, RANTES, MCP-1, ABCD-1, CCR1, CCR5, CCR7

Chemokines

↑ LFA-1, ICAM-1, VCAM-1, E-selectin, P-selectin, VLA-4

Adhesion Molecules

**Figure 2** Potential role of CD40 and CD40L on cytokines, adhesion molecules, chemokines, growth factors, metalloproteinases, and coagulation factors (Adopted from Ref. 86)

CI 1.51 to 5.35; P = 0.001 (Figure 3) [94]. Furthermore, in this study, patients with elevated sCD40L obtained the most benefit from abciximab compared to those with low sCD40L levels. In another study, Varo et al. studied 195 patients with death, myocardial infarction, or new progressive congestive heart failure with 195 age and sex matched controls from the OPUS-TIMI 16 trial [95]. After adjusting for CRP and troponin I (cTnI), levels of sCD40L remained associated with death, myocardial infarction, and congestive heart failure. Interestingly, patients with elevations of both sCD40L and cTnI had increased risk of death, MI, or composite of death/MI/CHF compared with patients with low cTnI and sCD40L. Levels of sCD40L have also been predictive in healthy patients. In a nested case-control study by Schonbeck et al., high plasma sCD40L in healthy women was associated with increased incidence of MI, stroke, or cardiovascular death [96]. In addition, levels of sCD40L have also been shown to be elevated in hypercholestrolemic patients [97].

*Limitations of sCD40L as an Inflammatory Marker for ACS*

As noted earlier for CRP, similar limitations exist for sCD40L. As of now, sCD40L has not met the criteria set forth by the Guide to Clinical Preventive Services, and its accuracy, reliability, and likelihood of beneficial intervention has not been established. However,

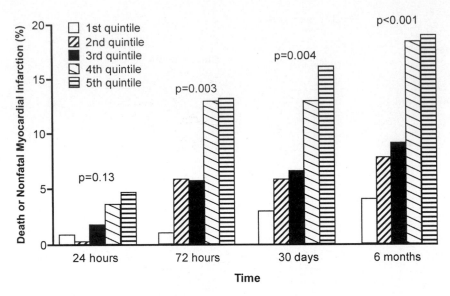

**Figure 3** Association between sCD40L levels and clinical endpoints at 24 hours, 72 hours, 30 days, and 6 months among 544 patients with ACS (From Ref. 94)

the scientific bases for its role in acute coronary syndrome is very strong and new data is emerging. Future clinical studies are indicated to assess the value of measuring sCD40L in different patient populations. Furthermore, as the availability of assays that are cost effective and standardized improves, the clinical utility of sCD40L will become clearer. Current data is insufficient to support its routine measurement in patients presenting with acute coronary syndromes.

## Myeloperoxidase and Acute Coronary Syndromes

### Background

Myeloperoxidase (MPO) is an abundant heme protein secreted from activated neutrophils and monocytes [98]. MPO is present in certain subpopulations of tissue macrophages, such as within the shoulder regions of atherosclerotic lesions, particularly those prone to undergo fissuring or plaque rupture [99,100]. Monocytes use MPO as a catalyst to oxidize LDL, rendering it into an atherogenic form [101–103]. MPO catalytically consumes nitric oxide (NO) as a substrate, leading to protein nitration and possibly contributing to endothelial dysfunction [104,105]. Furthermore, MPO-generated oxidants activate matrix metalloproteases, potentially contributing to plaque destabilization and rupture [106]. In addition, genetic studies link MPO to atherosclerosis development, since MPO deficient subjects have decreased rates of coronary artery disease, and individuals with a polymorphism linked to decreased MPO expression are protected from development of atherosclerosis as monitored by coronary angiography (odd ratio [OR] = 0.13) [107,108].

### Myeloperoxidase Mediated Oxidation Reactions

Leukocytes use MPO as part of normal host defenses against invading pathogens. MPO amplifies the oxidative potential of hydrogen peroxide by generating reactive oxidants

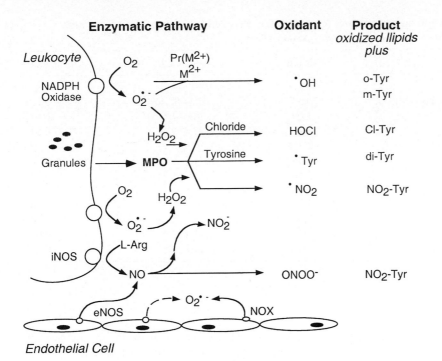

**Figure 4** Scheme of enzymatic pathways used by leukocytes and vascular wall cells for generating reactive oxidants and diffusible radical species. Each of the oxidation pathways and reactive oxidant species noted has the potential to initiate lipid peroxidation. eNOS indicates endothelial NO synthase; $H_2O_2$, hydrogen peroxide; HOCl, hypochlorous acid; iNOS, inducible NO synthase; L-Arg, L-arginine, $M^{2+}$, redox-active metal ion; $m$-Tyr, meta-tyrosine; MPO, myeloperoxidase; $\cdot NO_2$, nitrogen dioxide; $NO_2^-$, nitrite; NOX, NAD(P)H oxidase of vascular endothelial cells; $O_2$, molecular oxygen; $\cdot O_2^-$, superoxide anion; $\cdot OH$, hydroxyl radical; $ONOO^-$, peroxynitrite; $Pr(M^{2+})$, protein-bound redox-active metal ion; and $\cdot Tyr$, tyrosyl radical (From Ref. 109)

and microbicidal species such as hypochlorous acid (bleach), tyrosyl radical, and nitrogen dioxide (through oxidation of chloride, tyrosine, and the nitric oxide metabolite nitrite, respectively) (Figure 4) [103]. These reactive species oxidatively modify protein and lipid targets in diseased artery walls. Numerous oxidation products generated by MPO are enriched in human atheroma and LDL recovered from diseased arteries such as chlorotyrosine, nitrotyrosine and dityrosine [104–106]. In recent studies, MPO-generated reactive nitrogen species have been shown to promote peroxidation of endogenous lipids and conversion of LDL into atherogenic forms. Furthermore, we have shown that serum nitrotyrosine levels, a specific marker for protein modification by nitric oxide-derived oxidants, are associated with CAD presence and are modulated by statin therapy [109,110].

*Myeloperoxidase, Oxidant Stress Markers, and Acute Coronary Syndromes*

In 2001, Zhang et al. showed for the first time that MPO levels were associated with CAD as quantified by coronary angiography. Patients with established CAD (n = 158) and healthy subjects (n = 178) without significant angiographic evidence of CAD were sequentially enrolled in a study where Leukocyte-MPO levels were examined along with

**Table 3**  **Multivariate Analysis for Association Between Leukocyte-MPO Level and Angiographic Evidence of Coronary Artery Disease**

|  | Odds ratio | 95% CI | P Value |
|---|---|---|---|
| *Model 1* | | | |
| Myeloperoxidase (MPO) | 20.3 | (7.9–52.1) | <0.001 |
| Age | 1.09 | (1.06–1.12) | <0.001 |
| Diabetes | 3.4 | (1.3–9.1) | 0.01 |
| Hypertension | 1.7 | (0.9–3.1) | 0.08 |
| Smoking | 3.4 | (1.7–6.9) | <0.001 |
| WBC | 1.10 | (1.02–1.21) | 0.04 |
| *Model 2* | | | |
| Myeloperoxidase (MPO) | 15.4 | (4.6–52.0) | <0.001 |
| Framingham risk score | 1.3 | (1.1–1.4) | <0.001 |
| WBC | 1.2 | (1.1–1.4) | 0.003 |
| CRP | 2.3 | (1.8–3.5) | <0.001 |

(Adapted from Ref 107)

conventional cardiovascular disease risk factors [111]. The results of the leukocyte-MPO multivariable analyses comparing the upper vs. the lowest quartile of leukocyte-MPO are shown in Table 3. MPO levels served as strong independent predictors of CAD status with 4th quartile odds ratios ranging from 15–20, depending on the multiregression model used.

The diagnostic and prognostic value of plasma MPO levels in ACS were recently assessed in 604 conseqative patients presenting to the emergency room with chest pain [85]. Patients with MPO levels in the upper quartile compared to first quartile had significant increase in 30 days and 6 months major adverse cardiac outcomes. MPO levels at baseline were predictive of incident myocardial infarction at presentation in all patients, and even in those individuals with initial negative troponin at presentation (Figure 5).

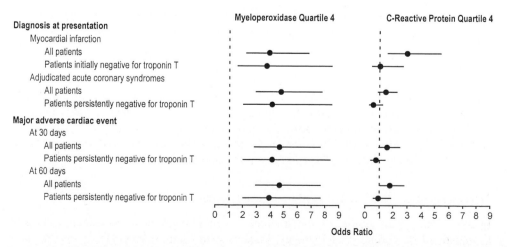

**Figure 5**  Fourth versus first quartile odds ratio and 95% confidence interval of major adverse cardiac events for myeloperoxidase and C-reactive protein levels (Adopted from Ref. 85).

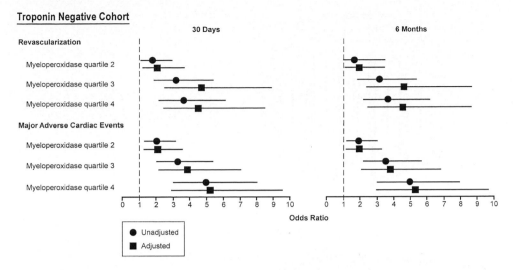

**Figure 6** Risks of revascularization and major adverse cardiac events among patients who were consistently negative for troponin T, according to base-line myeloperoxidase levels (From Ref. 85).

Within the persistantly negative troponin cohort, MPO remained predictive of cardiac risks over the ensuing 1-month and 6-month intervals, even following adjustments for traditional cardiac risk factors, CRP, electrocardiogram (EKG) changes consistent with ischemia, and history of CAD or revascularization (Figure 6). These results indicated that MPO levels may identify a group of patients with vulnerable plaque who initially present with negative troponin levels but subsequently suffer a cardiac event.

In an independent study, similar results were recently observed by Baldus et al. examining the prognostic value of serum levels of MPO in patients with acute coronary syndromes [112]. They followed 1,090 patients from the CAPTURE trial with recurrent chest pain at rest with EKG changes. The primary outcomes were death and nonfatal MI at 6 months. In this study, patients with elevated MPO levels ($> 350 \ \mu g/L$) were at significantly greater risk of death and MI (adjusted hazard ratio, 2.25; 95% CI 1.32 to 3.82; p = 0.003). More importantly, in patients with persistantly negative troponin on admission, MPO levels predicted 6 month composite endpoint of death and nonfatal MI (adjusted hazard ratio, 7.48; 95% CI 1.98 to 28.29; p = 0.001) (Figure 7) [85]. Thus, in two recent independent studies, MPO levels also had significant additive predictive value when used in conjunction with troponin levels or CRP in the setting of patients with chest pain or acute coronary syndromes. Remarkably, CRP was not a predictor of near-term risks in patients in these studies (Figure 5). Patients with elevated MPO levels benefited most from abciximab therapy compared to those with lower levels [112].

### Limitations of MPO as an Inflammatory Marker for ACS

The major limitation of MPO is its relatively new entrance into the field as a potential prognostic marker in patients with acute coronary syndromes. Despite the dramatic findings thus far with this marker, it cannot yet be recommended as a routine screening test in patients presenting with chest pain of suspected cardiac origin. The many links between

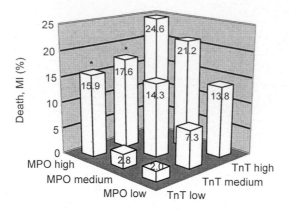

* P<0.01 versus MPO low

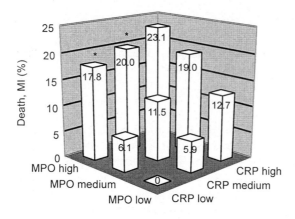

* P<0.001 versus MPO low

**Figure 7** Predictive value of myeloperoxidase for clinical endpoints according to troponin T levels (**A**) and C-reactive protein levels (**B**) (From Ref. 112).

MPO and its oxidant-generating activities and cardiovascular disease make this marker a strong candidate for future widespread use. A critical enabling step will be the development of approved diagnostic tests for MPO in clinical studies, since at present it is only available for research purposes.

## Other Potential Inflammatory Markers

A number of other inflammatory markers have been identified; however, many lack repro-ducibility, stability, and commercial availability. Fibrinogen and SAA are two acute phase reactants that have been most widely studied. To date, a number of studies have assessed the association between acute phase reactants and acute coronary syndromes [45,47,49,50,56]. However, the reults have not been consistent. For example, Liuzzo et al. assessed the association between CRP and SAA with in-hospital MI or death in patients with chronic stable angina, severe unstable angina, and acute MI [45]. In this study, elevated CRP and SAA were strong predictors of adverse outcome in patients with unstable angina. However, in a separate study by Haverkate et al., SAA was not a significant factor in predicting coronary events in 2,121 patients that were followed for 2 years [48]. Similar contradictory results have been seen with fibrinogen. For example, Toss et al. found a strong association between fibrinogen and worse clinical outcome in 965 patients with unstable angina or non–Q-wave MI [49]. However, Montalescot et al. did not find any association between fibrinogen levels and composite end point of death, MI, recurrent angina, or revascularization at 14 and 30 days in patients with unstable angina or non–Q-wave MI [56]. At the present time, the utilization of fibrinogen or SAA as an inflammatory marker in the setting of acute coronary syndromes is unclear.

A number of inflammatory cytokines (Interleukin [IL]-6 [113,114], IL-1 [114], IL-10 [115], and tumor necrosis factor [TNF-α][??] [116]) and adhesion molecules (Soluble vascular cell adhesion molecule [sVCAM-1] [117], Soluble Intracellular adhesion molecule (sICAM-1) [117–119], SE-selectin [117], sP-selectin) have also been identified as potential biomarkers in acute coronary syndrome patients. IL-6 is an inflammatory cytokine that stimulates the liver to release a number of acute phase reactants, including CRP. Although, there is a direct correlation between CRP and IL-6, Ridker et al. showed that IL-6 predicts the risk of future MI even after adjusting for CRP levels. [120]. In another study of 3,489 patients, plasma IL-6 levels ($\geq 5$ ng/L) were significantly associated with mortality. Furthermore, increased IL-6 levels identified the patients that obtained the most benefit from an invasive approach [121].

Tumor necrosis factor α (TNF-α) is also correlated with CRP. In a case control study of 272 patients from the CARE trial, individuals with elevated TNF-α were significantly at higher risk of cardiovascular death or recurrent MI [122]. Various integrins, immunoglobulins, and selectins have been suggested to possess potential clinical value independent of CRP or IL-6. In a study by Ridker et al. from the women's health study, sICAM-1 levels were predictive of cardiovascular events even after adjusting for CRP, IL-6, and other markers [70]. However, given the lack of stability and reproducibility, data on these markers of inflammation are lagging. Future sensitive assays may provide a venue to utilize these markers in the setting of acute coronary syndromes.

More recently, a number of protease related inflammatory markers such as pregnancy-associated plasma protein A (PAPP-A) have been investigated in patients with acute coronary syndromes. PAPP-A is a zinc-binding metalloproteinase which is found in both sexes [123]. Bayes-Genis et al. measured plasma levels of PAPP-A in patients with acute myocardial infarction, unstable angina, stable angina, and controls. PAPP-A was significantly higher in unstable angina or myocardial infarction patients compared to those with stable angina or controls (p < 0.001) [124]. Future studies assessing the prognostic value of PAPP-A in patients is warranted.

## CDC/AHA GUIDELINES FOR INFLAMMATORY MARKERS AND CARDIOVASCULAR DISEASE

In 2002, a workshop entitled ''CDC/AHA Workshop on Inflammatory Markers and Cardiovascular Disease: Application to Clinical and Public Health Practice'' convened in Atlanta, Georgia, to address the growing number of publications relating inflammatory markers to cardiovascular disease [125]. The goals of this workshop were to identify the best available test, define patients who should be tested, identify conditions in which the test would be useful, and implement the criteria used to define high risk. CRP was chosen as the inflammatory marker of choice at present for cardiovascular risk stratification. However, the relatively early stage of research on most alternative inflammatory markers, including their lack of commercialization as clinical diagnostics, was noted to limit their use at present. Promising new markers like MPO and sCD40L will likely herald a new era in acute cardiovascular risk stratification as further studies and commercial availability of these tests improve.

## CDC/AHA Recommended Use of Inflammatory Markers in Clinical Practice

*Indications for Measuring CRP*

Based on recent guidelines, CRP should not be measured in individuals with underlying infectious or inflammatory conditions for the purpose of risk stratification. For standardization of reporting, results of CRP assays should be reported in mg/L. In order to reduce within individual variability, it is recommended that two fasting or nonfasting assays be performed at least two weeks apart, the average of which should give a stable result. For levels greater than 10 mg/L, a search for a secondary inflammatory source should be initiated. The result of this test should then be discarded and CRP levels measured again in approximately two weeks. The following cutpoints were suggested; a CRP level of less than 1.0 mg/L is considered low risk, 1.0 to 3.0 mg/L as intermediate risk, and greater than 3.0 mg/L high risk. These cutpoints are based on the distribution of CRP in over 40,000 persons, from over 15 populations.

*Who Should be Tested*

The Writing Group endorsed the optional use of CRP in patients with 10% to 20% risk of coronary heart disease (CHD) over 10 years, the so-called intermediate risk group. The test was recommended for physicians who may need more information in order to guide their decision in regard to further diagnostic testing or therapy. According to the Writing Group, routine measurement of CRP in individuals with 10-year risk of greater than 20% would not be beneficial, since these individuals already qualify as CHD risk equivalent and require aggressive medical therapy. It is not currently recommended that treatment be guided by targeting a goal CRP level.

*Can Inflammation be Treated*

The results of Air Force/Texas Coronary Atherosclerosis Prevention Study (AFCAPS/ TexCAPS) trial of lovastatin, and the physician's Health Study of aspirin vs. placebo, both suggest that patients with elevated CRP levels gain the largest absolute risk reduction from these treatments [126,127]. However, to date, there are no randomized studies that have assessed the clinical benefit of reducing inflammation in the setting of acute coronary syndromes. Two ongoing trials, Clopidogrel for High Atherothrombotic Risk and Ischemic Stabilization, Management, and Avoidance (CHARISMA), and Justification for the Use of Statins in Primary Prevention, an Intervention Trial Evaluating Rosuvastatin (JUPI-TER), will attempt to answer some of these questions [128]. However, clinical trials that treat inflammation in the setting of acute coronary syndromes are lacking.

## CONCLUSION

The recent guidelines issued by the AHA/CDC Working Group are a dramatic advancement in the new paradigm of global risk assessment. However, despite the preponderance of basic and clinical data linking inflammation to atherogenesis, and the strong association between inflammatory markers and cardiovascular risk, randomized trials that test the arterial inflammation hypothesis, are lacking.

The field of cardiology has seen a significant shift in the past 10–15 years. We now understand that the atherosclerotic plaque is not merely a deposit of inert lipid, rather it is a biologically active complex environment [129]. It therefore seems highly probable that novel markers of inflammation and thrombosis will one day be utilized as wide-spread screening tools to identify the vulnerable patient before a coronary event occurs.

## REFERENCES

1. Lusis AJ. Atherosclerosis. Nature 2000;407(6801):233–241.
2. Libby P, Ridker PM, Maseri A. Inflammation and atherosclerosis. Circulation 2002;105(9): 1135–1143.
3. Qiao JH, Fishbein MC. The severity of coronary atherosclerosis at sites of plaque rupture with occlusive thrombosis. J Am Coll Cardiol 1991;17(5):1138–1142.
4. Giroud D, Li JM, Urban P, Meier B, Rutishauer W. Relation of the site of acute myocardial infarction to the most severe coronary arterial stenosis at prior angiography. Am J Cardiol 1992;69(8):729–732.
5. Rioufol G, Finet G, Ginon I, Andre-Fouet X, Rossi R, Vialle E, Desjoyaux E, Convert G, Huret JF, Tabib A. Multiple atherosclerotic plaque rupture in acute coronary syndrome: a three-vessel intravascular ultrasound study. Circulation 2002;106(7):804–808.
6. Burke AP, Tracy RP, Kolodgie F, Malcom GT, Zieske A, Kutys R, Pestaner J, Smialek J, Virmani R. Elevated C-reactive protein values and atherosclerosis in sudden coronary death: association with different pathologies. Circulation 2002;105(17):2019–2023.
7. Buffon A, Biasucci LM, Liuzzo G, D'Onofrio G, Crea F, Maseri A. Widespread coronary inflammation in unstable angina. N Engl J Med 2002;347(1):5–12.
8. Hazen SL. Oxidation and atherosclerosis. Free Radic Biol Med 2000;28(12):1683–1684.
9. Steinberg D, Parthasarathy S, Carew TE, Khoo JC, Witztum JL. Beyond cholesterol. Modifications of low-density lipoprotein that increase its atherogenicity. N Engl J Med 1989;320(14): 915–924.
10. Chisolm GM, Hazen SL, Fox PL, Cathcart MK. The oxidation of lipoproteins by monocytes-macrophages. Biochemical and biological mechanisms. J Biol Chem 1999;274(37): 25959–25962.
11. Chisolm GM, Steinberg D. The oxidative modification hypothesis of atherogenesis: an overview. Free Radic Biol Med 2000;28(12):1815–1826.
12. Hulthe J, Fagerberg B. Circulating oxidized LDL is associated with subclinical atherosclerosis development and inflammatory cytokines (AIR Study). Arterioscler Thromb Vasc Biol 2002; 22(7):1162–1167.
13. Huber J, Boechzelt H, Karten B, Surboeck M, Bochkov VN, Binder BR, Sattler W, Leitinger N. Oxidized cholesteryl linoleates stimulate endothelial cells to bind monocytes via the extracellular signal-regulated kinase 1/2 pathway. Arterioscler Thromb Vasc Biol 2002;22(4): 581–586.
14. Yamada Y, Doi T, Hamakubo T, Kodama T. Scavenger receptor family proteins: roles for atherosclerosis, host defence and disorders of the central nervous system. Cell Mol Life Sci 1998;54(7):628–640.
15. Ross R. Atherosclerosis—an inflammatory disease. N Engl J Med 1999;340(2):115–126.
16. Mach F, Schonbeck U, Libby P. CD40 signaling in vascular cells: a key role in atherosclerosis? Atherosclerosis 1998;137(Suppl:):S89–95.
17. Bhatt DL, Topol EJ. Scientific and therapeutic advances in antiplatelet therapy. Nat Rev Drug Discov 2003;2(1):15–28.
18. Binder CJ, Chang MK, Shaw PX, Miller YI, Hartvigsen K, Dewan A, Witztum JL. Innate and acquired immunity in atherogenesis. Nat Med 2002;8(11):1218–1226.

19. Hansson GK. Cell-mediated immunity in atherosclerosis. Curr Opin Lipidol 1997;8(5): 301–311.

20. Hansson GK, Holm J, Jonasson L. Detection of activated T lymphocytes in the human atherosclerotic plaque. Am J Pathol 1989;135(1):169–175.

21. van der Wal AC, Becker AE, van der Loos CM, Das PK. Site of intimal rupture or erosion of thrombosed coronary atherosclerotic plaques is characterized by an inflammatory process irrespective of the dominant plaque morphology. Circulation 1994;89(1):36–44.

22. Libby P. Atherosclerosis: the new view. Sci Am 2002;286(5):46–55.

23. Libby P. Current concepts of the pathogenesis of the acute coronary syndromes. Circulation 2001;104(3):365–372.

24. Fu X, Kassim SY, Parks WC, Heinecke JW. Hypochlorous acid generated by myeloperoxidase modifies adjacent tryptophan and glycine residues in the catalytic domain of matrix metalloproteinase-7 (matrilysin): an oxidative mechanism for restraining proteolytic activity during inflammation. J Biol Chem 2003;278(31):28403–28409.

25. Fu X, Kassim SY, Parks WC, Heinecke JW. Hypochlorous acid oxygenates the cysteine switch domain of pro-matrilysin (MMP-7). A mechanism for matrix metalloproteinase activation and atherosclerotic plaque rupture by myeloperoxidase. J Biol Chem 2001;276(44): 41279–41287.

26. Askari AT, Brennan ML, Zhou X, Drinko J, Morehead A, Thomas JD, Topol EJ, Hazen SL, Penn MS. Myeloperoxidase and plasminogen activator inhibitor 1 play a central role in ventricular remodeling after myocardial infarction. J Exp Med 2003;197(5):615–624.

27. Tillet WS, Francis TJ. Serologic reactions in pneumonia with a non-protein somatic fraction of pneumococcus. J Exp Med 1930;52:561.

28. Pepys MB, Hirschfield GM. C-reactive protein: a critical update. J Clin Invest 2003;111(12): 1805–1812.

29. Jones SA, Novick D, Horiuchi S, Yamamoto N, Szalai AJ, Fuller GM. C-reactive protein: a physiological activator of interleukin 6 receptor shedding. J Exp Med 1999;189(3):599–604.

30. Cermak J, Key NS, Bach RR, Balla J, Jacob HS, Vercellotti GM. C-reactive protein induces human peripheral blood monocytes to synthesize tissue factor. Blood 1993;82(2):513–520.

31. Ballou SP, Lozanski G. Induction of inflammatory cytokine release from cultured human monocytes by C-reactive protein. Cytokine 1992;4(5):361–368.

32. Zouki C, Beauchamp M, Baron C, Filep JG. Prevention of In vitro neutrophil adhesion to endothelial cells through shedding of L-selectin by C-reactive protein and peptides derived from C-reactive protein. J Clin Invest 1997;100(3):522–529.

33. Gershov D, Kim S, Brot N, Elkon KB. C-Reactive protein binds to apoptotic cells, protects the cells from assembly of the terminal complement components, and sustains an antiinflammatory innate immune response: implications for systemic autoimmunity. J Exp Med 2000; 192(9):1353–1364.

34. Shishehbor MH, Bhatt DL, Topol EJ. Using C-reactive protein to assess cardiovascular disease risk. Cleve Clin J Med 2003;70(7):634–640.

35. Keaney JF, Vita JA. The value of inflammation for predicting unstable angina. N Engl J Med 2002;347(1):55–57.

36. Mosca L. C-reactive protein—to screen or not to screen? N Engl J Med 2002;347(20): 1615–1617.

37. Mold C, Gewurz H, Du Clos TW. Regulation of complement activation by C-reactive protein. Immunopharmacology 1999;42(1–3):23–30.

38. Pasceri V, Willerson JT, Yeh ET. Direct proinflammatory effect of C-reactive protein on human endothelial cells. Circulation 2000;102(18):2165–2168.

39. Nakajima T, Schulte S, Warrington KJ, Kopecky SL, Frye RL, Goronzy JJ, Weyand CM. T-cell-mediated lysis of endothelial cells in acute coronary syndromes. Circulation 2002; 105(5):570–575.

40. Nakagomi A, Freedman SB, Geczy CL. Interferon-gamma and lipopolysaccharide potentiate monocyte tissue factor induction by C-reactive protein: relationship with age, sex, and hormone replacement treatment. Circulation 2000;101(15):1785–1791.

41. Verma S, Wang CH, Li SH, Dumont AS, Fedak PW, Badiwala MV, Dhillon B, Weisel RD, Li RK, Mickle DA, Stewart DJ. A self-fulfilling prophecy: C-reactive protein attenuates nitric oxide production and inhibits angiogenesis. Circulation 2002;106(8):913–919.

42. Venugopal SK, Devaraj S, Yuhanna I, Shaul P, Jialal I. Demonstration that C-reactive protein decreases eNOS expression and bioactivity in human aortic endothelial cells. Circulation 2002;106(12):1439–1441.

43. Devaraj S, Xu DY, Jialal I. C-reactive protein increases plasminogen activator inhibitor-1 expression and activity in human aortic endothelial cells: implications for the metabolic syndrome and atherothrombosis. Circulation 2003;107(3):398–404.

44. Jarvisalo MJ, Harmoinen A, Hakanen M, Paakkunainen U, Viikari J, Hartiala J, Lehtimaki T, Simell O, Raitakari OT. Elevated serum C-reactive protein levels and early arterial changes in healthy children. Arterioscler Thromb Vasc Biol 2002;22(8):1323–1328.

45. Liuzzo G, Biasucci LM, Gallimore JR, Grillo RL, Rebuzzi AG, Pepys MB, Maseri A. The prognostic value of C-reactive protein and serum amyloid a protein in severe unstable angina. N Engl J Med 1994;331(7):417–424.

46. Morrow DA, Rifai N, Antman EM, Weiner DL, McCabe CH, Cannon CP, Braunwald E. C-reactive protein is a potent predictor of mortality independently of and in combination with troponin T in acute coronary syndromes: a TIMI 11A substudy. Thrombolysis in Myocardial Infarction. J Am Coll Cardiol 1998;31(7):1460–1465.

47. Lindahl B, Toss H, Siegbahn A, Venge P, Wallentin L. Markers of myocardial damage and inflammation in relation to long-term mortality in unstable coronary artery disease. FRISC Study Group. Fragmin during Instability in Coronary Artery Disease. N Engl J Med 2000; 343(16):1139–1147.

48. Haverkate F, Thompson SG, Pyke SD, Gallimore JR, Pepys MB. Production of C-reactive protein and risk of coronary events in stable and unstable angina. European Concerted Action on Thrombosis and Disabilities Angina Pectoris Study Group. Lancet 1997;349(9050): 462–466.

49. Toss H, Lindahl B, Siegbahn A, Wallentin L. Prognostic influence of increased fibrinogen and C-reactive protein levels in unstable coronary artery disease. FRISC Study Group. Fragmin during Instability in Coronary Artery Disease. Circulation 1997;96(12):4204–4210.

50. Biasucci LM, Liuzzo G, Grillo RL, Caligiuri G, Rebuzzi AG, Buffon A, Summaria F, Ginnetti F, Fadda G, Maseri A. Elevated levels of C-reactive protein at discharge in patients with unstable angina predict recurrent instability. Circulation 1999;99(7):855–860.

51. Mueller C, Buettner HJ, Hodgson JM, Marsch S, Perruchoud AP, Roskamm H, Neumann FJ. Inflammation and long-term mortality after non-ST elevation acute coronary syndrome treated with a very early invasive strategy in 1042 consecutive patients. Circulation 2002; 105(12):1412–1415.

52. Heeschen C, Hamm CW, Bruemmer J, Simoons ML. Predictive value of C-reactive protein and troponin T in patients with unstable angina: a comparative analysis. CAPTURE Investigators. Chimeric c7E3 AntiPlatelet Therapy in Unstable angina REfractory to standard treatment trial. J Am Coll Cardiol 2000;35(6):1535–1542.

53. James SK, Lindahl B, Siegbahn A, Stridsberg M, Venge P, Armstrong P, Barnathan ES, Califf R, Topol EJ, Simoons ML, Wallentin L. N-terminal pro-brain natriuretic peptide and other risk markers for the separate prediction of mortality and subsequent myocardial infarction in patients with unstable coronary artery disease: a Global Utilization of Strategies To Open occluded arteries (GUSTO)-IV substudy. Circulation 2003;108(3):275–281.

54. Sabatine MS, Morrow DA, de Lemos JA, Gibson CM, Murphy SA, Rifai N, McCabe C, Antman EM, Cannon CP, Braunwald E. Multimarker approach to risk stratification in non-ST elevation acute coronary syndromes: simultaneous assessment of troponin I, C-reactive protein, and B-type natriuretic peptide. Circulation 2002;105(15):1760–1763.

55. Oltrona L, Ardissino D, Merlini PA, Spinola A, Chiodo F, Pezzano A. C-reactive protein elevation and early outcome in patients with unstable angina pectoris. Am J Cardiol 1997; 80(8):1002–1006.

56. Montalescot G, Philippe F, Ankri A, Vicaut E, Bearez E, Poulard JE, Carrie D, Flammang D, Dutoit A, Carayon A, Jardel C, Chevrot M, Bastard JP, Bigonzi F, Thomas D. Early

increase of von Willebrand factor predicts adverse outcome in unstable coronary artery disease: beneficial effects of enoxaparin. French Investigators of the ESSENCE Trial. Circulation 1998;98(4):294–299.

57. Chew DP, Bhatt DL, Robbins MA, Penn MS, Schneider JP, Lauer MS, Topol EJ, Ellis SG. Incremental prognostic value of elevated baseline C-reactive protein among established markers of risk in percutaneous coronary intervention. Circulation 2001;104(9):992–997.

58. Buffon A, Liuzzo G, Biasucci LM, Pasqualetti P, Ramazzotti V, Rebuzzi AG, Crea F, Maseri A. Preprocedural serum levels of C-reactive protein predict early complications and late restenosis after coronary angioplasty. J Am Coll Cardiol 1999;34(5):1512–1521.

59. Versaci F, Gaspardone A, Tomai F, Crea F, Chiariello L, Gioffre PA. Predictive value of C-reactive protein in patients with unstable angina pectoris undergoing coronary artery stent implantation. Am J Cardiol 2000;85(1):92–95, A98.

60. Almagor M, Keren A, Banai S. Increased C-reactive protein level after coronary stent implantation in patients with stable coronary artery disease. Am Heart J 2003;145(2):248–253.

61. Lenderink T, Boersma E, Heeschen C, Vahanian A, de Boer MJ, Umans V, van den Brand MJ, Hamm CW, Simoons ML. Elevated troponin T and C-reactive protein predict impaired outcome for 4 years in patients with refractory unstable angina, and troponin T predicts benefit of treatment with abciximab in combination with PTCA. Eur Heart J 2003;24(1): 77–85.

62. Chan AW, Bhatt DL, Chew DP, Reginelli J, Schneider JP, Topol EJ, Ellis SG. Relation of inflammation and benefit of statins after percutaneous coronary interventions. Circulation 2003;107(13):1750–1756.

63. de Winter RJ, Heyde GS, Koch KT, Fischer J, van Straalen JP, Bax M, Schotborgh CE, Mulder KJ, Sanders GT, Piek JJ, Tijssen JG. The prognostic value of pre-procedural plasma C-reactive protein in patients undergoing elective coronary angioplasty. Eur Heart J 2002; 23(12):960–966.

64. Chew DP, Bhatt DL, Robbins MA, Mukherjee D, Roffi M, Schneider JP, Topol EJ, Ellis SG. Effect of clopidogrel added to aspirin before percutaneous coronary intervention on the risk associated with C-reactive protein. Am J Cardiol 2001;88(6):672–674.

65. Tracy RP, Lemaitre RN, Psaty BM, Ives DG, Evans RW, Cushman M, Meilahn EN, Kuller LH. Relationship of C-reactive protein to risk of cardiovascular disease in the elderly. Results from the Cardiovascular Health Study and the Rural Health Promotion Project. Arterioscler Thromb Vasc Biol 1997;17(6):1121–1127.

66. Danesh J, Whincup P, Walker M, Lennon L, Thomson A, Appleby P, Gallimore JR, Pepys MB. Low grade inflammation and coronary heart disease: prospective study and updated meta-analyses. BMJ 2000;321(7255):199–204.

67. Ridker PM. High-sensitivity C-reactive protein: potential adjunct for global risk assessment in the primary prevention of cardiovascular disease. Circulation 2001;103(13):1813–1818.

68. Ridker PM. Role of inflammatory biomarkers in prediction of coronary heart disease. Lancet 2001;358(9286):946–948.

69. Ridker PM, Glynn RJ, Hennekens CH. C-reactive protein adds to the predictive value of total and HDL cholesterol in determining risk of first myocardial infarction. Circulation 1998; 97(20):2007–2011.

70. Ridker PM, Hennekens CH, Buring JE, Rifai N. C-reactive protein and other markers of inflammation in the prediction of cardiovascular disease in women. N Engl J Med 2000; 342(12):836–843.

71. Ridker PM, Rifai N, Rose L, Buring JE, Cook NR. Comparison of C-reactive protein and low-density lipoprotein cholesterol levels in the prediction of first cardiovascular events. N Engl J Med 2002;347(20):1557–1565.

72. Ridker PM, Rifai N, Clearfield M, Downs JR, Weis SE, Miles JS, Gotto AM. Measurement of C-reactive protein for the targeting of statin therapy in the primary prevention of acute coronary events. N Engl J Med 2001;344(26):1959–1965.

73. Ridker PM, Stampfer MJ, Rifai N. Novel risk factors for systemic atherosclerosis: a comparison of C-reactive protein, fibrinogen, homocysteine, lipoprotein(a), and standard cholesterol screening as predictors of peripheral arterial disease. JAMA 2001;285(19):2481–2485.

74. Albert CM, Ma J, Rifai N, Stampfer MJ, Ridker PM. Prospective study of C-reactive protein, homocysteine, and plasma lipid levels as predictors of sudden cardiac death. Circulation 2002;105(22):2595–2599.

75. Koenig W, Sund M, Frohlich M, Fischer HG, Lowel H, Doring A, Hutchinson WL, Pepys MB. C-Reactive protein, a sensitive marker of inflammation, predicts future risk of coronary heart disease in initially healthy middle-aged men: results from the MONICA (Monitoring Trends and Determinants in Cardiovascular Disease) Augsburg Cohort Study, 1984 to 1992. Circulation 1999;99(2):237–242.

76. Luc G, Bard JM, Juhan-Vague I, Ferrieres J, Evans A, Amouyel P, Arveiler D, Fruchart JC, Ducimetiere P. C-Reactive Protein, Interleukin-6, and Fibrinogen as Predictors of Coronary Heart Disease: The PRIME Study. Arterioscler Thromb Vasc Biol 2003;23(7):1255–1261.

77. Kuller LH, Tracy RP, Shaten J, Meilahn EN. Relation of C-reactive protein and coronary heart disease in the MRFIT nested case-control study. Multiple Risk Factor Intervention Trial. Am J Epidemiol 1996;144(6):537–547.

78. Roivainen M, Viik-Kajander M, Palosuo T, Toivanen P, Leinonen M, Saikku P, Tenkanen L, Manninen V, Hovi T, Manttari M. Infections, inflammation, and the risk of coronary heart disease. Circulation 2000;101(3):252–257.

79. Pradhan AD, Manson JE, Rifai N, Buring JE, Ridker PM. C-reactive protein, interleukin 6, and risk of developing type 2 diabetes mellitus. JAMA 2001;286(3):327–334.

80. Lowe GD, Yarnell JW, Rumley A, Bainton D, Sweetnam PM. C-reactive protein, fibrin D-dimer, and incident ischemic heart disease in the Speedwell study: are inflammation and fibrin turnover linked in pathogenesis? Arterioscler Thromb Vasc Biol 2001;21(4):603–610.

81. Packard CJ, O'Reilly DS, Caslake MJ, McMahon AD, Ford I, Cooney J, Macphee CH, Suckling KE, Krishna M, Wilkinson FE, Rumley A, Lowe GD. Lipoprotein-associated phospholipase A2 as an independent predictor of coronary heart disease. West of Scotland Coronary Prevention Study Group. N Engl J Med 2000;343(16):1148–1155.

82. Kushner I, Sehgal AR. Is high-sensitivity C-reactive protein an effective screening test for cardiovascular risk? Arch Intern Med 2002;162(8):867–869.

83. Levinson SS, Elin RJ. What is C-reactive protein telling us about coronary artery disease? Arch Intern Med 2002;162(4):389–392.

84. Biasucci LM, Liuzzo G, Colizzi C, Rizzello V. Clinical use of C-reactive protein for the prognostic stratification of patients with ischemic heart disease. Ital Heart J 2001;2(3): 164–171.

85. Brennan ML, Penn MS, Van Lente F, Nambi V, Shishehbor MH, Aviles RJ, Goormastic M, Pepoy ML, McErlean ES, Topol EJ, Nissen SE, Hazen SL. Prognostic value of myeloperoxidase in patients with chest pain. N Engl J Med 2003;349(17):1595–1604.

86. Schonbeck U, Libby P. CD40 signaling and plaque instability. Circ Res 2001;89(12): 1092–1103.

87. Clark LB, Foy TM, Noelle RJ. CD40 and its ligand. Adv Immunol 1996;63:43–78.

88. Grewal IS, Flavell RA. CD40 and CD154 in cell-mediated immunity. Annu Rev Immunol 1998;16:111–135.

89. Celi A, Pellegrini G, Lorenzet R, De Blasi A, Ready N, Furie BC, Furie B. P-selectin induces the expression of tissue factor on monocytes. Proc Natl Acad Sci USA 1994;91(19): 8767–8771.

90. Rinder HM, Bonan JL, Rinder CS, Ault KA, Smith BR. Dynamics of leukocyte-platelet adhesion in whole blood. Blood 1991;78(7):1730–1737.

91. Henn V, Slupsky JR, Grafe M, Anagnostopoulos I, Forster R, Muller-Berghaus G, Kroczek RA. CD40 ligand on activated platelets triggers an inflammatory reaction of endothelial cells. Nature 1998;391(6667):591–594.

92. Schonbeck U, Mach F, Sukhova GK, Herman M, Graber P, Kehry MR, Libby P. CD40 ligation induces tissue factor expression in human vascular smooth muscle cells. Am J Pathol 2000;156(1):7–14.

93. Aukrust P, Muller F, Ueland T, Berget T, Aaser E, Brunsvig A, Solum NO, Forfang K, Froland SS, Gullestad L. Enhanced levels of soluble and membrane-bound CD40 ligand in

patients with unstable angina. Possible reflection of T lymphocyte and platelet involvement in the pathogenesis of acute coronary syndromes. Circulation 1999;100(6):614–620.

94. Heeschen C, Dimmeler S, Hamm CW, van den Brand MJ, Boersma E, Zeiher AM, Simoons ML. Soluble CD40 ligand in acute coronary syndromes. N Engl J Med 2003;348(12): 1104–1111.

95. Varo N, de Lemos JA, Libby P, Morrow DA, Murphy SA, Nuzzo R, Gibson CM, Cannon CP, Braunwald E, Schonbeck U. Soluble CD40L: risk prediction after acute coronary syndromes. Circulation 2003;108(9):1049–1052.

96. Schonbeck U, Varo N, Libby P, Buring J, Ridker PM. Soluble CD40L and cardiovascular risk in women. Circulation 2001;104(19):2266–2268.

97. Garlichs CD, John S, Schmeisser A, Eskafi S, Stumpf C, Karl M, Goppelt-Struebe M, Schmieder R, Daniel WG. Upregulation of CD40 and CD40 ligand (CD154) in patients with moderate hypercholesterolemia. Circulation 2001;104(20):2395–2400.

98. Brennan ML, Hazen SL. Emerging role of myeloperoxidase and oxidant stress markers in cardiovascular risk assessment. Curr Opin Lipidol 2003;14(4):353–359.

99. Daugherty A, Dunn JL, Rateri DL, Heinecke JW. Myeloperoxidase, a catalyst for lipoprotein oxidation, is expressed in human atherosclerotic lesions. J Clin Invest 1994;94(1):437–444.

100. Sugiyama S, Okada Y, Sukhova GK, Virmani R, Heinecke JW, Libby P. Macrophage myeloperoxidase regulation by granulocyte macrophage colony-stimulating factor in human atherosclerosis and implications in acute coronary syndromes. Am J Pathol 2001;158(3):879–891.

101. Podrez EA, Schmitt D, Hoff HF, Hazen SL. Myeloperoxidase-generated reactive nitrogen species convert LDL into an atherogenic form in vitro. J Clin Invest 1999;103(11):1547–1560.

102. Podrez EA, Febbraio M, Sheibani N, Schmitt D, Silverstein RL, Hajjar DP, Cohen PA, Frazier WA, Hoff HF, Hazen SL. Macrophage scavenger receptor CD36 is the major receptor for LDL modified by monocyte-generated reactive nitrogen species. J Clin Invest 2000;105(8): 1095–1108.

103. Podrez EA, Abu-Soud HM, Hazen SL. Myeloperoxidase-generated oxidants and atherosclerosis. Free Radic Biol Med 2000;28(12):1717–1725.

104. Abu-Soud HM, Hazen SL. Nitric oxide is a physiological substrate for mammalian peroxidases. J Biol Chem 2000;275(48):37524–37532.

105. Abu-Soud HM, Hazen SL. Nitric oxide modulates the catalytic activity of myeloperoxidase. J Biol Chem 2000;275(8):5425–5430.

106. Peppin GJ, Weiss SJ. Activation of the endogenous metalloproteinase, gelatinase, by triggered human neutrophils. Proc Natl Acad Sci USA 1986;83(12):4322–4326.

107. Pecoits-Filho R, Stenvinkel P, Marchlewska A, Heimburger O, Barany P, Hoff CM, Holmes CJ, Suliman M, Lindholm B, Schalling M, Nordfors L. A functional variant of the myeloperoxidase gene is associated with cardiovascular disease in end-stage renal disease patients. Kidney Int Suppl 2003(84):S172–176.

108. Nikpoor B, Turecki G, Fournier C, Theroux P, Rouleau GA. A functional myeloperoxidase polymorphic variant is associated with coronary artery disease in French-Canadians. Am Heart J 2001;142(2):336–339.

109. Shishehbor MH, Brennan ML, Aviles RJ, Fu X, Penn MS, Sprecher DL, Hazen SL. Statins promote potent systemic antioxidant effects through specific inflammatory pathways. Circulation 2003;108(4):426–431.

110. Shishehbor MH, Aviles RJ, Brennan ML, Fu X, Goormastic M, Pearce GL, Gokce N, Keaney JF, Penn MS, Sprecher DL, Vita JA, Hazen SL. Association of nitrotyrosine levels with cardiovascular disease and modulation by statin therapy. JAMA 2003;289(13):1675–1680.

111. Zhang R, Brennan ML, Fu X, Aviles RJ, Pearce GL, Penn MS, Topol EJ, Sprecher DL, Hazen SL. Association between myeloperoxidase levels and risk of coronary artery disease. JAMA 2001;286(17):2136–2142.

112. Baldus S, Heeschen C, Meinertz T, Zeiher AM, Eiserich JP, Munzel T, Simoons ML, Hamm CW. Myeloperoxidase serum levels predict risk in patients with acute coronary syndromes. Circulation 2003;108(12):1440–1445.

113. Woods A, Brull DJ, Humphries SE, Montgomery HE. Genetics of inflammation and risk of coronary artery disease: the central role of interleukin-6. Eur Heart J 2000;21(19):1574–1583.

114. Biasucci LM, Liuzzo G, Fantuzzi G, Caligiuri G, Rebuzzi AG, Ginnetti F, Dinarello CA, Maseri A. Increasing levels of interleukin (IL)-1Ra and IL-6 during the first 2 days of hospitalization in unstable angina are associated with increased risk of in-hospital coronary events. Circulation 1999;99(16):2079–2084.

115. Smith DA, Irving SD, Sheldon J, Cole D, Kaski JC. Serum levels of the antiinflammatory cytokine interleukin-10 are decreased in patients with unstable angina. Circulation 2001; 104(7):746–749.

116. Appels A. Inflammation and the mental state before an acute coronary event. Ann Med 1999; 31(Suppl):41–44.

117. Blankenberg S, Rupprecht HJ, Bickel C, Peetz D, Hafner G, Tiret L, Meyer J. Circulating cell adhesion molecules and death in patients with coronary artery disease. Circulation 2001; 104(12):1336–1342.

118. Haught WH, Mansour M, Rothlein R, Kishimoto TK, Mainolfi EA, Hendricks JB, Hendricks C, Mehta JL. Alterations in circulating intercellular adhesion molecule-1 and L-selection: further evidence for chronic inflammation in ischemic heart disease. Am Heart J 1996;132(1 Pt 1):1–8.

119. Ogawa H, Yasue H, Miyao Y, Sakamoto T, Soejima H, Nishiyama K, Kaikita K, Suefuji H, Misumi K, Takazoe K, Kugiyama K, Yoshimura M. Plasma soluble intercellular adhesion molecule-1 levels in coronary circulation in patients with unstable angina. Am J Cardiol 1999;83(1):38–42.

120. Ridker PM, Rifai N, Stampfer MJ, Hennekens CH. Plasma concentration of interleukin-6 and the risk of future myocardial infarction among apparently healthy men. Circulation 2000; 101(15):1767–1772.

121. Lindmark E, Diderholm E, Wallentin L, Siegbahn A. Relationship between interleukin 6 and mortality in patients with unstable coronary artery disease: effects of an early invasive or noninvasive strategy. JAMA 2001;286(17):2107–2113.

122. Ridker PM, Rifai N, Pfeffer M, Sacks F, Lepage S, Braunwald E. Elevation of tumor necrosis factor-alpha and increased risk of recurrent coronary events after myocardial infarction. Circulation 2000;101(18):2149–2153.

123. Lawrence JB, Oxvig C, Overgaard MT, Sottrup-Jensen L, Gleich GJ, Hays LG, Yates JR, Conover CA. The insulin-like growth factor (IGF)-dependent IGF binding protein-4 protease secreted by human fibroblasts is pregnancy-associated plasma protein-A. Proc Natl Acad Sci USA 1999;96(6):3149–3153.

124. Bayes-Genis A, Conover CA, Overgaard MT, Bailey KR, Christiansen M, Holmes DR, Virmani R, Oxvig C, Schwartz RS. Pregnancy-associated plasma protein A as a marker of acute coronary syndromes. N Engl J Med 2001;345(14):1022–1029.

125. Pearson TA, Mensah GA, Alexander RW, Anderson JL, Cannon RO, Criqui M, Fadl YY, Fortmann SP, Hong Y, Myers GL, Rifai N, Smith SC, Taubert K, Tracy RP, Vinicor F. Markers of inflammation and cardiovascular disease: application to clinical and public health practice: a statement for healthcare professionals from the centers for disease control and prevention and the american heart association. Circulation 2003;107(3):499–511.

126. Ridker PM, Rifai N, Pfeffer MA, Sacks F, Braunwald E. Long-term effects of pravastatin on plasma concentration of C-reactive protein. The Cholesterol and Recurrent Events (CARE) Investigators. Circulation 1999;100(3):230–235.

127. Ridker PM, Cushman M, Stampfer MJ, Tracy RP, Hennekens CH. Inflammation, aspirin, and the risk of cardiovascular disease in apparently healthy men. N Engl J Med 1997;336(14): 973–979.

128. Ridker PM. Should statin therapy be considered for patients with elevated C-reactive protein? The need for a definitive clinical trial. Eur Heart J 2001;22(23):2135–2137.

129. Nissen SE, Tsunoda T, Tuzcu EM, Schoenhagen P, Cooper CJ, Yasin M, Eaton GM, Lauer MA, Sheldon WS, Grines CL, Halpern S, Crowe T, Blankenship JC, Kerensky R. Effect of recombinant ApoA-I Milano on coronary atherosclerosis in patients with acute coronary syndromes: a randomized controlled trial. JAMA 2003;290(17):2292–2300.

# 17

# Early Invasive Vs. Early Conservative Strategies for Acute Coronary Syndromes

**Philippe L. L'Allier**
*Department of Medicine, Montreal Heart Institute (P.L.L.)*

**Michael A. Lincoff**
*Department of Cardiovascular Medicine, Cleveland Clinic Foundation (A.M.L.)*

## INTRODUCTION

Acute coronary syndromes (ACS) are a continuum of clinical entities that range from accelerated angina to acute myocardial infarction. The present chapter will use this term to designate unstable angina (UA) and non–Q-wave myocardial infarction (MI), excluding acute MI with ST segment elevation and/or Q-waves.

Acute coronary syndromes share a common pathophysiology, based on underlying atherosclerotic changes, plaque vulnerability to erosion or rupture, and consequent initiation of the coagulation cascade and thrombus formation followed by infarction and disease progression. Understanding the basic processes involved is fundamental to design an integrated treatment strategy.

The optimal treatment strategy has been the subject of heated debate. Recent reports of more favorable outcomes with better anticoagulants such as low molecular weight heparins [1–3], direct antithrombins [4,5] and antiplatelet agents—platelet glycoprotein (GP) IIb/IIIa blockers [6,7], and P2Y12 blockers [8]— have addressed some of the issues relating to the underlying thrombotic substrate and are specifically discussed in Chapters 17–20. The present chapter will focus on the relative merits of early invasive vs. early conservative strategies with regard to angiography and revascularization, and on the integration of new data to define an optimal approach to the treatment of ACS.

## UNDERSTANDING THE TREATMENT OPTIONS AND THEIR RELATIVE MERITS

When caring for patients with ACS, physicians are faced with conditions that may vary considerably with regard to disease severity and prognosis. Patients with mildly progressive anginal symptoms and minimal coronary disease have very favorable outcomes when compared with patients with rest pain, electrocardiographic changes, and evidence of myocardial necrosis (elevated serum troponin, creatinine kinase). Refining definitions and classifications for unstable angina has been one of many challenges in the evaluation of new therapies, partially explaining diverging results in clinical trials.

Opinions are polarized around two approaches to ACS: early conservative and early invasive strategies. This polarization arises from differing interpretations of the need for and timing of revascularization procedures following a course of optimal medical therapy. Most of the controversy relates to the delicate balance between the unacceptable event rates (death, reinfarction, urgent revascularization, rehospitalization, etc.) associated with medical management alone, the documented excess in adverse events associated with revascularization procedures in the acute setting from early trials, and patient quality of life.

## Early Conservative Strategy

This approach is based on the assumption that most patients can be stabilized with a short course of intensive medical therapy, following which only patients with significant residual ischemia or symptoms despite optimal medical therapy (failed medical therapy) are referred for catheterization and revascularization. This strategy relies heavily on the sensitivity and specificity of noninvasive stress testing (with or without imaging) to identify high-risk patients with significant residual ischemia that are known to derive maximal benefit from revascularization. It has the advantages of avoiding the risks of revascularization in the acute setting and the costs of such procedures (although a significant proportion of these patients eventually need rehospitalization for angiography and revascularization during medium term follow-up). On the other hand, length of stay may be considerably longer and patients with unrecognized high-risk anatomies may not receive attention and appropriate treatment. Furthermore, contemporary ACS trials have confirmed incomplete plaque stabilization, at best, with medical therapy alone as death or reinfarction at 30 days occurs in 8–15% (depending on baseline characteristics and entry criteria), and refractory angina in approximately 25%, with most of these events occurring after hospital discharge. In fact, although the risk of adverse outcome is higher in the first days to weeks, events continue to occur at a significant rate months after the index hospitalization. Despite a 20% reduction in the composite endpoint of death or reinfarction with new platelet GP IIb/IIIa receptor blockers (30 days), low molecular weight heparins (14 days), and clopidogrel (12 months) the absolute event rate in the treatment groups is still unacceptably high and other means of improving outcomes are needed [1,2,6–8].

## Early Invasive Strategy

This approach is based on the assumption that patients with ACS cannot be adequately stabilized and symptomatically improved by medical therapy alone. Angiography with the intention to revascularize whenever possible is central to this strategy. Patients are brought to the angiographic suite and studied as soon as possible after diagnosis. Percutaneous coronary interventions (PCI) or coronary artery bypass grafting (CABG) are performed ad hoc or shortly thereafter if possible. This strategy relies on the safety and efficacy of coronary angiography and revascularization procedures in the acute setting. Proponents of this strategy believe that the "early procedural hazard" described in early trials is largely offset by easier and faster initial patient management, better symptomatic relief, greater decrease in subacute events, and possibly better survival. Angiography plays a role in risk stratification, mainly by identifying patients with left main disease, severe three-vessel disease, or multivessel disease, and decreased left ventricular function, all of which benefit from aggressive myocardial revascularization. Angiography also reliably identifies patients with no or minimal disease who can be discharged early with a very good prognosis and who do not significantly benefit from extensive long-term medical therapy. This approach is becoming increasingly attractive due to recent developments in adjunctive pharmacotherapy with platelet GP IIb/IIIa inhibitors which have been shown to decrease procedural and provide long-term protection against ischemic complications following PCI [9–15], and cost containment issues [16].

## DEDICATED RANDOMIZED CONTROL TRIALS

Five randomized control clinical trials that were specifically designed to compare an early invasive with an early conservative strategy will be discussed hereafter. They can be divided in two categories based on their therapeutic interventions and results: early clinical trials (TIMI III B, VANQWISH) and contemporary trials (FRISC II, TACTICS-TIMI 18, RITA 3).

### Thrombolysis in Myocardial Infarction (TIMI) III B Study

This landmark multinational/multicenter study, published a decade ago (1994), was designed to determine the effect of a fibrinolytic agent added to conventional medical therapies and to compare an early invasive management strategy to a more conservative early strategy in patients with UA and non–Q-wave MI [17]. Inclusion criteria for study entry were ischemic symptoms at rest within 24 hours of study enrollment and accompanied by objective evidence of ischemic heart disease.

Between October 1989 and June 1992, 1425 patients were randomly assigned by a two-by-two factorial design to treatment with t-PA or placebo as well as to an early invasive or early conservative strategy. By protocol, baseline medical therapy consisted of bed rest, oxygen, metoprolol, diltiazem, and isosorbide dinitrate. Patients were to receive intravenous heparin and 325-mg aspirin was to be given on the second day and administered daily for at least for one year.

The early invasive strategy (n = 740) called for coronary angiography within 18–48 hours after randomization. Revascularization (as complete as possible) was to be performed at the time of catheterization or as soon as possible thereafter (within 6 weeks for CABG).

The early conservative strategy (n = 733) called for medical management alone unless failure of such therapy had occurred according to strict prespecified criteria. The primary endpoint of the study was the composite of death, reinfarction, or unsatisfactory exercise treadmill test at 6 weeks. Analyses for different subgroups were prespecified and included 6-week death or reinfarction for patients with unstable angina vs. non-Q myocardial infarction, age younger than 65 years vs. older than 65 years, and ST-T changes.

Of the patients assigned to the early invasive strategy, 98% underwent catheterization before 6 weeks (median of 1.5 days after randomization, 0.1% after discharge). Revascularization was performed in a total of 61% of cases (38% by PCI, 25% by CABG). Of the patients assigned to the early conservative strategy, 64% underwent unplanned cardiac catheterization (median of 7.1 days, 10% after discharge). Revascularization was performed in 49% (26% by PCI, 24% by CABG). Importantly, there was no difference between treatment groups in procedural success or complication rates (death, infarction, emergency CABG, or abrupt closure).

The primary endpoint of the study was reached in 16.2% of patients in the early invasive group, vs. 18.1% in the early conservative group (p = 0.33). Specifically, death occurred in 2.4% vs. 2.5%, and nonfatal myocardial infarction occurred in 5.1% vs 5.7%, respectively (p = ns) at 6 weeks. Importantly, length of initial hospital stay (10.2 days vs. 10.9 days, p = 0.01), percentage of patients requiring rehospitalization (7.8% vs. 14.1%, p<0.001) and the total number of days of rehospitalization per treatment group (365 vs. 930, p<0.001) at 6 weeks, were all significantly lower with the early invasive strategy.

By one year [18], cumulative angiography and revascularization rates were higher in the early invasive (99% and 64% vs. 73% and 58%, p<0.001), although angioplasty rates were only slightly different (39% vs. 32%, p<0.001), and rates of bypass grafting by 1 year were identical (30% in each group). Clinical outcomes (death/non-fatal MI) were not statistically different in the two groups (10.8% vs. 12.2%, in the invasive and conservative groups, respectively), but patients in the early invasive strategy were rehospitalized less frequently (26% vs. 33%, p<0.001). It was concluded that the early invasive strategy provided more rapid relief of angina, without excess in the risk of death or myocardial infarction.

The results of the TIMI III B trial may be largely inapplicable to contemporary practice due to a number of limitations. First, these results were obtained in the context of 50% of patients receiving fibrinolytic therapy shortly before revascularization procedures, and it has been established that such therapy activates platelets and provides an unfavorable milieu to perform PCI or CABG. Second, the difference in the rates of revascularization was small and therefore may have decreased the power of the study to detect a difference in outcome. Third, coronary stents and platelet GP IIb/IIIa receptor inhibitors, which have been shown to yield better and more durable acute results and decrease peri-PCI and long-term ischemic complications, respectively, were not routinely used. Furthermore, CABG and anesthesiology techniques have also evolved to be safer and more appropriate for ACS patients [19].

## Veterans Affairs Non-Q Wave Infarction Strategies in Hospital (VANQWISH) Trial

Patients (n = 920) with acute non-Q MI (ischemic discomfort and creatinine kinase MB isoenzyme elevation) were enrolled at 17 centers between April 1993 and December 1995 [20]. Patients were randomly assigned to an early invasive or an early conservative strategy within 24–72 hours of onset of symptoms. Patients in both groups received 325-mg aspirin daily and diltiazem CD 180–300 mg daily. Patients could also receive any other standard medical therapy during hospitalization (including beta-blockers, ACE inhibitors, heparin, and nitrates).

The early invasive strategy (n = 462) specified coronary angiography soon after randomization. Importantly, however, the protocol did not require early myocardial revascularization. Patients assigned to the early conservative strategy (n = 458) underwent radionucleotide ventriculography as the initial noninvasive test, followed by predischarge exercise treadmill test (symptom-limited) with perfusion imaging. Failure of medical therapy and consequent angiography/revascularization in this group was strictly defined per protocol.

A total of 96% of patients assigned to the early invasive strategy underwent angiography (median time from randomization 2 days, 98% predischarge), although revascularization was performed in only 44% of those patients (median time from randomization 8 days, 48% by PCI, 47% by CABG, and 5% by both). In patients assigned to the early conservative strategy, 48% underwent angiography (median time from randomization 14 days, 48% predischarge), and 33% received a revascularization procedure (median time from randomization 24.5 days, 36% by PCI, 57% by CABG, and 7% by both).

The primary endpoint of the study was the combination of death from any cause or recurrent nonfatal infarction during a minimum of 12 months of follow-up. This endpoint was reached in 26.9% vs. 29.9% in the conservative and invasive groups, respectively (hazard ratio 0.87, 95% confidence interval 0.68–1.10, p = 0.35) during a mean follow-up of 23 months. There were 59 vs. 80 deaths in the conservative vs. invasive groups, respectively (hazard ratio 0.72, 95% confidence interval 0.51–1.01). There were no significant differences between groups in the incidence of reinfarction during follow-up. It was concluded that most patients with non-Q MI did not benefit from routine, early invasive management and that a conservative, ischemia-guided initial approach was both safe and effective.

Four important findings are noteworthy for the interpretation of the results of the VANQWISH study. First, procedural details were not reported for either PCI or CABG (angiographic success, abrupt or threatened closures, emergency CABG, number of grafts, completeness of revascularization, use of abciximab and stents, etc.). Second, 30-day mortality following CABG was reported to be 11.6%, an unexpectedly high rate in this group while there was no excess mortality in the PCI treated patients. Third, the extent of symptomatic relief, which is often recognized as an important endpoint in the evaluation of strategies to treat ACS was not reported. Fourth, as might have been expected with a protocol that did not recommend revascularization per se, the absolute revascularization rate (44%) in the invasive arm is regarded by many as insufficient in light of contemporary standards and technical expertise. In effect, more than half of patients in this group were subjected to the risks of angiography without the benefits of revascularization and many deaths in the invasive arm occurred in this subgroup of patients. Furthermore, the differential between the two treatment arms in revascularization rates (44% vs. 33%) may also be insufficient to fully evaluate an invasive vs. conservative strategy. As is the case with the TIMI III B study, results of VANQWISH are difficult to incorporate into contemporary practice.

## Fragmin and Fast Revascularization During Instability in Coronary Artery Disease (FRISC) II

The FRISC II trial was designed to compare an early invasive with a noninvasive strategy in patients with unstable coronary artery disease superimposed upon an intensive background antithrombotic medical regimen: aspirin for all patients and dalteparin vs. unfractionated heparin according to the second randomization of the two-by-two factorial design, other drugs were given at the discretion of the investigators, use of abciximab was encouraged during PCI, and ticlopidine was recommended for 3–4 weeks following stenting. Patients (n = 2457) were recruited between June 1996 and May 1998 [21].

Patients were eligible for randomization if they had increasing or rest symptoms of ischemia or if myocardial infarction was suspected, with the last anginal episode within 48 hours of hospitalization. Myocardial ischemia was to be accompanied by ECG changes (ST depression $\geq$0.1 mV or T wave inversion $\geq$ 0.1 mV) or by elevated biochemical markers of myocardial damage (CK-MB>0.6 ug/L, troponin T>0.1 ug/L, or qualitative troponin T test positive).

In the invasive arms, the aim was to perform all revascularization procedures within 7 days of initiation of open label treatment with dalteparin or unfractionnated heparin (admission). Patients therefore underwent coronary angiography within a few days of randomization, and revascularization was recommended in all patients with a 70% stenosis or greater of any artery supplying a significant amount of myocardium. Percutaneous procedures were recommended if there were 1 or 2 diseased vessels and CABG was recommended if there was left main or 3-vessel disease.

In the noninvasive strategy, angiography was permitted for refractory or recurrent angina despite maximally tolerated medical therapy or severe ischemia on a symptom-limited exercise test before discharge.

Of the patients assigned to the invasive strategy, 98% underwent angiography (median 4 days after initiation of open label therapy, 96% within 7 days), and a total of 47% of patients assigned to the noninvasive strategy underwent unplanned angiography (median 17 days after initiation of open label therapy, 10% within 7 days). Seventy-seven percent of patients underwent a revascularization procedure as part of the invasive strategy (55% with PCI at a median of 4 days after initiation of treatment, 45% with CABG at a median of 7 days after initiation of treatment) vs. 37% in the noninvasive strategy (49% with PCI at a median of 16.5 days after initiation of treatment, 51% with CABG at a median of 28 days after initiation of treatment).

Results of PCI were not different in the invasive vs. noninvasive arms: mean number of treated segments 1.35 vs. 1.34 and successfully treated segments 95% vs. 91%, respectively. Procedural characteristics were also very similar, particularly with regard to rate of stenting 61% vs. 70% and rate of abciximab use 10% vs. 10%.

The primary composite endpoint of death or MI by 6 months was reached in 9.4% of patients assigned to the invasive strategy and in 12.1% of patients assigned to the noninvasive strategy (risk ratio 0.78, 95% confidence interval 0.62–0.98, p = 0.031). Individual endpoints were also less frequent in the invasive group, with death rates of 1.9% vs. 2.9% (p = 0.10) and reinfarction rates of 7.8% vs. 10.1% (p = 0.045) respectively (Fig. 1). There was an approximate 50% relative reduction in anginal symptoms in the invasive compared with the noninvasive group, and a corresponding difference in the Canadian Cardiovascular Society score for angina. Furthermore, the need for readmission was halved in the invasive group due to the lower incidence of incapacitating angina or recurring unstable angina or myocardial infarction. At 1 year, 2.2% of patients in the invasive group and 3.9% in the noninvasive group had died (risk ratio 0.57 [95% CI 0.36–0.90], p = 0.016), and 8.6% vs. 11.6% had myocardial infarction (0.74 [0.59–0.94], p = 0.015). There were also reductions in readmission (37% vs. 57%; 0.67 [0.62–0.72]), and revascularization after the initial admission (7.5% vs. 31%; 0.24 [0.20–0.30]). The authors therefore concluded that an invasive approach should be the preferred strategy in

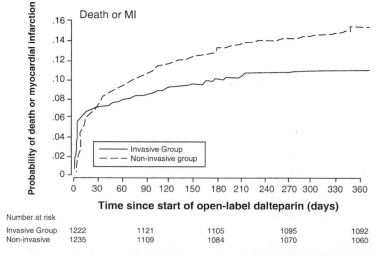

**Figure 1** FRISC II: Probability of death or MI in invasive and conservative groups. (From Ref. 21)

patients with unstable coronary-artery disease and signs of ischemia on electrocardiography or raised levels of biochemical markers of myocardial damage.

## Comparison of Early Invasive and Conservative Strategies in Patients with Unstable Coronary Syndromes Treated with the Glycoprotein IIb/IIIa Inhibitor Tirofiban (TACTICS-TIMI 18)

Patients (n = 2220) with unstable angina and myocardial infarction without ST-segment elevation who had electrocardiographic evidence of changes in the ST segment or T-wave, elevated levels of cardiac markers, a history of coronary artery disease, or all three findings were enrolled in this trial designed to compare an early invasive to an early conservative (selectively invasive) initial strategy with background potent platelet aggregation inhibition with the GP IIb/IIIa inhibitor tirofiban [22]. All patients were also treated with aspirin and heparin. The recommended medical therapy included beta-blockers, nitrates, and lipid lowering agents and was given to the vast majority of patients. Tirofiban was available for all PCIs performed during follow-up.

In the invasive arm, the aim was to perform coronary angiography within 4–48 hours and revascularization when appropriate on the basis of coronary anatomic findings. In the noninvasive strategy, angiography and revascularization were permitted for refractory or recurrent angina despite maximally tolerated medical therapy or severe ischemia on noninvasive testing before discharge (prespecified criteria).

Of the patients assigned to the invasive strategy, 97% underwent angiography during initial hospitalization (median 22 hours after randomization), and a total of 51% of patients assigned to the noninvasive strategy underwent unplanned angiography during initial hospitalization (median 79 hours after randomization). Sixty percent of patients underwent a revascularization procedure as part of the invasive strategy (41% with PCI at a median of 25 hours, 20% with CABG at a median of 89 hours) vs. 36% in the noninvasive strategy (24% with PCI at a median of 93 hours, 13% with CABG at a median of 144 hours). By 6 months, the total rate of revascularization had increased by 1% vs. 8% in the invasive and conservative groups respectively. Procedural characteristics were very similar with regard to stent use (83% vs. 86%) but rates of tirofiban use were different, 94% vs. 59%, despite its availability for all PCIs, in the invasive and conservative groups respectively.

The primary end point was a composite of death, nonfatal myocardial infarction, and rehospitalization for an acute coronary syndrome at six months (Fig. 2). The rate of

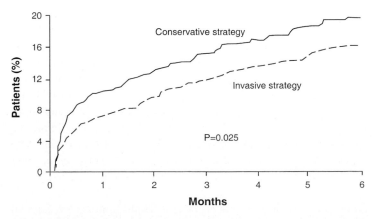

**Figure 2** TACTICS-TIMI 18: Cumulative incidence of death, MI, or rehospitalization for acute coronary syndrome in invasive and conservative groups. (From Ref. 22)

the primary end point was 15.9% with use of the early invasive strategy and 19.4% with use of the conservative strategy (odds ratio, 0.78; 95% confidence interval, 0.62 to 0.97; P = 0.025). The rate of death or nonfatal myocardial infarction at six months was similarly reduced (7.3 % vs. 9.5 %; odds ratio, 0.74; 95% confidence interval, 0.54 to 1.00; P<0.05). The authors therefore concluded that in patients with unstable angina and myocardial infarction without ST-segment elevation who were treated with the glycoprotein IIb/IIIa inhibitor tirofiban, the use of an early invasive strategy significantly reduced the incidence of major cardiac events. These data were also interpreted as supportive of a policy involving broader use of the early inhibition of glycoprotein IIb/IIIa in combination with an early invasive strategy in such patients.

### Interventional Vs. Conservative Treatment for Patients with Unstable Angina or non-ST-elevation Myocardial Infarction: The British Heart Foundation RITA 3 Randomized Trial

Patients (n = 1810) with non-ST-elevation acute coronary syndromes who had suspected cardiac chest pain at rest, documented evidence of coronary artery disease (acute or chronic) based on ECG criteria, or a previous angiogram were enrolled in this trial designed to test the hypothesis that routine, early angiography with myocardial revascularization (as clinically indicated) is better than a conservative strategy [23]. By contrast with FRISC II and TACTICS-TIMI 18 in which the threshold for myocardial infarction differed between those undergoing revascularization and those treated conservatively, RITA 3 used a common definition irrespective of treatment allocation. All patients were also treated with aspirin and heparin. The recommended medical therapy included beta-blockers and aspirin unless contraindicated and the anti-thrombin therapy was enoxaparin for all patients per protocol. Other medications (including GP IIb/IIIa inhibitors and thienopyridines) were left at the treating physician's discretion.

In the invasive arm, the aim was to perform coronary angiography as soon as possible (ideally within 72 hours of randomization) and revascularization when appropriate on the basis of coronary anatomic findings (vessels with lesion at least 70% cross-sectional stenoses or left main stenosis of at least 50%). In the noninvasive strategy, angiography and revascularization were permitted for refractory or recurrent angina despite maximally tolerated medical therapy or severe ischemia on noninvasive testing before discharge (prespecified criteria).

Of the patients assigned to the invasive strategy, 96% underwent angiography during initial hospitalization (median 2 days after randomization), and a total of 16% of patients assigned to the noninvasive strategy underwent unplanned angiography during initial hospitalization (median 79 hours after randomization). Forty-four percent of patients underwent a revascularization procedure as part of the invasive strategy (33% with PCI at a median of 3 days, 12% with CABG at a median of 22 days) vs. 10% in the noninvasive strategy (7% with PCI at a median of 93 hours, 4% with CABG at a median of 144 hours). By 1 year, the total rate of revascularization had increased to 57% vs. 28% in the invasive and conservative groups respectively. Procedural characteristics were very similar with regard to stent use (88% vs. 90%) and a quarter of PCI patients were treated with a GP IIb/IIIa inhibitor.

The primary endpoints were: (a) the combined rate of death, nonfatal myocardial infarction, or refractory angina at 4 months and (b) the combined rate of death or nonfatal MI at 1 year. The predefined endpoint at 4 months occurred in significantly less patients

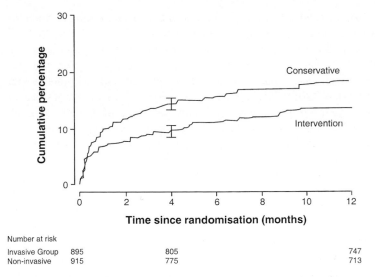

**Figure 3** RITA 3: Cumulative risk of death, MI, or refractory angina in invasive and conservative groups. (From Ref. 23)

in the intervention group as compared with the conservative group (9.6% vs. 14.5%, risk ratio 0.66, 95% CI [0.51,0.85], p0.001) (Fig. 3). This difference remained significant at 1 year (risk ratio 0.72, 95% CI [0.58, 0.90], p = 0.003). Intervention halved the likelihood of death, MI, refractory angina, or further revascularization. The predefined 1-year primary endpoint occurred in a similar proportion of patients in both groups (7.6% vs. 8.3%, p = NS). However, if the new definition of MI agreed upon by the ESC/AHA is used, there was a highly significant difference between the 2 groups favoring intervention (12.5% vs. 17.1%, risk ratio 0.73, 95% CI [0.59, 0.92], p = 0.007). The authors concluded that in patients presenting with unstable coronary-artery disease, an interventional strategy is preferable to a conservative strategy, mainly because of the halving of refractory or severe angina, and with no increased risk of death or myocardial infarction.

## Summary

The TIMI III B trial [17] confirmed that despite the use of fibrinolytic therapy in 50% of patients, the absence of stent usage and potent anti-platelet therapy, an early invasive strategy for ACS without ST segment elevation was safe and provided more rapid and more effective symptomatic relief, lowering the need for rehospitalization. In addition, subgroup analysis revealed that the higher risk patients (ECG changes, elevated cardiac enzymes, female gender, and age greater than 65 years) tended to benefit the most for an early aggressive strategy. Subsequently the VANQWISH trial [20] reported that most patients with non-Q wave MI did not benefit from routine angiography, and that a conservative, ischemia-driven strategy was both safe and effective when the endpoint of death or reinfarction during 23 months follow-up is considered. When interpreting these results, it is important to note the very low revascularization rates in the early invasive group (many deaths in this group occurred in patients that were not revascularized), the similar revascularization rates in both groups and the disturbingly high 30-day mortality following CABG. The much more favorable results with an early invasive strategy in the contemporary FRISC II [21], TACTICS-TIMI 18 [22], and RITA 3 [23] trials relative to TIMI III B and VANQWISH are likely explained by the greater absolute difference in revascularization rates in the invasive and noninvasive groups, the higher use of stents during PCI, the lower surgical mortality, and the use of GP IIb/IIIa during PCI (although heterogenous across trials: 10%, 94%, 25% respectively) (Table 1). As such, the early invasive strategies used in these 3 trials are much more representative of contemporary clinical practice than those of either TIMI IIIB or VANQWISH. Furthermore, it is likely that these results can be improved with increasing use of potent platelet inhibition in light of its very favorable interaction with PCIs [24,25]. Indeed, the early hazard associated with early revascularization disappeared when tirofiban was used to inhibit platelet aggregation (upstream and intraprocedural) in TACTICS-TIMI 18. In addition, there appears to be a gradient of benefit of routine coronary angiography with increasing risk at presentation [26]. This was specifically evaluated in the TACTICS-TIMI 18 trial in which the TIMI risk score [27] was used to stratify patients according to their short-term risk at randomization. Benefits (primary endpoint) of an early invasive strategy were observed in patients at intermediate-risk (16.1% for invasive vs. 20.3% for conservative) and high-risk (19.5% vs. 30.6%) in this trial, while outcomes were similar in patients at low-risk (12.8% vs. 11.8). Patients with elevated troponin T (16.4% vs. 24.5%) or ST segment changes (16.4% vs. 26.3%) also benefited particularly from early referral for angiography and revascularization, a finding that was also observed in the FRISC II trial [28]. Of note, patients with previous bypass surgery were excluded from these trials, so that the optimal treatment strategy in this patient population remains to be defined. However, based on the results of FRISC II, TACTICS-TIMI 18, and RITA 3, all patients with acute coronary syndromes, except those at low risk or with contraindication to angiography, derive clinical benefit from an early invasive strategy.

## TECHNICAL ASPECTS OF PCI AND ADJUNCTIVE PHARMACOTHERAPY

Technical aspects of PCI have considerably evolved in recent years. The most important change may have been the use of metallic stents in most clinical situations. The use of such stents allowed interventional cardiologists to expand the indications of PCI to more complex anatomies through better immediate- and long-term results as compared with balloon angioplasty [29]. Furthermore, with better understanding of the role of platelets in the pathophysiology of subacute stent thrombosis, this complication is now largely avoided with the use of the combination of thienopyridine agents and aspirin even in situations previously considered an absolute contraindication to stenting such as acute coronary syndromes. Indeed, stents were shown to improve outcomes when used in the setting of primary percutaneous coronary intervention for acute MI [30]. Although there are no dedicated trials of stenting vs. balloon angioplasty in the context of ACS without ST segment elevation, it is logical to extend the findings of the acute myocardial infarction trials to this population [30–31]. Recently, drug-eluting stents (sirolimus and paclitaxel) have been shown to substantially decrease restenosis rates across a wide spectrum of lesion types [32,33]. This benefit may eventually be extended to ACS patients, further improving outcomes in these patients and widening the gap between early invasive and early conservative strategies, although rates of stent thrombosis are currently under scrutiny by the US Food and Drug Administration. Other new devices also have the potential to improve the safety of early PCI. They include distal emboli protection and thrombectomy devices. As these are perfected, they might become part of the arsenal used to further prevent ischemic complications associated with PCI.

**Table 1** Randomized Control Trials of Early Invasive versus Conservative Strategy in Acute Coronary Syndromes

| Trial | Strategy | Index hospitalization revascularization rate (%) | End of study revascularization rate (%) | % stent use | % GPIIb/IIIa inhibitor use | Time to angiogram (days) | Study duration | Primary endpoint (%) |
|---|---|---|---|---|---|---|---|---|
| TIMI IIIB (17) | Invasive | 61 | 64 | negligible | 0 | 1.5 | 6 weeks | 16.2* |
| (n = 1473) | Conservative | 49 | 58 | negligible | 0 | 7.1 | 6 weeks | 18.1* |
| VANQWISH (20) | Invasive | N/A | 44 | negligible | negligible | 2 | 23 months | 29.9** |
| (n = 920) | Conservative | N/A | 33 | negligible | negligible | 14 | 23 months | 26.9** |
| FRISC II (21) | Invasive | 71 | 77 | 61 | 10 | 4 | 6 months | 9.4*** |
| (n = 2457) | Conservative | 9 | 37 | 70 | 10 | 16.5 | 6 months | 12.1*** |
| TACTICS-TIMI 18 (22) | Invasive | 60 | 61 | 83 | 94 | 0.9 | 6 months | 15.9**** |
| (n = 2220) | Conservative | 36 | 44 | 86 | 59 | 3.3 | 6 months | 19.4**** |
| RITA 3 (23) | Invasive | 44 | 57 | 88 | 25 | 2 | 12 months | 12.5***** |
| (n = 1810) | Conservative | 10 | 28 | 90 | 25 | N/A | 12 months | 17.1***** |

* TIMI IIIB: Death, MI, or unsatisfactory exercise treadmill test (p = ns)
** VANQWISH: Death or MI (p = ns)
*** FRISC II: Death or MI (p = 0.03)
**** TACTICS-TIMI 18: death/non-fatal MI/re-hospitalization for ACS at 6 months (p = 0.025)
***** RITA (co-primary): death/mi 12 months (ESC/ACC MI definition) (p = 0.007)

Therapeutic agents designed to block platelet GP IIb/IIIa receptors have been shown to decrease ischemic complications associated with PCI and to improve outcomes in ACS in large-scale clinical trials. Specifically, when used empirically in ACS, there is a trend toward better treatment effect if PCI is performed. In addition, subgroup analyses of interventional trials have suggested that clinical benefits from GP IIb/IIIa antagonists are greatest among patients with ACS [34]. Overall, platelet GP IIb/IIIa inhibitors particularly improve outcomes in high-risk patients with ACS undergoing PCI [35]. They are efficacious to stabilize patients during the initial phase of treatment and suppress the early hazard associated with revascularization procedures. These agents are therefore expected to enhance any benefit associated with an early invasive strategy and become an integral part of such a strategy, as was the case in TACTICS-TIMI 18.

The combination of clopidogrel (a platelet ADP-receptor blocker) and aspirin was recently shown to decrease the combined endpoint of cardiovascular death, MI, or stroke during a median follow-up of 9 months after ACS when compared with aspirin (9.3% vs. 11.4%, RR 0.80, p<0.001) [8]. Patients randomized in this trial were at moderate- to high-risk. Although, the trial design did not include randomization to an early invasive vs. an early conservative strategy, a significant proportion of patients underwent PCI during the index hospitalization. Patients assigned to the combination of clopidogrel and aspirin had a 30% risk reduction with regard to the primary endpoint of cardiovascular death, nonfatal MI or urgent target vessel revascularization at 30 days (4.5% vs. 6.4%, p=0.03), suggesting that this combination therapy has favorable interactions with PCI in the setting of ACS when given for a median of 6 days before PCI [24]. However, recent interventional trials have found opposing results with regard to the benefit of clopidogrel pretreatment. Indeed, post hoc analyses from the EPISTENT and TARGET trials have suggested an additional benefit of pretreatment in addition to intraprocedural platelet GP IIb/IIIa inhibition (intravenous) [36,37]. The CREDO trial, which was designed to address the question, did not show pretreatment benefit except in non-prespecified subgroups [38]. These results may be explained by differences in the length of pretreatment and patient characteristics. Whether this treatment can be integrated to an early invasive strategy remains to be proven in light of discordant results from randomized control trials. Of note, patients pretreated with clopidogrel are at increased risk of bleeding if they undergo CABG within 5 days of the last dose. It is therefore currently recommended that these patients be subjected to a 5-day waiting period to minimize bleeding complications, lengthening hospital stay, and risking instability in the interim.

## UNRESOLVED ISSUES

Although the weight of evidence favors an early invasive approach for all ACS patients except those at low-risk, there remain unresolved issues. The more pressing relate to: (a) the optimal period of pretreatment or stabilization before angiography and revascularization, (b) the extent of revascularization (culprit lesion vs. complete revascularization), and (c) the choice of platelet GP IIb/IIIa inhibitor.

In early retrospective studies of angioplasty in ACS, patients pretreated with heparin for several days and patients who had their procedure more than 2 weeks after initiation of treatment had a lower rate of periprocedural complications. However, these studies were inherently flawed by an important selection bias with only the more stable patients tolerating pretreatment. Evidence from a meta-analysis of GP IIb/IIIa inhibitors trials in ACS has recently become available regarding the pretreatment before PCI [39]. Most angiography and PCI in these trials were performed a few days after randomization, allowing for outcomes assessment in the window between hospitalization and PCI. It was reported that a significant number of events occurred (2.9% vs. 4.3%, in the GP IIb/IIIa inhibitor and placebo groups respectively, p = 0.001) during the first 72 hours while an even larger number of events occurred at the time of PCI. Although results from the meta-analysis convincingly demonstrated an early benefit of GP IIb/IIIa inhibition (before PCI), most of the benefit was seen at the time of PCI (4.9 vs. 8.0%, p = 0.001). An important question remained: would a prolonged potent antithrombotic pretreatment improve outcomes or would an even earlier referral for PCI limit the number of events occurring while waiting for revascularization. This question was specifically addressed in the "Evaluation of Prolonged Antithrombotic Pretreatment ("Cooling-Off" Strategy) Before Intervention in Patients with Unstable Coronary Syndromes" [40]. Patients (n = 410) were randomly allocated to antithrombotic pretreatment for 3 to 5 days or to early intervention after pretreatment for less than 6 hours. In both groups, antithrombotic pretreatment consisted of intravenous unfractionated heparin, aspirin, oral clopidogrel, and intravenous tirofiban. The composite of large nonfatal myocardial infarction or death from any cause at 30 days was the primary endpoint. The primary end point was reached in 11.6% (3 deaths, 21 infarctions) of the group receiving prolonged antithrombotic pretreatment and in 5.9% (no deaths, 12 infarctions) of the group receiving early intervention (relative risk 1.96, 95% confidence interval [1.01–3.82]; p = 0.04) (Fig. 4). This outcome was attributable to events occurring before catheterization; after catheterization, both groups incurred 11 events each (p = 0.92). The authors concluded that in patients with unstable coronary syndromes, deferral of intervention for prolonged antithrombotic pretreatment does not improve the outcome compared with immediate intervention accompanied by intense antiplatelet treatment.

Another important issue is the optimal revascularization strategy per se. There are two main strategies available in this regard: (a) treating the culprit lesion only in the acute setting, taking into consideration the patient's previous clinical status, and factoring in the added risk of multivessel interventions, and (b) attempting complete revascularization with the expectation of providing optimal symptomatic relief and possibly improving survival in some subgroups of patients. No randomized data is available to address this issue. From nonrandomized studies, it appears that revascularization of the culprit lesion only provides adequate symptomatic relief in most of these patients while minimizing procedural risks. However, as procedural risk diminishes over time with improved equipment and adjunctive therapy, this assessment may become outdated. Furthermore, certain subgroups of patients appear to particularly benefit from more complete revascularization (severe three vessel disease, low ejection fraction, two vessel disease including proximal left anterior descending artery, and diabetics).

A recent comparison between tirofiban (small molecule GP IIb/IIIa inhibitor) and abciximab (monoclonal antibody GP IIb/IIIa inhibitor) was performed in the context of PCI [41]. This trial showed better outcomes at 30 days with abciximab suggesting superiority of this agent to protect against PCI-related ischemic complications, especially in patients with ACS [42]. As mentioned previously, tirofiban was used as an integral part of an early invasive strategy in TACTICS-TIMI 18, which showed superiority of this strategy possibly by preventing pre-PCI events in addition to peri-PCI events. However, it has become clear from the GUSTO-IV trial that abciximab cannot simply be given upstream in place of tirofiban in this setting (no benefit of prolonged abciximab therapy in low-intermediate risk patients mostly treated medically) [43]. In addition, eptifibatide has not been formally studied as part of an early invasive strategy although this drug was shown to improve clinical outcomes in intermediate/high-risk ACS patients [7] and those undergoing PCI (no high-risk ACS patients were enrolled in the ESPRIT interventional trial) [14]. Therefore,

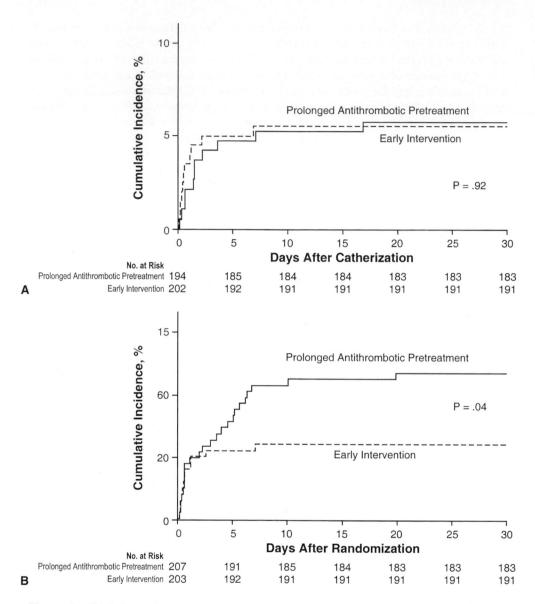

**Figure 4** ISAR-Cool: Cumulative incidence of death or MI at 30 days (**Panel A**) and at 30 days after catheterization (**Panel B**) according to randomization to prolonged antithrombotic pretreatment or early intervention. (From Ref. 40)

it is unknown whether "upstream administration" of tirofiban/eptifibatide or "in-lab" administration of abciximab at the time of PCI is preferable The answer probably lies in the evaluation of the delay before angiography and PCI: if the expected delay is longer than a few hours, administration of tirofiban/eptifibatide has theoretical merits whereas if the expected delay is less than a few hours, administration of abciximab may be preferable.

The interaction between gender and treatment effect has been evaluated in four studies designed to compare early invasive vs. early conservative strategies. Subgroup analyses from FRSC II and RITA 3 have suggested that the benefits associated with an early invasive strategy were limited to men and that women did not derive similar benefits, while in TACTICS-TIMI 18 there was no difference between men and women. The reasons behind these differences are not entirely clear. They might be explained in part by heterogeneity within the female population with regard to baseline risk profiles (diabetes, normal angiograms, troponin elevations, type of ECG changes, etc.) or statistical chance, and the ACC/AHA recommendations do not suggest a different therapeutic approach based on gender [44,45].

## INTEGRATED APPROACH

The ultimate goals of therapy in ACS are to improve survival, limit progression to myocardial infarction, and improve quality of life—anginal symptoms, anxiety, and rehospitalization. A suggested management algorithm for these patients based on contemporary clinical data is as follows. Patients should undergo risk stratification early after admission using recognized contemporary predictors of unfavorable outcomes (physical examination, ECG, biochemical markers of disease severity such as CK-MB, troponin, CRP, etc). If moderate to high-risk patients are candidates for revascularization, they should undergo angiography as early as possible with the intent to perform PCI (with concomitant potent antiplatelet therapy) or CABG revascularization if feasible (as clinical benefits are most likely related to revascularization, not angiography per se). The revascularization procedure of choice will depend on patient/physician preference, coronary anatomy, and expertise; complete revascularization seems an appropriate goal, but should be weighed against the inherent risks. For patients at lower risk, the optimal strategy possibly involves a short stabilization period of medical therapy followed by noninvasive testing, leading to an ischemia-guided revascularization strategy, minimizing the early hazard of revascularization in patients without significant myocardium at risk and/or symptoms.

## CONCLUSIONS AND FUTURE IMPLICATIONS

When assessing the best therapeutic strategy for patients with ACS, it is crucial to identify the true goals of therapy. These goals should definitely include patient-related outcomes, but also practical management issues (resource utilization, length of stay, costs, etc.). In this context, the objective evidence favors an early invasive strategy for patients at moderate- to high-risk when considering death, myocardial infarction, residual symptoms, and rehospitalization. Furthermore, with the increasing use of the stents, platelet GP IIb/IIIa inhibitors, thienopyridines, better anticoagulants (low molecular weight heparins, direct thrombin inhibitors), and potentially emboli protection devices, the benefits associated with an early invasive strategy will likely increase.

## REFERENCES

1. Cohen M, Demers C, Gurfinkel EP, Turpie AG, Fromell GJ, Goodman S, Langer A, Califf RM, Fox KA, Premmereur J, Bigonzi F. A comparison of low-molecular-weight heparin with unfractionated heparin for unstable coronary artery disease. Efficacy and Safety of Subcutaneous Enoxaparin in Non-Q-Wave Coronary Events Study Group. N Engl J Med 1997;337: 447–452.
2. Antman EM, McCabe CH, Gurfinkel EP, Turpie AG, Bernink PJ, Salein D, Bayes De Luna A, Fox K, Lablanche JM, Radley D, Premmereur J, Braunwald E. Enoxaparin prevents death

and cardiac ischemic events in unstable angina/non-Q-wave myocardial infarction. Results of the thrombolysis in myocardial infarction (TIMI) 11B trial. Circulation 1999;100:1593–1601.

3.  Goodman SG, Cohen M, Bigonzi F, Gurfinkel EP, Radley DR, Le Iouer V, Fromell GJ, Demers C, Turpie AG, Califf RM, Fox KA, Langer A. Randomized trial of low molecular weight heparin (enoxaparin) vs. unfractionated heparin for unstable coronary artery disease: one-year results of the ESSENCE Study. Efficacy and Safety of Subcutaneous Enoxaparin in Non-Q Wave Coronary Events. J Am Coll Cardiol 2000;36:693–698.

4.  Effects of recombinant hirudin (lepirudin) compared with heparin on death, myocardial infarction, refractory angina, and revascularisation procedures in patients with acute myocardial ischaemia without ST elevation: a randomised trial. Organisation to Assess Strategies for Ischemic Syndromes (OASIS-2) Investigators. Lancet 1999;353:429–438.

5.  Lincoff AM, Bittl JA, Harrington RA, Feit F, Kleiman NS, Jackman JD, Sarembock IJ, Cohen DJ, Spriggs D, Ebrahimi R, Keren G, Carr J, Cohen EA, Betriu A, Desmet W, Kereiakes DJ, Rutsch W, Wilcox RG, de Feyter PJ, Vahanian A, Topol EJ. Bivalirudin and provisional glycoprotein IIb/IIIa blockade compared with heparin and planned glycoprotein IIb/IIIa blockade during percutaneous coronary intervention: REPLACE-2 randomized trial. JAMA 2003; 289:853–863.

6.  Inhibition of the platelet glycoprotein IIb/IIIa receptor with tirofiban in unstable angina and non-Q-wave myocardial infarction. Platelet Receptor Inhibition in Ischemic Syndrome Management in Patients Limited by Unstable Signs and Symptoms (PRISM-PLUS) Study Investigators. N Engl J Med 1998;338:1488–1497.

7.  Inhibition of platelet glycoprotein IIb/IIIa with eptifibatide in patients with acute coronary syndromes. The PURSUIT Trial Investigators. Platelet Glycoprotein IIb/IIIa in Unstable Angina: Receptor Suppression Using Integrilin Therapy. N Engl J Med 1998;339:436–443.

8.  Yusuf S, Zhao F, Mehta SR, Chrolavicius S, Tognoni G, Fox KK. Effects of clopidogrel in addition to aspirin in patients with acute coronary syndromes without ST-segment elevation. N Engl J Med 2001;345:494–502.

9.  Use of a monoclonal antibody directed against the platelet glycoprotein IIb/IIIa receptor in high-risk coronary angioplasty. The EPIC Investigation. N Engl J Med 1994;330:956–961.

10. Platelet glycoprotein IIb/IIIa receptor blockade and low-dose heparin during percutaneous coronary revascularization. The EPILOG Investigators. N Engl J Med 1997;336:1689–1696.

11. Topol EJ, Lincoff AM, Kereiakes DJ, Kleiman NS, Cohen EA, Ferguson JJ, Tcheng JE, Sapp S, Califf RM. Multi-year follow-up of abciximab therapy in three randomized, placebo-controlled trials of percutaneous coronary revascularization. Am J Med 2002;113:1–6.

12. Randomised placebo-controlled and balloon-angioplasty-controlled trial to assess safety of coronary stenting with use of platelet glycoprotein-IIb/IIIa blockade. The EPISTENT Investigators. Evaluation of Platelet IIb/IIIa Inhibitor for Stenting. Lancet 1998;352:87–92.

13. Topol EJ, Mark DB, Lincoff AM, Cohen E, Burton J, Kleiman N, Talley D, Sapp S, Booth J, Cabot CF, Anderson KM, Califf RM. Outcomes at 1 year and economic implications of platelet glycoprotein IIb/IIIa blockade in patients undergoing coronary stenting: results from a multicentre randomised trial. EPISTENT Investigators. Evaluation of Platelet IIb/IIIa Inhibitor for Stenting. Lancet 1999;354:2019–2024.

14. Novel dosing regimen of eptifibatide in planned coronary stent implantation (ESPRIT): a randomised, placebo-controlled trial. Lancet 2000;356:2037–2044.

15. O'Shea JC, Buller CE, Cantor WJ, Chandler AB, Cohen EA, Cohen DJ, Gilchrist IC, Kleiman NS, Labinaz M, Madan M, Hafley GE, Califf RM, Kitt MM, Strony J, Tcheng JE. Long-term efficacy of platelet glycoprotein IIb/IIIa integrin blockade with eptifibatide in coronary stent intervention. JAMA 2002;287:618–621.

16. Mahoney EM, Jurkovitz CT, Chu H, Becker ER, Culler S, Kosinski AS, Robertson DH, Alexander C, Nag S, Cook JR, Demopoulos LA, DiBattiste PM, Cannon CP, Weintraub WS. Cost and cost-effectiveness of an early invasive vs conservative strategy for the treatment of unstable angina and non-ST-segment elevation myocardial infarction. JAMA 2002;288: 1851–1858.

17. Effects of tissue plasminogen activator and a comparison of early invasive and conservative strategies in unstable angina and non-Q-wave myocardial infarction. Results of the TIMI IIIB Trial. Thrombolysis in Myocardial Ischemia. Circulation 1994;89:1545–1556.

18. Anderson HV, Cannon CP, Stone PH, Williams DO, McCabe CH, Knatterud GL, Thompson B, Willerson JT, Braunwald E. One-year results of the Thrombolysis in Myocardial Infarction (TIMI) IIIB clinical trial. A randomized comparison of tissue-type plasminogen activator vs. placebo and early invasive vs. early conservative strategies in unstable angina and non-Q wave myocardial infarction. J Am Coll Cardiol 1995;26:1643–1650.

19. Favaloro RG. Landmarks in the development of coronary artery bypass surgery. Circulation 1998;98:466–478.

20. Boden WE, O'Rourke RA, Crawford MH, Blaustein AS, Deedwania PC, Zoble RG, Wexler LF, Kleiger RE, Pepine CJ, Ferry DR, Chow BK, Lavori PW. Outcomes in patients with acute non-Q-wave myocardial infarction randomly assigned to an invasive as compared with a conservative management strategy. Veterans Affairs Non-Q-Wave Infarction Strategies in Hospital (VANQWISH) Trial Investigators. N Engl J Med 1998;338:1785–1792.

21. Invasive compared with noninvasivetreatment in unstable coronary-artery disease: FRISC II prospective randomised multicentre study. FRagmin and Fast Revascularisation during InStability in Coronary artery disease Investigators. Lancet 1999;354:708–715.

22. Cannon CP, Weintraub WS, Demopoulos LA, Vicari R, Frey MJ, Lakkis N, Neumann FJ, Robertson DH, DeLucca PT, DiBattiste PM, Gibson CM, Braunwald E. Comparison of early invasive and conservative strategies in patients with unstable coronary syndromes treated with the glycoprotein IIb/IIIa inhibitor tirofiban. N Engl J Med 2001;344:1879–1887.

23. Fox KA, Poole-Wilson PA, Henderson RA, Clayton TC, Chamberlain DA, Shaw TR, Wheatley DJ, Pocock SJ. Interventional vs. conservative treatment for patients with unstable angina or non-ST-elevation myocardial infarction: the British Heart Foundation RITA 3 randomised trial. Randomized Intervention Trial of unstable Angina. Lancet 2002;360:743–751.

24. Mehta SR, Yusuf S, Peters RJ, Bertrand ME, Lewis BS, Natarajan MK, Malmberg K, Rupprecht H, Zhao F, Chrolavicius S, Copland I, Fox KA. Effects of pretreatment with clopidogrel and aspirin followed by long-term therapy in patients undergoing percutaneous coronary intervention: the PCI-CURE study. Lancet 2001;358:527–533.

25. Roffi M, Chew DP, Mukherjee D, Bhatt DL, White JA, Moliterno DJ, Heeschen C, Hamm CW, Robbins MA, Kleiman NS, Theroux P, White HD, Topol EJ. Platelet glycoprotein IIb/IIIa inhibition in acute coronary syndromes. Gradient of benefit related to the revascularization strategy. Eur Heart J 2002;23:1441–1448.

26. Solomon DH, Stone PH, Glynn RJ, Ganz DA, Gibson CM, Tracy R, Avorn J. Use of risk stratification to identify patients with unstable angina likeliest to benefit from an invasive vs. conservative management strategy. J Am Coll Cardiol 2001;38:969–976.

27. Antman EM, Cohen M, Bernink PJ, McCabe CH, Horacek T, Papuchis G, Mautner B, Corbalan R, Radley D, Braunwald E. The TIMI risk score for unstable angina/non-ST elevation MI: A method for prognostication and therapeutic decision making. JAMA 2000;284:835–842.

28. Diderholm E, Andren B, Frostfeldt G, Genberg M, Jernberg T, Lagerqvist B, Lindahl B, Wallentin L. ST depression in ECG at entry indicates severe coronary lesions and large benefits of an early invasive treatment strategy in unstable coronary artery disease; the FRISC II ECG substudy. The Fast Revascularisation during InStability in Coronary artery disease. Eur Heart J 2002;23:41–49.

29. Cura FA, Bhatt DL, Lincoff AM, Kapadia SR, L'Allier PL, Ziada KM, Wolski KE, Moliterno DJ, Brener SJ, Ellis SG, Topol EJ. Pronounced benefit of coronary stenting and adjunctive platelet glycoprotein IIb/IIIa inhibition in complex atherosclerotic lesions. Circulation 2000;102:28–34.

30. Stone GW, Grines CL, Cox DA, Garcia E, Tcheng JE, Griffin JJ, Guagliumi G, Stuckey T, Turco M, Carroll JD, Rutherford BD, Lansky AJ. Comparison of angioplasty with stenting, with or without abciximab, in acute myocardial infarction. N Engl J Med 2002;346:957–966.

31. Zhu MM, Feit A, Chadow H, Alam M, Kwan T, Clark LT. Primary stent implantation compared with primary balloon angioplasty for acute myocardial infarction: a meta-analysis of randomized clinical trials. Am J Cardiol 2001;88:297–301.

32. Moses JW, Leon MB, Popma JJ, Fitzgerald PJ, Holmes DR, O'Shaughnessy C, Caputo RP, Kereiakes DJ, Williams DO, Teirstein PS, Jaeger JL, Kuntz RE. Sirolimus-eluting stents vs.

standard stents in patients with stenosis in a native coronary artery. N Engl J Med 2003;349: 1315–1323.

33. Colombo A, Drzewiecki J, Banning A, Grube E, Hauptmann K, Silber S, Dudek D, Fort S, Schiele F, Zmudka K, Guagliumi G, Russell ME. Randomized study to assess the effectiveness of slow- and moderate-release polymer-based paclitaxel-eluting stents for coronary artery lesions. Circulation 2003;108:788–794.

34. Lincoff AM, Califf RM, Anderson KM, Weisman HF, Aguirre FV, Kleiman NS, Harrington RA, Topol EJ. Evidence for prevention of death and myocardial infarction with platelet membrane glycoprotein IIb/IIIa receptor blockade by abciximab (c7E3 Fab) among patients with unstable angina undergoing percutaneous coronary revascularization. EPIC Investigators.Evaluation of 7E3 in Preventing Ischemic Complications. J Am Coll Cardiol 1997;30:149–156.

35. Kereiakes DJ, Lincoff AM, Anderson KM, Achenbach R, Patel K, Barnathan E, Califf RM, Topol EJ. Abciximab survival advantage following percutaneous coronary intervention is predicted by clinical risk profile. Am J Cardiol 2002;90:628–630.

36. Steinhubl SR, Ellis SG, Wolski K, Lincoff AM, Topol EJ. Ticlopidine pretreatment before coronary stenting is associated with sustained decrease in adverse cardiac events: data from the Evaluation of Platelet IIb/IIIa Inhibitor for Stenting (EPISTENT) Trial. Circulation 2001; 103:14031–409.

37. Chan AW, Moliterno DJ, Berger PB, Stone GW, DiBattiste PM, Yakubov SL, Sapp SK, Wolski K, Bhatt DL, Topol EJ. Triple antiplatelet therapy during percutaneous coronary intervention is associated with improved outcomes including one-year survival: results from the Do Tirofiban and ReoProGive Similar Efficacy Outcome Trial (TARGET). J Am Coll Cardiol 2003;42: 1188–1195.

38. Steinhubl SR, Berger PB, Mann JT, Fry ET, DeLago A, Wilmer C, Topol EJ. Early and sustained dual oral antiplatelet therapy following percutaneous coronary intervention: a randomized controlled trial. JAMA 2002;288:2411–2420.

39. Boersma E, Harrington RA, Moliterno DJ, White H, Theroux P, Van de Werf F, de Torbal A, Armstrong PW, Wallentin LC, Wilcox RG, Simes J, Califf RM, Topol EJ, Simoons ML. Platelet glycoprotein IIb/IIIa inhibitors in acute coronary syndromes: a meta-analysis of all major randomised clinical trials. Lancet 2002;359:189–198.

40. Neumann FJ, Kastrati A, Pogatsa-Murray G, Mehilli J, Bollwein H, Bestehorn HP, Schmitt C, Seyfarth M, Dirschinger J, Schomig A. Evaluation of prolonged antithrombotic pretreatment (''cooling-off'' strategy) before intervention in patients with unstable coronary syndromes: a randomized controlled trial. JAMA 2003;290:1593–1599.

41. Topol EJ, Moliterno DJ, Herrmann HC, Powers ER, Grines CL, Cohen DJ, Cohen EA, Bertrand M, Neumann FJ, Stone GW, DiBattiste PM, Demopoulos L. Comparison of two platelet glycoprotein IIb/IIIa inhibitors, tirofiban and abciximab, for the prevention of ischemic events with percutaneous coronary revascularization. N Engl J Med 2001;344:1888–1894.

42. Stone GW, Moliterno DJ, Bertrand M, Neumann FJ, Herrmann HC, Powers ER, Grines CL, Moses JW, Cohen DJ, Cohen EA, Cohen M, Wolski K, DiBattiste PM, Topol EJ. Impact of clinical syndrome acuity on the differential response to 2 glycoprotein IIb/IIIa inhibitors in patients undergoing coronary stenting: the TARGET Trial. Circulation 2002;105:2347–2354.

43. Simoons ML. Effect of glycoprotein IIb/IIIa receptor blocker abciximab on outcome in patients with acute coronary syndromes without early coronary revascularisation: the GUSTO IV-ACS randomised trial. Lancet 2001;357:1915–1924.

44. Hochman JS, Tamis-Holland JE. Acute coronary syndromes: does sex matter?. JAMA 2002; 288:3161–3164.

45. Braunwald E, Antman EM, Beasley JW, Califf RM, Cheitlin MD, Hochman JS, Jones RH, Kereiakes D, Kupersmith J, Levin TN, Pepine CJ, Schaeffer JW, Smith EE, Steward DE, Theroux P, Gibbons RJ, Alpert JS, Faxon DP, Fuster V, Gregoratos G, Hiratzka LF, Jacobs AK, Smith SC. ACC/AHA guideline update for the management of patients with unstable angina and non-ST-segment elevation myocardial infarction--2002: summary article: a report of the American College of Cardiology/American Heart Association Task Force on Practice Guidelines (Committee on the Management of Patients With Unstable Angina). Circulation 2002;106:1893–1900.

# 18

## Intravenous Platelet Glycoprotein IIb/IIIa Inhibitors for Acute Coronary Syndromes

**Hitinder S. Gurm and Eric J. Topol**
*The Cleveland Clinic Foundation*
*Cleveland, Ohio, U.S.A*

### INTRODUCTION

Coronary artery disease is increasing in prevalence and is the leading cause of death and disability worldwide [1]. Clinically manifest coronary artery disease may present as stable angina, acute coronary syndrome, or sudden cardiac death. Acute coronary syndromes encompass patients who have evidence of myonecrosis, or are felt to be at high risk of myonecrosis in the immediate future, and thus include patients with unstable angina (USA), non-ST elevation myocardial infarction (NSTEMI), and ST elevation myocardial infarction (STEMI) [2–5].

Patients with ACS have one or more of the following underlying etiologies: (a) a non-occlusive or an occlusive thrombus on a preexisting plaque, (b) vasoconstriction or dynamic obstruction, (c) progressive mechanical obstruction, (d) inflammation, and (e) secondary unstable angina [6,7]. The inciting event in this cascade is typically plaque disruption, which with its attendant superimposed thrombosis and associated vasoconstriction impairs coronary blood flow and may be complicated by distal embolization [8,9]. Work done in the 1970s demonstrated that platelets play a key role in unstable plaque with aggregation and release of vasoconstrictors contributing to further worsening of the ischemic cascade. Autopsy studies by Falk demonstrated a layered structure of the coronary thrombus suggesting episodes of thrombosis with progressive luminal encroachment and a final occlusive thrombus in a majority of patients with myocardial infarction (MI) [8]. Furthermore, he demonstrated that patients had evidence of platelet micro-embolization distal to the thrombus suggesting a period of thrombus instability and spontaneous recanalization. Based on this and corroborating evidence, it was recognized that platelet inhibition would provide therapeutic value in ACS and this in turn lead to the early investigations and the consequent widespread use of aspirin and heparin in ACS [10].

The current body of knowledge supports a central role for platelets in coronary thrombosis. Exposure of the subendothelial matrix subsequent to arterial injury or plaque rupture triggers platelet adherence to the subendothelial collagen. Adhesion of platelets to the subendothelium is followed by platelet activation that in turn leads to further platelet recruitment and platelet aggregation. Platelet aggregation is dependent on platelet fibrinogen interaction and is mediated via the glycoprotein (GP) IIb/IIIa receptor. The GP

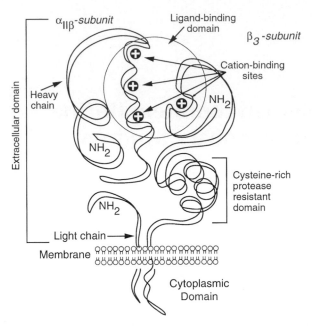

**Figure 1**   Schematic depiction of the $\alpha_{IIb}\beta_3$ (GP IIb/IIIa) integrin. (From Ref. 19)

IIb/IIIa receptor is a member of the integrin family of adhesion molecules that are found on virtually all cell surfaces and mediate myriad physiological functions (Fig. 1) [11–14]. The GP IIb/IIIa receptor is most abundant on platelet surface with over 50,000 to 80,000 copies per platelet [15]. This receptor is usually in a ligand non-receptive phase with limited receptor function on the surface of the unstimulated platelet. Platelet stimulation induces conformational changes in the receptor along with an increase in the number of receptors on the platelet surface. The activated GP IIb/IIIa receptor has a very high affinity for fibrinogen and acts to cross-link other activated platelets thus forming the platelet plug (Figure 2). In contrast to being the final common pathway in platelet aggregation, GP IIb/IIIa receptor does not play a key role in platelet adhesion. Recent studies suggest that in addition to its role in thrombosis, GP IIb/IIIa is also involved in inflammatory processes via its interaction with CD40 ligand [16]. Full inhibition of GP IIb/IIIa prevents shedding of (soluble) sCD40 ligand from activated platelets. Outside-in signaling by GP IIb/IIIa following platelet aggregation is associated with release of pro-inflammatory content of the alpha granules (TGF-beta, PF4, RANTES, P–selectin, etc.) thus contributing to vascular inflammation [17]. Given its central role in platelet aggregation, GP IIb/IIIa receptor provides an ideal target for blocking platelet aggregation associated with ACS.

There are currently three commercially available intravenous GP IIb/IIIa inhibitors, abciximab, eptifibatide and tirofiban. These have been extensively studied in the setting of ACS and percutaneous coronary intervention.

## PHARMACOLOGY OF THE INTRAVENOUS PLATELET GP IIB/IIA RECEPTOR INHIBITORS

Three parenteral agents abciximab (ReoPro, Eli Lilly, Indianapolis, IN), eptifibatide (Integrilin, COR Therapeutics, South San Francisco, CA), and tirofiban (Aggrastat, Guilford

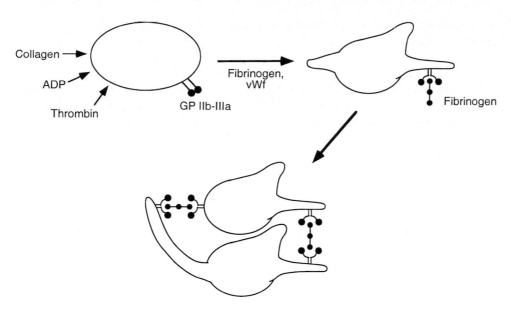

**Figure 2**   Illustration of key events that occur during the processes of platelet activation and aggregation. In the presence of agonists such as collagen, adenosine diphosphate (ADP) and thrombin, platelet activation leads to changes in platelet shape and activation of the GP IIb/IIIa receptor. Activated GP IIb/IIIa receptors bind mainly fibrinogen and this adhesive protein forms bridges between adjacent platelets—the principal mechanism resulting in platelet aggregation and formation of the advancing platelet plug. (From Ref. 17a)

Pharmaceuticals, Baltimore, MD) are currently approved for clinical use (albeit for different specific indications) by the US Food and Drug Administration. The first to reach the clinical arena, abciximab, is a monoclonal antibody directed against the GP IIb/IIIa integrin [18]. Unlike the small molecule agents, abciximab interacts with the GP IIb/IIIa receptor at sites distinct from the ligand-binding RGD sequence site, and probably exerts its inhibitory effect by steric hindrance [19]. Abciximab also binds the $\alpha_v\beta_3$ integrin (a vitronectin receptor) suggesting that it is the $\beta_3$ (GP IIIa) subunit that contains conformational epitopes involved in ligand-receptor binding [20,21]. The antibody has unique pharmacokinetics, with the majority of the drug cleared from plasma within 25 minutes, but much slower clearance from the body with a catabolic half-life up to 7 hours [22].Yet, platelet-associated abciximab can still be detected in the circulation for more than 14 days after cessation of infusion, in part related to its high affinity for the receptor [23].Throughout this time, the drug remains evenly distributed among the population of circulating platelets. With an average period of platelet circulation of about 7 days, it appears that abciximab molecules can freely dissociate and re-associate with GP IIb/IIIa as the turnover of platelets in the circulation continues, thus prolonging the ''biological'' half-life of the drug. Both preclinical studies and pharmacodynamic evaluation in patients have set the range of less than 80% inhibition of platelet aggregation as the target for effective anti-platelet activity. The appropriateness of this target has been validated by the clinical trials demonstrating both efficacy and safety with this level of platelet inhibition.

Synthetic peptides and small molecule GP IIb/IIIa antagonists were developed because of concerns regarding potential immunogenicity lack of reversibility and cost of the monoclonal antibody agents. These contain the RGD sequence (or a variant of it) and occupy the RGD binding site of the GP IIb/IIIa receptor. The so-called KGD peptide GP IIb/IIIa receptor inhibitor, eptifibatide, has a lysine residue substituted for the arginine in the RGD sequence, while lamifiban (Hoffmann-La Roche, Basel, Switzerland) and tirofiban are small molecule GP IIb/IIIa receptor antagonists based on the RGD motif. Unlike abciximab, these small molecule agents are specific for GP IIb/IIIa without any appreciable binding to other integrins such as $\alpha_v\beta_3$ [19]. Because of their small size, these drugs are also much less likely to induce an antibody response than abciximab. They have a high affinity for GP IIb/IIIa, but not as strong as abciximab, and are rapidly eliminated from the circulation once the infusion is stopped. Thus, they have the "biological" profile of short-acting agents whose effects on platelet aggregation rapidly dissipate (within 4 hours) once the drug infusion is terminated.

For eptifibatide, approximately 25% of the drug molecules in plasma are protein bound, leaving the remaining 75% to constitute the pool of pharmacologically active drug. The stoichiometry of both eptifibatide and tirofiban is greater than 100 molecules of drug per GP IIb/IIIa receptor needed to achieve full platelet inhibition. This compares with a stoichiometry of 1.5 molecules of abciximab for each receptor. Eptifibatide has an elimination half-life of 2.5 hours, with the majority of the drug eliminated through renal mechanisms. Approximately 65% of tirofiban molecules end up bound to plasma proteins, with a half-life for that drug of around 2.0 hours. As with eptifibatide, the main route of excretion is through the renal tract. Plasma clearance of both eptifibatide and tirofiban is likely to be affected by significant renal impairment and the doses of these drugs should be adjusted where creatinine clearance is reduced.

## CLINICAL TRIALS IN ACS

The role of GP IIb/IIIa inhibitors in ACS has been defined in the setting of both conservative and early invasive therapy. The use of these agents as part of the medical regimen was evaluated in six large randomized clinical trials. Table 1 and Table 2 provide a comparison of the major GP IIb/IIIa inhibitor trials in ACS. The clinical trial experience with each agent in ACS is summarized in the following sections.

### Abciximab

Abciximab was the first GP IIb/IIIa inhibitor to undergo clinical evaluation. It was initially evaluated for adjunctive use in PCI. The Evaluation of 7E3 for the Prevention of Ischaemic Complications (EPIC) trial enrolled 2099 patients undergoing high-risk angioplasty in the setting of acute evolving myocardial infarction, unstable angina or high-risk clinical or angiographic characteristics [24]. Patients were randomized to receive a placebo, a bolus (0.25mg/kg) of abciximab or a bolus and infusion (10μg/minute for 12 hours) of abciximab. The majority (90%) of patients in EPIC underwent isolated percutaneous transluminal coronary balloon angioplasty (PTCA), with the remainder undergoing directional coronary atherectomy (DCA) or both PTCA and DCA. The Evaluation in PTCA to Improve Long-Term Outcome with Abciximab GP IIb/IIIa blockade (EPILOG) study enrolled 2792 patients undergoing urgent or elective PCI [25]. Patients were randomized to placebo, abciximab (0.25mg/kg bolus, followed by 0.125 ug/kg/min infusion to maximum 10ug/min for 12 hours) and low dose heparin, or abciximab bolus and infusion and standard dose heparin. The evaluation of Platelet IIb/IIIa Inhibitor for Stenting (EPISTENT) enrolled 2399 patients undergoing PCI for elective or urgent indications [26]. Patients were randomized to stent plus placebo with standard dose heparin (100 units/kg bolus), stent

**Table 1**  Trial Design and Patient Population From Six Major Randomized Trials of GP IIb/IIIa Receptor Blockade in Unstable Angina or Non-ST Elevation Myocardial Infarction

| Trial | Agent | Number of Patients | Entry Criteria | Co-Administration of Heparin | Angiography and Revascularization | Primary Endpoint |
|---|---|---|---|---|---|---|
| PUSUIT | Eptifibatide | 10,948 | CP at rest within 24hrs, and either ECG changes or CK-MB rise | Heparin use encouraged, but not randomized | At discretion of attending physician | Death of MI at 30 days |
| PRISM PLUS | Tirofiban | 1,915 | CP at rest or minimal exertion within 12 hrs, and either ECG changes or CK-MB rise | Yes | Deferred for 48 hrs then performed during study drug infusion | Death, MI or refractory ischemia at 7 days |
| PRISM | Tirofiban | 3,232 | CP at rest or minimal exertion within 12 hrs, and either ECG changes or CK-MB rise or history of coronary disease or positive stress test | No | Discouraged | Death, MI or refractory ischemia at 48 hrs |
| PARAGON A | Lamifiban | 2,282 | CP at rest within 12 hrs, and ECG changes | Randomized | Discouraged | Death or MI at 30 days |
| GUSTO IV | Abciximab | 7800 | Angina within 24 hrs, and either elevated troponin I or T or transient or persistent ST depression on the ECG | Yes | Discouraged during and within 12 hours of study drug infusion | Death or MI at 30 days |
| PARAGON B | Lamifiban | 5225 | CP at rest within 12 hrs, and either elevated troponin I or T or CK-MB or ECG changes | Yes | At discretion of attending physician | Death, MI or severe recurrent ischemia at 30 days |

Abbreviations: CF = chest pain, CK-MB = creatine kinase MB isoenzyme fraction, MI = myocardial infarction.
ECG changes include ST segment depression, T wave inversion or transient ST segment elevation

**Table 2** Short and Medium-Term Clinical Outcomes From Six Major Randomized Trials of GP IIb/IIIa Receptor Blockade in Unstable Angina or Non-ST Elevation Myocardial Infarction

| | 48–96 Hours | | | 30 Days | | | 6–12 Months | | |
|---|---|---|---|---|---|---|---|---|---|
| | Death | MI | Death or MI | Death | MI | Death or MI | Death | MI | Death or MI |
| **PURSUIT** | | | | | | | | | |
| Placebo (n=4739) | 1.2 | 8.3 | 9.1 | 3.7 | 13.5 | 15.7 | 6.2 | 15.7 | 19.0 |
| Eptifibatide (n=4722) | 0.9 | 7.1 | 7.6 | 3.5 | 12.6 | 14.2 | 6.4 | 14.7 | 17.9 |
| **PRISM PLUS** | | | | | | | | | |
| Heparin (n=797) | 0.3 | 2.6 | 2.6 | 4.5 | 9.2 | 11.9 | 7.0 | 10.5 | 15.3 |
| Tirofiban + heparin (n=773) | 0.1 | 0.9 | 0.9 | 3.6 | 6.6 | 8.7 | 6.9 | 8.3 | 12.3 |
| **PRISM** | | | | | | | | | |
| Heparin (n=1616) | 0.4 | 1.4 | 1.4 | 3.6 | 4.3 | 7.1 | – | – | – |
| Tirofiban (n=1616) | 0.2 | 0.9 | 0.9 | 2.3 | 4.1 | 5.8 | – | – | – |
| **PARAGON A** | | | | | | | | | |
| Placebo (n=758) | 0.5 | 3.3 | 3.7 | 2.9 | 10.6 | 11.7 | 6.6 | 14.3 | 17.9 |
| Lamifiban (low-dose) (n=755) | 0.3 | 3.5 | 3.5 | 3.0 | 9.4 | 10.6 | 5.2 | 10.8 | 13.7 |
| Lamifiban (high-dose) (n=769) | 0.4 | 2.5 | 2.6 | 3.6 | 10.9 | 12.0 | 6.8 | 12.9 | 16.4 |
| **GUSTO IV** | | | | | | | (1 year) | | |
| Placebo (n=2598) | 0.3 | 1.3 | 1.5 | 3.9 | 5.1 | 8.0 | 7.8 | – | – |
| Abciximab 24 hours (n=2590) | 0.7 | 1.3 | 1.9 | 3.4 | 5.6 | 8.2 | 8.2 | – | – |
| Abciximab 48 hours (n=2612) | 0.9 | 1.4 | 2.2 | 4.3 | 5.9 | 9.1 | 9.0 | – | – |
| **PARAGON B** | | | | | | | | | |
| Placebo (n=2569) | – | – | – | 3.3 | 9.8 | 11.5 | – | – | – |
| Lamifiban (n=2600) | – | – | – | 2.9 | 8.8 | 10.6 | – | – | – |

plus abciximab with low dose heparin, or balloon angioplasty plus abciximab with low dose heparin. All three trials demonstrated a consistent reduction in early and late mortality, periprocedural MI, and the need for urgent revascularization. While the benefit of abciximab was evident across all subgroups, patients with ACS appeared to derive an enhanced benefit from it. In the EPIC trial among the 489 patients who had a diagnosis of unstable angina, the magnitude of the risk reduction with abciximab was greater than among other patients without unstable angina for the end points of death (interaction: $p = 0.008$ at 30 days, $p = 0.002$ at 6 months) and MI (interaction: $p = 0.004$ at 30 days, $p = 0.003$ at 6 months) [27]. Compared with placebo, the bolus and infusion of abciximab resulted in a 62% reduction in the rate of the primary end point composite of death, MI or urgent repeat revascularization within 30 days of randomization (12.8% vs. 4.8%, $p = 0.012$) among patients with unstable angina. By 6 months, cumulative death and MI were further reduced by abciximab (6.6% vs. 1.8%, $p = 0.018$ and 11.1% vs. 2.4%, $p = 0.002$, respectively). This mortality benefit in ACS patients was preserved at 3 years [28]. In a pooled analysis of the EPIC, EPILOG, and EPISTENT trials the one-year incidence of death or MI was reduced from 13.2% to 6.7% ($P < 0.001$) among patients with ACS compared to a reduction from 13.1% to 9.0% ($P < 0.001$) among those with stable coronary artery disease. While no interaction analysis was reported, the findings appear consistent with earlier data in that the benefit of abciximab appears to be enhanced in ACS.

The use of abciximab in patients undergoing PCI for refractory unstable angina was evaluated in the CAPTURE trial [29]. Patients with ongoing chest pain associated with ECG changes on heparin and intravenous nitroglycerine who underwent angiography and had a lesion suitable for angioplasty were enrolled into the study. All patients were randomized to receive abciximab (0.25 mg/kg bolus and 10ug/min infusion) or placebo for 18–24 hours before angioplasty and continued for 1 hour after angioplasty. All patients received aspirin, and heparin was continued until 1 hour after PTCA. The primary endpoint was death, MI, or urgent intervention for ischemia during the initial hospitalization and within 30 days. The CAPTURE trial was discontinued after the third interim analysis revealed significant benefit in favor of abciximab. The 30-day composite endpoint occurred among 15.9% of the patients in the placebo group compared to 11.3% in the abciximab group ($P = 0.012$). The endpoint was predominantly driven by a reduction in MI (8.2% vs. 4.1%, $P = 0.002$). The reduction in MI occurred both before (2.1% vs. 0.6%, $P = 0.029$) and during PCI (5.5% vs. 2.6%, $P = 0.009$). Serum troponin levels at enrollment were available in 890 patients. The six-month cumulative death or MI rate was 23.9 % among patients with elevated troponin T levels, as compared with 7.5 % among patients without elevated troponin levels ($P < 0.001$). Use of abciximab was associated with a 68% relative reduction in the rate of death or MI at 6 months and reduced the incidence of the six-month event rates down to 9.5 percent for patients with elevated troponin T levels and 9.4 percent for those without elevated levels [30]. A recent analysis from this study suggests that sCD40 ligand levels may provide further guidance in choosing patients that derive enhanced benefits from abciximab. Six months ischemia endpoints were markedly increased in patients with elevated sCD40L levels. The increased risk in patients with elevated soluble CD40 ligand levels was significantly reduced by treatment with abciximab (adjusted hazard ratio as compared with those receiving placebo, 0.37; 95% CI, 0.20 – 0.68; $P = 0.001$), whereas there was no significant treatment effect of abciximab in patients with low levels of soluble CD40 ligand [31]. Angiographic data from the study revealed that use of abciximab was associated with resolution of thrombus in 43% of the patients compared to 22% of those randomized to placebo ($P = 0.033$). Furthermore, the reduction in clinical endpoints occurred in those with complex lesion morphology.

Further support for the use of abciximab in patients undergoing PCI for ACS has come from TARGET (Do Tirofiban and Reopro Give Similar Efficacy Trial). In this randomized comparison of tirofiban and abciximab in patients undergoing PCI, use of tirofiban was associated with a higher 30-day composite of death, MI, or urgent revascularization (9.3% vs. 6.3%, hazard ratio 1.49, 95% CI 1.15–1.93, P value for interaction 0.016) while no difference in outcome of patients with stable disease was seen [32]. The use of abciximab was associated with a 32% reduction in MI at 30 days and 27% at 6 months in patients with ACS (P < 0.01) [33,34]. It has been hypothesized that this difference may relate in part to use of a low dose of tirofiban and further trials to answer this question are being planned.

While the use of abciximab in ACS patients undergoing PCI has been clearly established, paradoxically the drug has not shown any benefit in patients receiving it as part of medical therapy in patients treated conservatively. The GUSTO IV trial randomized 7800 patients with chest pain and either ST-segment depression or raised troponin concentrations to placebo, abciximab bolus and 24 hour infusion, or abciximab bolus and 48 hour infusion [35]. All patients received aspirin and either unfractionated or low-molecular-weight heparin. At 30 days, 209 (8.0%) patients on placebo, 212 (8.2%) on 24-hour abciximab, and 238 (9.1%) on 48-hour abciximab were dead or had suffered a MI (odds ratio 1.0 [95% CI 0.83–1.24], for difference between placebo and 24 hour abciximab, and 1.1 [0.94–1.39] for difference between placebo and 48 hour abciximab). Mortality was significantly higher during the 48 hours while the study drug was being administered among patients randomized to abciximab [36]. Furthermore, unlike the PCI population, use of abciximab did not provide any survival benefit at 1 year. In subgroups of patients with low cardiac troponin or elevated C-reactive protein, abciximab use was associated with a paradoxical excess mortality [37]. The authors believe that the pro-inflammatory features of abciximab during the extended infusion stage, such as promoting the shedding of sCD40L, account for this unexpected, paradoxical increase in mortality. At sub-threshold IIb/IIIa blockade, this is akin to the problems encountered with the oral IIb/IIIa inhibitor programs.

Based on results of these trials, the use of abciximab in patients not considered for PCI cannot be advocated while there is clear evidence supporting its use in ACS patients coming to PCI. Indeed, it may be considered the agent of choice in patients undergoing PCI for ACS if they have not already received a GP IIb/IIIa inhibitor. There are, however, no convincing data to support switching patients who are on a small molecule GP IIb/IIIa inhibitor prior to PCI to abciximab at time of the procedure. Since typically the coronary anatomy is unknown before the angiogram is performed, the use of abciximab can be hard to justify for medical management in the precatheterization phase, however its strong efficacy may be the foundation for deferring the use of this particular agent until the coronary anatomy is defined.

## Lamifiban

Lamifiban is a nonpeptide, small molecule, highly specific GP IIb/IIIa inhibitor. It was first evaluated in 365 unstable angina patients in the Canadian Lamifiban Study [38]. Four different doses of lamifiban were tested. Aspirin was administered to all patients while heparin was given to 28%. Lamifiban reduced the risk of death, nonfatal myocardial infarction, or the need for an urgent revascularization during the infusion period from 8.1% to 3.3% (P = .04). At 1 month, death or nonfatal infarction occurred in 8.1% of patients with placebo and in 2.5% of patients with the two high doses (P = .03). The PARAGON A study subsequently tested the promise of this agent in a cohort of 2282 patients with USA/NSTEMI ACS [39]. Patients were randomly assigned to one of the 5 arms: lamifiban, low-dose (1 microg/min) with and without heparin, high-dose (5 microg/min) with and without heparin, or standard therapy (placebo and heparin). All patients received aspirin. The composite primary end point of death or nonfatal MI at 30 days occurred in 11.7% of those receiving standard therapy, 10.6% receiving low-dose lamifiban, and 12.0% receiving high-dose lamifiban (P = 0.668). By 6 months, this composite was lowest (13.7%) for those assigned to low-dose lamifiban (P = 0.027) and intermediate (16.4%) for those assigned to high-dose lamifiban (P = 0.450) compared with control (17.9%). A post hoc analysis of data from 810 patients in whom lamifiban levels were measured suggested a significant correlation between drug levels and outcome. Since lamifiban is excreted renally and has no known metabolite, PARAGON B trial adjusted dosing according to renal function. The study randomized 5225 patients with ACS to receive lamifiban dose adjusted for renal function or placebo in addition to aspirin or heparin. There was no difference in the composite of death, MI, or severe recurrent ischemia at 30 days between the two groups. Lamifiban levels were prospectively measured and those with targeted levels (>18ng/ml) did not show any difference in outcome compared to those not achieving the therapeutic level [40]. Although it has been a useful proof of a concept clinical development program, lamifiban is not commercially available.

## Tirofiban

The role of tirofiban as part of medical therapy of ACS has been evaluated in two large randomized controlled trials, PRISM and PRISM PLUS. The PRISM study enrolled ACS patients presenting with chest pain at rest or accelerating chest pain within 24 hours of randomization [41]. Coronary artery disease had to be manifested by one of the following three: (a) electrocardiographic evidence of myocardial ischemia in two contiguous leads during an episode of chest pain with new ST-segment depression of 0.1 mV or new T-wave inversion, or transient ST-segment elevation, (b) elevated cardiac-enzyme levels, or (c) a history of myocardial infarction, percutaneous revascularization more than six months earlier, coronary surgery more than one month earlier, a positive stress test, or 50 % narrowing of a major coronary artery on a previous coronary angiogram. Patients were randomized to receive tirofiban (0.6 μg per kilogram of body weight per minute for 30 minutes, followed by 0.15 μg per kilogram per minute for 47.5 hours) or heparin. Angiography and revascularization in the first 48 hours were discouraged with recommendation to stop study drug infusion in the event of such a procedure. In contradistinction to other trials, the primary end point was a composite of death, myocardial infarction, or refractory ischemia at the end of the 48-hour infusion. A secondary end point was death, myocardial infarction, or refractory ischemia at seven days although patients were followed for 30 days, and the composite end point (with the addition of readmission for unstable angina) and its components were analyzed at 30 days in a predefined analysis. Tirofiban arm had a significant reduction in the primary endpoint at 48 hours (3.8 % vs. 5.6%, P = 0.01) No difference was noted in the composite end points at 7 days or 30 days. The 30-day mortality in the tirofiban arm was 2.3% as compared with 3.6% in the heparin group (P = 0.02).

The PRISM PLUS study enrolled 1915 patients with ACS to one of the three arms: only tirofiban (0.6 μg per kilogram of body weight per minute for 30 minutes, followed by an infusion of 0.15 μg per kilogram per minute), tirofiban (0.4 μg per kilogram per minute for 30 minutes, followed by an infusion of 0.1 μg per kilogram per minute) plus adjusted-dose heparin, or only adjusted-dose heparin [42]. The tirofiban only arm was prematurely terminated secondary to an increase in 7-day mortality. The composite primary end point consisted of death, MI, or refractory ischemia within seven days after randomization. The primary endpoint occurred in 12.9 % of patients in the tirofiban plus heparin arm compared to 17.9% in the heparin only arm (P = 0.004, RR 0.68, 95 % CI 0.53–0.88). This reduction in events was maintained at 30 days (18.5 percent vs. 22.3 percent, P = 0.03) and at 6 months (27.7 percent vs. 32.1 percent, P = 0.02). Furthermore tirofiban and heparin reduced MI or death at seven days, (4.9% in the tirofiban-plus-heparin group vs. 8.3% in the heparin-only group' P = 0.006), 30 days (8.7 % vs. 11.9 %, P = 0.03), and at 6 months (12.3 % vs. 15.3 %, P = 0.06). Angioplasty was performed in one-third of the patients and they appeared to derive particular benefit from pretreatment with tirofiban plus heparin. These patients had a 46 percent reduction in cardiac ischemic events after angioplasty, including a 43% reduction in the composite end point of death or MI (Fig. 3a). Conversely, the beneficial effect of combination therapy with tirofiban and heparin became evident within the initial 48 hours, which due to being a protocol mandated procedure-free period required by the protocol suggests benefits independent of and in addition to revascularization (Fig. 3b).

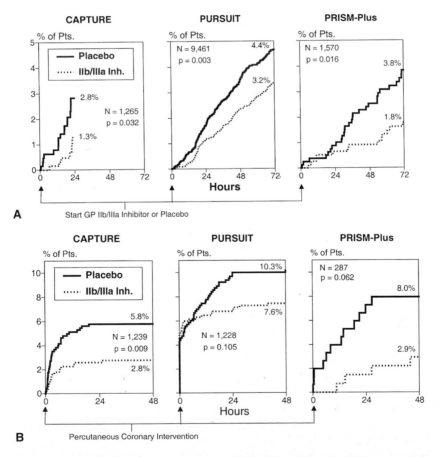

**Figure 3** (A) Kaplan-Meier curves showing the cumulative incidence of death or non-fatal myocardial infarction during the initial period of pharmacological therapy until time of percutaneous coronary intervention or coronary artery bypass surgery, if performed, from the CAPTURE, PURSUIT and PRISM-PLUS trials. (**B**) Kaplan-Meier curves showing the cumulative incidence of death or non-fatal myocardial infarction among patients undergoing percutaneous coronary intervention in the 48 hour period after the procedure. Patients received study medication during and for a short period after the procedure.

While the use of tirofiban appeared to be inferior to abciximab when started during PCI in patients with ACS in the TARGET trial, two recent studies provide indirect evidence for its use as initial medical therapy followed by continued use during PCI. Both TACTICS-TIMI 18 [43] and ISAR-COOL [44] (discussion following) trials used tirofiban as the GP IIb/IIIa inhibitor of choice in their therapeutic armamentarium.

## Eptifibatide

Eptifibatide, a cyclic heptapeptide, is another small molecule reversible inhibitor of GP IIb/IIIa. It was initially evaluated in ACS in a study of 227 patients with unstable angina. In this dose finding study, use of high dose eptifibatide was associated with a lower incidence and duration of ischemia on holter monitoring [45]. The PURSUIT (Platelet Glycoprotein IIb/IIIa in Unstable Angina: receptor Suppression Using Integrilin Therapy) investigators randomized 10,948 patients with ACS to receive high dose eptifibatide (a bolus of 180 ug/kg followed by an infusion of 2.0 ug/kg/minute), low dose eptifibatide (a bolus of 180 ug/kg followed by an infusion of 1.3 ug/kg/minute), or placebo [46]. All patients received aspirin, and heparin was dosed to achieve an APTT between 50–70 seconds. The low dose eptifibatide arm was discontinued per protocol after safety of the high dose arm was confirmed (after enrollment of 3218 patients). The primary end point, a composite of death and nonfatal MI at 30 days, was reduced from 15.7% in the placebo arm to 14.2% in the eptifibatide group. The benefit of eptifibatide was enhanced in patients undergoing early revascularization (31% relative reduction, 11.6% vs. 16.7%, P = 0.01) compared to the patients that did not undergo early intervention (7% relative reduction (14.5% vs. 15.6%, P = 0.23). Even in patients that underwent early revascularization there was a 3.8% absolute reduction in events (P < 0.001) seen in the time window between enrollment and before PTCA. The benefit of eptifibatide was consistent across most groups except in females and those enrolled in Latin America and eastern Europe. While the reasons for these differences may relate to differing clinical practice, the study was underpowered to detect outcomes in small subgroups. This issue was addressed at greater length by the meta-analysis that followed the publication of these trials.

While eptifibatide appeared to have enhanced benefits in patients receiving aggressive invasive therapy in PURSUIT, there is additional data supporting the use of this agent in ACS patients. In the ESPRIT trial, among ACS patients randomized to eptifibatide, there was a 47% relative reduction in the composite endpoint of death, MI, or urgent target vessel revascularization at 48 hours compared to a 25% relative reduction in those with stable angina. The number of patients with ACS was however small and this data cannot be used to compare the greater body of experience with tirofiban and abciximab.

## META-ANALYSIS OF GP IIB/IIIA INHIBITORS

The clinical trials of GP IIb/IIIa inhibition individually provide useful data with respect to their efficacy and safety but many questions regarding efficacy in subgroups as well as optimal patient selection are best answered by analysis of the entire body of available literature. There have been a few independently performed analyses of the large clinical trials of GP IIb/IIIa inhibition in ACS.

Boersma and colleagues pooled individual patient data from PRISM, PRISM-PLUS, PARAGON-A, PURSUIT, PARAGON-B, and GUSTO IV, ACS trials and evaluated the risks and benefits of GP IIb/IIIa inhibitors in ACS. Further by pooling individual patient data, they were able to evaluate the outcome at same time point for all studies.

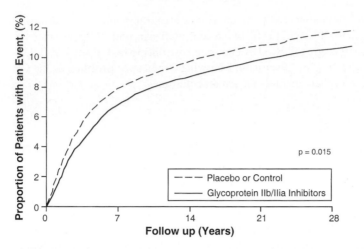

**Figure 4**  Kaplan Meier curve of death or MI among the entire cohort by randomization arm. (From Ref. 47a)

The studies differed with respect to definitions of MI and major bleeding, however the authors chose to use the individual study end point to adjudicate endpoint rather than redefining them with a common endpoint.

　　Their entire data set had 31,402 patients enrolled from 41 countries. There were no baseline differences between patients randomized to placebo or GP IIb/IIIa inhibitor. Of the entire cohort 46% had elevation in CK-MB isoenzyme, 56% had ST depression while 80 % had one of the two features. The authors evaluated outcome at 5 days and 30 days. No difference in mortality was noted across the two arms while there was a significant reduction in the incidence of non-fatal MI, or composite of death, or MI (Fig. 4). This reduction in events was evident early but there was no further reduction in events between day 5 and 30. Conversely no attenuation of the beneficial effect was seen during this time period. Subgroup analysis revealed that the effects of glycoprotein IIb/IIIa inhibitors were consistent across multiple subgroups (Figure 5). An enhanced benefit was seen in patients with elevated baseline troponin (discussion following). A significant interaction was noted between gender and the benefit of GP IIb/IIIa inhibitors. While in men there was clear benefit of GP IIb/IIIa inhibition the point estimate suggested the potential of an adverse outcome in women. The sex difference in outcome disappeared once troponin status was added to the multivariable model. It is possible that enrollment of women with no signifi-cant coronary artery disease into some of the trials may have diluted the demonstration of a treatment effect.

　　Roffi and colleagues also carried out two meta-analysis of these trials (discussion following) aimed at defining the subgroups that seemed to benefit the most from GP IIb/IIIa inhibition. The first demonstrated a clear survival benefit in diabetics [47] while the second demonstrated a gradient of benefit with the maximal benefit in those treated with an aggressive revascularization strategy [48].

## SELECT SUBGROUPS AND CLINICAL SUBTYPES

### Diabetes

Diabetics have indication of increased platelet reactivity [49–53] and appear to derive an enhanced benefit from GP IIb/IIIa platelet receptor antagonists [47,54–56]. Diabetics have

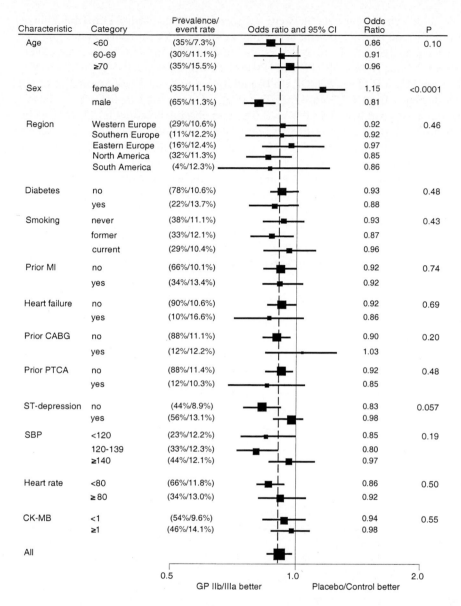

**Figure 5**   Odds of 30 day death and MI of patient subgroups defined by clinical characteristics. (From Ref. 47a)

evidence of increased platelet activation [50,53], adhesiveness and aggregability [51], and greater expression of platelet GP IIb/IIIa, thrombospondin, and P selectin [52]. While all patients appeared to benefit from peri-procedural abciximab, the diabetic substudy of Platelet IIb/IIIa Inhibitor for Stenting trial (EPISTENT) suggested an enhanced outcome in diabetics randomized to abciximab [56]. Combined analysis from 3 major PCI trials suggested a marked 1-year mortality benefit of abciximab in diabetics undergoing percutaneous coronary artery intervention [55]. Based on these lines of evidence, potent platelet inhibition may be of particular benefit in diabetic patients presenting with acute coronary syndromes although similar benefits were not seen in patients with STEMI randomized to receive half dose fibrinolytic and abciximab in GUSTO V. Roffi and colleagues performed a meta-analysis of the diabetic populations enrolled in the 6 large-scale platelet GP IIb/IIIa inhibitor ACS trials (PRISM, PRISM-PLUS, PARAGON A, PARAGON B, PURSUIT, and GUSTO IV) [47]. GP IIb/IIIa inhibition reduced 30-day mortality among the 6458 diabetics from 6.2% to 4.6% (OR 0.74; 95% CI 0.59 to 0.92; P = 0.007). Conversely, no survival benefit (3.0% vs. 3.0%) was observed among the 23,072 nondiabetic patients (Fig. 6). The interaction between platelet GP IIb/IIIa inhibition and diabetic status was statistically significant (P = 0.036). Among 1279 diabetic patients undergoing percutaneous coronary intervention (PCI) during index hospitalization, the use of these agents was associated with a mortality reduction at 30 days from 4.0% to 1.2% (OR 0.30; 95% CI 0.14 to 0.69; P = 0.002). Further it would appear that the excellent outcomes of

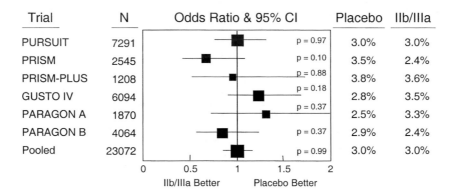

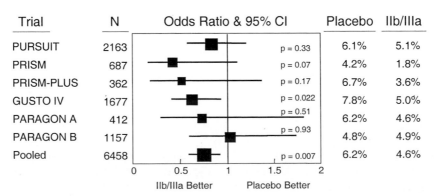

**Figure 6**  Impact of GP IIb/IIIa inhibitors on 30 day mortality in nondiabetics (a) or diabetics with ACS. Values to left of 1.0 indicate a survival benefit of platelet GP IIb/IIIa inhibition. (From Ref. 47)

PCI in diabetics as witnessed in the recent trials were obtained with triple anti-platelet therapy (aspirin, clopidogrel, and GP IIb/IIIa inhibitor) [57]. Indeed unlike GP IIb/IIIa inhibitors, clopidogrel has not demonstrated any enhanced benefits in diabetics [58]. These data help further define a subset that appears to derive greater benefit from GP IIb/IIIa inhibitors.

## Troponin

A major change in definition of ACS has been incorporation of troponin in defining NSTEMI [2,5]. Elevated troponin is regarded as a marker of microvascular obstruction and attendant myonecrosis. The underlying etiology is often platelet microthrombi that embolize distally from a ruptured plaque and hence these patients are theoretically likely to benefit from GP IIb/IIIa inhibition. Multiple studies have demonstrated an increase hazard of mortality and morbidity in association with elevated troponin in ACS patients [59–63]. As a post hoc analysis evaluating the efficacy of GP IIb/IIIa inhibitors in patients who have elevated troponin levels, Hamm and colleagues stratified patients in CAPTURE trial according to their baseline troponin levels [64]. The incidence of death or non-fatal MI at 6 months among patients receiving placebo was 23.9% among patients with elevated troponin vs. 7.5% among those with normal troponin. Treatment with abciximab was associated with a reduction in event rate among the troponin positive to 9.5% (RR 0.32, 95% CI, 0.14 − 0.62; P = 0.002). The lower event rates in patients receiving abciximab were attributable primarily to a reduction in the rate of MI (OR, 0.23; 95% CI, 0.12 − 0.49; P<0.001). In patients without elevated troponin T levels, abciximab therapy did not impact on the incidence of death or MI at 6 months (OR, 1.26; 95% CI, 0.74 − 2.31; P = 0.47). Similar data were reported from the PRISM study [65]. The investigators stratified patients according to those with elevated troponin T or I. The 30-day death or MI was markedly influenced by troponin status (13.0% for troponin-I-positive vs. 4.9% for troponin-I-negative patients p < 0.0001). Use of Tirofiban was associated with a reduction in both death (HR 0.25 [95% CI 0.09–0.68], p = 0.004) and MI (HR, 0.37 [95% CI 0.16–0.84], p = 0.01). This benefit was seen in both medically managed patients as well as those undergoing revascularization. There was no benefit of treatment in troponin-I-negative patients. Newby and colleagues prospectively enrolled 1160 patients in the PARAGON B trial in a troponin substudy [66]. Almost 40% of the patients were troponin positive at baseline and this cohort had a higher rate of adverse events [66]. Lamifiban was associated with significant reduction in the composite of death, MI, or severe ischemia (from 19.4% to 11.0%, P = 0.01) among TnT-positive patients but not among TnT-negative patients (11.2% for placebo vs. 10.8% for lamifiban, P = 0.86). The effect of troponin status was readdressed by the meta-analysis by Boersma and colleagues. Troponin status was available in 35% of their cohort. Among those with elevated troponin the risk of death or MI at 30 days was reduced from 12.0% to 10.3% with GP IIb/IIIa inhibitors while no difference in outcome of those with troponin negative status was seen (6.2% vs. 7.0%). Troponin status thus provides a useful marker to the clinician identifying patients that clearly benefit from GP IIb/IIIa inhibitors in ACS.

## INVASIVE THERAPY AND IIB/IIIA

The role of aggressive revascularization in the management of ACS is discussed at greater length in Chapter 16. As discussed earlier, the benefit of GP IIb/IIIa inhibitors appear to be greater in patients undergoing early revascularization. Roffi and colleagues analyzed a cohort of 29,570 patients enrolled in the IIb/IIIa ACS trials to assess the relative efficacy of GP IIb/IIIa inhibition based on the revascularization strategy. While not randomized, there was a clear gradient of benefit, with a 26% reduction in death or MI at 30 days in patients undergoing PCI while on a GP IIb/IIIa inhibitor (P = 0.02), a 13% reduction if PCI was performed after discontinuation of the drug (P = 0.17), and a 5% reduction in those medically managed (Fig. 7) [48]. An accompanying editorial calculated the numbers needed to treat with GP IIb/IIIa inhibition to prevent 1 death or MI as 32 if patients underwent PCI vs. 250 if the patients were medically treated [67]. The benefits of an early invasive approach have been tested in two landmark studies. The TIMI-TACTIC 18 study enrolled 2220 patients with ACS to early invasive vs. conservative therapy. All patients received tirofiban [43]. This study demonstrated a 22% reduction in the primary endpoint of death, MI, and rehospitalization for ACS at 6 months and a 26% reduction in death and MI. This was the first study to demonstrate a better outcome with invasive therapy and this was felt in part to relate to a lowering of periprocedural complications by tirofiban. The ISAR-COOL trial randomized 410 patients to either immediate intervention or medical therapy for delayed intervention [44]. All patients received aggressive antiplatelet therapy in the form of aspirin, clopidogrel, and tirofiban. The early intervention arm had a lower incidence of MI compared to those randomized to delayed intervention (Fig. 8). ISAR-COOL trial was the first to test the benefit of aggressive antiplatelet therapy and early PCI in ACS, a mode of practice that has come to be followed in the United States. These trials provide support for aggressive revascularization strategy on a background of a medical regimen including GP IIb/IIIa inhibitors. The pivotal role of GP IIb/IIIa inhibition in such a strategy becomes more evident when one compares the trials not using GP IIb/IIIa inhibitors such as FRISC II [68] where a slight excess of early myocardial infarctions was associated with aggressive revascularization a phenomenon not seen in TACTICS-TIMI 18 and thus likely related to the platelet passivation achieved by tirofiban.

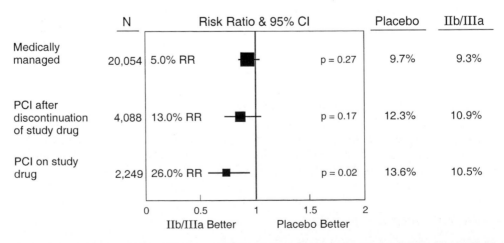

**Figure 7**  Odds of 30-day death or myocardial infarction: with 95% confidence intervals and P values according to revascularisation strategy among 29,570 patients. (From Ref. 48)

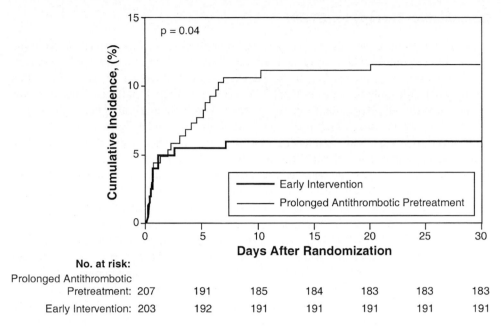

**No. at risk:**

| | | | | | | | |
|---|---|---|---|---|---|---|---|
| Prolonged Antithrombotic Pretreatment: | 207 | 191 | 185 | 184 | 183 | 183 | 183 |
| Early Intervention: | 203 | 192 | 191 | 191 | 191 | 191 | 191 |

**Figure 8** Cumulative incidence of death and myocardial infarction at 30 days among patients randomised to early intervention vs. prolonged antithrombotic therapy. (From Ref. 44)

## SAFETY

The major adverse effect of GP IIb/IIIa inhibitors is bleeding. While minor bleeding was commonly seen in all the trials, the incidence of major bleeding varied from 4.7% in the abciximab arm of GUSTO IV to 1.0% in the high dose lamifiban arm of PARAGON A. Combining the data from the six major trials the incidence of major bleeding was 2.4% in the GP IIb/IIIa arm compared to 1.4% in the placebo arm—translating into a 64% relative increase in a hazard of major bleeding. It is unclear if the risk of bleeding is higher with any particular agent. When the analysis was restricted to patients enrolled in the small molecule GP IIb/IIIa trials, the absolute incidence was lower (1.6%) although the relative hazard remained unchanged (64%) given the low risk of bleeding in the placebo arm (1%). No difference in the incidence of stroke or intracranial bleeding was noted. Bleeding was predominantly a function of invasive procedures with femoral access site bleeding being most common and most severe bleeding being associated with CABG. Subsequent data have emerged suggesting that the risk of CABG associated bleeding in patients with ACS is not substantially increased with GP IIb/IIIa inhibitors while there seems to be a reduction in the incidence of major adverse cardiac events in the peri-operative period [69].

## GP IIB/IIIA INHIBITION IN STEMI

Unlike the data in the setting of non-STEMI and PCI, among the available GP IIb/IIIa inhibitors only abciximab has been studied at length in the setting of STEMI. GP IIb/IIIa inhibition has been studied as adjunct to both mechanical and thrombolytic reperfusion.

## Combination Therapy for STEMI

Development of thrombolysis was a major step in improving outcome in STEMI. Multiple studies have demonstrated a significant survival advantage with thrombolysis especially when provided early after presentation. Despite its clinical success, it was evident that thrombolysis was able to achieve TIMI-3 flow in only 50% of patients. Further it was realized that thrombolytic agents may be associated with paradoxical platelet stimulation and resultant aggregation which may contribute to microvascular dysfunction and an increased propensity for reinfarction (Fig. 9) [70]. It was therefore hoped that by providing potent platelet inhibition with GP IIb/IIIa inhibition, further improvements in macro and microvascular flow would be obtained and translate into a survival advantage [71–73].

Combination therapy with GP IIb/IIIa inhibitors and fibrinolytics was evaluated in several pilot studies and was favorable enough to lead to larger clinical trials. In the Integrelin to Manage Platelet aggregation to combat Thrombosis in Acute Myocardial Infarction (IMPACT-AMI) [74] patients were randomized to receive eptifibatide or placebo in addition to alteplase. Significant improvement in TIMI-3 flow at 90 minutes was observed with combination therapy although the study was underpowered to detect differences in clinical endpoints. Similar early and enhanced myocardial perfusion was seen with combination of abciximab and tissue plasminogen activator [75] in TIMI-14 (Figure 10) and with eptifibatide and tissue plasminogen activator in INTRO AMI trial [76].

The clinical impact of the combination therapy was tested in two large clinical trials. In GUSTO V, 16,588 patients with ST elevation MI were randomly assigned to receive reteplase (two 10 U boluses 30 min. apart), or the combination of abciximab (infusion of 0.25 mg/kg bolus and 0.125 μg/kg per min, maximum of 10 μg/min) infusion for 12 hours plus half-dose reteplase (two boluses of 5 U, 30 min. apart) [77]. The primary endpoint of the study was all cause mortality at 30 days. There was no difference in the primary endpoint with 5.9% deaths in reteplase arm and 5.6% in the combination arm. There was a significant reduction in the rates of any

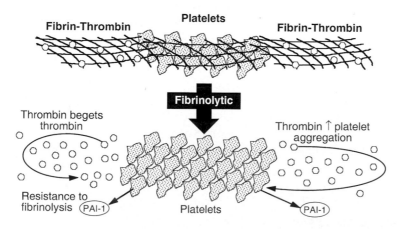

**Figure 9** Schematic illustration of the prothrombotic effects of fibrinolytic therapy. With fibrinolysis, thrombin, previously bound to clot, is re-exposed to the circulation. Thrombin is a potent platelet agonist and promotes further platelet aggregation. Platelets themselves are resistant to fibrinolytic agents. (From Ref. 70)

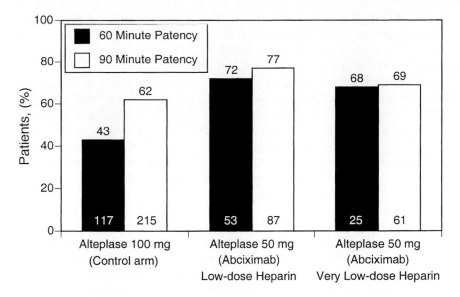

**Figure 10**  Percentage of patients with TIMI grade 3 flow at 60 minutes and 90 minutes in the TIMI-14 trial. The control group of alteplase 100 mg in accelerated dose regimen is compared with the regimens of alteplase 50 mg over 60 minutes, abciximab and either low-dose heparin (60 U/kg bolus and infusion of 7U/kg per hour) or very low-dose heparin (30 U/kg bolus and infusion of 4U/kg per hour). Significant increases in TIMI grade 3 flow rates were evident in the 50 mg alteplase, abciximab and low-dose heparin regimen at 60 and 90 minutes, compared with the control arm (* $p = 0.0009$, ** $p = 0.01$).

complications of MI and in the rate of reinfarction, recurrent ischemia, and ventricular fibrillation. These patients were followed for one year and no difference in mortality was noted across the two arms (8.4% vs. 8.4%) [78]. There was an increase in the risk of major bleeding which occurred in 1.1% of the patients in the combination arm compared to 0.5% of those in the reteplase arm.

The Assessment of the Safety and Efficacy of a New Thrombolytic-3 (ASSENT-3) investigators randomized 6095 patients to either full-dose tenecteplase and enoxaparin, half-dose tenecteplase with low-dose unfractionated heparin and abciximab, or full dose tenecteplase with unfractionated heparin [79]. The study had an efficacy endpoint (the composites of 30-day mortality, in-hospital reinfarction, or in-hospital refractory ischemia), and an efficacy plus safety endpoint (the composites of 30-day mortality, in-hospital reinfarction, in-hospital refractory ischemia, in-hospital intracranial hemorrhage, or in-hospital major bleeding complications). The best outcome was seen in the enoxaparin group with the efficacy endpoint in 11.4% vs. 15.4% in the heparin and 15.4% in the abciximab arm. Major bleeding occurred in 4.3% of the patients in the abciximab arm, 3.0% in the enoxaparin arm, and 2.2% in the heparin arm.

Thus, combination therapy, while providing a key reduction in secondary endpoints, is associated with no mortality benefit over standard fibrinolytic therapy and carries the cost of added bleeding risk. Given the failure of the secondary endpoint reduction to translate into a survival benefit at one year, and the increased propensity for bleeding complications, it is unlikely that combination therapy, as tested in these trials, will be incorporated in clinical practice.

The use of GP IIb/IIIa inhibitors in primary PCI is more established. Five studies have evaluated the role of GP IIb/IIIa inhibition in setting of primary PCI. In the ReoPro and Primary PTCA Organization and Randomized Trial (RAPPORT) of adjunctive GP IIb/IIIa receptor inhibition during infarct angioplasty, a total of 483 patients with evolving MI were assigned to either a bolus and 12 hour infusion of abciximab or a matching placebo [80]. Abciximab significantly reduced the incidence of death, reinfarction, or urgent TVR at 7 days (9.9% vs. 3.3%, P = 0.003), 30 days (11.2% vs. 5.8%, P = 0.03), and at 6 months (17.8% vs. 11.6%, P = 0.05) The Intracoronary Stenting and Antithrombotic Regimen-2 (ISAR-2) evaluated the impact of abciximab on restenosis after stenting performed in the setting of acute STEMI. While no difference was observed in the rate of restenosis, there was reduction in the composite of death, recurrent MI, and target lesion revascularization at 30 days (10.5% vs. 5.0%, P = 0.038).

Abciximab before Direct Angioplasty and Stenting in Myocardial Infarction Regarding Acute and Long-Term Follow-up (ADMIRAL) trial randomized 300 patients undergoing primary PCI with stenting for STEMI to abciximab or placebo [81]. The study demonstrated a reduction in the composite of death, MI, or urgent revascularization at 30 days from 14.6% in placebo arm to 6.0% in the abciximab arm (P = 0.01). Abciximab was administered in most patients prior to arrival in the catheterization laboratory and this was associated with TIMI-3 flow in 16.8% of the patients (vs. 5.4% in the placebo arm)

The Controlled Abciximab and Device Investigation to Lower Late Angioplasty Complications (CADILLAC) was the largest study evaluating abciximab in setting of primary PCI [82]. Patients were randomized in a two-by-two factorial design to angioplasty or stenting and abciximab or placebo. This trial did not demonstrate a difference in death, MI, or TIMI flow rate with abciximab. Eisenberg and Jamal pooled data from these four trials and divided them into those that used angioplasty with bail out stents vs. those that used stenting as the primary interventional strategy [71]. Use of abciximab was associated with a reduction in the composite of death MI and TVR at 30 days and 6 months in both groups. This endpoint was predominantly driven by TVR with one TVR prevented at 30 days for every 37 patients treated with abciximab.

The data providing convincing evidence for use of abciximab for primary PCI in STEMI comes from the recently published The Abciximab and Carbostent Evaluation (ACE) Trial. The study randomized 400 patients undergoing stenting for acute STEMI to abciximab or placebo. Randomization to abciximab reduced the composite of death, reinfarction, target vessel revascularization (TVR), and stroke at one month (primary endpoint) from 10.5% to 4.5% (P = 0.023). While the final TIMI blood flow was similar, abciximab use was associated with greater and earlier ST segment resolution and reduction of infarct size on scintigraphic analysis. More importantly, this improvement in microcirculation was associated with a significant reduction in the composite of death and MI at 6 months (5.5% vs. 13.5%, P = 0.006) [83]. One-year follow up from this trial demonstrates that this survival benefit is maintained long-term (5.1% vs. 10.7%, P = 0.040, David Antoniucci, personal communication).

The combined body of data on abciximab in primary PCI was reviewed in an editorial accompanying the ACE trial [84]. The pooled analysis from these 5 trials demonstrated a reduction in death at 30 days from 3.1% to 2.3%, in death and MI from 4.8% to 3.2%, and in death MI and TVR from 8.8% to 4.8% (Fig. 11). Thus the current body of literature supports the use of a catheter based reperfusion strategy on the background of early administration of abciximab.

Given that a major benefit of abciximab in ADMIRAL related to a better TIMI flow achieved at the time of angiography by early administration of the drug, the strategy of early administration of abciximab is being tested in the Facilitated Intervention with Enhanced

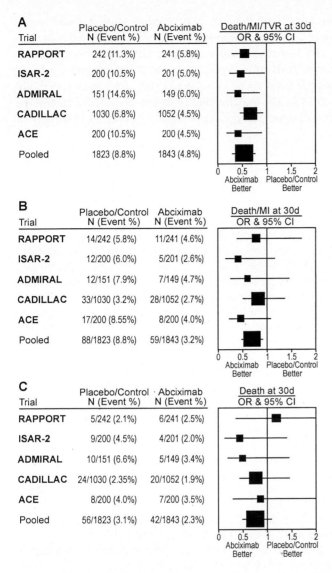

**Figure 11**  Odds of major adverse cardiac events in the 5 trials of abciximab for primary PCI. (**A**) Death, reinfarction and target vessel revascularization at 30 days. (**B**) Death or reinfarction at 30 days. (**C**) Death at 30 days. (From Ref. 84)

Reperfusion Speed to Stop Events (FINESSE) study [85]. This trial will further enhance our understanding of the role of GP IIb/IIIa inhibitors in a facilitated or rescue fashion with emergency coronary intervention.

## SUMMARY

GP IIb/IIIa inhibitors have been established as a major part of the therapeutic armamentarium available to a cardiologist in dealing with acute coronary syndromes. The last decade has witnessed an explosion of knowledge that has defined their role across the entire spectrum of ACS. Their proven benefit in diabetics and in those with elevated troponin serves to provide an easy tool for their appropriate therapeutic use in patients with USA/NSTEMI. The recently published trials firmly establish GP IIb/IIIa inhibition as pivotal for PCI performed for non-STEMI ACS. At the other end of the spectrum, patients with STEMI clearly stand to benefit from abciximab therapy used for primary PCI. GP IIb/IIIa inhibitors provide a useful tool for the clinician to improve clinical outcome by assuaging the activated platelets and have thus become integral to the modern therapy of ACS.

## REFERENCES

1. http://www.cdc.gov/nchs/data/lifetables/life89_1_4.pdf (accessed March10, 2003).
2. Braunwald E, Antman EM, Beasley JW, Califf RM, Cheitlin MD, Hochman JS, Jones RH, Kereiakes D, Kupersmith J, Levin TN, Pepine CJ, Schaeffer JW, Smith EE, Steward DE, Theroux P, Alpert JS, Eagle KA, Faxon DP, Fuster V, Gardner TJ, Gregoratos G, Russell RO, Smith SC. ACC/AHA guidelines for the management of patients with unstable angina and non-ST-segment elevation myocardial infarction. A report of the American College of Cardiology/American Heart Association Task Force on Practice Guidelines (Committee on the Management of Patients With Unstable Angina). J Am Coll Cardiol 2000;36:970–1062.
3. Braunwald E. Unstable angina. A classification. Circulation 1989;80:410–414.
4. Braunwald E, Califf RM, Cannon CP, Fox KA, Fuster V, Gibler WB, Harrington RA, King SB, Kleiman NS, Theroux P, Topol EJ, Van de Werf F, White HD, Willerson JT. Redefining medical treatment in the management of unstable angina. Am J Med. 2000;108:41–53.
5. Braunwald E, Antman EM, Beasley JW, Califf RM, Cheitlin MD, Hochman JS, Jones RH, Kereiakes D, Kupersmith J, Levin TN, Pepine CJ, Schaeffer JW, Smith EE, Steward DE, Theroux P, Gibbons RJ, Alpert JS, Eagle KA, Faxon DP, Fuster V, Gardner TJ, Gregoratos G, Russell RO, Smith SC. ACC/AHA guidelines for the management of patients with unstable angina and non-ST-segment elevation myocardial infarction: executive summary and recommendations. A report of the American College of Cardiology/American Heart Association task force on practice guidelines (committee on the management of patients with unstable angina). Circulation 2000;102:1193–1209.
6. Fuster V, Badimon L, Badimon JJ, Chesebro JH. The pathogenesis of coronary artery disease and the acute coronary syndromes (2). N Engl J Med 1992;326:310–318.
7. Fuster V, Badimon L, Badimon JJ, Chesebro JH. The pathogenesis of coronary artery disease and the acute coronary syndromes (1). N Engl J Med 1992;326:242–250.
8. Falk E. Unstable angina with fatal outcome: dynamic coronary thrombosis leading to infarction and/or sudden death. Autopsy evidence of recurrent mural thrombosis with peripheral embolization culminating in total vascular occlusion. Circulation 1985;71:699–708.
9. Davies MJ, Thomas AC. Plaque fissuring—the cause of acute myocardial infarction, sudden ischaemic death, and crescendo angina. Br Heart J 1985;53:363–373.
10. Theroux P, Ouimet H, McCans J, Latour JG, Joly P, Levy G, Pelletier E, Juneau M, Stasiak J, deGuise Pet al. Aspirin, heparin, or both to treat acute unstable angina. N Engl J Med 1988;319:1105–1111.
11. Hynes RO. Integrins: versatility, modulation, and signaling in cell adhesion. Cell 1992;69:11–25.
12. Tamkun JW, DeSimone DW, Fonda D, Patel RS, Buck C, Horwitz AF, Hynes RO. Structure of integrin, a glycoprotein involved in the transmembrane linkage between fibronectin and actin. Cell 1986;46:271–282.
13. Hynes RO. Integrins: a family of cell surface receptors. Cell 1987;48:549–554.
14. Parise LV. The structure and function of platelet integrins. Curr Opin Cell Biol 1989;1:947–952.

15. Wagner CL, Mascelli MA, Neblock DS, Weisman HF, Coller BS, Jordan RE. Analysis of GP IIb/IIIa receptor number by quantification of 7E3 binding to human platelets. Blood 1996; 88:907–914.

16. Henn V, Slupsky JR, Grafe M, Anagnostopoulos I, Forster R, Muller-Berghaus G, Kroczek RA. CD40 ligand on activated platelets triggers an inflammatory reaction of endothelial cells. Nature 1998;391:591–594.

17. Carroll RC, Wang XF, Lanza F, Steiner B, Kouns WC. Blocking platelet aggregation inhibits thromboxane A2 formation by low dose agonists but does not inhibit phosphorylation and activation of cytosolic phospholipase A2. Thromb Res 1997;88:109–125.

17a. Phillips DR. et al. Clinical pharmacology of eptifibatide. Am J Cardiol 1997; 80(4A): 11B–20B.

18. Coller BS. A new murine monoclonal antibody reports an activation-dependent change in the conformation and/or microenvironment of the platelet glycoprotein IIb/IIIa complex. J Clin Invest 1985;76:101–118.

19. Topol EJ, Byzova TV, Plow EF. Platelet GPIIb-IIIa blockers. Lancet 1999;353:227–231.

20. Kleiman NS. Pharmacokinetics and pharmacodynamics of glycoprotein IIb-IIIa inhibitors. Am Heart J 1999;138:263–275.

21. Kleiman NS. GP IIb/IIIa antagonists. Clinical experience and potential uses in cardiology. Drugs R D 1999;1:361–370.

22. Kleiman NS, Raizner AE, Jordan R, Wang AL, Norton D, Mace KF, Joshi A, Coller BS, Weisman HF. Differential inhibition of platelet aggregation induced by adenosine diphosphate or a thrombin receptor-activating peptide in patients treated with bolus chimeric 7E3 Fab: implications for inhibition of the internal pool of GP IIb/IIIa receptors. J Am Coll Cardiol 1995;26:1665–1671.

23. Mascelli MA, Lance ET, Damaraju L, Wagner CL, Weisman HF, Jordan RE. Pharmacodynamic profile of short-term abciximab treatment demonstrates prolonged platelet inhibition with gradual recovery from GP IIb/IIIa receptor blockade. Circulation 1998;97:1680–1688.

24. EPIC investigators. Use of a monoclonal antibody directed against the platelet glycoprotein IIb/IIIa receptor in high-risk coronary angioplasty. The EPIC Investigation. N Engl J Med 1994;330:956–961.

25. EPILOG investigators. Platelet glycoprotein IIb/IIIa receptor blockade and low-dose heparin during percutaneous coronary revascularization. The EPILOG Investigators. N Engl J Med 1997;336:1689–1696.

26. EPISTENT investigators. Randomised placebo-controlled and balloon-angioplasty-controlled trial to assess safety of coronary stenting with use of platelet glycoprotein- IIb/IIIa blockade. The EPISTENT Investigators. Evaluation of Platelet IIb/IIIa Inhibitor for Stenting. Lancet 1998;352:87–92.

27. Lincoff AM, Califf RM, Anderson KM, Weisman HF, Aguirre FV, Kleiman NS, Harrington RA, Topol EJ. Evidence for prevention of death and myocardial infarction with platelet membrane glycoprotein IIb/IIIa receptor blockade by abciximab (c7E3 Fab) among patients with unstable angina undergoing percutaneous coronary revascularization. EPIC Investigators. Evaluation of 7E3 in Preventing Ischemic Complications. J Am Coll Cardiol 1997;30: 149–156.

28. Topol EJ, Ferguson JJ, Weisman HF, Tcheng JE, Ellis SG, Kleiman NS, Ivanhoe RJ, Wang AL, Miller DP, Anderson KM, Califf RM. Long-term protection from myocardial ischemic events in a randomized trial of brief integrin beta3 blockade with percutaneous coronary intervention. EPIC Investigator Group. Evaluation of Platelet IIb/IIIa Inhibition for Prevention of Ischemic Complication. JAMA 1997;278:479–484.

29. CAPTURE investigators. Randomised placebo-controlled trial of abciximab before and during coronary intervention in refractory unstable angina: the CAPTURE Study. Lancet 1997;349: 1429–1435.

30. Hamm CW, Heeschen C, Goldmann B, Vahanian A, Adgey J, Miguel CM, Rutsch W, Berger J, Kootstra J, Simoons ML. Benefit of abciximab in patients with refractory unstable angina in relation to serum troponin T levels. c7E3 Fab Antiplatelet Therapy in Unstable Refractory Angina (CAPTURE) Study Investigators. N Engl J Med 1999;340:1623–1629.

31. Heeschen C, Dimmeler S, Hamm CW, van den Brand MJ, Boersma E, Zeiher AM, Simoons ML. Soluble CD40 ligand in acute coronary syndromes. N Engl J Med 2003;348:1104–1111.

32. Topol EJ, Moliterno DJ, Herrmann HC, Powers ER, Grines CL, Cohen DJ, Cohen EA, Bertrand M, Neumann FJ, Stone GW, DiBattiste PM, Demopoulos L. Comparison of two platelet glycoprotein IIb/IIIa inhibitors, tirofiban and abciximab, for the prevention of ischemic events with percutaneous coronary revascularization. N Engl J Med 2001;344: 1888–1894.

33. Moliterno DJ, Yakubov SJ, DiBattiste PM, Herrmann HC, Stone GW, Macaya C, Neumann FJ, Ardissino D, Bassand JP, Borzi L, Yeung AC, Harris KA, Demopoulos LA, Topol EJ. Outcomes at 6 months for the direct comparison of tirofiban and abciximab during percutaneous coronary revascularisation with stent placement: the TARGET follow-up study. Lancet 2002;360:355–360.

34. Stone GW, Moliterno DJ, Bertrand M, Neumann FJ, Herrmann HC, Powers ER, Grines CL, Moses JW, Cohen DJ, Cohen EA, Cohen M, Wolski K, DiBattiste PM, Topol EJ. Impact of clinical syndrome acuity on the differential response to 2 glycoprotein IIb/IIIa inhibitors in patients undergoing coronary stenting: the TARGET Trial. Circulation 2002;105:2347–2354.

35. Simoons ML. Effect of glycoprotein IIb/IIIa receptor blocker abciximab on outcome in patients with acute coronary syndromes without early coronary revascularisation: the GUSTO IV-ACS randomised trial. Lancet 2001;357:1915–1924.

36. Quinn MJ, Plow EF, Topol EJ. Platelet glycoprotein IIb/IIIa inhibitors: recognition of a two-edged sword?. Circulation 2002;106:379–85.

37. Ottervanger JP, Armstrong P, Barnathan ES, Boersma E, Cooper JS, Ohman EM, James S, Topol E, Wallentin L, Simoons ML. Long-term results after the glycoprotein IIb/IIIa inhibitor abciximab in unstable angina: one-year survival in the GUSTO IV-ACS (Global Use of Strategies To Open Occluded Coronary Arteries IV--Acute Coronary Syndrome) Trial. Circulation 2003;107:437–442.

38. Theroux P, Kouz S, Roy L, Knudtson ML, Diodati JG, Marquis JF, Nasmith J, Fung AY, Boudreault JR, Delage F, Dupuis R, Kells C, Bokslag M, Steiner B, Rapold HJ. Platelet membrane receptor glycoprotein IIb/IIIa antagonism in unstable angina. The Canadian Lamifiban Study. Circulation 1996;94:899–905.

39. PARAGON investigators. International, randomized, controlled trial of lamifiban (a platelet glycoprotein IIb/IIIa inhibitor), heparin, or both in unstable angina. The PARAGON Investigators. Platelet IIb/IIIa Antagonism for the Reduction of Acute coronary syndrome events in a Global Organization Network. Circulation 1998;97:2386–2395.

40. PARAGON B investigators. Randomized, placebo-controlled trial of titrated intravenous lamifiban for acute coronary syndromes. Circulation 2002;105:316–321.

41. PRISM investigators. A comparison of aspirin plus tirofiban with aspirin plus heparin for unstable angina. Platelet Receptor Inhibition in Ischemic Syndrome Management (PRISM) Study Investigators. N Engl J Med 1998;338:1498–1505.

42. PRISM-PLUS investigators. Inhibition of the platelet glycoprotein IIb/IIIa receptor with tirofiban in unstable angina and non-Q-wave myocardial infarction. Platelet Receptor Inhibition in Ischemic Syndrome Management in Patients Limited by Unstable Signs and Symptoms (PRISM-PLUS) Study Investigators. N Engl J Med 1998;338:1488–1497.

43. Cannon CP, Weintraub WS, Demopoulos LA, Vicari R, Frey MJ, Lakkis N, Neumann FJ, Robertson DH, DeLucca PT, DiBattiste PM, Gibson CM, Braunwald E. Comparison of early invasive and conservative strategies in patients with unstable coronary syndromes treated with the glycoprotein IIb/IIIa inhibitor tirofiban. N Engl J Med 2001;344:1879–1887.

44. Neumann FJ, Kastrati A, Pogatsa-Murray G, Mehilli J, Bollwein H, Bestehorn HP, Schmitt C, Seyfarth M, Dirschinger J, Schomig A. Evaluation of prolonged antithrombotic pretreatment (''cooling-off'' strategy) before intervention in patients with unstable coronary syndromes: a randomized controlled trial. JAMA 2003;290:1593–1599.

45. Schulman SP, Goldschmidt-Clermont PJ, Topol EJ, Califf RM, Navetta FI, Willerson JT, Chandra NC, Guerci AD, Ferguson JJ, Harrington RA, Lincoff AM, Yakubov SJ, Bray PF, Bahr RD, Wolfe CL, Yock PG, Anderson HV, Nygaard TW, Mason SJ, Effron MB, Fat-

terpacker A, Raskin S, Smith J, Brashears L, Gottdiener P, du Mee C, Kitt MM, Gerstenblith G. Effects of integrelin, a platelet glycoprotein IIb/IIIa receptor antagonist, in unstable angina. A randomized multicenter trial. Circulation 1996;94:2083–2089.

46.  PURSUIT investigators. Inhibition of platelet glycoprotein IIb/IIIa with eptifibatide in patients with acute coronary syndromes. The PURSUIT Trial Investigators. Platelet Glycoprotein IIb/IIIa in Unstable Angina: Receptor Suppression Using Integrilin Therapy. N Engl J Med 1998; 339:436–443.

47.  Roffi M, Chew DP, Mukherjee D, Bhatt DL, White JA, Heeschen C, Hamm CW, Moliterno DJ, Califf RM, White HD, Kleiman NS, Theroux P, Topol EJ. Platelet glycoprotein IIb/IIIa inhibitors reduce mortality in diabetic patients with non-ST-segment-elevation acute coronary syndromes. Circulation 2001;104:2767–2771.

47a. Boersma E, Harrington R, Moliterno D, et al. Platelet glycoprotein IIb/IIIa inhibitors in acute coronary syndromes: a meta-analysis of all major randomized clinical trials. Lancet 2002; 359:189–198.

48.  Roffi M, Chew DP, Mukherjee D, Bhatt DL, White JA, Moliterno DJ, Heeschen C, Hamm CW, Robbins MA, Kleiman NS, Theroux P, White HD, Topol EJ. Platelet glycoprotein IIb/IIIa inhibition in acute coronary syndromes. Gradient of benefit related to the revascularization strategy. Eur Heart J 2002;23:1441–1418.

49.  Marso SP, Mak KH, Topol EJ. Diabetes mellitus: biological determinants of atherosclerosis and restenosis. Semin Interv Cardiol 1999;4(1):29–143.

50.  Davi G, Catalano I, Averna M, Notarbartolo A, Strano A, Ciabattoni G, Patrono C. Thromboxane biosynthesis and platelet function in type II diabetes mellitus. N Engl J Med 1990;322: 1769–1774.

51.  Knobler H, Savion N, Shenkman B, Kotev-Emeth S, Varon D. Shear-induced platelet adhesion and aggregation on subendothelium are increased in diabetic patients. Thromb Res 1998;90: 181–190.

52.  Tschoepe D, Rauch U, Schwippert B. Platelet-leukocyte-cross-talk in diabetes mellitus. Horm Metab Res 1997;29:631–635.

53.  Davi G, Violi F, Catalano I, Giammarresi C, Putignano E, Nicolosi G, Barbagallo M, Notarbartolo A. Increased plasminogen activator inhibitor antigen levels in diabetic patients with stable angina. Blood Coagul Fibrinolysis 1991;2:41–45.

54.  Cho L, Marso SP, Bhatt DL, Topol EJ. Optimizing percutaneous coronary revascularization in diabetic women: analysis from the EPISTENT trial. J Womens Health Gend Based Med 2000;9:741–746.

55.  Bhatt DL, Marso SP, Lincoff AM, Wolski KE, Ellis SG, Topol EJ. Abciximab reduces mortality in diabetics following percutaneous coronary intervention. J Am Coll Cardiol 2000; 35:922–928.

56.  Marso SP, Lincoff AM, Ellis SG, Bhatt DL, Tanguay JF, Kleiman NS, Hammoud T, Booth JE, Sapp SK, Topol EJ. Optimizing the percutaneous interventional outcomes for patients with diabetes mellitus: results of the EPISTENT (Evaluation of platelet IIb/IIIa inhibitor for stenting trial) diabetic substudy. Circulation 1999;100:2477–2484.

57.  Roffi M, Topol E. Percutaneous coronary intervention in diabetic patients with non-ST-segment elevation acute coronary syndrome. Eur Heart J 2004:(in press).

58.  Yusuf S, Zhao F, Mehta SR, Chrolavicius S, Tognoni G, Fox KK. Effects of clopidogrel in addition to aspirin in patients with acute coronary syndromes without ST-segment elevation. N Engl J Med 2001;345:494–502.

59.  Hamm CW, Ravkilde J, Gerhardt W, Jorgensen P, Peheim E, Ljungdahl L, Goldmann B, Katus HA. The prognostic value of serum troponin T in unstable angina. N Engl J Med 1992; 327:146–150.

60.  Wu AH, Abbas SA, Green S, Pearsall L, Dhakam S, Azar R, Onoroski M, Senaie A, McKay RG, Waters D. Prognostic value of cardiac troponin T in unstable angina pectoris. Am J Cardiol 1995;76:970–972.

61.  Seino Y, Tomita Y, Takano T, Hayakawa H. Early identification of cardiac events with serum troponin T in patients with unstable angina. Lancet 1993;342:1236–1237.

62. Stubbs P, Collinson P, Moseley D, Greenwood T, Noble M. Prognostic significance of admission troponin T concentrations in patients with myocardial infarction. Circulation 1996;94:1291–1297.

63. Antman EM, Tanasijevic MJ, Thompson B, Schactman M, McCabe CH, Cannon CP, Fischer GA, Fung AY, Thompson C, Wybenga D, Braunwald E. Cardiac-specific troponin I levels to predict the risk of mortality in patients with acute coronary syndromes. N Engl J Med 1996;335:1342–1349.

64. Hamm CW, Heeschen C, Goldmann B, Vahanian A, Adgey J, Miguel CM, Rutsch W, Berger J, Kootstra J, Simoons ML. Benefit of abciximab in patients with refractory unstable angina in relation to serum troponin T levels. c7E3 Fab Antiplatelet Therapy in Unstable Refractory Angina (CAPTURE) Study Investigators. N Engl J Med 1999;340:1623–1629.

65. Heeschen C, Hamm CW, Goldmann B, Deu A, Langenbrink L, White HD. Troponin concentrations for stratification of patients with acute coronary syndromes in relation to therapeutic efficacy of tirofiban. PRISM Study Investigators. Platelet Receptor Inhibition in Ischemic Syndrome Management. Lancet 1999;354:1757–1762.

66. Newby LK, Ohman EM, Christenson RH, Moliterno DJ, Harrington RA, White HD, Armstrong PW, Van De Werf F, Pfisterer M, Hasselblad V, Califf RM, Topol EJ. Benefit of glycoprotein IIb/IIIa inhibition in patients with acute coronary syndromes and troponin t-positive status: the paragon-B troponin T substudy. Circulation 2001;103:2891–2896.

67. Antman EM. 'I can see clearly now': a new view on the use of IV GP IIb/IIIa inhibitors in acute coronary syndromes. Eur Heart J 2002;23:1408–1411.

68. FRISC II investigators. Invasive compared with non-invasive treatment in unstable coronary-artery disease: FRISC II prospective randomised multicentre study. FRagmin and Fast Revascularisation during InStability in Coronary artery disease Investigators. Lancet 1999;354:708–715.

69. Marso SP, Bhatt DL, Roe MT, Houghtaling PL, Labinaz M, Kleiman NS, Dyke C, Simmoons ML, Califf RM, Harrington RA, Topol EJ. Enhanced efficacy of eptifibatide administration in patients with acute coronary syndrome requiring in-hospital coronary artery bypass grafting. PURSUIT Investigators. Circulation 2000;102:2952–2958.

70. Topol EJ. Toward a new frontier in myocardial reperfusion therapy: emerging platelet preeminence. Circulation 1998;97:211–218.

71. Eisenberg MJ, Jamal S. Glycoprotein IIb/IIIa inhibition in the setting of acute ST-segment elevation myocardial infarction. J Am Coll Cardiol 2003;42:1–6.

72. Vivekananthan DP, Moliterno DJ. Glycoprotein IIb/IIIa combination therapy in acute myocardial infarction: tailoring therapies to optimize outcome. J Thromb Thrombolysis 2002;13:35–39.

73. Vivekananthan DP, Patel VB, Moliterno DJ. Glycoprotein IIb/IIIa antagonism and fibrinolytic therapy for acute myocardial infarction. J Interv Cardiol 2002;15:131–139.

74. Ohman EM, Kleiman NS, Gacioch G, Worley SJ, Navetta FI, Talley JD, Anderson HV, Ellis SG, Cohen MD, Spriggs D, Miller M, Kereiakes D, Yakubov S, Kitt MM, Sigmon KN, Califf RM, Krucoff MW, Topol EJ. Combined accelerated tissue-plasminogen activator and platelet glycoprotein IIb/IIIa integrin receptor blockade with Integrilin in acute myocardial infarction. Results of a randomized, placebo-controlled, dose-ranging trial. IMPACT-AMI Investigators. Circulation 1997;95:846–854.

75. Antman EM, Giugliano RP, Gibson CM, McCabe CH, Coussement P, Kleiman NS, Vahanian A, Adgey AA, Menown I, Rupprecht HJ, Van der Wieken R, Ducas J, Scherer J, Anderson K, Van de Werf F, Braunwald E. Abciximab facilitates the rate and extent of thrombolysis: results of the thrombolysis in myocardial infarction (TIMI) 14 trial. The TIMI 14 Investigators. Circulation 1999;99:2720–2732.

76. Brener SJ, Zeymer U, Adgey AA, Vrobel TR, Ellis SG, Neuhaus KL, Juran N, Ivanc TB, Ohman EM, Strony J, Kitt M, Topol EJ. Eptifibatide and low-dose tissue plasminogen activator in acute myocardial infarction: the integrilin and low-dose thrombolysis in acute myocardial infarction (INTRO AMI) trial. J Am Coll Cardiol 2002;39:377–386.

77. Topol EJ. Reperfusion therapy for acute myocardial infarction with fibrinolytic therapy or combination reduced fibrinolytic therapy and platelet glycoprotein IIb/IIIa inhibition: the GUSTO V randomised trial. Lancet 2001;357:1905–1914.

78. Lincoff AM, Califf RM, Van de Werf F, Willerson JT, White HD, Armstrong PW, Guetta V, Gibler WB, Hochman JS, Bode C, Vahanian A, Steg PG, Ardissino D, Savonitto S, Bar F, Sadowski Z, Betriu A, Booth JE, Wolski K, Waller M, Topol EJ. Mortality at 1 year with combination platelet glycoprotein IIb/IIIa inhibition and reduced-dose fibrinolytic therapy vs conventional fibrinolytic therapy for acute myocardial infarction: GUSTO V randomized trial. JAMA 2002;288:2130–2135.

79. ASSENT-3 investigators. Efficacy and safety of tenecteplase in combination with enoxaparin, abciximab, or unfractionated heparin: the ASSENT-3 randomised trial in acute myocardial infarction. Lancet 2001;358:605–613.

80. Brener SJ, Barr LA, Burchenal JE, Katz S, George BS, Jones AA, Cohen ED, Gainey PC, White HJ, Cheek HB, Moses JW, Moliterno DJ, Effron MB, Topol EJ. Randomized, placebo-controlled trial of platelet glycoprotein IIb/IIIa blockade with primary angioplasty for acute myocardial infarction. ReoPro and Primary PTCA Organization and Randomized Trial (RAPPORT) Investigators. Circulation 1998;98:734–741.

81. Montalescot G, Barragan P, Wittenberg O, Ecollan P, Elhadad S, Villain P, Boulenc JM, Morice MC, Maillard L, Pansieri M, Choussat R, Pinton P. Platelet glycoprotein IIb/IIIa inhibition with coronary stenting for acute myocardial infarction. N Engl J Med 2001;344: 1895–1903.

82. Stone GW, Grines CL, Cox DA, Garcia E, Tcheng JE, Griffin JJ, Guagliumi G, Stuckey T, Turco M, Carroll JD, Rutherford BD, Lansky AJ. Comparison of angioplasty with stenting, with or without abciximab, in acute myocardial infarction. N Engl J Med 2002;346:957–966.

83. Antoniucci D, Rodriguez A, Hempel A, Valenti R, Migliorini A, Vigo F, Parodi G, Fernandez-Pereira C, Moschi G, Bartorelli A, Santoro GM, Bolognese L, Colombo A. A randomized trial comparing primary infarct artery stenting with or without abciximab in acute myocardial infarction. J Am Coll Cardiol 2003;42:1879–1885.

84. Topol EJ, Neumann FJ, Montalescot G. A preferred reperfusion strategy for acute myocardial infarction. J Am Coll Cardiol 2003;42:1886–1889.

85. Topol EJ. Current status and future prospects for acute myocardial infarction therapy. Circulation 2003;108:III6–13.

# 19

# The Role of P2Y12 Blockade in Acute Coronary Syndromes and in the Catheterization Laboratory

**Peter Berger**
*Duke University Medical Center Duke Clinical Research Institute*
*Durham, North Carolina, U.S.A.*

## INTRODUCTION

In most cases, myocardial infarction and stroke, and often sudden death, are caused by arterial thrombosis. Antiplatelet drugs may reduce the occurrence of arterial thrombosis, particularly among patients with vascular disease who are at increased risk for arterial thrombosis. Oral antiplatelet drugs including aspirin, the thienopyridines, a class of drugs that currently includes only ticlopidine and clopidogrel, and cilostazol, a selective inhibitor of cyclic AMP phosphodiesterase, are used more and more frequently for the prevention of ischemic events in a wide variety of clinical settings. Several oral platelet glycoprotein (GP) IIb/IIIa inhibitors have been studied in randomized trials involving tens of thousands of patients; the results of these trials have been uniformly disappointing, resulting in an increase in mortality when analyzed in aggregate. These drugs will not be discussed in this chapter.

The following review will focus solely on the thienopyridines for the prevention and treatment of vascular events in patients with coronary artery disease.

## THE THIENOPYRIDINES: TICLOPIDINE AND CLOPIDOGREL

Ticlopidine, approved for use in the United States in 1991, and clopidogrel, approved in March 1998, are the only two members of the thienopyridines class of drugs currently available for use. The chemical structure and function of ticlopidine and clopidogrel are similar. However, clopidogrel has a carboxymethyl side group that ticlopidine does not, and no common metabolites of the two drugs have been identified. Both drugs exert their effects through an irreversible interaction with the P2Y12 adenosine 5′-diphosphate (ADP) receptor on platelets, one of the 3 identified ADP receptors on the surface of platelets, which results in the blockade of these receptors for the life of the platelet [1–3]. This prevents up-regulation of the platelet GP IIb/IIIa receptor, reducing fibrinogen binding to these receptors. ADP-receptor blockade also reduces thrombosis due to sheer stress and abolishes cyclic flow variations, and prolongs the bleeding time by approximately two-fold. Both ticlopidine and clopidogrel inhibit vascular smooth muscle contraction in rabbits and rats in response to endothelin and serotonin, and inhibit platelet-induced expression of tissue factor in endothelial cells, although the clinical relevance of these latter actions in humans remains unclear [4]. Neither ticlopidine nor clopidogrel influences heparin activity, affects the partial thromboplastin time, or affects the activated clotting time. Despite the similarities between ticlopidine and clopidogrel, however, there are important differences between the two drugs.

## Ticlopidine

Ticlopidine itself is not active, but it is metabolized to active metabolites by the liver [5]. Although peak levels of ticlopidine's active metabolite are reached within 2 hours, it takes ticlopidine between 5 and 7 days to achieve maximal platelet inhibition [5]. The reasons for the delay in antiplatelet effect have not been elucidated.

### Secondary Prevention Trials

Ticlopidine has been studied in 39 randomized placebo-controlled trials in which a total of 6,528 patients with vascular disease were enrolled for the prevention of vascular death, myocardial infarction, or stroke trials (Fig. 1) [6]. Meta-analysis reveals that ticlopidine reduced the frequency of the combined endpoint of vascular death, infarction, and stroke in these trials by 33% [6]. In one trial, enrollment was limited to patients with unstable angina [7]. In that trial, ticlopidine with conventional therapy was compared with conventional therapy alone, but aspirin was not routinely administered to patients in either arm, by study design. Ticlopidine reduced the frequency of vascular death and nonfatal myocardial infarction by 46% (13.6% vs. 7.3%, p = 0.009).

Ticlopidine has been compared with aspirin in 3 randomized trials in which 3,471 patients with either a stroke or a transient ischemic attack were enrolled [6]. Meta-analysis

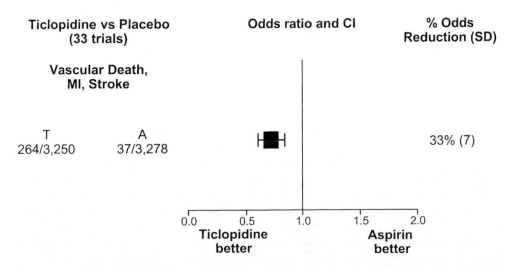

**Figure 1** Meta-analysis of the reduction in adverse vascular events seen in randomized trials comparing ticlopidine with placebo in which patients with stroke or transient ischemic attacks were enrolled. (From Ref. 6)

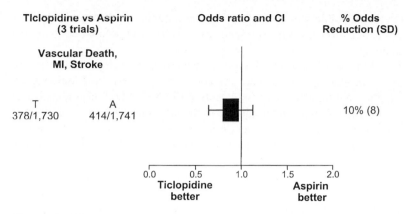

**Figure 2**   Meta-analysis of randomized trials comparing ticlopidine with aspirin in which patients with vascular disease were enrolled. (From Ref. 6)

revealed a 10% reduction in the frequency of the combined endpoint of vascular death, infarction, and stroke by ticlopidine compared with aspirin (Fig. 2) [6].

### In the Catheterization Laboratory

Two placebo-controlled randomized trials evaluated the efficacy of ticlopidine in patients undergoing balloon angioplasty who were not on aspirin [8,9]. In both studies, ticlopidine significantly reduced the frequency of acute vessel closure [8,9].

Little is known about whether aspirin combined with ticlopidine is more effective among patients undergoing balloon angioplasty than aspirin alone. Two retrospective studies suggested it does not [10,11]. In the Total Occlusion Study of Canada (TOSCA) trial, 410 patients with a coronary occlusion were randomly assigned to receive more than 1 heparin-coated Palmaz-Schatz coronary stent or treatment with balloon angioplasty alone [10]. Patients treated with balloon angioplasty alone received either aspirin and ticlopidine or aspirin alone, according to physician preference. The combination of aspirin and ticlopidine did not reduce the frequency of reocclusion or restenosis at six months, or adverse clinical events at one year. Although there were important differences in the baseline clinical, angiographic, and procedural characteristics among the two groups of patients, multivariate analysis used to adjust for these differences did not suggest benefit from adding ticlopidine to aspirin. An analysis of patients undergoing balloon angioplasty in the treatment of acute myocardial infarction in the STENT-PAMI trial revealed similar results [11]. These two retrospective studies are certainly not definitive. Subsequent to the performance of these two studies, a postrandomization subgroup analysis of patients enrolled in the CURE trial who underwent PCI by physician preference did suggest benefit from a thienopyridine (clopidogrel) in the approximately 20% of patients undergoing PCI in whom a stent was not used [12]. Clopidogrel had been administered a median of 10 days before PCI was performed in that study. The PCI-CURE substudy was far larger than the other two retrospective analyses and provides the best data addressing the issue of whether a thienopyridine, specifically clopidogrel (in contrast to the other two studies in which ticlopidine was used) prior to PCI is beneficial even when a stent is not placed, suggesting that it is.

### Ticlopidine and Coronary Stents

Six randomized trials have compared the combined use of aspirin and ticlopidine with aspirin alone, or aspirin with coumadin, in patients undergoing coronary stent placement

[13–18]. Aspirin and ticlopidine was the most effective regimen in all 6 trials (Fig. 3). Hemorrhagic complications were also less frequent with aspirin and ticlopidine than with aspirin and coumadin.

While aspirin and ticlopidine were both more efficacious and safe than aspirin and coumadin or aspirin alone among patients receiving coronary stents, the Full Anticoagulation vs. Ticlopidine plus Aspirin after Stent Implantation (FANTASTIC) trial revealed an important limitation of therapy with ticlopidine [17]. In FANTASTIC, the first dose of ticlopidine was administered on the day of stent implantation; pretreatment was not performed. The results of the trial reveal that stent thrombosis actually occurred more frequently in the 24 hours after stent placement among patients receiving ticlopidine than those receiving intravenous heparin while coumadin was being initiated (2.4% vs. 0.4%, respectively, p = 0.06). Subsequent to 24 hours, the frequency of stent thrombosis was reduced in the ticlopidine-treated patients, and the cumulative occurrence of stent thrombosis tended to be less in the ticlopidine patients (2.8% vs. 3.9%, p = NS). However, the trial indicates that when ticlopidine is first initiated the day of stent placement, as it frequently is in clinical practice, ticlopidine appears to provide insufficient antiplatelet inhibition for at least the first 24 hours after stent placement.

A hematological study of patients undergoing stent implantation randomly assigned to receive aspirin alone, ticlopidine alone, or aspirin and ticlopidine (with the first dose of ticlopidine administered on the day of the procedure in both ticlopidine arms) confirms the inadequate platelet inhibition in the ticlopidine arm early after stent placement. In that study, platelet aggregation and fibrinogen binding to GP IIb/IIIa receptors were most inhibited on the 7th and 14th days after stent placement in the group receiving aspirin and ticlopidine [19]. However, in the 24 hours following stent implantation, platelet aggregation and fibrinogen binding were similar in the three groups, which may explain ticlopi-

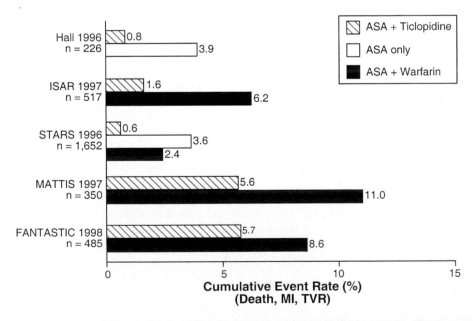

**Figure 3**  Results from the six randomized trials in which aspirin and ticlopidine were compared with either aspirin or aspirin and coumadin in patients following coronary stent placement.

dinc's inability to prevent stent thrombosis early after stent placement when pretreatment with ticlopidine has not been performed.

*Side Effects of Ticlopidine*

In many of the trials evaluating ticlopidine in patients with vascular disease, ticlopidine caused side effects, such as nausea, diarrhea, and rash, requiring discontinuation in as many as 20% of patients. The most serious side effects of ticlopidine, neutropenia and thrombotic thrombocytopenic purpura (TTP), are less frequent. Neutropenia occurs in approximately 1% to 3% of patients and can be life threatening; TTP which occurs much less frequently, perhaps in as few as 0.03% of patients, is fatal in 25% to 50% of cases [20]. Mortality from TTP is reduced if plasmapheresis is initiated rapidly. Because of these potentially lethal hematologic side effects and the need to make a diagnosis and begin treatment rapidly, blood counts should be examined serially in the first several months of ticlopidine use, the period during which these side effects are most likely to occur.

*Duration of Ticlopidine Therapy in Stent Patients*

Based on the six randomized trials showing that ticlopidine, with aspirin, is the most efficacious therapy following stent placement to prevent stent thrombosis, and based on the increasing frequency with which stents are placed during percutaneous revascularization procedures, the frequency with which ticlopidine is prescribed grew enormously. In an attempt to reduce not only the frequent minor side effects of ticlopidine but especially the risk of life-threatening neutropenia and TTP, studies were performed of the safety and efficacy of administering ticlopidine for only 2 weeks after stent placement. Neutropenia is exceedingly rare during 2 weeks or less of therapy; TTP does occur with less than 2 weeks of ticlopidine therapy, although less frequently than after longer periods of therapy.

In a study of 827 consecutive patients at the Mayo Clinic in whom ticlopidine was discontinued on the 14th day after stent placement, 1.6% of patients suffered an adverse event (including death, myocardial infarction, or the need for a repeat angioplasty procedure or bypass surgery) in the first 14 days after stent placement, while ticlopidine was being administered [21]. However, stent thrombosis did not occur in the 15th through 30th days after stent placement, after ticlopidine had been discontinued [21]. The ninety-five percent confidence intervals for stent thrombosis, given no observed cases in 817 patents, range from 0–0.5%, suggesting that the risk of late stent thrombosis was less than the combined incidence of neutropenia and TTP when ticlopidine is given for 30 days. The investigators concluded that in patients undergoing stent implantation treated with ticlopidine, ticlopidine should be administered for only 14 days. In a subsequent substudy of the ATLAST (Antiplatelet Therapy Alone vs. Lovenox Plus Antiplatelet Therapy in Patients at Increased Risk of Stent Thrombosis) trial, 1,102 patients at increased risk of stent thrombosis who did not receive a platelet GP IIb/IIIa inhibitor were randomized to receive either enoxaparin or placebo subcutaneously for 2 weeks; all patients received ticlopidine for only 2 weeks [22]. In the third and fourth weeks after enrollment, after ticlopidine had been discontinued, there was one definite case of stent thrombosis and two possible cases, for a frequency of definite or possible stent thrombosis of 0.27% (95% confidence intervals 0.06–0.77). These data indicate that although longer periods of treatment with a thienopyridine may well be helpful in terms of reducing events other than stent thrombosis, they do not appear to be required to reduce the frequency of stent thrombosis in the 15–30 days after placement of a bare metal stent.

*Consequences of the Slow Onset of Action of Ticlopidine*

**Stent thrombosis.**    Although limiting the duration of therapy of ticlopidine to two weeks after stent placement eliminates neutropenia and significantly reduces the frequency of TTP, there remains problems associated with ticlopidine not only due to its frequent nonlethal side effects, but related to the slow onset of action of ticlopidine, as described above. Most percutaneous revascularization procedures are not planned for days in advance of the procedure, precluding pretreatment of patients with ticlopidine before a stent procedure. A study from Mayo Clinic suggests that more complete platelet inhibition from a thienopyridine at the time of stent placement may decrease the risk of stent thrombosis [23]. Wilson et al. compared the frequency and timing of stent thrombosis rate in patients treated with aspirin and coumadin to that in patients treated with aspirin and ticlopidine. In the aspirin and coumadin patients, the median time to stent thrombosis was 4 days. In contrast, in the aspirin and ticlopidine patients, the median time to stent thrombosis was 12 hours, during the time that maximal platelet inhibition with a thienopyridine has not yet occurred. Stent thrombosis was very rare after the first day. These data suggest that more complete platelet inhibition at the time of the stent procedure might reduce the risk of early stent thrombosis.

A study from Schomig et al. also suggests that the slow onset of action of ticlopidine may well be important. These investigators examined their first 2,833 patients who received coronary stents. Initially, patients were treated with aspirin and coumadin; subsequent patients were treated with aspirin and ticlopidine [24]. Although the group who received aspirin and coumadin had a 5-fold greater frequency of stent thrombosis, stent thrombosis was as likely to occur in the first day after stent placement in patients treated with heparin while coumadin was being initiated as it was in patients treated with ticlopidine. That stent thrombosis was most likely to occur in the first day of stent placement in the ticlopidine cohort, and less likely to occur subsequently when platelet aggregation was more inhibited by ticlopidine, also suggests that more complete platelet inhibition by a thienopyridine at the time of stent placement might reduce the risk of stent thrombosis.

**Procedural infarction.**    Data from Steinhubl and others at Cleveland Clinic indicate that more complete platelet inhibition from ticlopidine at the time of stent placement procedure might reduce the frequency of procedural myocardial infarction [25]. These investigators studied 175 patients undergoing elective stent placement patients and found that among patients who had received ticlopidine more than 3 days prior to the stent implantation procedure, the frequency of myocardial infarction (defined as any elevation of creatinine phosphokinase above normal with an elevation of CK-MB) was only 11%. If ticlopidine was administered for 1–2 days prior to stent placement, the frequency of myocardial infarction was 17%. If ticlopidine was first administered the day of the procedure, as is the practice at most hospitals where unplanned procedures are common, 29% of patients suffered a procedural myocardial infarction.

A second study by Steinhubl et al. also supports the theory that more complete platelet inhibition reduces procedural myocardial infarction [26]. In the EPISTENT trial, 2,399 patients requiring a percutaneous coronary intervention were randomly assigned to undergo coronary stent placement with aspirin and ticlopidine without a platelet GP IIb/IIIa inhibitor; stent placement with aspirin, ticlopidine, and the GP IIb/IIIa inhibitor abciximab; or balloon angioplasty with aspirin and abciximab [27]. Although by study protocol patients were to receive pretreatment with ticlopidine whenever possible, only about one-half of patients were pretreated with ticlopidine for more than 24 hours. A retrospective analysis indicated that the frequency of the combined endpoint of death, myocardial infarction, or urgent target vessel revascularization within 30 days after enrollment was significantly lower among stent patients who received pretreatment with ticlopidine [26]. The reduction in the combined endpoint was driven by a reduction in procedural myocardial infarction. The addition of abciximab further reduced the frequency of adverse events among stent patients, even among those pretreated with ticlopidine, but the risk reduction from ticlopidine pretreatment was approximately equal to the reduction in risk seen with abciximab. These data indicate that pretreatment with a thienopyridine may reduce procedural myocardial infarction, although they also indicate that the reduction in procedural myocardial infarction achieved with a thienopyridine is less than the reduction that can be achieved with abciximab.

These limitations of ticlopidine—its frequent side effects, the need to monitor blood counts during its administration, and its slow onset of action—stimulated interest in the more recently developed thienopyridine, clopidogrel.

## Clopidogrel

Clopidogrel is a thienopyridine closely related to ticlopidine in chemical structure and function [3]. Despite the similarities, no common metabolites of the two drugs have yet been identified. All metabolites of clopidogrel that have been identified contain a carboxymethyl side group that metabolites of ticlopidine lack.

Like ticlopidine, clopidogrel itself is not believed to be active; clopidogrel is metabolized by the liver to other compounds that account for its activity [3,28]. Peak levels of the metabolite that accounts for its antiplatelet effect are reached in approximately 1 hour; however, like ticlopidine, it takes approximately 5 days to achieve maximal platelet inhibition from clopidogrel when no loading dose is administered.

*Secondary Prevention*

A dose-finding study of clopidogrel found that 75 mg per day achieved greater steady-state inhibition of platelets to $5\mu M$ ADP than did lower doses; doses higher than 75 mg/day did not achieve greater platelet inhibition (Fig. 4) [29]. A dose of 75 mg per day achieved the same degree of platelet inhibition as ticlopidine 250 mg twice daily.

On the basis of the dose-finding study, a daily dose of 75 mg of clopidogrel was used in the CAPRIE trial in which 19,185 patients, one third of whom had peripheral vascular disease, one third cerebrovascular disease, and one third coronary artery disease, were enrolled [30]. Patients were randomly assigned to receive clopidogrel 75 mg per day or aspirin 325 mg per day in addition to their other medications. After 3 years of follow-up, patients receiving clopidogrel had a slightly though statistically significantly 8.7% lower rate of death, myocardial infarction, or ischemic stroke (p = 0.043) (Fig. 5). The risk reduction of 8.7% was small in absolute terms, corresponding to 0.5% fewer events per year. Perhaps the most impressive finding in CAPRIE was the infrequency with which side effects required that the study drug be discontinued (Table 1). Clopidogrel was discontinued because of side effects slightly less frequently than aspirin, even though only aspirin-tolerant patients were included in CAPRIE [30].

When the same endpoints are examined as were examined in the previously published meta-analysis of the 3 randomized trials comparing ticlopidine and aspirin—vascular death, nonfatal myocardial infarction, or any stroke—the risk reduction achieved with clopidogrel in CAPRIE was 10%, the same risk reduction seen with ticlopidine in the meta-analysis of trials comparing ticlopidine and aspirin [31]. Therefore, not only is the amount of ex-vivo inhibition of platelet aggregation with clopidogrel the same as is

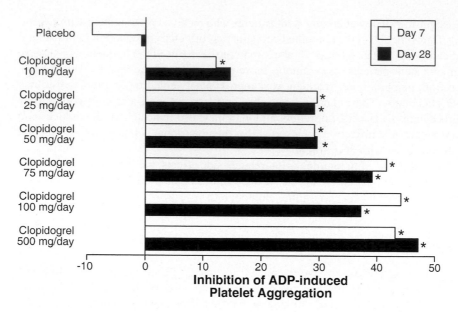

**Figure 4** Results from a dose-ranging study in which clopidogrel 75 mg per day achieved greater steady-state inhibition of platelets than lower doses of clopidogrel, and the same degree of platelet inhibition as ticlopidine 250 mg twice daily. (From Ref. 29)

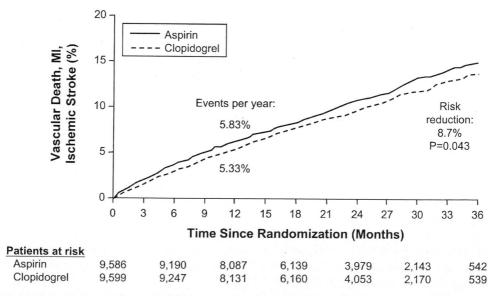

**Figure 5** Results of the CAPRIE study. The 8.7% reduction in the risk of death, hemorrhagic stroke, and nonfatal myocardial infarction with clopidogrel over aspirin during 3 years of follow-up corresponded to 0.5% fewer events per year. (Modified from Ref. 30.)

**Table 1**　Frequency of Side Effects Requiring Permanent Discontinuation of Study Drug in CAPRIE. Discontinuation of Study Drug Tended To Be More Frequent Among Patients Taking Aspirin Than Clopidogrel in the Study, Even Though Only Patients Believed Tolerant of Aspirin Were Eligible for Inclusion

| | Study Drug Permanently Discontinued | | | |
| | Clopidogrel n = 9,599 | | Aspirin n = 9,586 | |
| Adverse Experience | No. | % | No. | % |
| --- | --- | --- | --- | --- |
| Rash | 86 | 0.90 | 39 | 0.41* |
| Diarrhea | 40 | 0.42 | 26 | 0.27 |
| Indigestion/nausea/vomiting | 182 | 1.90 | 231 | 2.41* |
| Any bleeding disorder | 115 | 1.20 | 131 | 1.27 |
| Intracranial hemorrhage | 20 | 0.21 | 32 | 0.33 |
| Gastrointestinal hemorrhage | 50 | 0.52 | 89 | 0.93* |
| Abnormal liver function | 22 | 0.23 | 28 | 0.29 |
| | | 5.3 | | 6.0 |

* Statistically significant, $P < 0.05$
(From Ref. 30)

achieved with ticlopidine, but the reduction in adverse events with clopidogrel is also identical to the reduction with ticlopidine.

The benefits of clopidogrel in the CAPRIE trial are probably not sufficient to recommend that patients currently on aspirin be switched to clopidogrel. The results of CAPRIE do, however, indicate that in patients with vascular disease intolerant of aspirin, clopidogrel is the antiplatelet treatment of choice, and it should be continued indefinitely (a position endorsed by the American Heart Association and American College of Cardiology) [32]. The excellent safety profile of clopidogrel in CAPRIE also raises questions not addressed by the study, such as whether clopidogrel should be administered to patients who suffer a myocardial infarction or develop an acute coronary syndrome while on aspirin, or to patients at very high risk of myocardial infarction or death due to severe atherosclerosis, perhaps involving all three coronary arteries and perhaps the peripheral and cerebral circulations. It is also raises the question whether clopidogrel should be administered to patients with biochemical evidence of aspirin resistance, which has been reported to exist in between 5 and 40% of patients, depending on how it is defined [33–35]. The available studies do suggest a greater frequency of thrombotic events in such patients, and it has been hypothesized that such patients may derive particular benefit from a thienopyridine [36–39].

The Clopidogrel in Unstable Angina (CURE) study examined many of these issues. In CURE, 12,562 patients admitted to the hospital for treatment of an acute coronary syndrome were randomly assigned to combination therapy with aspirin and clopidogrel vs. aspirin and placebo [40]. Only sites that generally pursue a noninvasive evaluation in such patients and infrequently perform coronary angiography were permitted to participate in the trial. The results of the trial revealed that the primary endpoint, a combined endpoint of vascular death, myocardial infarction, and stroke were reduced by 20% (11.47 vs. 9.28%, p = 0.00005) (Fig. 6). Although there was a significant increase in the risk of bleeding associated with clopidogrel, most people believe that the benefits exceeded the risks in this study.

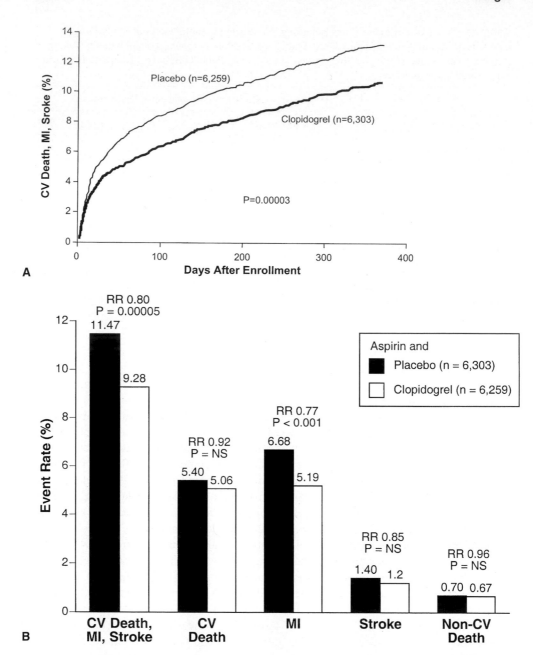

**Figure 6** The CURE Study. (**A**) The frequency of vascular death, non-fatal myocardial infarction, and stroke were reduced with dual antiplatelet therapy, and the event curves appear to be diverging during the year following study entry. (**B**) Not only the primary end-point but also all of its individual components were lower when clopidogrel was combined with aspirin. Not only vascular death but all cause death tend to be lower with dual antiplatelet therapy.

A subsequent subgroup analysis of this study revealed that the risk reduction was approximately similar in high-, intermediate-, and low-risk patients [41]. The absolute reduction in events was greatest among high-risk patients since such patients had the highest event rate. However, benefit from dual antiplatelet therapy with aspirin and clopidogrel was seen in all subgroups reported.

Another large trial of dual antiplatelet therapy with aspirin and clopidogrel is underway, the Clopidogrel for High Atherothrombotic Risk and Ischemic Stabilization, Management and Avoidance (CHARISMA) trial. In it, patients with stable coronary, peripheral, or cerebrovascular are being randomized to aspirin and clopidogrel vs. aspirin and placebo. Enrollment of patients (n = 15,200) has been completed; the trial will not be terminated until a certain number of events are reached in the overall trial, and follow-up is expected to last several years.

## Clopidogrel in the Catheterization Laboratory

The available data suggest that clopidogrel and ticlopidine have equivalent antiplatelet activity [29]. However, there are reasons to believe that clopidogrel might be more effective than ticlopidine in patients undergoing coronary revascularization procedures. Since maximal platelet inhibition is not achieved until at least 5 days of treatment with ticlopidine, a 500 mg loading dose of ticlopidine is usually administered in order to slightly speed the onset of platelet inhibition. Larger loading doses of ticlopidine frequently cause nausea and vomiting and are not recommended. Clopidogrel 75 mg, administered once daily, also takes at least 5 days to achieve maximal platelet inhibition but, in contrast to ticlopidine, large loading doses are well tolerated. A 375 mg dose of clopidogrel produced 60% platelet inhibition in healthy volunteers at 90 minutes in response to 5 μM ADP, and maximal platelet inhibition was achieved within 6 hours [42].

## Clopidogrel in Patients Undergoing Stent Placement

Based on the data indicating that clopidogrel and ticlopidine produce equivalent ex-vivo platelet inhibition [29], an equivalent reduction in adverse events among patients with vascular disease when compared with aspirin [31], and that both appeared to be very effective in animal models at reducing stent thrombosis [43,44], many laboratories changed their practice and began administering clopidogrel in place of ticlopidine to patients undergoing coronary stent procedures. In most cases, a 300 mg dose of clopidogrel was administered immediately before or after the implantation procedure, when pretreatment was not possible, and 75 mg per day had been continued for 14–30 days. Data from 4 randomized trials, all relatively small, and several observational analyses have been published [45–57].

## Randomized trials

In the Clopidogrel Aspirin Stent International Cooperative Study (CLASSICS) trial performed in Europe, 1020 stent patients were randomly assigned to receive clopidogrel with a 300 mg loading dose followed by 75 mg per day for 28 days; clopidogrel 75 mg without a loading dose followed by 75 mg per day for 28 days; or ticlopidine 250 mg followed by 250 mg twice daily for 28 days [43]. The initial dose of a thienopyridine was administered between one and six hours after stent placement, limiting the benefit one might hope to see from the most rapidly-acting regimen, clopidogrel with a 300 mg loading dose. The result of the trial indicated that clopidogrel, with or without a loading dose, was better tolerated than ticlopidine. Paradoxically, a 300 mg loading dose of clopidogrel was better tolerated than a 75 mg dose of clopidogrel with respect to side effects, which can only be attributed to chance. Although the study was sized to detect a difference in side effects and was too small to detect a difference in the frequency of stent thrombosis or other major adverse events, the frequency of such events was similar in all 3 arms: 0.9% in the ticlopidine arm, 1.5% in the arm that received an initial dose of 75 mg of clopidogrel, and 1.2% in the group that received clopidogrel with a 300 mg loading dose, a difference of one event between each of the groups, p = NS for all comparisons.

In the second randomized trial, a single center study from Barnes Hospital in St. Louis, Ticlid or Plavix Post-Stents (TOPPS), 1000 stent patients were randomly assigned to receive a 300 mg loading dose of clopidogrel followed by 75 mg per day for 14 days or 500 mg loading dose of ticlopidine followed by 250 mg twice daily for 14 days [44]. The initial dose of study drug was administered within 2 hours after stent placement. An intravenous platelet GP IIb/IIIa inhibitor was administered to 48% of patients in the trial. The results of an interim analysis including the first 941 patients enrolled in the trial reveal that the frequency of stent thrombosis within 24 hours of stent placement was 0.62% in the ticlopidine arm vs. 0.66% in the clopidogrel arm (p = 0.93). The frequency of stent thrombosis in the subsequent 29 days was 0.82% in the ticlopidine arm vs. 1.10% in the clopidogrel arm (p = 0.66). The frequency of death, stent thrombosis, or need for a repeat target lesion revascularization procedure was 3.49% in the ticlopidine arm vs. 2.64% in the clopidogrel arm (p = 0.45).

In the third randomized trial comparing clopidogrel and ticlopidine, this one from Germany, 700 stent patients were randomly assigned to receive a clopidogrel 75 mg per day without a loading dose, or a 500 mg loading dose of ticlopidine, followed by 250 mg twice daily, for 4 weeks [45]. The initial dose of study drug was administered within 1 hour after stent placement. The results of the study indicate that the frequency of a major adverse event (death, myocardial infarction, stent thrombosis, or need for a repeat target lesion revascularization procedure) was 1.7% in the ticlopidine arm vs. 3.1% in the clopidogrel arm (p = 0.24). Stent thrombosis occurred in 0.6% of patients in the ticlopidine arm vs. 2.0 % in the clopidogrel arm (p = 0.10).

A fourth randomized trial compared a 300 mg loading dose of clopidogrel followed by 75 mg daily for 4 weeks with ticlopidine 250 twice daily for 4 weeks without a loading dose [46]. Only 68 patients were enrolled in this very small trial.

Meta-analysis of the three large randomized trials and registries reveals that the frequency of stent thrombosis, and the frequency of any major ischemic event, has tended to be lower in the clopidogrel cohort than the comparator ticlopidine groups in nearly all of these retrospective studies (Fig. 7) [58]. The observational studies which generally suggest superiority of clopidogrel over ticlopidine are limited, since newer generation stents have become available and are generally superior in at least some way over the older stents, and operator experience has increased. However, taken together, the results of these registries along with the randomized trials suggest that clopidogrel is associated with a very low frequency of stent thrombosis and other ischemic events, and there is nothing to suggest that the outcome of stent patients treated with clopidogrel is inferior to that of patients treated with ticlopidine.

The data, in aggregate, suggest that clopidogrel is at least equivalent to ticlopidine in preventing stent thrombosis and procedural infarction. Whether clopidogrel is superior to ticlopidine given its rapid onset of action remains unproven. However, clopidogrel has nonetheless completely replaced ticlopidine in the United States and around the world wherever both drugs are available, both in and out of the catheterization laboratory, because

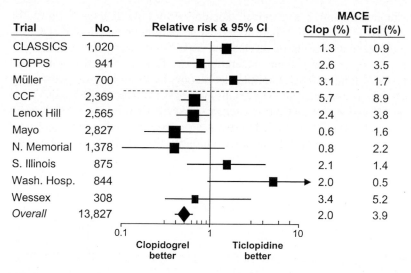

| Trial | No. | Relative risk & 95% CI | MACE Clop (%) | Ticl (%) |
|-------|-----|------------------------|---------------|----------|
| CLASSICS | 1,020 | | 1.3 | 0.9 |
| TOPPS | 941 | | 2.6 | 3.5 |
| Müller | 700 | | 3.1 | 1.7 |
| CCF | 2,369 | | 5.7 | 8.9 |
| Lenox Hill | 2,565 | | 2.4 | 3.8 |
| Mayo | 2,827 | | 0.6 | 1.6 |
| N. Memorial | 1,378 | | 0.8 | 2.2 |
| S. Illinois | 875 | | 2.1 | 1.4 |
| Wash. Hosp. | 844 | | 2.0 | 0.5 |
| Wessex | 308 | | 3.4 | 5.2 |
| Overall | 13,827 | | 2.0 | 3.9 |

0.1    1    10

Clopidogrel better     Ticlopidine better

**Figure 7** Data from randomized trials and registries in which patients treated with clopido-grel were compared with patients who had received ticlopidine. Different regimens were examined in each of the randomized trials and in many of the registries, and many different definitions of endpoints were used. Nonetheless, the data indicate a low rate of stent throm-bosis and other major adverse events among stent patients treated with clopidogrel.

frequent side effects such as nausea, vomiting, diarrhea, and rare potentially fatal side effects, such as neutropenia and TTP, are far fewer than with clopidogrel.

With over 22 million patients treated with clopidogrel, TTP has been reported via postmarketing surveillance to have occurred in 70 patients. Many were on other drugs reported to be associated with the development of TTP, and causality has not been proven in most of these patients (personal conversation, Melvin Blumenthal, Bristol-Myers-Squibb). Although postmarketing surveillance nearly always suffers from underreporting, this ap-proximate frequency of roughly 3.2 cases of TTP per million patients treated with clopido-grel appears similar to the background frequency of TTP in the general population which is approximately 4 per million patients. Clopidogrel also replaced ticlopidine because it is approximately 30% less expensive than ticlopidine (United States wholesale prices). The cost of clopidogrel is further reduced by not needing to monitor blood counts in patients receiving the drug, as is required every 2 weeks for the first 3 months of treatment with ticlopidine.

*Pretreatment and Duration of Treatment with Clopidogrel and PCI*

The Clopidogrel for Reduction of Events During Extended Observation (CREDO) trial tested the hypothesis that more complete inhibition with a thienopyridine at the time of a percutaneous revascularization procedure is beneficial. It also examined the most appropriate duration of therapy with a thienopyridine after a percutaneous revascularization procedure. In CREDO, 2116 patients undergoing percutaneous revascularization (with or without a stent) were randomly assigned to receive a 300 mg loading dose of clopidogrel about 3 hours before the procedure vs. clopidogrel 75 mg per day beginning immediately before the procedure [59]. Patients assigned to the clopidogrel 300 mg loading dose re-ceived clopidogrel 75 mg per day for 1 year (along with aspirin) whereas patients assigned to clopidogrel without a loading dose received clopidogrel for only 28 days, followed by placebo for 11 months, with aspirin. There were two primary endpoints in CREDO; the first evaluated the potential benefits of the loading dose by assessing the frequency of adverse events at 28 days among patients undergoing PCI. The second primary endpoint assessed the benefits of long-term dual antiplatelet therapy by examining one year event rates using an intention-to-treat analysis. The results at 28 days revealed an 18.5% reduction in vascular death, MI and stroke that did not reach statistical significance (6.8 vs. 8.3% no pretreatment, p = 0.23) (Fig. 8) [59]. However, a prespecified subgroup analysis of patients undergoing PCI more than 6 hours after administration of the loading dose, the

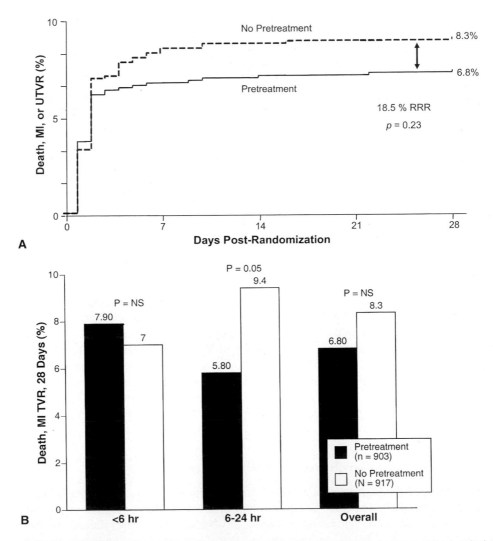

**Figure 8**  Results of the CREDO trial at 28 days. Panel A: Thrombotic events tended to occur less frequently among stent patients who received a loading dose of clopidogrel, but the difference did not come close to reaching significance. Panel B: When patients pretreated more and less than 6 hours before stent placement, were analyzed separately, it can be seen that only patients pretreated more than 6 hours before stent placement had a reduction in adverse events.

time required for a 300 mg loading dose of clopidogrel to achieve it's full antiplatelet effect assessed by light transmission aggregometry, revealed that there was significant reduction in adverse events with pretreatment more than 6 hours before the procedure (5.8% vs. 9.4% no pretreatment, p = 0.05). There was no evidence of benefit from pretreatment when it was administered less than 6 hours prior to PCI (7.9 vs. 7.0% no pretreatment, p = NS) [59].

A subsequent analysis of CREDO revealed that although in vitro data had indicated that 6 hours was sufficient to allow time to achieve maximal inhibition of aggregation, no benefit from pretreatment was seen unless administered 15 hours before PCI (Fig. 9) [60]. Since light-transmission aggregometry had suggested that maximal inhibition of aggregation was achieved only 6 hours after administration of a 300 mg loading dose, these data raise the question of whether ex vivo aggregation studies correlate with clinical outcomes and can be used as a surrogate for clinical data, and suggest that they cannot.

The results of the second primary endpoint in the CREDO trial, the frequency of death, nonfatal myocardial infarction, and stroke at 1 year in all patients using an intention-to-treat analysis, revealed a 26.9% reduction in these events with prolonged clopidogrel therapy (8.5 vs. 11.5, p = 0.02) [59]. Since patients were not rerandomized after 28 days, the study is confounded in the possibility that the lesser frequency of events at one year were in part related to the loading dose administered to all patients in the prolonged clopidogrel arm and no patients in the other arm. However, analysis of the frequency of events in the two groups during the first 28 days and the subsequent 11 months suggests that the apparent reduction in events in the arm of CREDO in which both a loading dose and long-term therapy were administered was unlikely to be the result of the loading dose, and that indeed, long-term therapy is likely beneficial after a planned PCI procedure, as it was among patients admitted with an acute coronary syndrome in CURE (Fig. 10).

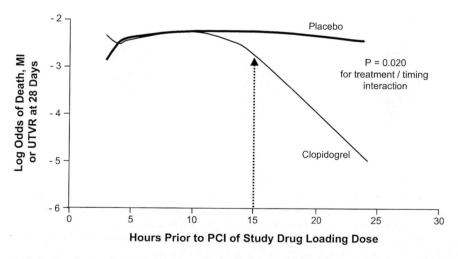

**Figure 9** Analysis of the duration of pretreatment in CREDO and the reduction in ischemic events at 28 days suggests that 15 hours of pretreatment is necessary for clinical benefit to be achieved. No such reduction in events was seen with increasing duration of pretreatment with placebo, suggesting that enrollment bias does not account for the observation. Light transmission aggregometry data had suggested that peak inhibition of aggregation was achieved within 6 hours.

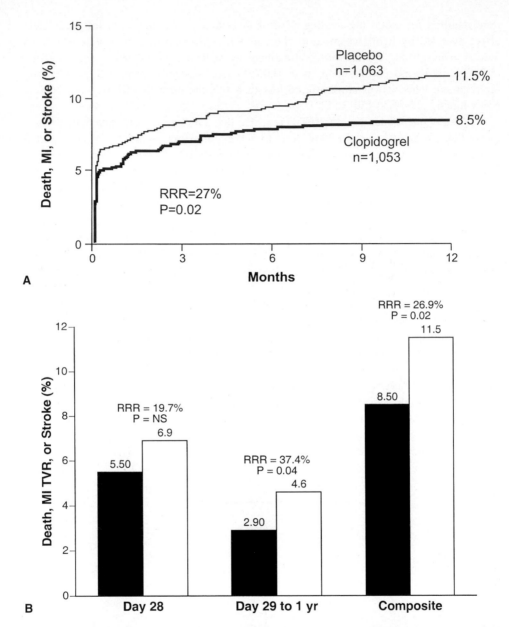

**Figure 10**   Results of the CREDO trial at 1 year. (**A**) Event curves reveal a lower frequency of death, non-fatal infarction, and stroke among patients randomized to a loading dose of clopidogrel, and treatment with clopidogrel for one year, vs. clopidogrel without a loading dose, and treatment for only 28 days. (**B**) The frequency of events was reduced between the two arms not only before the first 28 days, but also between 28 days and one year, suggesting that confounding resulting from the initial difference in treatment the two groups received does not account for the difference in events at 1 year.

*The Most Appropriate Loading Dose of Clopidogrel*

The choice of a 300-mg loading dose of clopidogrel in CLASSICS and all the subsequent studies was largely arbitrary. Data indicate that larger loading doses of clopidogrel act more rapidly, are well tolerated, and have the potential to reduce adverse events when administered shortly before unplanned PCI procedures, and perhaps during other high-risk periods. Peyrou et al. examined stable patients with coronary disease and found that loading doses larger than 300 mg were increasingly rapid acting up to loading doses of 525 mg; a 675 mg loading dose was only slightly although not significantly more rapid than a loading dose of 525 mg [61]. Loading doses of 525 and 675 mg were able to achieve the maximal antiplatelet effect able to be achieved with clopidogrel within 2 hours of administration assessed by light transmission aggregometry [61].

A group of investigators in Munich also found that maximal inhibition of aggregation was achieved within 2 hours with a 600 mg loading dose [62]. These investigators then changed their clinical practice and examined the clinical outcome of 870 patients undergoing PCI after a 600 mg loading dose (followed by 75 twice a day until discharge) with a prior cohort of 864 patients who had received ticlopidine prior to PCI. The results suggested significantly fewer adverse events with the 600 mg loading dose but, perhaps more importantly, did not identify any adverse reactions resulting from such a large loading dose or any drug–drug interactions [63].

Following this observational study, the same group of investigators performed a randomized trial, the ISAR-COOL study, in which all patients received 600 mg of clopidogrel, along with aspirin and heparin and the IIb/IIIa inhibitor tirofiban [64]. Half of the patients were randomized to undergo coronary angiography within 6 hours, and half were treated with medical therapy for at least 72 hours in the hope that antithrombotic and antiplatelet therapy would ''cool off'' the active coronary lesion and reduce thrombotic events at the time of a percutaneous coronary intervention. The results showed that performing angioplasty and revascularization within 6 hours was associated with fewer events, not more (Fig. 11) [64]. With respect to the large loading dose of clopidogrel, the 600 mg loading dose of clopidogrel appeared to be well tolerated without apparent side effects.

Subsequently, the ISAR-REACT trial, in which as in ISAR-COOL all patients received 600 mg of clopidogrel a minimum of 2 hours before undergoing PCI with stent placement; half were then randomized to receive the IIb/IIIa inhibitor abciximab, and half received placebo (Fig. 12) [65]. Only low- to intermediate-risk patients were included in the trial; patients with insulin dependent diabetes and a recent infarction (within 2 weeks) were excluded. Patients with noninsulin dependent diabetes were included in the trial and made up 20% of the patient population. The results indicated that the addition of abciximab to these patients did not procedure any apparent clinical benefit at 30 days (Fig. 12). Although all patients received the 600 mg loading dose, precluding any direct lessons that can be learned from such a large loading dose, again, no adverse effects from the 600 mg loading dose of clopidogrel were identified, suggesting safety of this large loading dose. Furthermore, the fact that this study was the first study of PCI patients to indicate no additional benefit from a IIb/IIIa inhibitor, and the first in which all patients had achieved maximal inhibition from clopidogrel suggests, as did CREDO, that pretreatment with a large enough loading dose to achieve maximal inhibition before PCI is probably beneficial. Additional trials are underway examining whether abciximab provides added benefit in higher risk patients, such as those with insulin dependent diabetes mellitus (ISAR-SWEET) and positive biomarkers (ISAR-REACT 2) undergoing PCI after pretreatment with clopidogrel. Although ISAR-REACT was neither designed nor able to detect benefit from a larger than traditional loading dose of clopidogrel, the study has led to a change in clinical

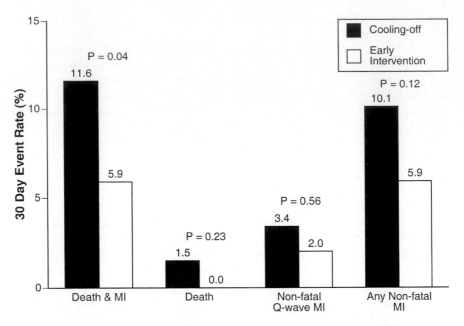

**Figure 11** The results of the ISAR-COOL trial reveal that among patients treated with aspirin, 600 mg of clopidogrel, tirofiban, and heparin, proceeding rapidly to coronary angiography (within 6 hours) improves outcome when compared with delaying angiography for at least 3 days in order to "cool patients off."

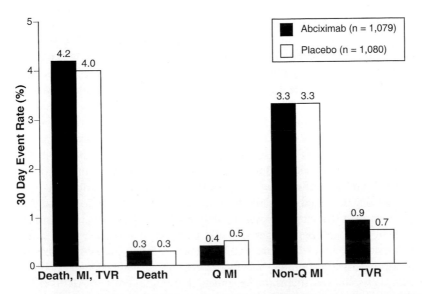

**Figure 12** The ISAR-REACT Trial. In this trial, among low- to intermediate-risk patients treated with aspirin and clopidogrel 600 mg at least 2 hours before stent placement, there was no added benefit from abciximab at 30 days.

practice by many physicians who now administer 600 mg of clopidogrel to patients in whom PCI is planned within 15–24 hours to permit the achievement of maximal inhibition of aggregation. Patients in whom PCI is planned greater than 24 hours in advance need only receive a 300 mg loading dose of clopidogrel.

*Operative Risk of Bleeding*

The main reason that all patients who are either admitted to the hospital for an acute coronary syndrome or in whom coronary angiography is planned for any reason to not receive clopidogrel is because of the fear of an increased risk of bleeding should the patient need to undergo coronary artery bypass surgery within 5 to 7 days, the time required for the platelet function to return to baseline after cessation of clopidogrel. Several observational studies have suggested a 4- to 10-fold increase in severe postoperative bleeding requiring an operation when CABG is performed on a patient receiving a thienopyridine [66–68]. Such studies are inherently limited in that the sicker patients generally proceed more rapidly to CABG, introducing bias into such retrospective analyses. However, even after adjustment for all measured variables and exclusion of patients undergoing emergency surgery, the studies indicate a significant increase in the risk of major postoperative bleeding.

The best data indicating the increased risk of bleeding when surgery is performed on a thienopyridine comes from a randomized trial, the CURE trial [40]. Among the 912 patients in whom a study drug had been given within the 5 days prior to CABG, there was a 50% increase in the risk of life threatening or major bleeding among patients who had received clopidogrel (9.6 vs. 6.3% in patients receiving placebo, p = 0.06.) It is likely that the risk would be less if clopidogrel were administered 5 days before CABG and much greater if administered the day of CABG. Newer P2Y12 inhibitors are being developed with a more rapid offset of action so that these drugs need not be withheld in case a patient does require CABG within 5 days. Until such thienopyridines are available, many believe that patients undergoing coronary angiography in whom surgical anatomy is anticipated and in whom surgery would be performed within 5 days ought not to receive clopidogrel prior to a diagnostic angiogram. In others, clopidogrel ought to be administered to permit achievement of maximal inhibition of platelet aggregation if PCI is performed within hours of the diagnostic angiogram.

*Clopidogrel Resistance*

As is the case with aspirin, many studies have shown that certain patients fail to respond to clopidogrel on platelet function tests as most patients do. Some have termed this clopidogrel resistance. There are no good data to suggest that such patients are at increased risk of thrombotic complications, though one small study did reveal a slightly greater frequency of stent thrombosis among such patients. To further evaluate the true frequency of this phenomenon, Serebrauny et al. analyzed several different patient populations that had previously been extensively studied [69]. These investigators suggested the term hyporesponders rather than patients truly resistant to the drug be used, since there are few examples in pharmacology in which patients are believed to respond fully or not at all to a given drug; most patients respond to a drug to a greater or lesser extent. These investigators, suggested defining hyporesponsiveness as a response less than two standard deviations from the mean, which would lead to a 4.2% frequency of hyporesponsiveness among the 544 patients in the study, less than many much smaller studies had reported using differing definitions [69]. Whether such patients are at increased risk of ischemic events, as may be the case with patients "resistant" to aspirin, is unknown.

*Unanswered Questions About Clopidogrel*

There remain important unanswered questions about the thienopyridines: does pretreatment with clopidogrel obviate the need for abciximab in high-risk patients as it appears to in lower risk patients? What is the optimal loading dose of clopidogrel? Are aspirin and clopidogrel more effective than aspirin alone in patients with stable coronary disease, or with important risk factors for coronary disease, as it is in patients with an acute coronary syndrome? Will new P2Y12 inhibitors be developed with more rapid onset and offset of action, permitting the universal treatment of patients with unstable coronary disease regardless of the possible need for urgent coronary artery bypass surgery? Ongoing studies should provide the answer to all of these questions in the next few years.

## SUMMARY

For more than 100 years, aspirin was the only oral antiplatelet agent available for the primary and secondary prevention of myocardial infarction and for patients undergoing percutaneous coronary revascularization procedures. Then, ticlopidine became available and further improved clinical outcome, both in and out of the catheterization laboratory. Now, clopidogrel has become the thienopyridine of choice for most if not all indications. Ongoing studies of dual antiplatelet therapy in patients with stable coronary disease and studies of newer P2Y12 receptor blockers, both intravenous and oral, with more desirable pharmacokinetic features in certain clinical situations including a more rapid onset of action and quicker recovery of platelet function will further define the role of P2Y12 inhibitors in preventing adverse events in patients undergoing percutaneous revascularization procedures acute coronary syndromes, and with stable coronary disease as well.

## REFERENCES

1. Savi P, Herbert JM. ADP receptors on platelets and ADP-selective antiaggregating agents. Medicinal Research Reviews 1996;16(2):159–179.
2. Mills DC, Puri R, Hu CJ, et al. Clopidogrel inhibits the binding of ADP analogues to the receptor mediating inhibition of platelet adenylate cyclase. Arteriosclerosis & Thrombosis 1992;12(4):430–436.
3. Coukell AJ, Markham A. Clopidogrel. Drugs 1997;54(5):745–750.
4. Yang LH, Fareed J. Vasomodulatory action of clopidogrel and ticlopidine. Thrombosis Research 1997;86(6):479–491.
5. Puri RN, Colman RW. ADP-induced platelet activation. Critical Reviews in Biochemistry and Molecular Biology 1997;3:437–502.
6. Antiplatelet Trialists' Collaboration. Collaborative overview of randomised trials of antiplatelet therapy–I: Prevention of death, myocardial infarction, and stroke by prolonged antiplatelet therapy in various categories of patient.
7. Balsano F, Rizzon P, Violi F, Scrutinio D, Cimminiello C, Aguglia F, Pasotti C, Rudelli G. and the Studio della nell'Angina Instabile Group. Antiplatelet treatment with ticlopidine in unstable angina. A controlled multicenter clinical trial. Circulation 1990;82:17–26.
8. White CW, Chaitman B, Knudson ML, Chisholm RJ. and the Ticlopidine Study Group. Antiplatelet agents are effective in reducing the acute ischemic complications of angioplasty but do not prevent restenosis: results from the ticlopidine trial. Coronary Artery Disease. Circulation 1991;2:757–767.
9. Bertrand ME, Allain H, LaBlanche JM. on behalf of the Investigators of the TACT Study. Results of a randomized trial of ticlopidine vs. placebo for prevention of acute closure and

restenosis after coronary angioplasty (PTCA); The TACT study. Circulation 1990;82(suppl III):III–190.

10. Morice SP, Lefevre T, Grines C, Mattos L, den Heuvel PV, Nobuyoshi M, van der Giessen W, Brodie B, Katz S. Antiplatelet treatment with ticlopidine and aspirin does not prevent major adverse cardiac events in acute myocardial infarction patients treated with balloon alone. Results from the Stent PAMI Trial. Circulation 1998;98(suppl I):I–572 (Abstract).

11. Berger PB, Dzavik V, Al-Rashdan I, Penn IM, Zidar JP, Catellier D, Buller CE. Does ticlopidine reduce reocclusion after successful balloon angioplasty of coronary occlusions? Insights from TOSCA. J Am Coll Cardiol 1999;33:40A (abstract).

12. Mehta SR, Yusuf S, Peters RJ, Bertrand ME, Lewis BS, Natarajan MK, Malmberg K, Rupprecht H, Zhao F, Chrolavicius S, Copland I, Fox KA. Clopidogrel in Unstable angina to prevent Recurrent Events trial (CURE) Investigators. Effects of pretreatment with clopidogrel and aspirin followed by long-term therapy in patients undergoing percutaneous coronary intervention: the PCI-CURE study. Lancet. 2001;358:527–33.

13. Hall P, Nakamura S, Maiello L, Itoh A, Blengino S, Martini G, Ferraro M, Colombo A. A randomized comparison of combined ticlopidine and aspirin therapy vs. aspirin therapy alone after successful intravascular ultrasound-guided stent implantation. Circulation 1996;93(2):215–222.

14. Urban P, Macaya C, Rupprecht HJ, Kiemeneij F, Emanuelsson H, Fontanelli A, Pieper M, Wesseling T, Sagnard L. Randomized evaluation of anticoagulation vs. antiplatelet therapy after coronary stent implantation in high-risk patients: the multicenter aspirin and ticlopidine trial after intracoronary stenting (MATTIS). Circulation 1998;98(20):2126–2132.

15. Schomig A, Neumann FJ, Kastrati A, Schuhlen H, Blasini R, Hadamitzky M, Walter H, Zitzmann-Roth EM, Richardt G, Alt E, Schmitt C, Ulm K. A randomized comparison of antiplatelet and anticoagulant therapy after the placement of coronary-artery stents. New Engl J Med 1996;334(17):1084–1089.

16. Leon MB, Baim DS, Popma JJ, Gordon PC, Cutlip DE, Ho KK, Giambartolomei A, Diver DJ, Lasorda DM, Williams DO, Pocock SJ, Kuntz RE. A clinical trial comparing three antithrombotic-drug regimens after coronary-artery stenting. Stent Anticoagulation Restenosis Study Investigators. New Engl J Med 1998;339(23):1665–1671.

17. Bertrand ME, Legrand V, Boland J, Fleck E, Bonnier J, Emmanuelson H, Vrolix M, Missault L, Chierchia S, Casaccia M, Niccoli L, Oto A, White C, Webb-Peploe M, Van Belle E, McFadden EP. Randomized multicenter comparison of conventional anticoagulation vs. antiplatelet therapy in unplanned and elective coronary stenting. The full anticoagulation vs. aspirin and ticlopidine (FANTASTIC) study. Circulation 1998;98(16):1597–1603.

18. Foussas S, Alexopoulos D, Steefanadis C, Olympios C, Voudris V, Hatzimiltiadis S, Sionis D, Vavouranakis E, Vrahatis A, Fakiolas C, Pissimisis E, Stefanidis A, Zairis M, Pavlides G, Vitakis S, Louridas G, Cokkinos D, Toutouzas P. Antiplatelet is superior to anticoagulant treatment after coronary stenting: fewer coronary and other events within 30 days after stenting. Angiology 2000;51:289–294.

19. Rupprecht HJ, Darius H, Borkowski U, Voigtlander T, Nowak B, Genth S, Meyer J. Comparison of antiplatelet effects of aspirin, ticlopidine, or their combination after stent implantation. Circulation 1998;97(11):1046–1052.

20. Steinhubl SR, Tan WA, Foody JM, Topol EJ. for the EPISTENT Investigators. Incidence and clinical course of thrombotic thrombocytopenic purpura due to ticlopidine following coronary stenting. JAMA 1999;281:806–810.

21. Berger PB, Bell MR, Grill DE, Melby S, Holmes DR. Safety and efficacy of ticlopidine for only two weeks after successful intracoronary stent placement. Circulation 1999;99:248–253.

22. Berger PB, Mahaffey KW, Buller CE, Meier SJ, Batchelor W, Zidar JP. Safety of only 2 weeks of ticlopidine therapy in patients at increased risk of coronary stent thrombosis: results from the ATLAST (Antiplatelet Therapy vs. Antiplatelet Therapy Alone in Patients at Increased Risk of Stent Thrombosis) Trial. Circulation 1999;100(18):I–152.

23. Wilson S, Rihal CS, Bell MR, Holmes DRJ, Berger PB. Timing of coronary stent thrombosis in patients treated with ticlopidine and aspirin. Am J Cardiol 1999;83:1006–1011.

24. Schuhlen H, Kastrati A, Pache J, Dirschinger J, Schomig A. Incidence of thrombotic occlusion and major adverse cardiac events between two and four weeks after coronary stent placement: analysis of 5678 patients with a four week ticlopidine regimen. J Am Coll Cardiol 2001;37: 2066–2073.

25. Steinhubl SR, Lauer MS, Mukherjee DP, Moliterno DJ, Lincoff AM, Ellis SG, Topol EJ. The duration of pretreatment with ticlopidine prior to stenting is associated with the risk of procedure-related non-Q-wave myocardial infarctions. J Am Coll Cardiol 1998;32(5):1366–1370.

26. Steinhubl S, Ellis SG, Wolski K, Lincoff AM, Topol EJ. Ticlopidine pretreatment before stenting is associated with sustained decrease in adverse cardiac events: data from the Evaluation of Platelet IIb/IIIa Inhibitor for Stenting (EPISTENT) trial. Circulation 2001;103: 1403–1409.

27. The EPISTENT Investigators. Randomised placebo-controlled and balloon-angioplasty-controlled trial to assess safety of coronary stenting with use of platelet glycoprotein-IIb/IIIa blockade. Evaluation of Platelet IIb/IIIa Inhibitor for Stenting. Lancet 1998;352(9122):87–92.

28. Savi P, Pereeillo JM, Uzabriaga MF, Combalbert J, Picard C, Maffrand JP, Pascal M, Herbert LM. Identification and biological activity of the active metabolite of clopidogrel. Thromb Haemost 2000;84(5):891–896.

29. Boneu B, Destelle G. Platelet anti-aggregating activity and tolerance of clopidogrel in atherosclerotic patients. Thrombosis & Haemostasis 1996;76(6):939–943.

30. CAPRIE Steering Committee. A randomised, blinded, trial of clopidogrel vs. aspirin in patients at risk of ischaemic events (CAPRIE). Lancet 1996;348(9038):1329–1339.

31. Easton JD. Net benefit of clopidogrel over aspirin for the prevention of atherothrombotic events. Cerebrovascular Disease 1998;8(suppl 4):46.

32. Gibbons RJ, Chatterjee KD, Daley J, Douglas JS, Fihn SD, Gardin JM, Grunwald MA, Levy D, Lytle BW, O'Rourke RA, Schafer WP, Williams SV. ACC/AHA/ACP-ASIM guidelines for the management of patients with chronic stable angina: executive summary and recommendations: a report of the American College of Cardiology/American Heart Association Task Force on Practice Guidelines (Committee on Management of Patients With Chronic Stable Angina). Circulation 1999;99:2829–2848.

33. Helgason CM, Tortorice KL, Winkler SR, Penney DW, Schuler JJ, McClelland TJ, Brace LD. Aspirin response and failure in cerebral infarction. Stroke 1993;24(3):345–350.

34. Helgason CM, Bolin KM, Hoff JA, Penney DW, Schuler JJ, McClelland TJ, Brace LD. Development of aspirin resistance in persons with previous ischemic stroke. Stroke 1994;25(12): 2331–2336.

35. Buchanan MR, Brister SJ. Individual variation in the effects of ASA on platelet function: implications for the use of ASA clinically. Canadian J of Cardiology 1995;11(3):221–227.

36. Grotemeyer KH, Scharafinski HW, Husstedt IW. Two-year follow-up of aspirin responder and aspirin non responders. A pilot-study including 180 post-stroke patients. Thrombosis Research 1993;71(5):397–403.

37. Buchanan MR, Hirsh J. Effect of aspirin on hemostasis and thrombosis. New England & Regional Allergy Proceedings 1986;7(1):26–31.

38. Mueller MR, Salat A, Stangl P, Murabito M, Pulaki S, Boehm D, Koppensteiner R, Ergun E, Mittlboeck M, Schreiner W, Losert U, Wolner E. Variable platelet response to low-dose ASA and the risk of limb deterioration in patients submitted to peripheral arterial angioplasty. Thromb Haemost 1997;78:1003–1007.

39. Gum P, Kottke-Marchant K, Welsh PA, White J, Topol EJ. A prospective, blinded determination of the natural history of aspirin resistance among stable patients with cardiovascular disease. J Am Coll Cardiol 2003;41:961–965.

40. Yusuf S, Zhao F, Mehta SR, Chrolavicius S, Tognoni G, Fox KK. The Clopidogrel in Unstable Angina to Prevent Recurrent Events Trial Investigators. Effects of clopidogrel in addition to aspirin in patients with acute coronary syndromes without ST-segment elevation. N Engl J Med 2001;345:494–502.

41. Yusuf S, Mehta SR, Zhao F, Gersh BJ, Commerford PJ, Blumenthal M, Budaj A, Wittlinger T, Fox KA. Clopidogrel in Unstable angina to prevent Recurrent Events Trial Investigators.

Early and late effects of clopidogrel in patients with acute coronary syndromes. Circulation. 2003;107:966–72.

42. Bachmann F, Savic M, Hauert J, Geudelin B, Kieflfer G, Cariou R. Rapid onset of inhibition of ADP-induced platelet aggregation by a loading dose of clopidogrel. Eur Heart J 1996:263A.

43. Makkar RR, Eigler NL, Kaul S, Frimerman A, Nakamura M, Shah PK, Forrester JS, Herbert JM, Litvack F. Effects of clopidogrel, aspirin and combined therapy in a porcine ex vivo model of high-shear induced stent thrombosis. Euro Heart J 1998;19:1538–1546.

44. Harker LA, Marzec UM, Kelly AB, Chronos NR, Sundell IB, Hanson SR, Herbert JM. Clopidogrel inhibition of stent, graft, and vascular thrombogenesis with antithrombotic enhancement by aspirin in nonhuman primates. Circulation 1998;1998:2461–2469.

45. Bertrand M, Rupprecht H, Urban P, Gershlick A. Investigators. Double-blind study of the safety of clopidogrel with and without a loading dose in combination with aspirin compared with ticlopidine in combination with aspirin after coronary stenting : the clopidogrel aspirin stent international cooperative study (CLASSICS). Circulation 2000;102(6):624–629.

46. Taniuchi M, Kurz HI, Lasala JM. Randomized comparison of ticlopidine and clopidogrel after intracoronary stent implantation in a broad patient population. Circulation 2001;104:539–543.

47. Mueller C, Buttner HJ, Ptererson J, Roskamm H. A randomized comparison of clopidogrel and aspirin vs. ticlopidine and aspirin after the placement of coronary-artery stents. Circulation 2000;101:590–593.

48. Piamsomboon C, Laothavorn P, Chatlaong B, Saguanwong S, Nasawadi C, Tanprasert P, Leelaprute M, Intayakorn U, Amornsak N. Effectivenss of clopidogrel and aspirin vs. ticlopidine and aspirin after coronary stent implantation: 1 and 6 month follow-up. J Med Association Thailand 2001;84:1701–1707.

49. Berger PB, Bell MR, Rihal CS, Ting H, Barsness G, Garratt K, Bellot V, Mathew V, Melby S, Hammes L, Grill D, Holmes DR Jr. Clopidogrel vs. ticlopidine after intracoronary stent placement. J Am Coll Cardiol 1999;34:1891–1894.

50. Wang X, Oetgen M, Maida R, Lawrence E, Peters MJ, Zucker D, Cohen N, Moussa I, Iyer S, Kreps E, Collins M, Roubin G, Colombo A, Moses J. The effectiveness of the combination of Plavix and aspirin vs. Ticlid and aspirin after coronary stent implantation. J Am Coll Cardiol 1999;33:13A.

51. Moussa I, Maida R, DeGregorio J, Chui M, Cohen N, Collins M. Prospective experience with clopidogrel use after coronary stent implantation in 1100 consecutive patients. Circulation 1999;100(suppl I):I–379 (abstract).

52. Berger P, Clopidogrel vs. ticlopidine after coronary stent placement, Presented at the Transcatheter Therapeutics conference, October, 1999, Washington D.C..

53. Mehran R, Dangas G, Ticlopidine vs. clopidogrel in patients receiving coronary stents, Presented at the Transcatheter Therapeutics Course, Washington D.C., October, 1999.

54. L'Allier PL, Aronow HD, Cura FA, et al. Short term mortality lower with clopidogrel than ticlopidine following coronary artery stenting. J Am Coll Cardiol 2000;35(suppl A):66A.

55. Mishkel GJ, Aguirre FV, Ligon RW, Rocha-Singh KJ, Lucore CL. Clopidogrel as adjunctive antiplatelet therapy during coronary stenting. J Am Coll Cardiol 1999;34:1884–1890.

56. Calver AL, Blows LJ, Dawkins KD, Gray HH, Morgan JM, Simpson IA. The use of clopidogrel instead of ticlopidine after intra-coronary stent insertion: initial results in stents of ≤ 3 mm in diameter. Eur Heart J 1999;20:529 (abstract).

57. Plucinski DA, Scheltema K, Krusmark J, Panchyshyn N. A comparison of clopidogrel to ticlopidine therapy for the prevention of major adverse cardiac events at thirty days and six months following coronary stent implantation. J Am Coll Cardiol 2000;35(suppl A):67A.

58. Bhatt DL, Bertrand ME, Berger PB, L'Allier PP, Moussa I, Moses JW, Dangas G, Taniuchi M, Lasala JM, Holmes DR, Ellis SG, Topol EJ. Meta-analysis of randomized and registry comparisons of ticlopidine with clopidogrel after stenting. J Am Coll Cardiol 2002;39:9–14.

59. Steinhubl SR, Berger PB, Mann JT, Fry ETA, DeLago A, Wilmer C, Topol EJ. for the CREDO Investigators. Early and sustained dual oral antiplatelet therapy following percutaneous coronary intervention. A randomized controlled trial. JAMA 2002;288(19):2411–2420.

60. Steinhubl SR, Darrah S, Brennan D, McErlean E, Berger PB, Topol EJ. Optimal duration of pretreatment with clopidogrel prior to PCI: Data from the CREDO trial. Circulation 2003; 108(suppl IV):1742 (Abstract).

61. Peyrou V, Leimback ME, Marzec UM, Chronos NRA, King SB, Harker LA, Spencer BKing. Single-dose clopidogrel inhibition of platelet adenosine diphosphate receptor function in patients with atherosclerotic coronary artery disease. Submitted.

62. Pache J, Kastrati A, Mehilli J, Gawaz M, Neumann FJ, Seyfarth M, Hall D, Braun S, Dirschinger J, Schomig A. Clopidogrel therapy in patients undergoing coronary stenting: Value of a high-loading-dose regimen. Catheter Cardiovasc Interv 2002;55:43641.

63. Müller I, Seyfarth M, Rudiger S, Wolf B, Pogatsa-Murray G, Schomig A, Gawaz M. Effect of a high loading dose of clopidogrel on platelet function in patients undergoing coronary stent placement. Heart 2001;85(9):2–93.

64. Neumann FJ, Kastrati A, Pogatsa-Murray G, Mehilli J, Bollwein H, Bestehorn H-P, Schmitt C, Seyfarth M, Dirschinger J, Schomig A. Evvaluation of prolonged antithrombotic pretreatment (''cooling-off'' strategy) before intervention in patients with unstable coronary syndromes. A randomized controlled trial. JAMA 2003;298:1593–1599.

65. Kastrati A, Mehilli J, Schuhlen H, Dirschinger J, Dotzer F, ten Berg J, Neumann FJ, Bollwein H, Volmer C, Gawaz M, Berger PB, Schomig A. for the intracoronary stenting and antithrombotic regimen-rapid early action for coronary treatment study investigators. A double-blind, placebo-controlled, randomized trial evaluating the glycoprotein IIb/IIIa inhibitor Abciximab in patients undergoing elective percutaneous coronary interventions after pretreatment with a high loading dose of clopidogrel. New Engl J Med 2004;350:232–238.

66. Hongo RH, Ley J, Dick SE, Rupsa RY. The effect of clopidogrel in combination with aspirin when given before coronary artery bypass grafting. J Am Coll Cardiol 2002;40:231–237.

67. Yende S, Wunderink RG. Effect of clopidogrel on bleeding after coronary artery bypass surgery. Crit Care Med 2001;29:2271–2275.

68. Ray JG, Deniz S, Olivieri A, Pollex E, Vermeulen MJ, Alexander KS, Cain DJ, Cybulsky I, Hamielec CM. Increased blood product use among coronary artery bypass patients prescribed preoperative aspirin and clopidogrel. BMC Cardiovasc Disord 2003;3:3.

69. Serebruany VL, Steinhubl SR, Berger PB, Malinin AI, Bhatt DL, Topol EJ. Variability in platelet responsiveness to clopidogrel among 544 individuals. Submitted.

# 20
# Dosing and Aspirin

**Steven R. Steinhubl**
*Associate Professor of Medicine, University of Kentucky*
*Lexington, Kentucky, U.S.A*

## INTRODUCTION

The medicinal use of salycilic acid was first documented in the time of Hippocrates [1] and was studied in clinical trials as early as 1763 [2]. Acetylsalicylic acid (ASA), or aspirin, was originally synthesized in 1897 by Felix Hoffman, a chemist at Friedr Bayer & Company, as a more palatable formulation of this widely used pain reliever [3]. Although it was initially sold to pharmacists in 250 gm bottles, with patients being dispensed 1 gm of the powder in a paper bag, imitators and adulterated versions of the powder led to the development by Bayer of an aspirin pill in 1900 [4]. In the United States, this was a 5-grain (approximately 325 mg) pill; the dose still most commonly used today.

Paul Gibson, in 1948, first proposed that salicylic acid might be useful in the treatment of coronary thrombosis [5], and the following year presented case reports detailing the success of aspirin in the treatment of angina [6]. In 1953 L. L. Craven, a general practitioner who noticed that his tonsillectomy patients experienced increased bleeding after using aspirin for pain relief, was the next to suggest, and then study the use of aspirin in the prevention of ''coronary occlusion'' [7]. However, it took another 30 years before the striking clinical benefit of aspirin in the treatment of patients with an acute coronary syndrome was conclusively confirmed through multiple randomized trials.

Today, there is no drug that has been more thoroughly researched than aspirin. The central role of aspirin therapy in the treatment of all aspects of cardiovascular disease has been well established through the study of hundreds of thousands of patients in hundreds of placebo-controlled clinical trials [8]. Despite this, and likely related to its unique history as a familiar pain-reliever prior to being established as a life-saving platelet inhibitor, there remain surprisingly wide gaps in our knowledge of how to best utilize aspirin in the individual patient. In particular, questions regarding the optimal dose, and whether it is the same for everyone, have been the subject of debate for decades now. In this chapter, the data supporting the role of aspirin in the treatment of patients with an acute coronary syndrome, with a particular emphasis on the data regarding dosage and interindividual variability in response, will be presented.

## ASPIRIN IN THE TREATMENT OF ACUTE CORONARY SYNDROMS

The beneficial role of aspirin in the acute and long-term treatment of patients presenting with a non–ST-elevation acute coronary syndrome has been conclusively proven through four randomized trials (Table 1). The first of these, the Veterans Administration Cooperative Study was a double blind randomized trial initiated in 1974 [9]. Using 324 mg of a buffered aspirin dissolved in water (Alka-Seltzer, Miles Laboratories, Elkhart, Indiana) or matching placebo, they evaluated the effect of 12 weeks of daily therapy in patients within 51 hours of presenting to a hospital with symptoms of unstable angina. Treatment with aspirin was found to decrease the risk of death or acute myocardial infarction by 51% (5.0% vs. 10.1%, p = 0.0005). Although treatment as well as controlled medical care was discontinued at 12 weeks, the mortality benefit in the aspirin treated patients persisted at one year (5.5% vs. 9.6%, P = 0.008).

The first randomized, placebo-controlled study that evaluated long-term aspirin therapy in patients with unstable angina was the Canadian Multicenter Trial [10]. In this trial 555 patients were randomized to one of four possible therapies: aspirin (325 mg four times daily), sulfinpyrazone, a weak inhibitor of platelet cyclooxygenase (200 mg four times daily), both, or neither for 2 years. At a mean follow-up of 18 months there was no decrease in the rate of MI or cardiac death between those receiving sulfinpyrazone alone and those receiving placebo. Aspirin treated patients on the other hand had a 51% risk reduction (8.6% vs. 17.0%, P = 0.008) for this combined endpoint compared with nonaspirin treated patients.

The Research Group on Instability in Coronary Artery Disease (RISC) trial was the first to evaluate the addition of the anticoagulant heparin to aspirin in the treatment of unstable angina [11]. Seven hundred and ninety-six men were randomized to aspirin 75 mg daily, intravenous heparin four times a day for five days, both, or neither. Patients were enrolled up to 72 hours after hospital admission, with treatment started a median of 33 hours after admission. The incidence of death or MI was evaluated at 5 days, 1 month, and 3 months. While intermittent (4 times daily) intravenous heparin alone had no affect on the combined endpoint, aspirin therapy significantly reduced the risk of death or MI compared with placebo. At 5 days the risk ratio was 0.43 (95% confidence interval (CI) 0.21–0.91, P = 0.033), at 1 month 0.31 (95% CI 0.18–0.53, P<0.0001), and at 3 months 0.36 (95% CI 0.23–0.57, P<0.0001). The combination of aspirin and heparin had the same benefit as aspirin alone. A follow-up report by this study group confirmed that daily aspirin for 1 year maintained a significant benefit over placebo with a risk ratio of 0.52 (95% CI 0.37–0.72, P = 0.0001) [12].

Theroux and colleagues also evaluated the effectiveness of aspirin, heparin, or its combination compared with placebo [13]. Unlike the delayed treatment allowed in previous studies, patients were randomized promptly following admission to the emergency room. Aspirin was given as 325 mg twice daily, whereas heparin was infused intravenously at 1000 units per hour. Study endpoints were evaluated early, at the time long-term care was decided, which was a mean of 6 days following admission. The incidence of myocardial infarction was 11.9% in those receiving placebo compared with 3.3% in patients treated with aspirin alone (risk ratio 0.29, 95% CI 0.08–0.80, P = 0.012). Unlike the results of the RISC Study Group, a combination of heparin and aspirin, as well as heparin alone were of even more benefit than aspirin alone. Importantly, clustering of events soon after therapy was stopped in patients who received heparin alone, thought to be related to reactivation, and was prevented with concomitant aspirin therapy [14].

All the above trials included only patients with unstable angina or non–ST-segment-elevation myocardial infarctions (MI). The Second International Study of Infarct Survival (ISIS-2) unequivocally established the beneficial role of aspirin in another critically important subgroup of acute coronary syndrome patients; those experiencing an ST-segment-elevation MI [15]. In this trial 17,187 patients, admitted within 24 hours after the onset

**Table 1** Trials of Aspirin vs. Placebo in Acute Coronary Syndromes

| Trial | Years | Number of Patients | Treatment | Time Limit for Study Entry Following Admission | Follow-up | % Death and MI | | Risk Reduction (%) | P Value |
|---|---|---|---|---|---|---|---|---|---|
| | | | | | | Placebo | Treatment | | |
| **VA Cooperative Study (9)** | 1974–81 | 1266 | ASA 324 mg daily | 51 hours | 12 weeks | 10.1 | 5.0 | 51 | 0.0005 |
| **Canadian Multi-center Trial (10)** | 1979–83 | 555 | ASA 325 mg 4 × daily | 8 days | 18 months (mean) | 17.0 | 8.6 | 51 | 0.008 |
| **RISC Group (11)** | 1985–88 | 796 | ASA 75 mg daily | 72 hours | 90 days | 17.1 | 6.5 | 62 | <0.0001 |
| **Theroux (13)** | 1986–88 | 479 | ASA 325 mg twice daily | As soon as possible after ER presentation | 6±3 days (mean ± SD) | 12.0 | 3.3 | 72 | 0.01 |
| | | | | | | **% Vascular Death** | | | |
| **ISIS-2 (15)** | 1985–87 | 17,187 | 162.5 mg daily | Within 24 hours of onset of pain | 35 days | 9.4 | 11.8 | 23 | <0.00001 |

VA: Veterans Administration
RISC: Research Group on Instability in Coronary Artery Disease
ISIS-2: Second International Study of Infarct Survival

of a suspected acute myocardial infarction, were randomized to streptokinase (1.5 MU) alone, aspirin (162.5 mg daily for 30 days) alone, both, or neither. Patients receiving aspirin alone experienced a significant 23% relative reduction in vascular mortality during the 5 weeks following admission compared with those receiving placebo tablets (9.4% vs. 11.8%, p<0.00001), with randomization to streptokinase being associated with a similar 25% reduction in 5-week mortality (9.2% for streptokinase vs. 12.0% for placebo infusion, p<0.00001). The greatest benefit however was found in patients treated with the combination of aspirin plus streptokinase. This cohort experienced a 42% reduction in vascular mortality compared to placebo allocated patients (8.0% vs. 13.2%, p<0.00001), and was significantly better than either active therapy alone.

## ASPIRIN DOSING

Worldwide consumption of aspirin in the year 2000 was approximately 350 tons, or the equivalent of almost 100 billion tablets. It is estimated by the Centers for Disease Control that 26 million individuals in the United States take a daily aspirin for the primary or secondary prevention of the thrombotic complications of atherosclerotic cardiovascular disease. Although in general aspirin is a very well tolerated drug, like all medications it carries a risk of significant side effects [16]. With so many individuals receiving chronic aspirin therapy to treat and prevent a disease process that has such important global implications as atherothrombotic disease does, the importance of optimizing its clinical benefits and minimizing its risks is clear. Utilizing a dose of aspirin that decreases side effects but does not diminish efficacy is a critical step towards accomplishing this.

Placebo-controlled trials that have confirmed the benefit of aspirin in the treatment of acute coronary syndromes utilized doses ranging from 75 mg to 1300 mg daily. Clinical trials in other patient populations have evaluated doses as low as 30 mg, and as high as 1500 mg daily. In the United States, professional labeling by the Food and Drug Administration recommends doses ranging from 50 mg to 1300 mg daily for the treatment of the multiple clinical manifestations of atherosclerotic disease. Because of this, there remains substantial controversy and debate regarding just what the "correct" dose of aspirin is.

## Mechanism of Action

The beneficial, as well as detrimental effects of aspirin are believed to be primarily due to interference with the biosynthesis of prostanoids; in particular thromboxane $A_2$ ($TXA_2$) and prostacyclins. Aspirin specifically and irreversibly inhibits platelet cyclooxygenase-1 (COX-1, also known as prostaglandin H synthase-1) through the acetylation of the amino acid serine at position 529 [17], thereby preventing arachidonic acid access to the COX-1 catalytic site through steric hindrance [18]. By inhibiting COX-1, the platelet is unable to synthesize $PGH_2$, which is then unable to be converted to $TXA_2$ via the enzyme thromboxane synthase. Because the nonnucleated platelets lack the biosynthetic capabilities necessary to synthesize new protein, the aspirin-induced defect cannot be repaired for the 8–10 day life span of the platelet. Due to platelet turnover, about 10% of platelet COX activity is recovered daily following cessation of aspirin therapy [19]. Therefore, up to 10 days may be required for complete recovery of platelet COX activity, however, it may require only 20% of normal COX activity in order to have normal hemostasis [20].

COX-1 is constitutively expressed in almost all cells and plays an important role beyond platelet $TXA_2$ production; of particular importance, gastric mucosal protection through prostacyclin $PGE_2$ and endothelial cell production of prostacyclin $PGI_2$, which is a vasodilator and inhibitor of platelet aggregation. However, unlike platelets, gastric mucosal and endothelial cells possess the biosynthetic machinery necessary to produce new enzyme, and therefore recover their ability to synthesize prostacyclin within a few hours after aspirin. COX-2, a second cyclooxygenase isoenzyme which is not routinely present in most cells, but is rapidly inducible by inflammatory stimuli, is less effected by aspirin as it is 170-fold less potent of an inhibitor of COX-2 than COX-1 [21]. Whereas in the presence of aspirin COX-1 activity is completely inhibited, COX-2 is still able to convert arachidonic acid to 15-R-hydroxyeicosatetraenoic acid (15-R-HETE) [22].

The role of inflammation in the progression and clinical manifestations of atherosclerosis is now well established [23]. Therefore, it has been postulated that aspirin's anti-inflammatory properties may explain at least part of the mechanism of its clinical benefit [24]. However, with aspirin's much greater selectivity for COX-1, and the central role of COX-2 in inflammation, doses necessary to achieve measurable anti-inflammatory effects are much higher than that routinely utilized clinically, with some studies suggesting the need for several grams of aspirin in order to achieve adequate anti-inflammatory effects [25]. Consistent with this lack of a direct anti-inflammatory effect at clinically effective doses are the conflicting results from several studies analyzing the influence of aspirin on high-sensitivity C-reactive protein (hsCRP), with most finding no effect [26–33].

## Pharmacokinetics and Pharmacodynamics

After oral dosing, aspirin is rapidly absorbed in the stomach and upper intestine. Acetylation of platelet COX-1 begins to occur in the portal circulation prior to any measurable levels systemically, making the measurement of plasma levels an incomplete measure of efficacy [34]. Nonetheless, peak plasma levels are achieved rapidly, within about 30 minutes, followed by a rapid clearance with a half-life of 15–20 minutes [34,35]. The systemic bioavailability of aspirin is approximately 50% for single oral doses ranging from 20 mg to 1300 mg [34].

Multiple methods of measuring the platelet inhibitory effects of aspirin have been studied, leading to sometimes conflicting results. Unfortunately, no one measure of aspirin's affect on platelets has yet been reliably proven to correlate with the clinical efficacy of aspirin, and therefore there is no "gold-standard" measure of aspirin's pharmacodynamics. However, the ability of aspirin to inhibit $TXA_2$ production, as measured by decreases in levels of its stable metabolite, thromboxane $B_2$ ($TXB_2$) is one method that has been frequently utilized and is consistent with its mechanism of action.

### Acute Dosing

A wide range of aspirin doses, preparations, and methods of ingestion have been evaluated in order to determine the best way to rapidly achieve maximal antiplatelet effects in the acute setting. In one study that evaluated the acute antiplatelet effects of a 40 mg, 100 mg, 300 mg and 500 mg dose of aspirin, the 300 mg and 500 mg doses were found to achieve equal levels of inhibition of all measures of platelet function two hours following ingestion [36], suggesting that when a noncoated aspirin pill is swallowed whole that doses greater than 300 mg do not influence the rate at which maximal antiplatelet effects are achieved. Aspirin absorption and the onset of antiplatelet activity are significantly shortened however by chewing an aspirin, or drinking solubilized aspirin (e.g., Alka-Seltzer). A study of 12 volunteers compared 325 mg of buffered aspirin, either chewed or swallowed, with Alka-Seltzer [37]. Chewing the pill or drinking the solution maximally inhibited serum $TXB_2$ within 20–30 minutes, whereas just swallowing the pill required

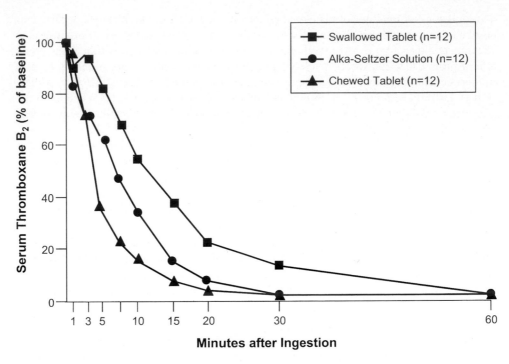

**Figure 1** Mean levels of serum thromboxane $B_2$ measured 3–60 minutes after aspirin ingestion in 12 volunteers. Buffered aspirin, 325 mg, was either swallowed whole, chewed then swallowed, or a 4 ounce solution of Alka-Seltzer containing 325 mg of aspirin was swallowed. (Modified from Ref. 37)

approximately 60 minutes (Fig. 1). In another study of 18 volunteers, chewing an 81 mg, 162 mg, and 324 mg aspirin pill lead to equivalent reduction in $TXB_2$ production, but maximal inhibition by 15 minutes after ingestion was achieved in all volunteers only after the 162 mg and 324 mg doses [38]. The results of these and other studies [39,40] suggest that in order to achieve the maximal effects of aspirin most rapidly (approximately 15 minutes), at least 162 mg should be chewed and swallowed.

*Chronic Dosing*

Due to its irreversible inactivation of platelet COX-1, and the lack of de novo synthesis of new COX-1 by platelets, the affect of chronic aspirin dosing is cumulative. Therefore, once complete inhibition of COX-1 is achieved only minimal doses of aspirin are required to assure adequate acetylation of the fraction (approximately 10%) of new platelets entering the circulation daily. Because of this, daily doses of as little as 30 mg have been shown to be all that is required to completely inhibit serum $TXB_2$ production (Fig. 2) [20].

## Aspirin Dose-Effect Clinical Data

Even though ex-vivo pharmacodynamic studies suggest that as little as 30 mg of aspirin daily is adequate to maximize the antiplatelet effects of aspirin, doses 2- to 10-fold this are routinely utilized clinically, with some even advocating doses 50-times this for select patient [41,42]. Although no dose of aspirin has been shown to inhibit platelet thromboxane

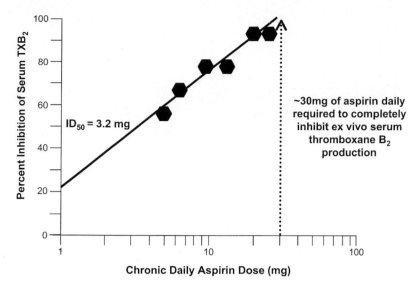

**Figure 2** Percent inhibition of serum thromboxane $B_2$ production after 1 month of chronic daily dosing in 4 volunteers. A daily dose of aspirin of 3.2 mg was needed to inhibit serum thromboxane $B_2$ production by 50%, whereas approximately 30 mg daily was required for near complete inhibition. (Modified from Ref. 20)

production to a greater degree than 30 mg daily, several nonthromboxane-related effects of aspirin could potentially contribute to its beneficial effects in the treatment and prevention of atherothrombotic disease. Therefore the results of clinical trials rather than ex vivo or in vitro studies should be utilized when determining the optimal aspirin dose in various clinical settings.

*Efficacy*

A number of large, blinded, controlled trials have directly studied the clinical efficacy of different doses of aspirin, and several meta-analyses have attempted to evaluate the relative risk reduction of different aspirin doses used in numerous placebo-controlled trials. The one constant finding among all of these studies has been the lack of any relationship between increasing aspirin dose and improved efficacy. In fact, the trend in benefit has almost uniformly favored lower doses.

Trials directly comparing the efficacy of different doses of aspirin have included patients with virtually every clinical manifestation of atherosclerotic disease—stroke, transient ischemic attack (TIA), percutaneous coronary and peripheral interventions, carotid endarterectomy, and myocardial infarction (MI). As shown in Table 2, together these trials have included nearly 10,000 patients and have studied doses ranging from 30 mg to 1500 mg daily [43,44,54,63–65]. In no trial was a significant benefit of higher doses of aspirin found, and in most trials the lowest event rates were realized in those patients randomized to the low-dose aspirin arms. In one trial of 2,849 patients scheduled for endarterectomy, the ACE (ASA and Carotid Endarterectomy) trial, patients randomized to lower doses of aspirin (81 mg or 325 mg) experienced a significantly lower rate of the combined endpoint of death, MI, or stroke compared with those patients randomized to higher doses (650mg or 1300mg) (6.4% vs. 8.4%, p = 0.03) [43]. The best trial of long-term therapy comparing

**Table 2**  Trials Studying the Effect of Different Doses of Aspirin on Clinical Outcomes

| Trial | Number of Patients | Study Population | Aspirin Doses Studied | Mean Follow-Up | Primary Endpoint | Percent with Primary Endpoint |
|---|---|---|---|---|---|---|
| **UK-TIA Trial (54)** | 2435 | TIA or minor stroke | Placebo<br>300 mg daily<br>600 mg twice daily | 4 years | Vascular Death, MI or Major Stroke | Placebo 22.9%<br>300 mg 20.1%<br>1200 mg 19.9% |
| **Dutch-TIA Trial (44)** | 3131 | TIA or minor stroke | 30 mg daily<br>283 mg daily | 2.6 years | Vascular Death, MI or Stroke | 30 mg 14.7%<br>283 mg 15.2% |
| **ACE Trial (43)** | 2849 | Scheduled for carotid endarterectomy | 81 mg daily<br>325 mg daily<br>325 mg twice daily<br>650 mg twice daily | 3 months | Vascular Death, MI or Stroke | 81 mg + 325 mg 6.2%<br>650 mg + 1300 mg 8.4%<br>(p=0.03)* |
| **Cottbus Reinfarction Study (63)** | 701 | Following acute myocardial infarction | 30 mg daily<br>60 mg daily<br>1000 mg daily | 2 years | Death and re-infarction) | 30 mg 11.2%<br>60 mg 10.6%<br>1000 mg 18.0% |
| **Ranke (64)** | 359 | Following peripheral angioplasty | 50 mg daily<br>300 mg three times a day | 35 weeks | Restenosis | 50 mg 16.2%<br>900 mg 15.1% |
| **Mufson (65)** | 495 | Scheduled for coronary angioplasty | 80 mg daily<br>1500 mg daily | Post-angioplasty | Death, MI or urgent revascularization | 80 mg 7.2%<br>1500 mg 7.6% |

TIA: Transient ischemic attack
ACE: ASA Carotid Endarterectomy
* all other comparisons between aspirin doses were not statistically significant.

**Table 3** Indirect Comparison of Aspirin Doses and Reduction in Vascular
Events from the Antithrombotic Trialists' Collaboration (8)

| Daily Aspirin Dose | Number of Trials | Number of Patients | Percent Odds Reduction ($\pm$SE) |
|---|---|---|---|
| 500 mg to 1500 mg | 34 | 22,451 | 19% ($\pm$3) |
| 160 mg to 325 mg | 19 | 26,513 | 26% ($\pm$3) |
| 75 mg to 150 mg | 12 | 6,776 | 32% ($\pm$6) |
| < 75 mg | 3 | 3,655 | 13% ($\pm$8) |

a somewhat contemporary dose and a very low dose of aspirin is the Dutch-TIA trial [44]. In this trial 3,131 individuals following a TIA or minor stroke were randomized to either 283 mg or 30 mg of aspirin daily. The incidence of vascular death, MI, or stroke after a mean of 2.6 years of follow-up was similar in the two groups (14.7% vs. 15.2% for 30mg vs. 283mg, p = NS).

Several meta-analyses have indirectly compared the dose-related relative risk reduction of aspirin from placebo-controlled trials. In one recent analysis specifically focused on 5,228 patients in 11 randomized clinical trials who were randomized to aspirin or placebo following a TIA or stroke, similar efficacy was found for all doses ranging from 50–1500 mg daily [45]. Results from the Antithrombotic Trialists' Collaboration, which included all placebo-controlled aspirin trials found a similar lack of relationship between dose and efficacy (Table 3) [8]. In this analysis the greatest risk reduction was found in those placebo-controlled trials utilizing a 75 mg to 150 mg dose of aspirin, whereas the small number of trials using less than 75 mg seemed to suggest a smaller effect, although the confidence intervals were wide.

The observational results of two recent, large-scale clinical trials are also consistent with the lack of any increase in benefit with higher doses of aspirin. In the BRAVO (Blockade of the Glycoprotein IIb/IIIa Receptor to Avoid Vascular Occlusion) trial 9,190 patients with vascular disease were randomized to one of two doses of the glycoprotein (GP) IIb/IIIa antagonist lotrafiban or placebo in addition to aspirin at doses ranging from 75 mg to 325 mg daily, the aspirin dose being at the discretion of the physician [46]. Among those patients randomized to placebo, 2,410 patients received 75 mg to162 mg daily and 2,179 were treated with more than 162 mg daily. No difference in the combined endpoint of all cause mortality, MI, or stroke was found between these 2 cohorts with a median follow-up of 366 days (Fig. 3). Interestingly though, even though lower doses of aspirin were in general associated with a lower incidence of vascular events, only higher dose aspirin was associated with significantly lower mortality in the multivariate model. The CURE (Clopidogrel in Unstable angina to prevent Recurrent Events) trial is another recent trial that allowed for the evaluation of any potential dose response of aspirin [47]. In this trial 12,562 patients with a non–ST-elevation acute coronary syndrome were randomized to clopidogrel or matching placebo on top of chronic aspirin therapy of 75 mg to 325 mg daily, again at the discretion of the investigator. In patients randomized to either active therapy or placebo, the lowest event rates tended to be in those patients treated with less than 100 mg daily (Fig. 3).

*Adverse Effects*

The major risk of NSAID therapy, including aspirin, is the risk of bleeding. Although the antiplatelet effects of aspirin likely contributes to some increase in the risk of bleeding,

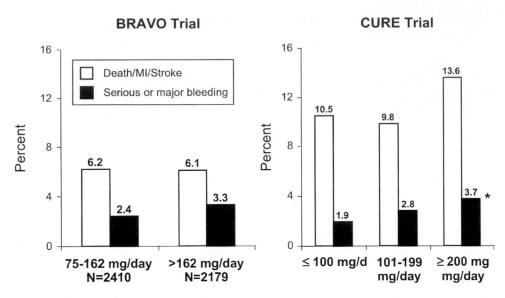

**Figure 3**  Observational results from the placebo arms (i.e., aspirin alone) arms of the BRAVO (Blockade of the Glycoprotein IIb/IIIa Receptor to Avoid Vascular Occlusion) and CURE (Clopidogrel in Unstable angina to prevent Recurrent Events) trials. Efficacy end-points were all cause death, myocardial infarction, or stoke in BRAVO, and cardiovascular death, myocardial infarction. or stroke in CURE. Bleeding was identified as Serious in BRAVO or Major in CURE. * Difference in bleeding risk with increasing aspirin dose in CURE was statistically significant (p = 0.0001).

as highlighted by a risk increase of hemorrhagic stroke in 12 patients for every 10,000 persons treated [48], the majority of increased bleeding is due to a gastrointestinal (GI) etiology. Overall, NSAID users have a 2- to 3-fold increased risk of GI bleeding, an 8-fold increased risk of GI surgery, and a 5-fold increased risk of GI-related mortality [49]. Although this increase in risk is often thought to be primarily related to nonaspirin NSAIDs, a recent evaluation of patients hospitalized for ulcer bleeding found that low-dose aspirin therapy was responsible for as much ulcer bleeding as all other NSAIDs combined [50].

Through the inhibition of COX-1 in gastric mucosal cells aspirin decreases the production of cytoprotective prostacyclins. The influence of aspirin on gastric prostacyclin levels is dose-dependent with almost 50% inhibition at just 30 mg daily, but maximal inhibition requiring approximately 1300 mg daily (Fig. 4) [51]. Consistent with these data, there is no conventional dose of aspirin that has been found to be free from the risk of ulcer bleeding. In a case-control study of patients admitted with a bleeding ulcer, the odds ratio was increased for all doses of aspirin [52]. Treatment with a 75 mg daily dose of aspirin was associated with an odds ratio of 2.3 for a bleeding ulcer (95% confidence interval 1.2 to 4.4), whereas a 300 mg daily increased the odds ratio by over 50% to 3.9 (95% confidence interval 2.5 to 6.3). Importantly, enteric-coating or buffered aspirin preparations do not influence the risk of major upper-GI bleeding [53].

Consistent with the pharmacodynamic and observational studies of patients with ulcer bleeding, the trials that directly compared different doses of aspirin for cardiovascular preventive therapy also found an increased risk in all GI side effects, and in particular GI bleeding with increased doses of aspirin. In the UK-TIA trial the odds ratio for a gastroin-

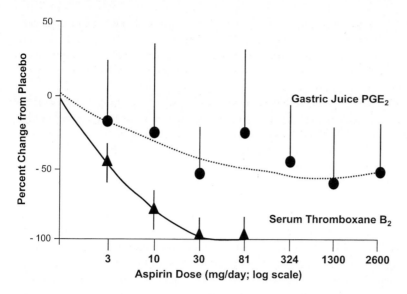

**Figure 4** Dose-related inhibitory effects of aspirin on gastric juice prostacyclin (PGE$_2$) levels and serum thromboxane B$_2$levels. (From Ref. 51)

testinal hemorrhage was 2.57 (95% CI 1.20–5.53) in those randomized to 300 mg of aspirin daily compared with placebo, whereas the odds ratio for those randomized to 1200 mg daily compared to 300 mg daily was 1.62 (95%CI 0.94–2.79) [54]. In the Dutch-TIA trial a similar trend towards less bleeding was found in the 30 mg group compared with the 283 mg group (2.6% vs. 3.2%) [44]. The observational data from the BRAVO and CURE trials also demonstrated an increased risk of bleeding with increasing doses of aspirin, even when doses no higher than 325 mg were utilized (Fig. 3) [46,47].

Based on the observed dose-dependent risk of bleeding, and the potential 40–50% reduction in this risk suggested by several trials when aspirin doses of less than 100 mg daily are used instead of doses greater than 300 mg daily, minimizing the aspirin dose to the least required to maintain efficacy would be expect to have a substantial impact on the morbidity and mortality associated with GI bleeding.

## INTERPATIENT VARIABILITY IN ASPIRIN EFFECTS

Wide interpatient variability in response to aspirin has been recognized for almost 40 years; even longer than its clinical benefit has been appreciated [55]. Since that time, numerous small studies using a wide variety of ex vivo determinants of aspirin responsiveness have consistently found substantial variability in individuals' responses to aspirin, with several suggesting a correlation with clinical outcomes and ex vivo aspirin ''nonresponsiveness'' or ''resistance''—a relationship which has yet to be proven in adequately powered, large-scale, prospective clinical trials. Identifying patients as either a ''responder'' or as a ''nonresponder'' suggests a dichotomous response that is quite different from what would be expected based on the multiple genetic and environmental factors that influence platelet responsiveness [56–58]. The limitations of such a classification are highlighted by the results of studies that have attempted to correlate some ex vivo measure of aspirin responsiveness to clinical outcomes. Three studies that were able to find a significant correlation between some measure of aspirin responsiveness and clinical outcomes identified as few as 5%, and as many as 75% of patients as achieving an inadequate response to aspirin, despite including similar patient populations [59–61]. Others have been unable to find any difference in clinical outcomes in patients prospectively labeled as "responders" or "nonresponders" [62].

Although it has been suggested that increasing the dose of aspirin can overcome an inadequate response to aspirin [41,42], the clinical data do not currently support this contention. While it is possible that a subgroup of patients may benefit from higher doses of aspirin, in order to reconcile this hypothesis with the clinical data one would have to assume there is an equal-sized subgroup that is put at greater risk of thrombotic events by receiving a higher dose of aspirin. If such a subgroup exists we are unable to identify it at this time.

Clearly, the available data are consistent with wide variability among individuals in response to aspirin. However, until clinical trials are carried out that are able to identify some measure of aspirin's effect on platelets that correlates with clinical outcomes, which then allow for changes in therapy that improve outcomes, the routine evaluation of patient responsiveness to aspirin is not warranted. Several trials designed to fill this important void in our understanding of aspirin therapy are currently being planned.

## SUMMARY AND FUTURE DIRECTION

There is no drug that is used by a greater number of people worldwide than aspirin. Although, in general, it is safe when it is used in such a large population even a low overall incidence of side effects can have a substantial impact in terms of absolute numbers of patients effected. A clear association between an increase in aspirin dose and the risk of adverse events has been confirmed in multiple studies. However, a similar relationship has not been shown for conventionally utilized cardiovascular protective doses of aspirin. This would suggest that following the rapid, acute inhibition of platelet COX-1 with a 160 to 325 mg chewed dose of aspirin, every effort should be made to minimize the chronic dose. Currently, the data are most supportive of a 75 or 81 mg daily dose, although further study is clearly needed.

The greatest challenge for the future is to determine the optimal method for identifying the best antiplatelet regimen for the individual patient. The ability to routinely assess a clinically relevant measure of platelet function during treatment with aspirin or any other antiplatelet therapy will be central to accomplishing this.

## REFERENCES

1.   Schindler PE. Aspirin therapy. NY: Walker and Company, 1978.
2.   Stone E. An account of the success of the bark of the willow in the cure of agues. Philos Trans R Soc Lond [Biol] 1763;53:195–200.
3.   Mann CC, Plummer ML. The aspirin wars: Money, medicine and 100 years of rampant competition. NY: Alfred A. Knopf Inc., 1991.
4.   Zundorf U. 100 years aspirin. The future has just begun. Leverkusen: Bayer AG, 1997.
5.   Gibson P. Salicylic acid for coronary thrombosis? Lancet 1948;1:965.
6.   Gibson PC. Aspirin in the treatment of vascular diseases. Lancet 1949;2:1172–1174.
7.   Craven LL. Experiences with aspirin (acetylsalicylic acid) in the nonspecific prophylaxis of coronary thrombosis. Mississippi Valley Medical Journal 1953;75:38–44.

8. Antithrombotic Trialists C. Collaborative meta-analysis of randomised trials of antiplatelet therapy for prevention of death, myocardial infarction, and stroke in high risk patients. [erratum appears in bmj 2002 jan 19;324(7330):141]. BMJ 2002;324:71–86.

9. Lewis HD, Davis JW, Archibald DG, Steinke WE, Smitherman TC, Doherty JE, Schnaper HW, LeWinter MM, Linares E, Pouget JM, Sabharwal SC, Chesler E, Demots H. Protective effects of aspirin against acute myocardial infarction and death in men with unstable angina: Results of a veterans administration cooperative study. N Eng J Med 1983;309:396–403.

10. Cairns JA, Gent M, Singer J, Finnie KJ, Frogatt GM, Holder DA, Jablonsky G, Kostuk WJ, Melendez LJ, Myers MG, Sackett DL, Sealey BJ, Tanser PH. Aspirin, sulfinpyrazone, or both in unstable angina. N Engl J Med 1985;313:1369–1375.

11. The RISC Group. Risk of myocardial infarction and death during treatment with low dose aspirin and intravenous heparin in men with unstable coronary artery disease. Lancet 1990; 336:827–830.

12. Wallentin LC. and the RISC Group. Aspirin (75 mg/day) after an episode of unstable coronary artery disease: Long-term effects on the risk of myocardial infarction, occurrence of severe angina and the need for revascularization. J Am Coll Cardiol 1991;18:1587–1593.

13. Théroux P, Ouimet H, McCans J, Latour J, Joly P, Levy G, Pelletier E, Juneau M, Stasiak J, de Guise P, Pelletier GB, Rinzler D, Waters DD. Aspirin, heparin, or both to treat acute unstable angina. N Engl J Med 1988;319:1105–1111.

14. Théroux P, Waters D, Lam J, Juneau M, McCans J. Reactivation of unstable angina after the discontinuation of heparin. N Engl J Med 1992;327:141–145.

15. ISIS-2 (Second International Study of Infarct Survival) Collaborative Group. Randomized trial of intravenous streptokinase, oral aspirin, both, or neither among 17,187 cases of suspected acute myocardial infarction; isis-2. Lancet 1988:349–360.

16. Tramer MR. Aspirin, like all other drugs, is a poison. BMJ 2000;321:1170–1171.

17. Roth G, Stanford N, Majerus P. Acetylation of prostaglandin synthase by aspirin. Proc Nat Acad Sci USA 1975;72:3073–3076.

18. Loll P, Picot D, Garavito R. The structural basis for aspirin activity inferred from the crystal structure of inactivated prostaglandin $h_2$ synthase. Nature (Struct Biol) 1995;2:637–643.

19. Burch J, Stanford N, Majerus P. Inhibition of platelet prostaglandin synthase by oral aspirin. J Clin Invest 1979;61:314–319.

20. Patrono C, Ciabattoni G, Patrignani P, Pugliese F, Filabozzi P, Catella F, Davi G, Forni L. Clinical pharmacology of platelet cyclooxygenase inhibition. Circulation 1985;72:1177–1184.

21. Vane JR, Bakhle YS, Botting RM. Cyclooxygenases 1 and 2. Ann Rev Pharmacol Toxicol 1998;38:97–120.

22. Smith WL, DeWitt DL. Biochemistry of prostaglandin endoperoxide h synthase-1 and synthase-2 and their differential susceptibility to nonsteroidal anti-inflammatory drugs. Semin Nephrol 1995;15:179–194.

23. Libby P, Ridker PM, Maseri A. Inflammation and atherosclerosis.[comment]. Circulation 2002; 105:1135–1143.

24. Ridker PM, Cushman M, Stampfer MJ, Tracy RP, Hennekens CH. Inflammation, aspirin, and the risk of cardiovascular disease in apparently healthy men. N Engl J Med 1997;336:973–979.

25. Voisard R, Fischer R, Osswald M, Voglic S, Baur R, Susa M, Koenig W, Hombach V. Aspirin (5 mmol/l) inhibits leukocyte attack and triggered reactive cell proliferation in a 3d human coronary in vitro model. Circulation 2001;103:1688–1694.

26. Feng D, Tracy RP, Lipinska I, Murillo J, McKenna C, Tofler GH. Effect of short-term aspirin use on c-reactive protein. J Thromb Thrombolysis 2000;9:37–41.

27. Kennon S, Price CP, Mills PG, Ranjadayalan K, Cooper J, Clarke H, Timmis AD. The effect of aspirin on c-reactive protein as a marker of risk in unstable angina. J Am Coll Cardiol 2001;37:1266–1270.

28. Feldman M, Jialal I, Devaraj S, Cryer B. Effects of low-dose aspirin on serum c-reactive protein and thromboxane b2 concentrations: A placebo-controlled study using a highly sensitive c-reactive protein assay. J Am Coll Cardiol 2001;37:2036–2041.

29. Kim SB, Lee SK, Min WK, Chi HS, Park JS. Lack of effects of low-dose aspirin on high-sensitivity c-reactive protein, hemostatic factors, and troponin t in capd patients. Perit Dial Int 2002;22:721–723.

30. Azar RR, Klayme S, Germanos M, Kassab R, Tawm S, Aboujaoude S, Naman R. Effects of aspirin (325 mg/day) on serum high-sensitivity c-reactive protein, cytokines, and adhesion molecules in healthy volunteers. Am J Cardiol 2003;92:236–239.

31. Takeda T, Hoshida S, Nishino M, Tanouchi J, Otsu K, Hori M. Relationship between effects of statins, aspirin and angiotensin ii modulators on high-sensitive c-reactive protein levels. Atherosclerosis 2003;169:155–158.

32. Eidelman RS, Lamas GA, Hennekens CH, Ridker PM. Aspirin, postmenopausal hormones, and c-reactive protein. Arch Intern Med 2002;162:480–481.

33. Ikonomidis I, Andreotti F, Economou E, Stefanadis C, Toutouzas P, Nihoyannopoulos P. Increased proinflammatory cytokines in patients with chronic stable angina and their reduction by aspirin. Circulation 1999;100:793–798.

34. Pedersen AK, FitzGerald GA. Dose-related kinetics of aspirin. Presystemic acetylation of platelet cyclooxygenase. N Eng J Med 1984;311:1206–1211.

35. Benedek IH, Joshi AS, Pieniaszek HJ, King S-YP, Kornhauser DM. Variability in the pharmacokinetics and pharmicodynamics of low dose aspirin in healthy male volunteers. J Clin Pharmacol 1995;35:1181–1186.

36. Buerke M, Pittroff W, Meyer J, Darius H. Aspirin therapy: Optimized platelet inhibition with different loading and maintenance doses. Am Heart J 1995;130:465–472.

37. Feldman M, Cryer B. Aspirin absorption rates and platelet inhibition times with 325-mg buffered aspirin tablets (chewed or swallowed intact) and with buffered aspirin solution. Am J Cardiol 1999;84:404–409.

38. Dabaghi SF, Kamat SG, Payne J, Marks GF, Roberts R, Schafer AI, Kleiman NS. Effects of low-dose aspirin on in vitro platelet aggregation in the early minutes after ingestion in normal subjects. Am J Cardiol 1994;74:720–723.

39. Patrignani P, Filabozzi P, Patrono C. Selective cumulative inhibition of platelet thromboxane production by low-dose aspirin in healthy subjects. J Clin Invest 1982;69:1366–1372.

40. Weksler BB, Tack-Goldman K, Subramanian VA, Gay WA. Cumulative inhibitory effect of low-dose aspirin on vascular prostacyclin and platelet thromboxane production in patients with atherosclerosis. Circulation 1985;71:332–340.

41. Alberts M, Bergman D, Molner E, Jovanovic B, Ushiwata I, Teruya J. Antiplatelet effect of aspirin in patients with cerebrovascular disease. Stroke 2004;35:175–178.

42. Helgason CM, Bolin KM, Hoff JA, Winkler SR, Mangat A, Tortorice KL, Brace LD. Development of aspirin resistance in persons with previous ischemic stroke. Stroke 1994;25: 2331–2336.

43. Taylor DW, Barnett HJM, Haynes RB, Ferguson GG, Sackett DL, Thorpe KE, Simard D, Silver FL, Hachinski V, Clagett GP, Barnes R, Spence JD. for the ASA and Carotid Endarterectomy (ACE) Trial Collaborators. Low-dose and high-dose acetylsalicylic acid for patients undergoing carotid endarterectomy: A romdomised controlled trial. Lancet 1999;353: 2179–2184.

44. The Dutch TIA Study Group. A comparison of two doses of aspirin (30 mg vs. 283 mg a day) in patients after transient ischemic attack or minor ischemic stroke. N Engl J Med 1991;325: 1261–1266.

45. Johnson E, Lanes S, Wentworth C, Satterfield M, Abebe B, Dicker L. A metaregression analysis of the dose-response effect of aspirin on stroke. Arch Intern Med 1999;159:1248–1253.

46. Topol EJ, Easton D, Harrington RA, Amarenco P, Califf RM, Graffagnino C, Davis S, Diener HC, Ferguson J, Fitzgerald D, Granett J, Shuaib A, Koudstaal PJ, Theroux P, Van de Werf F, Sigmon K, Pieper K, Vallee M, Willerson JT. Randomized, double-blind, placebo-controlled, international trial of the oral iib/iiia antagonist lotrafiban in coronary and cerebrovascular disease. Circulation 2003;108:399–406.

47. Peters RJ, Mehta SR, Fox KA, Zhao F, Lewis BS, Kopecky SL, Diaz R, Commerford PJ, Valentin V, Yusuf S. Clopidogrel in Unstable angina to prevent Recurrent Events (CURE)Trial Investigators. Effects of aspirin dose when used alone or in combination with clopidogrel in patients with acute coronary syndromes: Observations from the clopidogrel in unstable angina to prevent recurrent events (cure) study. Circulation 2003;108:1682–1687.

48.  He J, Whelton P, Vu B, Klag M. Aspirin and risk of hemorrhagic stroke. A meta-analysis of randomized controlled trials. JAMA 1998;280:1930–1935.
49.  Gabriel SE, Jaakkimainen L, Bombardier C. Risk of serious gastrointestinal complications related to nonsteroidal anti-inflammatory drugs: A meta-analysis. Ann Intern Med 1991;115: 787–796.
50.  Stack WA, Atherton JC, Hawkey G, Logan RFA, Hawkey CJ. Interactions between helicobacter pylori and other risk factors for peptic ulcer bleeding. Aliment Pharmacol Ther 2002; 16:497–506.
51.  Lee M, Cryer B, Feldman M. Dose effects of aspirin on gastric prostaglandins and stomach mucosal injury. Annals of Internal Medicine 1994;120:184–189.
52.  Weil J, Colin-Jones D, Langman M, Lawson D, Logan R, Murphy M, Rawlins M, Vessey M, Wainwright P. Prophylactic aspirin and risk of peptic ulcer bleeding. Br Med J 1995;310: 827–830.
53.  Kelly J, Kaufman DW, Jurgelon J, Sheehan J, Koff R, Shapiro S. Risk of aspirin-associated major upper-gastrointestinal bleeding with enteric-coated or buffered product. Lancet 1996; 348:1413–1416.
54.  UK-TIA study Group. The united kingdom transient ischemic attack (uk-tia) aspirin trial: Final results. J Neurol Neurosurg Psychiatry 1991;54:1044–1054.
55.  Quick AJ. Salicylates and bleeding: The aspirin tolerance test. Am J Med Sci 1966;252: 265–269.
56.  Karnicki K, Owen WG, Miller RS, McBane RD. Factors contributing to individual propensity for arterial thrombosis. Arteriosclerosis, Thrombosis & Vascular Biology 2002;22:1495–1499.
57.  Michelson AD, Furman MI, Goldschmidt-Clermont P, Mascelli MA, Hendrix C, Coleman L, Hamlington J, Barnard MR, Kickler T, Christie DJ, Kundu S, Bray PF. Platelet gp iiia pla polymorphisms display different sensitivities to agonists. Circulation 2000;101:1013–1018.
58.  Cooke GE, Bray PF, Hamlington JD, Pham DM, Goldschmidt-Clermont PJ. Pla2 polymorphism and efficacy of aspirin. Lancet 1998;351:1253.
59.  Grotemeyer K-H, Scharafinski H-W, Husstedt I-W. Two-year follow-up of aspirin responder and aspirin non-responder. A pilot study including 180 post-stroke patients. Thrombosis Research 1993;71:397–403.
60.  Gum P, Kottke-Marchant K, Welsh PA, White J, Topol EJ. A prospective, blinded determination of the natural hisotry of aspirin resistance among stable patients with cardiovascular disease. J Am Coll Cardial 2003;41:961–965.
61.  Eikelboom JW, Hirsh J, Weitz JI, Johnston M, Yi Q, Yusuf S. Aspirin-resistant thromboxane biosynthesis and the risk of myocardial infarction, stroke, or cardiovascular death in patients at high risk for cardiovascular events. Circulation 2002;105:1650–1655.
62.  Gum P, Kottke-Marchant K, Welsh PA, White J, Topol EJ. Determination of the natural history of aspirin resistance among stable patients with cardiovascular disease. J Am Coll Cardiol 2003;42:1336–1337.
63.  Hoffman W, Forster W. Two year cottbus reinfarction study with 30 mg aspirin per day. Prostaglandins Leukotrienes and Essential Fatty Acids 1991;44:159–169.
64.  Ranke C, Creutzig A, Luska G, Wagner H-H, Galanski M, Bode-Boger S, Frolich J, Avenarius H-J, Hecker H, Alexander K. Controlled trial of high- versus low-dose aspirin treatment after percutaneous transluminla angioplasty in patients with peripheral vascular disease. Clin Investig 1994;72:673–680.
65.  Mufson L, Black A, Roubin G, Wilentz J, Mead S, McFarland K, Weintraub WS, Douglas JS, King SB. A randomized trial of aspirin in ptca: Effect of high vs. Low dose aspirin on major complications and restenosis.[abstract]. J Am Coll Cardial 1988;11:236A.

# 21

# Antithrombin Therapy in Acute Coronary Syndromes

**Albrecht Vogt**
*Medizinische Klinik II Klinikum Kassel*
*Kassel, Germany*

## INTRODUCTION

Thrombin plays a pivotal role in platelet-mediated thrombosis associated with atheromatous plaque rupture in patients with acute coronary syndromes. Thrombin inhibition is, therefore, a basic therapeutic goal in this setting, together with thrombolysis and platelet inhibition.

## HEPARIN

Heparin is a mixture of glycosaminglycans with an average molecular weight of 12,000 to 15,000. Heparin interacts with antithrombin III to inhibit the coagulation factors Xa and IXa, but especially thrombin. Inhibition of thrombin occurs via the formation of a ternary complex of heparin, antithrombin III, and thrombin. Low-molecular weight (LMW) heparin is produced by depolymerization of standard heparin into polysaccharide fragments with a molecular weight of 4000 to 6500. The advantage of LMW heparin is a better bioavailability after subcutaneous injection, being close to 100% compared to 30% for standard heparin. The plasma half-life is two to four times that of standard heparin. The anticoagulant effect of LMW heparin is mostly due to inhibition of factor Xa [1].

### Unfractionated Heparin in Unstable Angina and Non–Q-Wave Myocardial Infarction

Patients with unstable angina tend to have an activated coagulation system and especially heightened thrombin activity, which is associated with an early unfavourable outcome [2,3,4,5]. Therefore, heparin has become a standard treatment for unstable angina and non–Q-wave myocardial infarction. Its efficacy has been well documented in terms of prevention of definite transmural myocardial infarction and death, reducing the need for urgent revascularization, and reducing the incidence of recurrent myocardial ischemia (Table 1) [6–12]. Most studies applied a dose regimen with an intravenous bolus of 5000 IU followed by an infusion of 1000 IU/h adjusted to a target aPTT around two times the

**Table 1** Heparin in Unstable Angina

| Study | No. patients | Heparin | Controls | Enpoints/efficacy |
|---|---|---|---|---|
| Telford 1988 (9) | 214 | 4 × 5000 IU IV | Placebo | MI 3% vs. 15% |
| Théroux 1988 (10) | 479 | a) IV (aPTT 1.2–2 × control)<br>b) IV + 2 × 325 mg ASS | c) 2 × 325 mg ASS<br>d) Placebo | Refractory angina/death/MI a) 9.3%; b) 11.5%; c) 16.5%; d) 26.3% |
| RISC 1990 (12) | 796 | a) 4 × 5000 bolus IV<br>b) a + 1 × 75 mg ASS | c) 1 × 75 mg ASS<br>d) Placebo | MI/death 5 days : a) 5.6%; b) 1.4%; c) 3.7%; d) 6.0% |
| Théroux 1993 (11) | 484 | IV (aPTT 1.5–2.5 × control) | 2 × 325 mg ASS | MI 0.8% vs. 3.7% |
| Cohen 1994 (6) | 214 | IV (aPTT 2-fold) + ASS, contd. Warfarin | 1 × 162.5 mg ASS | Re-ischemia/MI/death 10.5% vs. 27% |
| Holdright 1994 (7) | 285 | IV (aPTT 1.5–2.5 × control) + ASS 1 × 150 mg | 1 × 150 mg ASS | MI/death 27.3 vs. 30.5% Ischemia (Holter) no diff. |
| Serneri 1995 (8) | 108 | IV or SC + ASS (aPTT 1.5 to 2-fold) | 1 × 325 mg ASS | Re-ischemia reduced by IV and SC heparin |

control value. Dosing heparin by a weight-based nomogram instead of the standard doses results in a more reliable anticoagulation with respect to the target aPTT [13]. The clinical advantage of this technically more complex regime has, however, not been demonstrated. Intermittent intravenous bolus injections of heparin were effective in one study [9] but did not prevent myocardial infarction or episodes of myocardial ischemia in two others [12,14]. The Thrombolysis in Myocardial Infarction (TIMI) study group recommended a target aPTT of 45 to 60 seconds according to the results of the TIMI-3 study [15]. A more aggressive anticoagulation did not seem to result in further reduction of ischemic events.

Treatment with heparin is certainly superior to placebo and very probably better than aspirin alone [6,8,10,11]. It seems reasonable to combine heparin with aspirin, since platelet inhibition is desirable in acute coronary syndromes and, moreover, heparin might enhance platelet function in unstable angina [16]. The combination is widely used, but there is no proof evidence of a clinical benefit over heparin alone. While there was no significant difference in the incidence of ischemic events, the incidence of serious bleedings was 3.3% in patients treated with heparin and aspirin vs. 1.7% in those on heparin only [17].

The vast majority of patients with unstable angina can be stabilized initially by maximal drug therapy including heparin and a combination of antianginal drugs; only 8.8% had truly refractory unstable angina in a cohort of 125 patients [18]. Pretreatment of unstable angina patients with heparin over 3 days was reported to markedly reduce the incidence of major ischemic complications of a subsequent angioplasty procedure as compared to an immediate angioplasty [19]. This early hazard of coronary angioplasty in acute coronary syndromes, however, can be overcome by simultaneous treatment with glycoprotein IIb/IIIa receptor antagonists [20]. Therefore, early angioplasty without prolonged medical pretreatment becomes more widely used in unstable angina, especially in high-risk patients with elevated troponin levels.

## Low Molecular-Weight Heparin in Unstable Angina and Non–Q-Wave Myocardial Infarction

Low molecular-weight (LMW) heparin can be easily applied by SC injections and obviates the need of close monitoring of the aPTT. Dalteparin was shown to be more effective in unstable angina than aspirin alone to prevent ischemic events [21]. Several studies have been performed to compare various preparations of LMW heparin given subcutaneously with IV standard heparin guided by aPTT values (Table 2). Dalteparin and nadroparin were equally effective as standard heparin, while enoxaparin 1 mg/kg BID proved to be superior in the ESSENCE and TIMI 11B studies [22,23]. A meta-analysis of these two studies revealed about 20% reduction of definite transmural myocardial infarction and death in patients with unstable angina or non–Q-wave myocardial infarction by this regimen of enoxaparin as compared to standard heparin [24], and this benefit persisted after one year [25]. It is unclear yet why enoxaparin but not dalteparin or nadroparin was more effective than standard heparin. Enoxaparin has the smallest molecule size, the longest plasma half-life, and the most selective effect on factor Xa of these preparations [26]. Whether these differences are clinically important could only be tested by head-to-head comparisons of enoxaparin with other LMW heparins.

Full-dose intravenous heparin as well as subcutaneous LMW heparin may both give rise to a rebound after cessation of treatment [27,21]. The reason for this is unclear. It is probably not due to depletion of antithrombin III [28], but there is a transient rise in thrombin activity and activated protein C [29]. It may well be that treatment with heparin over 2–7 days is too short to allow for healing of the underlying coronary plaque fissure. The rebound seems to be avoided when heparin is given in combination with aspirin. Fourteen of 107 patients given heparin alone had reactivation of unstable angina after discontinuation vs. only 5 of 100 similar patients with concomitant aspirin treatment [27].

The necessary duration of therapy with heparin or LMW heparin has not been defined. Several trials tested prolonged treatment with LMW heparin after hospital discharge [21,22,30,31], but the results were mostly negative with respect to the prevention of clinical events whether or not the patients had coronary angioplasty. This is surprising, since the duration of initial treatment in these studies of only 2–8 days is probably too short to passivate the underlying complicated coronary lesion. Only the FRISC-II study demonstrated a reduction of ischemic events by prolonged treatment with dalteparin in patients treated conservatively for approximately 2 months, but thereafter the benefit dissipated and was no more significant after 6 months [30,32]. Presently, the majority of patients with unstable angina is treated invasively with coronary stenting, and these patients routinely receive combination antiplatelet therapy with aspirin and clopidogrel thereafter. The addition of prolonged LMW heparin is unusual today.

## Unfractionated Heparin as Adjunct to Thrombolysis in Acute Myocardial Infarction

Plasminogen activators cause a paradoxically increased local thrombin generation [33]. This hypercoagulable state is associated with elevated plasma fibrinogen levels [34], an increase in thrombin-antithrombin-III complexes and in prothrombin fragments [35], and a partial resistance to heparin [36]. It seems reasonable, therefore, to combine thrombolytic treatment with adjunctive anticoagulation to improve early infarct vessel patency and

**Table 2** Low-Molecular Weight Heparin SC in Unstable Angina

| Study | No. patients | Heparin dose SC | Controls | Endpoints / efficacy |
|---|---|---|---|---|
| Correia 1995 (109) | 314 | 160 or 320 IU/kg/day | Heparin IV by aPTT | Death/MI no difference |
| Gurfinkel 1995 (110) | 219 | a) 214 IU/kg BID + 1 × 200 mg ASS | b) 1 × 200 mg ASS<br>c) Hep. IV (aPTT 2-fold) + ASS | MI/Reischemia/urgent revasc.<br>a) 22.1%; b) 58.9%; c) 60.0% |
| FRISC 1996 (21) | 1506 | 120 IU/kg BID + ASS | ASS | Death/MI 1.8 vs. 4.8%<br>Urgent revasc. 0.4% vs. 1.2% |
| ESSENCE 1997 (23) | 3171 | 1 mg/kg BID + ASS | Heparin IV, aPTT 55–85 sec | Death/MI/rec. AP 19.8 vs. 23.3% |
| FRIC 1997 (111) | 1482 | 120 IU/kh BID + ASS | Heparin IV, aPTT 1.5-fold | Death/MI/rec. AP 9.3% vs. 7.6% |
| TIMI 11B 1999 (22) | 3910 | 1 mg/kg BID + ASS | Heparin IV, aPTT 1.5–2.5 × control | Death/MI/revasc. 12.4% vs. 14.5% |
| FRAXIS 1999 (112) | 3468 | 87 IU/kg BID (6 or 14 days) | Heparin IV, aPTT 1.5–2.5 × control | Death/MI/rec. AP Heparin 18.1%,<br>LMW 6d 17.8%, LMW 14d<br>20.0% |
| INTERACT 2002 (113) | 746 | 1 mg/kg BID + ASS + Eptifibatide | Heparin IV, aPTT 2-fold control +<br>ASS + Eptifibatide | Death/MI 5.0% vs. 9.0%<br>Major bleeding 1.1% vs. 3.8% |
| A To Z 2002 | 3987 | 1 mg/kg BID + ASS + Tirofiban | Heparin IV, aPTT 2-fold control +<br>ASS + Tirofiban | Death/MI/refract. Ischemia 8.4%<br>vs. 9.4% |

prevent reocclusion. However, the available controlled clinical studies of adjunctive heparin in acute myocardial infarction treated with thrombolysis do not clearly support its routine use to improve the clinical outcome [37].

Most clearly the need of adjunctive heparin has been demonstrated when alteplase is given as thrombolytic agent [38–40]. In one study, the patency of infarct vessels in subgroups with optimal, suboptimal, and inadequate anticoagulation was 90%, 80%, and 72%, respectively, at angiography 2–5 days after thrombolysis with alteplase [41]. While the aPTT during heparin treatment correlated positively with infarct vessel patency at 18 hours after alteplase, there was no correlation with late reocclusion [42]. Infarct vessel patency was also improved by an initial bolus of 5000 IU heparin before thrombolysis with saruplase; angiography after 6–12 hours showed an open infarct vessel in 78.6% of the pretreated patients vs. 56.5% of those receiving heparin only after thrombolysis [43]. The clinical outcome after thrombolysis for acute myocardial infarction with streptokinase, alteplase, or anistreplase, however, was not improved by adjunctive heparin SC in the mega-trials GISSI-2 and ISIS-3 (Table 3) [44,45]. Furthermore, in GISSI-2, the 6-month survival rates as well as the incidence of reinfarction were not different in patients with or without initial SC heparin treatment [46].

GUSTO-I was the first trial to demonstrate a survival benefit of thrombolysis with alteplase vs. streptokinase in acute myocardial infarction [47], which was not seen in the preceding mega-trials GISSI-2 and ISIS-3 [44,45]. The difference is probably due to the front-loaded dosing of alteplase and to adjunctive full-dose heparin treatment in GUSTO but the relative importance of these cannot be estimated. The optimal intensity of anticoagulation is in the range of aPTT values of 50–70 seconds. Those patients had the lowest 30-day mortality, stroke, and bleeding rates in GUSTO-I [48]. Interestingly, reinfarction was more common among patients with higher aPTT values, and there was a clustering of reinfarction in the first 10 hours after discontinuation of heparin [48]. This may reflect a comparable rebound as seen in the treatment of unstable angina with heparin.

Left ventricular mural thrombi occur in about one-third of patients with anterior myocardial infarction [49–52]. Subcutaneous heparin treatment with $2 \times 12,500$ IU was effective against left ventricular thrombus formation as compared to low-dose treatment with $2 \times 5000$ IU; in this randomized study left ventricular thrombi were observed in 11% vs. 32% ($P = .0004$) [53]. In a subgroup of GISSI-2, however, the incidence of echocardiographically detected left ventricular thrombi was similar in patients with and without $2 \times 12,500$ IU heparin [54]. Full-dose heparin followed by oral anticoagulants was investigated in two small controlled studies in patients with first anterior myocardial infarction. Anticoagulants were effective against left ventricular thrombus formation in one study [55,56], but without any effect in the other [57]. In the Fragmin in Acute Myocardial Infarction (FRAMI) study, subcutaneous dalteparin started 8 hours after thrombolysis with streptokinase in patients with acute anterior myocardial infarction provided a significant reduction in left ventricular thrombus formation 9 days after the acute event. However, this benefit was obtained at the expense of a higher bleeding risk (major hemorrhage 2.9% vs. 0.3%, p = 0.006) [58].

When alteplase is given as thrombolytic agent in acute myocardial infarction, adjunctive heparin should be added aiming at an aPTT of 50–70 sec. No benefit has been convincingly demonstrated of IV heparin as adjunct to streptokinase and anistreplase, and SC heparin seems not to be effective at all.

## Low-Molecular Weight Heparin as Adjunct to Thrombolysis in Acute Myocardial Infarction

Triggered by the encouraging results of LMW in unstable angina pectoris, only recently LMW heparin has been investigated as adjunct to thrombolysis in acute myocardial infarc-

**Table 3** Megatrials of Heparin as Adjunct to Thrombolysis in AMI

| Study | No.pts. | Heparin | Controls | Death (%) | Reinfarction (%) | Major bleeds (%) |
|---|---|---|---|---|---|---|
| GISSI-2 (44) | 12,490 | 12,500 IU SC BID + ASS beginning after 12 h | No heparin, SK or t-PA lysis | 8.3 vs. 9.3 | 1.9 vs. 2.3 | 1.0 vs. 0.6 |
| ISIS-3 (45) | 41,299 | 12,500 IU SC BID + ASS beginning after 4 h | No heparin, SK, t-PA, or APSAC lysis | 10.3 vs. 10.6 | 3.2 vs. 3.5 | Noncerebral 1.0 vs. 0.8; cerebral 0.6 vs. 0.4 |
| GUSTO-I (47) | 20,251 | 12,500 IU SC BID + ASS beginning after 4 h | Heparin IV, aPTT 60–85 sec | 7.2 vs. 7.4 | 3.4 vs. 4.0 | Noncerebral 0.3 vs. 0.5; cerebral 0.5 vs. 0.5 |
| ASSENT-3 (61) | 4078 | Enoxaparin 30 mg/kg IV + 1 mg/kg SC BID | Heparin IV, aPTT 50–70 sec. | 5.4 vs. 6.0 | 2.7 vs. 4.2 | Noncerebral 3.0 vs. 2.2 cerebral 0.9 vs. 0.9 |

tion. Enoxaparin was started with a bolus of 30 mg IV followed by 1 mg/kg BID for at least 3 days, while the control group received unfractionated heparin aiming at an aPTT 2- to 2.5-fold the control value. Complete perfusion of the infarct vessel 90 minutes after treatment was seen in 52.9% vs. 47.6% of the patients. Control angiograms after 5–7 days showed reocclusion (from TIMI-grade 3 to grade 0/1) in 3.1% vs. 9.1% [59]. This study was designed and did clearly demonstrate the noninferiority of LMW as compared to standard heparin. The ENTIRE-TIMI 23 study investigated enoxaparin verus unfractionated heparin as adjunct to full-dose tenecteplase or half-dose tenecteplase with abciximab [60]. Angiographic patency rates were similar, but there were less ischemic events within 30 days in the enoxaparin-treated patients without increased bleeding risk.

The clinical efficacy of LMW heparin was shown by the Assessment of the Safety and Efficacy of a New Thrombolytic Regimen (ASSENT-3) study [61]. Patients with acute myocardial infarction (less than 12 hours) treated by bolus thrombolysis with tenecteplase were randomly assigned to an IV bolus of 30 mg enoxaparin followed by 1 mg/kg SC BID for a maximum of 7 days (n = 2040), or unfractionated heparin aimed at an aPTT of 50–70 seconds for 48 hours (n = 2038). A third group received half-dose tenecteplase together with abciximab over 12 hours (n = 2017). The primary endpoint was the combined incidence of 30-day mortality, in-hospital reinfarction, or in-hospital refractory ischemia. This endpoint was reached in 11.4% in the group treated with LMW heparin vs. 15.4% in the standard heparin group, the relative risk was 0.74 (95%-CI 0.63–0.87). The efficacy of enoxaparin was the same as in the group treated with abciximab (Fig. 1). There was no excess bleeding with enoxaparin as compared to standard heparin (intracranial hemorrhage 0.9% in all groups, major bleeding other than intracranial 3.0% enoxaparin vs. 2.2% unfractionated heparin). By analysis of the ST-segment resolution in ASSENT-3 it was concluded that the combination of half-dose tenecteplase with abciximab elicited more rapid and complete reperfusion, while the combination with enoxaparin led

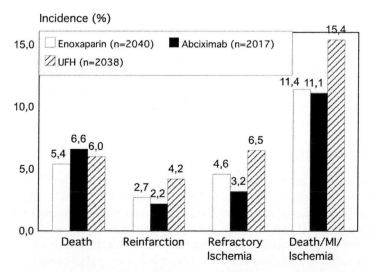

**Figure 1** Efficacy of enoxaparin as adjunct to tenecteplase in acute myocardial infarction, data from ASSENT-3. With respect to the combined endpoint of 30-day mortality, in-hospital reinfarction, or in-hospital refractory ischemia, enoxaparin is as effective as abciximab (with half-dose thrombolysis), and more effective than unfractionated heparin (UFH). The improved efficacy is mainly due to the prevention of reinfarction and reischemia.

to more stable coronary patency [62]. In a parallel study, ASSENT-3 PLUS, the same treatment was given to 1639 patients in the prehospital setting [63]. The efficacy endpoint was reached in 14.2% of the enoxaparin treated patients vs. 17.4 of those on unfractionated heparin (p = 0.08), but stroke increased to 2.9% vs. 1.3% (p = 0.026). An increase in intracranial hemorrhage was seen in patients older than 75 years of age. Therefore, the investigators discouraged the use of enoxaparin as adjunct to tenecteplase in the prehospital setting.

As in unstable angina, the necessary duration of treatment with heparin after myocardial infarction is unknown. The ASSENT-PLUS study randomized 439 patients with AMI treated with alteplase to dalteparin 120 IU SC BID for 4–7 days or unfractionated heparin IV. An angiogram between day 4 and hospital discharge showed overall higher TIMI-flow in the infarct vessel in the dalteparin-group (p = 0.016), but the difference for complete perfusion with TIMI-grade 3 was not significant. Reinfarction occurred less often in the dalteparin group during treatment, but there was a raised risk of events after cessation reflecting a possible rebound eliminating any long-term gain [64].

## Fondaparinux

Fondaparinux is a novel synthetic pentasaccharide which selectively inhibits factor X. It has a plasma half-life of 15 hours, with linear pharmacokinetics and low intraindividual and interindividual variability, thus allowing once daily administration without laboratory monitoring [65]. Recent studies in patients undergoing major orthopaedic surgery have shown a significant reduction of venous thrombosis by 2.5 mg Fondaparinux once daily SC as compared to enoxaparin [66–68]. In patients with acute myocardial infarction treated with alteplase, fondaparinux yielded a similar early coronary patency and a trend to less reocclusion when compared to unfractionated heparin [69]. In a dose finding study, 1138 patients with non–ST-elevation acute coronary syndromes received four different doses of Fondaparinux (2.5, 4, 8, or 12 mg once daily SC), and a control group was treated with 1 mg/kg enoxaparin SC BID. The primary efficacy endpoint of death, myocardial infarction, or recurrent ischemia occurred in 27.9%, 35.9%, 34.7%, and 30.3% of the four Fondaparinux dose groups and in 35.7% of the patients on enoxaparin [70]. The lowest event rates were observed in the group receiving only 2.5 mg Fondaparinux, which was significantly lower than for enoxaparin in the perprotocol analysis, but not in the intention-to-treat analysis. This dose was therefore recommended to be evaluated in further large-scale studies to define the clinical role of this novel drug.

## DIRECT THROMBIN INHIBITORS

Heparin inhibits thrombin only in the presence of antithrombin III as cofactor. The first available direct thrombin inhibitor was hirudin, a polypeptide of 65 amino acids which binds directly to thrombin forming an irreversible complex. In contrast to heparin, hirudin inhibits also clot-bound thrombin. Direct thrombin inhibitors have been shown to elicit a more stable and predictable anticoagulation than heparin [71]. A meta-analysis of all major studies of direct thrombin inhibitors in acute coronary syndromes and percutaneous coronary interventions demonstrated a small but statistically significant advantage over heparin [72]. The combined incidence of death or reinfarction by 30 days was 7.4% vs. 8.2% (p = 0.02), and there was no excess of intracranial bleedings. A specific advantage of all direct thrombin inhibitors vs. heparin is their inability to induce severe thrombocytopenia, which side effect is not uncommon with heparin especially if given for prolonged periods of time. Patients with known heparin-induced thrombocytopenia (HIT) may only be treated with direct thrombin inhibitors.

## Hirudin

Hirudin has been tested in patients with the whole spectrum of acute coronary syndromes in the GUSTO-II study. GUSTO-IIa was terminated early because of an excess of intracranial bleeding occurring in 1.3% of patients treated with 0.6 mg/kg bolus followed by 0.2 mg/kg/h infusion without aPTT-adjustment, as compared to 0.7% of the control group treated with heparin adjusted to an aPTT of 60 to 90 seconds [73]. The study was reinitiated as GUSTO IIb with reduced doses of both anticoagulants. Hirudin was given as 0.1 mg/kg bolus followed by an infusion of 0.1 mg/kg/h, and the aPTT was adjusted to 60 to 85 seconds in both treatment groups [74]. The study enrolled 12,142 patients of whom 8011 had unstable angina without ST-elevation and did not receive thrombolysis. Confirming earlier results [71,75], the patients treated with hirudin had less fluctuation of the aPTT values than those on heparin. The combined incidence of death and myocardial infarction was 8.3% in the hirudin group and 9.1% in the heparin group. This small and statistically nonsiginificant difference was mainly due to the prevention of myocardial infarction (5.6% vs. 6.4%), whereas the death rates were similar (3.75 vs. 3.9%). The Organization to Assess Strategies for Ischemic Syndromes (OASIS-2) study in 10,141 patients with unstable angina or non–Q-wave myocardial infarction demonstrated a small advantage of hirudin over heparin with 3.6% vs. 4.2% (p = 0,077) of the patients suffering death or myocardial infarction within 7 days [76]. In the doses tested, hirudin seems to be marginally better than heparin with respect to the clinical outcome of patients with unstable angina.

Three large-scale trials designed to investigate hirudin in relatively high doses as adjunct to thrombolysis for acute myocardial infarction were terminated early because of an excess of intracranial hemorrhages [73,77,78]. Of note, the high incidence of cerebral bleedings was not specific for hirudin, but the heparin-treated patients had also unexpectedly high bleeding rates. As compared to the earlier GUSTO-I study [47] using approximately 20% lower average doses of heparin, the bleeding risk was particularly high in patients treated with streptokinase irrespective of the anticoagulant given. The TIMI-9 and GUSTO-II studies were reinitiated with markedly lower doses of hirudin and the aPTT values were targeted at lower values also in the heparin groups. Both studies exhibited bleeding rates in the usually expected range for thrombolytic treatment of acute myocardial infarction, and the risk was similar for hirudin and heparin [79,74]. However, overall there was no advantage of hirudin over heparin to prevent death or reinfarction.

Therefore, the studies performed on hirudin in acute coronary syndromes do not show a relevant clinical benefit over heparin despite some pharmacological advantages. Presently, hirudin is only used in patients with heparin-induced thrombocytopenia as an alternative to heparin.

## Bivalirudin

Bivalirudin (formerly called Hirulog) is a dodecapeptide derived from hirudin. It binds to the active catalytic site of thrombin via a Phe-Pro-Arg linker molecule. Like hirudin, hirulog inhibits free as well as clot-bound thrombin [80]. A recent meta-analysis of 6 studies performed until 1999 concluded that bivalirudin is at least as effective as heparin in ischemic heart disease, with clearly superior safety [81].

The TIMI-7 trial investigated bivalirudin to treat unstable angina in 410 patients randomized to four groups of constant infusions over 72 hours with 0.02 to 1.0 mg/kg/h

[82]. All patients received 325 mg aspirin. The primary endpoint was unsatisfactory out-come by 72 hours defined as death, myocardial infarction, rapid clinical deterioration, or reischemia at rest occurred in 6.2% to 11.4% of the four groups without significant between-group differences. However, the secondary endpoint of in-hospital death or nonfa-tal myocardial infarction occurred in 10% of the patients in the lowest dose group vs. 3.2% of those treated with the three higher doses (p = 0.008). The subsequent TIMI-8 trial was undertaken to compare the clinical efficacy of bivalirudin vs. unfractionated heparin in patients with unstable angina and non–ST-elevation myocardial infarction [83]. This trial was terminated after enrollment of 133 of the planned 5,320 patients since the sponsor withdrew support. The preliminary results were promising (Table 4).

Four studies compared bivalirudin to heparin as adjunct to thrombolysis with strepto-kinase in patients with acute myocardial infarction. In an angiographic pilot study of 45 patients hirulog yielded a higher 90-minute patency rate of 77% vs. 47% of the patients treated with heparin (p<0.05). No reocclusions were seen at control angiography per-formed 4–7 days later [84]. Théroux et al. [85] randomized 68 patients treated with strepto-kinase and aspirin for acute myocardial infarction to hirulog 0.5 mg/kh/h over 12 hours followed by 0.1 mg/kg/h (low dose), hirulog 1.0 mg/kg/h followed by placebo (high dose), or standard heparin treatment. At 90 min angiogram TIMI-grade 3 flow of the infarct vessel was found in 85%, 61%, and 31% of the low-dose, high-dose, and heparin groups, respectively (p = 0.008). In the Hirulog Early Reperfusion Occlusion (HERO) trial of 412 patients treated with streptokinase for AMI, TIMI-grade 3 flow of the infarct artery was achieved in 46% and 48% of patients treated with low- or high-dose hirulog, vs. only 35% of patients treated with adjunctive heparin [86]. The combined incidence of death, shock, or reinfarction by day 35 was 12.5% and 14.0% in the hirulog groups vs. 18.0% in the heparin-treated patients (n.s.), major bleeding occurred in 14% and 19% with hirulog and in 28% with heparin. These promising angiographic and clinical results gave rise to the subsequent HERO-2 study with 30-day mortality as the primary endpoint [87]. 17,073 patients with ST-elevation myocardial infarction treated with streptokinase were random-ized to bivalirudin or heparin. The mortality by 30 days was 10.8% vs. 10.9%, and the mortality rates adjusted for baseline factors were 10.5% vs. 10.9% (n.s.). There were, however, fewer in-hospital reinfarctions in the bivalirudin group (2.8% vs. 3.6%, p = 0.005). Severe bleeding occurred in 0.7% of the bivalirudin-treated patients vs. 0.5% with heparin (p = 0.07), and intracranial bleeding in 0.6% vs. 0.4% (p = 0.09). Taking these results together, hirulog yields better early patency rates of the infarct vessels than heparin when given as adjunct to streptokinase without an increased bleeding risk. The mortality was not reduced despite some reduction of early reinfarctions.

Bivalirudin during coronary angioplasty was investigated in a study of 4,098 patients with interventions for unstable or postinfarction angina [88]. Bivalirudin did not reduce the incidence of ischemic complications, but the bleeding risk was significantly lower on bivalirudin with 3.8% as compared to 9.8% with heparin. In the prospectively stratified subgroup of 704 patients with postinfarction angina, hirulog reduced the incidence of death, myocardial infarction, or abrupt vessel closure to 9.1% vs. 14.2% in the heparin control group. After six months of follow-up, however, the rate of death, myocardial infarction, or repeat revascularization was similar in both groups. This study was performed before the widespread use of coronary stents and of glycoprotein (GP) IIb/IIIa inhibitors, which might attenuate the advantages of bivalirudin. After a promising pilot study of 268 patients [89], the REPLACE-2 trial compared bivalirudin and provisional GP IIb/IIIa inhibitors with heparin and planned GP IIb/IIIa blockade during elective or urgent percuta-neous coronary interventions in 6,010 patients from October 2001 to August 2002 [90]. Patients were randomly assigned to intravenous bivalirudin (0.75 mg/kg bolus plus 1.75

**Table 4** Heparin-Controlled Trials of Bivalirudin

| Study | Indication | No.pts. | Bivalirudin mg/kg | Heparin IU | Ischemic events |
|---|---|---|---|---|---|
| TIMI-8 (83) | UAP / Non-Q-MI | 133 | 0.1 bolus + 0.25 / h | 70/kg Bolus + 15 / kg / h | Death/MI 14 day 2.9% vs. 9.2% |
| Bittl et al. (88) | Angioplasty for UAP | 4098 | 1,0 bolus + 2.5/h × 4h, then 0.2/h | 175/kg Bolus + 15 / kg / h | In-hosp.death 0.4% vs. 0.2%, MI 3.2% vs. 3.9% |
| Théroux et al. (85) | Acute MI, SK-lysis | 116 | No bolus, 0.5/kg | 5000 Bolus + 1000/h | In-hosp. death/MI 8.1% vs. 10.3% |
| HERO-1 (86) | Acute MI, SK lysis | 412 | 0.125 or 0.25 bolus + 0.25/h × 12h, then 0.125 or 0.25/h | 5000 Bolus + 1000–1200 / h | 35 day death/shock/re-MI 12.5%/14% vs. 18% |
| HERO-2 (87) | Acute MI, SK-lysis | 17,073 | 0.25 bolus + 0.5/h × 12h, then 0.25/h | 5000 Bolus + 800–1000 / h | 30-day death 10.5% vs. 10.9%, death or Re-MI 12.6% vs. 13.6% |
| REPLACE-2 (91) | Angioplasty | 6010 | 0.75 bolus + 1.75/h during interv. | 65 / kg Bolus + GP-IIb/IIIa-blocker | 30-day death/MI/revasc 7.1% vs. 7.6% |

mg/kg/h during the procedure) or a bolus of 65 U/kg unfractionated heparin together with abciximab or eptifibatide. Provisional GP IIb/IIIa blockade was given to 7.2% of the patients on bivalirudin. The primary composite endpoint of 30-day mortality, myocardial infarction, urgent repeat revascularization, or in-hospital major bleeding occurred in 9.2% of the bivalirudin group vs. 10.0% in the heparin group (n.s.). Thus, the study satisfied prespecified statistical criteria for noninferiority of bivalirudin as compared to heparin plus planned GP IIb/IIIa-blockade. The bleeding risk was lower in the bivalirudin group. As compared to patients of two earlier studies treated with heparin only during coronary stenting [91,92], bivalirudin was significantly superior to prevent ischemic events and reduce the bleeding risk.

Taken together, the reported trials on bivalirudin demonstrate at least equal efficacy as compared to heparin in the conservative and interventional treatment of acute coronary syndromes with an improved safety reflected by lower bleeding risk.

## Argatroban, Efegatran, and Inogatran

Argatroban is a synthetic arginin derivative binding to a hydrophobic pocket near the active catalytic site of thrombin [93]. Like other direct thrombin inhibitors, argatroban inhibits also clot-bound thrombin since it does not bind to the fibrin binding site [94,95]. In contrast to hirudin and bivalirudin, thrombin inhibition by argatroban is reversible [96]. Thrombolysis by alteplase was enhanced by argatroban, and reocclusion after t-PA lysis was prevented in various experimental models of arterial thrombosis [97–100]. The Myocardial Infarction Novastan and TPA (MINT) study compared two doses of argatroban with unfractionated heparin in 125 patients treated with alteplase for acute myocardial infarction [101]. TIMI grade 3 flow of the infarct related artery was achieved after 90 minutes in 42.1% by heparin, and in 56.5% and 58.7% by low- and high-dose argatroban (n.s.). In patients presenting after more than 3 hours, TIMI-grade 3 flow was significantly more often seen in the argatroban group than in the control patients on heparin (57.1% vs. 20.0%, p = 0.03). Major bleeding was observed in 10.0% of heparin, and in 2.6% and 4.3% of low-dose and high-dose argatroban patients, respectively.

In unstable angina, argatroban caused a dose-dependent increase of aPTT and a decrease of fibrinopeptide A, reflecting potent thrombin inhibition. However, 5.8 hours (± 2.6 hours) after cessation of the infusion, 9 of 43 patients experienced an episode of unstable angina [102]. This rebound phenomenon was significantly correlated to higher argatroban doses.

Another novel synthetic direct thrombin inhibitor, inogatran, was tested in 1,209 patients with unstable angina in comparison to IV heparin [103]. Inogatran was given in three dose groups increasing the aPTT values by 1.3- to 1.8-fold control. The rate of death or myocardial infarction was 7.6% to 9.0% in the inogatran-treated patients without evidence of a dose dependency vs. 5.9% in the heparin-treated control group. Interestingly, a later analysis of this study demonstrated ischemic events to be associated with higher aPTT values in the inogatran-treated patients, while no such association was observed with heparin [104]. This emphasizes the poorly defined optimal aPTT time range during treatment with direct thrombin inhibitors in acute coronary syndromes. Inogatran, like argatroban, seems to give rise to a rebound after cessation of therapy [105].

Efegatran is a tripeptide direct thrombin inhibitor inhibiting fibrin formation as well as thrombin-induced platelet aggregation. Efegatran markedly prolongs the thrombin time with only modest effects on the aPTT [106]. In patients with unstable angina, efegatran elicited more stable prolongation of the aPTT than heparin, but the incidence of ischemic events was similar in patients treated with three different doses of efegatran and the control group on heparin [107]. Efegatran was also tested adjunct to streptokinase in patients with acute myocardial infarction. The dose of 0.5 mg/kg/h achieved no better coronary patency at 90-minutes angiogram than heparin and alteplase in the control group [108]. Moreover, major bleeding occurred in 23% of the efegatran-treated patients vs. 11% of those treated with heparin and t-PA. The authors concluded that there is no indication that this experimental treatment can achieve better clinical outcome.

## SUMMARY

Antithrombin therapy is of utmost importance in all types of acute coronary syndromes. In unstable angina pectoris the standard treatment consists of intravenous heparin given as a bolus of 5000 IU followed by an infusion of 1000 IU/h adjusted to an aPTT of 50 to 70 seconds. An alternative and at least equally effective treatment is subcutaneous application of LMW heparin, the best data exists for enoxaparin given BID in a dose of 1 mg/kg. The direct thrombin inhibitors are only marginally more effective than heparin, but bivalirudin has a better safety profile and therefore provides a net clinical benefit over heparin. This is especially true for patients with acute coronary syndromes treated interventionally, where bivalirudin with provisional GP IIb/IIIa inhibitors was equally effective as heparin with planned GP IIb/IIIa-blockade.

In acute myocardial infarction treated with alteplase, full-dose heparin should be given as adjunct to enhance thrombolysis and prevent reocclusion. With tenecteplase given as thrombolytic, enoxaparin is more effective than unfractionated heparin. The combination of enoxaparin with tenecteplase was equally effective as half-dose tenecteplase with abciximab. Though not explicitly tested, the combination with low-molecular weight heparin might also be the strategy of choice when alteplase is used. With streptokinase or other nonfibrin-specific plasminogen activators, there is no proven benefit of adjunctive heparin therapy or other thrombin inhibitors. Bivalirudin as adjunct to streptokinase does improve the early infarct vessel patency, but there is no reduction in mortality or bleeding risk. Hirudin enhances thrombolysis by alteplase as measured by angiography, but the clinical outcome was not improved.

## REFERENCES

1. Wallentin L. Low molecular weight heparins: a valuable tool in the treatment of acute coronary syndromes. Eur Heart J 1996;17:1470–1476.
2. Wilson JM, Dougherty KG, Ellis KO, Ferguson JJ, Blumenthal RS, Brinker JA. Activated clotting times in acute coronary syndromes and percutaneous transluminal coronary angioplasty. Catheter Cardiovasc Diagn 1995;34:1–7.
3. Fuchs J, Pinhas A, Davidson E, Rotenberg Z, Agmon J, Weinberger I. Plasma viscosity, fibrinogen and haematocrit in the course of unstable angina. Eur Heart J 1990;11:1029–1032.
4. Ardissino D, Merlini PA, Gamba G, Barberis P, Demicheli G, Testa S, Colombi E, Poli A, Fetiveau R, Montemartini C. Thrombin activity and early outcome in unstable angina pectoris. Circulation 1996;93:1634–1639.
5. Merlini PA, Ardissino D, Oltrona L, Broccolino M, Coppola R, Mannucci PM. Heightened thrombin formation but normal plasma levels of activated factor VII in patients with acute coronary syndromes. Arterioscler Thromb Vasc Biol 1995;15:1675–1679.
6. Cohen M, Adams PC, Parry G, Xiong J, Chamberlain D, Wieczorek I, Fox KAA, Chesebro JH, Strain J, Keller C, Kelly A, Lancaster G, Ali J, Kronmal R, Fuster V. Combination antithrombotic therapy in unstable rest angina and non-Q-wave infarction in nonprior aspirin users: Primary end points analysis from the ATACS trial. Circulation 1994;89:81–88.

7.  Holdright D, Patel D, Cunningham D, Thomas R, Hubbard W, Hendry G, Sutton G, Fox K. Comparison of the effect of heparin and aspirin vs. aspirin alone on transient myocardial ischemia and in-hospital prognosis in patients with unstable angina. J Am Coll Cardiol 1994; 24:39–45.

8.  Serneri GGN, Modesti PA, Gensini GF, Branzi A, Melanari G, Poggesi L, Rostagno C, Tamburini C, Carnovali M, Magnani B. Randomised comparison of subcutaneous heparin, intravenous heparin, and aspirin in unstable angina. Lancet 1995;345:1201–1204.

9.  Telford AM, Wilson C. Trial of heparin vs. atenolol in prevention of myocardial infarction in intermediate coronary syndrome. Lancet 1981;I:1225–1228.

10. Theroux P, Ouimet H, McCans J, Latour JG, Joly P, Levy G, Pelletier E, Juneau M, Stasiak J, DeGuise P, Pelletier GB, Rinzler D, Waters DD. Aspirin, heparin, or both to treat acute unstable angina. New Engl J Med 1988;319:1105–1111.

11. Theroux P, Waters D, Qiu S, McCans J, de Guise P, Juneau M. Aspirin vs. heparin to prevent myocardial infarction during the acute phase of unstable angina. Circulation 1993; 88:2045–2048.

12. Wallentin L. Risk of myocardial infarction and death during treatment with low dose aspirin and intravenous heparin in men with unstable coronary artery disease. Lancet 1990;336: 827–830.

13. Raschke RA, Reilly BM, Guidry JR, Fontana JR, Srinivas S. The weight-based heparin dosing nomogram compared with a 'standard care' nomogram: A randomized controlled trial. Ann Intern Med 1993;119:874–881.

14. Neri Serneri GG, Gensini GF, Poggesi L, Trotta F, Modesti PA, Boddi M, Ieri A, Margheri M, Casolo GC, Bini M, Rostagno C, Cranovali M, Abbate R. Effect of heparin, aspirin, or alteplase in reduction of myocardial ischaemia in refractory unstable angina. Lancet 1990; 335:615–618.

15. Becker RC, Cannon CP, Tracy RP, Thompson B, Bovill EG, Desvigne NP, Randall AMY, Knatterud G, Braunwald E. Relation between systemic anticoagulation as determined by activated partial thromboplastin time and heparin measurements and in-hospital clinical events in unstable angina and non-Q wave myocardial infarction. Am Heart J 1996;131:421–433.

16. Berglund U, Wallentin L. Influence on platelet function by heparin in men with unstable coronary artery disease. Thromb Haemostasis 1991;66:648–651.

17. Théroux P, Quimet H, McCans J, Latour JG, Joly P, Lévy G, Pelletier E, Juneau M, Stasiak J, DeGuise P, Pelletier GB, Rinzler D, Waters DD. Aspirin, heparin, or both to treat acute unstable angina. N Engl J Med 1988;17:1105–1111.

18. Grambow DW, Topol EJ. Effect of maximal medical therapy on refractoriness of unstable angina pectoris. Am J Cardiol 1992;70:577–581.

19. Arai H, Saito S, Kim K, Aoki N, Hatano K, Hirashima O. Delayed catheter intervention for unstable angina pectoris. Jpn J Intervent Cardiol 1995;10:157–162.

20. Cannon CP, Weintraub WS, Demopoulos LA, Vicari R, Frey MJ, Lakkis N, Neumann FJ, Robertson DH, DeLucca PT, DiBattiste PM, Gibson CM, Braunwald E. TACTICS-TIMI 18 investigators. Comparison of early invasive and conservative strategies in patients with unstable coronary syndromes treated with the glycoprotein IIb/IIIa inhibitor tirofiban. N Engl J Med 2001;344:1879–1887.

21. Wallentin L. FRISC study group. Low-molecular-weight heparin during instability in coronary artery disease. Lancet 1996;347:561–568.

22. Antman EM, McCabe CH, Gurfinkel EP, Turpie AGG, Bernink PJLM, Salein D, Bayes de Luna A, Fox K, Lablanche J-M, Radley D, Premmereur J, Braunwald E. TIMI 11B investigators. Enoxaparin prevents death and cardiac ischemic events in unstable angina/non-Q-wave myocardial infarction. Results of the Thrombolysis In Myocardial Infarction (TIMI) 11B trial. Circulation 1999;100:1593–1601.

23. Cohen M, Demers C, Gurfinkel EP, Turpie AGG, Fromell G, Goodman S, Langer A, Califf RM, Fox KAA, Premmereur J, Bigonzi F. A comparison of low-molecular-weight heparin with unfractionated heparin for unstable coronary artery disease. N Engl J Med 1997;337: 447–452.

24. Antman EM, Cohen M, Radley D, McCabe C, Rush J, Premmereur J, Braunwald E. for the TIMI 11B and ESSENCE investigators. Assessment of the treatment effect of enoxaparin for unstable angina/non-Q-wave myocardial infarction. TIMI 11B - ESSENCE meta-analysis. Circulation 1999;100:1602–1608.

25. Antman EM, Cohen M, McCabe C, Goodman SG, Murphy SA, Braunwald E. TIMI 11B and ESSENCE investigators. Enoxaparin is superior to unfractionated heparin for preventing clinical events at 1-year follow-up of TIMI 11B and ESSENCE. Eur Heart J 2002;23:264–268.

26. Collignon F, Frydman A, Caplain H, Ozoux ML, Le Roux Y, Bouthier J, Thebault JJ. Comparison of the pharmacokinetic profiles of three low molecular mass heparins – dalteparin, enoxaparin and nadroparin – administered subcutaneously in healthy volunteers (doses for prevention of thromboembolism). Thromb Haemost 1995;73:630–640.

27. Theroux P, Waters D, Lam J, Juneau M, McCans J. Reactivation of unstable angina after the discontinuation of heparin. New Engl J Med 1992;327:141–145.

28. Lidon RM, Theroux P, Robitaille D. Antithrombin-III plasma activity during and after prolonged use of heparin in unstable angina. Thromb Res 1993;72:23–32.

29. Granger CB, Miller JM, Bovill EG, Gruber A, Tracy RP, Krucoff MW, Green C, Berrios E, Harrington RA, Ohman EM, Califf RM. Rebound increase in thrombin generation and activity after cessation of intravenous heparin in patients with acute coronary syndromes. Circulation 1995;91:1929–1935.

30. FRISC II Investigators. Long-term low-molecular mass heparin in unstable coronary-artery disease: FRISC II prospective randomised multicentre study. Lancet 1999;354:701–707.

31. Jang IK, Gold HK, Leinbach RC, Rivera AG, Fallon JT, Bunting S, Collen D. Persistent inhibition of arterial thrombosis by a 1-hour intravenous infusion of argatroban, a selective thrombin inhibitor. Coron Artery Dis 1992;3:407–414.

32. FRISC II Investigators. Invasive compared with non-invasive treatment in unstable coronary-artery disease: FRISC II prospective randomised multicentre study. Lancet 1999;354: 708–715.

33. Aronson DL, Chang P, Kessler CM. Platelet-dependent thrombin generation after in vitro fibrinolytic treatment. Circulation 1992;85:1706–1712.

34. Vila V, Reganon E, Aznar J, Lacueva V, Ruano M, Laiz B. Hypercoagulable state after thrombolytic therapy in patients with acute myocardial infarction (AMI) treated with streptokinase. Thromb Res 1990;57:783–794.

35. Hoffmann JJML, Michels HR, Windeler J, Gunzler WA. Plasma markers of thrombin activity during coronary thrombolytic therapy with saruplase or urokinase: No prediction of reinfarction. Fibrinolysis 1993;7:330–334.

36. Zahger D, Maaravi Y, Matzner Y, Gilon D, Gotsman MS, Weiss AT. Partial resistance to anticoagulation after streptokinase treatment for acute myocardial infarction. Am J Cardiol 1990;66:28–30.

37. Mahaffey KW, Granger CB, Collins R, O'Connor CM. Overview of randomized trials of intravenous heparin in patients with acute myocardial infarction treated with thrombolytic therapy. Am J Cardiol 1996;77:551–556.

38. Bleich SD, Nichols TC, Schumacher RR, Cooke DH, Tate DA, Teichman SL. Effect of heparin on coronary arterial patency after thrombolysis with tissue plasminogen activator in acute myocardial infarction. Am J Cardiol 1990;66:1412–1417.

39. De Bono DP, Simoons ML, Tijssen J, Arnold AER, Betriu A, Burgersdijk C, Lopez Bescos L, Mueller E, Pfisterer M, Van de Werf F, Zijlstra F, Verstraete M. Effect of early intravenous heparin on coronary patency, infarct size, and bleeding complications after alteplase thrombolysis: Results of a randomised double blind European Cooperative Study Group trial. Br Heart J 1992;67:122–128.

40. Hsia J, Hamilton WP, Kleiman N, Roberts R, Chaitman BR, Ross AM. A comparison between heparin and low-dose aspirin as adjunctive therapy with tissue plasminogen activator for acute myocardial infarction. New Engl J Med 1990;323:1433–1437.

41. Arnout J, Simoons M, De Bono D, Rapold HJ, Collen D, Verstraete M. Correlation between level of heparinization and patency of the infarct-related coronary artery after treatment of acute myocardial infarction with alteplase (rt-PA). J Am Coll Cardiol 1992;20:513–519.

42. Hsia J, Kleiman N, Aguirre F, Chaitman BR, Roberts R, Ross AM. Heparin-induced prolonga-
    tion of partial thromboplastin time after thrombolysis: Relation to coronary artery patency.
    J Am Coll Cardiol 1992;20:31–35.
43. Tebbe U, Windeler J, Boesl I, Hoffmann H, Wojcik J, Ashmawy M, Schwarz ER, Von
    Loewis Of Menar P, Rosemeyer P, Hopkins G, Barth H. Thrombolysis with recombinant
    unglycosylated single-chain urokinase-type plasminogen activator (Saruplase) in acute myo-
    cardial infarction: Influence of heparin on early patency rate (LIMITS study). J Am Coll
    Cardiol 1995;26:365–373.
44. Gruppo Italiano per lo Studio della Sopravvivenza nell'Infarto Miocardico. GISSI-2: A facto-
    rial randomised trial of alteplase vs. streptokinase and heparin vs. no heparin among 12,490
    patients with acute myocardial infarction. Lancet 1990;336:65–71.
45. ISIS-3 (Third international study of infarct survival) collaborative group. ISIS-3: A randomi-
    sed comparison of streptokinase vs tissue plasminogen activator vs anistreplase and of aspirin
    plus heparin vs aspirin alone among 41,299 cases of suspected acute myocardial infarction.
    Lancet 1992;339:753–770.
46. Gruppo Italiano per lo Studiodella Sopravvivenza nell'Infarto Miocardico (GISSI-2). Six-
    month survival in 20 891 patients with acute myocardial infarction randomized between
    alteplase and streptokinase with or without heparin. Eur Heart J 1992;13:1692–1697.
47. GUSTO-I investigators. An international randomized trial comparing four thrombolytic strate-
    gies for acute myocardial infarction. New Engl J Med 1993;329:673–682.
48. Granger CB, Hirsh J, Califf RM, Col J, White HD, Betriu A, Woodlief LH, Lee KL, Bovill
    EG, Simes RJ, Topol EJ. Activated partial thromboplastin time and outcome after thrombo-
    lytic therapy for acute myocardial infarction: Results from the GUSTO-I trial. Circulation
    1996;93:870–878.
49. Funke Kupper AJ, Verheugt FWA, Peels CH, Galema TW, Den Hollander W, Roos JP.
    Effect of low dose acetylsalicylic acid on the frequency and hematologic activity of left
    ventricular thrombus in anterior wall acute myocardial infarction. Am J Cardiol 1989;63:
    917–920.
50. Jugdutt BI, Sivaram CA, Wortman C, Trudell C, Penner P. Prospective two-dimensional
    echocardiographic evaluation of left ventricular thrombus and embolism after acute myocar-
    dial infarction. J Am Coll Cardiol 1989;13:554–564.
51. Keren A, Goldberg S, Gottlieb S, Klein J, Schuger C, Medina A, Tzivoni D, Stern S. Natural
    history of left ventricular thrombi: Their appearance and resolution in the posthospitalization
    period of acute myocardial infarction. J Am Coll Cardiol 1990;15:790–800.
52. Nihoyannopoulos P, Smith GC, Maseri A, Foale RA. The natural history of left ventricular
    thrombus in myocardial infarction: A rationale in support of masterly inactivity. J Am Coll
    Cardiol 1989;14:903–911.
53. Turpie AGG, Robinson JG, Doyle DJ, Mulji AS, Mishkel GJ, Sealey BJ, Cairns JA, Skingley
    L, Hirsh J, Gent M. Comparison of high-dose with low-dose subcutaneous heparin to prevent
    left ventricular mural thrombosis in patients with acute transmural anterior myocardial infarc-
    tion. New Engl J Med 1989;320:352–357.
54. Vecchio C, Chiarella F, Lupi G, Bellotti P, Domenicucci S. Left ventricular thrombus in
    anterior acute myocardial infarction after thrombolysis: A GISSI-2 connected study. Circula-
    tion 1991;84:512–519.
55. Johannessen KA, Nordrehaug JE, Von der Lippe G. Left ventricular thrombi after short-term
    high-dose anticoagulants in acute myocardial infarction. Eur Heart J 1987;8:975–980.
56. Nordrehaug JE, Johannessen KA, Von der Lippe G. Usefulness of high dose anticoagulants
    in preventing left ventricular thrombus in acute myocardial infarction. Am J Cardiol 1985;
    55:1491–1493.
57. Arvan S, Boscha K. Prophylactic anticoagulation for left ventricular thrombi after acute
    myocardial infarction: A prospective randomized trial. Am Heart J 1987;113:688–693.
58. Kontny F, Dale J, Abildgaard U, Pedersen TR. FRAMI study group. Randomized trial of
    low molecular weight heparin (dalteparin) in prevention of left ventricular thrombus formation
    and arterial embolism after acute myocardial infarction: the Fragmin in Acute Myocardial
    Infarction (FRAMI) study. J Am Coll Cardiol 1997;30:962–969.

59. Ross AM, Molhock GP, Lundergan C, Knudtson ML, Draoui Y, Regalado L, Le Louer V, Bigonzi F, Schwartz W, De Jong E, Coyne K. Randomized comparison of enoxaparin, a low-molecular-weight heparin, with unfractionated heparin adjunctive to recombinant tissue plasminogen activator thrombolysis and aspirin (HART II). Circulation 2001;104:648–652.

60. Antman EM, Louwerenburg HW, Baars HF, Wesdorp JCL, Hamer B, Bassand JP, Bigonzi F, Pisapia G, Gibson CM, Heidbuchel H, Braunwald E, Van de Werf F. for the ENTIRE-TIMI. Enoxaparin as Adjunctive Antithrombin Therapy for ST-Elevation Myocardial Infarction: Results of the ENTIRE-Thrombolysis in Myocardial Infarction (TIMI) 23 Trial. Circulation 2002;105:1642–1649.

61. ASSENT-3 investigators. Efficacy and safety of tenecteplase in combination with enoxaparin, abciximab, or unfractionated heparin: the ASSENT-3 randomised trial in acute myocardial infarction. Lancet 2001;358:605–613.

62. Armstrong PW, Wagner G, Goodman SG, Van de Werf F, Granger CB, Wallentin L, Fu Y. ST segment resolution in ASSENT 3: insights into the role of three different treatment strategies for acute myocardial infarction. Eur Heart J 2003;24:1515–1522.

63. Wallentin L, Goldstein P, Armstrong PW, Granger CB, Adgey AA, Arntz HR, Bogaerts K, Lindahl B, Makijarvi M, Verheugt FW, Van de Werf F. Efficacy and safety of tenecteplase in combination with the low-molecular weight enoxaparin or unfractionated heparin in the prehospital setting: the Assessment of Safety and Efficacy of a New Thrombolytic Regimen (ASSENT)-3 Plus randomized trial in acute myocardial infarction. Circulation 2003;108: 135–142.

64. Wallentin L, Bergstrand L, Dellborg M, Fellenius C, Granger CB, Lindahl B, Lins LE, Nilsson G, Pehrsson K, Siegbahn A, Swahn E. Low molecular weight heparin (dalteparin) compared to unfractionated heparin as adjunct to rt-PA (alteplase) for improvement of coronary artery patency in acute myocardial infarction - the ASSENT Plus study. Eur Heart J 2003;24: 897–908.

65. Bauer KA. Fondaparinux sodium : a selective inhibitor of factor Xa. Am J Health Syst Pharm 2001;58(Suppl.2):S14–S17.

66. Bauer KA, Eriksson BI, Lassen MR, Turpie AGG. steering committee of the Pentasaccharide in Major Knee Surgery study. Fondaparinux compared with enoxaparin for the prevention of venous thromboembolism after elective major knee surgery. N Engl J Med 2001;345: 1305–1310.

67. Eriksson BI, Bauer KA, Lassen MR, Turpie AGG. steering committee of the Pentasaccharide in Hip-Fracture Surgery study. Fondaparinux compared with enoxaparin for the prevention of venous thromboembolism after hip-fracture surgery. N Engl J Med 2001;345:1298–1304.

68. Turpie AGG, Gallus AS, Hoek JA. Pentasaccharide Investigators. A synthetic pentasaccharide for the prevention of deep vein thrombosis after total hip replacement. N Engl J Med 2001; 344:619–625.

69. Coussement PK, Bassand JP, Convens C, Vrolix M, Boland J, Grollier G, Michels R, Vahanian A, Vanderheyden M, Rupprecht H-J, Van de Werf F. A synthetic factor-Xa inhibitor (ORG31540/SR9017A) as an adjunct to fibrinolysis in acute myocardial infarction. The PENTALYSE study. Eur Heart J 2001;22:1716–1724.

70. Gardien M, Boland J, Lensing AWA, Bobbink IWG, Ruzyllo W, Klootwijk P, Umans VAWM, Vahanian A, Van de Werf F, Zeymer U, Simoons ML. PENTUA-investigators. A dose finding study of fondaparinux in patients with non ST-segment elevation acute coronary syndromes: the PENTUA study. J Am Coll Cardiol 2004;43:2183–2190.

71. Topol EJ, Fuster V, Harrington RA, Califf RM, Kleiman NS, Kereiakes DJ, Cohen M, Chapekis A, Gold HK, Tannenbaum MA, Rao AK, Debowey D, Schwartz D, Henis M, Chesebro J. Recombinant hirudin for unstable angina pectoris: A multicenter, randomized angiographic trial. Circulation 1994;89:1557 1566.

72. The Direct Thrombin Inhibitor Trialists' Collaborative GroupYusuf SDirect thrombin inhibitors in acute coronary syndromes: principal results of a meta-analysis based on individual patients' data. Lancet 2002;359:294–302.

73. GUSTO IIa Investigators. Randomized trial of intravenous heparin vs. recombinant hirudin for acute coronary syndromes. Circulation 1994;90:1631–1637.

74. GUSTO IIb investigators. A comparison of recombinant hirudin with heparin for the treatment of acute coronary syndromes. N Engl J Med 1996;335:775–782.

75. Zeymer U, von Essen R, Tebbe U, Niederer W, Mäurer W, Vogt A, Neuhaus KL. Frequency of ''optimal anticoagulation'' for acute myocardial infarction after thrombolysis with front-loaded recombinant tissue-type plasminogen activator and conjunctive therapy with recombinant hirudin (HBW 023). Am J Cardiol 1995;76:997–1001.

76. Organisation to Assess Strategies for Ischemic Syndromes (OASIS-2) Investigators. Effects of recombinant hirudin (lepirudin) compared with heparin on death, myocardial infarction, refractory angina, and revascularisation procedures in patients with acute myocardial ischaemia without ST elevation: a randomised trial. Lancet 1999;353:429–438.

77. Antman EM. TIMI 9A Investigators. Hirudin in acute myocardial infarction. Safety report from the thrombolysis and thrombin inhibition in myocardial infarction (TIMI) 9A trial. Circulation 1994;90:1624–1630.

78. Neuhaus KL, V Essen R, Tebbe U, Jessel A, Heinrichs H, Mäurer W, Döring W, Harmjanz D, Kötter V, Kalhammer E, Simon H, Horacek T. Safety observations from the pilot phase of the randomized r- hirudin for improvement of thrombolysis (HIT-III) study: A study of the Arbeitsgemeinschaft Leitender Kardiologischer Krankenhausarzte (ALKK). Circulation 1994;90:1638–1642.

79. Antman EM. TIMI 9B investigators. Hirudin in acute myocardial infarction. Thrombolysis and thrombin inhibition in myocardial infarction (TIMI) 9B trial. Circulation 1996;94:911–921.

80. Topol EJ. Novel antithrombotic approaches to coronary artery disease. Am J Cardiol 1995;75:27B–33B.

81. Kong DF, Topol EJ, Bittl JA, White HD, Théroux P, Hasselblad V, Califf RM. Clinical outcomes of bivalirudin for ischemic heart disease. Circulation 1999;100:2049–2053.

82. Braunwald E, Fuchs J, Cannon CP, Antman EM, McCabe CH, DeFeo Fraulini T, Sollecito B, Wallman L, Tudor G, Williams DO, Sharaf B, Ferreira P, Miele N, Chaitman B, Stocke K, Hennekens C, Kelton J, Friesinger GC, Gersh B. Hirulog in the treatment of unstable angina: Results of the thrombin inhibition in myocardial ischemia (TIMI) 7 trial. Circulation 1995;92:727–733.

83. Antman EM, McCabe CH, Braunwald E. Bivalirudin as a replacement for unfractionated heparin in unstable angina / non-ST elevation myocardial infarction: observations from the TIMI 8 trial. Am Heart J 2002;143:189–192.

84. Lidón RM, Théroux P, Lespérance J, Adelman B, Bonan R, Duval D, Lévesque J. A pilot, early angiographic patency study using a direct thrombin inhibitor as adjunctive therapy to streptokinase in acute myocardial infarction. Circulation 1994;89:1567–1572.

85. Theroux P, Perez Villa F, Waters D, Lesperance J, Shabani F, Bonan R. Randomized double-blind comparison of two doses of Hirulog with heparin as adjunctive therapy to streptokinase to promote early patency of the infarct- related artery in acute myocardial infarction. Circulation 1995;91:2132–2139.

86. White HD, Aylward PE, Frey MJ, Adgey AAJ, Nair R, Hillis WS, Shalev Y, Brown MA, French JK, Collins R, Maraganore J, Adelman B. HERO trial investigators. Randomized, double-blind comparison of hirulog vs. heparin in patients receiving streptokinase and aspirin for acute myocardial infarction (HERO). Circulation 1997;96:2155–2161.

87. HERO-2 Trial Investigators. Thrombin-specific anticoagulation with bivalirudin vs. heparin in patients receiving fibrinolytic therapy for acute myocardial infarction: the HERO-2 randomised trial. Lancet 2001;358:1855–1863.

88. Bittl JA, Strony J, Brinker JA, Ahmed WH, Meckel CR, Chaitman BR, Maraganore J, Deutsch E, Adelman B. Treatment with bivalirudin (hirulog) as compared with heparin during coronary angioplasty for unstable or postinfarction angina. New Engl J Med 1995;333:764–769.

89. Lincoff AM, Kleiman NS, Kottke Marchant K, Maierson ES, Maresh K, Wolski KE, Topol EJ. Bivalirudin with planned or provisional abciximab vs. low-dose heparin and abciximab during percutaneous coronary revascularization: results of the Comparison of Abciximab Complications with Hirulog for Ischemic Events Trial (CACHET). Am Heart J 2002;143:847–853.

90. Lincoff AM, Bittl JA, Harrington RA, Feit F, Kleiman NS, Jackman JD, Sarembock IJ, Cohen DJ, Spriggs D, Ebrahimi R, Keren G, Carr J, Cohen EA, Betriu A, Desmet W, Kereiakes D, Rutsch W, Wilcox R, De Feyter P, Vahanian A, Topol EJ. REPLACE-2 investigators. Bivalirudin and provisional glycoprotein IIb/IIIa blockade compared with heparin and planned gycoprotein IIb/IIIa blockade during percutaneous coronary intervention. REPLACE-2 randomized trial. JAMA 2003;289:853–863.

91. ESPRIT investigators. Novel dosing regimen of eptifibatide in planned coronary stent implantation (ESPRIT): a randomised, placebo-controlled trial. Lancet 2000;356:2037–2044.

92. EPISTENT investigators. Randomised placebo-controlled and balloon-angioplasty-controlled trial to assess safety of coronary stenting with use of platelet glycoprotein-IIb/IIIa blockade. Lancet 1998;352:87–92.

93. Okamoto S, Hijikata A. Potent inhibition of thrombin by the newly synthesized arginine derivative no. 805. The importance of stereostructure of its hydrophobic carboxamide portion. Biochem Biophys Res Commun 1981;101:440–445.

94. Hogg PJ, Jackson CM. Fibrin monomer protects thrombin from inactivation by heparin-antithrombin III: implications for heparin efficacy. Proc Natl Acad Sci USA 1989;86:3619–3623.

95. Lunven C, Gauffeny C, Lecoffre C, O'Brien DP, Roome NO, Berry CN. Inhibition by argatroban, a specific thrombin inhibitor, of platelet activation by fibrin clot-associated thrombin. Thromb Haemost 1996;75:154–160.

96. Callas DD, Hoppensteadt D, Fareed J. Comparative studies on the anticoagulant and protease generation inhibitory actions of newly developed site-directed thrombin inhibitor drugs. Efegatran registered , argatroban, hirulog, and hirudin. Semin Thromb Hemost 1995;21:177–183.

97. Fitzgerald DJ, Fitzgerald GA. Role of thrombin and thromboxane A-2 in reocclusion following coronary thrombolysis with tissue-type plasminogen activator. Proc Natl Acad Sci USA 1989;86:7585–7589.

98. Jang IK, Gold HK, Leinbach RC, Fallon JT, Collen D. In vivo thrombin inhibition enhances and sustains arterial recanalization with recombinant tissue-type plasminogen activator. Circ Res 1990;67:1552–1561.

99. Mellott MJ, Connolly TM, York SJ, Bush LR. Prevention of reocclusion by MCI-9038, a thrombin inhibitor, following t-PA-induced thrombolysis in a canine model of femoral arterial thrombosis. Thromb Haemostasis 1990;64:526–534.

100. Yasuda T, Gold HK, Yaoita H, Leinbach RC, Guerrero JL, Jang IK, Holt R, Fallon JT, Collen D. Comparative effects of aspirin, a synthetic thrombin inhibitor and a monoclonal antiplatelet glycoprotein IIb/IIIa antibody on coronary artery reperfusion, reocclusion and bleeding with recombinant tissue-type plasminogen activator in a canine preparation. J Am Coll Cardiol 1990;16:714–722.

101. Jang IK, Brown DF, Giugliano RP, Anderson HV, Losordo D, Nicolau JC, Dutra OP, Bazzino O, Viamonte VM, Norbady R, Liprandi AS, Massey TJ, Dinsmore R, Schwarz RPJ. A multicenter, randomized study of argatroban vs. heparin as adjunct to tissue plasminogen activator (TPA) in acute myocardial infarction: myocardial infarction with novastan and TPA (MINT) study. J Am Coll Cardiol 1999;33:1879–1885.

102. Gold HK, Torres FW, Garabedian HD, Werner W, Jang IK, Khan A, Hagstrom JN, Yasuda T, Leinbach RC, Newell JB, Bovill EG, Stump DC, Collen D. Evidence for a rebound coagulation phenomenon after cessation of a 4-hour infusion of a specific thrombin inhibitor in patients with unstable angina pectoris. J Am Coll Cardiol 1993;21:1039–1047.

103. Thrombin inhibition in myocardial ischemia (TRIM) study group. A low molecular weight, selective thrombin inhibitor, inogatran, vs heparin, in unstable coronary artery disease in 1209 patients. Eur Heart J 1997;18:1416–1425.

104. Oldgren J, Linder R, Grip L, Siegbahn A, Wallentin L. Activated partial thromboplastin time and clinical outcome after thrombin inhibition in unstable coronary artery disease. Eur Heart J 1999;20:1657–1666.

105. Andersen K, Dellborg M, Emanuelsson H, Grip L, Swedberg K. Thrombin inhibition with inogatran for unstable angina pectoris: evidence for reactivated ischaemia after cessation of short-term treatment. Coron Artery Dis 1996;7:673–681.

106. Ohman EM, Slovak JP, Anderson RL, Grossman WJ, Barbeau GR, Butler JF, Frey MJ, Talley DJ, Leimberger JD, Scherer JC, Kleiman NS. PRIME group. Potent inhibition of thrombin with efegatran in combination with tPA in acute myocardial infarction: results of a multicenter randomized dose ranging trial. Circulation 1996;94(Suppl.I):I-430–I-430.

107. Klootwijk P, Lenderink T, Meij S, Boersma E, Melkert R, Umans VAWM, Stibbe J, Müller EJ, Poortermans KJ, Deckers JW, Simoons ML. Anticoagulant properties, clinical efficacy and safety of efegatran, a direct thrombin inhibitor, in patients with unstable angina. Eur Heart J 1999;20:1101–1111.

108. Fung AY, Lorch G, Cambier PA, Hansen D, Titus BG, Martin JS, Lee JJ, Every NR, Hallstein NN, Stock-Novack D, Scherer J, Weaver WD. Efegatran sulfate as an adjunct to streptokinase vs. heparin as an adjunct to tissue plasminogen activator in patients with acute myocardial infarction. ESCALAT study. Am Heart J 1999;138:696–704.

109. Correia LC, Neubauer C, Azevedo A, Ribeiro F, Braga J, Passos LC, Teixeira M, Matos M, Aires V, Souza V, Rocha M, Camara E, Pericles Esteves J. The role of low molecular weight heparin in unstable angina, acute myocardial infarction and post-elective percutaneous transluminal coronary angioplasty. Arq Bras Cardiol 1995;65:475–478.

110. Gurfinkel EP, Manos EJ, Mejail RI, Cerda MA, Duronto EA, Garcia CN, Daroca AM, Mautner B. Low molecular weight heparin vs. regular heparin or aspirin in the treatment of unstable angina and silent ischemia. J Am Coll Cardiol 1995;26:313–318.

111. Klein W, Buchwald A, Hillis SE, Monrad S, Sanz G, Turpie AGG, Van der Meer J, Olaisson E, Undeland S, Ludwig K. FRIC investigators. Comparison of low-molecular-weight heparin with unfractionated heparin acutely and with placebo for 6 weeks in the management of unstable coronary artery disease. Fragmin in Unstable Coronary Artery Disease Study (FRIC). Circulation 1997;96:61–68.

112. FRAX.I.S.study group. Comparison of two treatment durations (6 days and 14 days) of a low molecular weight heparin with a 6-day treatment of unfractionated heparin in the initial management of unstable angina or non-Q wave myocardial infarction: FRAX.I.S. (FRAXiparin in Ischaemic Syndrome). Eur Heart J 1999;20:1553–1562.

113. Goodman SG, Fitchett D, Armstrong PW, Tan M, Langer A. for the Integrilin and Enoxaparin Randomized Assessment of Acute Coronary Syndrome Treatment (INTERACT) Trial Investigators. Randomized evaluation of the safety and efficacy of enoxaparin vs. unfractionated heparin in high-risk patients with non-ST-segment elevation acute coronary syndromes receiving the glycoprotein IIb/IIIa inhibitor eptifibatide. Circulation 2003;107:238–244.

# 22
# Bedside Anticoagulant Testing

**Jacqueline Saw**
*The Cleveland Clinic Foundation*
*Cleveland, Ohio, U.S.A.*

**David J. Moliterno**
*University of Kentucky*
*Lexington, Kentucky, U.S.A.*

## INTRODUCTION

Anticoagulants are central in the management of both atherothrombotic arterial and venous disorders. Unfractionated heparin (UFH) is currently the most widely used intravenous anticoagulant, but its dominance is progressively being supplanted by low molecular-weight heparins (LMWH) and direct thrombin inhibitors. Nevertheless, at this juncture, the prevalence of UFH use necessitates knowledge of monitoring its anticoagulant effect, especially in the setting where high doses are required for therapeutic efficacy. Unfortunately, UFH has a relatively narrow therapeutic window, thus setting the premise for the monitoring of anticoagulant activity to optimize efficacy while maintaining safety. In this chapter, we will specifically review the role of bedside anticoagulant monitoring devices of antithrombin activity. There is considerably less need for routine anticoagulant monitoring of LMWH and direct thrombin inhibitors, given their more favorable pharmacokinetics; these will be briefly discussed as well.

## RATIONALE FOR ANTICOAGULANT MONITORING

Data from sentinel anticoagulant and thrombolytic trials have enhanced our understanding of the importance of achieving an optimal anticoagulant level with UFH during acute coronary syndromes (ACS). For example, the GUSTO-I (Global Utilization of Streptokinase and t-PA for Occluded Coronary Arteries) trial in the early 1990s showed a linear relationship between activated partial thromboplastin time (aPTT) and the risk of hemorrhage when aPTT was more than 70 seconds. Each 10-second increase in aPTT was associated with an approximate 1% absolute increase in moderate or severe hemorrhage, and a 0.07% increase in intracranial hemorrhage (Fig. 1a and 1b) [1]. There was also an association with higher mortality when aPTT was less than 50 seconds or greater than 75 seconds (Fig. 1c). Furthermore, in the GUSTO-IIa trial, the 20% higher dose of heparin used (resulting in a 5–10 second higher aPTT) compared with GUSTO-I was associated

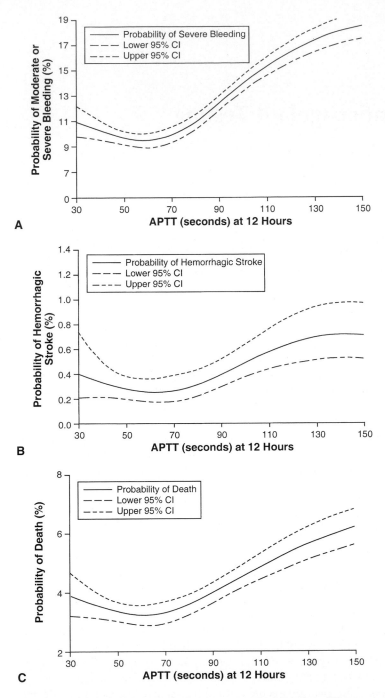

**Figure 1** Probability of (**A**) moderate or severe bleeding, (**B**) intracranial hemorrhage, and (**C**) 30-day mortality according to aPTT at 12 hours after enrollment among patients on IV heparin in the GUSTO I trial. Dotted lines represent 95% confidence intervals. (From Ref. 1)

**Table 1** Heparin Adjustment Nomogram for Standard Laboratory
Reagents With a Mean Control aPTT of 26–36 seconds

| aPTT (s) | Bolus dose (U) | Stop infusion (min) | Rate change (ml/h) | Repeat aPTT |
|---|---|---|---|---|
| <4 0 | 3000 | 0 | + 2 | 6h |
| 40–49 | 0 | 0 | + 1 | 6h |
| 50–75 | 0 | 0 | 0 (no change) | Next AM |
| 76–85 | 0 | 0 | − 1 | Next AM |
| 86–100 | 0 | 30 | − 2 | 6h |
| 101–150 | 0 | 60 | − 3 | 6h |
| >150 | 0 | 60 | − 6 | 6h |

Heparin infusion concentration = 50 U/mL. Target aPTT = 50–70s (for the CoaguChek
  Plus bedside monitor, target aPTT is 60–85 seconds, and the nomogram should be
  modified accordingly).(From Ref. 5)

with double the risk of intracranial hemorrhage among patients given thrombolytics [2].
This incidence was reduced with the subsequent lowering of heparin dose in the GUSTO-
IIb trial, whereby the aPTT at 12 hours was 65 seconds (compared with 85 seconds
in GUSTO-IIa) among thrombolytic-treated patients, and this decreased the intracranial
hemorrhage rate by half to 0.6% [3]. Likewise, in the TIMI-9B (Thrombolysis and Thrombin Inhibition in Myocardial Infarction) trial, a reduction of intracranial hemorrhage risk
was seen with reduction of anticoagulant doses [4]. Accordingly, the American College
of Cardiology/American Heart Association (ACC/AHA) altered the guidelines for the
management of acute myocardial infarction (AMI) in 1999 to lower UFH dose to 60 u/
kg bolus followed by 12 u/kg/hr to target an aPTT of 50–70 seconds, in the setting of
thrombolytic therapy [5]. This guideline also included a nomogram for titrating heparin
dose for management of AMI (Table 1).

In the setting of non–ST-segment elevation MI (NSTEMI) ACS, a lower range of
aPTT was also sufficient for optimal reduction of ischemic events. In an analysis of the
TIMI-3B study, aggressive anticoagulation with heparin to achieve aPTTs greater than
2.0 times control did not offer additional clinical benefit compared with lower aPTT levels
(1.5 to 2.0 times control) among patients with NSTEMI ACS receiving intravenous heparin
and oral aspirin. Thus, these data translate to an optimal standard aPTT range of approximately 50–70 seconds during management of patients with ACS. An even lower range
may be acceptable when antithrombins are used in combination with potent antiplatelet
therapies (e.g., platelet glycoprotein IIb/IIIa inhibitors) though this has not been well
characterized for medically-treated patients.

## PROBLEMS WITH TRADTIONAL CENTRAL LABORATORY METHODS

The standard method for monitoring heparin anticoagulation is the aPTT, a test that reflects
the inhibitory effect of heparin on the intrinsic coagulation pathway, thrombin, factor Xa,
and factor IXa. The therapeutic aPTT range was originally based on a rabbit jugular
venous thrombosis model [6], in which an aPTT greater than or equal to 1.5 times control
(corresponding to an anti-Xa level of 0.2 U/ml) prevented thrombus extension. APTT
determination is usually made in a central laboratory on citrated plasma, using one of

several commercially available instruments and one of many reagents, each with a different range of control values and a different aPTT-heparin level sensitivity relationship. Using a central laboratory involves multiple steps, including venipuncture, transport to the lab, centrifugation, batching, testing, and communication of results back to the care provider. Each of these steps can contribute to substantial delays in providing aPTT results to the care provider. In fact, this delay is typically about 2 hours. In 1992, data were collected on 60 aPTT samples ordered ''STAT'' and showed a 45 minute delay from the time of blood draw to receipt of the sample in the laboratory, and an additional 80 min until the results were available to the clinician (unpublished data) (Fig. 2). Data collected on 272 aPTT values in the cardiac care unit at the University of Massachusetts showed a mean time of 2 hours and 6 minutes [7], with 36 minutes from sample acquisition until arrival in the laboratory. A survey of 79 hospitals that participated in the GUSTO-I trial and collected data on 387 aPTTs showed the mean time from blood draw until aPTT availability at 1 hour and 46 minutes [8]. Because patients with ACS are at risk for acute life-threatening thrombosis and serious hemorrhage, any unnecessary delay in obtaining a standard central laboratory aPTT could compromise patient care.

In addition to the delay, aPTTs obtained from a central laboratory are subject to both artifact related to the sampling technique and handling, as well as considerable variability between different laboratory reagents and laboratories. Sources of sampling artifact include a difficult or poor venipuncture, collection of insufficient blood, delay between sampling and measurement of results, and incomplete centrifugation [9–11]. Therefore, even in a laboratory with controlled conditions in which the aPTT is precise, accurate and reproducible (low coefficient of variation), the aPTT may poorly reflect the level of anticoagulation in the patient due to variations related to events prior to the sample actually being tested

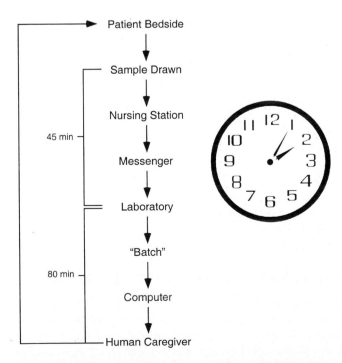

**Figure 2** Delays in obtaining the aPTT by standard laboratory methods. Data are derived from 60 "STAT" samples from the Duke Cardiac Care Unit in 1992.

[12]. Moreover, there is substantial variability among different laboratories, related to differences between reagent-instrument combinations [13], different reagents [14], and even among different batches of the same reagent [15]. In one study [14], seven commercially available reagents were tested; the average amount of heparin required to double the baseline aPTT varied by twofold. In spite of efforts to do so, the hematology and laboratory societies have been unable to institute a standard aPTT measure [16], analogous to the International Normalized Ratio for the prothrombin time. Brill-Edwards and colleagues studied five different reagents and found that the aPTT ratio corresponding to a heparin level of 0.2 U/ml by protamine titration varied from 1.8 to 4.2 [17]. Based on these results, many hospitals have established a target aPTT range based on a target heparin level of 0.2 to 0.4 U/ml by protamine titration or 0.3 to 0.7 U/ml by anti-Xa activity. Unfortunately, many hospitals have performed this range-finding by adding known amounts of heparin in vitro to a plasma pool, which can systematically underestimate the aPTT range needed in vivo [17].

Thus, while central laboratory aPTT remains the gold standard for measuring UFH's effects, the limitations to current methods are important. In addition to the typically long delay in obtaining the laboratory values, there is a substantial lack of consistency in the relationship of aPTT to heparin level between different laboratories and between different time periods in the same laboratory. Moreover, there is a lack of data to indicate whether aPTT, heparin level, or some other guide to adjusting dose is associated with the best patient outcomes. These issues are also present for assays of LMWH, which primarily assay the drug's anti-Xa effect.

## BEDSIDE "POINT-OF-CARE" TESTING

Technologies that enable rapid determination of laboratory values at the patient bedside—so called point-of-care (POC) testing—have required health care providers to decide when these methods provide an overall advantage in patient care and when they should therefore supplant traditional central laboratory testing. Typically, there is a trade-off when using POC testing of lower accuracy, less rigorous quality control, and higher cost per sample for more rapid and convenient determination of the result (Table 2). When time and convenience are more important than a particulary high degree of accuracy (for example with routine blood glucose monitoring in diabetics), POC testing has been widely adopted. There has been a general trend towards the use of more POC testing, although

**Table 2** Advantages and Disadvantages of Bedside "Point-of-Care" Testing

| Advantages | Disadvantages |
|---|---|
| Rapid determination of results | Generally less accurate and reproducible |
| More convenient | Generally more costly per sample |
| Less nursing time in awaiting and retrieving results | More difficult to implement quality control |
| | More difficult to bill for |
| | Requires training more ancillary personnel |
| | More difficult to archive and integrate results into hospital information systems |

both regulatory requirements of the Clinical Laboratory Improvement Amendments of 1988 [18] and concern in the laboratory pathology community that loss of quality control may result in decreased quality of care [19] have limited the spread of bedside testing. POC testing raises logistic issues of training more individuals in the use of the chosen system, developing means of quality control, incorporating results into patient records and hospital information systems, and tracking use for billing purposes.

Currently, there are numerous POC devices available in the United States designed to measure a variety of hemostatic parameters (Table 3). Most instruments available can measure multiple coagulation parameters (i.e., activated clotting time [ACT], aPTT, prothrombin time [PT]) depending on the cartridge selected. In the realm of interventional cardiology, where management of ACS patients undergoing percutaneous coronary interventions (PCI) is frequent, assessment of adequate anticoagulation with thrombin inhibitors is particularly relevant. Such POC devices are also valuable in cardiovascular surgical operating rooms, critical care units, emergency rooms, dialysis centers, and anticoagulation clinics. We will review the various devices available for measuring anticoagulant effects of UFH, LMWH (specifically enoxaparin), and direct thrombin inhibitors (e.g., bivalirudin). It is important to realize that different devices often yield different numbers with the same blood sample (e.g., different ACT levels on separate POC machines) (Fig. 3) [20]. Furthermore, the ACT target varies depending on the type of procedures performed; cardiovascular surgery often requires an ACT target greater than 400–600 seconds, PCI requires an ACT of 250–350 seconds (depending on the use of glycoprotein [GP] IIb/IIIa inhibitors), patients on dialysis and extracorporeal membrane oxygenators require lower target ACT levels of approximately 180–200 seconds, and the appropriate ACT level to remove arterial sheaths is generally less than 175 seconds.

**Table 3**  Point-of-Care Anticoagulant Monitoring Devices

| Device | Main tests | Clot formation setting |
|---|---|---|
| Hemochron Tube Techonology (e.g. Response, 401) | ACT, PT, aPTT | Blood clots in a tube inserted with magnet, and rotated in a magnetic field |
| Hemochron Cuvette Technology (e.g. Junior II, Signature, Signature+) | ACT+, LR-ACT, PT, aPTT | Forced movement of unclotted blood through a narrow channel |
| Hemotec ACT II, Hepcon HMS | HR-ACT, LR-ACT, HMS, PT, aPTT | Mechanical plunger in and out of blood sample wells |
| Rapidpoint Coag | HMT, PT, aPTT, Enox, ECT | Chamber with paramagnetic iron particles with oscillating magnetic field |
| i-STAT | ACT | Electromechanical biosensor of thrombin conversion which produces an electroactive compound |
| CoaguChek | ACT, PT, aPTT | Capillary flow of unclotted blood |
| Actalyke | ACT, MAX-ACT, PT, aPTT | Two-point electromagnetic detection of blood clot in a tube |

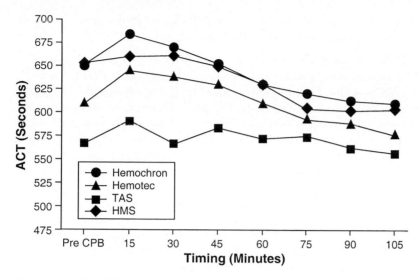

**Figure 3** The different ACT levels obtained with several point-of-care ACT measuring instruments based on the same samples of patients undergoing cardiopulmonary bypass. (From Ref. 20)

## Devices for Monitoring Unfractionated Heparin

*Hemochron Whole Blood Coagulation Systems (International Technidyne Corporation, USA)*

The Hemochron instruments have been available for 30 years to measure whole-blood ACT, representing the traditional gold-standard of bedside ACT measurement. In addition, a variety of other coagulant tests can be measured: aPTT, PT, thrombin time (TT), fibrinogen, etc. (Table 3). This company produces two types of instruments that either uses a tube or cuvette platform. The first type of machine uses 3 kinds of tubes that either contains celite, kaolin, or glass beads (e.g., Hemochron Response, Hemochron 401). The second type of machine (cuvette-based) uses cartridges preloaded with silica, kaolin, and phospholipid (e.g., Hemochron Junior II, Hemochron Junior Signature and Signature +). The tube-based machine requires approximately 2 ml of whole blood collected in the glass tubes, followed by manual shaking of the tube to mix the blood. The tube is then placed in a heating chamber (37° C) and rotated in a magnetic field. When blood clots, the magnet that was inserted inside the tube is displaced, activating a switch. The time taken for the clot to displace the magnet a given distance is recorded as the clotting time. The cuvette-based machine is a microcoagulation system that uses a disposable cuvette on which a drop of fresh whole blood is placed. In the cartridge, blood comes into contact with kaolin and platelet factor substitute reagent to induce clotting. The unclotted blood is mechanically moved back and forth through a capillary, and clotting is detected as cessation of flow by a change in light transmission. Different types of cuvettes can be separately purchased to measure ACT (ACT-LR or ACT +), aPTT, or PT. The ACT+ cuvettes are unaffected by aprotinin and correlate linearly with in vitro heparin levels of 1.0–6.0 IU/ml [21]. A study by Jaryno et al. showed that the Hemochron Response (a third generation Hemochron POC whole blood coagulation analyzer) is reliable and equivalent to the Hemochron standard in clinical applications [22].

*Hemotec Automated Coagulation Timer (™ACT) II & ™Hepcon Hemostasis
Management System (HMS) Devices (Medtronic Hemotec Inc)*

The ™Hepcon HMS is a microprocessor clot-timing instrument, capable of measuring
ACT, whole blood heparin concentration, and heparin dose-response. Different cartridges
can be used depending on the measurements desired (e.g., High-Range ACT, Heparin
Assay, and Heparin Dose Response cartridges). The whole blood (about 400 µl) samples
are placed in both wells of a cartridge containing kaolin as activator. An automated plunger
is then mechanically dipped in and out of the blood samples. As the sample clots, a fibrin
web forms which impedes the descent rate of the plunger. This rate change is detected
by optical photocells, and the clotting time is defined as the time to reach a prespecified
threshold of drop in plunger descent rate. The ™ACT II device uses the same principle,
with the added advantage of being a portable POC system. A frequently quoted study by
Despotis et al. showed that the heparin levels measured by the Hepcon device correlated
well with laboratory-measured plasma heparin levels, both before and during cardiopulmonary bypass (r = 0.95), unlike the weak correlation between ACT levels (r = 0.34–0.59)
and plasma heparin levels during cardiopulmonary bypass [23].

*Thrombolytic Assessment System / Rapidpoint™ Coag (PharmaNetics Inc,
Morrisville, NC)*

The ™Rapidoint Coag machine uses disposable test cards (e.g., the Heparin Management
Test [™HMT] card) containing small paramagnetic iron oxide particles (PIOP) in a flat
capillary reaction chamber with reagents (e.g., celite). When one drop of whole blood
(citrated or noncitrated) is added to the test card, the sample (approximately 30µL) is
drawn into the reaction chamber dissolving the dry reagents. The PIOP begin to oscillate
in a magnetic field, which slow down when blood clotting commences, and eventually
stop moving when the clot entraps the particles. This movement is detected by an infrared
photosensor, which records the test completion time when the rate of PIOP movement
drops. The ™HMT card can measure a broad range of heparin levels (1–10 U/ml). In fact,
the ™HMT levels have been reported to have better correlation with heparin levels and
anti-Xa levels compared with ACT levels (24,25). Among 53 patients undergoing cardiac
surgery, Fitch et al. found that ™HMT had a strong correlation with the Hemochron
measured ACT (r = 0.899; p < 0.001). Furthermore, the ™HMT had a significantly
stronger correlation with anti-Xa activity than the ACT (r = 0.82 for ™HMT r = 0.72
for ACT; p < 0.01) [24]. Tsimikas et al. compared the HMT levels to the Hemotec
measured ACT, and found significant correlation (r = 0.77; p < 0.001) for patients
undergoing PCI [26]. The effective range of the ™HMT test is from 50–850 seconds
(normal range is 89–169 seconds for citrated blood, and 76–195 seconds for noncitrated
blood) [27]. Similarly, the PT and aPTT test cards can be used with the ™Rapidpoint
Coag device to monitor PT and aPTT levels, respectively.

*i-STAT Analyzer (Abbott Laboratories, USA)*

This bedside analyzer uses disposable cartridges, and is capable of measuring numerous
laboratory tests, including electrolytes, creatinine, glucose, blood gases, and ACT levels.
It uses celite proloaded cartridges to measure ACT of whole blood samples. The analyzer
uses an electromechanical microminiaturized sensor based on silicon chip semiconductor
technology. The ACT cartridge contains preloaded celite, which activates the whole blood
sample to convert to a thrombin substrate. The electromechanical biosensor detects this
conversion, which produces an electroactive compound that is detected amperometrically.

A recent study by Paniccia et al. showed that the ACT values from the i-STAT device are relatively comparable to those obtained from the Hemachron 401 device among 165 blood samples of patients undergoing cardiopulmonary bypass or hemodialysis. They found good correlation between anti-Xa activity and i-STAT ACTs ($r^2 = 0.79$; $p < 0.001$) and Hemochron ACTs ($r^2 = 0.69$; $p < 0.001$) [28]. However, the i-STAT ACT is not currently cleared for low ACT range applications.

### ™CoaguChek System (Roche Diagnostics Corporation, Indianapolis, IN)

The ™CoaguChek is a portable hand-held instrument that can measure PT, aPTT, and ACT levels using disposable cartridges. A single drop of whole blood (from fingerstick puncture or venipuncture) is placed onto the cartridge which is preloaded with celite. The blood clotting time is determined by sensing the cessation of blood flow through a capillary channel via laser photometry (detecting a change in light scatter from red blood cells). The laser beam through the blood sample is blocked when blood clots, and this time is registered by the instrument. However, this system cannot measure ACT levels greater than 500 seconds, and thus is not as applicable during cardiovascular surgery [29]. The aPTT levels obtained with this device have conflicting correlation with central laboratory measured aPTT. Ferring et al. studied 233 samples from surgical intensive care patients following surgery, and found poor correlation of aPTT levels obtained from the CoaguChek device vs. central laboratory measurement ($r^2 = 0.077$) [30]. On the other hand, Ansell et al. reported that the aPTT measurement from this device correlated well (0.79–0.83) with standard laboratory measurement in 319 subjects [31]. However, this system may be useful for home monitoring of PT levels for patients taking coumadin [32].

### Actalyke Activated Clotting Time System (Helena Laboratories, Allen Park, MI)

The Actalyke is a simple bedside heparin monitoring system that uses the whole-blood ACT method. It uses test tubes preloaded with reagents, which are cross-compatible with the Hemochron system. Similar to the Hemochron system, it uses magnetic-displacement clot detection. However, it uses two-point clot detection, which enables detection of clot at early fibrin formation, minimizing testing error and nonheparin related prolongation. In addition to the celite ACT test, this system also can perform the new MAX-ACT measurement, which utilizes tubes that are preloaded with multiple activators (celite, ka-olin, and glass beads). These particular tubes maximally convert all Factor XII to XIIa for greatest heparin specificity, and may be less susceptible to changes associated with hypothermia and hemodilution as experienced with the traditional celite-ACT methods. A study by Levyi et al. showed that Hemochron ACT and MAX-ACT did not differ during normothermia, but did during hypothermia, with ACT significantly longer than MAX-ACT ($p = 0.009$) [33].

## Devices For Monitoring Low Molecular-Weight Heparin

LMWH are increasingly replacing UFH for the prevention and treatment of both arterial and venous thrombotic disorders. Several clinical trials have demonstrated the equivalence or superiority of LMWH over UFH for the treatment of coronary artery disease and venous thromboembolism. In particular, enoxaparin has consistently been proven safe and effica-cious compared to UFH or placebo in medical therapy trials [34–38]. Unlike UFH whereby the aPTT and ACT are routinely used to monitor its anticoagulant activity, LMWH does not appreciably affect these measurements [39]. Central laboratory anti-Xa assays are available to measure LMWH activity, but are relatively expensive and require long turn-around times, precluding their practical use during PCI or acute care settings. Until recently, the lack of a rapid and convenient measurement of enoxaparin anticoagulant activity has contributed to the reluctance of some clinicians in using this agent during PCI or surgical procedures. The recent availability of a POC assay, ᵀᴹRapidpoint ENOX, to specifically evaluate clotting times in response to enoxaparin will hopefully enhance the use of LMWH in these settings.

### ᵀᴹRapidpoint ENOX test (PharmaNetics Inc, Morrisville, NC)

The Rapidpoint ENOX test is a 1-step assay, whereby all the components necessary to measure enoxaparin clotting time (aside from the patient's sample) are included in the test card's reaction chamber, to be used in conjunction with the ᵀᴹRapidpoint Coag analyzer. A drop of the blood sample (approximately 35 μl) is manually added to the sample well on the front of the test card. The test sample is then drawn into a reaction chamber via capillary action, rehydrating reagents and stimulating PIOP to move by an oscillating magnetic field in the test chamber. A specific factor Xa activator then rapidly activates factor X which initiates the clotting process, with formation of fibrin strands that attach to and impede iron particles movements. An infrared optical system monitors particle movement and indicates when a preset reduction in movement is achieved (corresponding to the test's endpoint which is reported in seconds). The ᵀᴹENOX test card is optimized for use with enoxaparin (clotting time range of 50–700 seconds), and should not be used to monitor UFH or other LMWH. Platelet inhibitors and thrombolytic agents do not affect the ᵀᴹENOX test; however, direct thrombin inhibitors have significant effects. ᵀᴹENOX times ranged from 106–160 seconds (mean ± 2 SD) in 120 normal volunteers, and from 70–180 seconds (mean ± 2 SD) among 166 unanticoagulated patients using citrated samples [40]. A study by Saw et al. demonstrated that the ᵀᴹRapidpoint ENOX times correlated strongly to anti-Xa activities measured by the ᵀᴹStachrom Heparin Assays ([r = 0.89, p < 0.001] for citrated whole blood [Fig. 4a], and [r = 0.82, p < 0.001] for noncitrated whole blood [Fig. 4b]) among 332 samples from 166 patients who received enoxaparin for the prevention of deep venous thrombosis or as treatment during ACS or PCI [41].

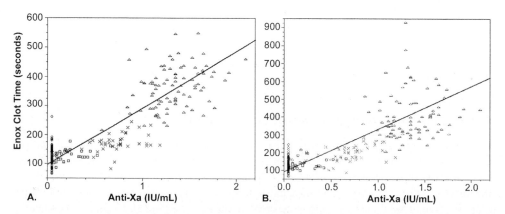

**Figure 4**  Bivariate fit of ENOX times by anti-Xa activities for 332 samples of (**A**) citrated whole-blood, and (**B**) noncitrated whole-blood. (From Ref. 41)

## Devices for Monitoring Direct Thrombin Inhibitors

Direct thrombin inhibitors do not require a cofactor to antagonize thrombin activity; thus they directly inhibit thrombin's activity on fibrinogen and also attenuate thrombin-induced platelet aggregation. Hirudin and its analogs (e.g., bivalirudin) have numerous other advantages over UFH, and are increasingly being used for ACS and PCI, especially for patients with heparin-induced thrombocytopenia (HIT). In fact, bivalirudin was approved by the US Food and Drug Administration in 2000 for patients with unstable angina undergoing PCI. Several PCI studies evaluating the procedural use of direct thrombin inhibitors have been completed [42–49], which together included over 13,000 patients and showed these agents to be safe and at least as effective at minimizing acute ischemic events as heparin, while lowering bleeding events. In the most recent REPLACE-2 trial (Randomized Evaluation in PCI Linking Angiomax to reduce Clinical Events) [50] which enrolled 6,010 patients, bivalirudin with provisional GP IIb/IIIa blockade (given to 7.2% of patients) was shown to be noninferior to the combination of heparin plus routine GP IIb/IIIa blockade during PCI (30-day secondary composite endpoint of death, MI or urgent revascularization were 7.6% bivalirudin and 7.1% heparin plus GP IIb/IIIa blockade). Thus, it is anticipated that the use of direct thrombin inhibitors will increase dramatically, particularly during PCI, so will the need to monitor the anticoagulant activity of these agents.

Anticoagulation levels with hirudins can be measured accurately with chromogenic-based substrate assays or the ecarin clotting times (ECT). Unfortunately, the aPTT is inadequate for monitoring hirudin levels since the correlation is linear only for hirudin concentrations up to 1 mg/L (low normal therapeutic range) (Fig. 5) [51]. Furthermore, there is limited linear correlation between the ACT and hirudin plasma levels, with high levels of hirudin concentrations (greater than 2 mg/L) associated with ACT levels beyond the detection limit [52]. Bivalirudin does appreciably affect aPTT, prothrombin, and thrombin times in a dose-dependent manner, though over a limited range. Fortunately, the ECT provides a more accurate measurement of direct thrombin inhibitor activity than ACT. This test utilizes ecarin (from the venom of *Echis carinatus*) to convert prothrombin to

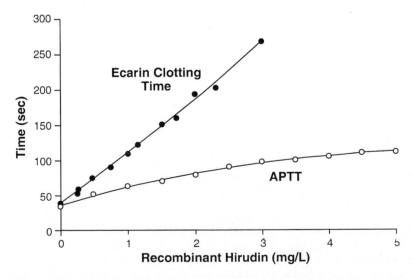

**Figure 5** Dose-response curves of aPTT and ECT (ecarin clotting time) to hirudin concentration. (From Ref. 51)

meizothrombin, which then catalyzes the conversion of fibrinogen to fibrin (which is inhibited by direct thrombin inhibitors) [53]. A new POC assay capable of measuring ECT was recently developed by PharmaNetics Inc.

*Thrombolytic Assessment System (TAS) Ecarin Clotting Time (ECT) Test Cards (PharmaNetics Inc, Morrisville, NC)*

The TAS ECT test card was recently authorized by the US Federal Law for use in determining the anticoagulant effect of recombinant hirudin (r-hirudin) (Refludan) during cardiopulmonary bypass in patients who have HIT. This test card is a 2-step test that requires the patient's citrated whole blood sample to be first diluted with pooled normal human plasma. The diluted sample is then added to a prewarmed ECT test card, which contains the dry ecarin (protein prothrombin activator from *Echi carinatus* venom) reagent and PIOP. Ecarin catalyzes the hydrolytic cleavage of the human prothrombin molecule, generating thrombin without the release of any zymogen fragment. Hirudin (and low molecular-weight synthetic thrombin inhibitors) inhibits the formation of this form of thrombin (meizothrombin). The use of ecarin to activate prothrombin bypasses the coagulation cascade (activation of factors V-XII), and thus a deficiency in any of these factors will not be reflected in the results. The ECT is measured in a similar fashion as the ᵀᴹENOX test cards deposited in the ᵀᴹRapidpoint Coag analyzer, by assessing the movements of the PIOP in an oscillating magnetic field. This instrument reports the ECT in seconds, and is sensitive to r-hirudin to 100 ng/ml. The normal range in 120 normal patients was between 41.6 and 55.3 seconds (mean + 2 standard deviations) [54]. This test card has also been reliably used in patients receiving bivalirudin. Among 64 patients (263 samples) undergoing PCI at the Cleveland Clinic who received procedural bivalirudin, Cho et al. showed that the TAS ECT correlated strongly (r = 0.9) with bivalirudin concentration (anti-IIa levels), whereas the Hemochron measured ACT levels only moderately correlated with anti-IIa levels (r = 0.71) (Fig. 6) [55]. The same group subsequently evaluated a larger PCI population (170 patients, 784 samples) in a multi-center study, and found that citrated ECT, noncitrated ECT, and ACT correlated well with bivalirudin concentrations (0.96, 0.93, and 0.90, respectively). However, samples collected at therapeutic bivalirudin levels had overall lower correlation with bivalirudin concentration; although the correlation

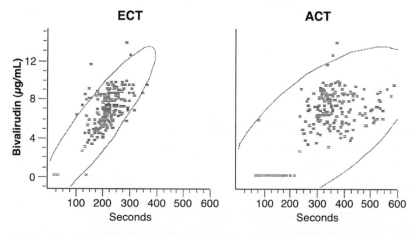

**Figure 6**  Correlation of ECT and ACT to anti-IIa levels in 263 samples from patients undergoing PCI who received bivalirudin at the Cleveland Clinic. (From Ref. 55)

appear better with ECT (correlation 0.75 with citrated, and 0.59 with noncitrated samples) than ACT (correlation 0.37) [56]. The use of bivalirudin during cardiopulmonary bypass is not currently accepted, although Koster et al. reported a successful case with the use of the TAS ECT to monitor procedural bivalirudin anticoagulation in a patient with HIT [57].

## RATIONALE FOR USING ACT TO MEASURE HEPARIN EFFECT DURING PCI

Since the early days of PCI, high dose intravenous heparin has been used to prevent thrombosis related to both transient obstruction of coronary flow as well as endothelial disruption. Similar to cardiopulmonary bypass surgery, the doses and levels of heparin used during coronary intervention are above the level at which the heparin-aPTT response curve allows discrimination, and therefore the ACT has become the standard monitoring test. Because rapid turnaround time is essential to document the degree of anticoagulation and proceed expeditiously with the procedure, the ACT has evolved as a test used locally in the catheterization laboratory. Of the devices currently available (described earlier), the two most commonly used devices to measure ACT are the Hemochron and HemoTec instruments, both of which use whole blood and provide results within minutes. However, the two tests vary substantially, with the ACT from the Hemochron being approximately 50 seconds longer than from the HemoTec [58].

Although there are no randomized studies specifically comparing different levels of heparin during PCI, a number of observational studies prior to widespread use of GP IIb/IIIa inhibitors have found that the degree of heparin effect as measured by the procedural ACT is associated with risk of thrombotic complications [59–62]. Each showed that lower ACTs are associated with greater risk of complications. One study compared 103 patients who died or had emergency bypass surgery with 400 uncomplicated patients, and found that the ACT, measured with the HemoTec device, was 60 to 80 seconds lower among patients with complications [60]. Another study compared 63 patients with abrupt closure to 124 controls matched for other predictors of abrupt closure. The median ACT, measured with the Hemochron device, was 30 to 40 seconds shorter among patients with abrupt closure, and abrupt closure risk was twice as high with an ACT of 300 compared to 400 [61]. These two studies have led to the recommendation that heparin be titrated to an ACT of at least 300 (HemoTec) to 350 (Hemochron) seconds before angioplasty [63].

When abciximab is administered with heparin, the use of a less aggressive heparin regimen (less than or equal to 70 U/kg with an ACT of at least 200 seconds) in the EPILOG (Evaluation in PTCA to Improve Long-term Outcome with abciximab GP IIb/IIIa blockade) [64] study reduced bleeding complications without any loss of efficacy compared to the EPIC (Evaluation of c7E3 Fab in the Prevention of Ischemic Complications) trial [65]. Thus, a lower-dose heparin regimen is recommended when GP IIb/IIIa inhibitors are coadministered [64,66]. Moreover, in the presence of abciximab, the relationship of heparin dose and ACT is altered, such that after adjusting for patient weight, the ACT is prolonged by approximately 10% on average by abciximab [67]. In contrast, there is minimal to no effect on the ACT level with concomitant use of eptifibatide or tirofiban with heparin. Dauerman et al. measured ACT levels after eptifibatide boluses with both the ™CoaguChek and Hemochron 801 devices in 70 patients, and found that eptifibatide does not significantly prolong the ACT in patients undergoing PCI [68]. In a post hoc analysis of the TARGET (Tirofiban And Reopro Give similar Efficacy outcomes Trial) study, Casserly et al. showed no difference in the peak ACT level among those randomized to abciximab or tirofiban when receiving lower dose heparin (50 U/kg). However, ACT level was not measured pre-tirofiban and post-tirofiban administration to specifically address the effect of tirofiban on ACT [69].

## EXPERINCE WITH BEDSIDE ANTICOAGULANT MONITORING IN CLINICAL TRIALS OF PCI

Since the widespread availability of POC ACT monitoring devices, it has become routine to measure ACT during PCI when UFH is used. Thus, numerous randomized PCI trials assessing novel antithrombotic and antiplatelet agents have peak ACT levels available for comparison. Chew et al. pooled 6 large randomized PCI trials (EPIC [65], EPILOG [64], EPISTENT [Evaluation of Platelet IIb/IIIa Inhibitor for STENTing] [70], IMPACT-II [Integrilin to Minimize Platelet Aggregation and Coronary Thrombosis] [71], RAPPORT [Reopro and Primary PTCA Organization and Randomized Trial] [72], and HAS [Hirudin Angioplasty Study] [73]) and correlated peak ACT levels to clinical outcomes [74]. The 5216 patients who had ACT levels available around device deployment were grouped according to their peak ACT at 25-second intervals, from 275 to 475 seconds. The majority of ACT levels were measured with the Hemochron device (95%), with a small proportion measured by the Hemotec device (5%). The incidence of death, MI, or any revascularization and bleeding (major or minor) complications at 7 days were calculated for each group and compared. When UFH is used alone, 7-day ischemic complications were lower among patients with higher ACT levels. The lowest events were observed for ACT values between 350–375 seconds, though more bleeding complications were noted (Fig. 7). Importantly, patients receiving both abciximab and UFH had increased bleeding risks with higher ACT levels, and no incremental benefit of ischemic endpoint reduction with ACT beyond 250 seconds (Fig. 8). Thus, the target ACT level should be lower (approximately 250 seconds) when GP IIb/IIIa inhibitors are coadministered with UFH during PCI.

The correlation of ™ENOX clotting time to clinical outcomes was recently addressed by the ELECT (Evaluating ENOX Clotting Times) study [75]. This study prospectively analyzed 445 patients receiving subcutaneous or intravenous enoxaparin during PCI, measuring the ™Rapidpoint ENOX time and correlating to clinical outcomes. The mean procedural ™ENOX time was similar for patients with or without an ischemic event (in-hospital composite of death, MI, and urgent target vessel revascularization) (461 seconds and 429 seconds, respectively). The nadir event rate was observed for ™ENOX times approximately 300–350 seconds (Figure 9), however, no significant association between ischemic events and ™ENOX times was seen using logistic regression (p = 0.222). During sheath removal, increasing ™ENOX time was correlated to any bleeding (p = 0.01). From this study and, in conjunction with the suggested anti-Xa level of 0.8 to 1.8 IU/ml while using enoxaparin for PCI [76–79], Moliterno et al. recommended an ENOX® time range of 250–450 seconds for PCI, and less than 200–250 seconds for arterial sheath removal [75].

## EXPERINCE WITH BEDSIDE APTT MONITORING IN CLINICAL TRIALS OF ACS

### ™CoaguChek Plus

In the 41,000 patient GUSTO-I trial, a prospective observational study was performed to evaluate patient outcomes according to the method of anticoagulant monitoring. Each participating investigator was given the option of using the ™CoaguChek Plus monitor vs. central laboratory measured aPTT. Of the 28,172 patients treated with intravenous heparin who had at least one aPTT determined, 1713 patients had all aPTT measurements

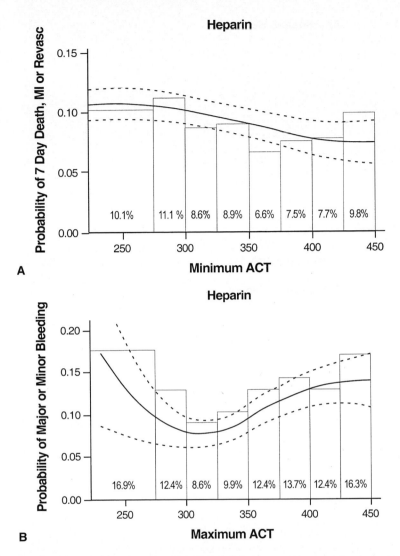

**Figure 7** Correlation between ACT levels with the use of heparin to clinical endpoints. (**A**) Relationship between minimum ACT and 7d ischemic events (death, MI or revascularization). (**B**) Relationship between maximum ACT and 7d major or minor bleeding events. (From Ref. 74)

by the ™CoaguChek Plus monitor [80]. Patients who had bedside monitoring were more likely to be in the target aPTT range at 24 hours (26% vs. 22%), had lower rates of bleeding, less of a drop from baseline to nadir hematocrit, less need for transfusion, a tendency towards slightly higher reinfarction rate, and tendency to lower mortality (Table 4). These data support the concept that bedside aPTT monitoring can provide a standardized, safe and effective approach towards anticoagulation.

### Hemochron Jr.

The PARAGON Trial [81] randomized 2282 patients with unstable angina to the intravenous GP IIb/IIIa blocker lamifiban, with and without intravenous heparin, or placebo with

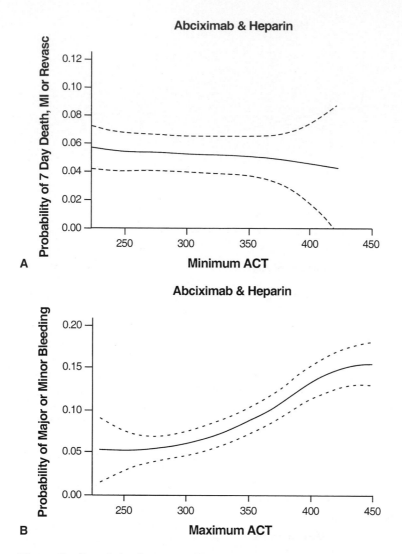

**Figure 8** Correlation between ACT level with the use of abciximab and heparin to clinical endpoints. (**A**) Relationship between minimum ACT and 7d ischemic events (death, MI or revascularization). (**B**) Relationship between maximum ACT and 7d major or minor bleeding events. (From Ref. 74)

intravenous heparin. APTT monitoring and heparin adjustment were achieved using the Hemochron Jr. bedside aPTT monitor and a blinded, computerized system of using the aPTT results (in an encrypted code) to determine heparin adjustment (target aPTT was 50–70 seconds). The median aPTT of the 758 patients randomized to the heparin control group was 62 seconds at 6 hours, and 50 seconds (25th to 75th percentile, 40 to 63 seconds) at 24 hours [82], ranges that compared favorably with standard care approaches of heparin adjustment (Table 5). Bleeding rates in the heparin control arm (5.5%) were likewise favorable compared with historical controls. Thus, the PARAGON experience shows that a bedside monitor, used with an automated blinded system of heparin adjustment, can achieve consistent therapeutic aPTT levels and low bleeding rates.

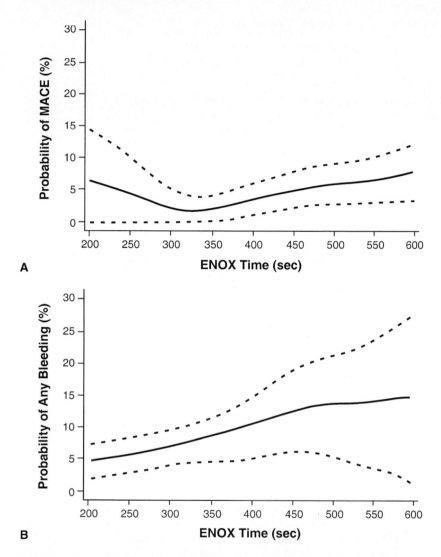

**Figure 9** Results from the ELECT trial, reproduced with permission from reference [75]. (**A**) Correlation of ENOX time to major adverse cardiac events (MACE), in-hospital death, myocardial infarction, or urgent target vessel revascularization. (**B**) Correlation of ENOX time to any bleeding events.

## SUMMARY

It has been well established that antithrombotic therapy for the acute phase of coronary syndromes has potential for substantial benefit in preventing thrombotic complications while at the same time predisposing to serious hemorrhage. The concept that sophisticated, precise, and rapid monitoring of the effects of anticoagulants will be critical to optimize the benefit/risk ratio is the basis for the need for bedside anticoagulation testing. Although both observational and small randomized studies have suggested that bedside testing is associated with improved outcome, until more definitive outcome studies are performed to show that the additional cost, loss of precision and challenge of quality control are

**Table 4**   Clinical Events by Monitoring Equipment in the GUSTO I Trial

|  | CoaguChek aPTT (n = 1713) | Standard aPTT (n = 26,459) | *P* |
|---|---|---|---|
| Mortality |  |  |  |
| 30 days (unadjusted) | 4.3% | 4.8% | 0.33 |
| 30 days (adjusted[a]) | 4.3% | 4.8% | 0.27 |
| 1 year | 7.1% | 7.7% | 0.38 |
| Reinfarction | 4.9% | 4.1% | 0.14 |
| Bleeding |  |  |  |
| Moderate | 9.6% | 11.8% | 0.01 |
| Severe | 0.7% | 1.2% | 0.07 |
| Moderate or severe | 10..4% | 13.0% | .001 |
| RBC transfusion | 7% | 11% | <0.001 |
| Drop in hematocrit (%) | 5.5 ± 5.2 | 6.7 ± 5.8 | <0.001 |
| Stroke |  |  |  |
| Hemorrhagic | 0.7% | 0.7% | 0.80 |
| Overall | 1.3% | 1.4% | 0.71 |

[a] Adjusted for important baseline predictors of mortality following acute myocardial infarction. (From Ref. 80)

warranted, it will be difficult to change practice so that bedside testing for management of acute coronary syndromes becomes the dominant strategy.

In the setting of percutaneous coronary interventions, bedside ACT monitoring is now considered the standard of care during administration of unfractionated heparin. Numerous devices are currently available for the bedside measurements of ACT, along with

**Table 5**   Target and Achieved aPTT Ranges According to Monitoring Method in Clinical Trials of Acute Coronary Syndromes Among Patients Treated with Intravenous Heparin

|  | GUSTO-I, Central laboratory | GUSTO-I, CoaguChek Plus | TIMI-5, CoaguChek Plus | GUSTO-II, Central laboratory | PARAGON, Hemochron Jr. |
|---|---|---|---|---|---|
| *n* | 25,766 | 1713 | 84 | 2868 | 758 |
| Patient population | ST elevation, thrombolytic treated | ST elevation, thrombolytic treated | ST elevation, thrombolytic treated | Unstable angina/ non-Q-wave MI | Unstable angina/non -Q-wave MI |
| Nomogram | Yes | Yes | Yes | Yes | Computer-automated |
| Target aPTT | 60–85 sec | 65–90 sec | 60–90 sec | 60–85 sec | 50–70 sec |
| Actual aPTT at 24 hours | 62 (47, 88) | 71 (52,103) | 63 (48,75) | 61 (50,75) | 50 (−0,63) |
| Moderate or severe bleeding | 13.0% | 10.4% | 23%[a] | 8.4% | 5.5% |

[a] All patients underwent early angiography.

other hemostatic parameters. The device choice will depend on the clinical setting and different pharmacologic regimens necessitate different ACT target levels. There is no clear winner at this juncture given the absence of large-scale studies correlating devices and their measurements to clinical outcomes. With PCI anticoagulation polypharmacy and the flat dose-response relationship of ACT to ischemic events, some argue that no monitoring is needed and that low levels of anticoagulation should be routinely targeted. The emergence of new point-of-care assays to measure low molecular-weight heparin and direct thrombin inhibitor anticoagulant effects will likely aid the gradual transition in utilizing these agents during PCI. As new antithrombotic approaches are developed, establishing the optimal methods of dosing and monitoring, including at the patient's bedside, may be as important as which agents are used.

# REFERENCES

1.  Granger CB, Hirsch J, Califf RM, Col J, White HD, Betriu A, Woodlief LH, Lee KL, Bovill EG, Simes RJ, Topol EJ. Activated partial thromboplastin time and outcome after thrombolytic therapy for acute myocardial infarction: results from the GUSTO-I trial. Circulation 1996;93: 870–878.
2.  Randomized trial of intravenous heparin vs. recombinant hirudin for acute coronary syndromes. The Global Use of Strategies to Open Occluded Coronary Arteries (GUSTO) IIa Investigators. Circulation 1994;90:1631–1637.
3.  A clinical trial comparing primary coronary angioplasty with tissue plasminogen activator for acute myocardial infarction. The Global Use of Strategies to Open Occluded Coronary Arteries in Acute Coronary Syndromes (GUSTO IIb) Angioplasty Substudy Investigators. N Engl J Med 1997;336:1621–1628.
4.  Antman EM. Hirudin in acute myocardial infarction. Thrombolysis and Thrombin Inhibition in Myocardial Infarction (TIMI) 9B trial. Circulation 1996;94:911–921.
5.  Ryan TJ, Antman EM, Brooks NH, Hillis LD, Hiratzka LF, Rapaport E, Riegel B, Russell RO, Smith EE 3rd, Weaver WD, Gibbon RJ, Alpert JS, Eagle KA, Gardner TJ, Garson A Jr, Gregoratos G, Ryan TJ, Smith SC Jr. 1999 update: ACC/AHA guidelines for the management of patients with acute myocardial infarction. A report of the American College of Cardiology/ American Heart Association Task Force on Practice Guidelines (Committee on Management of Acute Myocardial Infarction). J Am Coll Cardiol 1999;34:890–911.
6.  Chiu HM, Hirsh J, Yung WL, Regoeczi E, Gent M. Relationship between the anticoagulant and antithrombotic effects of heparin in experimental venous thrombosis. Blood 1977;49: 171–184.
7.  Becker RC, Cyr J, Corrao JM, Ball SP. Bedside coagulation monitoring in heparin-treated patients with active thromboembolic disease: a coronary care unit experience. Am Heart J 1994;128:719–723.
8.  GUSTO Gazette. 1992;2.
9.  Peterson P, Gottfried EL. The effects of inaccurate blood sample volume on prothrombin time (PT) and activated partial thromboplastin time (aPTT). Thromb Haemost 1982;47:101–103.
10. Thomson J. Pre-test variables in blood coagulation testing. In: Thomson J, Ed. Blood Coagulation and Hemostasis, A Practical Guide. New York: Churchill Livingstone, 1985:340–369.
11. Brandt JT, Triplett DA. Laboratory monitoring of heparin. Effect of reagents and instruments on the activated partial thromboplastin time. Am J Clin Pathol 1981;76:530–537.
12. Watts NB. Reproducibility (precision) in alternate site testing. A clinician's perspective. Arch Pathol Lab Med 1995;119:914–917.
13. D'Angelo A, Seveso MP, D'Angelo SV, Gilardoni F, Dettori AG, Bonini P. Effect of clot-detection methods and reagents on activated partial thromboplastin time (APTT). Implications in heparin monitoring by APTT. Am J Clin Pathol 1990;94:297–306.
14. Bjornsson TD, Nash PV. Variability in heparin sensitivity of APTT reagents. Am J Clin Pathol 1986;86:199–204.

15. Shojania AM, Tetreault J, Turnbull G. The variations between heparin sensitivity of different lots of activated partial thromboplastin time reagent produced by the same manufacturer. Am J Clin Pathol 1988;89:19–23.

16. Poller L, Thomson J, Taberner D. Use of the activated partial thromboplastin time for monitoring heparin therapy: problems and possible solutions. Res Clin Lab 1989;19:363–370.

17. Brill-Edwards P, Ginsberg JS, Johnston M, Hirsh J. Establishing a therapeutic range for heparin therapy. Ann Intern Med 1993;119:104–109.

18. Ehrmeyer SS, Laessig RH. The relationship of intralaboratory bias and imprecision on laboratories' ability to meet medical usefulness limits. Am J Clin Pathol 1988;89:14–18.

19. Howanitz PJ. College of American Pathologists Conference XXVIII on alternate site testing. What must we now do? Arch Pathol Lab Med 1995;119:979–983.

20. Huffman S. Presented at the AmSECT Meeting (abstract). 1998.

21. Pan C, Jobes D, Van Riper D, Ogilby JD, Lin C, Horrow J, Blumenthal R, Mendoza N, La Duca F. Modified microsample ACT test for heparin monitoring. J Extracorpor Technol 1996; 28:16–20.

22. Jaryno S, Bennett K, Loder C, Zucker ML, Pan CM, LaDuca FM. Validation of a new whole blood coagulation monitoring system. J Extra Corpor Technol 2002;34:271–275.

23. Despotis GJ, Summerfield AL, Joist JH, Goodnough LT, Santoro SA, Spitznagel E, Cox JL, Lappas DG. Comparison of activated coagulation time and whole blood heparin measurements with laboratory plasma anti-Xa heparin concentration in patients having cardiac operations. J Thorac Cardiovasc Surg 1994;108:1076–1082.

24. Fitch JC, Geary KL, Mirto GP, Byrne DW, Hines RL. Heparin management test vs. activated coagulation time during cardiovascular surgery: correlation with anti-Xa activity. J Cardiothorac Vasc Anesth 1999;13:53–57.

25. Gibbs NM, Weightman WM, Thackray NM, Michalopoulos N. Evaluation of the TAS coagulation analyzer for monitoring heparin effect in cardiac surgical patients. J Cardiothorac Vasc Anesth 1998;12:536–541.

26. Tsimikas S, Beyer R, Hassankhani A. Relationship between the heparin management test and the HemoTec activated clotting time in patients undergoing percutaneous coronary intervention. J Thromb Thrombolysis 2001;11:217–221.

27. HMT Test Cards Insert. http://www.pharmanetics.com/pdfs/pi/1900032.05.pdf, 2002.

28. Paniccia R, Fedi S, Carbonetto F, Noferi D, Conti P, Bandinelli B, Giusti B, Evangelisti L, Pretelli P, Palmarini MF, Abbate R, Prisco D. Evaluation of a new point-of-care celite-activated clotting time analyzer in different clinical settings. The i-STAT celite-activated clotting time test. Anesthesiology 2003 99:54–59.

29. Giavarina D, Carta M, Fabbri A, Manfredi J, Gasparotto E, Soffiati G. Monitoring high-dose heparin levels by ACT and HMT during extracorporeal Circulation: diagnostic accuracy of three compact monitors. Perfusion 2002;17:23–26.

30. Ferring M, Reber G, de Moerloose P, Merlani P, Diby M, Ricou B. Point of care and central laboratory determinations of the aPTT are not interchangeable in surgical intensive care patients. Can J Anaesth 2001;48:1155–1160.

31. Ansell J, Tiarks C, Hirsh J, McGehee W, Adler D, Weibert R. Measurement of the activated partial thromboplastin time from a capillary (fingerstick) sample of whole blood. A new method for monitoring heparin therapy. Am J Clin Pathol 1991;95:222–227.

32. Anderson DR, Harrison L, Hirsh J. Evaluation of a portable prothrombin time monitor for home use by patients who require long-term oral anticoagulant therapy. Arch Intern Med 1993; 153:1441–1447.

33. Leyvi G, Shore-Lesserson L, Harrington D, Vela-Cantos F, Hossain S. An investigation of a new activated clotting time "MAX-ACT" in patients undergoing extracorporeal Circulation. Anesth Analg 2001;92:578–583.

34. Cohen M, Demers C, Gurfinkel E, Turpie AG, Fromell GJ, Goodman S, Langer A, Califf RM, Fox KA, Premmereur J, Bigonzi F. A comparison of low-molecular-weight heparin with unfractionated heparin for unstable coronary artery disease. N Engl J Med 1997;337:447–452.

35. Antman E, McCabe C, Gurfinkel E, Turpie AG, Bernink PJ, Salien D, Bayes De Luna A, Fox K, Lablanche JM, Radley D, Premmereur J, Braunwald E. Enoxaparin prevents death and

cardiac ischemic events in unstable angina/non-Q-wave myocardial infarction: results of the thrombolysis in myocardial infarction (TIMI) 11B trial. Circulation 1999;100:1593–601.

36. The ASSENT-3 Investigators. Efficacy and safety of tenecteplase in combination with enoxaparin, abciximab, or unfractionated heparin: the ASSENT-3 randomised trial in acute myocardial infarction. Lancet 2001;358:605–613.

37. Levine M, Gent M, Hirsh J, Leclerc J, Anderson D, Weitz J, Ginsberg J, Turpie AG, Demers C, Kovacs M. A comparison of low-molecular-weight heparin administered primarily at home with unfractionated heparin administered in the hospital for proximal deep-vein thrombosis. N Engl J Med 1996;334:677–681.

38. Samama M, Cohen A, Darmon J, Desjardins L, Eldor A, Janbon C, Leizorovicz A, Nguyen H, Olsson CG, Turpie AG, Weisslinger N. A comparison of enoxaparin with placebo for the prevention of venous thromboembolism in acutely ill medical patients. N Engl J Med 1999; 341:793–800.

39. Linkins L, Julian J, Rischke J, Hirsh J, Weitz J. In vitro comparison of the effect of heparin, enoxaparin and fondaparinux on tests of coagulation. Thromb Res 2002;107:241–244.

40. ENOX package insert. http://enoxtest.com/pdfs/enoxpackageinsert.pdf, 2003.

41. Saw J, Kereiakes D, Mahaffey K, Applegale RJ, Braden GA, Brent BN, Brodie BR, Groce JB, Levine GN, Leya F, Moliterno DJ. Evaluation of a Novel Point-of-Care Enoxaparin Monitor with Central Laboratory Anti-Xa Levels. Thrombosis Research, 2003.

42. van den Bos AA, Deckers JW, Heyndrickx GR, Laarman GJ, Suryapranata H, Zijlstra F, Close P, Rijnierse JJ, Buller HR, Serruys PW. Safety and efficacy of recombinant hirudin (CGP 39 393) vs. heparin in patients with stable angina undergoing coronary angioplasty. Circulation 1993;88:2058–2066.

43. Topol EJ, Bonan R, Jewitt D, Sigwart U, Kakkar W, Rothman M, de Bono D, Ferguson J, Willerson JT, Strony J, Ganz P, Cohen MD, Raymond R, Fox I, Maraganore J, Adelman B. Use of a direct antithrombin, hirulog, in place of heparin during coronary angioplasty. Circulation 1993;87:1622–1629.

44. Rupprecht HJ, Terres W, Ozbek C, Luz M, Jessel A, Hafner G, vom Dahl J, Kromer EP, Prellwitz W, Meyer J. Recombinant hirudin (HBW 023) prevents troponin T release after coronary angioplasty in patients with unstable angina. J Am Coll Cardiol 1995;26:1637–1642.

45. Serruys PW, Herrman JP, Simon R, Rutsch W, Bode C, Laarman GJ, Van Dijk R, van den Bos AA, Umans VA, Fox KA, Close P, Deckers JW, for The Helvetica Investigators. A comparison of hirudin with heparin in the prevention of restenosis after coronary angioplasty. Helvetica Investigators. N Engl J Med 1995;333:757–763.

46. Bittl JA, Strony J, Brinker JA, Ahmed WH, Meckel CR, Chaitman BR, Maraganore J, Deutsch E, Adelman B. Treatment with bivalirudin (Hirulog) as compared with heparin during coronary angioplasty for unstable or postinfarction angina. Hirulog Angioplasty Study Investigators. N Engl J Med 1995;333:764–769.

47. The Global Use of Strategies to Open Occluded Coronary Arteries in Acute Coronary Syndromes (GUSTO IIb) Angioplasty Substudy Investigators. A clinical trial comparing primary coronary angioplasty with tissue plasminogen activator for acute myocardial infarction. N Engl J Med 1997;336:1621–1628.

48. Lewis BE, Matthai W, Grassman ED, Leya FS, Fareed J, Walenga JM, Wrona L, Rangel Y, Joffrion JL, Whitlow PL, McKeever LS. Results of phase 2/3 trial of argatroban anticoagulation during PTCA of patients with heparin-induced thrombocytopenia (HIT). Circulation 1997; 96:I-217.

49. Lincoff A, Kleiman N, Kottke-Marchant K, Maierson ES, Maresh K, Wolski KE, Topol EJ. Bivalirudin with planned or provisional abciximab vs. low-dose heparin and abciximab during percutaneous coronary revascularization: results of the Comparison of Abciximab Complications with Hirulog for Ischemic Events Trial (CACHET). American Heart Journal 2002;143: 847–853.

50. Lincoff A, Bittl J, Harrington R, Feit F, Kleiman NS, Jackman JD, Saremback IJ, Cohen DJ, Spriggs D, Ebrahimi R, Keren G, Carr J, Cohen EA, Betriu A, Desmet W, Kereiakes DJ, Rutsch W, Wilcox RG, de Feyter PJ, Vahanian A, Topol EJ, REPLACE-2 Investigators.

Bivalirudin and provisional glycoprotein IIb/IIIa blockade compared with heparin and planned glycoprotein IIb/IIIa blockade during percutaneous coronary intervention. JAMA 2003 289: 853–863.

51. Hafner G, Roser M, Nauck M. Methods for the monitoring of direct thrombin inhibitors. Semin Thromb Hemost 2002;28:425–430.

52. Despotis GJ, Hogue CW, Saleem R, Bigham M, Skhubas N, Apostolidou I, Qayum A, Joist JH. The relationship between hirudin and activated clotting time: implications for patients with heparin-induced thrombocytopenia undergoing cardiac surgery. Anesth Analg 2001;93:28–32.

53. Cho L, Kottke-Marchant K, Lincoff AM, Roffi M, Reginelli JP, Kaldus T, Moliterno DJ. Correlation of point-of-care ecarin clotting time vs. activated clotting time with bivalirudin concentrations. Am J Cardiol 2003;91:1110–1113.

54. TAS ECT Test Cards Insert. http://www.pharmanetics.com/pdfs/inserts/1800520.05.pdf, 2002.

55. Cho L, Kottke-Marchant K, Lincoff AM, Roffi M, Reginelli JP, Kaldus T, Moliterno DJ. Correlation of point-of-care ecarin clotting time vs. activated clotting time with bivalirudin concentrations. Am J Cardiol 2003;91:1110–1113.

56. Casserly I, Kereiakes D, Gray W, Gibson PH, Lauer MA, Reginelli JP, Moliterno DJ. Point-of-care ecarin clotting time versus activated clotting time in correlation with bivalirudin concentration. Thrombosis Research 2004;113:115–121.

57. Koster A, Chew D, Grundel M, Bauer M, Kuppe H, Spiess BD. Bivalirudin monitored with the ecarin clotting time for anticoagulation during cardiopulmonary bypass. Anesth Analg 2003;96:383–386.

58. Avendano A, Ferguson JJ. Comparison of Hemochron and HemoTec activated coagulation time target values during percutaneous transluminal coronary angioplasty. J Am Coll Cardiol 1994;23:907–910.

59. McGarry TF, Gottlieb RS, Morganroth J, Zelenkofske SL, Kasparian H, Duca PR, Lester RM, Kreulen TH. The relationship of anticoagulation level and complications after successful percutaneous transluminal coronary angioplasty. Am Heart J 1992;123:1445–1451.

60. Ferguson JJ, Dougherty KG, Gaos CM, Bush HS, Marsh KC, Leachman DR. Relation between procedural activated coagulation time and outcome after percutaneous transluminal coronary angioplasty. J Am Coll Cardiol 1994;23:1061–1065.

61. Narins CR, Hillegass WB, Nelson CL, Tcheng JE, Harrington RA, Phillips HR, Stacks RS, Califf RM. Relation between activated clotting time during angioplasty and abrupt closure. Circulation 1996;93:667–671.

62. Bittl JA, Ahmed WH. Relation between abrupt vessel closure and the anticoagulant response to heparin or bivalirudin during coronary angioplasty. Am J Cardiol 1998;82:50P–56P.

63. Popma JJ, Coller BS, Ohman EM, Bittl JA, Weitz J, Kuntz RE, Leon MB. Antithrombotic therapy in patients undergoing coronary angioplasty. Chest 1995;108:486S–501S.

64. The EPILOG Investigators. Platelet glycoprotein IIb/IIIa receptor blockade and low dose heparin during percutaneous coronary revascularization. N Engl J Med 1997;336:1689–1696.

65. The EPIC Investigators. Use of a monoclonal antibody directed against the platelet glycoprotein IIb/IIIa receptor in high-risk coronary angioplasty. N Engl J Med 1994;330:956–61.

66. Lincoff AM, Tcheng JE, Califf RM, Bass T, Popma JJ, Teirstein PS, Kleiman NS, Hattel LJ, Anderson HV, Ferguson JJ, Cabot CF, Anderson KM, Berdan LG, Musco MH, Weisman HF, Topol EJ. Standard vs. low-dose weight-adjusted heparin in patients treated with the platelet glycoprotein IIb/IIIa receptor antibody fragment abciximab (c7E3 Fab) during percutaneous coronary revascularization. PROLOG Investigators. Am J Cardiol 1997;79:286–291.

67. Moliterno DJ, Califf RM, Aguirre FV, Anderson K, Sigmon KH, Weisman HF, Topol EJ. Effect of platelet glycoprotein IIb/IIIa integrin blockade on activated clotting time during percutaneous transluminal coronary angioplasty or directional atherectomy (the EPIC trial). Evaluation of c7E3 Fab in the Prevention of Ischemic Complications trial. Am J Cardiol 1995; 75:559–562.

68. Dauerman HL, Ball SA, Goldberg RJ, Desourdy MA, Furman MI. Activated clotting times in the setting of eptifibatide use during percutaneous coronary intervention. J Thromb Thrombolysis 2002;13:127–132.

69. Casserly IP, Topol EJ, Jia G, Lange RA, Hamm C, Meier B, DiBattiste PM, Lakkis N, Chew DP, Stone GW, Cohen DJ, Moliterno DJ. Effect of abciximab vs. tirofiban on activated clotting time during percutaneous intervention and its relation to clinical outcomes--observations from the TARGET trial. Am J Cardiol 2003;92:125–129.

70. The EPISTENT Investigators. Randomized placebo-controlled and balloon angioplasty controlled trial to assess safety of coronary stenting with use of platelet glycoprotein IIb/IIIa blockade. Lancet 1998;352:87–92.

71. The IMPACT-II Investigators. Randomized, placebo-controlled trial of effect of eptifibatide on complications of percutaneous coronary intervention: IMPACT-II. Lancet 1997;349: 1422–1428.

72. Brener S, Barr L, Burchenal J, Katz S, George BS, Jones AA, Cohen ED, Gainey PC, White H, Cheek HB, Moses JW, Moliterno DJ, Effron MB, Topol EJ. Randomized, placebo-controlled trial of platelet glycoprotein IIb/IIIa blockade with primary angioplasty for acute myocardial infarction. Circulation 1998;98:734–741.

73. Bittl JA, Strony J, Brinker JA, Ahmed WH, Meckel CR, Chaitman BR, Maraganore J, Deutsch E, Adelman B. Treatment with bivalirudin (Hirulog) as compared with heparin during coronary angioplasty for unstable or postinfarction angina. Hirulog Angioplasty Study Investigators. N Engl J Med 1995;333:764–769.

74. Chew D, Bhatt D, Lincoff A, Moliterno DJ, Brener SJ, Wolski KE, Topol EJ. Defining the optimal activated clotting time during percutaneous coronary intervention. Aggregate results from 6 randomized, controlled trials. Circulation 2001;103:961–966.

75. Moliterno D, Hermiller J, Kereiakes D, Yow E, Applegate RI, Braden GA, Dippel EJ, Furman MI, Grimes CL, Kleiman NS, Levine GN, MANN T 3rd, Nair RN, Stine RA, Yacubov SJ, Tcheng JE, ELECT Investigators. A Novel Point-of-Care Enoxaparin Monitor for Use During Percutaneous Coronary Intervention Results of the Evaluating Enoxaparin Clotting Times (ELECT) Study. J Am Coll Cardiol 2003;42:1132–1139.

76. Collet J, Montalescot G, Lison L, Choussat R, Ankri A, Drobinski G, Sotirov I, Thomas D. Percutaneous coronary intervention after subcutaneous enoxaparin pretreatment in patients with unstable angina pectoris. Circulation 2001;103:658–663.

77. Kereiakes D, Kleiman N, Fry E, Mwawasi G, Lengerich R, Maresh K, Burkert ML, Aquilina JW, Deloof M, Broderick TM, Shimshak TM. Dalteparin in combination with abciximab during percutaneous coronary intervention. Am Heart J 2001;141:348–352.

78. Martin J, Fry E, Serano A. Pharmacokinetic study of enoxaparin in patients undergoing coronary intervention after treatment with subcutaneous enoxaparin in acute coronary syndromes: the PEPCI Study [abstr]. Eur Heart J 2001;22(suppl):14.

79. Choussat R, Montalescot G, Collet J, Vicaut E, Ankri A, Gallois V, Drobinski G, Sotirov I, Thomas D. A unique, low dose of intravenous enoxaparin in elective percutaneous coronary intervention. J Am Coll Cardiol 2002;40:1943–1950.

80. Zabel KM, Granger CB, Becker RC, Bouill EG, Hirsh J, Aylward PE, Topol EJ. Use of bedside activated partial thromboplastin time monitor to adjust heparin dosing after thrombolysis for acute myocardial infarction: results of GUSTO-I. Global Utilization of Streptokinase and TPA for Occluded Coronary Arteries. Am Heart J 1998;136:868–76.

81. The PARAGON Investigators. International, randomized, controlled trial of lamifiban (a platelet glycoprotein IIb/IIIa inhibitor), heparin, or both in unstable angina. Circulation 1998;97: 2386–2395.

82. Newby LK, Harrington RA, Bhapkar MV, Van de Werf F, Hochman JS, Granger CB, Simes RJ, Davis GG, Topol EJ, Califf RM, Moliterno DJ, PARAGON A Investigators. An automated strategy for bedside aPTT determination and unfractionated heparin infusion adjustment in acute coronary syndromes: insights from PARAGON A. J Thromb Thrombolysis 2002;14: 33 42.

# 23
# Bedside Platelet Monitoring

**Debabrata Mukherjee**
*University of Michigan*
*Ann Arbor, Michigan*

**David J. Moliterno**
*Cleveland Clinic Foundation*
*Cleveland, Ohio*

## INTRODUCTION

Platelet tests measure the functional capacity of platelets to adhere, activate, aggregate, and secrete. The goal of platelet function testing is to provide information about the platelet contributions to the risk of thrombotic or hemorrhagic events. Important clinical questions in acute coronary syndromes are whether an antiplatelet agent is having the desired effect on platelet inhibition (efficacy) and whether the patient has sufficient residual platelet function to avoid bleeding (safety). While the role of aspirin and thienopyridines is well established in management of coronary artery disease and in the setting of coronary interventions continued refinement in dosing and patient response continues. Likewise, the last decade has demonstrated the unequivocal efficacy of intravenously administered platelet glycoprotein (GP) IIb/IIIa antagonists in the management of acute coronary syndromes and in the setting of percutaneous interventions.

Twenty-five years ago, an important insight into the molecular basis for platelet aggregation was provided by the discovery that two major membrane glycoprotein bands, GP II and GP III, were missing from the surface of thrombasthenic platelets [1]. To date, more than 100,000 patients with ischemic heart disease have been treated in clinical trials with a new class of potent and highly effective antiplatelet agents, specifically targeting this IIb/IIIa receptor [2]. Three such parenteral drugs have been licensed by the US Food and Drug Administration (abciximab, eptifibatide, and tirofiban) and have been tested for two different clinical indications, percutaneous coronary interventions, and acute coronary syndromes.

## IIB/IIIA EFFICACY

In patients with acute coronary syndromes, GP IIb/IIIa inhibitors have shown a pronounced reduction in the 30-day composite endpoint of death, non fatal myocardial infarction, or urgent revascularization. The greatest benefit was seen among patients with positive troponin and those undergoing early percutaneous coronary intervention (PCI) [3]. Three-year follow-up of the patients who entered the first placebo-controlled PCI trial (EPIC) with an acute coronary syndrome demonstrated a 60% decrease in mortality among those receiving abciximab [4]. The most impressive effect of mortality reduction with GP IIb/IIIa was reported in EPISTENT with a 58% reduction in 1-year mortality among stented patients treated with abciximab [5]. Empiric treatment (i.e., not necessarily associated with PCI) with eptifibatide or tirofiban for unstable angina or non–Q-MI has been shown to reduce death or myocardial infarction by 10–35%, and the effects are persistent at 6 months [6,7]. The ESPRIT trial tested the hypothesis that a new double-bolus dose of eptifibatide (two boluses of 180 μg/kg bolus 10 minutes apart and an infusion of 2 μg/kg/min) would improve outcome among patients undergoing PCI with coronary stenting [8]. Previously, a lower dose of 135 μg/kg bolus followed by a 0.5 μg/kg/min continuous infusion for 20 to 24 hours had been shown to be less effective [9]. Of the 2,064 patients enrolled in the ESPRIT trial, 1,024 were randomly assigned to placebo and 1,040 received eptifibatide and 372 (18%) had an acute coronary syndrome. The primary endpoint was the composite of death, MI, urgent TVR, and thrombotic bailout GP IIb/IIIa inhibitor at 48 hours, and the secondary end point was the composite of death, MI, and urgent target vessel TVR at 30 days. In the ESPRIT trial, patients treated with eptifibatide had a 37% relative risk reduction (10.5% vs. 6.6%; 95% confidence interval, 0.47 to 0.84; P = 0.002) in the primary end point and 35% risk reduction (10.5% vs. 6.8%; confidence interval, 0.49 to 0.87; P = 0.003) in the secondary end point. These impressive benefits using a higher dosing regimen of eptifibatide were not only present in the setting of contemporary treatment strategies including thienopyridines and coronary stents, but they were also maintained through 12 months of follow-up [8]. The TARGET trial tested the noninferiority of tirofiban compared to abciximab among patients expected to undergo PCI with coronary stenting [10]. Of all patients enrolled in the trial, 63% presented with acute coronary syndromes. The primary endpoint of the study was a composite of 30-day death, nonfatal MI, or urgent target-vessel revascularization. This head-to-head comparison between tirofiban and abciximab showed that treatment with abciximab among patients undergoing PCI with coronary stenting was significantly better at 30 days. The incidence of the primary endpoint was lower among patients treated with abciximab (6.0% vs. 7.6%; P = 0.038). Important prespecified subgroup analyses included patients with acute coronary syndromes and there was a 32% risk reduction among patients presenting with acute coronary syndromes (hazard ratio, 1.49; 95% confidence interval, 1.15 to 1.93) [10]. Several groups have demonstrated that the current bolus dosing of tirofiban in patients undergoing coronary intervention for unstable angina is suboptimal with less than a third of the patients achieving greater than or equal to 80% platelet aggregation inhibition [11,12]. There remains significant variability in efficacy among the studies. The GOLD study demonstrated that the extent of percent platelet inhibition was strongly and independently associated with the composite ischemic end point with an odds ratio of 0.44 for those achieving greater than 95% inhibition (P = .019) [13].

Both eptifibatide [14] and tirofiban [6,7] have been shown to be beneficial in the medical management of patients with acute coronary syndromes, however abciximab has not been shown to have any significant benefit [15]. It remains unclear how much of the apparent difference in efficacy among the agents is related to the clinical setting or trial design or drug itself or the extent and duration of antiplatelet effect. It has been postulated that the protracted inhibition afforded by the antibody fragment or its binding to other integrins may explain some of the interagent differences in clinical outcome.

## IIB/IIIA SAFETY

In early PCI trials, GP IIb/IIIa blockade was associated with a higher rate of bleeding complications [16,17]. This was subsequently learned to be due to excessive and prolonged concurrent heparin administration and delayed sheath removal. Thus, later trials which incorporated reduced weight-adjusted heparin regimens and earlier sheath removal demonstrated no excess in major bleeding as compared with placebo [5,7,9]. However, there remains an increase in minor bleeding with these agents, and it is conceivable that "optimal dosing" of the GP IIb/IIIa antagonist would further reduce bleeding complications. Previous studies have suggested that more than 80% of GP IIb/IIIa receptors must be occupied for the antagonist to block thrombus formation, and that receptor blockade more than 90% may increase the risk of bleeding [18]. Likewise, the frequency of thrombocytopenia (less than 100,000 platelets/$\mu$L) is low with the intravenously used GP IIb/IIIa agents (approximately 1%), but better titration of the dosage used may further minimize this side effect.

In addition to abciximab (Reopro, c7E3), two low molecular-weight GP IIb/IIIa antagonists patterned on the arginine-glycine-asparatic acid (RGD) recognition sequence have also shown benefit in the prevention and treatment of ischemic thrombotic coronary artery disease. Correlative studies of the antithrombotic effects of 7E3 compared with its effects on bleeding time, platelet aggregation, and GP IIb/IIIa receptor blockade were performed prior to clinical studies with abciximab [19–21]. These studies provided information for dosing for the first phase III study (EPIC) [16]. Similar preclinical studies have been reported with the other GP IIb/IIIa antagonists [22,23]. The rapid off rates of the low molecular-weight compounds as compared with abciximab made it technically more difficult to directly and accurately assess GP IIb/IIIa receptor blockade with these agents, but binding studies have been reported with fluorescent and radiolabeled compounds [24,25]. The pharmacokinetics for the synthetic peptide and the nonpeptide GP IIb/IIIa antagonists differ from that of the monoclonal antibody. These small-molecule compounds are renally excreted, and dosage infusion rates likely need to be adjusted in patients with significant renal insufficiency.

## CURRENT QUESTIONS

The widespread use of GP IIb/IIIa antagonists as therapeutic agents, the varied results from their clinical trials, and known interpatient variability has raised several important questions:

- What is the extent of interindividual variability in dose-response (blockade of platelet aggregation) with the current weight-adjusted GP IIb/IIIa bolus?
- Is variability in dose-response associated with clinical (ischemic or bleeding) events?
- Could patient-specific bolus dosing (beyond weight adjustment) improve efficacy or safety of therapy?
- Is there interpatient or intrapatient variability in platelet blockade over time (i.e., during the drug infusion period)?
- Could monitoring and adjustment of the drug infusion improve outcome?
- Are there differences among drugs in this class (antibody, peptides, nonpeptides) regarding predictability of response?
- What is the optimal target to measure: plasma drug levels, number of IIb/IIIa receptors occupied, percentage of IIb/IIIa receptors blocked, or extent of aggregation inhibition?
- What is the best agonist (collagen, ADP, TRAP) and at what concentration (1 $\mu$M, 10 $\mu$M, 20 $\mu$M) for the assay?

- Would a functional assay (e.g., clot formation in whole blood) be more clinically relevant than a platelet-specific (platelet rich plasma) assay?
- Can an ideal assay be developed which is rapid, simple, accurate and inexpensive?

## PLATELET RECEPTOR AGONISTS

Platelet activation can be induced by a variety of chemical and mechanical methods that work through several distinct intracellular pathways (Fig. 1). Recognition of these pathways and their associated receptors and ligands is important in assessing platelet function. Agonists are classified as weak or strong with strong agonists leading to platelet degranulation, exteriorization of GP IIb/IIIa receptors and release of fibrinogen from the alpha granules. Several agonists are shown in Figure 1. Historically, adenosine diphosphate (ADP) has been the agonist most commonly used for turbidimetric aggregation studies. The aggregatory response to ADP is concentration dependent. Aggregation in response to low concentrations of ADP (1–5 μM) is spontaneously reversible, whereas aggregation induced by higher concentrations (10–20 μM) is not [26]. Most physiological studies of congenital platelet defects have been performed using concentrations of 1–5 μM ADP or less [27,28]. Studies of GP IIb/IIIa antagonists have required more intense stimulation of the platelets in order to discriminate among doses and have been conducted using concentrations of 10–20 μM [29,30).

The strength of collagen as an agonist also depends on the concentration used. The relevance of collagen as an agonist stems from the abundance of collagen in the subendothelium and exposure at the time of arterial injury. Unlike ADP-induced aggregation, aggregation in response to collagen is sensitive to the effects of aspirin. The use of collagen as an agonist is limited by variability between production lots that occurs at the time of harvest. Arachidonic acid and thromboxane $A_2$ are weak platelet agonists that are completely inhibited by aspirin. Arachidonic acid-induced platelet aggregation is sometimes used to assess compliance with aspirin therapy.

Thrombin is the most potent platelet agonist and in addition to stimulating aggregation, it also stimulates platelet degranulation. The use of α-thrombin as a platelet agonist

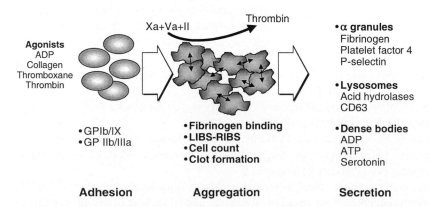

**Figure 1**   Platelets can respond to over 100 different agonists. When they do, they activate and may aggregate releasing vasoconstrictors, inhibitors of thrombolysis, and growth factors. Importantly, thrombin is generated on the platelet lipid-rich surface.

has been well accepted. However, thrombin-induced platelet aggregation has several limitations including lot-to-lot variability, storage requirements, and thrombin's ability to activate the clotting cascade and thus interfere with the assay. Recently, a thrombin receptor agonist peptide (TRAP) has been used in place of thrombin to allow activation of platelets through the thrombin receptor without activating the clotting cascade. As such, TRAP does not suffer from the limitations affecting the use of thrombin and the peptide can be produced inexpensively. The substitution of isoserine for serine has led to the development of iso-TRAP, which is more resistant than TRAP to degradation by the plasma enzyme aminopeptidase and yields more reproducible results [31]. When aggregation to ADP or collagen is blocked, stimulation with TRAP is able to recruit more activated receptors to the platelet surface and can still produce aggregation [32,33]. Increasing the plasma concentration of GP IIb/IIIa antagonist can further block this aggregation [32]. TRAP is thus useful for discriminating effects of higher doses of GP IIb/IIIa antagonists when ADP-induced aggregation appears to be inhibited maximally. It is commonly used in concentrations of 5–10 μM.

## GP IIB/IIIA ANTAGONIST PHARMACODYNAMICS

The dose response curves of GP IIb/IIIa antagonists are generally considered steep. Figure 2 shows receptor blockade and platelet aggregation response to 5 μM of ADP in subjects

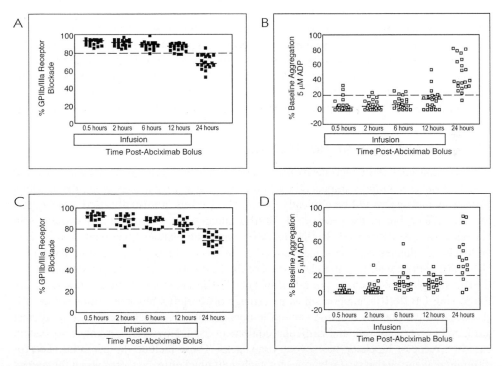

**Figure 2**   GP IIb/IIIa receptor blockade (**A** and **C**) and platelet aggregation response to 5 μmol/L ADP (**B** and **D**) of subjects who received 0.25-mg/kg bolus and 12-hour infusion of abciximab. Degrees of GP IIb/IIIa receptor blockade and platelet aggregation are expressed as percent of baseline values. Symbols represent individual subject values; solid lines, median values; and dashed line, 80% blockade of both GP IIb/IIIa receptors and aggregation. A and B, Test subjects who received 10 μg/min (non-weight-adjusted; n = 24) infusion regimen. (From Ref. 33a)

who received 0.25 mg/kg bolus and 12-hour infusion of abciximab. There is little inhibition of platelet aggregation initiated by ADP and similar antagonists until more than 50% of the receptors are blocked [20,34]. At a greater than 80% GP IIb/IIIa receptor blockade, platelet aggregation with conventional agonists is nearly abolished [20,34]. However, giving an additional dose of either antibody 10E5 or 7E3 (both of which block IIb/IIIa), to animals that already have complete inhibition of platelet aggregation, causes further prolongation of bleeding time results demonstrating that the additional antibody has functional consequences which are not detected by turbidimetric aggregometry [35].

For acute GP IIb/IIIa inhibition during coronary interventions, monitoring may not be necessary if a dosing regimen consistently achieves adequate receptor blockade in all patients and if there is no increase in clinical hemorrhage in patients having the greatest receptor blockade. Previous studies of the pharmacokinetics of abciximab support the hypothesis that most, but not all, patients achieve and sustain greater than or equal to 80% threshold level with the current dose of 0.25 mg/kg bolus and infusion of either 10 µg/min or 0.125 µg/kg/min [29,36,37]. However, some individual variations in receptor blockade have been observed [29,37,38], and as demonstrated by Mascelli et al. [36], mean GP IIb/IIIa receptor blockade was approximately 80% at 6 and 12 hours after therapy was initiated, so some patients were below this level. The theoretical peak whole-blood level of abciximab exceeds the amount of antibody required to fully saturate the GP IIb/IIIa receptors on a normal number of circulating platelets by approximately two-fold. Despite this, it is plausible that patients with thrombocytosis or more activated receptors per platelet will not achieve as high a degree of receptor blockade as patients with normal platelet counts. A systematic assessment of the effects of elevated platelet counts on the efficacy of abciximab would be desirable and dose adjustments have the potential to improve efficacy. Assessment of receptor blockade after discontinuation of GP IIb/IIIa may also be important in determining the return of normal platelet function. This information can help physicians decide whether platelet transfusions or more time for renal clearance is necessary before surgery or other invasive procedures. In general, there is little hemostatic compromise at receptor blockade levels less than 50%.

## GP IIB/IIIA ANTAGONIST MONITORING

An important question which needs to be answered is the optimum way to monitor GP IIb/IIIa dose to potentially impact clinical outcome. Table 1 lists some scenarios in which platelet monitoring would be clinically useful. Drug levels are usually used as surrogate for drug effect, but in the case of GP IIb/IIIa antagonists, interindividual variations in platelet count, density of GP IIb/IIIa receptors, intrinsic platelet functional competence, or levels of platelet cofactors may affect the response to a given plasma level of a GP IIb/IIIa antagonist. It is not clear whether the best parameter is the percentage of GP IIb/IIIa receptors blocked or the effect of GP IIb/IIIa antagonism on platelet function. Expressing GP IIb/IIIa antagonism as percentage of receptors blocked avoids some variables that affect platelet function such as anticoagulant use, platelet preparation, agonist used, end point measured, and particular equipment used. However, a monitoring system based on receptor blockade has several drawbacks. These include the potential need for different reagents and assay techniques for each individual drug, concerns about the impact of variability in drug uptake by platelets on the result of binding studies, need for expensive equipment, and technical expertise with the current assays used. The original correlation between receptor blockade and inhibition of platelet function were based on studies of apparently normal individuals, and extrapolation of these data to a wider population of patients with chronic illnesses that may affect platelet functioning, and other concurrent medications may not be justified.

**Table 1** List of Scenarios in Which Platelet Monitoring Would be Clinically Useful

Patient
    Confirm 80% aggregation inhibition
        Prior to PCI
        In patients with refractory ischemia on IIb/IIIa inhibitors
        Interruption of intravenous therapy
        Abnormal platelet count
        Renal insufficiency
        High or low body-weight
Clinical
    Bleeding
        Confirm excess inhibition
        Guidance during reversal of therapy
    Emergent Surgery
        Confirm 50% aggregation inhibition
        Guidance to reverse therapy if needed
Other
    Drug-specific
        Switching among intravenous agents
        Combination with other antiplatelet/anticoagulants
        Aspirin resistance
        Clopidogrel – CYP3A4 interaction

Using a ''functional'' platelet assay to monitor GP IIb/IIIa therapy has the advantage of directly assessing the goal of therapy as well as integrating the effects of nearly all the variables listed above. For example, standard doses of a GP IIb/IIIa antagonist may be excessive in patients with low platelet counts, on other medications which affect platelet function, or illnesses that may affect platelet function. Another major advantage of a ''functional assay'' is that a single assay may be applicable to monitor the available GP IIb/IIIa antagonists.

Conventional turbidimetric platelet aggregometry using citrated platelet-rich plasma is the most accepted and widely used method of testing platelet function but involves sample preparation, extensive quality control, operator experience and expensive equipment. Also, the calcium chelation caused by citrate anticoagulation may artifactually enhance the inhibition observed with some GP IIb/IIIa antagonists such as eptifibatide [39]. Citrate chelation reduces the $Ca^{2+}$ concentration of PRP to 40 to 50 $\mu$mol/L, partially removing Ca2+ from the divalent cation binding sites on GP IIb/IIIa. Although the reduced $Ca^{2+}$ lowers the affinity of fibrinogen for GP IIb/IIIa on the surface of activated platelets, sufficient binding persists to allow for platelet aggregation. Reduced $Ca^{2+}$ simultaneously increases the binding of eptifibatide, possibly because eptifibatide and $Ca^{2+}$ occupy overlapping sites on GP IIb/IIIa. The increased binding of eptifibatide to GP IIb/IIIa and the decreased binding of fibrinogen together serve to increase the inhibitory activity of eptifibatide.

The characteristics of an ideal platelet function assay includes the requirements of a small amount of whole blood, the requirement of minimal processing or pipetting, and the availability of accurate results within a few minutes. Table 2 shows the desired characteristics of an ideal test. For obvious reasons, undiluted whole blood is preferable for bedside testing rather than PRP as it involves an extra processing step. Tests, which involve

**Table 2**   Characteristics
of an Ideal Platelet Assay

- Whole blood
- No pipetting or exposure
- No reagent preparation
- Small sample
- Small device (POCT)
- Ease of use
- Automated
- Quick
- Inexpensive
- Easily interpretable
- Accurate
- Reliable
- Reproducible

dilution of whole blood, may not accurately measure inhibition due to low-molecular agents with rapid GP IIb-IIIa off rates. There is currently no test, which fulfills all the criteria for an ideal test. There is also no certain gold standard against which other tests can be compared and little data regarding clinical outcomes using the currently available tests.

## PLATELET FUNCTION TEST

Table 3 lists the currently available platelet function tests, their substrates and principles of assessment.

### Ivy Bleeding Time

Bleeding time evaluates primary hemostasis (platelet adhesion, release reaction, aggregation and primary plug formation) and assesses an overall functional ability of platelets to form a thrombus.

**Table 3**   List of the Commonly Available Platelet Function Assays, Their Substrate, and Principles of Assessment

|                              | Whole blood | Platelet rich plasma (PRP) | Pont-of-care test | Principle             |
| ---------------------------- | ----------- | -------------------------- | ----------------- | --------------------- |
| Ivy bleeding time            | Y           |                            | +                 | Primary hemostasis    |
| Light transmission aggregometry |         | Y                          |                   | Aggregation           |
| Flow cytometry               | Y           |                            |                   | Activation            |
| Thromboelastograph           | Y           |                            |                   | Clot strength         |
| PFA-100                      | Y           |                            | +                 | Primary hemostasis    |
| Clot signature analyzer      | Y           |                            | +                 | Adhesion, Aggregation |
| Plateletworks                | Y           |                            | +                 | Aggregation           |
| Rapid Platelet Function assay | Y          |                            | +                 | Aggregation           |

This is a rapid, noninvasive test that can assess overall platelet function. However, the test requires a dedicated technologist and can take up to 30 minutes to perform. Also the accuracy, validity, and predictability of this test are not proven. A number of other patient and technique-related factors may affect bleeding time. The normal range of bleeding time is 7–10 minutes.

## Light Transmission Aggregometry

This is the most commonly practiced assay of platelet function. Instruments used with this technique include the Chrono-Log (Havertown, PA), Bio-Data (Hatboro, PA), Payton-Scientific (Buffalo, NY) and Helena Laboratories (Beaumont, TX). For this assay platelet rich plasma (PRP) and platelet poor plasma (PPP) are prepared from citrated blood, pipetted into matched cuvettes, placed in the appropriate positions in the instrument and equilibrated at 37°C. The instrument is calibrated so that the amount of light transmitted through the PPP is defined as 100% aggregation and light transmitted through unstimulated PRP is defined as 0% aggregation. In some laboratories, platelet count in the PRP is adjusted by the addition of PPP to achieve a standardized count between 250,000 and 350,000/μL [40]. Aggregation is initiated by adding a measured aliquot of platelet agonist such as ADP, collagen, or epinephrine. Stirring is achieved by means of a magnetic stirbar and the change in light transmitted through the PRP monitored. As aggregation proceeds, large platelet aggregates form, turbidity decreases, and light transmitted through the sample is increased. The light received through the sample is converted into electrical signals, amplified and recorded. Results are expressed as percentage of aggregation. Figure 3 illustrates the principles of this assay.

*Clinical Utility*

This widely available method has been used for more than 30 years. This method can be standardized, is well accepted, and has been most widely used for clinical correlation. The process however, is laborious, time consuming, and limited by the optical quality of the PRP. The centrifugation step involved in the procedure may also modulate platelet behavior

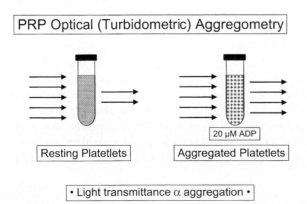

**Figure 3** In photo-optical turbidimetric aggregometry, as platelets aggregate more light is able to pass through the sample and this light is converted into an electrical signal.

as a subpopulation of platelets may be lost during centrifugation. Hospitals may standardize their tests differently, and it is often somewhat difficult to compare results from one clinical site with those of another using this test. Clinical areas of variation in procedure include PRP (preparation, centrifugation), use of adjusted or unadjusted platelet count, cuvette size, stirbar speed, choice of agonist or agonist concentration, paper speed and use of aggregation vs. slope of aggregation as the primary end-point. This method is useful in detecting platelet function defects in patients with congenital or acquired bleeding disorders. This assay has been used for phase II studies for drug development of GP IIb/IIIa inhibitors and can be used clinically, although it is time consuming. A rapid assay using this principle yet limiting pitfalls of variability, would be ideal.

## Flow Cytometry

Flow cytometry can rapidly measure specific characteristics of a large number of individual platelets. In response to agonists such as thrombin, collagen, or ADP, a spectrum of specific activation-dependent modifications of platelet surface antigens can be detected. This process leads to an intracellular signal transduction cascade involving ion fluxes and activation of the cytoskeleton. The end result is secretion of endosomes, which causes reorganization and conformational changes of surface receptor expression through inside-out signaling. Platelet activation also leads to an altered expression of already constitutively expressed surface glycoproteins. Increased numbers of GP IIb/IIIa complexes and reduced numbers of GP Ib-IX complexes result from bidirectional trafficking of these glycoproteins between the cell surface, the surface-connected canalicular system and intracellular storage. Inside-out signaling leads to conformational changes of GP IIb-IIIa complexes, exposing conformation-dependent activation epitopes with high affinity for their ligands. The release reaction of platelets is associated with the neoexpression of a-granule glycoproteins such as CD62P or CD63. Thus measuring the expression of these antigens on circulating platelets reflects not only the activation state of the platelets but also the extent to which secretion has occurred.

Flow cytometry is a sensitive and rapid research-specific tool for the study of both inherited and acquired platelet disorders by quantitation of the surface expression of the principal adhesion and aggregation receptors (GPIb-IX, GP IIb/IIIa) and of secreted platelet proteins (CD62P, CD63, thrombospondin, fibrinogen). Conformational changes in platelet glycoproteins, especially GP IIb/IIIa, can be measured using monoclonal antibodies recognizing receptor-induced binding sites (RIBS) on the ligand, or ligand-induced binding sites (LIBS) on the receptor. Increased amount of platelet-bound ligands such as fibrinogen, von Willebrand Factor, P-selectin, or thrombospondin can be quantified using ligand-directed antibodies.

To perform cytometry platelets are labeled with a fluorescent-conjugated monoclonal antibody and placed in the flow chamber. The cells are passed at a rate of 1,000 to 10,000 cells per minute through the focused light beam of a laser. Exposure of labeled cells to light at the excitation wavelength results in emitted fluorescence, which is detected and processed along with the forward and side light scattering properties of the cell. Activation state of circulating platelets is assessed with an activation-dependent monoclonal antibody. Such antibodies bind strongly to activated platelets and weakly or undetectably to unstimulated platelets. The number of fluorescent platelets is directly related to the activation of the pathway being assessed.

### Clinical Utility

In addition to the benefits of whole blood analysis and a small amount of blood required, the minimal handling of samples needed prevents artifactual in vitro platelet activation.

Also, with this assay both the activation state and the reactivity of platelets can be assessed. The disadvantages include the need for expensive equipment, and a dedicated technologist. Flow cytometry is helpful in assessing specific platelet functions, activity, and hyperreactivity. Thus, this test can be used to monitor the inhibition of the GP IIb/IIIa receptor by specific antagonists, but its use is mainly limited to use as a research tool.

## Thromboelastography

Thromboelastography measures clot strength [41]. A clot is allowed to form between a cup and a sensing device (pin suspended from a torsion wire). Platelet participation in clot retraction results in increased fibrin rigidity. In this device, Figure 4a (Thromboelastograph Coagulation analyzer, Haemoscope, Morton Grove, IL), the cup is oscillated and the transduction of the oscillatory movement to the torsion wire is measured and represented graphically. The measurement is most directly related to the physical properties of the clot. Several parameters, reflecting different stages of clot development are measured as shown in Figure 4b. The strength of a clot is graphically represented over time as a characteristic cigar shaped curve. The five parameters of the thromboelastograph tracing: R, K, alpha angle, MA and MA60, measures different stages of a clot development. R is the time from initiation of the test to the initial fibrin formation. K is a measure of the time from the beginning of clot formation until the amplitude of thromboelastogram reaches 20 mm, and represents the dynamics of clot formation. Alpha angle is the angle between the line in the middle of the tracing and the line tangential to the developing body of the tracing. Alpha angle represents the kinetcs of fibrin buildup and cross-linking. MA is the maximum amplitude of movement and reflects the strength of the clot, which is dependent on the number and function of platelets and its interaction with fibrin. MA60 measures the rate of amplitude reduction 60 minutes after MA and represents the stability of the clot. Platelet function is evaluated at physiologic calcium concentrations and under maximal thrombin generation. The test is allowed to run until clot lysis or retraction occurs, which can take up to one hour.

### Clinical Utility

This method uses whole blood and assesses multiple components of thrombosis. However, the method requires considerable time, is cumbersome and requires pipetting. Recently a modified thromboelastographic method was described for monitoring heparinized patients receiving abciximab [42]. Addition of abciximab in vitro resulted in a linearly dose-dependent reduction in clot strength and platelet force. The method currently available is unlikely to be applicable to rapid point-of-care testing.

## PFA-100 Analyzer

The Dade Behring (Miami, FL) platelet function analyzer (PFA-100) evaluates primary hemostasis through platelet-platelet interaction as whole blood flows under shear stress conditions through an aperture [43]. The instrument (Fig. 5) uses citrated whole blood which is drawn by means of a vacuum through a capillary tube producing high shear forces and then through a precisely defined aperture in a membrane that has been coated with either collagen and epinephrine or collagen and ADP. The platelets adhere and aggregate at the aperture until it is occluded, and the results reported as a closure time. The testing process takes about ten minutes. Occlusion is blocked by antibodies directed at GP Ib, vWF, GP IIb/IIIa, as well as RGD containing peptides, which suggests a critical

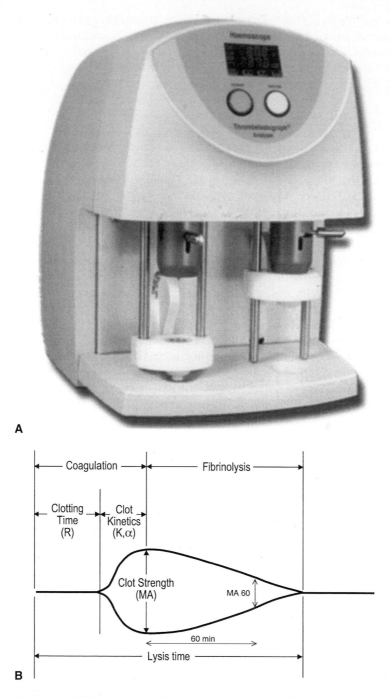

**Figure 4** (**A**) The thromboelastograph instrument. (**B**) The five parameters of the thromboelastograph tracing: R, K, Alpha-angle, MA, and MA60 which measures different stages of clot development.

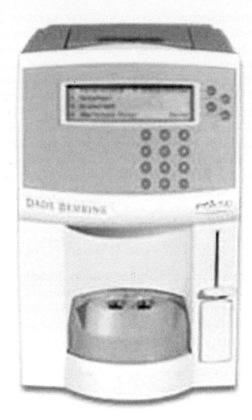

A

## Platelet Function Analyzer (PFA-100)

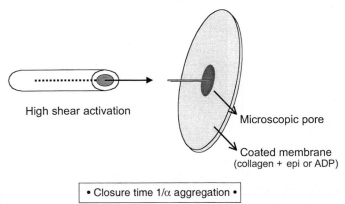

High shear activation

Microscopic pore

Coated membrane
(collagen + epi or ADP)

• Closure time 1/α aggregation •

B

**Figure 5** (**A**) The Platelet Function Analyzer (PFA-100) instrument. (**B**) The PFA-100 Analyzer uses citrated whole blood which is drawn by means of a vacuum through a capillary tube producing high shear forces and then through a precisely defined aperture in a membrane that has been coated with either collagen and epinephrine or collagen and ADP. The platelets adhere and aggregate at the aperture until it is occluded, and the results reported as a closure time.

role for these molecules. A polyclonal antifibrinogen antibody did not permit occlusion, presumably because of the high shear rate involved. The proposed molecular mechanism evaluated in this system: initial binding of vWF by GP Ib followed by GP IIb/IIIa-dependent binding of vWF and possibly collagen is distinct from that of fibrinogen mediated platelet aggregation. This distinction may have clinical relevance because different GP IIb/IIIa inhibitors may preferentially block binding of vWF over fibrinogen or vice-versa. Blood can be collected in routine vacutainer tubes, and can be kept in room temperature for up to 4 hours. The instrument can run two tests in sequence. With the two test cartridges, the dysfunction of platelets caused by aspirin can be detected as a prolonged closure time with collagen/epinephrine cartridge but normal with collagen/ADP cartridge. This is a high shear system generating capillary shear rates on the order of 4000–5000 reciprocal seconds. A constant vacuum of 40 mBar is maintained in the system that mimics the pressure in a microcapillary in the human body.

*Clinical Utility*

This assay evaluates multiple factors involved in primary hemostasis similar to the template bleeding time without the incisional variability. It uses whole blood, is simple to perform, and is quick and automatic. The normal closure time is 100 seconds and the instrument can detect a closure time of up to 300 seconds, so this assay has a limited range. Its usefulness in monitoring GP IIb/IIIa therapy requires further study, but in general the closure times are increased well beyond 300 seconds with GP IIb/IIIa antagonists. The PFA-100 with the collagen-ADP cartridge correlates well with optical aggregometry at lower levels of aggregation inhibition (Fig. 6).

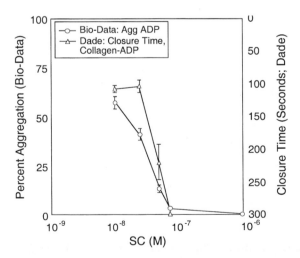

**Figure 6** Closure time (collagen-ADP membrane) and ADP-induced aggregation in PRP. Concentrations of SC ranging from 10−8 to 10−6 mol/L were added to citrated blood samples and added to test cartridge. Sample was through capillary under high shear flow conditions. Sample then passed through aperture in membrane coated with collagen and ADP. Instrument determined time required for occlusion of aperture (closure time). PRP was prepared from same samples by differential centrifugation and ADP-induced aggregation measured The PFA-100 with the collagen-ADP cartridge correlates well with optical aggregometry at lower levels of aggregation. (From Ref. 44a)

## Clot Signature Analyzer

This assay measures several aspects of platelet function and clotting properties. The instrument Clot Signature Analyzer, Figure 7a (Xylum Corporation, Scarsdale, NY), has a collagen channel to simulate the exposure of blood to thrombogenic subendothelial tissue. Blood is perfused over the collagen fiber at a high shear rate (approximately $6200 \text{ s}^{-1}$). Platelets activated by collagen adhere and aggregate to form a thrombus. The clot signature analyzer (CSA) has a punch channel that provides information on platelet function (Fig. 7b). While blood flows through the channel, the channel is punched by a 0.15 mm needle resulting in two fine holes. A high shear rate at the punch point promotes platelet adhesion to the injury site and recruitment of activated platelets and resultant aggregation at the site. A growing fibrin clot gradually occludes the pathway, resulting in reduction of the flow as evidenced by decrease in the pressure. Pressure in millimeters of mercury is plotted against time for both channels to produce a clot signature.

*Clinical Utility*

This is an automated assay that uses whole nonanticoagulated blood under conditions of physiologic flow and temperature. It evaluates both platelet activation and aggregation. These ideal features are somewhat offset since the current instrument is rather large for routine use, and interpretation of the results is complex.

## Plateletworks

Plateletworks (Helena Laboratories, Beumont, TX) is an in vitro diagnostic screening assay for the determination of percentage of platelet aggregation or percentage of platelet inhibition in fresh whole blood samples. The change in platelet count due to activation and aggregation of functional platelets is measured using an electronic impedance-based cell counter. The Plateletworks methodology is an adaptation of platelet aggregometry that is relatively simple, inexpensive, and quick to perform (results are available in about five minutes). This two-step method involves using an automated cell counter to measure total platelet count in a whole blood sample and then to reassess the number of platelets on a second sample that has been exposed to a known platelet agonist. The agonist will stimulate those platelets which are functional to aggregate into clumps, and they will not be counted as platelets in the second sample. The difference in the platelet count between samples one and two provides a direct measurement of platelet aggregation. Platelets rendered inactive or nonfunctional by antiplatelet agents are considered inhibited. The Plateletworks results may be expressed as percent inhibition.

$$\frac{\text{Agonist Platelet Count}}{\text{Baseline Platelet Count}} \times 100 = \text{Inhibition}$$

*Clinical Utility*

The validity of the Plateletworks assay is dependent on the accuracy of the platelet counts obtained. Multiple factors may potentially interfere with the accuracy of the platelet count when performed on an automated cell counter. Therefore, platelet counts obtained should be scrutinized in light of the patient's clinical circumstance and previous platelet count results. This assay has been used clinically to determine the degree of platelet aggregation inhibition with GP IIb/IIIa antagonists [11,44] and with clopidogrel [45,46].

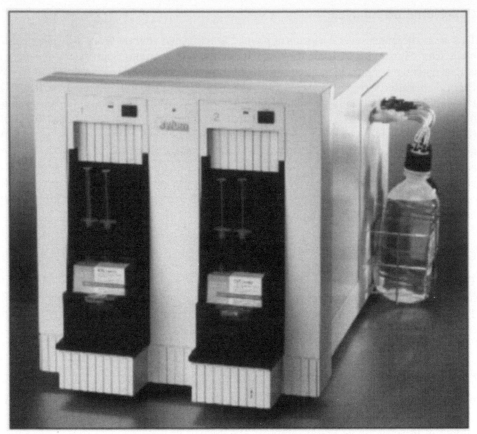

## Clot Signature Analysis (CSA)

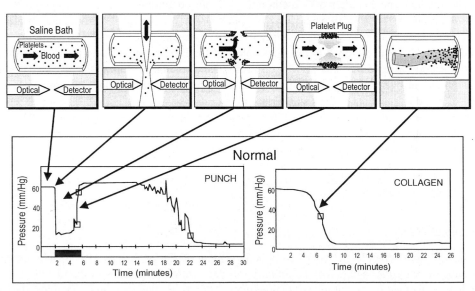

**Figure 7** (**A**) The Clot Signature Analyzer. (**B**) Principle of the Clot Signature Analyzer. The Clot Signature Analyzer has a punch channel that provides information on platelet function.

## Rapid Platelet Function Assay

The *Ultegra*-RPFA (Accumetrics, San Diego, CA) is an automated, whole-blood, cartridge-based, point-of-care device that allows for the rapid and reproducible evaluation of platelet function in patients treated with GP IIb/IIIa inhibitors (Fig. 8). It is designed to assess platelet function utilizing the ability of activated platelets to bind fibrinogen [47]. Fibrinogen-coated polystyrene microparticles agglutinate in whole blood in proportion to the number of unblocked platelet GP IIb/IIIa receptors. Pharmacologic blockade of GP IIb/IIIa receptors prevents this interaction and therefore diminishes agglutination in proportion to the degree of receptor blockade achieved. Because the speed of bead agglutination is more rapid and reproducible if platelets are activated, the thrombin receptor-activating peptide iso-TRAP ([iso-S]FLLRN) is incorporated into the assay.

Blood samples are obtained in either a standard citrate blood tube, or if eptifibatide is the agent being used, PPACK (Phe-Pro-Arg chloromethyl ketone) is utilized for the anticoagulant instead of citrate. The tube is inserted into a disposable plastic cartridge and the blood is automatically drawn into 2 sample channels containing lyophilized iso-TRAP and fibrinogen-coated beads. The sample is then mixed for 70 seconds by the movement of a steel ball driven by a microprocessor. The light absorbance of the sample is measured 16 times per second by an automated detector. As the platelets interact with the fibrinogen-coated beads resulting in agglutination, there is a progressive increase in light transmission. The rate of agglutination is quantified as the slope of the change of absorbance over a fixed time interval and reported as millivolts per 10 seconds (mV/10sec). An individual patient's pre-GP IIb/IIIa inhibitor baseline slope is retained in memory and all additional specimens are reported as the raw slope as well as a percentage of the baseline slope.

*Clinical Utility*

The *Ultegra*-RPFA has several advantages over turbidimetric aggregometry, including: (a) use of whole blood, thus avoiding the need for sample preparation and eliminating

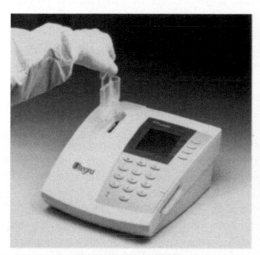
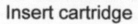
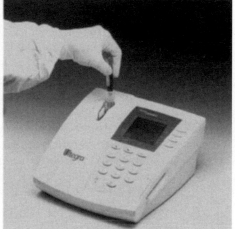

Insert cartridge          Insert Vaccutainer

**Figure 8**   The Rapid Platelet Function Analyzer (™Ultegra) device.

variables in sample preparation, (b) semiautomated format, which avoids operator errors and subjective endpoint assessments, (c) rapid test completion, (d) digital readout, and (e) duplicate analysis to minimize random errors. Studies involving simultaneous measurement of platelet function measured by RPFA and turbidimetric platelet aggregometry induced by 20 µM ADP of samples treated in vivo with increasing doses of abciximab demonstrated a close correlation between the results ($r^2 = 0.95$), as well as between the RPFA results and the percentage of unblocked GP IIb/IIIa receptors assessed directly by radiolabeled monoclonal antibody binding ($r^2 = 0.96$). Similarly, the mean difference in measurements between RPFA and aggregometry was only negative 4% ($\pm 4\%$ SD) and the mean difference in measurements between RPFA and free GP IIb/IIIa receptors was negative 2% ($\pm 6\%$ SD) [48]. A functional assay such as RPFA provides information on the total effect of the agents on platelet function, independent of the agent, and so provides a measure that is likely to be biologically relevant. The disadvantages of RPFA are that it requires a baseline sample comparison, and a specific agonist.

## CLINICAL STUDIES

Several clinical studies have considered platelet function assays and optimal GP IIb/IIIa blockade [12,38,49,50]. These include the PARADISE [38] and the GOLD [49] studies. The PARADISE study involved 100 patients and demonstrated substantial interpatient variability in response to standard, weight-adjusted abciximab. Almost all patients achieved more than 80% of platelet inhibition after an abciximab bolus, but approximately 13% of patients did not maintain this level of inhibition during the infusion. Even a wider range of variability was noted after the termination of the infusion. Although this study was not designed to evaluate clinical outcomes, systematic measuring of postprocedural myocardial enzymes was carried out. Of the 13 patients with platelet function inhibited by less than 80% at 8 hours, six (46%) had an adverse cardiac event. This is in comparison with only five (7%) events among 75 patients with more than 80% inhibition at 8 hours (P < .001). Although not a predefined objective of the study, these results are consistent with the hypothesis that a specific level of platelet inhibition must be maintained to prevent thrombotic complications associated with PCI.

The GOLD study [49] prospectively enrolled 469 patients undergoing elective PCI with adjunctive GP IIb/IIIa therapy. The Rapid Platelet Function Assay (RPFA) device was used to assess percentage of Inhibition of Platelet Aggregation (IPA) at baseline, during PCI, and serially after PCI. The occurrence of death, myocardial infarction, or urgent target revascularization was correlated to the extent of IPA percent during the procedure. Specifically, the incidence of this composite ischemic outcome occurred in 14.4% of patients whose platelets were less than 95% inhibited vs. 6.4% for those whose platelets were greater than 95% inhibited (P = 0.006). A multivariable model was performed on this data set and showed that the extent of percent IPA was strongly and independently correlated to the ischemic end point composite with an odds ratio of 0.44 for those achieving greater than 95% IPA (P = .019). (Figure 9)

In the Do Tirofiban And Reopro Give similar Efficacy outcome Trial (TARGET), a lower 30-day incidence of the combined end point of death, myocardial infarction, and urgent target vessel revascularization was seen in patients treated with abciximab compared with those who received tirofiban [10]. Kabbani et al. studied whether the difference observed reflected suboptimal inhibition of platelet aggregation during the first 2 hours after initiation of treatment with tirofiban using flow cytometry and light transmission aggregometry (51). The inhibition of maximal aggregation was greater 15–60 minutes

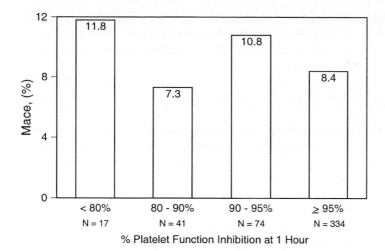

**Figure 9** Data from the GOLD study showing incidence of major adverse cardiac events (MACE) and percent GP IIb/IIIa inhibition. (From Ref. 49)

after onset of treatment with abciximab than with tirofiban when aggregation was induced by 20 M adenosine diphosphate. The average inhibition of maximal aggregation ranged from 90% to 94% from 15 to 45 minutes after initiation of treatment with abciximab and from 61% to 66% after initiation of tirofiban (p < 0.001 at 15, 30, and 45 minutes) [51]. Similarly Herrmann et al. demonstrated that that the dose of tirofiban used in TARGET may not have fully inhibited platelet aggregation at the key time point near the initial balloon inflation [52]. These findings may potentially explain improved clinical outcomes at 30-days with abciximab compared to tirofiban in the TARGET trial. Soffer et al. [11] used the Plateletworks assay to validate that the current bolus dosing of tirofiban in patients undergoing coronary intervention for unstable angina results in inadequate platelet inhibition The pharmacology of higher dose eptifibatide in percutaneous coronary intervention (the PRIDE study) using light transmission aggregometry revealed that double-bolus of eptifibatide at 180 μg/kg bolus followed by a 2.0 μg/kg/min infusion at steady state consistently achieved more than 80% inhibition of platelet aggregation [53]. With the single-bolus regimen, however, there was an early loss of the inhibition of platelet aggregation before steady state was reached. The double-bolus regimen was associated with improved clinical outcomes [54]. The lack of benefit of abciximab in the GUSTO IV study may potentially be due to the lack of sustained platelet inhibition in patients with acute coronary syndrome with the current infusion regimen.

Mukherjee et al. reported several illustrative cases in which platelet monitoring with the Ultegra Rapid Platelet Function Assay was used to guide dosing of a GP IIb/IIIa inhibitor for coronary and peripheral intervention among patients at increased bleeding risk [55]. While GP IIb/IIIa inhibitors are not currently indicated for patients with thrombocytopenia or those on oral anticoagulants, the case series demonstrated that these agents may be used safely and effectively in some of these patients with reduction of GP IIb/IIIa dosage and monitoring of IPΛ% [55].

In summary, GP IIb/IIIa antagonists are becoming the standard of care for patients undergoing PCI and those with ACS. As such, there are many scenarios related to the patient, clinical situation, or other phenomenon whereby monitoring the extent of platelet aggregation inhibition would be useful. Outcome data are becoming available suggesting that a specific extent of %IPA may be optimal. With evolution of monitoring techniques, the hope is that this class of drug can be extended to more patients without increasing bleeding rates. Among those currently receiving therapy, monitoring may not only improve efficacy but also reduce adverse events.

## Aspirin Resistance

Despite proven benefit of aspirin in patients with coronary artery disease there is evidence that a subset of patients may not benefit from aspirin therapy. There are no drugs that are 100% effective, but there appears an identifiable subset of patients in whom aspirin is less efficacious and these individuals are considered aspirin resistant. Gum et al. [56] demonstrated that among patients with cardiac disease, 5–9% are aspirin resistant, and an additional 23% are aspirin semiresponders. Previous studies have demonstrated a significantly higher vascular event rate in aspirin nonresponders [57]. The availability of safe and effective alternate antiplatelet therapy makes the identification of these individuals with bedside platelet monitoring clinically relevant.

## Clopidogrel-Statin Interaction

A recent study suggested that statins metabolized by CYP3A4 such as atorvastatin, may significantly attenuate platelet aggregation inhibition by clopidogrel [46]. Such potential drug interactions with clopidogrel may be particularly important to recognize in patients diagnosed with acute coronary syndromes where clopidogrel may be prescribed for 9 to 12 months. Because many drugs are metabolized by CYP3A4, it is likely that other drugs may affect the efficacy of clopidogrel, making it even more important to determine whether platelet aggregation inhibition targets are being met in individual patients by point-of-care platelet function testing.

## Clopidogrel Resistance Assays

The assessment of platelet inhibitory effect of clopidogrel can be made using flow cytometry [58,59], light transmission aggregometry [60,61] or the Plateletworks assay [45,46]. The agonist used for these assays is ADP. These studies illustrated the variable platelet inhibitory response to the standard administered dose of clopidogrel. These observations, irrespective of the methodology chosen to detect inhibition suggest that the response to clopidogrel therapy is heterogeneous with significant patient variability and resistance in some individuals [60].

## SUMMARY

The use of parenteral platelet GP IIb/IIIa antagonists has been consistently shown to reduce the risk of thrombotic complications in the setting of acute coronary syndrome and PCI. However, many important issues remain unresolved regarding these agents. The ability to rapidly and reproducibly monitor the effects of these agents in individual patients is likely important to optimizing their use. For example, if via monitoring a similarly well-controlled and maintained therapeutic level of IIb/IIIa blockade were obtained using several different agents (antibody vs. small molecule peptidomimetics), more similar clinical outcome may be obtained. The recognition of aspirin resistance in a significant proportion of patients, the interindividual variation in clopidogrel effect and the potential of clopidogrel–CYP3A4 interaction and the availability of alternative effective therapeutic agents for both these scenarios makes recognition of these individuals clinically relevant. CD40, a 48-kDa phosphorylated transmembrane glycoprotein belonging to the TNF receptor superfamily has been described on platelets. Recent studies support a role for CD40-mediated platelet activation in thrombosis, inflammation, and atherosclerosis [62]. Furthermore, elevation of soluble CD40 ligand levels in patients with acute coronary syndrome appears to be associated with an increased risk of cardiovascular events [63]. Elevation of soluble CD40 ligand may identify a subgroup of patients at high-risk who are likely to benefit from antiplatelet treatment with abciximab [63]. Soluble CD40 ligand levels may be used to identify higher degree of platelet reactivity in the future and target these high-risk patients for more effective platelet inhibition.

## REFERENCES

1. Nurden AT, Caen JP. An abnormal platelet glycoprotein pattern in three cases of Glanzmann's thrombasthenia. Br J Haematol 1974;28:253–260.
2. Topol EJ, Byzova TV, Plow EF. Platelet GPIIb-IIIa blockers. Lancet 1999;353:227–231.
3. Boersma E, Harrington RA, Moliterno DJ, White H, Theroux P, Van de Werf F, de Torbal A, Armstrong PW, Wallentin LC, Wilcox RG, Simes J, Califf RM, Topol EJ, Simoons ML. Platelet glycoprotein IIb/IIIa inhibitors in acute coronary syndromes: a meta-analysis of all major randomised clinical trials. Lancet 2002;359:189–198.
4. Topol EJ, Ferguson JJ, Weisman HF, Tcheng JE, Ellis SG, Kleiman NS, Ivanhoe RJ, Wang AL, Miller DP, Anderson KM, Califf RM. Long-term protection from myocardial ischemic events in a randomized trial of brief integrin beta3 blockade with percutaneous coronary intervention. EPIC Investigator Group. Evaluation of Platelet IIb/IIIa Inhibition for Prevention of Ischemic Complication. JAMA 1997;278:479–484.
5. Randomised placebo-controlled and balloon-angioplasty-controlled trial to assess safety of coronary stenting with use of platelet glycoprotein- IIb/IIIa blockade. The EPISTENT Investigators. Evaluation of Platelet IIb/IIIa Inhibitor for Stenting. Lancet 1998;352:87–92.
6. A comparison of aspirin plus tirofiban with aspirin plus heparin for unstable angina. Platelet Receptor Inhibition in Ischemic Syndrome Management (PRISM) Study Investigators. N Engl J Med 1998;338:1498–1505.
7. Inhibition of the platelet glycoprotein IIb/IIIa receptor with tirofiban in unstable angina and non-Q-wave myocardial infarction. Platelet Receptor Inhibition in Ischemic Syndrome Management in Patients Limited by Unstable Signs and Symptoms (PRISM-PLUS) Study Investigators. N Engl J Med 1998;338:1488–1497.
8. O'Shea JC, Buller CE, Cantor WJ, Chandler AB, Cohen EA, Cohen DJ, Gilchrist IC, Kleiman NS, Labinaz M, Madan M, Hafley GE, Califf RM, Kitt MM, Strony J, Tcheng JE. Long-term efficacy of platelet glycoprotein IIb/IIIa integrin blockade with eptifibatide in coronary stent intervention. JAMA 2002;287:618–621.
9. Randomised placebo-controlled trial of effect of eptifibatide on complications of percutaneous coronary intervention: IMPACT-II. Integrilin to Minimise Platelet Aggregation and Coronary Thrombosis-II. Lancet 1997;349:1422–1428.
10. Topol EJ, Moliterno DJ, Herrmann HC, Powers ER, Grines CL, Cohen DJ, Cohen EA, Bertrand M, Neumann FJ, Stone GW, DiBattiste PM, Demopoulos L; TARGET Investigators. Comparison of two platelet glycoprotein IIb/IIIa inhibitors, tirofiban and abciximab, for the prevention of ischemic events with percutaneous coronary revascularization. N Engl J Med 2001; 344:1888–1894.
11. Soffer D, Moussa I, Karatepe M, Harjai KJ, Boura J, Dixon SR, Grines CL, O'Neill WW, Roubin GS, Moses JW. Suboptimal inhibition of platelet aggregation following tirofiban bolus in patients undergoing percutaneous coronary intervention for unstable angina pectoris. Am J Cardiol 2003;91:872–875.

12. Kereiakes DJ, Broderick TM, Roth EM, Whang D, Shimshak T, Runyon JP, Hattemer C, Schneider J, Lacock P, Mueller M, Abbottsmith CW. Time course, magnitude, and consistency of platelet inhibition by abciximab, tirofiban, or eptifibatide in patients with unstable angina pectoris undergoing percutaneous coronary intervention. Am J Cardiol 1999;84:391–395.
13. Steinhubl SR, Talley JD, Braden GA, Tcheng JE, Casterella PJ, Moliterno DJ, Navetta FI, Berger PB, Popma JJ, Dangas G, Gallo R, Sane DC, Saucedo JF, Jia G, Lincoff AM, Theroux P, Holmes DR, Teirstein PS, Kereiakes DJ. A prospective multicenter study to determine the optimal level of platelet inhibition with GP IIb/ IIIa inhibitors in patients undergoing coronary intervention - The GOLD study. J Am Coll Cardiol 2000;35(2):44A.
14. Lincoff A, Califf R, Topol E. Platelet glycoprotein IIb/IIIa receptor blockade in coronary artery disease. J Am Coll Cardiol 2000;35:1103–1115.
15. Simoons ML. Effect of glycoprotein IIb/IIIa receptor blocker abciximab on outcome in patients with acute coronary syndromes without early coronary revascularisation: the GUSTO IV-ACS randomised trial. Lancet 2001;357:1915–1924.
16. Use of a monoclonal antibody directed against the platelet glycoprotein IIb/IIIa receptor in high-risk coronary angioplasty. The EPIC Investigation. N Engl J Med 1994;330:956–961.
17. Randomised placebo-controlled trial of abciximab before and during coronary intervention in refractory unstable angina: the CAPTURE Study. Lancet 1997;349:1429–1435.
18. Chong PH. Glycoprotein IIb/IIIa receptor antagonists in the management of cardiovascular diseases. Am J Health Syst Pharm 1998;55:2363–2386.
19. Gold HK, Gimple LW, Yasuda T, Leinbach RC, Werner W, Holt R, Jordan R, Berger H, Collen D, Coller BS. Pharmacodynamic study of F(ab′)2 fragments of murine monoclonal antibody 7E3 directed against human platelet glycoprotein IIb/IIIa in patients with unstable angina pectoris. J Clin Invest 1990;86:651–659.
20. Coller BS, Scudder LE, Beer J, Gold HK, Folts JD, Cavagnaro J, Jordan R, Wagner C, Iuliucci J, Knight D. Monoclonal antibodies to platelet glycoprotein IIb/IIIa as antithrombotic agents. Ann N Y Acad Sci 1991;614:193–213.
21. Wagner CL, Mascelli MA, Neblock DS, Weisman HF, Coller BS, Jordan RE. Analysis of GPIIb/IIIa receptor number by quantification of 7E3 binding to human platelets. Blood 1996; 88:907–914.
22. Barrett JS, Murphy G, Peerlinck K, De Lepeleire I, Gould RJ, Panebianco D, Hand E, Deckmyn H, Vermylen J, Arnout J. Pharmacokinetics and pharmacodynamics of MK-383, a selective non- peptide platelet glycoprotein-IIb/IIIa receptor antagonist, in healthy men. Clin Pharmacol Ther 1994;56:377–388.
23. Harrington RA, Kleiman NS, Kottke-Marchant K, Lincoff AM, Tcheng JE, Sigmon KN, Joseph D, Rios G, Trainor K, Rose D. Immediate and reversible platelet inhibition after intravenous administration of a peptide glycoprotein IIb/IIIa inhibitor during percutaneous coronary intervention. Am J Cardiol 1995;76:1222–1227.
24. Tsao PW, Bozarth JM, Jackson SA, Forsythe MS, Flint SK, Mousa SA. Platelet GPIIb/IIIa receptor occupancy studies using a novel fluoresceinated cyclic Arg-Gly-Asp peptide. Thromb Res 1995;77:543–556.
25. Bednar B, Cunningham ME, McQueney PA, Egbertson MS, Askew BC, Bednar RA, Hartman GD, Gould RJ. Flow cytometric measurement of kinetic and equilibrium binding parameters of arginine-glycine-aspartic acid ligands in binding to glycoprotein IIb/IIIa on platelets. Cytometry 1997;28:58–65.
26. Cardinal DC, Flower RJ. The electronic aggregometer: a novel device for assessing platelet behavior in blood. J Pharmacol Methods 1980;3:135–158.
27. Di Minno G, Cerbone AM, Mattioli PL, Turco S, Iovine C, Mancini M. Functionally thrombasthenic state in normal platelets following the administration of ticlopidine. J Clin Invest 1985;75:328–338.
28. Kuzniar J, Splawinska B, Malinga K, Mazurek AP, Splawinski J. Pharmacodynamics of ticlopidine: relation between dose and time of administration to platelet inhibition. Int J Clin Pharmacol Ther 1996;34:357–361.
29. Tcheng JE, Ellis SG, George BS, Kereiakes DJ, Kleiman NS, Talley JD, Wang AL, Weisman HF, Califf RM, Topol EJ. Pharmacodynamics of chimeric glycoprotein IIb/IIIa integrin antiplatelet antibody Fab 7E3 in high-risk coronary angioplasty. Circulation 1994;90:1757–1764.

30. Kereiakes DJ, Kleiman N, Ferguson JJ, Runyon JP, Broderick TM, Higby NA, Martin LH, Hantsbarger G, McDonald S, Anders RJ. Sustained platelet glycoprotein IIb/IIIa blockade with oral xemilofiban in 170 patients after coronary stent deployment. Circulation 1997;96: 1117–1121.

31. Coller BS, Springer KT, Scudder LE, Kutok JL, Ceruso M, Prestwich GD. Substituting isoserine for serine in the thrombin receptor activation peptide SFLLRN confers resistance to aminopeptidase M-induced cleavage and inactivation. J Biol Chem 1993;268:20741–20743.

32. Kleiman NS, Raizner AE, Jordan R, Wang AL, Norton D, Mace KF, Joshi A, Coller BS, Weisman HF. Differential inhibition of platelet aggregation induced by adenosine diphosphate or a thrombin receptor-activating peptide in patients treated with bolus chimeric 7E3 Fab: implications for inhibition of the internal pool of GPIIb/IIIa receptors. J Am Coll Cardiol 1995;26:1665–1671.

33. Theroux P, Kouz S, Roy L, Knudtson ML, Diodati JG, Marquis JF, Nasmith J, Fung AY, Boudreault JR, Delage F, Dupuis R, Kells C, Bokslag M, Steiner B, Rapold HJ. Platelet membrane receptor glycoprotein IIb/IIIa antagonism in unstable angina. The Canadian Lamifiban Study [see comments]. Circulation 1996;94:899–905.

33a. Mascelli MA, Lance ET, Damaraju L, Wagner CL, Weisman HF, Jordan RE. Pharmacodynamic profile of short-term abciximab treatment demonstrates prolonged platelet inhibition with gradual recovery from GPIIb-IIIa receptor blockade. Circulation 1998; 97(17)1680–1688.

34. Coller BS, Peerschke EI, Scudder LE, Sullivan CA. A murine monoclonal antibody that completely blocks the binding of fibrinogen to platelets produces a thrombasthenic-like state in normal platelets and binds to glycoproteins IIb and/or IIIa. J Clin Invest 1983;72:325–38.

35. Coller BS, Folts JD, Smith SR, Scudder LE, Jordan R. Abolition of in vivo platelet thrombus formation in primates with monoclonal antibodies to the platelet GPIIb/IIIa receptor. Correlation with bleeding time, platelet aggregation, and blockade of GPIIb/IIIa receptors [see comments]. Circulation 1989;80:1766–1774.

36. Mascelli MA, Worley S, Veriabo NJ, Lance ET, Mack S, Schaible T, Weisman HF, Jordan RE. Rapid assessment of platelet function with a modified whole-blood aggregometer in percutaneous transluminal coronary angioplasty patients receiving anti-GP IIb/IIIa therapy [see comments]. Circulation 1997;96:3860–3866.

37. Simoons ML, de Boer MJ, van den Brand MJ, van Miltenburg AJ, Hoorntje JC, Heyndrickx GR, van der Wieken LR, de Bono D, Rutsch W, Schaible TF. Randomized trial of a GPIIb/IIIa platelet receptor blocker in refractory unstable angina. European Cooperative Study Group. Circulation 1994;89:596–603.

38. Steinhubl SR, Kottke-Marchant K, Moliterno DJ, Rosenthal ML, Godfrey NK, Coller BS, Topol EJ, Lincoff AM. Attainment and maintenance of platelet inhibition through standard dosing of abciximab in diabetic and nondiabetic patients undergoing percutaneous coronary intervention. Circulation 1999;100:1977–1982.

39. Phillips DR, Teng W, Arfsten A, Nannizzi-Alaimo L, White MM, Longhurst C, Shattil SJ, Randolph A, Jakubowski JA, Jennings LK, Scarborough RM. Effect of Ca2 + on GP IIb-IIIa interactions with integrilin: enhanced GP IIb-IIIa binding and inhibition of platelet aggregation by reductions in the concentration of ionized calcium in plasma anticoagulated with citrate. Circulation 1997;96:1488–1494.

40. Berkowitz SD, Frelinger AL, Hillman RS. Progress in point-of-care laboratory testing for assessing platelet function. Am Heart J 1998;136:S51–65.

41. Mallett SV, Cox DJ. Thrombelastography [see comments]. Br J Anaesth 1992;69:307–313.

42. Greilich PE, Alving BM, O'Neill KL, Chang AS, Reid TJ. A modified thromboelastographic method for monitoring c7E3 Fab in heparinized patients. Anesth Analg 1997;84:31–38.

43. Mammen EF, Comp PC, Gosselin R, Greenberg C, Hoots WK, Kessler CM, Larkin EC, Liles D, Nugent DJ. PFA-100 system: a new method for assessment of platelet dysfunction. Semin Thromb Hemost 1998;24:195–202.

44. Soffer D, O'Neill WW, Harjai KJ, Dixon SR, Boura B, Safian RD, Grines CL, Moussa I, Roubin GS, Moses JW. Inter-Assay Variability in the Degree of Platelet Inhibition Following GPIIb/IIIa Receptor Blockade in Patients Undergoing Coronary Intervention: A Comparison of Three Different Point-of-Care Assays. J Am Coll Cardiol 2002;39:887–892.

44a. Nicholson NS, Panzer-Knodle SG, Haas NF, Taite BB, Szalony JA, Page JD, Feigan LP, Lansky DM, Salyers AK. Assessment of platelet function assays. Am Heart J 1998; 135: s170–178.

45. Soffer D, Moussa I, Harjai KJ, Boura JA, Dixon SR, Grines CL, O'Neil WW, Roubin GS, Moses JW. Impact of angina class on inhibition of platelet aggregation following clopidogrel loading in patients undergoing coronary intervention: do we need more aggressive dosing regimens in unstable angina? Catheter Cardiovasc Interv 2003;59:21–25.

46. Lau WC, Waskell LA, Watkins PB, Neer CJ, Horowitz K, Hopp AS, Tait AR, Carville DG, Guyer KE, Bates ER. Atorvastatin reduces the ability of clopidogrel to inhibit platelet aggregation: a new drug-drug interaction. Circulation 2003;107:32–37.

47. Coller BS, Lang D, Scudder LE. Rapid and simple platelet function assay to assess glycoprotein IIb/IIIa receptor blockade. Circulation 1997;95:860–867.

48. Smith JW, Steinhubl SR, Lincoff AM, Coleman JC, Lee TT, Hillman RS, Coller BS. Rapid platelet-function assay: an automated and quantitative cartridge- based method. Circulation 1999;99:620–625.

49. Steinhubl SR, Talley JD, Braden GA, Tcheng JE, Casterella PJ, Moliterno DJ, Navetta FI, Berger PB, Popma JJ, Dangas G, Gallo R, Sane DC, Saucedo JF, Jia G, Lincoff AM, Theroux P, Holmes DR, Teirstein PS, Kereiakes DJ. Point-of-care measured platelet inhibition correlates with a reduced risk of an adverse cardiac event after percutaneous coronary intervention: results of the GOLD (AU-Assessing Ultegra) multicenter study. Circulation 2001;103: 2572–2578.

50. Kereiakes DJ, Mueller M, Howard W, Lacock P, Anderson LC, Broderick TM, Roth EM, Whang DD, Abbottsmith CW. Efficacy of abciximab induced platelet blockade using a rapid point of care assay. J Thromb Thrombolysis 1999;7:265–276.

51. Kabbani SS, Aggarwal A, Terrien EF, DiBattiste PM, Sobel BE, Schneider DJ. Suboptimal early inhibition of platelets by treatment with tirofiban and implications for coronary interventions. Am J Cardiol 2002;89:647–650.

52. Herrmann HC, Swierkosz TA, Kapoor S, Tardiff DC, DiBattiste PM, Hirshfeld JW, Klugherz BD, Kolansky DM, Magness K, Valettas N, Wilensky RL. Comparison of degree of platelet inhibition by abciximab vs. tirofiban in patients with unstable angina pectoris and non-Q-wave myocardial infarction undergoing percutaneous coronary intervention. Am J Cardiol 2002;89:1293–1297.

53. Tcheng JE, Talley JD, O'Shea JC, Gilchrist IC, Kleiman NS, Grines CL, Davidson CJ, Lincoff AM, Califf RM, Jennings LK, Kitt MM, Lorenz TJ. Clinical pharmacology of higher dose eptifibatide in percutaneous coronary intervention (the PRIDE study). Am J Cardiol 2001; 88:1097–1102.

54. O'Shea JC, Hafley GE, Greenberg S, Hasselblad V, Lorenz TJ, Kitt MM, Strony J, Tcheng JE, ESPIRIT Investigators. Platelet glycoprotein IIb/IIIa integrin blockade with eptifibatide in coronary stent intervention: the ESPRIT trial: a randomized controlled trial. JAMA 2001; 285:2468–2473.

55. Mukherjee D, Chew DP, Robbins M, Yadav JS, Raymond RE, Moliterno DJ. Clinical application of procedural platelet monitoring during percutaneous coronary intervention among patients at increased bleeding risk. J Thromb Thrombolysis 2001;11:151–154.

56. Gum PA, Kottke-Marchant K, Poggio ED, Gurm H, Welsh PA, Brooks L, Sapp SK, Topol EJ. Profile and prevalence of aspirin resistance in patients with cardiovascular disease. Am J Cardiol 2001;88:230–235.

57. Grotemeyer KH, Scharafinski HW, Husstedt IW. Two-year follow-up of aspirin responder and aspirin non responder. A pilot-study including 180 post-stroke patients. Thromb Res 1993;71:397–403.

58. Barragan P, Bouvier JL, Roquebert PO, Macaluso G, Commeau P, Comet B, Lafont A, Camoin L, Walter U, Eigenthaler M. Resistance to thienopyridines: Clinical detection of coronary stent thrombosis by monitoring of vasodilator-stimulated phosphoprotein phosphorylation. Catheter Cardiovasc Interv 2003;59:295–302.

59. Jaremo P, Lindahl TL, Fransson SG, Richter A. Individual variations of platelet inhibition after loading doses of clopidogrel. J Intern Med 2002;252:233–238.

60. Gurbel PA, Bliden KP, Hiatt BL, O'Connor CM. Clopidogrel for coronary stenting: response variability, drug resistance, and the effect of pretreatment platelet reactivity. Circulation 2003; 107:2908–2913.

61. Gurbel PA, Bliden KP. Durability of platelet inhibition by clopidogrel. Am J Cardiol 2003; 91:1123–1125.

62. Inwald DP, McDowall A, Peters MJ, Callard RE, Klein NJ. CD40 is constitutively expressed on platelets and provides a novel mechanism for platelet activation. Circ Res 2003;92: 1041–1048.

63. Heeschen C, Dimmeler S, Hamm CW, van den Brand MJ, Boersma E, Zeiher AM, et al. Soluble CD40 ligand in acute coronary syndromes. N Engl J Med 2003;348:1104–1111.

# 24

# Statins and Plaque Stabilization

**Michael Miller and Robert A. Vogel**
*University of Maryland School of Medicine*
*Baltimore, Maryland, U.S.A.*

## INTRODUCTION

Dyslipidemia contributes substantially to the development and clinical expression of atherosclerosis, especially in the coronary *Circulation* [1–10]. Considerable evidence suggests that cholesterol lowering stabilizes atherosclerotic plaques and reduces CHD events, including all-cause mortality [11–37]. Those at highest risk of recurrent CHD events, notably diabetics and subjects with pre-existing CHD benefit the most from cholesterol lowering [16–21,128–129,132]. Angiographic or ultrasound trials of hypolipidemic therapy have shown a reduction in disease progression with aggressive compared with moderate treatment [38–95]. Large primary and secondary prevention event trials have demonstrated significant reductions in cardiovascular events in patients with a wide range of cholesterol levels [96–133]. These findings suggest that aggressive lipid management can accomplish the same treatment goals as traditional antianginal and interventional therapy, specifically reductions in anginal frequency, exercise intolerance, CHD events, and mortality [14,120–122,125–129,132,134]. This chapter reviews the pathophysiology and impact of hypolipidemic therapy on atherosclerosis [135–172] and vascular biology [173–241] and outlines the lipid management for coronary artery disease patients [242–337], including those undergoing interventional procedures.

## PATHOPHYSIOLOGY OF ATHEROSCLEROSIS

The early stages of coronary atherosclerosis is characterized by endothelial dysfunction, intimal lipid, monocyte and T lymphocyte accumulation with inflammation leading to the migration and proliferation of smooth muscle cells and elaboration of collagen and matrix [135–172]. In its more advanced stages, this process is punctuated by acute episodes of plaque disruption, thrombosis, and vessel reorganization, which underlie the clinical syndromes of unstable angina and acute myocardial infarction [140,143,146,147,151,153]. The disease generally begins during the second decade of life [6,10] and remains asymptomatic until significant lumenal compromise develops or sudden occlusion occurs. In the former circumstance, stable exertional angina may be the presenting symptom, although this occurs in only 12% to 26% of men and 47% of women [5,7]. Unstable angina, urgent need for coronary revascularization, acute myocardial infarction, and sudden death together make up the majority of the initial presenting symptoms of coronary heart disease. Important early pathophysiological processes include endothelial dysfunction [173–213] caused by coronary risk factors, mechanical trauma, and possibly infections (*Chlamydia pneumoniae*, CMV, and herpes viruses), and the progressive modification of LDL, predominantly by oxidation [137,142,148,150]. Once atherosclerotic plaques develop, the combined factors of local plaque inflammation [146,156], dissolution of internal plaque collagen, and vasomotion lead to plaque disruption, with ensuing partial or complete vessel thrombosis [135,140,141]. Cholesterol lowering has been shown to slow the progression of coronary atherosclerosis and reduce plaque rupture [38–71,77,78,80]. It also decreases thrombogenicity and platelet adhesion to the denuded or ruptured vessel wall [25,26,33–35]. Beyond its effects on the atherosclerotic process, improvements in endothelial function are thought to decrease the ischemic manifestations of coronary artery disease by increasing flow-mediated vasodilation at both the conduit and arteriolar vessel level [22,27,28,30,31,36,37].

## Endothelial Pathway

Two processes play key roles in the initiation of atherosclerosis: endothelial dysfunction and lipid accumulation and modification (Fig. 1) [19,137,141,142,174,192,199,201, 202,205,207]. The endothelium is a major regulator of vasoactivity, vessel growth, aggregation of platelets, adhesion of monocytes, inflammation, immune responses, plaque remodeling, thrombosis, and fibrinolysis (Fig. 2) [19,173,177,179,182,193,207]. Endothelium-derived relaxing factors in conduit and resistance vessels include nitric oxide (NO) or an NO adduct, prostacyclin, and hyperpolarizing factor which operate through the intermediate signaling mechanisms of cyclic-GMP, cyclic-AMP, and $K^+$ channels, respectively [183,186]. Endothelium-mediated or activated vasocontrictors include endothelin-1, angiotensin II, thromboxane, prostacyclin-$H_2$ and oxygen free radicals. Endothelin-1 also potentiates renin and catecholamines. The endothelium also expresses several monocyte adhesion molecules and coagulation altering factors [19,179]. These factors are released in response to endothelium-dependent stimuli, such as acetylcholine, serotonin, thrombin, and blood flow shear. Normal endothelium pre-

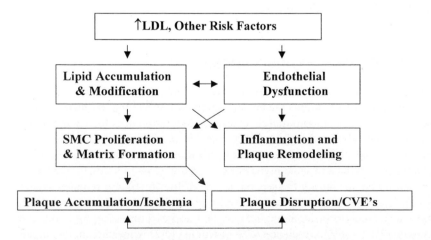

**Figure 1**  The pathogenesis of coronary atherosclerosis. CVE's = cardiovascular events, LDL = low-density lipoprotein, SMC = smooth muscle cell.

Functions | Products
--- | ---

Functions
Vasodilation:
Thrombolysis & A/C:
Platelet disaggregation:
SMC growth inhibition:
Lipoprotein metabolism:

Products
NO, PGI$_2$, EDHF
tPA, heparan sulfate
NO, PGI$_2$
NO
LPL

Anti-atherogenic

Pro-atherogenic

Vasoconstriction:
Monocyte/platelet adhesion:
Inflammation:
SMC growth factors:
Coagulation:

ET-1, ACE (A-II), TxA$_2$, PGH$_2$
ICAM-1, VCAM-1, P-Selectin
free radicals, IL-1, IL-6, TNF-$\alpha$
PDGF, b-FGF, IGF, TGF, CSF
PAI-1, TF, vWF, protein S

**Figure 2** Anti- and proatherogenic regulatory functions and products of the endothelium. A-II = angiotensin-II, ACE = angiotensin converting enzyme, A/C = anticoagulation, b-FGF = basic fibroblast growth factor, CSF = colony stimulating factor, EDHF = endothelium-derived hyperpolarizing factor, ET-1 = endothelin-1, ICAM-1 = intercellular adhesion molecule-1, IGF = insulin-like growth factor, IL-1 = interleukin-1, IL-6 = interleukin-6, LPL = lipoprotein lipase, NO = nitric oxide, PAI-1 = platelet activator inhibitor-1, PDGF = platelet derived growth factor, PGH$_2$ = prostaglandin-H$_2$, PGI$_2$ = prostacyclin, SMC = smooth muscle cell, TF = tissue factor, TGF = transforming growth factor, TNF-$\alpha$ = tumor necrosing factor-$\alpha$, tPA = tissue plasminogen inhibitor, TXA$_2$ = thromboxane-A$_2$, VCAM-1 = vascular cell adhesion molecule-1, vWF = von Willebrand factor.

vents the development of atherosclerosis by promoting vasodilation, inhibiting smooth muscle cell proliferation, decreasing platelet and monocyte adhesion, and increasing thrombolysis (increased tPA:PAI-1). Experimental studies have demonstrated that NO synthesis inhibition (L-NAME) accelerates the development of atherosclerosis, whereas increasing NO availability (L-arginine) retards its development, at least for a period of several weeks [194,195]. While a correlation has been reported between brachial vasoreactivity and severity of coronary disease [208], several reports suggest that clinical events occur more frequently in patients with the least endothelial-dependent vasodilation, even in the absence of disparity in extent of coronary artery stenosis [214–216].

All major coronary risk factors (both modifiable and immutable) are associated with endothelial dysfunction [178,181,184,189,193,201,205,207]. Several mechanism have been postulated for the decrease in NO availability with hypercholesterolemia, including increased production of oxygen free radicals (predominantly superoxide anion) which rapidly combine with and deactivate nitric oxide, producing the toxic peroxynitrite radical (Fig. 3). Abnormal G protein signaling, and decreased NO production, possibly through reduced NO synthase expression caused by oxidized LDL also reduce NO availability [190,205,207]. Other postulated mechanisms include reduced microdomain availability of the substrate L-arginine, increased asymmetric dimethylarginine (ADMA), reduced tetrahydobiopterin (NO synthase cofactor), and increased activity of caveolin, a membrane inhibitor of NO synthase. Nitric oxide deactivation and endothelial dysfunction result in increased vasocontriction, smooth muscle cell proliferation, platelet aggregation, monocyte adhesion, inflammation, metalloproteinase and tissue factor production, and decreased fibrinolysis, all of which are important factors in the development of atherosclerosis, plaque

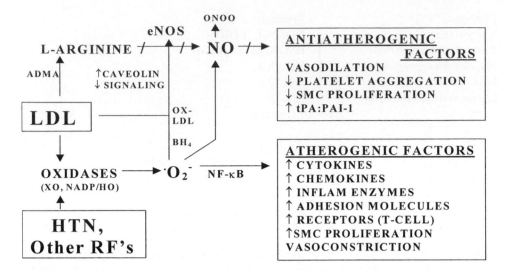

**Figure 3** The endothelial dysfunction pathways by which risk factors lead to atherosclerosis. ADMA = asymmetric dimethylarginine, BH4 = tetrahydrobiopterin, eNOS = endothelium nitric oxide synthase, HTN = hypertension, LDL = low-density lipoprotein, NADP/HO = nicotinamide adenine dinucleotide phosphate oxidase, NF-κB = nuclear factor-κB, NO = nitric oxide, ONOO· = perioxynitrite radical, OX-LDL = oxidized low-density lipoprotein, PAI-1 = platelet activator inhibitor-1, RF's = risk factors, SMC = smooth muscle cell, tPA = tissue plasminogen inhibitor, XO = xanthine oxidase.

rupture, and vessel thrombosis. The vasoregulatory aspect of endothelial function can be assessed in the coronary *Circulation* using intracoronary infusions of acetylcholine, serotonin, or substance P and in the brachial *Circulation* using a postocclusion hyperemic vasodilation (flow-mediated) or forearm plethysmographic assessment of blood flow following cholinergic stimulation. Normal responses to these stimuli are manifest as vasodilation, whereas endothelial dysfunction is associated with reduced vasodilation or vasoconstriction [174,176,177,180,182,184,187,200,205,207]. Vasoregulation is, however, spatially variable, distal and smaller vessels generally being more reactive [185,196–198]. Endothelial dysfunction is thought to be an important component in the pathophysiology of coronary ischemia. In the presence of endothelial dysfunction, clinical stimuli such as exercise-induced hyperemia, cold exposure, and emotional stress have been shown to result in vasoconstriction in the stenotic regions [199]. Resistance vessel endothelial dysfunction also contributes to ischemia [21,27,30,35,36]. The measurement of soluble adhesion molecules and systemic inflammatory markers (e.g., C-reactive protein) also reflect, in part, endothelial function [151,156,161–163,173].

The vast majority of clinical studies have reported significant or borderline improvements in coronary or brachial artery endothelial function with cholesterol lowering in subjects with and without coronary heart disease (Table 1) [217–241]. Initial subject cholesterol has ranged from 195 to 373 mg/dl. Endothelium-dependent vasodilation improves with low-density lipoprotein (LDL) cholesterol lowering to below 100 mg/dl [238]. Certain high-fat meals, hypertriglyceridemia, and elevated remnant particle levels have also been demonstrated to impair endothelial function, a phenomenon which appears to be caused by free radical release and can be reduced, at least short-term, by antioxidant vitamins, statins, folic acid, angiotensin receptor blockers, and ACE-inhibitors [204,206,

**Table 1** Effect of Cholesterol Lowering On Endothelial Function

| Study | Pts | Chol. | Circ. | Interv | Months | Result |
|---|---|---|---|---|---|---|
| Egashira[218] | CAD | 272 | CA | PRAVA | 6 | (+) |
| Treasure[219] | CAD | 226 | CA | LOVA | 6 | (+) |
| Anderson[200] | CAD | 209 | CA | LO/CH | 12 | (±) |
| | | | | LO/PROB | 12 | (+) |
| Seiler[224] | CAD | 300 | CA | BEZAFIB | 7 | (+) |
| Yeung[225] | CAD | 230 | CA | SIMVA | 6 | (−) |
| CARE[226] | CAD | 209 | FMV | PRAVA | 54 | (+) |
| Tamai[227] | CAD | 195 | FVR | APHER | 1 HR | (+) |
| O'Driscol[228] | CAD | 254 | FVR | SIMVA | 1 | (+) |
| Andrews[229] | CAD | 202 | FMV | GEM/NIA/CH | 30 | (−) |
| Dupuis[234] | CAD | 246 | FMV | PRAVA | 1.5 | (+) |
| Herrington[235] | CAD | 200 | FMV | LOVA | 1.5 | (+) |
| Yokoyama[237] | CAD | 263 | PET | VARIOUS | 6 | (+) |
| Vita[241] | CAD | 204 | CA | SIMVA | 6 | (−) |
| Shechter[238] | CAD | N/A | FMV | VARIOUS | N/A | (+) |
| Leung[217] | NL | 239 | CA | CH | 6 | (+) |
| Stroes[221] | NL | 354 | FVR | SIM/CO | 3 | (+) |
| Goode[222] | NL | 373 | EVR | UNSPEC | 10 | (+) |
| Vogel[223] | NL | 200 | FMV | SIMVA | 0.5–3 | (+) |
| DeMan[230] | NL | 1065 (TG) | FVR | ATORVA | 1.5 | (+) |
| Simons[231] | NL | 320 | FMV | SIMVA/CH | 7 | (+) |
| | | | | ATORVA | 7 | (+) |
| Vogel[232] | NL | 198 | FMV | PRAVA | 1 DAY | (−) |
| | | | | | 1 | (+) |
| John[233] | NL | 278 | FVR | FLUVA | 6 | (+) |
| John[239] | NL | 295 | FVR | CERIVA | 0.5 | (+) |
| Mullen[240] | DM | 189 | FMV | ATORVA | 1.5 | (+) |

APHER = apheresis, ATORVA = atorvastatin, BEZA = bezafibrate, CA = coronary artery, CAD = coronary artery disease, CERIVA = cerivastatin, CH = cholestyramine, CHOL = mean cholesterol (mg/dl), CIRC = *Circulation* studied, CO = colestipol, DM = diabetes mellitus, EVR = excised vascular ring, FLUVA = fluvastatin, GEM = gemfibrozil, INTERV = study intervention, LO = lovastatin, NIA = niacin, NL = normal, PET = positron emission tomography, PRAVA = pravastatin, PROB = probucol, SIMVA = simvastatin, TG = triglycerides, UNSPEC = unspecified, (+) = improvement, (±) = borderline, (−) = no improvement.

210–213]. Improvements in endothelium-dependent vasodilation have been demonstrated with antioxidant vitamins, B-complex vitamins, and estrogen and ACE-inhibitor administration [201,205,207]. Antioxidant vitamin administration has also been shown to reduce the endothelial expression of monocytes adhesion molecules in smokers [203]. In contrast to cholesterol lowering, the chronic administration of antioxidant vitamins, however, has not been shown to reduce cardiovascular events [288,300,320].

## Cholesterol Pathway

Cholesterol deposition (predominantly from LDL) and modification is the second major process initiating atherosclerosis [137,140–142]. Initially, LDL passes through the endothelial barrier by a process termed transcytosis. This process is accelerated by increased serum LDL and endothelial injury. Subintimal LDL may undergo progressive modification via glycosylation, oxidation, and acetylation. The former process may occur despite normal LDL concentrations in smokers and diabetics [165–167]. Similarly, enhanced LDL oxidation may occur in normolipidemics with low HDL because in addition to its role in reverse cholesterol transport, HDL bears the antioxidant paraoxonase which impedes LDL oxidation [145,168–170].

Minimally modified LDL is a potent inhibitor of endothelial function. Maximally modified LDL is recognized as foreign material by macrophages and taken up by the unregulated scavenger receptors, creating metabolically active foam cells. These express a number of growth factors and cytokines, which induce smooth muscle cell migration, proliferation, and matrix generation, leading to the formation of complex atheroma. Positive remodeling of the vessel wall in the form of abluminal dilation occurs in the majority of plaques during the development of early atherosclerosis without affecting the lumen (Fig. 4) [171]. As such, intravascular ultrasound (IVUS) rather than coronary arteriography may detect lesions in the vessel wall that occur prior to luminal encroachment.

Eventually, expansion of the atheroma exceeds this locally variable compensatory mechanism, leading to luminal narrowing and signifies advanced CAD, even in the absence

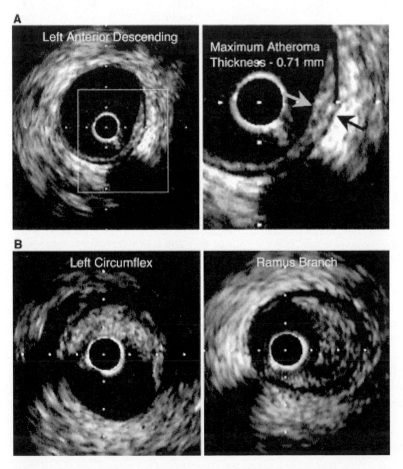

**Figure 4** (**A**) Example of atherosclerosis in LAD of 17-year-old man. Eccentric intimal thickening representing early atherosclerosis is evident. Note normal intima opposite diseased arc. Right, Magnified view of same lesion. (**B**) Evidence of advanced atherosclerosis in 32-year-old woman. (From Ref. 171)

of symptoms which generally do not become evident until luminal diameter exceeds 70% [135,141,149].

## Plaque Disruption and Inflammation

Cardiovascular events usually occur as a consequence of disruption or ulceration of "vulnerable" atheromas [141,146,147,152]. Hypercholesterolemia and cigarette smoking have been shown to be directly associated with plaque disruption and ulceration, respectively [151,153]. Plaque disruption is associated with variable degrees of intramural hemorrhage and luminal thrombosis. Incomplete luminal thrombosis may produce accelerated or unstable angina. Complete thrombosis may produce myocardial infarction if inadequate collaterals are present. Intramural hemorrhage and luminal thrombosis are important mechanisms for rapid progression of stenosis severity [140].

Vulnerable plaques tend to be eccentric and have large, soft (cholesterol ester), coalescent lipid pools, thin fibrous caps, and reduced internal plaque collagen [146,147,152]. They are generally of moderate severity and high elasticity. High concentrations of T lymphocytes, foam and mast cells, and cytokines have been identified in the region of plaque rupture, suggesting an inflammatory mechanism [156]. Vulnerable plaques are warmer, have lower pH, and are undergoing more oxidative stress than are stable plaques. The inflammatory process is often increased in the "shoulder" region of the plaque at the intersection of the atheroma and normal vessel wall. Through the elaboration of interferon-$\gamma$, T lymphocytes may suppress smooth muscle cell proliferation and induce foam cells to digest internal plaque collagen through the secretion of metalloproteinases [146]. Inflammation and vasoactivity are thought to be the predominate factors responsible for plaque instability. In contrast to plaque morphology (histologic and angiographic "complexity"), stenosis severity correlates poorly with vulnerability to plaque disruption [72–72,82,151]. The most severe stenosis is often not the site of plaque rupture, which usually occurs in intermediate-grade stenoses. High-grade stenoses (e.g., greater than 70%) are often associated with collaterals and may progress to total occlusion without accompanying myocardial infarction. Angiographic "complex" stenoses demonstrate more progression and are associated with acute ischemic events more commonly than smooth lesions [82]. Soluble adhesion molecules and systemic inflammatory markers are increased in patients with acute coronary syndromes and are predictive of subsequent cardiovascular event risk [155,156,161–164]. Elevations in inflammatory markers, such as C-reactive protein, also appear to predict greater benefit from cholesterol lowering (e.g., statin) therapy than in CAD subjects without active inflammation [164].

## Plaque Stabilization

In addition to improving endothelial function, cholesterol lowering stabilizes plaques by decreasing plaque inflammation and foam cell number and activity and by increasing plaque collagen matrix [79,146]. Normalization of diet in cholesterol-fed monkeys reduces macrophage number, increases collagen, and depletes and hardens plaque lipids, resulting in a smaller, stiffer atheroma and larger lumen. These changes theoretically reduce plaque vulnerability to disruption. In contrast to experimental studies, only modest degrees of regression, defined as lumenal increase, have been observed with clinical cholesterol lowering [75,76,79]. The lack of "regression" may be due to associated negative remodeling, which reduces expansion of the lumen, despite plaque regression. Reduced disease progression is associated with plaque stabilization because of the associated marked reduction in the incidence of cardiovascular events [77,82,86,87].

Disruption of lipid-rich plaques with ensuing intramural hemorrhage and luminal thrombosis accounts for 55–85% of acute ischemic events [135,137–140,147,154]. A second mechanism is thrombosis on superficial erosions of proteoglycan-rich and smooth muscle-cell rich plaques lacking a lipid core [151,153]. These lesions are more often seen in younger individuals, smokers, and women, and are associated with less luminal narrowing, calcification, macrophages, and T lymphocytes. For both plaque disruption and superficial erosions, the extent of luminal thrombosis depends on intramural concentrations of tissue factor and systemic factors, including Lp(a), platelet aggregability, fibrinogen, and other procoagulants. Cholesterol lowering has been shown to decrease platelet adhesion to denuded endothelium [25,26,33–35]. Decreasing LDL cholesterol also reduces the risk associated with increased Lp(a) [172].

## CLINICAL STUDIES

The landmark Framingham Heart (3.5), Seven Countries [2,8], and MRFIT [12] Studies firmly established that hypercholesterolemia is a major risk factor for cardiovascular morbidity and mortality. The Lipid Research Clinics Coronary Primary Prevention [96,97] and Helsinki Heart [98] Trials demonstrated significant reductions in cardiac events with cholesterol lowering in healthy subjects. Initially in 1987, and revised in 1993 and 2001, the Adult Treatment Panel of the National Cholesterol Education Program (NCEP) [254,255,297] published guidelines on testing and treating hypercholesterolemic patients which outlined a more intensive approach to cholesterol lowering than had been in practice [247]. During the late 1980s and early 1990s, several angiographic trials demonstrated reduced progression of coronary artery disease using lifestyle, drug, and surgical means for reducing cholesterol [38–70]. The latter trials commonly employed HMG-CoA reductase inhibitors (''statins'') reflecting their increasing clinical usage. Although these trials demonstrated statistically significant but modest anatomical benefit associated with cholesterol lowering, on average 48% reductions in major cardiovascular event rates were observed (Table 2) [16–22,75,79,110,111,117,118]. Since 1994, many large cardiovascular event trials have evaluated a wide range of high-risk groups, including subjects with stable and unstable angina as well as coronary risk equivalents. These studies have demonstrated remarkable consistency with the general improviso that aggressive cholesterol lowering reduces both cardiovascular morbidity and mortality. Overall survival benefits have also been observed in adequately powered trials: Scandinavian Simvastatin Survival Study [100–105], West of Scotland Coronary Prevention Study [106], Cholesterol and Recurrent Events Trial [107,108,113,114,118,119], Long-Term Intervention with Pravastatin in Ischemic Disease [116], Air Force Coronary Atherosclerosis Prevention Study/Texas Coronary Atherosclerosis Prevention Study [112,125], Veterans Affairs HDL Intervention Trial [121,126], and the Heart Protection Study [128,132]. Myocardial Ischemia Reduction with Aggressive Cholesterol Lowering [124], a large aggressive versus moderate cholesterol lowering angiographic trial (Post-CABG Trial [63,68,123]), and a small aggressive versus usual cholesterol lowering event trial (Atorvastatin versus Revascularization Trial [120]).

### Primary Prevention Trials

The strongest evidence that cholesterol is causally related to the development of coronary heart disease is derived from randomized, controlled primary, and secondary prevention clinical trials. The Lipid Research Clinics Coronary Primary Prevention Trial (LRC-CPPT) [96,97], studied 3,806 middle-aged men (35–59 years) without symptomatic coronary

**Table 2** Angiographic Changes and Clinical Cardiovascular Event Reductions in the Randomized Placebo-Controlled Cholesterol-Lowering Studies

| Trial | Angiographic change | | % Event reduction |
|---|---|---|---|
| | Treated pts | Control patients | |
| NHLBI[38,39] | 32%/7%* | 49%/7%* | 33 |
| CLAS I[41] | +0.35 %DS | +2.65 %DS | 25 |
| FATS[42] | −0.8 %DS ** | +2.1 %DS | 75 |
| SCOR[43] | −1.5 %DS | +0.8 %DS | (0/1) |
| LHT[44,67] | −3.1 %DS | +5.4 %DS | 44 |
| POSCH[45] | 55/6* | 85/4* | 35 |
| HEIDELBERG[46] | 28%/39%%* | 33%/6%* | 27 |
| STARS[47] | −1.5 %DS ** | +5.8 %DS | 75 |
| CLAS II[48] | −0.05 mm IMT | +0.05 mm IMT | 43 |
| MARS[49] | +1.6 %DS | +2.2 %DS | 24 |
| HARP[50] | −0.14 mm | −0.15 mm | 33 |
| MAAS[51] | +0.9 %DS | +3.6 %DS | 22 |
| SCRIP[52,58] | +0.3 %DS | +0.9 %DS | 50 |
| CCAIT[53] | +1.66 %DS | +2.89 %DS | 25 |
| PLAC I[55] | +0.67 %DS | +1.11 %DS | 38 |
| PLAC II[56] | +0.059 mm/year IMT | +0.068 mm/year IMT | 60 |
| ACAPS[57] | −0.009 mm IMT | +0.006 mm IMT | 64 |
| KAPS[59] | +0.017 mm/year IMT | +0.031 mm/year IMT | 40 |
| REGRESS[60] | +1.10 %DS | +3.26 %DS | 42 |
| BECAIT[61] | +1.70 %DS | +4.25 %DS | 77 |
| CIS[64] | −0.20 mm MLD | −0.58 mm MLD | 21 |
| LCAS[65] | −0.028 mm MLD | −0.100 mm MLD | 24 |
| LOCAT[66] | −0.04 mm MLD | −0.09 mm MLD | 0 |
| LIPID[69] | −0.014 mm IMT | + 0.048 mm IMT | 24 |
| SCAT[70] | −0.07 mm MLD | −0.14 mm MLD | 16 |
| HATS[75] | −0.04 % DS | +3.9% DS | 90 |

%DS = percent diameter stenosis
IMT = intima-media thickness
MLD = minimal lumen diameter
* patients with progression / patients with regression
** mean of two treatment groups

heart disease but with total cholesterol greater than 265 mg/dl. During the 7 year trial, cholestyramine 24 gm daily decreased total cholesterol 13% and LDL-cholesterol 20%. Definite coronary heart disease death occurred in 155 treated men and 187 control men (19% difference). Significant reductions were observed in angina (20%), positive exercise tests (25%), surgical revascularization (21%), and congestive heart failure (28%). The study found that cardiovascular events are reduced about 2% for every 1% reduction in cholesterol.

The Helsinki Heart Study [98] randomized 4,081 middle-aged (40–55 years) men with non-HDL cholesterol greater than 200 mg/dl. Gemfibrozil 600 mg twice daily resulted in decreases in total cholesterol (8%), LDL-cholesterol (8%), and triglycerides (35%) and an increase in HDL-cholesterol (10%). The treated population experienced 34% fewer cardiovascular events in this 5-year trial. In both the LRC-CPPT and the Helsinki Heart Study, no differences were observed in all-cause mortality.

Primary prevention trials have also employed HMG-CoA reductase inhibitors. The West of Scotland Coronary Prevention Study [106] randomized 6,695 men between the ages of 45 and 64 years with LDL-cholesterol greater than 155 mg/dl to either pravastatin 40 mg daily or placebo. Associated with the reductions in total cholesterol (20%) and LDL-cholesterol (26%), the primary end-point, coronary heart disease mortality and nonfatal myocardial infarction was reduced 31%. All-cause mortality, which fell 22% (p = 0.51), became statistically significant (p = 0.39) after adjustment for baseline risk factors.

The Air Force Coronary Atherosclerosis Prevention Study/Texas Coronary Atherosclerosis Prevention Study [112,125] randomized 6,605 healthy, middle-aged men and women with HDL-cholesterol less than 50 mg/dl, LDL-cholesterol 130–190 mg/dl, and an increased LDL-cholesterol to HDL-cholesterol level to lovastatin in stepwise dose to achieve LDL-cholesterol less than 110 mg/dl versus placebo. This 5-year study demonstrated a 36% reduction in death, myocardial infarction, or hospital admission for unstable angina (162 vs.105, P<0.001), which was evident by the end of the first year of the trial. Subsequent analysis has shown 45% and 44% risk reductions in those with HDL-cholesterol less than 35 mg/dl and 35–39 mg/dl, respectively, suggesting that healthy individuals with HDL-cholesterol less than 40 mg/dl and LDL-cholesterol greater than130 mg/dl benefit from treatment with an HMG-CoA reductase inhibitor. The majority of such individuals would not require treatment under the 1993 or 2001 NCEP guidelines, and the vast majority of these individuals remain under-treated at present.

Most recently, the ASCOT trial evaluated 10,305 hypertensive men and women (40–79 years) with CHD risk factors and total cholesterol less than 250 mg/dl. In addition to random assignment of a specific antihypertensive regimen, subjects were also randomized to either atorvastatin 10 mg/d or placebo. The 5 year study was prematurely stopped after a median 3.3 years because of the significant reduction in CHD event rates (36%) in the statin group who reduced LDL-cholesterol levels on average below 100 mg/dL. The results of this study support more intensive treatment (LDL less than 100 mg/dl) in hypertensive, subjects with multiple CHD risk factors even if they do not meet the NCEP designation of CHD equivalence [127].

## Angiographic Trials

During the past two decades, numerous randomized, controlled trials have investigated whether cholesterol lowering was associated with reduced rates of angiographic or ultrasonic progression of coronary or carotid atherosclerosis, respectively (Table 2) [38–71]. Cholesterol reduction in these trials was achieved by widely differing regimens including low-fat diet (LHT [44,67], STARS [47]), exercise (Heidelberg [46]), single drug (NHLBI-Type II [38,39], MARS [49], STARS [47], MAAS [51], CCAIT [53], PLAC-I [55], PLAC-II [56], ACAPS [57], KAPS [59], REGRESS [60], BECAIT [61], CIS [64], LCAS [65], LOCAT [66], LIPID [69], SCAT [70]), multiple drugs (CLAS-I [41], FATS [42], SCOR [43], CLAS-II [48], HARP [50], SCRIP [52,58], LCAS [65]), and partial ileal bypass surgery (POSCH [45]). Later trials consistently employed quantitative coronary arteriography and more commonly employed HMG-CoA reductase inhibitors reflecting their widespread clinical use (MARS, MAAS, CCAIT, PLAC-I, PLAC-II, REGRESS, CAPS, ACAPS, CIS, LCAS). Trials ranged from 1 to 10 years in duration and enrolled from 43 to 838 patients. All but one of the trials (HARP), undertaken in patients with the lowest cholesterol, demonstrated angiographic improvement in those randomized to lipid lowering in the form of less disease progression, more stability of existing lesions, fewer new lesions, fewer progressions to total occlusion, and/or more disease regression than in the control group. Although absolute differences in coronary luminal dimensions between the treatment and control groups were found to be significant but small (1–3%), on average this represented a 50–75% relative reduction in disease progression. The reduction in disease progression was associated with substantial decreases in cardiovascular events. Seven trials (LHT, FATS, STARS, SCOR, Heidelberg, CLAS-II, ACAPS) demonstrated an average minimal reduction in percent diameter stenosis or intima-media thickness. Although this finding suggests disease regression, the angiographic trials provided data only on luminal dimensions and are unable to provide data on changes in plaque volume. Preliminary intravascular ultrasound data however, suggests that cholesterol lowering reduces the atherosclerosis plaque area, even if luminal diameter is not increased. One recent 18 month trial (REVERSAL) of 502 hyperlipidemic subjects (mean age, 56 years, mean LDL, 150 mg/dl, mean triglycerides, 197 mg/dl) with CHD, found that high dose atorvastatin (80 mg/d) resulted in mean LDL lowering to 79 mg/dL although very minimal regression (0.4%) in plaque volume was identified by IVUS. In contrast, the use of pravastatin (40 mg/d) resulted in mean LDL of 110 mg/dL and 2.7% progression of plaque volume. These data reaffirm that intensive LDL cholesterol lowering retards progression of disease but do not appreciably regress coronary lesions [71].

## Secondary Prevention Trials

*Scandinavian Simvastatin Survival Study (4S)*

Although earlier event and angiographic secondary prevention trials had demonstrated reductions in cardiovascular events, this was the first to demonstrate reduction in all-cause mortality [100–105]. The 4S Study enrolled 4,444 men (81%) and women, aged 35 to 70 years with prior myocardial infarction (79%) and/or angina, initial cholesterol levels 213 to 310 mg/dl, and triglycerides less than 200 mg/dl. Simvastatin was administered at 20 or 40 mg/day with the intent to lower cholesterol below 200 mg/dl. Over the 5.4 year mean followup period, simvastatin lowered mean cholesterol from 260 to 189 mg/dl ( − 25%). A 30% reduction in all-cause mortality was observed (182 vs. 256 deaths, p = 0.0003). Significant reductions were also observed in myocardial infarction, need for coronary angioplasty or bypass surgery, stroke or transient ischemic attack, and hospitalizations. Of all the subgroups studied, diabetic patients received the greatest relative and absolute benefit (55% risk reduction). The risk of major cardiovascular events was reduced to the same extent at all initial cholesterol levels. Patients with either higher triglyceride and/or lower HDL-cholesterol levels appeared to derive more benefit. Both the magnitude of LDL-cholesterol decrease and on treatment LDL-cholesterol levels correlated with CV and mortality benefit. Cost-benefit analysis suggested a $3,000 to $10,000 cost per year saved [103,104,108,109].

*Cholesterol and Recurrent Events (CARE) Study*

The majority of coronary heart disease patients in the U.S. have "borderline" elevated cholesterol levels (mean 225 mg/dl) leading to the incorrect impression that they would not benefit from cholesterol lowering. The CARE Study [107,108,113,114,118,119] was designed to determine the value of cholesterol lowering (pravastatin 40 mg/day) in 4,159 men (86%) and women with a prior myocardial infarction and "average" cholesterol, i.e., less than 240 mg/dl. Mean lipid values for the patients studied were total cholesterol 209 mg/dl, LDL-cholesterol 139 mg/dl, HDL-cholesterol 39 mg/dl, and triglycerides 155 mg/dl. This mean cholesterol is almost equal to the American average (208 mg/dl). Pravastatin reduced total and LDL-cholesterol by 20% and 32%, respectively. Over the 5 years of the trial, the primary end-point, coronary heart disease mortality and nonfatal myocardial infarction was reduced from 274 in the control group to 212 in the pravastatin group ($-24\%$, p $=$ 0.003). As in the 4S Study, the need for coronary angioplasty or bypass surgery, episodes of unstable angina, and stroke were also reduced (13–31%). The CARE Trial results extend the important observations of the 4S Study to the majority of coronary heart disease patients in the U.S., including women.

### Long-Term Intervention with Pravastatin in Ischemic Disease (LIPID) Trial

The third large secondary prevention trial LIPID [116], conducted in Australia and New Zealand, enrolled 9,014 men and women with cholesterol 155 to 271 mg/dl. Treatment with pravastatin 40 mg/day reduced the primary end-point coronary heart disease mortality 24% (P<0.001). As observed in the other secondary prevention trials, stroke risk was reduced 19% [29,118]. In the LIPID trial, risk reduction was determined in prespecified tertiles of initial cholesterol. These secondary prevention trials generally demonstrated reduction in cardiovascular events as LDL cholesterol was reduced to less than 100 mg/dl (Fig. 5).

### Post-CABG Trial

Although the 4S and CARE Trials demonstrated clear benefits in secondary prevention populations over a wide range of initial cholesterol levels, they were not intended to assess the benefit afforded by different degrees of cholesterol lowering. The Post-CABG Trial [63,68,123] addressed this issue. Predominately an angiographic trial, it compared disease progression in 1,351 men (92%) and women who had undergone prior bypass surgery in a two-by-two factorial design trial of moderate versus aggressive cholesterol lowering and low-dose warfarin versus placebo administration. The moderately treated group had a mean LDL-cholesterol of 135 mg/dl compared with the aggressive cholesterol lowering group (statin $+/-$ bile acid sequestrant), in whom a mean LDL-cholesterol of 95 mg/dl coincided with less bypass graft disease progression than the moderate treatment group over 4 years. Long-term (7.5-year) cardiovascular event risk was reduced 24% (P<0.001), and mortality was reduced 35% in the aggressive treatment group. As such, this trial was the first to demonstrate additional benefit with intensive LDL lowering (e.g., less than 100 mg/dL) as recommended by the National Cholesterol Education Program (NCEP) [254,255,297].

### Atorvastatin versus Revascularization Trial (AVERT)

The findings of the Post-CABG trial were substantiated by the AVERT trial [120] which compared aggressive cholesterol reduction (atorvastatin 80 mg/day) to usual cholesterol reduction and angioplasty in 341 coronary heart disease subjects with stable mild angina. Atorvastatin reduced LDL-cholesterol from 144 to 77 mg/dl and the usual cholesterol lowering regimen from 147 to 119 mg/dl. The primary composite clinical end-point was reduced 36% in the aggressive treatment group, mostly due to reduced hospitalizations for unstable angina (p $=$ 0.048) and time to first event was significantly reduced (p<0.03). A present limitation of AVERT interpretation is the lack of generalizability of these findings as the study was performed before widespread stent deployment.

### The Myocardial Ischemia Reduction with Aggressive Cholesterol Lowering (MIRACL) Study

Prior to the MIRACL study, secondary prevention trials enrolled patients with stable CHD. In contrast, the MIRACL study assessed the 16-week effect of atorvastatin (80 mg/day)

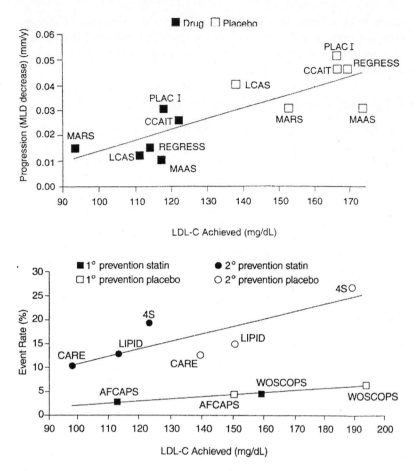

**Figure 5** Association between on-treatment LDL-cholesterol and cardiovascular events in primary prevention, secondary prevention and angiographic trials. 4S = Scandinavian Simvastatin Survival Study, AFCAPS = Air Force/Texas Coronary Atherosclerosis Prevention Study, CARE = Cholesterol and Recurrent Events trial, LIPID = Long-term Intervention with Pravastatin in Ischemic Disease trial, WOCOPS = West of Scotland Coronary Prevention Study. CCAIT = Canadian Coronary Atherosclerosis Intervention Trial, LCAS = Lipoprotein and Coronary Atherosclerosis Study, LDL-C = low-density lipoprotein cholesterol, MAAS = Multicentre Anti-Atheroma Study, MARS = Monitored Atherosclerosis Regression study, PLAC I = Pravastatin Limitation of Atherosclerosis in the Coronary Arteries, REGRESS = Regression Growth Evaluation Statin Study. (From Ref. 284)

in 3,086 men and women, 26–94 years of age presenting with acute coronary syndrome (unstable angina or non–Q-wave myocardial infarction [124]. Atorvastatin was started 1–4 days after admission and was given if cholesterol was less than 270 mg/dl. The initial mean total and LDL cholesterol levels were 206 and 124 mg/dl, respectively. Treated and control patients had LDL cholesterol levels of 72 and 135 mg/dl, respectively. At 16 weeks, the primary composite endpoint, death, nonfatal myocardial infarction, cardiac arrest and resuscitation, or hospitalization for angina was lowered 16% (14.8% vs. 17.4%) by atorvastatin (p = 0.048). Statistically significant benefit was found in the subgroup with below median initial LDL cholesterol (less than 121 mg/dl). An unexpected 50% reduction in stroke was also observed. This study highlights that early, intensive cholesterol lowering potentiates the reduction in inflammation [133] and improves the outcome of patients presenting with ACS, irrespective of baseline cholesterol level. Conversely, discontinuation of statin therapy in ACS patients who had been previously treated, may result in rebound increases in CHD event rates [134].

## Medical Research Council-Heart Protection Study (MRC-HPS)

The largest of all the clinical endpoint trials (n = 20,000), HPS was a 5 year study designed to evaluate the impact of statin (simvastatin) therapy in high-risk patients with or without antioxidant vitamins. Entry criteria included preexisting CHD, diabetes mellitus, other vascular disease, or treated hypertension. Significant reductions in overall mortality and CHD event rates (24–33%) were observed in essentially all high-risk subjects, including diabetics and with low baseline LDL cholesterol (e.g., less than 100 mg/dL) [128,132]. This study provided compelling evidence that all subjects with vascular disease should be treated with statin therapy irrespective of baseline LDL cholesterol and a revised policy statement regarding MRC-HPS and its application in the National Cholesterol Education Program is anticipated in 2004.

## Veterans Affairs HDL Intervention Trial (VA-HIT)

The VA-HIT trial [121,126,129] was designed to investigate the use of the fibrate, gemfibrozil, in normocholesterolemic CHD patients (mean age, 64 years, LDL-C, 111 mg/dl) with low HDL-cholesterol (e.g., less than 40 mg/dl). Gemfibrozil 600 mg twice daily increased HDL-cholesterol 6%, reduced triglycerides 31%, without affecting levels of LDL-cholesterol. The primary end-point, coronary heart disease mortality and nonfatal myocardial infarction was reduced 22% (P = 0.006). HDL cholesterol raising accounted for less than 25% of the benefit observed in the study with the highest on-treatment HDL-C evidencing the lowest event rates. The results were most favorable in the presence of diabetes or elevated plasma insulin [137].

## Bezafibrate Infarction Prevention (BIP) study

The BIP study, another secondary prevention study employing fibrate (bezafibrate) therapy, evaluated 3,090 subjects with different demographic and biochemical characteristics than in VA-HIT, namely younger age (mean = 60 yrs), higher baseline LDL-cholesterol (mean = 148 mg/dl), and fewer diabetes (10% vs. more than 25%) [130,131]. The data from this 6.2 year study found a nonsignificant 7.3% reduction in the primary endpoint, recurrent MI, or sudden cardiac death. However, subgroup analysis demonstrated a 40% reduction in the subgroup with baseline TG greater than or equal to 200 mg/dl [130]. These data suggest that fibrate therapy is not effective first line therapy, compared with statins in CHD subjects with mixed hyperlipidemia [324].

## TREATMENT GOALS

The NCEP Adult Treatment Panel recommendations [254,255,297] are based on measurements of LDL and HDL cholesterol and triglycerides which require fasting conditions. Dietary and drug management should be initiated as soon as the diagnoses of cardiovascular disease and dyslipidemia are established. For patients with established cardiovascular disease, diabetes, or coronary disease equivalent risk, the NCEP guidelines recommend that lipid management be undertaken with the primary goal of reducing

LDL cholesterol less than 100 mg/dl, and secondary goals of: reducing non-HDL cholesterol less than 130 mg/dl (or triglycerides less than 150 mg/dl) [285] followed by increasing HDL cholesterol greater than 40 mg/dl. The third report of the NCEP employs a global risk assessment table to prioritize primary prevention. With multiple risk factors, but without established CHD or its risk equivalent risk, the NCEP recommends treatment of LDL less than130 mg/dl. In healthy individuals without multiple risk factors (10-year risk less than 10%), the NCEP recommends LDL less than 160 mg/dl. Before therapy is initiated, the following secondary causes of dyslipidemia should be evaluated: hypothyroidism, diabetes mellitus, renal and hepatic disease, dysproteinemias, alcoholism, anorexia, porphyria, and pregnancy, and use of progestins, anabolic steroids, corticosteroids, diuretics, and beta-blockers. Lipid management should be based on multiple fasting lipoprotein determinations. It is estimated that 36 million Americans may benefit with cholesterol lowering drugs in comparison with the approximate 10 million American currently on therapy.

## Dietary Treatment

Most westernized individuals have elevated cholesterol levels because of excess saturated fat and calorie intake and inadequate physical activity levels. Some westernized societies, however, have particularly low rates of coronary heart disease. Examples include the Pacific Rim population, which consumes a low fat diet and the Mediterranean Region population, which consumes a high monounsaturated fat, fruit and vegetable diet. Low total fat, low saturated fat, and Mediterranean diets have been shown to reduce the progression of coronary disease and cardiovascular events [8,44,46,47,243,248,252,258,261–264, 267,270,274,275,290,298,299]. Dietary saturated fat reduces the activity of hepatic LDL receptors [138] and obesity leads to an overproduction of lipoproteins [139]. Dietary therapy remains the cornerstone of cholesterol reduction in primary prevention—especially for low-risk individuals [254,255,297]—and is an important addition to drug therapy in secondary prevention. In addition to improving cholesterol levels, appropriate diet can achieve weight loss and improve blood pressure, hyperglycemia, and insulin resistance.

The goals of diet are to achieve desirable body weight, serum lipids, insulin sensitivity, and vascular biology. Replacing saturated fat with monounsaturated and polyunsaturated fats reduces serum total and LDL-cholesterol [290,298,299]. The reduction in HDL-cholesterol caused by polyunsaturated fats may in part reflect upregulation of the SR-B1 receptor which receives free cholesterol directly from HDL and participates in reverse cholesterol transport (discussion following) [301]. In general, reductions in dietary saturated fat and calories are more effective in lowering cholesterol than is reducing dietary cholesterol. Although effective in reducing cholesterol, a high carbohydrate diet (greater than 60% of total calories) will often increase triglycerides [305].

Saturated and monounsaturated fats directly impair endothelial function through an oxidative stress mechanism in a manner similar to hypercholesterolemia [192,194 198–200]. The impairment is more pronounced in diabetic patients and is reduced by the concomitant consumption of antioxidant-rich fruits and vegetables [302]. This may explain the benefit of high dietary intake of antioxidants in the form of flavonoid-rich fruits and vegetables observed in the Seven Countries and Lyon Diet Heart studies [8,264].

The physician plays a pivotal role in suggesting and reinforcing dietary modification, but implementation is greatly assisted by dietitians and/or nurses [248,253–257, 259,261,265]. To lower LDL cholesterol, the NCEP recommend a diet containing: 25% to 35% of calories from fat, less than 7% of calories from saturated fat, and more than 200 mg per day of cholesterol. Examples of the cholesterol lowering potential of foods are: 15% by stanol and sterol ester margarines (2 gm per day), 10% by soy products containing 50 gm isoflavones per day, and 5% by oat bran containing 6 gm per day. The NCEP recommends the use of soluble fiber and stanol/sterol ester margarines to lower cholesterol. Importantly, 54% of Americans are currently more than 20% overweight [9]. Reduction in saturated and trans fats can be achieved by eating less meat, whole milk products, tropical oils (palm, coconut), and hydrogenated vegetable oils. The FDA has mandated that food labels contain the quantity of these dietary fats in food packages. Omega-3 fatty acids found in fish and vegetable oils, such as canola oil, have several vascular benefits, including improvements in endothelial function, membrane stabilization, reduction in platelet aggregability and reductions in triglycerides [209,243, 261–264,267,274,277]. One of two angiographic trials has demonstrated a reduction in disease progression with administration of fish oil [84,93]. The GISSI Study Group reported a 17% decrease in cardiovascular mortality with addition of omega-3 fatty acid (1 gm/day) in postmyocardial infarction patients, most of which was due to a decrease in sudden death (26%) [198]. Low-glycemic index, complex carbohydrate intake (e.g., especially soluble fiber) is strongly encouraged in a heart healthy diet. Moderate alcohol intake (1–2 oz/day) is associated with reduced cardiovascular risk and total mortality compared with either abstinence of heavier intake. Overall mortality is increased with more alcohol consumption, however, because of other alcohol related diseases, as well as increased hypertension and myocardial dysfunction [9]. Regular physical activity decreases weight, LDL-cholesterol, triglycerides, and the risk of myocardial infarction and sudden death and increases HDL-cholesterol, cardiovascular conditioning, and a sense of well being.

In contrast to the generally prudent recommendations of the NCEP, which produce approximately 5% reductions in cholesterol, the Mediterranean diet rich in fruits, vegetables, fish, pasta, and wine appears to offer a substantial advantage in reducing cardiovascular risk [261–264,267,274]. The Lyon Diet Heart Trial [274] demonstrated a 72% reduction in cardiovascular events and 60% in mortality with the following dietary advice: more bread, fruits, vegetables, and beans, less meat and whole-milk dairy products, and use of omega-3 enriched canola oil. An alternative approach is the very low fat diet (Pritikin, Ornish) [44,67] containing approximately 10% of calories from fat. Less long-term data is available of these diets, but small angiographic trials have reported angiographic disease regression in mean luminal diameter of 3% at 5 years. However, few patients and physicians are willing and/or able to implement these diets, in part due to palatability and the restriction of cardioprotective mono and polyunsaturates, particularly omega-3 fats. The current NCEP guidelines [297] recommend up to 35% calories from fat, but recommend minimizing, and if possible eliminating, saturates and trans fats.

## Physical Activity

Reduced physical activity is a major risk factor for cardiovascular disease, and is an essential component in the management of hypercholesterolemia. Myocardial infarction risk is reduced by: 50% by walking 30 minutes (about 1.5 miles) daily, 80% by vigorous activity once or twice weekly, 90% by vigorous activity 3 or 4 times weekly, and 98% by vigorous activity 5 or more times weekly [303,304]. Physical activity provides a number of salutary effects on the cardiovascular system and coronary risk factors, including decreases in blood pressure and heart rate and increases in HDL cholesterol. It also reduces triglycerides, increases insulin sensitivity, and promotes fibrinolysis. The combination of an exercise regimen (30 minutes of cycle ergometry daily to achieve 75% of age-predicted maximum heart rate) combined with a low-fat diet (less than 20% of calories from fat) has been demonstrated to reduce the progression of angiographic coronary artery disease and increase the frequency of disease regression. Subjective improvements in patients' sense of well-being and less depression have also been noted. Weight training appears to provide an additional 20–25% reduction in CHD events that is independent of aerobic activities [306]. The NCEP recommends at least 30 minutes of exercise daily.

## Drug Treatment

Drug treatment of hypercholesterolemia is generally more effective than dietary manipulation [9,252,268,278,279,282,289]. Drug therapy may be postponed in low-risk primary prevention patients for 3–6 months to allow patients to modify their diet. In contrast, secondary prevention and high-risk primary prevention patients should be started on both drug and dietary therapy as soon as hypercholesterolemia is identified [278,297]. Cholesterol modifying drugs can generally be divided into two classes, those which predominately lower LDL cholesterol (HMG-CoA reductase inhibitors or ''statins'' and bile acid sequestrants) and those which predominately lower triglycerides and increase HDL cholesterol (nicotinic acid and fibric acid derivatives) [9,297]. HMG-CoA reductase inhibitors secondarily increase HDL-cholesterol and lower triglycerides (Table 3). Higher doses of HMG-CoA reductase inhibitors are more effective in lowering triglycerides in hypertriglyceridemic subjects and in increasing HDL cholesterol in low HDL cholesterol subjects. In contrast, bile acid sequestrants may increase triglycerides, as can a high carbohydrate diet, alcohol, and estrogen. Intestinal absorption inhibitors reduce LDL 15–20% without raising triglycerides. Nicotinic acid is the most effective drug for increasing HDL cholesterol, and in higher doses (more than 1 gm/d) also decreases LDL cholesterol. The fibric acid derivatives are the most effective drugs for decreasing triglycerides.

### Statins: LDL-cholesterol lowering effects

The LDL cholesterol target goal set for CHD patients remains less than 100 mg/dl. Determinations of LDL-cholesterol require a fasting blood sample; transient reductions occur following MI, acute illness, and hospitalization [269]. HMG-CoA reductase inhibitors are the agents of first choice for elevated LDL-cholesterol because of their high effectiveness (25–60% LDL-cholesterol lowering) and infrequent side effects [251,260,271, 280,282,284,292,294,336]. This drug class inhibits cellular production of cholesterol, which increases the expression of hepatic LDL receptors. At present, six HMG-CoA reductase inhibitors are available in the US: atorvastatin, fluvastatin, lovastatin, pravastatin, rosuvastatin, and simvastatin. On average, doubling the dose of an HMG-CoA reductase

**Table 3**   Drug Effects on Lipoproteins

|                        | Total-C   | LDL-C     | HDL-C    | Trig      |
|------------------------|-----------|-----------|----------|-----------|
| HMG-CoA RIs            | ↓20–50%   | ↓20–60%   | ↑5–15%   | ↓7–30%    |
| Bile acid sequestrants | ↓10–20%   | ↓15–30%   | ↑3–5%    | ↑5–15%    |
| Fibric acid derivatives| ↓0–10%    | ↓0–10%    | ↑5–20%   | ↓20–50%   |
| Nicotinic acid:        | ↓10–20%   | ↓10–20%   | ↑15–35%  | ↓15–40%   |

C = cholesterol, HDL-C = high-density cholesterol, RI = LDL-C = low-density cholesterol, HMG-CoA RI = 3-hydroxy-3-methylglutaryl-coenzyme A reductase inhibitors, Trig = triglycerides

inhibitor will lower LDL-cholesterol an additional 6–7%. HMG-CoA reductase inhibitors are usually given once-a-day in the evening since most cholesterol is synthesized at night. Dividing the HMG-CoA reductase inhibitors into twice-a-day doses adds 2–4% cholesterol lowering (atorvastatin should be given only once-a-day at any time). After initiating an HMG-CoA reductase inhibitor, a lipid panel should be repeated in about 6 weeks and diet modification should again be reinforced. If the LDL-cholesterol goal is not reached, a higher dose or more potent statin should be considered. Alternatively, a second agent such as a cholesterol absorption inhibitor or bile acid sequestrant may be added. With combination therapy, it is now possible to achieve LDL-cholesterol reduction in the range of 60–70% in patients with polygenic hypercholesterolemia, the most common phenotype of elevated LDL-cholesterol.

*Statins: non LDL-cholesterol lowering effects*

In addition to inhibiting HMG-CoA reductase, statins block other intermediaries in the cholesterol biosynthetic pathway, including farnesyl pyrophosphate and geranylgeranylpyrophosphate (Fig. 6) [307]. This results in reduction in the isoprenylation of signaling G-proteins (e.g., RHO and RAS) that are important in cellular processing and posttranslational modification [307]. Inhibition in protein isoprenylation contributes to improvement in endothelial function as well as reduction in inflammation, smooth muscle cell hypertrophy and thrombogenicity (Fig. 7). While the clinical significance of these effects beyond lipid lowering is yet to be established, the strongest link between statins and LDL independent effects is on reduction of systemic inflammation as measured by C-reactive protein [308]. Additional salutary effects attributable to statins include reduction of calcific aortic stenosis [309], improvement in symptomatic CHF [310], and claudication [311]. Other

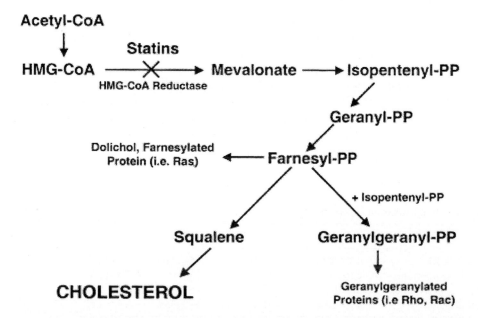

**Figure 6** Cholesterol biosynthetic pathway. Inhibition of 3-hydroxy-3-methylglutaryl coenzyme A (HMG-CoA) reductase by statins decreases the synthesis of isoprenoids and cholesterol. PP indicates pyrophosphate. (From Ref. 307)

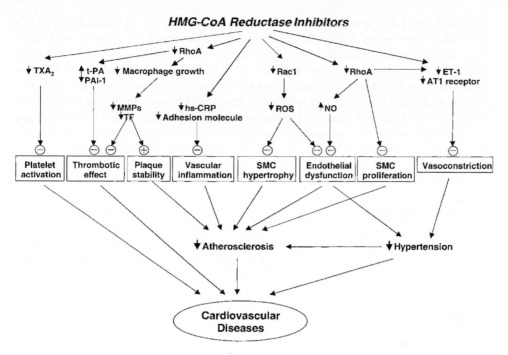

**Figure 7** Effects of statins on vascular wall cells. Summary of the cholesterol-independent effects of statins, which include improving endothelial function, inhibiting SMC proliferation and hypertrophy, enhancing the stability of atherosclerotic plaques, decreasing oxidative stress, preventing thrombotic responses, and attenuating vascular inflammation. ET-1 indicates endothelin-1; AT1 receptor, angiotensin type 1 receptor; TF, tissue factor; t-PA, tissue-type plasminogen activator; PAI-1, plasminogen activator inhibitor-1; and $TXA_2$, thromboxane $A_2$. (From Ref. 307)

cardiovascular areas under active investigation include neuroinflammatory (e.g., multiple sclerosis) and neurodegenerative disorders (e.g., Alzheimer's disease) [312].

HMG-CoA reductase inhibitors are generally well tolerated drugs. Infrequently, hepatocellular injury or myositis occur. HMG-CoA reductase inhibitors commonly produce minimal elevations in liver function tests and should not be discontinued unless values exceed three times normal upper limit. Increased alcohol intake should also be considered if abnormal liver function tests are observed. Hepatic dysfunction is reversible after drug discontinuation, and a lesser dose or another agent may be tried. Myositis (diffuse muscle pain and weakness) with markedly elevated CPK's (greater than 10 times upper normal limit) rarely occurs with HMG-CoA reductase inhibitors, although the frequency rises with concomitant use of gemfibrozil, immunosuppressive agents, macrolide antibiotics, and antifungal therapy [313]. In the extreme, rhabdomyolysis and renal failure occur. Conditions enhancing the likelihood of the latter include elderly age, female gender, reduced muscle mass, hypothyroidism, and renal insufficiency. In the absence of elevated CPK, myalgias may also present with bilateral and symmetric muscle (proximal greater than distal) involvement. Intercurrent illness may precipitate a transient episode. In these cases, statins are temporarily discontinued but may be reinitiated at a lower dose or changed to another class (e.g., cholesterol absorption inhibitors, bile acid sequestrants) following a short (1–2 weeks) wash out period.

Cholesterol absorption inhibitors represent a new class of agents that selectively reduce uptake of dietary and biliary cholesterol at the intestinal brush border membrane [314]. The prototype, ezetimibe and its glucoronide metabolite is active at the intestinal wall with minimal systemic absorption. This agent lowers LDL-cholesterol 15–20% and appears to be well tolerated. Mild gastrointestinal discomfort has been reported. The medication is available in one dose (10 mg) which may be taken anytime during the day with or without food. It may be used as monotherapy or in combination with statins. Reduction in triglycerides and C-reactive protein and HDL-cholesterol enhancement occurs when statin-ezetimibe combination is employed [315]. Clinical trials are underway to determine whether statin-ezetimibe combination may be more effective in reducing CHD events compared with statin monotherapy.

Bile acid sequestrants (cholestyramine, colestipol, colesevelam) increase cholesterol excretion by binding bile acids in the intestine during enterohepatic re*Circulation* [9,260,282]. These non-systemic agents lower LDL-cholesterol 10–25%. Gastrointestinal side effects (e.g., constipation, bloating, and flatulence) are less common with colesevelam or with low doses (8–12 gm divided daily) of other resins. They may also interfere with the absorption of other drugs, including coumadin and other cholesterol lowering agents. Patients should be advised to take other drugs at least 30 minutes before or wait 4 to 5 hours after taking cholestyramine or colestipol. A similar time restriction does not apply to colesevelam.

*HDL-Cholesterol*

Low HDL-cholesterol predicts initial cardiac events [242] and is the most common lipoprotein abnormality in CHD patients. In the setting of desirable total cholesterol (less than 200 mg/dl), the likelihood of low HDL ranges between 65–80% and is associated with a 2-fold increased rate of reinfarction and cardiovascular death [316]

With each 5 mg/dl below the median (45 mg/dl in men and 55 mg/dl in women), the rate of CHD events increases 25%. HDL is credited as a primary promoter of reverse cholesterol transport. It begins as a partially lipidated disc-like moiety that derives surface components (apolipoproteins and phopholipid) during the hydrolysis of triglyceride-rich lipoproteins derived from liver and intestine. These pre-β HDL particles avidly participate in the transport of cholesterol effluxed from extrahepatic cells (e.g., vascular wall macrophages) and are mediated by an ATP binding cassette transporter (ABCA1) (Fig. 8) [317]. Apolipoprotein A-I assists in esterification of cholesterol and the resulting cholesterol-enriched HDL particles may then transfer cholesteryl ester to lower density lipoproteins for hepatic uptake in exchange for triglyceride, a process mediated by cholesteryl ester transfer protein (CETP). Alternatively, HDL may anchor and deposit cholesterol in peripheral (e.g., steroidogenic) tissues for hormone production or directly taken into the liver for hepatic catabolism and ultimately, biliary excretion. While it has generally been accepted that high levels of HDL-cholesterol are cardioprotective, CHD that develops with high HDL-cholesterol may be a consequence of proinflammatory HDL particles [318]. In contrast, the risk of CHD with isolated low HDL-cholesterol (e.g., in the absence of other CHD risk factors) is not significantly elevated unless accompanied by additional factors, including triglyceride and LDL-C elevation. Primary isolated low HDL-cholesterol (less than 40 mg/dl in men and less than 50 mg/dl with TG less than 100 mg/dl) is common in young individuals but rare in the aged [319] as metabolic factors (e.g., weight gain, sedentary lifestyle) intervene to enhance the likelihood of concomitant hypertriglyceridemia. Subjects at highest risk include the triad of elevated LDL-cholesterol and triglycerides in association with low HDL-cholesterol [250].

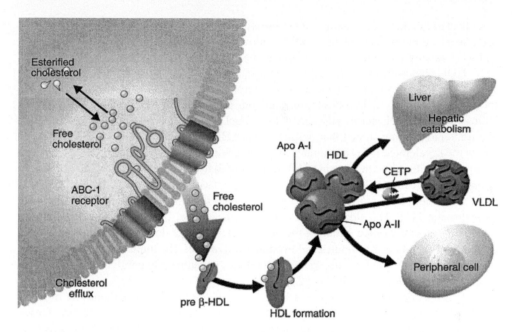

**Figure 8** Overview of reverse cholesterol transport. ABCA1 = adenosine triphosphate-binding cassette transporter-1; Apo = apolipoprotein; CETP = cholesterol-ester transfer protein; HDL = high-density lipoprotein; VLDL = very-low-density lipoprotein. (From Ref. 317)

The most promising data suggesting that regression of atherosclerosis may occur was the intravenous use of recombinant ApoAI Milano which after only 5 weekly injections demonstrated a 4% regression in plaque volume as measured by IVUS (Fig. 9). This study reaffirms prior clinical data where combination of LDL lowering (statin + bile acid sequestrant) and HDL raising therapies (niacin) resulted in the greatest regression [42].

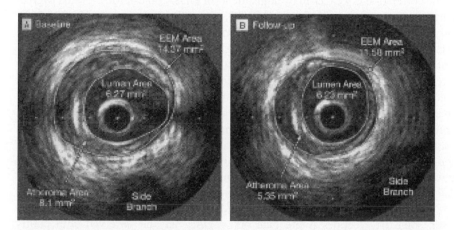

**Figure 9** apoAI Milano Example of atheroma regression in a patient who received high dose ETC-216. The atheroma area decreased from 8.1 to 5.35 mm2 with virtually change in lumen area. EEM indicates external elastic membrane. (From Ref. 337)

If replicated in larger scale studies, these promising preliminary data support the potential acute use of therapy that enhances RCT, followed by the combination of LDL lowering and RCT raising therapies to maximize CHD event reduction [337].

HDL-cholesterol is increased by exercise, alcohol, smoking cessation, estrogen, and weight loss [9]. A low fat diet and anabolic steroids lower HDL-cholesterol, although the former is useful for LDL-cholesterol reduction. Drugs are generally not as effective in increasing HDL-cholesterol as they are in lowering LDL-cholesterol [9,260,282,286]. Clinical trials have demonstrated that despite meager HDL-cholesterol raising, statin therapy blunts the accelerated CHD event rates in patients with low HDL-cholesterol [321]. While statins remain first line therapy in CHD subjects with low HDL-cholesterol, nicotinic acid is the most effective HDL-cholesterol raising agent (up to 30%). A delayed (15 year) reduction in all-cause mortality (11%) was observed with nicotinic acid in the Coronary Drug Project [11]. The side effects of flushing, headache, dyspepsia, and dry skin are common, especially when initiating the drug or increasing a dose. The use of nonenteric coated aspirin taken 30 minutes before niacin attenuates flushing. Nicotinic acid may precipitate a gouty attack in susceptible individuals, accentuate hyperglycemia and in rare cases lead to hepatic dysfunction [322].

If immediate release niacin is selected, low doses (50 mg bid) should be initiated with slow increases in titration to 1.0 to 1.5 gm bid. Alternatively, slow release (twice daily) or extended release (once daily) preparations are often better tolerated and effective.

Fibric acid derivatives (gemfibrozil, fenofibrate) are also useful in increasing HDL-cholesterol (5–10%) [281,282] particularly when accompanied by elevated triglycerides [323] and have been shown to reduce the progression of coronary artery disease and cardiovascular events (BECAIT [61], LOCAT [66], Helsinki Heart Study [98], VA-HIT [121,126]). These agents are generally well tolerated, but the concomitant use of an HMG-CoA reductase inhibitor and gemfibrozil increases the risk of myositis. Therefore, fenofibrate is now the agent of choice if combined with a statin. Fibric acid derivatives are recommended as second line therapy in CHD patients with low HDL-cholesterol (less than 40 mg/dl) and low LDL-cholesterol (less than 130 mg/dl) [121,281,282].

*Triglycerides*

Although the correlation is weakened by adjustment for HDL-cholesterol, elevated triglycerides remain an independent risk factor for CHD, especially in women [9,283,287,293]. Hypertriglyceridemia strongly predicts cardiovascular events in those with established cardiovascular disease and hypertriglyceridemic patients derive greater benefit from LDL-cholesterol lowering (4S Study [100–105]) and HDL-cholesterol raising therapies (Helsinki Heart Study [98]). Not unexpectedly, subjects with mixed dyslipidemia, characterized by elevated LDL-cholesterol and triglycerides in association with low HDL-cholesterol have high event rates which are reduced to a far greater extent with statin therapy compared with isolated high LDL-cholesterol, in whom event rates are considerably lower [324].

Postprandial rather than fasting hypertriglyceridemia may be more predictive of coronary disease risk [9] and increases in postprandial triglycerides have been shown to correlate with the transient endothelial dysfunction observed after a fatty meal [204,206]. The NCEP Adult Treatment Panel guidelines consider a fasting triglyceride more than150 mg/dl as borderline high and greater than 200 mg/dl as elevated [254,255,297]. The presence of very high triglycerides (more than 400 mg/dl) may be observed with poorly controlled diabetes mellitus, alcoholism, and renal insufficiency [293,325].

While the optimal fasting triglyceride has not been established there are data that support a cutpoint of less than 100 mg/dL [326–328]. However, there are limitations in measuring triglycerides which in part is related to inherent variability affected by caloric intake and blood volume. Therefore, to establish a more accurate baseline triglyceride level, a minimum of 3 measurements should be taken after an overnight (10-hour) fast and collected in the same postural position for a minimum of 10–15 minutes [329]. Still, triglycerides do not measure atherogenicity of triglyceride-rich particles and therefore other parameters (e.g., apoC3 levels and circulating remnant lipoproteins) [330] may in time enhance identification of subjects with mild-moderate elevation in triglycerides who are at highest risk of CHD events.

Hypertriglyceridemia should be initially managed by exclusion of secondary causes followed by lifestyle modification, including weight reduction, decreased dietary fat and alcohol, exercise, and smoking cessation. Estrogen, bile acid sequestrants, and very high carbohydrate diets increase triglycerides [9]. Fish oil is effective in reducing triglycerides (20–40%) and reduces cardiovascular events [209,243,261–264,274,277]. Fibric acid derivatives and nicotinic acid are the most effective drugs in lowering triglycerides (35%) [9,281,282]. HMG-CoA reductase inhibitors may also lower elevated triglycerides 20–30% with baseline levels exceeding 200 mg/dl.

*Mixed Dyslipidemia*

A reduced HDL-cholesterol combined with elevated triglycerides is frequently associated with small-dense LDL particles and is particularly atherogenic [9,92,95,160,272,273,276]. Mixed dyslipidemia may be associated with the metabolic syndrome, which is also comprised of visceral adiposity, impaired fasting glucose and hypertension. The current NCEP guidelines recommend a non-HDL (LDL cholesterol + VLDL cholesterol ) of less than 130 mg/dl for patients with mixed hyperlipidemia. Because triglycerides are derived using the formula VLDL-cholesterol/5, target goals are LDL cholesterol less than 100 mg/dl and triglycerides less than 150 mg/dl. Nicotinic acid and fibric acid derivatives are effective agents in normalizing LDL particle composition and changing the LDL pattern to less atherogenic (reduced susceptibility to oxidation), more buoyant LDL particles [157]. HMG-CoA reductase inhibitors decrease total particle number [158,159]. Therefore, mixed dyslipidemia is often managed with a combinations of an HMG-CoA reductase inhibitor and either nicotinic acid or a fibric acid derivative [282]. The risk of myositis with combined therapy is a potential concern, but is relatively uncommon in the absence of drug-drug interactions (e.g., immunosuppressive therapy), renal failure, and hypothyroidism [331].

**Treatment Gap**

Despite widespread lay and physician education programs stressing the importance of cholesterol management, many patients potentially benefiting from cholesterol lowering remain untreated [9,243–247,253,256,259,265,266,295]. Patients with vascular disease in general [295] and women in particular are under treated even when there is no difference compared to men in either extent or severity of CAD [332]. There also continues to be hesitancy toward the use of statin therapy among the aged, despite recent data demonstrating reduction in CHD events in octogenarians [333,334]. Several explanations have been proposed for this treatment gap including: lack of belief in the cholesterol hypothesis, confusion regarding guidelines, routine nature of cholesterol treatment, lack of knowledge of lifestyle and drug management, extended reliance on diet treatment, missed communication between generalists and specialists, concerns over adverse effects and/or expense of drug treatment, and poor reimbursement for cholesterol management [9,247,253,259,266].

In view of the overwhelming data demonstrating clinical benefit with lipid lowering therapies, there has been rising momentum toward in-hospital initiation of these agents which have yielded important dividends because earlier implementation of cardioprotective agents reduces clinical events and improves overall patient care [335].

## REFERENCES

1. Anitschkow N. Experimental atherosclerosis in animals. In Cowdry EV, Ed. Arteriosclerosis: A Survey of the Problem. New York: Macmillan, 1933:271–322.
2. Keys A, Araranis C, Blackburn HW, Van Buchem FS, Buzina R, Djordjevic BD, Dontas AS, Fidanza F, Karvonen VJ, Kimura N, Lekos D, Monti M, Puddu V, Taylor HL Epidemiologic studies related to coronary heart disease: Characteristics of men aged 40–59 in seven countries. Acta Med Scand Suppl. 1966;460:1–392.
3. Gordon T, Kannel WB. Premature mortality from coronary heart disease. Framinghan Heart Study. JAMA 1971;215:1617–1625.
4. AHA Committee Report. Risk factors and coronary heart disease. A statement for physicians. Circulation 1980;62:449A–455A.
5. Anderson M, Castelli WP, Levy D. Cholesterol and mortality: 30 years of follow-up from the Framingham Study. JAMA 1987;257:2176–2180.
6. Joseph A, Ackerman D, Talley JD, Johnstone JD, Kupersmith. Manifestations of coronary atherosclerosis in young trauma victims– an autopsy study. J Am Coll Cardiol. 1993 Aug; 22(2):459–67.
7. Thaulow E, Erikssen J, Sansvik L, Erikssen G, Jorgensen L, Cohn PF. Initial clinical presentation of cardiac disease in asymptomatic men with silent myocardial ischemia and angiographically documented coronary artery disease (the Oslo Ischemia study). Am J Cardiol. 1993;72:629–633.
8. Verschuren WMM, Jacobs DR, Bloemberg BP, Kromhout D, Menotti A, Aravanis C, Blackburn H, Buzina R, Dontas AS, Fidanza F. Serum total cholesterol and long–term coronary heart disease motality in different cultures. Twenty–five year follow up of the seven countries study. JAMA. 1995;274(2):131–6.
9. Miller M, Vogel R. The practice of coronary disease prevention. Baltimore: Williams and Wilkins, 1996:1–294.
10. Berenson GS, Srinivasan SR, Bao W, Newman WP 3rd, Tracey RE, Wattigney WA. Association between multiple cardiovascular risk factors and atherosclerosis in children and young adults: the Bogalusa Heart Study. N Engl J Med. 1998 Jun 4;338(23):1650–6.
11. Holme I. An analysis of randomized trials evaluating the effect of cholesterol reduction on total mortality and coronary heart disease incidence. Circulation 1990;82:1916–1924.
12. Rossouw J, Lewis B, Rifkind BM. The value of lowering cholesterol after myocardial infarction. N Engl J Med 1990;323:1112–1119.
13. The Multiple Risk Factor Intervention Trial Research Group. Mortality rates after 10.5 years for participants in the Multiple Risk Factor Intervention Trial. Findings related to a priori hypothesis of the trial. JAMA 1990;263:1795–1801.
14. Vogel RA. Comparative clinical consequences of aggressive lipid management, coronary angioplasty and bypass surgery in coronary disease. Am J Cardiol 1992;69:1229–1233.
15. Manson JE, Tosteson H, Ridker PM, Satterfield S, Herbert P, O'Connor GT, Buring JE, Hennekens CH. The primary prevention of myocardial infarction. N Engl J Med. 1992 May 21;326(21):1406–16.
16. LaRosa JC, Cleeman JI. Cholesterol lowering as a treatment for established coronary heart disease. Circulation 1992;85:1229–1235.
17. LaRosa JC. Cholesterol lowering, low cholesterol, and mortality. Am J Cardiol 1993;72: 776–786.

18. Stamler J, Stamler R, Brown WV, Gotto AM, Greenland P, Grundy S, Hegsted DM, Luepker RV, Neaton JD, Steinberg D. Serum cholesterol. Doing the right thing. Circulation. 1993Oct; 88(4 pt 1):1954–60.

19. Levine GN, Keaney JF, Vita JA. Medical progress: Cholesterol reduction in cardiovascular disease. N Engl J Med 1995;332:512–521.

20. Gotto AM. Lipid lowering, regression and coronary events. A review of the Interdisciplinary Council on Lipids and Cardiovascular Risk Intervention, seventh council meeting. Circulation 1995;92:646–656.

21. Gould AL, Rossouw JE, Santanello NC, Heyse JF, Furberg CD. Cholesterol reduction yields clinical benefit. A new look at old data. Circulation. 1995 Apr 15;91(8):2274–82.

22. Gould KL, Ornish D, Scherwitz L, Brown S, Edens RP, Hess MJ, Mullani N, Bolomey L, Dobbs F, Armstrong WT. Changes in myocardial perfusion abnormalities by positron emission tomography after long–term , intense risk factor modification. JAMA. 1995 Sep 20; 274(11):894–901.

23. Lacoste L, Lam JYT, Hung J, Letchacovski G, Solymoss CB, Waters D. Hyperlipidemia and coronary disease. Correction of the increased thrombogenic potential with cholesterol reduction. Circulation. 1995 Dec 1;92(11):3172–7.

24. Ganz P, Creager MA, Fang JC, McConnell MV, Lee RT, Libby P, Selwyn AP. Pathogenic mechanisms of atherosclerosis: effect of lipid lowering on the biology of atherosclerosis. Am J Med. 1996 Oct 8;101(4A):4A10S–16S.

25. Nofer JR, Tepel M, Kehrel B, Wierwille S, Walter M, Seedorf U, Zidek W, Assman G. Low–density lipoproteins inhibit the NA+/H+ antiport in human platelets. A novel mechanism enhancing platelet activity in hypercholesterolemia. Circulation. 1997 Mar 18;95(6):1370–7.

26. Rosenson RS, Tangney CC. Antiatherothromboic properties of statins. Implications for cardio-vascular event reduction. JAMA 1998;279:1643–1650.

27. Andrews TC, Raby K, Barry J, Naimi CL, Allred E, Ganz P, Selwyn AP. Effect of cholesterol reduction on myocardial ischemia in patients with coronary disease. Circulation. 1997 Jan 21;95(2):324–8.

28. van Boven AJ, Jukema JW, Zwinderman AH, Crijns HJ, Lie KI, Bruschke AV. Reduction of transient myocardial ischemia with pravastatin in addition to the conventional treatment in patients with angina pectoris. REGRESS study group. Circulation. 1996 Oct 1;94(7): 1503–5.

29. Crouse JR 3rd, Byington RP, Hoen HM, Furberg CD. Reductase inhibitor monotherapy and stroke prevention. Arch Intern Med. 1997 Jun 23;157(12):1305–10.

30. Pedersen TR, Kjekshus J, Pyorala K, Olsson AG, Cook TJ, Musliner TA, Tobert JA, Haghfelt T. Effect of simvastatin on ischemic signs and symptoms in the Scandinavian Simvastatin Survival Study (4S). Am J Cardiol. 1998 Feb 1;81(3):333–5.

31. Huggins GS, Pasternak RC, Alpert NM, Fischman AJ, Gewirtz H. Effects of short–term treatment of hyperlipidemia on coronary vasodilator function and myocardial perfusion in regions having substantial impairment of baseline vasodilator reserve. Circulation. 1998 Sep 29;98(13):1291–6.

32. Bustos C, Hernandez–Presa MA, Ortego M, Tunon J, Ortega L, Perez F, Diaz C, Hernandez G, Egido J. HMG–CoA reductase inhibition by atorvastatin reduces neointimal inflammation in a rabbit model of atherosclerosis. J Am Coll Cardiol. 1998 Dec;32(7):2057–64.

33. Szczeklik A, Musial J, Undas A, Gajewski P, Gora P, Swadzba J, Jankowski M. Inhibition of thrombin generation by simvastatin and lack of addictive effects of aspirin in patients with marked hypercholesterolemia. J Am Coll Cardiol. 1999 Apr;33(5):1286–93.

34. Dangas G, Badimon JJ, Smith DA, Unger AH, Levine D, Shao JH, Meraj P, Fier C, Fallon JT, Ambrose JA. Pravastatin therapy in hyperlipidemia: effects on thrombus formation and the systemic hemostatic profile. J Am Coll Cardiol. 1999 Apr;33(5):1294–304.

35. Kearney D, Fitsgerald D. The anti-thrombotic effects of statins. J Am Coll Cardiol 1999;33: 1305–1307.

36. Yokoyama I, Momomura S, Ohtake T, Yonekura K, Yang W, Kobayakawa N, Aoyagi T, Sugiura S, Yamada N, Ohtomo K, Sasaki Y, Omata M, Yazaki Y. Improvement of impaired

myocardial vasodilation due to diffuse coronary atherosclerosis in hypercholesterolemics after lipid–lowering therapy. Circulation. 1999 Jul 13;100(2):117–122.

37.  Baller D, Notomamiprodjo G, Gleichmann U, Holzinger J, Weise R, Lehmann J. Improvement in coronary reserve determined by positron emission tomography after 6 months of choles-terol–lowering therapy in patients with early stages of coronary atherosclerosis. Circulation. 1999 Jun 8;99(22):2871–5.

38.  Brensike JF, Levy RL, Kelsey SF, Passamani ER, Richardson JM, Loh IK, Stone NJ, Aldrich RF, Battaglini JW, Moriarty DJ. Effects of therapy with cholestyramine on progression coro-nary arteriosclerosis: results of the NHLBI Type II Coronary Intervention Study. Circulation. 1984 Feb;69(2):313–24.

39.  Levy RI, Brensike JF, Epstein SE, Kelsey SF, Passamani ER, Richardson JM, Loh IK, Stone NJ, Aldrich RF, Battaglini JW. The influence of changes in lipid values induced by cholestyramine and diet on progression of coronary artery disease: results of the NHLBI Type II coronary Intervention Study. Circulation. 1984 Feb;69(2):325–37.

40.  Arntzenius AC, Kromhout D, Barth JD, Reiber JH, Bruschke AV, Buis B, van Gent CM, Kempen–Voogd N, Strikewerda S, van der Velde EA. Diet, lipoproteins and the progression of coronary atherosclerosis. The Leiden Intervention Trial. N Engl J Med. 1985 Mar 28; 312(13):805–11.

41.  Cashin–Hemphill L, Mack WJ, Pogoda JM, Sanmarco ME, Azen SP, Blankenhorn DH. Beneficial effects of colestipol–niacin on coronary atherosclerosis. A 4–year follow–up. JAMA. 1990 Dec 19;264(23):3013–7.

42.  Brown G, Albers JJ, Fisher LD, Schaefer SM, Lin JT, Kaplan C, Zhao XQ, Bisson BD, Fitzpatrick VF, Dodge HT. Regression of coronary artery disease as a result of intensive lipid–lowering therapy in men with high levels of apolipoprotein B. N Engl J Med. 1990 Nov 8;323(19):1289–98.

43.  Kan JP, Malloy MJ, Ports TA, Phillips NR, Diehl JC, Havel RJ. Regression of coronary atherosclerosis during treatment of familial hypercholesterolemia with combined drug regi-men. JAMA. 1990 Dec 19;264(23):3007–12.

44.  Ornish D, Brown SE, Scherwitz LW, Billings JH, Armstrong WT, Ports TA, McLanahan SM, Kirkeeide RL, Brand RJ, Gould KL. Can lifestyle changes reverse coronary heart disease? The Lifestyle Heart Trial. Lancet. 1990 Jul 21;336(8708):129–33.

45.  Buchwald H, Varco RL, Matts JP, Long JM, Fitch LL, Campbell GS, Pearce MB, Yellin AE, Edmiston WA, Smink RD Jr. Effect of partial ileal bypass surgery on mortality and morbidity from coronary heart disease in patients with hypercholesterolemia. Report of the Program on the Surgical Control of Hyperlipidemias (POSCH). N Engl J Med 1990 Oct 4; 323(14):946–55.

46.  Schuler G, Hambrecht R, Schlierf G, Grunze M, Methfessel S, Hauer K, Kubler W. Myocar-dial perfusion and regression of coronary artery disease in patients on a regimen of intensive physical exercise and a low fat diet. J Am Coll Cardiol. 1992 Jan;19(1):34–42.

47.  Watts GF, Lewis B, Brunt JNH, Lewis ES, Coltart DJ, Smith LD, Mann JI, Swan AV. Effects on coronary artery disease of lipid–lowering diet or diet plus cholestyramine in th eSt. Thomas Atherosclerosis Regression Study (STARS). Lancet. 1992 Mar 7;339(8793):563–9.

48.  Blankenhorn DH, Selzer RH, Crawford DW, Barth JD, Liu CR, Liu CH, Mack WJ, Alaupovic P. Beneficial effects of colestipol–niacin therapy on the common carotid artery. Two and four year reduction of intima–media thickness measured by ultrasound. Circulation. 1993 Jul;88(1):20–8.

49.  Blankenhorn DH, Azen SP, Kransch DM, Mack WJ, Cashin–Hemphill L, Hodis HN, DeBoer LW, Mahrer PR, Marstellar MJ, Vailas LI. Coronary and angiographic changes with lovastatin therapy: the Monitored Atherosclerosis Regression Study (MARS). Ann Intern Med. 1993 Nov 15;119(10):969–76.

50.  Sacks FM, Parternak RC, Gibson CM, Rosner B, Stone PH. Effect on coronary atherosclerosis of decrease in plasma control concentration in normocholesterolemic patients. Lancet. 1994 Oct 29;344(8931):1182–6.

51.  MAAS Investigators. Effect of simvastatin on coronary atheroma: the Multicentre Anti-Ather-oma Study. Lancet 1994;344:633–638.

52. Haskell WL, Alderman EL, Fair JM, Maron DJ, Mackey SF, Superko HR, Williams PT, Johnstone IM, Champagne MA, Krauss RM. Effects of intensive multiple risk factor reduction on coronary atherosclerosis and clinical events in men and women with coronary artery disease. The Stanford Coronary Risk Intervention Project (SCRIP). Circulation. 1994 Mar; 89(3):975–90.

53. Waters D, Higginson L, Gladstone P, Kimball B, Le May M, Boccuzzi SJ, Lesperance J. Effects of monotherapy with an HMG–CoA reductase inhibitor on the progression of coronary atherosclerosis as assessed by serial quantitative arteriography. The Canadian Coronary Atherosclerosis Trial. Circulation. 1994 Mar;89(3):959–68.

54. Wallidus G, Erikson U, Olsson AG, Bergstrand L, Hadell K, Johansson J, Kaijser L, Lassvik C, Molgaard J, Nilsson S. The effect of probucol on femoral atherosclerosis: the Probucol Quantitative Regression Swedish Trial (PQRST). Am J Cardiol. 1994 Nov 1;74(9):875–83.

55. Pitt B, Mancini GBJ, Ellis SG, Rosman HS, Park JS, McGovern ME. Pravastatin limitation of atherosclerosis in the coronary arteries (PLAC–I): Reduction in atherosclerosis progression and clinical events. J Am Coll Cardiol. 1995 Nov1; 26(5):1133–9.

56. Crouse JR, Byington RP, Bond MG, Espeland MA, Craven TE, Sprinkle JW, McGovern ME, Furberg CD. Pravastatin, lipids and atherosclerosis in the carotid arteries (PLAC–II). Am J Cardiol. 1995 Mar 1;75(7):455–9.

57. Furberg CD, Adams HP, Applegate WB, Byington RP, Espeland MA, Hartwell T, Hunninghake DB, Lefkowitz DS, Probstfield J, Riley WA. Effect of lovastatin on early carotid atherosclerosis and cardiovascular events. Circulation. 1994 Oct;90(4):1679–87.

58. Gordon NF, English CD, Contractor AS, Salmon RD, Leighton RF, Franklin BA, Haskell WL. Effectiveness of three models for comprehensive cardiovascular disease risk reduction. Am J Cardiol 2002;89:1263–1268.

59. Salonen R, Nyyssonen K, Porkala E, Rummukainen J, Belder R, Park JS, Salonen JT. Kuopio Atherosclerosis Prevention Study (KAPS). A population–based primary prevention trial of the effect of LDL lowering on atherosclerosis progression of the carotid and femoral arteries. Circulation. 1995 Oct 1;92(7):1758–64.

60. Jukema JW, Bruschke AVG, van Boven AJ, Reiber JH, Bal ET, Zwinderman AH, Jansen H, Boerma GJ, van Rappard FM, Lie KI. Effects of lipid lowering by pravastatin on progression and regression of coronary artery disease in symptomatic men with normal to moderately elevated serum cholesterol levels. The Regression Growth EvaluationStudy (REGRESS). Circulation. 1995 May;91(10):2528–2540.

61. Ericsson CG, Hamsten A, Nilsson J, Grip L, Svane B, de Fair U. Angiographic assessment of effects of bezafibrate on progression of coronary artery disease in young male posinfarction patients. Lancet. 1996 Mar 30;347(9005):849–53.

62. Kroon AA, Aengevaeren WRM, van der Werf T, Uijen GJ, Reiber JH, Bruschke AV, Stalenhoef AF. LDL–apheresis atherosclerosis regression study (LAARS). Effect of aggressive versus conventional lipid lowering treatment on coronary atherosclerosis. Circulation. 1996 May 15;93(10):1826–35.

63. The Post Coronary Artery Bypass Graft Trial Investigators. The effect of aggressive lowering of low-density lipoprotein cholesterol levels and low-dose anticoagulation on obstructive changes in saphenous-vein coronary-artery bypass grafts. N Engl J Med 1997;336:153–162.

64. Bestehorn HP, Rensing UFE, Roskmann H, Betz P, Benesch L, Schemeitat K, Claus J, Mathes P, Kappenberger L, Wieland H, Neiss A. The effect of simvastatin on progression of coronary artery disease. The multicenter coronary intervention study (CIS). Eur Heart J. 1997 Feb; 18(2):226–34.

65. Herd JA, Ballantyne CM, Farmer JA, Ferguson JJ 3rd, Jones PH, West MS, Gould KL, Gotto AM Jr. Effects of fluvastatin on coronary atherosclerosis in patients with mild to moderate cholesterol elevations (lipoportein and coronary atherosclerosis study [LCAS]). Am J Cardiol. 1997 Aug 1;80(3): 278–86.

66. Frick MH, Syvanne M, Nieminen MS, Kauma H, Majahalme S, Virtanen V, Kesaniemi YA, Pasternack A, Taskinen MR. Prevention of the angiographic progression of coronary and vein graft atherosclerosis by Gemfibrozil after coronary bypass surgery in men with low levels of HDL cholesterol. Circulation. 1997 Oct 7;96(7):2137–43.

67. Ornish D, Schweritz LW, Billings JH, Brown SE, Gould KL, Merritt TA, Sparler S, Armstrong WT, Ports TA, Kirkeeide RL, Hogeboom C, Brand RJ. Intensive lifestyle changes for reversal of coronary heart disease. JAMA. 1998 Dec 16;280(23):2001–7.

68. Campeau L, Hunninghake DB, Knatterud GL, White CW, Domanski M, Forman SA, Forrester JS, Geller NL, Gobel FL, Herd JA, Hoogwerf BJ, Rosenberg Y. Aggressive cholesterol lowering delays saphenous vein graft atherosclerosis in women, the elderly and patients with associated risk factors. Circulation 1999 Jun 29;99(25):3241–7.

69. MacMahon S, Sharpe N, Gamble G, Hart H, Scott J, Simes J, White H. Effects of lowering average or below average cholesterol levels on the progression of carotid atherosclerosis. Results of the LIPID atherosclerosis sub–study. Circulation. 1998 May 12;97(18):1784–90.

70. Teo KK, Burton JR, Buller CE, Plante S, Catellier D, Tymchak W, Dzavik V, Taylor D, Yokoyama S, Montague TJ. Long–term effect of cholesterol lowering and angitensis converting enzyme inhibitor on coronary atherosclerosis. The simvastatin/enelapril coronary atherosclerosis trial (SCAT). Circulation. 2000 Oct 10;102(15):1748–54.

71. Nissen S. REVERSAL: A Study Comparing the Effects of Atorvastatin Versus Pravastatin on the Progression of Coronary Atherosclerotic Lesions as Measured by Intravascular ultrasound. Presented at the AHA Annual Scientific Late Breaking Sessions on November 12. Orlando, FL 2003.

72. Little WC, Constantinescu M, Applegate RJ, Kutcher MA, Burrows MT, Kahl FR, Santamore WP. Can coronary arteriography predict the site of a subsequent myocardial infarction in patients with mild–to–moderate coronary artery disease? Circulation. 1988 Nov;78(5 pt 1): 1157–66.

73. Ellis S, Alderman E, Cain K, Fisher L, Sanders W, Bourassa M. Prediction of risk on anterior myocardial infarction by lesion severity and measurement method of stenosis in the left anterior descending coronary distribution: a CASS Registry Study. J Am Coll Cardiol. 1988 May;11(5):908–16.

74. Giroud D, Li JM, Urban P, Meier B, Rutishauer W. Relation of the site of myocardial infarction to the most severe coronary arterial stenosis at prior angiography. Am J Cardiol. 1992 Mar 15;69(8):729–32.

75. Brown BG, Zhao XQ, Chait A, Fisher LD, Cheung MC, Morse JS, Dowdy AA, Marino EK, Bolson EL, Alaupovic P, Frohlich J, Albers JJ. Simvastatin and niacin, antioxidant vitamins, or the combination for the prevention of coronary disease. N Engl J Med 2001;345:1583–1592.

76. Phillips NR, Waters D, Havel RJ. Plasma lipoproteins and progression of coronary artery disease evaluated by angiography and clinical events. Circulation 1993;88:2762–2770.

77. Waters D, Craven TE, Lesperance J. Prognostic significance of coronary atherosclerosis. Circulation 1993;87:1067–1075.

78. Hodis HN, Mack WJ, Azen SP, Alaupovic P, Pogoda JM, Labree L, Hemphill LC, Kramsch DM, Blackenhorn DH. Triglyceride and cholesterol rich lipoproteins have a differential effect on mild/moderate and severe lesion progression as assessed by quantitative coronary angiography in a controlled trial of lovastatin. Circulation. 1994 Jul;90(1):42–9.

79. Brown BG, Maher VMG. Reversal of coronary heart disease by lipid-lowering therapy. Observations and pathological mechanisms. Circulation 1994;89:2928–2933.

80. Maher VMG. Clinics Program. The Lipid Research Clinics Coronary Primary Prevention Trial Result. I. Reduction in incidence of coronary heart disease. JAMA 1984;251:351–364.

81. Stewart BF, Brown BG, Zhao XQ, Hillger LA, Sniderman AD, Dowdy A, Fisher LD, Albers JJ. Benefits of lipid lowering therapy in men with elevated apolipoprotein B are not confined to those with very high low density lipoprotein cholesterol. Circulation. 1994 Mar 15;23(4): 899–906.

82. Kaski JC, Chester MR, Chen L, Katritsis D. Rapid angiographic progression of coronary artery disease in patients with angina pectoris. The role of complex stenosis morphology. Circulation 1995;92:2058–2065.

83. Sacks FM, Gibson M, Rosner B, Pasternack RC, Stone PH. The influence of pretreatment low density lipoprotein cholesterol concentrations on the effect of hypocholesterolemic therapy on coronary atherosclerosis in angiographic trials. Am J Cardiol. 1995 Sep 28;76(9):78C–85C.

84. Sacks FM, Stone PH, Gibson CM, Silverman DI, Rosner B, Pasternak RC. Controlled trial of fish oil for regression of human coronary atherosclerosis. J Am Cardiol. 1995 Jun;25(7): 1492–8.

85. Thompson GR, Hollyer J, Waters DD. Percentage change rather than plasma level of LDL-cholesterol determines therapeutic response in coronary heart disease. Curr Opin Lipidiol 1995;6:386–388.

86. Phillips NR, Waters D, Havel RJ. Plasma lipoproteins and progression of coronary artery disease evaluated by angiography and clinical events. Circulation 1993;88:2762–2770.

87. Azen SP, Mack WJ, Cashin–Hemphill L, LaBree L, Shircore AM, Selzer RH, Blackenhorn DH, Hodis HN. Progression of coronary artery disease predicts clinical coronary events. Long–term follow up from the Cholesterol Lowering Atherosclerosis Study. Circulation 1996 Jan 1;93(1):34–41.

88. Lamarche B, Tchernof A, Cantin B, Moorjani S, Dagenais GR, Lupien PJ, Despres JP. Small, dense, low–density, lipoprotein particles as a predictor of the risk of ischemic heart disease in men. Prospective results from the Quebec Cardiovascular Study. Circulation. 1997 Jan 7; 97(1):69–75.

89. Syvanne M, Nieminen MS, Frick H, Kauma H, Majahalme S, Virtanen V, Kesaniemi YA, Pasternack A, Ehnholm C, Taskinen MR. Associations between lipoproteins and the progression of coronary and vein graft atherosclerosis in a controlled trial with gemfibrizol in men with low baseline levels of HDL cholesterol. Circulation. 1998 Nov 10;98(19):1993–9.

90. Ruotolo G, Ericsson CG, Tetamanti C, Karpe F, Grip L, Svane B, Nilsson J, de Faire U, Hamsten A. Treatment effects of serum lipoprotein lipids, apolipoproteins and low density lipoprotein particle size and relationships of lipoprotein variables to progression of coronary artery disease in the bezafibrate coronary atherosclerosis intervention trial (BECAIT). J Am Coll Cardiol. 1998 Nov 15;32(6):1648–56.

91. Freedman DS, Otvos JD, Jeyarajah EJ, Barboriak JJ, Anderson AJ, Walker JA. Relation of lipoprotein subclasses as measured by proton nuclear magnetic resonance spectroscopy to coronary artery disease. Arteriscler Thromb Vasc Biol. 1998 Jul;18(7):1046–53.

92. Otvos J. Measurement of triglyceride-rich lipoproteins by nuclear magnetic resonance spectroscopy. Clin Card 1999;22(suppl II):II–21–II–27.

93. von Schacky C, Angerer P, Kothny W, Theisen K, Mudra H. The effect of dietary ω-3 fatty acids on coronary atherosclerosis. A randomized, double-blind, placebo-controlled trial. Ann Intern Med 1999;130:554–562.

94. Ballantyne CM, Her JA, Ferlic LL, Dunn JK, Farmer JA, Jones PH, Schein JR, Gotto AM Jr. Influence of low HDL on progression of coronary artery disease and response to fluvastatin therapy. Circulation. 1999 Feb 16;99(6):736–43.

95. Lamarche B, Tchernof A, Moorani Set al. Small, dense low-density lipoprotein particles as a predictor of the risk of ischemic heart disease in men. Prospective results from the Quebec Cardiovascular Study. Circulation 1997;95:69–75.

96. Lipid Research Clinics Program. The Lipid Research Clinics Coronary Primary Prevention Trial Result. I. Reduction in incidence of coronary heart disease. JAMA 1984;251:351–364.

97. Lipid Research Clinics Program. The Lipid Research Clinics Coronary Primary Prevention Trial Results. II. The relationship of reduction in incidence of coronary heart disease to cholesterol lowering. JAMA 1984;25:365–374.

98. Frick MH, Elo O, Haapa K, Heinonen OP, Helo P, Huttenen JK, Kaitaniemi P, Koskinen P, Manninen V. Helsinki Heart Study: Primary prevention trial with gemfibrizol in middle aged men with dyslipidemia. Safety of treatment, changes in risk factors and incidence of coronary heart disease. N Engl J Med. 1987 Nov 12;317(20):1237–45.

99. Byington RP, Jukema JW, Salonen JT, Pitt B, Bruschke AV, Hoen H, Furberg CD, Mancini GB. Reduction in cardiovascular events during pravastatin therapy. Pooled analysis of clinical events of the Pravastatin Atherosclerosis Intervention Program. Circulation 1995 Nov 1; 92(9):2419–25.

100. Scandinavian Simvastatin Survival Study Group. Randomised trial of cholesterol lowering in 4444 patients with coronary heart disease: the Scandinavian Simvastatin Survival Study (4S). Lancet 1994;344:1383–1389.

101. Kjekshus J, Pedersen TR. Reducing the risk of coronary events: Evidence from the Scandinavian Simvastatin Survival Study (4S). Am J Cardiol 1995;76:64C–68C.

102. Scandinavian Simvastatin Survival Study Group. Baseline serum cholesterol and treatment effect in the Scandinavian Simvastatin Survival Study (4S). Lancet 1995;345:1274–1275.

103. Pedersen TR, Kjekshus J, Berg K, Olsson AG, Wilhelmsen L, Wedel H, Pyorala K, Miettinen T, Haghfelt T, Faegerman O, Thorgeirsson G, Jonsson B, Schwartz JS. Cholesterol lowering and the use of healthcare resources. Results of the Scandinavian Simvastatin Survival Study. Circulation. 1996 May 15;93(10):1796–802.

104. Johanesson M, Jonsson B, Kjekshus J, Olsson AJ, Pedersen TR, Wedel H. Cost effectiveness of simvastatin to lower cholesterol levels in patients with coronary artery disease. N Engl J Med. 1997 Jan 30;336(5):332–6.

105. Pyorala K, Olsson AG, Pedersen TR, Kjekshus J, Faergeman O, Thorgeirsson G. Cholesterol lowering with simvastatin improves prognosis of diabetic patients with coronary heart disease. A subgroup analysis of the Scandinavian Simvastatin Survival Study. Diabetes Care. 1997 Apr;20(4):614–20.

106. Shepherd J, Cobbe SM, Ford I, Isles CG, Lorimer AR, MacFarlane PW, McKillop JH, Packard CJ. Prevention of coronary heart disease with pravastatin in men with hypercholesterolemia. West of Scotland Coronary Prevention Study Group. N Engl J Med. 1995 Nov 16;333(20):1301–7.

107. Sacks FM, Pfeffer MA, Moye LA, Rouleau JL, Rutherford JD, Cole TG, Brown L, Warnica JW, Arnold JM, Wun CC, Davis BR, Braunwald E. The effect of pravastatin on coronary events after myocardial infarction in patients with average cholesterol. N Engl J Med. 1996 Oct 3;335(14):1001–9.

108. Ashraf T, Hay JW, Pitt B, Wittels E, Crouse J, Davidson M, Furberg CD, Radican L. cost effectiveness of pravastatin in secondary prevention of coronary artery disease. Am J Cardiol. 1996 Aug 15; 78(4):409–14.

109. Hay JW, Wittels EH, Gotto AM. An economic evaluation of lovastatin for cholesterol lowering and coronary disease reduction. Am J Cardiol 1991;67:789–796.

110. Gotto AM. Results of recent large cholesterol-lowering trials and their implications for clinical management. Am J Cardiol 1997;79:1663–1669.

111. Vogel RA. Clinical implications of recent cholesterol lowering trials for the secondary prevention of coronary heart disease. Am J Managed Care 1997;3:S83–S92.

112. Downs JR, Clearfield M, Weiss S, Whitney E, Shapiro DR, Beere PA, Langendorfer A, Stein EA, Kruyer W, Gotto AM Jr. Primary prevention of acute coronary events with lovastatin in men and women with average cholesterol levels. Results of the AFCAPS/TexCAPS. JAMA. 1998;279:1615–1622.

113. Sacks FM, Moye LA, Davis BR, Cole TG, Rouleau JL, Nash DT, Pfeffer MA, Braunwald E. Relationship between plasma LDL concentrations during treatment wih pravastatin and recurrent coronary events in the cholesterol and recurrent events trial. Circulation. 1998 Apr 21;97(15):1446–52.

114. Goldberg RB, Mellies MJ, Sacks FM, Moye LA, Howard BV, Howard BJ, Davis BR, Cole TG, Pfeffer MA, Braunwald E. Cardiovascular events and their reduction with pravastatin in diabetic and glucose–intolerant myocardial infarction survivors with average cholesterol levels. Subgroup analysis in the cholesterol and recurrent events trial (CARE). Circulation. 1998 Dec 8;98(23):2513–9.

115. Esselstyn CB. A symposium: Summit on cholesterol and coronary disease. Am J Cardiol 1998;82:1T–87T.

116. The Long-Term Intervention with Pravastatin in Ischemic Disease (LIPID) Study Group. Prevention of cardiovascular events and death with pravastatin in patients with coronary heart disease and a broad range of initial cholesterol levels. N Engl J Med 1998;339:1349–1357.

117. Gould AL, Rossouw JE, Santanello NC, Heyse JF, Furberg CD. Cholesterol reduction yields clinical benefit: impact of statin trials. Circulation. 1998 Mar 17;97(10):946–52.

118. Plehn JF, Davis BR, Sacks FM, Rouleau JL, Pfeffer MA, Bernstein V, Cuddy TE, Moye LA, Piller LB, Rutherford J, Simpson LM, Braunwald E. Reduction of stroke incidence after

myocardial infarction with pravastatin. The cholesterol and recurrent events (CARE) study. Circulation. 1999;99:216–223.

119. Pfeffer MC, Sacks FM, Moye LA, East C, Goldman S, Nash DT, Rouleau JR, Rouleau JL, Sussex BA, Theroux P, Vanden Belt RJ, Braunwald E. Influence of baseline lipids on effectiveness of pravastatin in the CARE trial. J Am Coll Cardio. 1999 Jan; 33(1):125–30.

120. Pitt B, Watrs D, Brown WV, VAN Boven AJ, Schwartz L, Title LM, Eisenberg D, Shurzinski L, McCormick LS. Aggressive lipid lowering therapy compared with angioplasty in stable coronary artery disease. N Engl J Med. 1999. Jul 8;341(2):70–6.

121. Rubins HB, Robins SJ, Collins D, Fye CL, Anderson JW, Elam MB, Faas FH, Linares E, Schaefer EJ, Schectman G, Wilt TJ, Wittes J. Genfibrozil for the secondary prevention of coronary heart disease in men with low levels of high–density lipoprotein cholesterol. N Engl J Med. 1999 Aug 5;341(6):410–8.

122. LaRosa JC, He J, Vupputuri S. Effect of statins on risk of coronary disease. A meta-analysis of randomized controlled trials. JAMA 1999;282:2340–2346.

123. Knatterud GL, Rosenberg Y, Campeau L, Geller NL, Hunninghake DB, Forman SA, Forrester JS, Gobel FL, Herd JA, Hickey A, Hoogwerf BJ, Terrin ML, White C. Long–term effects on clinical outcomes of aggressive lowering of low–density lipoprotein levels and low–dose anticoagulation in the Post Coronary Artery Bypass Surgery Trial. Circulation. 2000 Jul 11; 102(2):157–65.

124. Schwartz GG, Olsson AG, Ezekowitz MD, Ganz P, Oliver MF, Waters D, Zeiher A, Chaitman BR, Leslie S, Stern T. Effects of atorvastatin on early recurrent ischemic events in acute coronary syndrome. The MIRACL study: a randomized controlled trial. JAMA. 2001 Apr 4;285(13):1711–8.

125. Gotto AM, Whitney E, Stein EA, Shapiro DR, Clearfield M, Weis S, Jou JY, Langendorfer A, Beere PA, Stamler J, Gotto AM Jr. Relationship between baseline and on treatment lipid parameters and first acute major coronary events in the Air Force/ Texas Coronary Atherosclerosis Prevention Study (AFCAPS/TexCAPS). Circulation. 2000 Feb 8;101(5):477–84.

126. Robins SJ, Collins D, Wittes JT, Papademetriou V, Deedwania PC, Schaefer EJ, McNamara JR, Kashyap ML, Hershman JM, Wexler LF, Rubins HB. Relation of Gemfibrozil treatment and lipid levels with major coronary events: VA–HIT: a randomized controlled trial. JAMA. 2001 Mar 28;285(12):1585–91.

127. Sever PS, Dahlof B, Poulter NR, Wedel H, Beevers G, Caulfield M, Collins R, Kjeldsen SE, Kristinsson A, McInnes GT, Mehlsen J, Nieminen M, O'Brien E, Ostergren J. ASCOT investigators. Prevention of coronary and stroke events with atorvastatin in hypertensive patients who have average or lower-than-average cholesterol concentrations, in the Anglo-Scandinavian Cardiac Outcomes Trial—Lipid Lowering Arm (ASCOT-LLA): a multicentre randomised controlled trial. Lancet 2003;361:1149–1158.

128. Heart Protection Study Collaborative Group. MRC/BHF Heart Protection Study of cholesterol lowering with simvastatin in 20,536 high-risk individuals: a randomised placebo-controlled trial. Lancet 2002;360:7–22.

129. Rubins HB, Robins SJ, Collins D, Nelson DB, Elam MB, Schaefer EJ, Faas FH, Anderson JW. Diabetes, plasma insulin, and cardiovascular disease: subgroup analysis from the Department of Veterans Affairs high-density lipoprotein intervention trial (VA-HIT). Arch Intern Med 2002;162:2597–2604.

130. Anonymous. Secondary prevention by raising HDL cholesterol and reducing triglycerides in patients with coronary artery disease: the Bezafibrate Infarction Prevention (BIP) study. Circulation 2000;102:21–27.

131. Miller M. Differentiating the effects of raising low levels of high-density lipoprotein cholesterol versus lowering normal triglycerides: further insights from the Veterans Affairs High-Density Lipoprotein Intervention Trial. Am J Cardiol 2000;86:23L–27L.

132. Collins R, Armitage J, Parish S, Sleigh P, Peto R. Heart Protection Study Collaborative Group. MRC/BHF Heart Protection Study of cholesterol-lowering with simvastatin in 5963 people with diabetes: a randomised placebo-controlled trial. Lancet 2003;361:2005–2016.

133. Kinlay S, Schwartz GG, Olsson AG, Rifai N, Leslie SJ, Sasiela WJ, Szarek M, Libby P, Ganz P. Myocardial Ischemia Reduction with Aggressive Cholesterol Lowering Study Investi-

gators. High-dose atorvastatin enhances the decline in inflammatory markers in patients with acute coronary syndromes in the MIRACL study. Circulation 2003;108:1560–1566.

134.  Heeschen C, Hamm CW, Laufs U, Snapinn S, Bohm M, White HD. Platelet Receptor Inhibition in Ischemic Syndrome Management (PRISM) Investigators. Withdrawal of statins increases event rates in patients with acute coronary syndromes. Circulation 2002;105: 1446–1452.

135.  Fuster V, Steele PM, Chesebro JH. Role of platelets and thrombosis in coronary atherosclerotic disease and sudden death. J Am Coll Cardiol 1986;5:175B–184B.

136.  Glagov S, Weisenberg E, Zarins CK, Stankunavicius R, Kolettis, GJ. Compensatory enlargement of human atherosclerotic coronary arteries. N Engl J Med. 1987 May 28;316(22): 1371–5.

137.  Steinberg D, Parthasarathy S, Carew TE, Khoo JC, Witztum JL. Beyond cholesterol. Modifications of low-density lipoprotein that increase its atherogenicity. N Engl J Med 1989;320: 915–924.

138.  Spady DK, Woollett LA, Dietschy JM. Regulation of plasma LDL-cholesterol levels by dietary cholesterol and fatty acids. Annu Rev Nutr 1993;13:355–381.

139.  Chan DC, Watts GF, Redgrave TG, Mori TA, Barrett PH. Apolipoprotein B-100 kinetics in visceral obesity: associations with plasma apolipoprotein C-III concentration. Metabolism 2002;51:1041–1046.

140.  Ip JH, Fuster V, Badimon L, Badimon J, Taubman MB, Chesebro JH. Syndromes of accelerated atherosclerosis: Role of vascular injury and smooth muscle cell proliferation. J Am Coll Cardiol. 1990 Jun;15(7):1667–87.

141.  Fuster V, Badimon L, Badimon JJ, Chesebro JH. The pathogenesis of coronary artery isease. N Engl J Med 1992;326:310–318.

142.  Witstum JL. Role of oxidized low density lipoprotein in atherosclerosis. Br Heart J 1993; 69(suppl):S12–S18.

143.  Stary HC, Chandler AB, Glagov JR, Guyton JR, Insull W Jr., Rosenfeld ME, Schaffer MA, Schwartz CJ, Wagner WD, Wissler RW. A definition of initial, fatty streak and intermediate lesions of atherosclerosis. A report from the Committee on Vascular Lesions of the Coucil on Arteriosclerosis. American Heart Association. Arterioscler Thromb. 1994 May;14(5):840–56.

144.  Clarkson TB, Pritchard RW, Morgan TM. Remodeling of coronary arteries in human and nonhuman primates. JAMA 1994;271:289–294.

145.  Segrest JP, Anantharamaiah GM. Pathogenesis of atherosclerosis. Curr Opinion Cardiol 1994; 9:404–410.

146.  Libby P. Molecular basis of the acute coronary syndromes. Circulation 1995;91:2844–2850.

147.  Falk E, Shah PK, Fuster V. Coronary plaque disruption. Circulation 1995;92:657–671.

148.  Grayston JT, Kuo C, Coulston AS, Campbell LA, Lawrence RD, Lee MJ, Strandness ED, Wang SP. Chlamydia pneumoniae (TWAR) in atherosclerosis of the carotid artery. Circulation. 1995Dec 15;92(12):3397–400.

149.  Nishioka T, Luo H, Eigler NL, Berglund H, Kim CJ, Siegel RJ. Contribution of inadequate compensatory enlargement to development of human coronary artery stenosis: An in vitro intravascular ultrasound study. J Am Coll Cardiol. 1996 Jun;27(7):1571–6.

150.  Zhou YF, Leon MB, Waclawiw MA, Popma JJ, Yu ZX, Finkel T, Epstein SE. Association between prior cytomegalovirus infection and the risk of restenosis after coronary atherectomy. N Engl J Med. 1996 Aug 29:335(9):624–30.

151.  Farb A, Burke AP, Tang AL, Liang TY, Mannan P, Smialek J, Virmani R. Coronary plaque erosion without rupture into a lipid core. A frequent cause of coronary thrombosis in sudden coronary death. Circulation. 1996 Apr 1;93(7):1354–63.

152.  Mann JM, Davies MJ. Vulnerable plaque. Relation of characteristics to degree of stenosis in human coronary arteries. Circulation 1996;94:928–931.

153.  Burke AP, Farb A, Malcom GT, Liang YH, Smialek J, Virmani R. coronary risk factors and plaque morphology in men with coronary disease who die suddenly. N Engl J Med. 1997 May 1;336(18):1276–82.

154.  Ridker PM, Cushman M, Stampfer MJ, Tracy RP, Hennekens CH. Inflammation, aspirin and the risk of cardiovascular disease in apparently healthy men. N Engl J Med. 1997 Apr 3; 336(14):973–9.

155. Ridker PM, Rifai N, Pfeffer MA, Sacks FM, Moye LA, Goldman S, Flaker GC, Brauwald E. inflammation, pravastatin and the risk of coronary events after myocardial infarction in patients with average cholesterol levels. Circulation. 1998 Sep 1;98(9):839–44.

156. Ross R. Atherosclerosis – an inflammatory disease. N Engl J Med 1999;340:115–126.

157. McKenney JM, McCormick LS, Schaefer EJ, Black DM, Watkins ML. Effect of niacin and atorvastatin on lipoprotein subclasses in patients with atherogenic dyslipidemia. Am J Cardiol 2001;88:270–274.

158. Rosenson RS, Otvos JD, Freedman DS. Relations of lipoprotein subclass levels and low-density lipoprotein size to progression of coronary artery disease in the Pravastatin Limitation of Atherosclerosis in the Coronary Arteries (PLAC-I) trial. Am J Cardiol 2002;90:89–94.

159. Miller M, Dolinar C, Cromwell W, Otvos JD. Effectiveness of high doses of simvastatin as monotherapy in mixed hyperlipidemia. Am J Cardiol 2001;87(2):232–234.

160. Freedman DS, Otvos JD, Jeyarajah EJ, Barboriak JJ, Anderson JJ, Walker JA. Relation of lipoprotein subclasses as measured by proton nuclear magnetic resonacnse spectroscopy to coronary artery disease. Arterioscler Thromb Vasc Biol 1998 Jul;18(7):1046–53.

161. Ridker PMEvaluating novel cardiovascular risk factors: can we better predict heart attacks?. Ann Intern Med 1999;97:2007–2011.

162. Alexander RW, Dzau VJ. Vascular biology. The past 50 years. Circulation 2000;102:IV-112–IV-116.

163. Ridker PM, Stampfer MJ, Rifai N. Novel risk factors for systemic atherosclerosis: a comparison of C-reactive protein, fibrinogen, homocysteine, lipoprotein(a), and standard screening as predictors of peripheral vascular disease. JAMA 2001;285:2481–2484.

164. Ridker PM. High-sensitivity C-reactive protein and cardiovascular risk: rationale for screening and primary prevention. Am J Cardiol. 2003;92(4B):17K–22K.

165. Kopprasch S, Pietzsch J, Kuhlisch E, Fuecker K, Temelkova-Kurktschiev T, Hanefeld M, Kuhne H. In vivo evidence for increased oxidation of circulating LDL in impaired glucose tolerance. Diabetes 2002;51:3102–3106.

166. Nicholl ID, Bucala R. Advanced glycation endproducts and cigarette smoking. Cell Mol Biol 1998;44:1025–1033.

167. Miyazaki A, Nakayama H, Horiuchi S. Scavenger receptors that recognize advanced glycation end products. Trends Cardiovasc Med 2002;12:258–262.

168. Mertens A, Holvoet P. Oxidized LDL and HDL: antagonists in atherothrombosis. FASEB J 2001;15:2073–2084.

169. Mackness MI, Mackness B, Durrington PN. Paraoxonase and coronary heart disease. Atheroscler Suppl 2002;3:49–55.

170. Jaouad L, Milochevitch C, Khalil A. PON1 paraoxonase activity is reduced during HDL oxidation and is an indicator of HDL antioxidant capacity. Free Radic Res 2003;37:77–83.

171. Tuzcu EM, Kapadia SR, Tutar E, Ziada KM, Hobbs RE, McCarthy PM, Young JB, Nissen SE. High prevalence of coronary atherosclerosis in asymptomatic teenagers and young adults: evidence from intravascular ultrasound. Circulation 2001;103:2705–2710.

172. Maher VM, Brown BG, Marcovina SM, Hillger LA, Zhao XQ, Albers JJ. Effects of lowering elevated LDL cholesterol on the cardiovascular risk of lipoprotein(a). JAMA 1995;274(22):1771–1774.

173. Furchgott RF, Zawadski JV. The obligatory role of endothelial cells in the relaxation of arterial smooth muscle by acetylcholine. Nature 1980;288:373–376.

174. Ludmer PL, Selwyn AP, Shook TL, Wayne RR, Mudge GH, Alexander RW, Ganz P. paradoxical vasoconstriction induced by acetylcholine in atherosclerotic coronary arteries. N Engl J Med. 1986 Oct 23;315(17):1046–51.

175. Osborne JA, Siegman MJ, Sedar AW, Mooers SU, Lefer AM. Lack of endothelium–dependent relaxation in coronary resistance arteries of cholesterol fed rabbits. Am J Physiol 1989 Mar;256(3 pt 1):C591–7.

176. Drexler H, Zeiher AM, Wollscjlager H, Meinertz T, Just H, Bonzel T. Flow–dependent coronary artery dilation in humans. Circulation. 1989 Sep;80(3):446–74.

177. Harrison DG. From isolated vessels to the catheterization laboratory. Studies of endothelial function in the coronary Circulation of humans. Circulation 1989;80:703–706.

178.  Vita JA, Treasure CB, Nabel EG, McLenachan JM, Fish RD, Yeung AC, Vekshtein VI, Selwyn AP, Ganz P. Coronary vasomotor responses to acetylcholine relates to risk factors for coronary artery disease. Circulation. 1990 Feb;81(2):491–7.

179.  Vane JR, Anggard EE, Botting RM. Regulatory functions of the vascular endothelium. N Engl J Med 1990;323:27–36.

180.  Creager MA, Cooke JP, Mendelsohn ME, Gallagher SJ, Coleman SM, Loscalzo J, Dzau VJ. Impaired vasodilation of forearm resistance vessels in hypercholestrolemic humans. J Clin Invest. 1990 Jul;86(1):228–34.

181.  Kuhn FE, Mohler ER, Reagan K, Satler LF, Lu DY, Racklet CE. Effects of high–density lipoprotein on acetylcholine–induced coronary vasoreactivity. Am J Cardiol. 1991 Dec 1; 68(15):1425–30.

182.  Lerman A, Burnett JC. Intact and altered endothelium in regulation of vasomotion. Circulation 1992;86(suppl III):III-12–III-19.

183.  Flavahan NA. Atherosclerosis or lipoprotein-induced endothelial dysfunction. Potential mechanisms underlying reduction in EDRF/nitric oxide activity. Circulation 1992;85:1927–1938.

184.  Celermajer DS, Sorenson KE, Gooch VM, Spiegelhalter DJ, Miller OI, Sullivan ID, Lloyd JK, Deanfield JE. Non–invasive detection of endothelial dysfunction in children and adults at risk of atherosclerosis. Lancet 1992 Nov 7;340(8828):1111–5.

185.  Vogel RA. Endothelium-dependent vasoregulation of coronary artery diameter and blood flow. Circulation 1993;88:325–327.

186.  Mocada S, Higgs A. The L-arginine-nitric oxide pathway. N Engl J Med 1993;329: 2002–2012.

187.  Lefroy DC, Crake T, Uren NG, Davies GJ, Maseri A. Effect of inhibition of nitric oxide synthesis on epicardial coronary artery caliber and coronary blood flow in humans. Circulation. Jul;88(1):43–54.

188.  Matsuda Y, Hirata K, Inoue N, Suematsu M, Kawashima S, Akita H, Yokoyama M. High density lipoprotein reverses inhibitory effect on oxidized low–density lipoprotein on endothelium–dependent arterial relaxation. Circ Res 1993 May;72(5):1103–9.

189.  Seiler C, Hess M, Buechi M, Suter TM, Krayenbuehl HP. Influence of serum cholesterol and other coronary risk factors on vasomotion of angiographically normal coronary arteries. Circulation. 1993 Nov;88(5 pt 1):2139–48.

190.  Ohara Y, Pederson TE, Harrison DG. Hypercholesterolemia increases endothelial superoxide production. J Clin Invest 1993;91:2546–2551.

191.  Reddy KG, Nair RN, Sheehan HM, Hodgson JM. Evidence that selective endothelial dysfunction may occur in the absence of angiographic or ultrasound atherosclerosis in patients with risk factors for atherosclerosis. J Am Coll Cardiol. 1994 Mar 15;23(4):833–43.

192.  Benzuly KH, Padgett RC, Kaul S, Piegors DJ, Armstrong ML, Heistad DD. Functional improvement precedes structural regression of atherosclerosis. Circulation 1994 Apr;89(4): 1810–8.

193.  Celermajer DS, Sorenson KE, Bull C, Robinson J, Deanfield JE. Endothelium–dependent dilation in the systemic arteries of asymptomatic subjects relates to coronary risk factors and their interaction. J Am Coll Cardiol. 1994 Nov 15;24(6):1468–74.

194.  Cayette AJ, Palacino JJ, Cohen RA. Chronic inhibition of nitric oxide production accelerates neointimal formation and impairs endothelial function in hypercholesterolemic rabbits. Arterioscler Thromb 1994;14:753–759.

195.  Hamon M, Vallet B, Bauters C, Wernert N, McFadden EP, LaBlanche JM, Dupuis B, Bertrand ME. Long–term administration of L–arginine reduces intimal thickening and enhances neoendothelium–dependent acetylcholine relaxation after arterial injury. Circulation. 1994 Sep; 90(3):1357–62.

196.  El–Tamimi H, Mansour M, Wargovich TJ, Hill JA, Kerensky RA, Conti CR, Pepine CJ. Constrictor and dilator responses to intra–coronary acetylcholine in adjacent segments of the same coronary artery in patients with coronary artery disease. Circulation. 1994 Jan;89(1): 45–51.

197.  Penny WF, Rockman H, Long J, Bhargava V, Carrigan K, Ibriham A, Shabetai R, Ross J Jr., Peterson KL. Heterogeneity of vasomotor response to acetylcholine along the human coronary artery. J Am Coll Cardiol. 1995 Apr;25(5):1046–55.

198. Kuo L, Davis MJ, Chilian WM. Longitudinal gradients for endothelium-dependent and independent vascular responses in the coronary microCirculation. Circulation 1995;92:518–525.

199. Zeiher AM, Krause T, Schachinger V, Minners J, Moser E. Impaired endothelium–dependent vasodilation of coronary resistance vessels is associated with exercise–induced myocardial ischemia. Circulation 1995 May 1;91(9):2345–52.

200. Shiode N, Nakayama K, Morishima N, Yamagata T, Matsuura H, Kajiyama G. Nitric oxide production by coronary conductance vessels in hypercholesterolemic patients. Am Heart J 1996 Jun;131(6):1051–7.

201. Glasser SP, Selwyn AP, Ganz P. Atherosclerosis: risk factors and the vascular endothelium. Am Heart J 1996;131:379–384.

202. Anderson TJ, Meredith IT, Charbonneau F, Yeung AC, Frei B, Selwyn AP, Ganz P. Endothelium–dependent coronary vasomotion relates to the susceptibility of LDL to oxidation in humans. Circulation. 1996 May 1;93(9):1647–50.

203. Weber C, Erl W, Weber K, Weber PC. Increased adhesiveness of isolated monocytes to endothelium is prevented by Vitamin C intake in smokers. Circulation 1996 Apr 15;93(8): 1488–92.

204. Vogel RA, Corretti MC, Plotnick GD. Effect of a single high-fat meal on endothelial function in healthy subjects. Am J Cardiol 1997;79:350–354.

205. Vogel RA. Coronary risk factors, endothelial function, and atherosclerosis: a review. Clin Cardiol 1997;20:426–432.

206. Plotnick GD, Corretti MC, Vogel RA. Antioxidant vitamins blunt the transient impairment of endothelium-dependent brachial artery vasoactivity following a fatty meal. JAMA 1997; 278:1682–1686.

207. Vogel RA, Corretti MC, Gellman J. Cholesterol, cholesterol lowering, and endothelial function. Progr Cardiovasc Dis 1998;41:117–136.

208. Kaku B, Mizuno S, Ohsato K, Murakami T, Moriuchi I, Arai Y, Nio Y, Hirase H, Nagata M, Takahashi Y, Ohnaka M. The correlation between coronary stenosis index and flow-mediated dilation of the brachial artery. Jpn Circ J 1998;62:425–430.

209. GISSI-Prevenzione Investigators. Dietary supplementation with n-3 polyunsaturated fatty acids and vitamin E after myocardial infarction: results of the GISSI-Prevenzione trial. Lancet 1999;354:447–455.

210. Djousse L, Ellison RC, McLennan CE, Cupples LA, Lapinska I, Tofler GH, Gokce N, Vita JA. Acute effects of a high fat meal with and without red wine on endothelial function in healthy subjects. Am J Cardiol. 1999;84:660–64.

211. Williams MJA, Sutherland WHF, McCormick MP, de Jong SS, Walker RJ, Wilkins GT. Impaired endothelial function following a meal rich in used cooking oil. J Am Coll Cardiol. 1999;33:1050–1055.

212. Wilmink HW, Banga JD, Hijmering M, Stroes ES, Rabelink TJ. Effect of angiotensin–converting enzyme inhibition and angiotensin II type 1 receptor anatagonism on postprandial endothelial function. J Am Coll Cardiol 1999;34:140–145.

213. Lewis TV, Dart AM, Chin-Dusting JPF. Endothelium-dependent relaxation by acetylcholine is impaired in hypertriglyceridemic humans with normal levels of plasma LDL cholesterol. J Am Coll Cardiol 1999;33:805–812.

214. Schachinger V, Britten M, Zeiher A. Impaired epicardial coronary vasoactivity predicts for adverse cardiovascular events during long-term follow-up. Circulation 1999;100:I-54.

215. Neunteufl T, Heher S, Katzenschlager R, Wolfl G, Kostner K, Maurer G, Weidinger F. Late prognosticvalue of flow–mediated dilation in the brachial artery of patients with chest pain. Am J Cardiol 2000;86:207–210.

216. Al Suwaidi J, Hamasaki S, Higano ST, Nishimura RA, Holmes DR Jr., Lerman A. Long–term follow up of patients with mild coronary artery disease and endothelial dysfunction. Circulation 2000;101:948–954.

217. Leung W-H, Lau C-P, Wong C-K. Beneficial effect of cholesterol-lowering therapy on coronary endothelium-dependent relaxation in hypercholesterolaemic patients. Lancet 1993;341: 1496–1500.

218. Egashira K, Hirooka Y, Kai H, Sugimachi M, Suzuki S, Inou T, Takeshita A. Reduction in serum cholesterol with pravastatin improves endothelium–dependent coronary vasomotion in patients with hypercholesterolemia. Circulation 1994;89:2519–2524.

219. Treasure CB, Klein JL, Weintraub WS, Talley JD, Stillabower ME, Kosinski AS, Zhang J, Boccuzzi SJ, Cedarholm JC, Alexander RW. Beneficial effects of cholesterol lowering therapy on the coronary endothelium in patients with coronary artery disease. N Engl J Med 1995; 332:481–487.

220. Anderson TJ, Meredith IT, Yeung AC, Frei B, Selwyn AP, Ganz P. The effect of cholesterol lowering and antioxidant therapy on endothelium–dependent coronary vasomotion. N Engl J Med 1995;332:488–493.

221. Stroes ESG, Koomans HA, de Bruin TWA, Rabelink TJ. Vascular function in the forearm in hypercholesterolemic patients off and on lipid lowering medication. Lancet 1995;346: 467–471.

222. Goode GK, Heagerty AM. In vitro responses of human peripheral small arteries in hypercholesterolemia and effects of therapy. Circulation 1995;91:2898–2903.

223. Vogel RA, Corretti MC, Plotnick GP. Changes in flow-mediated brachial artery vasoactivity with lowering of desirable cholesterol levels in healthy middle-aged men. Am J Cardiol 1996; 77:37–40.

224. Seiler C, Suter TM, Hess OM. Exercise-induced vasomotion of angiographically normal and stenotic coronary arteries improves after cholesterol-lowering drug therapy with bezafibrate. J Am Coll Cardiol 1995;26:1615–1622.

225. Yeung A, Hodgson JMCB, Winniford M. Assessment of coronary vascular reactivity after cholesterol lowering. Circulation 1996;94(Suppl 1):I402–abstract.

226. Drury J, Cohen JD, Veerendrababu B. brachial artery endothelium–dependent vasodilation in patients enrolled in the Cholesterol and Recurrent Events Study (CARE).Circulation 1996; 94 (Suppl I):I402 abstract.

227. Tamai O, Matsuoka H, Itabe H, Wada Y, Kohno K, Imaizumio T. Single LDL apheresis improves endothelium–dependent vasodilation in hypercholesterolemic humans. Circulation 1997; 95:76–82.

228. O'Driscoll G, Green D, Taylor RR. Simvastatin, an HMG-CoA reductase inhibitor, improves endothelial function within 1 month. Circulation 1997;95:1126–1131.

229. Andrews TC, Whitney EJ, Green G, Kalenian R, Personius BE. Effect of gemfibrizol + niacin + cholestyramine on endothelial function in patients with serum low–density lipoprotein cholesterol levels<160 mg/dl and high–density lipoprotein cholesterol levels<40 mg/dl. Am J Cardil 1997;80:831–835.

230. de Man FH, Weverling AW, Smelt AH. Impaired endothelium–dependent vasodilation in the forearm of patients with endogenous hypertriglyceridemia: reversal upon lipid–lowering therapy by atorvastatin. Circulation 1998;98:I–243.

231. Simons A, Sullivan D, Simons J, Celermajer DS, Effects of atorvastatin monotherapy and simvastatin plus cholestyramine on arterial endothelial function in patients with severe primary hypercholesterolemia. Atherosclerosis 1998;137:197–203.

232. Vogel RA, Corretti MC, Plotnick GD. The mechanism of improvement in endothelial function by pravastatin: Direct effect or through cholesterol lowering. J Am Coll Cardiol 1998;31: 60A.

233. John S, Schlaich M, Lagenfeld M, Weihprecht H, Schmitz G, Weidinger G, Schmieder RE. Increased bioavailability of nitric oxide after lipid–lowering therapy in hypercholesterolemic patients. A randomized, place–controlled, double–blind study. Circulation 1998;98: 2112–2116.

234. Dupuis J, Tardif JC, Cernacek P, Theroux P. Cholesterol reduction rapidly improves endothelial function after acute coronary syndromes. The RECIFE (Reduction of Cholesterol in Ischemia and Function of the Endothelium) trial. Circulation 1999;99:3227–3233.

235. Herrington DM, Werbel BL, Riley WA, Pusser BE, Morgan TM. Individual and combined effects of estrogen/ progestin therapy and lovastatin on lipids and flow–mediated vasodilation in postmenopausal women with coronary artery disease. J Am Coll Cardiol 1999;33: 2030–2037.

236. Vogel RA. Cholesterol lowering and endothelial function. Am J Med 1999;107:479–487.
237. Yokoyama I, Monomura S, Ohtake T, Yonekura K, Yang W, Kobayakawa N, Aoyagi T, Sugiura S, Yamada N, Otomo K, Sasaki Y, Omata M, Yazaki Y. Improvement of impaired myocardial vasodilation due to diffuse coronary atherosclerosis in hypercholesterolemics after lipid–lowering therapy. Circulation 1999;100:117–122.
238. Shechter M, Sharir M, Labrador MJ, Forrester J, Merz CN. Improvement in endothelial–dependentbrachial artery flow–mediated vasodilation with low–density lipoprotein levels <100 mg/dl. Am J Cardiol 2000;86:1256–1259.
239. John S, Jacobi J, Delles C. Rapid improvement of endothelial function after lipid–lowering therapy with cerivastatin within 2 weeks. J Am Coll Cardiol 2000;35:256A.
240. Mullen MJ, Wright D, Donald AE, Thorne S, Thomson H, Deanfield JE. Atorvastatin but not L–arginine improves endothelial function in type I diabetes mellitus. A double–blind study. J Am Coll Cardiol 2000;36:410–416.
241. Vita JA, Yeung AC, Winniford M, Hodgson JM, Treasure CB, Klein JL, Wern S, Kern M, Plotkin D, Shih WJ, Mitchel Y, Ganz P. Effect of cholesterol lowering therapy on coronary endothelial function in patients with coronary artery disease. Circulation 2000;102:846–851.
242. Abbott RD, Wilson PWK, Kannel WB, Castelli WP. High density lipoprotein cholesterol, total cholesterol screening and myocardial infarction - the Framingham experience. Arteriosclerosis 1988;8:207–211.
243. Burr ML, Fehily AM, Gilbert JF, Holliday RM, Sweetnam PM, Elwood PC, Deadman NM. Effects of changes in fat, fish and fiber intakes on death and myocardial infarction: Diet and Reinfarction Trial (DART). Lancet 1989:757–761.
244. Sueta CA, Massing MW, Chowdhury M, Biggs DP, Simpson RJ. Undertreatment of hyperlipidemia in patients with coronary artery disease and heart failure. J Card Fail 2003;9:36–41.
245. van Dam M, van Wissen S, Kastelein JJ. Declaring war on undertreatment: rationale for an aggressive approach to lowering cholesterol. J Cardiovasc Risk 2002;9:89–95.
246. Pearson TA. The undertreatment of LDL-cholesterol: addressing the challenge. Int J Cardiol 2000;74(Suppl 1):S23–28.
247. Cohen MV, Byrne MJ, Levine B, Gutowski T, Adelson R. Low rate of treatment of hypercholesterolemia by cardiologists in patients with suspected and proven coronary artery disease. Circulation 1991;83:1294–1304.
248. Wood PD, Stefanick ML, Williams PT, Haskell WL. The effects on plasma lipoproteins of a prudent weight–reducing diet with or without exercise in overweight men and women. N Eng J Med 1991; 325:461–466.
249. Manninen V, Tenkanen L, Koskinen P, Huttunen JK, Manttari M, Heinonen OP, Frick MH. Joint effects of serum triglyceride and LDL cholesterol and HDL concentrations on coronary heart disease risk in the Helsinki Heart Study. Implications for treatment. Circulation 1992; 85:37–45.
250. Assmann G, Schulte H. Relation of high-density lipoprotein cholesterol and triglycerides to incidence of atherosclerotic coronary artery disease (the PROCAM experience). Am J Cardiol 1992;70:733–737.
251. Levy RI, Troendle AJ, Fattu JM. A quarter century of drug treatment of dyslipoproteinemia, with a focus on the new HMG-CoA reductase inhibitor fluvastatin. Circulation 1993(suppl III):III-45–III-53.
252. Hunninghake DB, Stein EA, Dujovne CA, Harris WS, Feldman EB, Miller VT, Toberta JA, Laskarzewski PM, Quiter E, Held J. The efficacy of intensive dietary therapy alone or in combination with lovastatin in outpatients with hypercholesterolemia. N Engl J Med 1993; 328:1213–19.
253. Roberts WC. Getting cardiologists interested in lipids. Am J Cardiol 1993;72:744–745.
254. Expert Panel on Detection, Evaluation, and Treatment of High Blood Cholesterol in Adults. Summary of the second report of the National Cholesterol Education Program (NCEP) Expert Panel on Detection, Evaluation and Treatment of High Blood Cholesterol in Adults (Adult Treatment Panel II). JAMA 1993;269:3015–3023.
255. Grundy SM, Bilheimer D, Chait A. National cholesterol education program expert panel on detection, evaluation and treatment of high blood pressure in adults (Adult Treatment Panel II). Circulation 1994;89:1329–1448.

256. DeBusk RF, Miller NH, Superko HR, Dennis CA, Thomas RJ, Lew HT, Berger WE 3rd, Heller RS, Rompf J, Gee D. A case–management system for coronary risk factor modification after acute myocardial infarction. Ann Intern Med 1994;120:721–29.

257. Cupples ME, McKnight A. Randomized trial of health promotion in general practice for patients at high cardiovascular risk. Br Med J 1994;309:993–996.

258. Watts GF, Jackson P, Mandalia S, Brunt JN, Lewis ES, Coltart DJ, Lewis B. Nutrient intake and progression of coronary artery disease. Am J Cardiol 1994;73:328–32.

259. Miller M. Maximizing secondary prevention of CAD: A model program. J Myocard Ischemia 1995;7:166–169.

260. Havel RJ, Rapoport E. Drug therapy: management of primary hyperlipidemia. N Engl J Med 1995;332:1491–1498.

261. Renaud S, de Longeril M, Delaye J, Guidollet J, Jacquard F, Mamelle N, Martin J-L, Monjaud I, Salen P, Toubol P. Cretan mediterranean diet for prevention of coronary heart disease. Am J Clin Nutr 1995;61(suppl):1360S–1367S.

262. de Longeril M, Salen P, Martin J-L, Mamelle N, Monjaud I, Touboul P, Delaye J. Effect of a mediterranean type of diet on the rate of cardiovascular complications in patients with coronary artery disease. Insights into the cardioprotective effect of certain nutrients. J Am Coll Cardiol 1996;28:1103–1108.

263. de Longeril M, Salem P, Martin J-L, Monjaud I, Boucher P, Mamelle N. Mediterranean dietary pattern in a randomized trial. Prolonged survival and possibly reduced cancer rate. Arch Intern Med 1998;158:1181–1187.

264. de Longeril M, Salem P, Martin J-L, Monjaud I, Delaye J, Mamelle N. Mediterranean diet, traditional risk factors, and the rate of cardiovascular complications after myocardial infarction. Final report of the Lyon Diet Heart Study. Circulation 1999;99:779–785.

265. The Clinical Quality Improvement Network (CQUIN) Investigators. Low incidence of assessment and modification of risk factors in acute care patients with high risk for cardiovascular events, particularly among females and the elderly. Am J Cardiol 1995;76:570–573.

266. Nieto FJ, Alonso J, Chambless LE, Zhong M, Ceraso M, Romm FJ, Cooper L, Folsom AR, Szklo M. Population awareness and control of hypertension and hypercholesterolemia. The AtherosclerosisRisk in Communities Study. Arch Intern Med 1995;155:677–84.

267. Renaud S, de Longeril M, Guidollet J, Delaye J, Jacquard F, Mamelle N, Martin JL, Monjaud I, Salen P, Toubol P. Cretan Mediterranean diet for prevention of coronary heart disease. Am J Clin Nutr 1995;61(suppl):1360S–67S.

268. Nawrocki JW, Weiss SR, Davidson MH, Sprecher DL, Schwartz SL, Lupien PJ, Jones PH, Haber HE, Black DM. Reduction of LDL cholesterol by 25% to 60% in patients with primary hypercholesterolemia by atorvastatin, a new HMG–CoA reductase inhibitor. Arterioscler Thromb Vasc Biol 1995;15:678–82.

269. Van Dis F, Keilson LM, Rundell CA, Rawstron MW. Direct measurement of serum low–density lipoprotein cholesterol in patients with acute myocardial infarction on admission to the emergency room. Am J Cardiol 1996;77:1232–34.

270. Rimm EB, Ascherio A, Giovannucci E, Spiegelman D, Stampfer MJ, Willett WC. Vegetable, fruit and cereal fiber intake and risk of coronary heart disease among men. JAMA 1996;19:683–9.

271. Rackley CE. Monotherapy with HMG-CoA reductase inhibitors and secondary prevention in coronary artery disease. Clin Cardiol 1996;19:683–689.

272. Gardner CD, Fortman SP, Krauss RM. Association of small low-dense lipoprotein particles with the incidence of coronary artery disease in men and women. JAMA 1996;276:875–881.

273. Stampfer MJ, Krauss RM, Ma J, Blanche PJ, Holl LG, Sacks FM, Hennekens CH. A prospective study of triglyceride level, low–density lipoprotein particle diameter and risk of myocardial infarction. JAMA. 1996;276:882–8.

274. de Lorgeril M, Salen P, Martin JL, Mamelle N, Monjaud I, Touboul P, Delaye J. Effect of a Mediterranean type on diet on the rate of cardiovascular complications in patients with coronary artery disease. Insights into the cardioprotective effects of certain nutrients. J Am Coll Cardiol 1996;28:1103–8.

275. Rodriguez BL, Sharp DS, Abbott RD, Burchfiel CM, Masaki K, Chyou PH, Huang B, Yano K, Curb JD. Fish intake may limit the increase in risk of coronary heart disease morbidity and mortality among heavy smokers. The Honolulu Heart Program. Circulation 1996;94: 952–56.

276. Superko HR. Beyond LDL cholesterol reduction. Circulation 1996;94:2351–2354.

277. Daviglus ML, Stamler J, Orencia AJ, Dyer AR, Liu K, Greenland P, Walsh MK, Morris D, Shekelle RB. Fish consumption and the 30–year risk of fatal myocardial infarction. N Engl J Med 1997;336:1046–53.

278. Grunsy SM, Balady GJ, Criqui MH, Fletcher G, Greenland P, Hiratzka LF, Houston–Miller N, Kris–Etherton P, Krumholz HM, LaRosa J, Ockene IS, Pearson TA, Reed J, Smith SC Jr., Washington R. When to start cholesterol–lowering therapy in patients with coronary heart disease. A statement for the healthcare professionals from the Task Force on Risk Reduction. Circulation 1997;95:1683–5.

279. Gotto AM. Cholesterol management in theory and practice. Circulation 1997;96:4424–4430.

280. Grundy SM. Statin trials and goals of cholesterol-lowering therapy. Circulation 1998;97: 1436–1439.

281. Fruchart JC, Brewer HB, Leitersdorf E. Consensus for the use of fibrates in the treatment of dyslipidemia and coronary heart disease. Am J Cardiol 1998;81:912–917.

282. Knopf RH. Drug treatment of lipid disorders. N Engl J Med 1999;341:498–511.

283. Grundy SM. Hypertriglyceridemia, insulin resistance, and the metabolic syndrome. Am J Cardiol 1999;83:25F–29F.

284. Ballantyne CM. Low-density lipoproteins and risk for coronary artery disease. Am J Cardiol 1998;82:3Q–12Q.

285. Xydakis AM, Ballantyne CM. Role of non-high-density lipoprotein cholesterol in prevention of cardiovascular disease: updated evidence from clinical trials. Curr Opin Cardiol 2003;18: 503–509.

286. Kwiterovich PO. The antiatherogenic role of high-density lipoprotein cholesterol. Am J Cardiol 1998;82:13Q–21Q.

287. Krauss RM. Triglycerides and atherogenic lipoproteins: rationale for lipid management. Am J Med 1998;105(1A):58S–62S.

288. Gruppo Italiano per lo Studio Della Soprevvivenza nell'Infarto Miocardico. Dietary supplementaion with n-3 polyunsaturated fatty acids and vitamin E after myocardial infarction: results of the GISSI-Prevenzione trial. Lancet 1999;354:447–455.

289. Grundy SM. Cholesterol management in the era of managed care. Am J Cardiol 2000;85: 3A–9A.

290. Krauss RM, Eckel RH, Howard B, Appel LJ, Daniels SR, Deckelbaum RJ, Erdmand JW Jr., Kris–Etherton P, Goldberg IJ, Kotchen TA, Lichtenstein AH, Mitch WE, Mullis R, Robinson K, Wylie–Rosett J, St Jeor S, Suttie J, Tribble DL, Bazzarre TL. AHA dietary guidelines. Revision 2000: a statement for healthcare professionals from the Nutrition Committee of the American Heart Association. Circulation 2000;102:2284–99.

291. Wang PS, Solomon DH, Mogun MS, Avorn J. HMG CoA reductase inhibitors and the risk of hip fractures in the elderly. JAMA 2000;283:3211–3216.

292. Vaughan CJ, Gotto AM, Basson CT. The evolving role of statins in the management of atherosclerosis. J Am Coll Cardiol 2000;35:1–10.

293. Miller M. Current perspectives on the management of hypertriglyceridemia. Am Heart J 2000;140:232–240.

294. Hay JW, Yu WM, Ashraf T. Pharmacoeconomics of lipid-lowering agents for primary and secondary prevention of coronary artery disease. Pharmacoeconomics 2000;15:47–74.

295. Pearson TA, Laurora I, Chu H, Kafonek S. The lipid treatment assessment project (L-TAP): a multicenter survey to evaluate the percentages of dyslipidemic patients receiving lipid-lowering therapy and achieving low-density lipoprotein cholesterol goals. Arch Intern Med 2000;160:459–467.

296. Gotto AM. Low high-density lipoprotein as a risk factor in coronary heart disease. A working group report. Circulation 2001;103:2213–2218.

297. Expert Panel on Detection, Evaluation, and Treatment of High Blood Cholesterol. Executive summary of the third report of the National Cholesterol Education Program (NCEP) Expert Panel on Detection, Evaluation, and Treatment of High Blood Cholesterol in Adults (Adult Treatment Panel III). JAMA 2001;285:2486–2497.

298. Hu FB, Manson JE, Willett WC. Types of dietary fat and risk of coronary artery disease: a critical review. J Am Coll Nutr 2001;20:5–19.

299. Kris–Etherton P, Daniels SR, Eckel RH, Engler M, Howard BV, Krauss RM, Lichtenstein AH, Sacks F, St Jeor S, Stampfer M, Eckel RH, Grundy SM, Appel LJ, Byers T, Campos H, Cooney G, Denke MA, Kennedy E, Marckmann P, Pearson TA, Riccardi G, Ruddell LL, Rudrum M, Stein DT, Tracy RP, Ursine V, Vogel RA, Zock PL, Bazzarre TL, Clark J. Summary of the scientific conference on dietary fatty acids and cardiovascular health: conference summary from the nutrition committee of the American Heart Association. Circualtion 2001;103:1034–9.

300. The Heart Outcomes Prevention Evaluation Study Investigators. Vitamin E supplementation and cardiovascular events in high-risk patients. N Engl J Med 2000;342:154–60.

301. Spady DK, Kearney DM, Hobbs HH. Polyunsaturated fatty acids up-regulate hepatic scavenger receptor BI (SR-BI) expression and HDL cholesteryl ester uptake in the hamster. J Lipid Res 1999;40:1384–1394.

302. Plotnick GD, Corretti MC, Vogel RA. Effect of antioxidant vitamins on the transient impairment of endothelium-dependent brachial artery vasoactivity following a single high-fat meal. JAMA 1997;278:1682–1686.

303. Hakim AA, Curb D, Petrovich H, Rodriguez BL, Yano K, Ross GW, White LR, Abbott RD. Effects of walking on coronary heart disease in elderly men. The Honolulu Heart Program. Circulation 1999;100:9–13.

304. Mittleman MA, Maclure M, Tofler GH, Sherwood JB, Goldberg RJ, Muller JE. Triggering of acute myocardial infarction by heavy physical exertion. Protection against triggering by regular exertion. N Engl J Med. 1993;329:1677–83.

305. Kris-Etherton PM, Krummel D, Russell ME, Dreon D, Mackey S, Borchers J, Wood PD. The effect of diet on plasma lipids, lipoproteins, and coronary heart disease. J Am Diet Assoc 1988;88:1373–1400.

306. Tanasescu M, Leitzmann MF, Rimm EB, Willett WC, Stampfer MJ, Hu FB. Exercise type and intensity in relation to coronary heart disease in men. JAMA 2002;288:1994–2000.

307. Takemoto M, Liao JK. Pleiotropic effects of 3-hydroxy-3-methylglutaryl coenzyme a reductase inhibitors. Arterioscler Thromb Vasc Biol 2001;21:1712–1719.

308. Balk EM, Lau J, Goudas LC, Jordan HS, Kupelnick B, Kim LU, Karas RH. Effects of statins on nonlipid serum markers associated with cardiovascular disease: a systematic review. Ann Intern Med 2003 21;139:670–682.

309. Shavelle DM, Takasu J, Budoff MJ, Mao S, Zhao XQ, O'Brien KD. HMG CoA reductase inhibitor (statin) and aortic valve calcium. Lancet 2002;359:1125–1126.

310. Node K, Fujita M, Kitakaze M, Hori M, Liao JK. Short-term statin therapy improves cardiac function and symptoms in patients with idiopathic dilated cardiomyopathy. Circulation 2003; 108:839–843.

311. Mohler ER, Hiatt WR, Creager MA. Cholesterol reduction with atorvastatin improves walking distance in patients with peripheral arterial disease. Circulation 2003;108:1481–1486.

312. Stuve O, Youssef S, Steinman L, Zamvil SS. Statins as potential therapeutic agents in neuroinflammatory disorders. Curr Opin Neurol 2003;16:393–401.

313. Ballantyne CM, Corsini A, Davidson MH, Holdaas H, Jacobson TA, Leitersdorf E, Marz W, Reckless JP, Stein EA. Risk for myopathy with statin therapy in high-risk patients. Arch Intern Med 2003;163:553–564.

314. Turley SD, Dietschy JM. The intestinal absorption of biliary and dietary cholesterol as a drug target for lowering the plasma cholesterol level. Prev Cardiol 2003;6:29–33,64.

315. Ballantyne CM, Houri J, Notarbartolo A, Melani L, Lipka LJ, Suresh R, Sun S, LeBeaut AP, Sager PT, Veltri EP. Ezetimibe Study Group. Effect of ezetimibe coadministered with atorvastatin in 628 patients with primary hypercholesterolemia: a prospective, randomized, double-blind trial. Circulation 2003;107:2409–2415.

316. Miller M, Seidler A, Kwiterovich PO, Pearson TA. Long-term predictors of subsequent cardiovascular events with coronary artery disease and "desirable" levels of plasma total cholesterol. Circulation 1992;86:1165–1170.

317. Fruchart JC. Peroxisome proliferator-activated receptor-alpha activation and high-density lipoprotein metabolism. Am J Cardiol 2001;88:24N–29N.

318. Ansell BJ, Navab M, Hama S, Kamranpour N, Fonarow G, Hough G, Rahmani S, Mottahedeh RR, Dave R, Reddy ST, Fogelman AM. Inflammatory/anti–inflammatory properties of high–density lipoprotein distinguish patients from control subjects better than high–density lipoprotein cholesterol levels and are favorably affected by simvastatin treatment. Circulation 2003:online.

319. Miller M, Zhan M. Factors influencing coronary risk in low HDL syndromes. Atherosclerosis 2003;169:347–348.

320. Heart Protection Study Collaborative Group. MRC/BHF Heart Protection Study of antioxidant vitamin supplementation in 20,536 high-risk individuals: a randomised placebo-controlled trial. Lancet 2002;360:23–33.

321. Miller M. New developments in the treatment of low high-density lipoprotein cholesterol. Curr Atheroscler Rep 1999;1:24–30.

322. Miller M. Niacin as a component of combination therapy for dyslipidemia. Mayo Clin Proc 2003;78:735–742.

323. Miller M, Bachorik PS, McCrindle BW, Kwiterovich PO. Effect of gemfibrozil in men with primary isolated low high-density lipoprotein cholesterol: a randomized, double-blind, placebo-controlled, crossover study. Am J Med 1993;94:7–12.

324. Ballantyne CM, Olsson AG, Cook TJ, Mercuri MF, Pedersen TR, Kjekshus J. Influence of low high-density lipoprotein cholesterol and elevated triglyceride on coronary heart disease events and response to simvastatin therapy in 4S. Circulation 2001;104:3046–3051.

325. Prinsen BH, de Sain-van der Velden MG, de Koning EJ, Koomans HA, Berger R, Rabelink TJ. Hypertriglyceridemia in patients with chronic renal failure: possible mechanisms. Kidney Int Suppl 2003;84:S121–S124.

326. Miller M, Seidler A, Moalemi A, Pearson TA. Normal triglyceride levels and coronary artery disease events: the Baltimore Coronary Observational Long-Term Study. J Am Coll Cardiol 1998;31:1252–1257.

327. Miller M. The epidemiology of triglyceride as a coronary artery disease risk factor. Clin Cardiol 1999;22(Suppl II):1–6.

328. Miller M, Zhan M, Georgopoulos A. Effect of desirable fasting triglycerides on the postprandial response to dietary fat. J Investig Med 2003;51:50–55.

329. Miller M, Bachorik PS, Cloey TA. Normal variation of plasma lipoproteins: postural effects on plasma concentrations of lipids, lipoproteins, and apolipoproteins. Clin Chem 1992;38:569–574.

330. Brewer HB. Hypertriglyceridemia: changes in the plasma lipoproteins associated with an increased risk of cardiovascular disease. Am J Cardiol 1999;83(suppl 9B):3F–12F.

331. Ballantyne CM, Corsini A, Davidson MH, Holdaas H, Jacobson TA, Leitersdorf E, Marz W, Reckless JP, Stein EA. Risk for myopathy with statin therapy in high-risk patients. Arch Intern Med 2003;163:553–564.

332. Miller M, Byington R, Hunninghake D, Pitt B, Furberg CD. Sex bias and underutilization of lipid-lowering therapy in patients with coronary artery disease at academic medical centers in the United States and Canada. Prospective Randomized Evaluation of the Vascular Effects of Norvasc Trial (PREVENT) Investigators. Arch Intern Med 2000;160:343–347.

333. Chin-Dusting JP, Dart AM. Age and the treatment gap in the use of statins. Lancet 2003; 361:1925–1926.

334. Shepherd J, Blauw GJ, Murphy MB, Bollen EL, Buckley BM, Cobbe SM, Ford I, Gaw A, Hyland M, Jukema JW, Kamper AM, Macfarlane PW, Meinders AE, Norrie J, Packard CJ, Perry IJ, Stott DJ, Sweeney BJ, Twomey C, Westendorp RG. PROSPER study group. PROspective Study of Pravastatin in the Elderly at Risk. Pravastatin in elderly individuals at risk of vascular disease (PROSPER): a randomised controlled trial. Lancet 2002;360: 1623–1630.

335. Fonarow GC. The role of in-hospital initiation of cardiovascular protective therapies to improve treatment rates and clinical outcomes. Rev Cardiovasc Med 2003(Suppl 3):S37–S46.

336. Jones PH, Davidson MH, Stein EA, Bays HE, McKenney JM, Miller E, Cain VA, Blasetto JW. STELLAR Study Group. Comparison of the efficacy and safety of rosuvastatin versus atorvastatin, simvastatin, and pravastatin across doses (STELLAR* Trial). Am J Cardiol 2003;92:152–160.

337. Nissen SE, Tsunoda T, Tuzcu EM, Schoenhagen P, Cooper CJ, Yasin M, Eaton GM, Lauer MA, Sheldon WS, Grines CL, Halpern S, Crowe T, Blankenship JC, Kerensky R. Effect of recombinant ApoA-I Milano on coronary atherosclerosis in patients with acute coronary syndromes: a randomized controlled trial. JAMA 2003;290:2292–2300.

# 25

# Diabetes in Acute Coronary Syndrome

**Koon-Hou Mak**
*National Heart Centre*
*Singapore*

**Eric J. Topol**
*The Cleveland Clinic Foundation*
*Cleveland, Ohio, U.S.A.*

## INTRODUCTION

Diabetes is one of the most common chronic diseases with increased cardiovascular morbidity and mortality [1]. About 150 million worldwide are suffering from this condition and the number is expected to rise to 300 million by 2025. In the United States, more than 17 million people suffer from diabetes [2]. Among those older than 25 years of age, 450,000 Americans (or 19% of all deaths) died from its related complications in 1999, with cardiovascular disease and stroke accounting for approximately two-thirds of the deaths. Overall, diabetes is the sixth most common cause of death, with an age-adjusted mortality rate of 18.5 per 100,000 Americans in 1996. This figure is almost three-fold greater than deaths attributed to Human Immuno-deficiency Virus infection (HIV). Not unexpectedly, the total cost burden for this condition was estimated to be $132 billion in 2002, with about a third of the expenditure attributed to indirect cost such as temporary or permanent disability, and premature death [3]. Of the remaining $92 billion used for direct medical costs, approximately a fifth was employed for management of cardiovascular complications. In fact, the annual medical expenditure for a patient with diabetes was estimated to be 2.4 times higher than a nondiabetic. With a million new patients diagnosed with diabetes each year in the United States, the strain on financial and medical resources will continue to increase to an estimated amount of $192 billion by 2020.

With diabetes imposing such a large economic burden to society, the individual and the family, one key strategy that may potentially reduce healthcare expenditure and increase productivity is to minimize the occurrence of the accompanying complications. Although there has been considerable improvement in managing patients with coronary artery disease, adverse cardiovascular events remained heightened among patients with diabetes [4], even among those without clinical symptoms and especially for women [5,6]. Indeed, short- and long-term outcomes were also less favorable among patients with diabetes undergoing coronary revascularization procedures [7].

Consistently, mortality was higher among diabetics with acute ST-segment-elevation myocardial infarction (MI), even when they were treated with contemporary fibrinolytic regimen [8] or direct angioplasty [9]. Correspondingly, outcomes among patients with diabetes with a broad spectrum of acute coronary syndrome [10], including unstable angina and non–ST-segment-elevation myocardial infarction [11,12] remain considerably poorer than those without diabetes.

## CLINICAL OUTCOMES

### Mortality

Even during the prefibrinolytic therapy era, short- and long-term mortality are known to be considerably higher among patients with diabetes than those without diabetes [13–19]. Patients with diabetes are generally older [16–18], more likely to be women [17,18], and to have suffered from a previous MI [16,17] and poorer renal function [17]. These adverse characteristics were thought to have contributed to the lower likelihood of survival among diabetics.

Undoubtedly, administration of fibrinolytic agents for the treatment of acute ST-segment-elevation MI has been shown to improve survival [20,21]. As time progressed from the prefibrinolytic to fibrinolytic era, outcomes also became significantly better among MI patients with and without diabetes [22]. Indeed, the benefit was greater among those with diabetes with the administration of a fibrinolytic agent. The Fibrinolytic Therapy Trialists Group [23] reported that administration of a fibrinolytic agent saved 37 lives per 1000 patients with diabetes compared with only 15 lives per 1000 nondiabetic patients at 35 days. Nonetheless, mortality following MI among diabetics remained high, even in the current era of pharmacological reperfusion therapy. In a pooled analysis of almost 104,000 patients, short-term mortality was consistently higher among patients with diabetes (Fig. 1). Compared with nondiabetics, early mortality was about 66% higher for those with diabetes (95% confidence interval [CI], 1.57–1.77). Among diabetics, insulin treatment portended a considerably poorer outcome (odds ratio [OR], 1.34; 95% CI, 1.15–1.56). Several reasons which may have accounted for this disparity [24], including lower likelihood for receiving pharmacological reperfusion therapy [25,26]. Patients with diabetes may present later or more likely with atypical symptoms [8], delaying the institution of lifesaving reperfusion therapy [8,27,28]. Furthermore, there was an undue concern regarding intraocular hemorrhage. In fact, only one patient sustained a periorbital hematoma following a fall among 6,011 patients with diabetes receiving fibrinolysis in the Global Utilization of Streptokinase and Tissue Plasminogen Activator for Occluded Arteries (GUSTO-I) Trial [29]. Therefore, the risk for intraocular hemorrhage was not excessively high. In addition, patients with diabetes were less likely to receive optimal pharmacological therapy which may also have accounted for the poorer outcome [25,30].

After the acute phase of MI, the excess in mortality among patients with diabetes continued to diverge at 6 to 12 months following the acute event (Fig. 2). The Second International Study of Infarct Survival [31] reported that survival among those treated with streptokinase was approximately 3.1% lower for diabetics (87.9% vs. 91.0%) at 35 days. By the end of 4 years, this difference widened to 18.9% (59.3% vs. 78.2%). This trend was also observed in 2 Danish MI cohorts, with the mortality gap for diabetics increased as the duration of follow-up lengthened [32]. The mortality rate ratio rose from 1.17 at 30 days to 2.51 at 7 to 9 years following discharge in the Glostrup cohort. Correspondingly, the mortality rate ratio increased from 1.03 at 30 days to 1.74 at 4 to 6 years of follow-up in the Trandolapril Cardiac Evaluation (TRACE) trial.

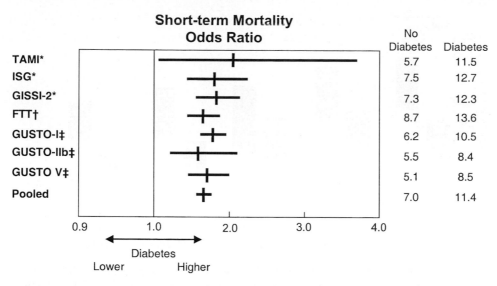

| | No Diabetes | Diabetes |
|---|---|---|
| TAMI* | 5.7 | 11.5 |
| ISG* | 7.5 | 12.7 |
| GISSI-2* | 7.3 | 12.3 |
| FTT† | 8.7 | 13.6 |
| GUSTO-I‡ | 6.2 | 10.5 |
| GUSTO-IIb‡ | 5.5 | 8.4 |
| GUSTO V‡ | 5.1 | 8.5 |
| Pooled | 7.0 | 11.4 |

**Figure 1**  Mortality and diabetes status in contemporary large randomized trials on fibrinolysis for acute ST-segment-elevation myocardial infarction. *In-hospital mortality; †35-day mortality; ‡30-day mortality. TAMI = Thrombolysis and Angioplasty in Myocardial Infarction [Ref. 37]; ISG = International Tissue Plasminogen Activator/ Streptokinase Mortality Trial [Ref. 38]; GISSI-2 = the Second Gruppo Italiano per lo Studio della Sopravvivenza nell'Infarto Micocardio Study [Ref. 39]; FTT = Fibrinolytic Therapy Trialists Collaborative Group [Ref. 23]; GUSTO-I = Global Utilization of Streptokinase and Tissue Plasminogen Activator for Occluded Coronary Arteries [Ref. 8]; GUSTO-IIb = The Global Strategies To Open Occluded Coronary Arteries in acute coronary syndromes study [Ref. 11]; GUSTO V = The Global Strategies To Open Occluded Coronary Arteries (GUSTO) V Trial [Ref. 66].

Likewise, among patients with non–ST-segment-elevation MI, short-term mortality remained higher for those with diabetes. Among 24,728 patients in 4 large randomized trials evaluating the efficacy of a variety of glycoprotein (GP) IIb/IIIa inhibitors [33–36], there were 5,409 (21.9%) with diabetes. Mortality at 30 days was considerably higher among diabetics (5.5% vs. 3.0%; $p < 0.001$) (Fig. 3). Similarly, in the Global Use of Strategies To Open Occluded Arteries in Acute Coronary Syndromes (GUSTO-IIb), among those with non–ST-segment-elevation MI, there were 1507 and 6503 patients with and without diabetes, respectively [11]. The 30-day mortality was significantly higher among diabetics (6.2% vs. 3.3%; $p < 0.0001$). By pooling these 5 studies, with a total of 32,738 patients, the likelihood of patients with diabetes dying at 30 days was 1.88 times (95% CI, 1.66–2.13) higher than nondiabetics. Besides clinical trials, the heightened mortality among patients with diabetes and unstable angina or non–Q-wave MI was also observed in contemporary practice. In an international registry of unstable angina and non–Q-wave MI, there were 1718 (21.4%) of 8013 patients who suffered from diabetes [10]. Although only about a fifth of the patients had an admitting diagnosis of non–Q-wave MI, the all-cause mortality at 2 years remained higher for those with diabetes (18% vs. 10%; $p < 0.001$), with an adjusted rate ratio of 1.57 (95% CI, 1.38–1.81).

## Other Clinical Outcomes

Patients with diabetes were more likely to suffer from complications following ST-segment-elevation MI during the in-hospital period [8,11,37–39], including heart failure (OR,

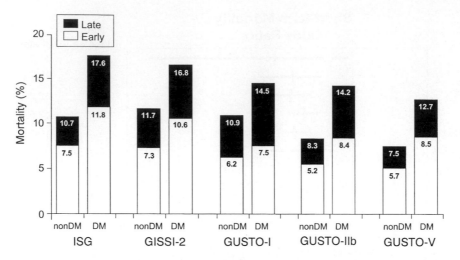

**Figure 2**  Early (30–35 days) and late (6–12 months) mortality following ST-segment-elevation myocardial infarction among patients with and without diabetes. NonDM = patients without diabetes; DM = patients with diabetes; ISG = International Tissue Plasminogen Activator/ Streptokinase Mortality Trial [Ref. 38]; GISSI-2 = the Second Gruppo Italiano per lo Studio della Sopravvivenza nell'Infarto Micocardio Study [Ref. 39]; GUSTO-I = Global Utilization of Streptokinase and Tissue Plasminogen Activator for Occluded Coronary Arteries [Ref. 8]; GUSTO-IIb = The Global Strategies To Open Occluded Coronary Arteries in acute coronary syndromes study [11]; GUSTO V = The Global Strategies To Open Occluded Coronary Arteries (GUSTO) V Trial [Ref. 66].

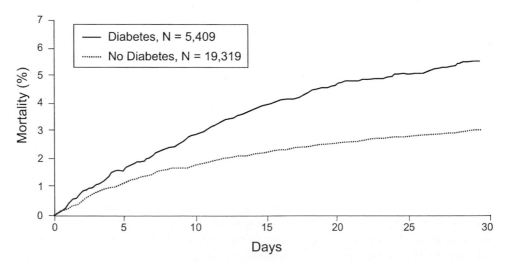

**Figure 3**  30-day mortality following unstable angina and non–ST-segment-elevation myocardial infarction among patients with and without diabetes. Data derived from Platelet IIb/IIIa Antagonism for the Reduction of Acute Coronary Syndrome Events in a Global Organization Network Trial (PARAGON-A) [Ref. 33], Platelet Glycoprotein IIb/IIIa in Unstable Angina: Receptor Suppression Integrilin Therapy (PURSUIT) [Ref. 34], PARAGON-B [Ref. 35], and the Global Utilization of Strategies To Open Occluded Coronary Arteries (GUSTO) IV trial [Ref. 36].

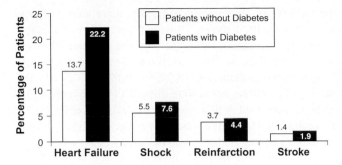

**Figure 4**  Clinical complications following ST-segment-elevation myocardial infarction. Data on heart failure were obtained as congestive heart failure [Ref. 8,39], pulmonary edema [Ref. 37], and Killip class 2 or greater [Ref. 38] from various trials. Sources of information for shock [Ref. 8,37–39], reinfarction [Ref. 8,11,37–39], and stroke [Ref. 8,37,38] differed.

1.80; 95% CI, 1.70–1.90), cardiogenic shock (OR, 1.40; 95% CI, 1.28–1.53), recurrent MI (OR, 1.23; 95% CI, 1.10–1.37), and stroke (OR, 1.43; 95% CI, 1.18–1.74) (Fig. 4). The clinical course of MI was more likely to be complicated by atrial fibrillation or atrioventricular conduction defects among patients with diabetes [8]. Notably, diabetics treated with insulin had a considerably poorer outcome, with a higher occurrence of heart failure (26.4% vs. 19.5%; p < 0.001), shock (8.4% vs. 6.8%; p = 0.01), and stroke (2.5% vs. 1.6%; p = 0.02) compared with noninsulin treated diabetics.

Similarly, adverse clinical outcomes were more likely to occur among patients with diabetes and unstable angina or non–Q-wave MI than nondiabetics. The Organization to Assess Strategies for Ischemic Syndromes (OASIS) Registry [10] reported that the rates of subsequent MI, stroke or heart failure were substantially higher after 2-year follow-up. After adjusting for baseline characteristics, the hazard ratios for the occurrence of MI, stroke, and heart failure were 1.34 (95% CI, 1.14–1.57), 1.45 (95% CI, 1.09–1.92), and 1.41 (95% CI, 1.26–1.60), respectively. With a considerably worse clinical outcome, a variety of approaches has been developed to improve the prognosis of patients with diabetes.

Several healthcare delivery and biological factors may have accounted for the deleterious outcome among patients with diabetes [7,24]. Although the exaggerated thrombogenic tendency did not result in impaired response to fibrinolysis or direct angioplasty, there was a trend towards a higher rate of angiographic reocclusion [40] and recurrent MI [8]. The lack of statistical significance may be partly attributed to the proportion of patients who died prior to scheduled angiography, which was 3 times higher for those with diabetes [40]. These patients who died were likely to suffer from angiographic reocclusion or recurrent MI. As silent MI may occur more frequently in diabetics, the rate could have been underestimated. Notwithstanding these limitations, the rate of ischemia was significantly higher among patients with diabetes (22% vs. 20%; p < 0.001) [8]. Other factors that could have accounted for the poorer outcomes among patients with diabetes include impairment of the recruitment of collateral circulation during acute closure of a vessel [41] and attenuation of the hyperkinetic response in the noninfarcted areas [40].

## EARLY INVASIVE STRATEGIES

### ST-segment-elevation Myocardial Infarction

Primary angioplasty has been clearly shown to be superior to fibrinolysis to achieve reperfusion in acute ST-segment-elevation MI to provide better short- and long-term survival [42].

Of 1,138 patients enrolled in the GUSTO-IIb Angioplasty Substudy, there were 177 who
suffered from diabetes [9]. Among those with diabetes, 78 were treated with accelerated
alteplase and 99 treated with angioplasty. The rates of successful angioplasty procedure were
similar between patients with and without diabetes. However, moderate to severe bleeding
complications were marginally higher among diabetics (18.2% vs. 9.1%; p = 0.07). Although 30-day mortality was not significantly higher among diabetics treated with angioplasty (9.1% vs. 6.4%), the rate of recurrent infarction was significantly lower (3.0% vs.
10.3%; p = 0.05). There was a favorable trend towards a lower occurrence of death, recurrent
infarction or disabling stroke at 30 days among patients with diabetes treated with angioplasty compared with alteplase (11.1% vs. 16.7%; adjusted OR, 0.70; 95% CI, 0.29 to 1.72).
However, there was little difference in the rate of death and recurrent infarction at 6 months
between these 2 therapeutic modalities. Conversely in another case-control study of diabetic
patients, 99 were treated with fibrinolytic therapy and 103 with angioplasty [43], the rate
of death or recurrent infarction was considerably lower among those receiving mechanical
reperfusion (17.5% vs. 31.3%; p = 0.02), with an adjusted rate ratio of 0.29 (95% CI, 0.15
to 0.57) (Fig. 5). In substudy of a randomized trial [44], there was a trend towards better
outcomes for primary angioplasty compared with prehosptial fibrinolysis. At 30 days, the
occurrence of death, MI or stroke was 5.8% in the angioplasty group and 21.7% in the fibrinolytic group (adjusted OR, 0.34; 95% CI, 0.1–1.1), with an interaction between diabetic status
and treatment strategy, favoring primary angioplasty.

Although patients with and without diabetes have similar procedural success rates
for direct coronary stenting and 30-day survival, those with diabetes were more likely to
suffer from stent thrombosis (18% vs. 1%; p = 0.003) [45]. At about a year, survival
was significantly lower for patients with diabetes (89% vs. 99%; p = 0.04). Of 3742
patients enrolled in the Primary Angioplasty in Myocardial Infarction (PAMI) trials [46],
there were 626 (17%) diabetics. While those with diabetes were less likely to undergo
direct angioplasty, procedural success rates were similar. However, in-hospital (4.6% vs.
2.6%; p = 0.005) and 6-month (8.1% vs. 4.2%; p < 0.0001) mortality were considerably

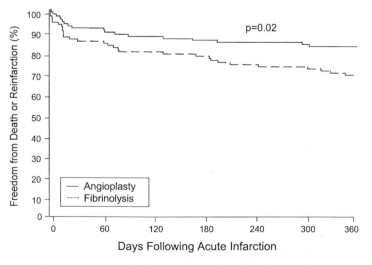

**Figure 5**   Kaplan-Meier plots showing freedom from death or reinfarction for patients with
diabetes treated with fibrinolysis or angioplasty at 12 months. (From Ref. 43)

higher for patients with diabetes. After adjusting for baseline characteristics, diabetes was independently associated with 6-month mortality (hazard ratio, 1.53; 95% CI, 1.03–2.26). Conversely, the Zwolle Myocardial Infarction Study Group [47] reported that 1-year mortality was not higher among diabetics after adjusting for differences in characteristics among 1791 patients undergoing primary angioplasty.

## Non–ST-segment-elevation Myocardial Infarction

While earlier studies failed to show benefits from an early invasive strategy for patients with unstable angina and non–ST-segment-elevation MI [48,49], more recent studies reported that an early invasive strategy improved outcomes in this group of patients [50–53]. From a broad timing of revascularization, ranging from a few [50,53] to less than 2 [51,52] days, with [51] and without [52] the use of GP IIb/IIIa inhibitors, and different low molecular weight heparins [50,53], an early invasive strategy reduced the occurrence of death or MI at 6 [51,52] to 12 [50,53] months (Fig. 6). From a total of 6,617 patients in these 4 randomized studies, the occurrences of death (3.2% vs. 5.1%; p < 0.001) or MI (5.1% vs. 8.2%; p < 0.001) were significantly lower for patients undergoing an early invasive strategy. Compared with those in the conservative strategy, the likelihood for death or MI (8.5% vs. 11.1%; p < 0.001) at 6 to 12 months was reduced substantially in the early invasive arm (OR, 0.74; 95% CI, 0.63–0.87). Although early angioplasty in patients with acute coronary syndromes without persistent ST-segment-elevation MI may reduce MI but the rate for 6-month repeat revascularization may be increased [54].

Patients with diabetes are likely to derive the benefits of early revascularization. Although diabetics have a poorer outcome among 1433 patients receiving early revasculari-

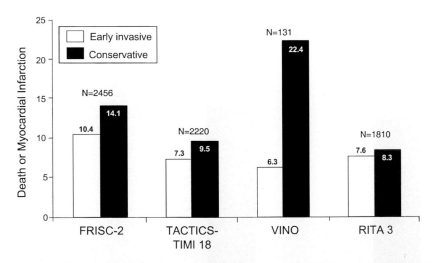

**Figure 6** Occurrence of death or myocardial infarction between early invasive or conservative strategies at 6 or 12 months following unstable angina or non–ST-segment-elevation myocardial infarction. FRISC-2 = Fast Revascularisation during Instability in Coronary artery disease invasive trial [Ref. 50]; TACTICS-TIMI 18 = Treat Angina with Aggrastat and Determine Cost of Therapy with an Invasive or Conservative Strategy – Thrombolysis in Myocardial Infarction 18 [Ref. 51]; VINO = Value of First Day Angiography/Angioplasty in Evolving Non-ST Segment Elevation Myocardial Infarction: an Open Multicenter Randomized Trial [Ref. 52]; RITA 3 = Randomized Intervention Trial of unstable Angina [Ref. 53].

zation within 24 hours of hospitalization, after adjusting for baseline characteristics, long-term mortality was comparable with nondiabetics [55]. In the FRISC II (Fast Revascularisation during Instability in Coronary artery disease) invasive trial [50], there were 298 (12.1%) patients with diabetes. Among these patients, the incidence of death or MI at 1 year was marginally lower among those randomized to the invasive strategy (20.8% vs. 29.9%), with a ratio of 0.70 (95% CI, 0.47–1.04). Correspondingly, in the TACTICS-TIMI 18 (Treat Angina with Aggrastat and Determine Cost of Therapy with an Invasive or Conservative Strategy–Thrombolysis in Myocardial Infarction 18) study [51], there were 613 (27.6%) patients with diabetes. At 6 months, those randomized to early invasive strategy were significantly less likely to suffer from death, MI or rehospitalization for an acute coronary syndrome (20.1% vs. 27.7%; OR, 0.66; 95% CI, 0.45–0.96; p = 0.036).

The issue of the intense prolonged antithrombotic treatment prior to coronary angiography and revascularization was evaluated in the Intracoronary Stenting With Antithrombotic Regimen Cooling-Off (ISAR-COOL) trial [56]. Of 410 patients enrolled, 207 were randomly assigned to receive 3 to 5 days of intense antithrombotic therapy consisting of aspirin, clopidogrel, heparin and tirofiban infusion, and another 203 to early intervention within 6 hours of admission. Notably, the occurrence of death or MI was considerably higher among those who had prolonged treatment (11.6% vs. 5.9%; p = 0.04). Patients with diabetes exhibited a similar trend (Fig. 7). Conversely, the Early or Late Intervention in unStable Angina (ELISA) pilot study [57] reported that a strategy of delaying angiography with pre-treatment with tirofiban was associated with an improved angiographic outcome. These patients had a smaller infarct size than those undergoing early angiography without GP IIb/IIIa blockade. However, there are several differences in the study protocol between ISAR-COOL and ELISA trials. In the ISAR-COOL trial, patients randomized to early angiography also received tirofiban and the procedure was performed substantially later in the intense antithrombotic group.

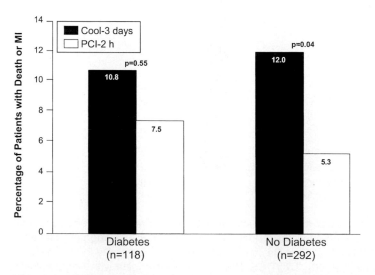

**Figure 7** The occurrence of death or myocardial infarction among patients randomized to prolonged antithrombotic therapy or early intervention in the ISAR-COOL. ISAR-COOL = Intracoronary Stenting With Antithrombotic Regimen Cooling-Off trial [Ref. 56]; MI = myocardial infarction; PCI = percutaneous coronary intervention.

## GLYCOPROTEIN IIb/IIIa BLOCKADE

While fibrinolytic therapy improves survival [23], several mechanistic pathways have been postulated to explain the failure in 45% to 50% of patients who do not achieve early and complete restoration of blood flow [58]. Of these, the prothrombotic effects of fibrinolytic agents and absence of a definitive strategy against platelets were considered to be the key elements for the deficiency of fibrinolytic agents. The discovery of GP IIb/IIIa receptors, the final common pathway for platelet aggregation, has resulted in the introduction of a new group of potent antiplatelet inhibitors [59]. Several large-scale randomized clinical trials have clearly shown the efficacy of this group of agents in a broad spectrum of patients with coronary artery disease [60]. The combination of GP IIb/IIIa inhibitors with various reperfusion regimens and antithrombotic agents for the treatment of patients with ST-segment-elevation and non–ST-segment-elevation MI, respectively, has also been extensively investigated.

## ST-segment-elevation Myocardial Infarction

Several experimental models of MI clearly showed the potential benefits of combination GP IIb/IIIa and fibrinolytic therapy, as evident by faster restoration of antegrade flow and prevention of re-occlusion [58]. Combination of a variety of fibrinolytic agents at full- or reduced-dose with either eptifibatide [61,62] and abciximab [63,64] have been shown to provide a greater proportion of patients with complete restoration of antegrade flow than the fibrinolytic agent alone. However, the favorable findings of these mechanistic studies were not corroborated by mortality reduction as evident from 2 large-scale randomized clinical trials [65,66]. The Assessment of the Safety and Efficacy of a New Thrombolytic Regimen (ASSENT)-3 trial studied the safety and efficacy of tenecteplase-tissue plasminogen activator with unfractionated heparin or enoxaparin and half-dose tenecteplase-tissue plasminogen activator with abciximab [65] and the GUSTO V trial compared the safety and efficacy of reteplase with half-dose reteplase plus abciximab [66]. Notably, in the ASSENT-3 trial, patients randomized to full-dose tenecteplase with enoxaparin or half-dose tenecteplase with abciximab were less likely to die at 30 days or suffer from in-hospital recurrent infarction or ischemia (11.4% and 11.1%) than those treated with full-dose tenecteplase with unfractionated heparin (15.4%; p < 0.0001). Of 20,643 patients studied, there was no difference in 30-day mortality (5.8% vs. 5.9%; p = 0.75) between patients treated with half-dose fibrinolytic agent with abciximab and full-dose fibrinolytic agent with unfractionated heparin. In the GUSTO V trial [66], there was little difference in 30-day mortality for patients with diabetes treated with reteplase or half-dose reteplase with abciximab (8.2% vs. 8.8%; p = 0.58) [66]. In contrast, the rates of recurrent MI (2.3% vs. 3.6%; p < 0.001) and recurrent ischemia (9.7% vs. 11.5%; p < 0.001) were substantially lower among those treated with abciximab, with an odds ratio of 0.62 (95% CI, 0.52–0.73) and 0.82 (95% CI, 0.75–0.90), respectively. The risk of major bleeding complications was significantly higher (1.5% vs. 0.8%; p < 0.001) (OR, 1.77; 95% CI, 1.36–2.31).

The role of GP IIb/IIIa blockers in patients undergoing direct angioplasty, with and without coronary stenting, for ST-segment elevation MI has also been evaluated [67–70]. Abciximab has been shown to improve microvascular perfusion and left ventricular function following coronary stenting for acute MI [71]. Taken together, with a total of 3,266 patients, there was no difference in the occurrence of death and recurrent MI at 30 days [72]. However, the rate of urgent target vessel revascularization (OR,

0.43; 95% CI, 0.28–0.66) and total target vessel revascularization (OR, 0.66; 95% CI, 0.48–0.91) were considerably lower. At the end of 6 months, only the difference in the rate of urgent target vessel revascularization remained statistically significant. To prevent an urgent target revascularization, 33 patients needed to be treated with GP IIb/IIIa inhibitors during direct angioplasty. While there was no information on patients with diabetes, the use of abciximab during elective angioplasty procedures was associated with better 1-year survival (2.5% vs. 4.5%; p = 0.03) [73].

## Non-ST-segment-elevation Myocardial Infarction

Several studies have been conducted to evaluate the efficacy and safety of GP IIb/IIIa blockade in the setting of unstable angina and non–ST-segment-elevation MI. In a meta-analysis based on individual patients of 6 large-scale randomized trials evaluating the efficacy of a variety of GP IIb/IIIa inhibitors with placebo or control, there were 31,402 patients [74]. The occurrence of death or MI at 30 days was substantially lower (OR, 0.91; 95% CI, 0.85–0.98) among patients treated with GP IIb/IIIa inhibitors (10.8% vs. 11.8%; p = 0.015) (Fig. 8). Importantly, for this outcome, the interaction product term for diabetes and treatment group in a logistic model adjusted for between-trial outcome differences was not significant (p = 0.48). Not unexpectedly, the risk of major bleeding complications was higher (OR, 1.64; 95% CI, 1.36–1.97) among those treated with GP IIb/IIIa inhibitors (2.4% vs. 1.4%; p < 0.0001).

Of these 6 trials, there were 6,458 (20.5%) patients with diabetes [75]. The use of GP IIb/IIIa inhibitors was associated with a considerable reduction in 30-day mortality, from 6.2% to 4.6% (OR, 0.74; 95% CI, 0.59–0.92; p = 0.007) (Fig. 9). This benefit was observed for both insulin treated and noninsulin treated patients. Of 1,279 diabetic patients undergoing percutaneous coronary intervention during the index hospitalization, the pooled mortality was 70% (OR, 0.30; 95% CI, 0.14–0.69) lower among those treated with GP IIb/IIIa inhibitors (1.2% vs. 4.0%; p = 0.002), which translated to one life saved for every thirty-six patients treated. Indeed, GP IIb/IIIa inhibitors have been shown to improve microvascular function among patients with unstable angina undergoing coronary intervention [76].

Despite the benefit afforded by GP IIb/IIIa inhibitors derived from several randomized clinical trials, these agents were not widely adopted into routine clinical practice.

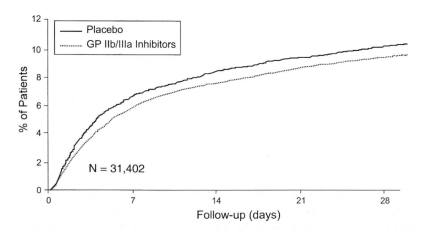

**Figure 8**   Occurrence of death or myocardial infarction within 30 days. GP = glycoprotein. (From Ref. 54)

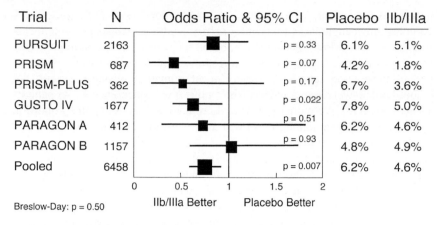

| Trial | N | Odds Ratio & 95% CI | | Placebo | IIb/IIIa |
|---|---|---|---|---|---|
| PURSUIT | 2163 | | p = 0.33 | 6.1% | 5.1% |
| PRISM | 687 | | p = 0.07 | 4.2% | 1.8% |
| PRISM-PLUS | 362 | | p = 0.17 | 6.7% | 3.6% |
| GUSTO IV | 1677 | | p = 0.022 | 7.8% | 5.0% |
| PARAGON A | 412 | | p = 0.51 | 6.2% | 4.6% |
| PARAGON B | 1157 | | p = 0.93 | 4.8% | 4.9% |
| Pooled | 6458 | | p = 0.007 | 6.2% | 4.6% |

Breslow-Day: p = 0.50    IIb/IIIa Better    Placebo Better

**Figure 9** Odds ratio and 95% confidence interval (CI) and corresponding p-values for treatment effect on 30-day mortality among diabetic patients with acute coronary syndromes. Values to the left of 1.0 indicate a survival benefit of platelet glycoprotein IIb/IIIa inhibition (IIb/IIIa) [Ref. 75]. (Reproduced with permission from the American Heart Association.)

The National Registry of Myocardial Infarction (NRMI) 4 enrolled 110,590 patients with non–ST-segment MI from 1,189 hospitals in the United States from July 2000 to July 2001 [77]. Of these, 60,770 (55%) patients were considered eligible for early administration of GP IIb/IIIa inhibitors. A total of 15,739 patients (25%) received a GP IIb/IIIa inhibitor within 24 hours of hospital admission, with a median time of 6 hours. Another 4,372 patients were treated with GP IIb/IIIa inhibitors after the first day, most commonly with percutaneous coronary intervention. The presence of diabetes was associated with a lower likelihood of early use of GP IIb/IIIa inhibitors (adjusted OR, 0.89; 95% CI, 0.85–0.94). After adjusting for patient risk, treatment propensity, provider factors and use of evidence-based medical therapies, patients receiving early GP IIb/IIIa inhibitors were less likely to die during the index hospitalization (OR, 0.88; 95% CI, 0.79–0.97).

## RESTORATION OF MYOCARDIAL PERFUSION

An emerging concept in the assessment of therapeutic modalities for the treatment of acute MI is the restoration of myocardial perfusion [58]. While earlier studies have stressed the importance of achieving normal antegrade coronary flow in the infarct-related artery, the ability to restore normal myocardial perfusion has been shown to further predict good outcomes in patients undergoing pharmacological [78] or mechanical [79] reperfusion strategies. Even among those with normal coronary antegrade perfusion following direct angioplasty, only 29% had normal myocardial blush [80]. Mortality at 1-year was lowest among those with normal myocardial perfusion (6.8%) compared with those with reduced (13.2%) or absent (18.3%) myocardial perfusion (p = 0.004). Interestingly, the presence of diabetes was not an adverse predictor for normal myocardial perfusion in this study.

Angiographic distal embolization during acute angioplasty for acute MI occurs in about 15% of patients and portends a poor outcome [81]. Furthermore, microvascular dysfunction occurs more frequently among patients with diabetes, even among those without clinical coronary atherosclerosis [82]. Therefore, preservation of the micro-circulation is even more critical for patients with diabetes. In a study conducted in 48 consecutive patients undergoing direct angioplasty for acute coronary syndrome, the lesion components that contribute to the "no-reflow" phenomenon, based on positron emission tomography at rest, during adenosine-induced hyperemia and response to cold pressor test, was determined [83]. The investigators reported a variety of atheromatous plaque materials, not just the thrombus burden, were associated with the "no-reflow" phenomenon. As patients with diabetes are known to have more extensive atheromatous disease [8], the proportion of diabetics tended to be higher among those with the "no-reflow" phenomenon in this study (66.7% vs. 37.8%; p = 0.1) [83].

Beyond angiographic and metabolic markers of restoration of microvasculature flow, resolution of ST-segment is another important characteristic for myocardial perfusion in patients treated with pharmacological or mechanical reperfusion therapies [84–86]. A series of clinical studies from the TIMI Study Group have reported similar rates of successful restoration of antegrade flow in patients with and without diabetes receiving pharmacological (55.4% vs. 59.0%) or adjunctive mechanical reperfusion (83.7% vs. 84.2%) therapies [87]. However, those with diabetes were less likely to have complete resolution of ST-segment resolution following fibrinolysis (38.6% vs. 49.2%; adjusted p-value = 0.04).

Conversely, another group of investigators found that diabetes was not a predictor for the "no-reflow" phenomenon using myocardial contrast echocardiography [88]. Instead, acute hyperglycemia (admission arterial blood sugar level greater than or equal to160 mg/dL or 8.9 mmol/L) was the strongest predictor (adjusted rate ratio, 12.1; 95% CI, 2.7–61.2) for the "no-reflow" phenomenon [89]. This adverse feature was associated with a larger infarct size and worse functional recovery (Fig. 10).

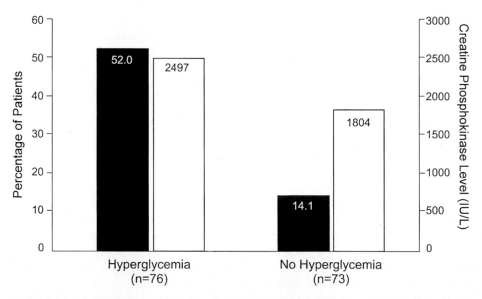

**Figure 10** Presence of "no-reflow" phenomenon and creatine phosphokinase level between patients with and without hyperglycemia [89]. Hyperglycemia = glucose level on admission ≥ 160 mg/dL (8.9 mmol/L). Left y-axis indicates the percentage of patients with "no-reflow" phenomenon (closed bar) and right y-axis indicates the level of creatine phosphokinase (open bar). The differences between the two groups for "no-reflow" phenomenon and creatine phosphokinase level were statistically significant, with p-values of < 0.0001 and 0.005, respectively.

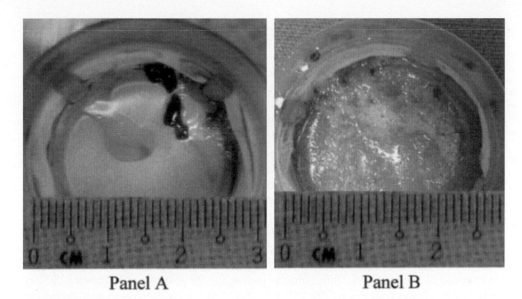

Panel A  Panel B

**Figure 11** The use of a distal protection device during direct angioplasty for acute myocardial infarction. (**A**) Initial aspiration consisted of mainly thrombotic material. (**B**) Subsequent aspiration following coronary stenting consisted of mainly whitish atheromatous debris.

Despite the controversy on the relationship between diabetes and acute hyperglycemia with the "no-reflow" phenomenon, restoration of myocardial perfusion is critical to improvement of outcomes. While GP IIb/IIIa inhibitors may reduce thrombotic complications [68,69], thrombectomy or distal protection devices may be more effective in preserving coronary micro-circulation during direct angioplasty for acute MI by preventing embolism of atheromatous debris. Recently, the preliminary results of a retrospective study suggested that a distal protection device is superior to abciximab in preserving myocardial perfusion among patients undergoing direct angioplasty for acute MI [90]. Prior to the angioplasty procedure, the presence of a patent infarct-related was greater among those treated with abciximab (37.5% vs. 18.7%; p = 0.027), but the proportion of patients with normal coronary flow at the end of the procedure was similar (85% vs. 83%; p = 0.32). However, those in the distal protection device group had an adjusted reduction of 12 corrected TIMI frame counts (95% CI, 5 to 18; p = 0.001). Furthermore, patients treated with a distal protection device were more likely to achieve a good myocardial blush score (adjusted OR, 3.0; 95% CI, 1.1–8.5; p = 0.039). Similar to the early study [83], during the initial aspiration, thrombus material was removed. However, following intervention, in particular, high-pressure inflation for coronary stenting, atheromatous debris was aspirated (Fig. 11).

## OPTIMAL GLYCEMIC CONTROL

Impaired glucose utilization may partly account for the adverse outcomes among patients with diabetes, especially during the acute phase of MI [91]. The ischemic insult followed by reperfusion injury has led several metabolic derangements, including increased lipolysis, cellular calcium overload, and relative intracellular potassium deficiency. These abnormalities formed part of the basis of glucose-insulin-potassium infusion regimens in the 1960s [92].

Several clinical trials have been conducted and by pooling 9 studies, administration of glucose-insulin-potassium infusion resulted in a relative reduction of 28% for in-hospital mortality [93]. Among those studies with sufficiently high concentration of glucose-insulin-potassium infusion, whereby free fatty acid levels were reduced, the relative reduction in mortality was even greater (48%). Conversely, in a randomized trial of 954 patients comparing between low-dose glucose-insulin-potassium with control, 35-day cardiac mortality (6.5% vs. 4.6%; p = 0.2) and adverse cardiac events (43.3% vs. 41.7%; p = 0.6) did not differ between those treated with and without glucose-insulin-potassium infusion [94]. Total mortality at 35 days was almost 2 times higher among those treated with glucose-insulin-potassium infusion (8.9% vs. 4.8%; p = 0.01). Similarly, glucose-insulin-potassium infusion did not improve survival among patients undergoing direct angioplasty for ST-segment-elevation MI [95]. Among 940 patients randomly assigned to glucose-insulin-potassium infusion for 8 to 12 hours or control, the 30-day mortality was similar (4.8% vs. 5.8%). Interestingly, among the 99 patients with diabetes, 30-day mortality was lower (rate ratio, 0.30; 95% CI, 0.06–1.56) in the glucose-insulin-potassium (4.0%) than control (12.2%; p = 0.16) group.

Likely, the dose and duration of infusion, and patient risk profile may be related to improved outcomes [96]. In the Diabetic Patients with Acute Myocardial Infarction (DIGAMI) study of 620 patients [97], 306 were randomly chosen to receive insulin-glucose followed by intensive subcutaneous insulin treatment and another 314 patients to conventional therapy. By 3 months, the glycosylated hemoglobin level was lower in the intensive treatment group (7.0% vs. 7.5%; p < 0.01). Correspondingly, there was a 29% relative reduction in 1-year mortality. Currently, an international randomized study evaluating the efficacy and safety of fondaparinux sodium versus control therapy and glucose-insulin-potassium infusion versus control in a broad spectrum of patients with acute ST-segment-elevation MI receiving either pharmacological or mechanical reperfusion strategies (Michelangelo: OASIS-6 Trial) is being conducted.

## ADJUNCTIVE PHARMACOLOGICAL THERAPY

### Oral Antiplatelet Therapy

The efficacy of antiplatelet therapy as a secondary prevention strategy for vascular diseases has been recently evaluated in a recent meta-analysis from the antiplatetet trialists, including patients with diabetes [98]. Overall, antiplatelet therapy reduced serious vascular events by about a quarter. Among 4,961 patients with diabetes from 9 trials, antiplatelet therapy was associated with a 7% proportional reduction in serious vascular events. Newer oral antiplatelet agents may confer greater protection against adverse vascular events. The Clopidogrel versus Aspirin in patients at Risk for Ischemic Events (CAPRIE) trial [99], which enrolled 19,185 patients with a history of recent stroke, MI, or peripheral vascular disease, reported a relative reduction of 8.7% in the occurrence of vascular death, MI, or stroke among those randomly allocated to clopidogrel compared with aspirin. Among 3,866 patients with diabetes in the CAPRIE, the annual event rate for vascular death, stroke, MI, or rehospitalization for ischemia or bleeding was considerably lower among those treated with clopidogrel (15.6% vs. 17.7%; p = 0.042), with an absolute reduction of 2.1% [100]. After adjusting for baseline characteristics, the use of clopidogrel, compared with aspirin, was associated with a 13% relative reduction of adverse vascular events among patients with diabetes. Of note, patients with diabetes treated with clopidogrel were less likely (rate ratio, 0.37; 95% CI, 0.04–0.59) to suffer from any bleeding complications than those treated with aspirin.

The efficacy of the long-term administration of aspirin plus clopidogrel was compared with aspirin alone in the Clopidogrel in Unstable Angina to Prevent Recurrent Events (CURE) trial [101]. Among 12,562 patients who presented within 24 hours of symptom onset were randomly assigned to receiving aspirin alone or aspirin plus clopidogrel. The combination of aspirin and clopidrogrel was associated with a lower likelihood (rate ratio, 0.80; 95% CI, 0.72–0.90; p < 0.001) for cardiovascular death, nonfatal MI, or stroke (9.3% vs. 11.4%). However, this benefit was accompanied by an increase in major bleeding complications (rate ratio, 1.38; 95% CI, 1.13–1.67) among those receiving dual antiplatelet therapy (3.7% vs. 2.7%; p = 0.001). There were 2,840 patients with diabetes, and the rates for the occurrence of adverse cardiovascular complications were marginally lower (OR, 0.83; 95% CI, 0.67–1.01) among those treated with aspirin plus clopidogrel than patients treated with aspirin alone (14.2% vs. 16.7%; p = 0.075).

In a substudy of the CURE trial, 2,658 patients underwent percutaneous coronary intervention on an average of 10 days following randomization [102]. Most patients (more than 80%) received open-label clopidogrel for 4 weeks. After which, patients continued on the allocated arm for a mean follow-up period of 8 months. The occurrence of cardiovascular death or MI was significantly lower (rate ratio, 0.75; 95% CI, 0.56–1.00; p = 0.047) among those treated with clopidogrel (8.0%) compared with placebo (6.0%). Of the 504 patients with diabetes, the relative reduction was substantially lower (rate ratio, 0.77; 95% CI, 0.48–1.22) for patients treated with long-term clopidogrel (16.5% vs. 12.9%). Similarly, among the 2,154 non-diabetics, the rate of cardiovascular death or recurrent MI was considerably lower (rate ratio, 0.66; 95% CI, 0.50–0.87) for patients treated with clopidogrel (7.9%) than placebo (11.7%). Whether the lack of benefit among patients with diabetes was attributed to a small number of patients or under-utilization of efficacious evidence-based medicine is unclear. Overall, only 24% of patients received GP IIb/IIIa inhibitors, and these agents were less likely administered among those randomized to the clopidogrel than placebo group (20.9% vs. 26.6%; p = 0.001).

## Beta-Blockers

Several studies have shown the efficacy of beta-blockers in improving survival following MI among patients [103], even for those with left ventricular dysfunction and heart failure [104]. Based on a meta-analysis of almost 55,000 patients, a variety of beta-blockers afforded a 23% relative reduction in long-term mortality [103]. Similarly, among 1,959 patients with left ventricular ejection fraction less than or equal to 40% with or without symptoms of heart failure, death, or MI occurred less frequently (hazard ratio, 0.71; 95% CI, 0.57–0.89) among those randomized to carvedilol (14%) than placebo (20%; p = 0.002) after a mean follow-up period of 1.3 years [104].

The benefits of beta-blockade were also observed among patients with diabetes [105,106]. After 5 years, the age-gender adjusted rate ratio for patients with diabetes receiving beta-blockers in the Augsburg MONICA (multinational monitoring of trends and determinants in cardiovascular disease) register was 0.62, comparable to those without diabetes [107]. Likewise, in the Cooperative Cardiovascular Project [108], there were 201,752 predominantly elderly patients with MI, of which 59,445 (29.5%) suffered from diabetes. The 2-year mortality was substantially lower (adjusted rate ratio, 0.64; 95% CI, 0.60–0.69) among those who received beta-blockers (17.0% vs. 26.6%). Importantly, the benefit was not accompanied by an increase in hospital admissions for diabetic complications, including hypoglycemia, hyperglycemia, or diabetic coma [109].

Even among patients receiving intensive insulin treatment, beta-blockers provided additional benefit [110]. In the subsequent multivariable analysis of the DIGAMI study, use of beta-blockers on discharge was associated with a striking reduction in 1-year mortality (rate ratio, 0.53; 95% CI, 0.36–0.78; p = 0.001), which was comparable to intensive insulin treatment (rate ratio, 0.65, 95% CI, 0.44–0.96; p = 0.03).

Despite the favorable effects of beta-blockade, patients with diabetes were less likely to receive the agent [111]. Among patients without contraindications for use of beta-blockers, the drug was not prescribed in 35% and 18% of patients with and without diabetes, respectively (p < 0.001). Likewise, in the Cooperative Cardiovascular Project [109], for 45,308 patients without contraindications for beta-blockade, administration of this agent was still lower among those with diabetes, with the rates for nondiabetics, noninsulin treated and insulin treated diabetics to be 51%, 48%, and 45%, respectively (p < 0.001). After adjusting for demographic and clinical parameters, both insulin treated (OR, 0.88; 95% CI, 0.82–0.96) and noninsulin treated (OR, 0.93; 95% CI, 0.88–0.98) patients with diabetes remained less likely to receive beta-blockers.

## Angiotensin-Converting Enzyme Inhibitors

The early use of angiotensin-converting enzyme inhibitors has been shown to improve survival over a broad range of patients with MI. A meta-analysis of 4 large trials with a total of 98,496 patients, the use of angiotensin-converting enzyme inhibitors was associated with a 7% (95% CI, 2%–11%; p < 0.004) relative reduction in 4- to 6-week mortality (7.1% vs. 7.6%) [112]. This effect translates to saving about 5 lives per 1000 patients treated. As patients with diabetes have a higher risk, the absolute benefit was even greater (17 vs. 3 lives saved per 1000 patients treated). However, the relative benefit between treated and placebo group was not statistically significant for patients with and without diabetes.

Several subgroup analyses of large clinical trials have shown that the efficacy of angiotensin-converting enzyme inhibitors among patients with diabetes and MI, and the benefit appeared to be greater than nondiabetics [113,114]. Among patients with diabetes and acute anterior MI in the Survival of Myocardial Infarction Long-term Evaluation (SMILE) study [113], the occurrence of 1-year mortality or severe congestive heart failure was significantly lower (rate ratio, 0.39; 95% CI, 0.18–84) following 6-week therapy of zofenopril compared with placebo (7.2% vs. 16.5%). Interestingly, the favorable effect was not observed among patients treated with beta-blockers. Similarly, the Gruppo Italiano per lo Studio della Sopravvivenza nell'Infarto Miocardico (GISSI-3) investigators [114] reported that patients with diabetes randomly allocated to early administration followed by 6 weeks of lisinopril was associated with a lower 6-week mortality than placebo (8.7% vs. 12.4%; OR, 0.68; 95% CI, 0.53–0.86). This translated to 37 ± 12 lives saved per 1000 treated patients. Importantly, the survival benefit in diabetics remained at 6 months (12.9% vs. 16.1%; OR, 0.77; 95% CI, 0.62–0.95). Unlike the SMILE study [113], the reduction in 6-week mortality was also observed in patients treated with intravenous beta-blockers (5.5% vs. 11.5%; p < 0.01) in the GISSI-3 trial [114].

Among patients with diabetes and left ventricular dysfunction, the use of trandolapril was associated with a significant improvement in long-term outcome [115]. Of 1,746 patients, 237 (13.6%) had diabetes in the TRACE study which enrolled patients with MI and left ventricular ejection less than or equal to 35%. After a mean follow-up of 26 months, mortality was significantly lower among those treated with trandolapril for diabetic (rate ratio, 0.64; 95% CI, 0.45–0.91) and nondiabetic (rate ratio, 0.82; 95% CI, 0.69–0.97) patients. The reduction in mortality was also observed after longer duration of follow-up. After adjusting for baseline characteristics and complications following MI, 26-month survival benefit was only observed among patients with diabetes (rate ratio, 0.72; 95% CI, 0.53–0.98). While the occurrence of severe heart failure was also reduced among patients with diabetes (rate ratio, 0.38; 95% CI, 0.21–0.67), this favorable effect was not observed among those without diabetes. Unlike the analysis for mortality, the interaction product term between use of trandolapril and diabetic status was significant for severe heart failure (p = 0.03).

In the Heart Outcomes Prevention Evaluation (HOPE) and microvascular, cardiovascular, and renal outcomes (MICRO) HOPE substudy, the benefits of long-term administration of ramipril in patients with diabetes was clearly demonstrated [116]. There were 3,577 patients with diabetes, aged older than 55 years, without clinical proteinuria, heart failure or left ventricular dysfunction, and 69% had previous cardiovascular disease. Patients assigned to ramipril was associated with a 25% relative reduction (95% CI, 12–36; p = 0.0004) in the composite endpoint of cardiovascular death, MI, or stroke after a median follow-up period of 4.5 years. Importantly, all-cause mortality (10.8% vs. 14.0%; p = 0.004), MI (10.2% vs. 12.9%; p = 0.01), stroke (4.2% vs. 6.1%; p = 0.007) occurred less frequently among those treated with ramipril, with relative reductions of 24% (95% CI, 8%–37%), 22% (95% CI, 6%–36%) and 33% (95% CI, 10%–50%), respectively.

## Angiotensin Receptor Antagonist

While angiotensin-converting enzyme inhibitors block the production of angiotensin II, there are other independent pathways that continue to generate this substance [117]. The level of angiotensin II was elevated in 50% of patients with heart failure who have been treated with angiotensin-converting enzyme inhibitors [118]. After a follow-up period of about 3 years, the occurrence of new heart failure or death was substantially higher among those with high angiotensin II levels. The identification of angiotensin II receptor, and subsequent development of pharmacological agents that specifically block its action, provides a rational basis for eliminating the adverse effects of angiotensin II [119]. However, the results of a large-scale clinical trial comparing the efficacy between captopril and losartan in high-risk patients following MI did not show that an angiotensin receptor blocker was not superior to an angiotensin converting enzyme inhibitor [120]. Of 5,477 patients with MI and clinical or echocardiographic features of left ventricular dysfunction, the mortality rates after a mean period of 2.7-year follow-up were 16% and 18% for those randomized to captopril or losartan, respectively (rate ratio, 1.13; 95% CI, 0.99–1.28; p = 0.07). The relationship was also observed among patients with diabetes. Currently, the Valsartan in Acute Myocardial Infarction (VALIANT) is being conducted [121]. The 14,500-patient trial has randomized patients to treatment with captopril, valsartan or both agents.

## Lipid Lowering Therapy

Several studies have shown the efficacy of lipid lowering therapy in preventing adverse cardiovascular events. Among patients with remote history (more than 3 months) of a coronary event, the use of statin was associated with a better outcome. In the Cholesterol and Recurrent Events (CARE) Trial [122], there were 586 (14.1%) patients with diabetes and a MI within 3–20 months. The low-density lipoprotein cholesterol levels were average (115–174 mg/dL or 2.94–4.45 mmol/L), and they were randomized to pravastatin 40 mg daily or placebo. The average follow-up duration was 5 years. In the Scandinavian Simvastatin Survival Study (4S) [123], there were 202 (4.5%) of patients with diabetes and previous MI (more than 6 months) or angina who were randomly allocated to simvastatin 20 mg daily or placebo. The serum total cholesterol for enrollment in this study was between 5.5 and 8.0 mmol/L (215 to 313 mg/dL), and the median follow-up period was 5.3 years. In the Long-Term Intervention with Pravastatin in Ischemic Disease (LIPID) [124], there were 1,077 (11.9%) patients with diabetes and previous MI or unstable angina (3–36 months) who were randomly assigned to pravastatin 40 mg daily or placebo. The serum cholesterol for enrollment in this study was between 4.0 and 7.0 mmol/L (156 and 273 mg/dL), and the median follow-up period was 6 years. In the Heart Protection Study (HPS) [125], there were 1981 (13.4%) patients with diabetes and previous coronary heart disease (including MI, coronary revascularization procedure, stable and unstable angina) who were randomized to simvastatin 40 mg daily or placebo. The mean total cholesterol and low-density–lipoprotein cholesterol levels for the entire cohort of patients with diabetes (n = 5963) were 5.7 (223) and 3.2 (125 mg/dL) mmol/L, respectively, with the mean duration of follow-up at 4.8 years.

The reduction of cholesterol was comparable between patients with and without diabetes [122–126]. Among these studies, patients with diabetes who received statins were less likely to suffer from coronary death or recurrent MI (OR, 0.73; 95% CI, 0.59–0.91), coronary revascularization procedures (OR, 0.71; 95% CI, 0.53–0.96), stroke (OR, 0.65; 95% CI, 0.46–0.92), a composite endpoint consisting of a variety of adverse cardiovascular events (OR, 0.77; 95% CI, 0.67–0.87) (Fig. 12).

Recent studies have shown the potential benefit of early administration of statins following an acute coronary event [127–129]. In the Swedish Myocardial Infarction Register [127], after adjusting for 43 covariants, including propensity score for statin use, 1-year mortality was lower for patients discharged with statin (3.7% vs. 5.0%; rate ratio, 0.75; 95% CI, 0.63–0.89; p = 0.001). Similarly, in the Myocardial Ischemia Reduction with Aggressive Cholesterol Lowering (MIRACL) study [128], high-dose (80 mg/d) atorvastatin was initiated within 24–96 hours following admission for unstable angina or non–Q-wave MI. The investigators reported a reduction in the occurrence of a composite endpoint, consisting of death, nonfatal MI, cardiac arrest, recurrent symptomatic myocardial ischemia with objective evidence and requiring emergency rehospitalization, at 16 weeks (14.8% vs. 17.4%; rate ratio, 0.84; 95% CI, 0.70–1.00; p = 0.048). By combining 2 large clinical trials on patients with unstable angina or non–ST-segment-elevation MI, there were 20,809 patients [129]. Those discharged with lipid lowering therapy were less likely to die at 6 months (1.7% vs. 3.5%; adjusted hazard ratio, 0.67; 95% CI, 0.48–0.95; p = 0.023). Among the 4,105 patients with diabetes, those receiving lipid lowering therapy also had a considerably lower 6-month mortality (2.7% vs. 5.9%; hazard ratio, 0.44; 0.29–0.68; p = 0.0002). Early administration after an acute coronary event may be particularly efficacious among patients with diabetes as endothelial function improves rapidly [130].

## EMERGING CONCEPTS

### Inflammatory Markers

Several studies have shown the role of inflammation and subsequent development of cardiovascular events in apparently healthy men [131,132] and women [133], and among patients with acute coronary syndromes [134–137]. Even among those who

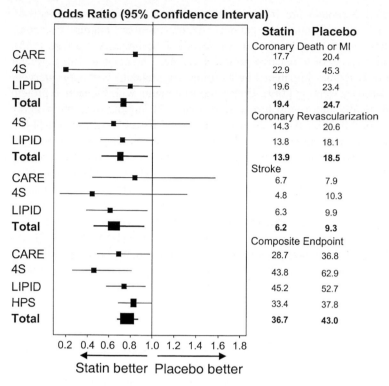

**Odds Ratio (95% Confidence Interval)**

| | Statin | Placebo |
|---|---|---|
| **Coronary Death or MI** | | |
| CARE | 17.7 | 20.4 |
| 4S | 22.9 | 45.3 |
| LIPID | 19.6 | 23.4 |
| **Total** | **19.4** | **24.7** |
| **Coronary Revascularization** | | |
| 4S | 14.3 | 20.6 |
| LIPID | 13.8 | 18.1 |
| **Total** | **13.9** | **18.5** |
| **Stroke** | | |
| CARE | 6.7 | 7.9 |
| 4S | 4.8 | 10.3 |
| LIPID | 6.3 | 9.9 |
| **Total** | **6.2** | **9.3** |
| **Composite Endpoint** | | |
| CARE | 28.7 | 36.8 |
| 4S | 43.8 | 62.9 |
| LIPID | 45.2 | 52.7 |
| HPS | 33.4 | 37.8 |
| **Total** | **36.7** | **43.0** |

0.2  0.4  0.6  0.8  1.0  1.2  1.4  1.6  1.8

Statin better   Placebo better

**Figure 12**  The effects of statins on patients with diabetes and remote history of cardio-vascular disease. Composite endpoint differed for each study: CARE = coronary death, MI and use of revascularization procedures ("expanded endpoint"); 4S = coronary death, hospital admission for a coronary event or revascularization procedure, stroke or peripheral vascular disease ("any atherosclerotic event"); LIPID = coronary death, MI and stroke ("any cardiovascular event"); HPS = coronary death, MI, stroke, coronary and non-coronary revascularization procedure ("major vascular event"). MI = myocardial infarction; CARE = Cholesterol and Recurrent Events Trial [Ref. 122]; 4S = Scandinavian Simvastatin Survival Study [123], LIPID = Long-term Intervention with Pravastatin in Ischemic Disease [Ref. 124], HPS = Heart Protection Study [Ref. 125].

received early revascularization for acute coronary syndromes, C-reactive protein was a predictor for short- and long-term mortality [138]. After adjusting for baseline characteristics, patient with levels more than 10 mg/L were 4.1 times (95% CI, 2.3–7.2) more likely to die after a mean follow-up of 20 months. Unlike what was previously thought of, the increase in inflammatory marker was unlikely to be related to infections [139]. Instead, elevated levels of C-reactive protein have been shown to enhance thrombosis, which may partly account for the adverse outcomes [140]. Furthermore, the predictive value of C-reactive protein appeared to be even stronger than low-density lipoprotein cholesterol for the first adverse cardiovascular event in asymptomatic women [141].

Diabetes has been associated with inflammation [142]. More recently, an increasing number of the components of the metabolic syndrome is correlated with raising levels of C-reactive protein [143]. Indeed, the level of C-reactive protein added prognostic information on patients with 4 or 5 components of the metabolic syndrome. Diabetes and levels of C-reactive protein are independent predictors for outcomes [136,144]. Early administration of a statin in patients with unstable angina or non Q-wave MI has been shown to reduce levels of several inflammatory markers [145].

Similarly, higher levels of C-reactive protein have been associated with a greater likelihood for adverse outcomes in patients undergoing percutaneous coronary intervention [146–148] or coronary stenting [149]. Compared to patients with C-reactive protein level less than 0.16 mg/dL, those with levels more than 1.10 mg/dL were more likely to suffer from death or MI at 30 days (adjusted OR, 3.68; 95% CI, 1.51–8.99) [146]. Statin therapy prior to the procedure may reduce adverse events [150]. Among patients with C-reactive levels more than 1.11 mg/dL, 1-year survival was lower in patients who were pre-treated with statins (5.7% vs. 14.8%; p = 0.009), with a propensity adjusted hazard of 0.44 (p = 0.039). Conversely, in another study [148], although patients who were pretreated with statin had a lower C-reactive protein level, use of statins were not associated with a reduction in ischemic complications. Despite these differences, high levels of inflammatory markers connote a poor outcome [147]. As such, part of the therapeutic strategy in improving outcomes of patients with diabetes and acute coronary syndromes may be aggressive lowering inflammation markers, particularly those scheduled for coronary revascularization procedures.

## Modulation of CD40 Ligand

Increasingly, the interaction between CD40 ligand (CD40L or CD154) with its receptor CD40 has been recognized as a key mediator in the inflammatory process of atherosclerosis [151]. The soluble form of CD40L (sCD40L) has been associated with unstable angina [152], and high levels following acute coronary syndromes have been associated with a greater likelihood for death, MI, or heart failure [153]. A novel group of insulin-sensitizing agents, thiazolidinediones, acts via the nuclear transcription factor peroxisome proliferator-activated receptor gamma (PPARγ) in controlling the expression of numerous genes. Recently, PPARγ agonists have been shown to reduce sCD40L levels in patients with diabetes in small clinical studies [154,155]. With these promising findings, larger trials are needed to determine if better outcomes are afforded by PPARγ agonists in patients with diabetes and acute coronary syndromes.

## Receptor Advanced Glycation End Products Blockade

The Receptor for Advanced Glycation End Products (RAGE) is found on macrophages, endothelial, smooth muscle, and neuronal cells and has been reported to be important in the development of atherosclerosis [156,157]. By blocking the interaction between advanced glycation end products and the receptor with a soluble form of RAGE in a diabetic apolipoprotein E-null mouse model, progression of atherosclerosis was arrested in established plaques [158]. The benefit was mediated through stabilization of vascular inflammation and collagen generation. Recently, the role of RAGE is being clarified in humans [159]. Among 60 patients who underwent carotid endarterectomy for asymptomatic carotid artery stenosis, 30 of them had diabetes. The investigators found that RAGE was found in higher amounts in diabetic plaques which correlated with a more inflammatory infiltrate and a greater expression of cyclooxygenase-2, microsomal prostaglandin synthetase type 1, and matrix metalloproteinases. Importantly, macrophages at the shoulder of the plaque contained the most RAGE, cyclooxygenase-2 and microsomal prostaglandin synthetase type 1. This distribution may have predisposed plaques to instability, and suggested that stringent glycemic control may prevent acute cardiovascular events. The current glucose paradox, whereby an intensive control of diabetes did not result in a reduction of macrovascular complications [160–162], could be attributed to a variety of reasons, including insufficient statistical power, relatively short study duration, adverse cardiovascular effects of sulphonylureas, and the control of other coronary risk factors.

## Drug-eluting Stents

The landscape of interventional cardiology has been revolutionized with the advent of drug-eluting stents. Both the sirolimus and paclitaxel eluting stents have been shown to be efficacious in preventing restenosis following an elective procedure [163–166]. Importantly, the benefits were extended to patients with diabetes. Indeed, the angiographic restenosis rates were substantially lower among patients treated with drug-eluting stents [166–169] (Fig. 13). Correspondingly, the repeat vessel revascularization rate was also lower. However, the value of using these devices on patients with acute coronary syndromes is unclear, especially with the concern that these patients already have endothelial disruption. Drug-eluting stents may impair healing and hence predispose to early thrombotic events. Recently, the Rapamycin-Eluting Stent Evaluated At Rotterdam Cardiology Hospital (RESEARCH) Registry noted that the early outcomes of implanting sirolimus-eluting stents in patients with acute coronary syndrome was comparable to stainless steel stent [169]. Whether this approach remains effective in a large clinical trial, and its relevance for patients with diabetes remain uncertain.

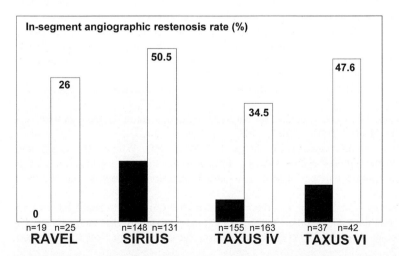

**Figure 13** In-segment Angiographic Rates for Patients with Diabetes Receiving Drug-eluting or Stainless Steel Coronary Stents. RAVEL = Randomized Double-Blind Study with the Sirolimus-Eluting Bx Velocity™ Balloon-Expandable Stent in the Treatment of Patients with De Novo Native Coronary Lesions Study (Ref. 166); SIRIUS = Sirolimus-Coated Bx Velocity™ Balloon-Expandable Stent in the Treatment of Patients with De Novo Coronary Artery Lesions (Ref. 167); TAXUS IV = The Pivotal, Prospective, Randomized Trial of the Slow-rate Release Polymer-based Paclitaxel-Eluting TAXUS™ Stent [Ref. 165]. TAXUS VI = A Randomized Trial of Moderate Rate Release Polymer-Based Paclitaxel-Eluting TAXUS™ Stent for Treatment of Longer Lesions [166]

## CONCLUSION

Despite significant advances in therapeutic modalities for patients with diabetes and acute coronary syndromes, morbidity and mortality remain heightened. Importantly, most of the effective approaches conferred an even greater benefit among patients with diabetes compared with nondiabetics. While the discovery of novel treatment strategies for this group of high-risk patients continues, the lack of adoption of efficacious evidence-based therapies is of great concern. Likely, psychosocial and socioeconomic factors, behavioral patterns of physicians and patients, together with a complex interplay of several other issues could have led to the failure in the delivery of optimal care. Nonetheless, patients with diabetes and acute coronary syndromes should be aggressively treated based on current treatment guidelines as we anticipate tomorrow's innovations to further reduce the burden of cardiovascular diseases.

## REFERENCES

1.  Stamler J, Vaccaro O, Neaton JD, Wentworth D. Diabetes, other risk factors, and 12-yr cardiovascular mortality for men screened in the Multiple Risk Factor Intervention Trial. Diabetes Care 1993;16:434–444.
2.  Centers for Disease Control and Prevention. National diabetes fact sheet: general information and national estimates on diabetes in the United States, 2000. Atlanta. GA: U.S. Department of Health and Human Services, Centers for Disease Control and Prevention, 2002.
3.  American Diabetes Association. Economic costs of diabetes n the U.S. in 2002. Diabetes Care 2003;26:917–932.
4.  Haffner SM, Lehto S, Rönnemaa T, Pyörälä K, Laakso M. Mortality from coronary heart disease in subjects with type 2 diabetes and in nondiabetic subjects with and without prior myocardial infarction. N Engl J Med 1998;330:229–234.
5.  Becker A, Bos G, de Vegt F, Kostense PJ, Dekker JM, Nijpels G, Heine RJ, Bouter LM, Stehouwer CDA. Cardiovascular events in type 2 diabetes: comparison in non-diabetic individuals without and with prior cardiovascular disease. 10-year follow-up of the Hoorn Study. Eur Heart J 2003;24:1406–1413.
6.  Mak K-H, Haffner SM. Diabetes abolishes the gender gap in coronary heart disease. Eur Heart J 2003;24:1385–1386.
7.  Mak K-H, Faxon DP. Clinical studies on coronary revascularization in patients with type 2 diabetes. Eur Heart J 2003;24:1087–1103.
8.  Mak KH, Moliterno DJ, Granger CB, Miller DP, White HD, Wilcox RG, Califf RM, Topol EJ. for the GUSTO-I Investigators. Influence of diabetes mellitus on clinical outcome in the thrombolytic era of acute myocardial infarction. J Am Coll Cardiol 1997; 30:171–179.
9.  Hasdai D, Granger CB, Srivatsa S, Criger DA, Ellis SG, Califf RM, Topol EJ, Holmes DR. Diabetes mellitus and outcome after primary coronary angioplasty for acute myocardial infarction: lessons from the GUSTO-IIb angioplasty substudy. J Am Coll Cardiol 2000; 35:1502–1512.
10. Malmberg K, Yusuf S, Gerstein HC, Brown J, Zhao F, Hunt D, Piegas L, Calvin J, Keltai M, Budaj A. for OASIS Registry Investigators. Impact of diabetes on long-term prognosis in patients with unstable angina and non-Q-wave myocardial infarction. Results of the OASIS (Organization to Assess Strategies for Ischemic Syndromes) Registry. Circulation 2000;102:1014–1019.
11. McGuire DK, Emanuelsson H, Granger CB, Ohman EM, Moliterno DJ, White HD, Ardissino D, Box JW, Califf RM, Topol EJ. for the GUSTO-IIb Investigators. Influence of diabetes mellitus on clinical outcomes across the spectrum of acute coronary syndromes. Findings from the GUSTO-IIb Study. Eur Heart J 2000;21:1750–1758.

12. Roffi M, Moliterno DJ, Meier B, Powers ER, Grines CL, DiBattiste PM, Herrmann HC, Bertrand M, Harris KE, Demopoulos LA, Topol EJ. for the TARGET Investigators. Impact of different platelet glycoprotein IIb/IIIa receptor inhibitors among diabetic patients undergoing percutaneous coronary intervention. Do Tirofiban and ReoPro Give Similar Efficacy Outcomes Trial (TARGET) 1-year follow-up. Circulation 2002;105:2730–2736.

13. Czyzk A, Krolewski AS, Szablowska S, Alot A, Kopczynski J. Clinical course of myocardial infarction among diabetic patients. Diabetes Care 1980;3:526–529.

14. Martin CA, Thompson PL, Armstrong BK, Hobbs MS, de Klerk N. Long-term prognosis after recovery from myocardial infarction: a nine year follow-up of the Perth Coronary Register. Circulation 1983;68:961–969.

15. Smith JW, Marcus FI, Serokman R. Prognosis of patients with diabetes mellitus after acute myocardial infarction. Am J Cardiol 1984;54:718–721.

16. Rytter L, Troelsen S, Beck-Nielsen H. Prevalence and mortality of acute myocardial infarction in patients with diabetes. Diabetes Care 1985;8:230–234.

17. Mølstad P, Nustad M. Acute myocardial infarction in diabetic patients. Acta Med Scand 1987;222:433–437.

18. Malmberg K, Rydén L. Myocardial infarction in patients with diabetes mellitus. Eur Heart J 1988;9:259–264.

19. Herlitz J, Malmberg K, Karlson BW, Rydén L, Hjalmarson Å. Mortality and morbidity during a five-year follow-up of diabetics with myocardial infarction. Acta Med Scand 1988;224:31–38.

20. GISSI. Effectiveness of intravenous thrombolytic treatment in acute myocardial infarction. Lancet 1986;1:397–402.

21. ISIS-2 (Second International Study on Infarct Survival) Collaborative Group. Randomised trial of intravenous streptokinase, oral aspirin, both, or neither among 17,187 cases of suspected acute myocardial infarction; ISIS-2. Lancet 1988;2:349–360.

22. Lynch M, Gammage MD, Lamb P, Nattrass M, Pentecost BL. Acute myocardial infarction in diabetic patients in the thrombolytic era. Diabet Med 1994;11:162–165.

23. Fibrinolytic Therapy Trialists' (FTT) Collaborative Group. Indications for fibrinolytic therapy in suspected acute myocardial infarction: collobarotive overview of early mortality and major morbidity results from all randomised trials of more than 1000 patients. Lancet 1994;343:311–322.

24. Mak KH, Topol EJ. Emerging concepts in the management of acute myocardial infarction in patients with acute myocardial infarction. J Am Coll Cardiol 2000;35:563–568.

25. Pfeffer MA, Moye LA, Braunwald E, Basta L, Brown EJ, Cuddy TE, Dagenais GR, Flaker GC, Geltman EM, Gersh BJ, Goldman S, Lamas GA, Packer M, Rouleau JL, Rutherford JD, Steingart RM, Werheimer JH. for the SAVE Investigators. Selection bias in the use of thrombolytic therapy in acute myocardial infarction. JAMA 1991;266: 528–532.

26. Vaur L, Danchin N, Hanania G, Cambou J, Lablanche J, Blanchard D, Clerson P, Gueret P. Management and short-term outcome of diabetic patients hospitalized for acute myocardial infarction: results of a nationwide French survey. Diabetes Metab 2003;29: 241–249.

27. The GISSI Avoidable Delay Study Group. Epidemiology of avoidable delay in the care of patients with acute myocardial infarction in Italy. A GISSI-generated study. Arch Intern Med 1995;155:1481–1488.

28. Newby LK, Rutsch WR, Califf RM, Simoons ML, Aylward PE, Armstrong PW, Woodlief LH, Lee KL, Topol EJ, Van de Werf F. Time from symptom onset to treatment and outcomes after thrombolytic therapy. GUSTO-1 Investigators. J Am Coll Cardiol 1996; 27:1646–1655.

29. Mahaffey KW, Granger CB, Toth CA, White HD, Stebbins AL, Barbash GI, Vahanian A, Topol EJ, Califf RM. for the GUSTO-I Investigators. Diabetic retinopathy should not be a contraindication to thrombolytic therapy for acute myocardial infarction: review of ocular hemorrhage incidence and location in the GUSTO-I trial. J Am Coll Cardiol 1997; 30:1606–1610.

30. Norhammar A, Malmberg K, Rydén L, Tornvall P, Stenestrand U, Wallentin L. for the Register of Information and Knowledge about Swedish Heart Intensive Care Admissions (RIKS-HIA). Under utilisation of evidence-based treatment partially explains for the unfavourable prognosis in diabetic patients with acute myocardial infarction. Eur Heart J 2003;24:838–844.

31. Baigent C, Collins R, Appleby P, Parish S, Sleight P, Peto R. on behalf of the ISIS-2 (Second International Study of Infarct Survival) Collaborative Group. ISIS-2: 10 year survival among patients with suspected acute myocardial infarction in randomised comparision of intravenous streptokinase, oral aspirin, both, or neither. BMJ 1998;316:1337–1343.

32. Melchior T, Køber L, Madsen CR, Seibæk M, Jensen GVH, Hildebrandt P, Torp-Pedersen C. on behalf of the TRACE Study Group. Acclerating impact of diabetes mellitus on mortality in the yearts following an acute myocardial infarction. Eur Heart J 1999;20: 973–978.

33. The PARAGON Investigators. International, randomized, controlled trial of lamifiban (a platelet glycoprotein IIb/IIIa inhibitor), heparin, or both in unstable angina. The PARAGON Investigators. Platelet IIb/IIIa Antagonism for the Reduction of Acute coronary syndrome events in a Global Organization Network. Circulation 1998;97:2386–2395.

34. The PURSUIT Investigators. Inhibition of platelet glycoprotein IIb/IIIa with eptifibatide in patients with acute coronary syndromes. The PURSUIT Trial Investigators. Platelet Glycoprotein IIb/IIIa in Unstable Angina: Receptor Suppression Using Integrilin Therapy. N Engl J Med 1998;339:436–443.

35. Moliterno DJ. Patient-specific dosing of IIb/IIIa antagonists during acute coronary syndromes: rationale and design of the PARAGON B study. The PARAGON B International Steering Committee. Am Heart J 2000;139:563–566.

36. Simoons ML. Effect of glycoprotein IIb/IIIa receptor blocker abciximab on outcome in patients with acute coronary syndromes without early coronary revascularisation: the GUSTO IV-ACS randomised trial. Lancet 2001;357:1915–1924.

37. Granger CB, Califf RM, Young S, Candela R, Samaha J, Worley S, Kereiakes DJ, Topol EJ. and the Thrombolysis and Angioplasty in Myocardial Infarction (TAMI) Study Group. Outcome of patients with diabetes mellitus and acute myocardial infarction treated with thrombolytic agents. J Am Coll Cardiol 1993;21:920–5.

38. Barbash GI, White HD, Modan M, Van de Werf F. and the Investigators of the International Tissue Plasminogen/Streptokinase Mortality Trial. Significance of diabetes mellitus in patients with acute myocardial infarction receiving thrombolytic agents. J Am Coll Cardiol 1993;22:707–713.

39. Zuanetti G, Latini R, Maggioni AP, Santoro L, Franzosi MG. on behalf of GISSI-2 Investigators. Influence of diabetes on mortality in acute myocardial infarction: data from the GISSI-2 study. J Am Coll Cardiol 1993;22:1788–1794.

40. Woodfield SL, Lundergan CF, Reiner JS, Greenhouse SW, Thomson MA, Rohrbeck SC, Deychak Y, Simoons ML, Califf RM, Topol EJ, Ross AM. for the GUSTO-I Investigators. Angiographic findings and outcome in diabetic opatients treated with thrombolytic therapy for myocardial infarction: the GUSTO-I experience. J Am Coll Cardiol 1996;28:1661–1669.

41. Werner GS, Richartz BM, Heinke S, Ferrari M, Figulla HR. Impaired acute collateral recruitment as a possible mechanism for increased cardiac adverse events in patients with diabetes mellitus. Eur Heart J 2003;24:1134–1142.

42. Keeley EC, Boura JA, Grines CL. Primary angioplasty versus intravenous thrombolytic therapy for acute myocardial infarction. Lancet 2003;361:13–20.

43. Hsu LF, Mak KH, Lau KW, Sim LL, Chan C, Koh TH, Chuah SC, Kam R, Ding ZP, Teo WS, Lim YL. Clinical outcomes of patients with diabetes mellitus and acute myocardial infarction treated with primary angioplasty or fibrinolysis. Heart 2002;88:260–265.

44. Bonnefoy E, Leborgne L, Dupouy P, Chabaud S, McFadden E, Steg G, Touboul P. Evidence that primary angioplasty is more effective than prehospital fibrinolysis in diabetics with acute myocardial infarction. A CAPTIM substudy [abstract]. Circulation 2002;106: II–698.

45. Silva JA, Ramee SR, White CJ, Collins TJ, Jenkins JS, Nunez E, Zhang S, Jain SP. Primary stenting in acute myocardial infarction: influence of diabetes mellitus in angiographic results and clinical outcome. Am Heart J 1999;138:446–455.

46. Harjai KJ, Stone GW, Boura J, Mattos L, Chandra H, Cox D, Grines L, O'Neill W, Grines C. Primary Angioplasty in Myocardial Infarction Investigators. Comparison of outcomes of diabetic and nondiabetic patients undergoing primary angioplasty for acute myocardial infarction. Am J Cardiol 2003;91:1041–1045.

47. Luca G, Suryapranata H, Zijlstra F, van't Hof AWJ, Hoorntje JCA, Gosselink ATM, Dambrink J-H, de Boer M-J. on behalf of the ZWOLLE Myocardial Infarction Study Group. Symptom-onset-to-balloon time and mortality in patients with acute myocardial infarction treated by primary angioplasty. J Am Coll Cardiol 2003;42:991–997.

48. Anderson HV, Cannon CP, Stone PH, Williams DO, McCabe CH, Knatterud GL, Thompson B, Willerson JT, Braunwald E. for the TIMI IIIB Investigators. One-year results of the Thrombolysis in Myocardial Infarction (TIMI) IIIB clinical trial. A randomized comparison of tissue-type plasminogen activator versus placebo and early invasive versus early conservative strategies in unstable angina and non-Q wave myocardial infarction. J Am Coll Cardiol 1995;26:1643–1650.

49. Boden WE, O'Rourke RA, Crawford MH, Blaustein AS, Deedwania PC, Zoble RG, Wexler LF, Kleiger RE, Pepine CJ, Ferry DR, Chow BK, Lavori PW. Outcomes in patients with acute non-Q-wave myocardial infarction randomly assigned to an invasive as compared with a conservative management strategy. Veterans Affairs Non-Q-Wave Infarction Strategies in Hospital (VANQWISH) Trial Investigators. N Engl J Med 1998;338:1785–1792.

50. Wallentin L, Lagerqvist B, Husted S, Kontny F, Stähle E, Swahn E. for the FRSIC II Investigators. Outcome at 1 year after an invasive compared with a non-invasive strategy in unstable coronary-artery disease: the FRISC II invasive randomised trial. Lancet 2000;356:9–16.

51. Cannon CP, Weintraub WS, Demopoulos LA, Vicari R, Frey MJ, Lakkis N, Neumann F-J, Robertson DH, DeLucca PT, DiBattiste PM, Gibson CM, Braunwald E. for the TACTICS-Thrombolysis in Myocardial Infarction 18 Investigators. Comparison of early invasive and conservative strategies in patients with unstable coronary syndromes treated with the glycoprotein IIb/IIIa inhibitor tirofiban. N Engl J Med 2001;344:1879–1887.

52. Spacek R, Widimsky P, Straka Z, Jiresova E, Dvorak J, Polasek R, Karel I, Jirmar R, Lisa L, Budesinsky T, Malek F, Stanka P. Value of first day angiography/angioplasty in evolving non-ST segment elevation myocardial infarction: an open multicenter randomized trial. The VINO Study. Eur Heart J 2002;23:230–238.

53. Fox KA, Poole-Wilson PA, Henderson RA, Clayton TC, Chamberlain DA, Shaw TR, Wheatley DJ, Pocock SJ. Randomized Intervention Trial of unstable Angina Investigators. Interventional versus conservative treatment for patients with unstable angina or non-ST-elevation myocardial infarction: the British Heart Foundation RITA 3 randomised trial. Randomized Intervention Trial of unstable Angina. Lancet 2002;360:743–751.

54. Ronner E, Boersma E, Laarman G-J, Somsen GA, Harrington RA, Deckers JW, Topol EJ, Califf RM, Simoons ML. Early angioplasty in acute coronary syndromes without persistent ST-segment elevation improves outcome but increases the need for six-month repeat revascularization. An analysis of the PURSUIT Trial. J Am Coll Cardiol 2002;39:1924–1929.

55. Mueller C, Neumann F-J, Roskamm H, Perruchoud AP, Buettner HJ. Impact of diabetes mellitus on long-term outcomes after non-ST-elevation acute coronary syndromes treated with very early revascularization [abstract]. J Am Coll Cardiol 2003;41:350A.

56. Neumann F-J, Kastrati A, Pogatsa-Murray G, Mehilli J, Bollwin H, Bestehorn H-P, Schimitt C, Seyfarth M, Dirschinger J, Schömig A. Evaluation of prolonged antithrombotic pretreatment ("Cooling-Off" strategy) before intervention in patients with unstable coronary syndromes. A randomized controlled trial. JAMA 2003;290:1593–1599.

57. van't Hof AWJ, de Vries ST, Dambrink J-HE, Miedema K, Suryapranata H, Hoorntje JCA, Gosselink M, Zijlstra F, de Boer M-J. A comparison of two invasive strategies in

patients with non-ST elevation acute coronary syndromes: results of the Early or Late Intervention in unStable Angina (ELISA) pilot study. 2b/3a upstream therapy and acute coronary syndromes. Eur Heart J 2003;24:1401–1405.

58. Topol EJ. Toward a new frontier in myocardial reperfusion therapy. Emerging platelet preeminence. Circulation 1998;97:211–218.

59. Coller BS. A new murine monoclonal antibody reports an activation-dependent change in the conformation and/or microenvironment of the platelet glycoprotein IIb/IIIa complex. J Clin Invest 1985;76:101–108.

60. Kong DF, Califf RM, Miller DP, Moliterno DJ, White HD, Harrington RA, Tcheng JE, Lincoff AM, Hasselblad V, Topol EJ. Clinical outcomes of therapeutic agents that block the platelet glycoprotein IIb/IIIa integrin in ischemic heart disease. Circulation 1998;98: 2829–2835.

61. Ohman EM, Kleiman NS, Gacioch G, Worley SJ, Navetta FI, Talley JD, Anderson HV, Ellis SG, Cohen MD, Spriggs D, Miller M, Kereiakes D, Yakubov S, Kitt MM, Sigmon KN, Califf RM, Krucoff MW, Topol EJ. Combined accelerated tissue-plasminogen activator and platelet glycoprotein IIb/IIIa integrin receptor blockade with Integrilin in acute myocardial infarction. Results of a randomized, placebo-controlled, dose-ranging trial. IMPACT-AMI Investigators. Circulation 1997;95:846–854.

62. Brener SJ, Zeymer U, Adgey AA, Vrobel TR, Ellis SG, Neuhaus KL, Juran N, Ivanc TB, Ohman EM, Strony J, Kitt M, Topol EJ. Eptifibatide and low-dose tissue plasminogen activator in acute myocardial infarction: the integrilin and low-dose thrombolysis in acute myocardial infarction (INTRO AMI) trial. J Am Coll Cardiol 2002;39:377–386.

63. Antman EM, Giugliano RP, Gibson CM, McCabe CH, Coussement P, Kleiman NS, Vahanian A, Adgey AAJ, Menown I, Rupprecht H-J, Van der Wieken R, Ducas J, Scherer J, Anderson K, Van de Werf F, Braunwald E. for the TIMI 14 Investigators. Abciximab facilitates the rate and extent of thrombolysis: results of the Thrombolysis In Myocardial Infarction (TIMI) 14 Trial. Circulation 1999;99:2720–2732.

64. Strategies for Patency Enhancement in the Emergency Department (SPEED) Group. Trial of Abciximab With and Without Low-Dose Reteplase for Acute Myocardial Infarction. Circulation 2000;101:2788–2794.

65. The Assessment of the Safety and Efficacy of a New Thrombolytic Regimen (ASSENT)-3 Investigators. Efficacy and safety of tenecteplase in combination with enoxaparin, abciximab, or unfractionated heparin: the ASSENT-3 randomised trial in acute myocardial infarction. Lancet 2001;358:605–613.

66. The GUSTO V Investigators. Reperfusion therapy for acute myocardial infarction with fibrinolytic therapy or combination reduced fibrinolytic therapy and platelet glycoprotein IIb/IIIa inhibition: the GUSTO V randomised trial. Lancet 2001;357:1905–1914.

67. Brener SJ, Barr LA, Burchenal JE, Katz S, George BS, Jones AA, Cohen ED, Gainey PC, White HJ, Cheek HB, Moses JW, Moliterno DJ, Effron MB, Topol EJ. Randomized, placebo-controlled trial of platelet glycoprotein IIb/IIIa blockade with primary angioplasty for acute myocardial infarction. ReoPro and Primary PTCA Organization and Randomized Trial (RAPPORT) Investigators. Circulation 1998;98:734–741.

68. Neumann F-J, Kastrati A, Schmitt C, Blasini R, Hadamitzky M, Mehilli J, Gawaz M, Schleef M, Seyfarth M, Dirschinger J, Schomig A. Effect of glycoprotein IIb/IIIa receptor blockade with abciximab on clinical and angiographic restenosis rate after the placement of coronary stents following acute myocardial infarction. J Am Coll Cardiol 2000;35: 915–921.

69. Montalescot G, Barragan P, Wittenberg O, Ecollan P, Elhadad S, Villain P, Boulenc J-M, Morice M-C, Maillard L, Choussat R, Pinton P. for the ADMIRAL Investigators. Platelet glycoprotein IIb/IIIa inhibition with coronary stenting for acute myocardial infarction. N Engl J Med 2001;344:1895–1903.

70. Stone GW, Grines CL, Cox DA, Garcia E, Tcheng JE, Griffin JJ, Guagliumi G, Stuckey T, Turco M, Carroll JD, Rutherford BD, Lanksy AJ. for the Controlled Abciximab and Device Investigation to Lower Late Angioplasty Complications (CADILLAC) Investigators.

Comparison of angioplasty with stenting, with or without abciximab, in acute myocardial infarction. N Engl J Med 2002;346:957–966.

71. Neumann F-J, Blasini R, Schmitt C, Alt E, Dirschinger J, Gawaz M, Kastrati A, Schömig A. Effect of glycoprotein IIb/IIIa receptor blockade on recovery of coronary flow and left ventricular function after the placement of coronary-artery stents in acute myocardial infarction. Circulation 1998;98:2695–2701.

72. Eisenberg MJ, JAMAl S. Glycoprotein IIb/IIIa inhibition in the setting of acute ST-segment elevation myocardial infarction. J Am Coll Cardiol 2003;42:1–6.

73. Bhatt DL, Marso SP, Lincoff AM, Wolski KE, Ellis SG, Topol EJ. Abciximab reduces mortality in diabetics following percutaneous coronary intervention. J Am Coll Cardiol 2000;35:922–928.

74. Boersma E, Harrington RA, Moliterno DJ, White H, Théroux P, Van de Werf F, de Torbal A, Armstrong PW, Wallentin LC, Wilcox RG, Simes J, Califf RM, Topol EJ. Platelet glycoprotein IIb/IIIa inhibitors in acute coronary syndromes: a meta-analysis of all major randomised clinical trials. Lancet 2002;359:189–198.

75. Roffi M, Chew DP, Mukherjee D, Bhatt DL, White JA, Heeschen C, Hamm CW, Moliterno DJ, Califf RM, White HD, Kleiman NS, Théroux P, Topol EJ. Platelet glycoprotein IIb/IIIa inhibitors reduce mortality in diabetic patients with non-ST-segment-elevation acute coronary syndromes. Circulation 2001;104:2767–2771.

76. Marzilli M, Sambuceti G, Testa R, Fedele S. Platelet glycoprotein IIb/IIIa receptor blockade and coronary resistance in unstable angina. J Am Coll Cardiol 2002;40:2102–2109.

77. Peterson ED, Pollack CV, Roe MT, Parsons LS, Littrell KA, Canto JG, Barron HV. for the National Registry of Myocardial Infarction (NRMI) 4. Early use of glycoprotein IIb/IIIa inhibition in non-ST-segment acute myocardial infarction: observations from the National Registry of Myocardial Infarction 4. J Am Coll Cardiol 2003;42:45–53.

78. Gibson CM, Cannon CP, Murphy SA, Ryan RA, Mesley R, Marble SJ, McCabe CH, Van de Werf F, Braunwald E. for the TIMI (Thrombolysis In Myocardial Infarction) Study Group. Relationship of TIMI myocardial perfusion grade to mortality after administration of thrombolytic drugs. Circulation 2000;101:125–130.

79. van't Hof AWJ, Liem A, Suryapranata H, Hoorntje JCA, de Boer M-J, Zijlstra F. on behalf of the Zwolle Myocardial Infarction Study Group. Angiographic assessment of myocardial reperfusion in patients treated with primary angioplasty for acute myocardial infarction. Myocardial Blush Grade. Circulation 1999;97:2302–2306.

80. Stone GW, Peterson MA, Lansky AJ, Dangas G, Mehran R, Leon MB. Impact of normalized myocardial perfusion after successful angioplasty in acute myocardial infarction. J Am Coll Cardiol 2002;39:591–599.

81. Henriques JPS, Zijlstra F, Ottervanger JP, de Boer M-J, van't Hof AWJ, Hoorntje JCA, Suryapranata H. Incidence and clinical significance of distal embolization during primary angioplasty for acute myocardial infarction. Eur Heart J 2002;23:1112–1117.

82. Di Carli MF, Janisse J, Grunberger G, Ager J. Role of chronic hyperglycemia in the pathogenesis of coronary microvascular dysfunction in diabetes. J Am Coll Cardiol 2003;41:1387–1393.

83. Kotani J, Nanto S, Mintz GS, Kitakaze M, Ohara T, Morozumi T, Nagata S, Hori M. Plaque gruel of atheromatous coronary lesion may contribute to the no-reflow phenomenon in patients with acute coronary syndrome. Circulation 2002;106:1672–1677.

84. Matetzky S, Freimark D, Chouraqui P, Novikov I, Agranat O, Rabinowitz B, Kaplinsky E, Hod H. The distinction between coronary and myocardial reperfusion after thrombolytic therapy by clinical markers of reperfusion. J Am Coll Cardiol 1998;32:1326–1330.

85. Angeja BG, Gunda M, Murphy SA, Sobel BE, Rundle AC, Syed M, Asfour A, Borzak S, Gourlay SG, Barron HV, Gibbons RJ, Gibson CM. for the LIMIT AMI Investigators. TIMI myocardial perfusion grade and ST segment resolution: association with infarct size as assessed by single photon emission computed tomography imaging. Circulation 2002;105:282–285.

86. Feldman LJ, Coste P, Furber A, Dupouy P, Slama MS, Monassier JP, Tron C, Lafont A, Faraggi M, Le Guludec D, Dubois-Rande JL, Steg PG. FRench Optimal STenting (FROST)-

2 Investigators. Incomplete resolution of ST-segment elevation is a marker of transient microcirculatory dysfunction after stenting for acute myocardial infarction. Circulation 2003;107: 2684–2689.

87. Angeja BG, de Lemos J, Murphy SA, Marble SJ, Antman EM, Cannon CP, Braunwald E, Gibson CM. for the TIMI Study Group. Impact of diabetes mellitus on epicardial and microvascular flow after fibrinolytic therapy. Am Heart J 2002;144:649–656.

88. Iwakura K, Ito H, Kawano S, Shintani Y, Yamamoto K, Kato A, Ikushima M, Tanaka K, Kitakaze M, Hori M, Higashino Y, Fujii K. Predictive factors for development of the no-reflow phenomenon in patients with reperfused anterior wall acute myocardial infarction. J Am Coll Cardiol 1999;38:472–477.

89. Iwakura K, Ito H, Ikushima M, Kawano S, Okamura A, Asano K, Kuroda T, Tanaka K, Masuyama T, Hori M, Fujii K. Association between hyperglycemia and the no-reflow phenomenon in patients with acute myocardial infarction. J Am Coll Cardiol 2003;41:1–7.

90. Mak K-H, Phay C, Kwok V, Wong A, Chan C, Koh T. Distal protection device is superior to glycoprotein IIb /IIIa blockade in restoring myocardial perfusion during percutaneous coronary intervention for acute myocardial infarction [abstract]. Circulation 2002;108: IV–674.

91. Depre C, Vanoverschelde J-LJ, Taegtmeyer H. Glucose for the heart. Circulation 1999;99: 578–588.

92. Sodi-Pallares D, Testelli MR, Fishleder BL. Effects of intravenous infusion of a potassium-glucose-insulin solution on electrocardiographic signs of myocardial infarction. Am J Cardiol 1962;9:166–181.

93. Fath-Ordoubadi F, Keatt KJ. Glucose-insulin-potassium therapy for treatment of acute myocardial infarction. An overview of randomized placebo-controlled trials. Circulation 1997; 96:1152–1156.

94. Ceremuzynski L, Budaj A, Czepiel A, Burzykowski T, Achremczyk P, Smielak-Korombel W, Maciejewicz J, Dziubinska J, Nartowicz E, Kawka-Urbanek T, Piotrowski W, Hanzlik J, Cieslinski A, Kawecka-Jaszcz K, Gessek J, Wrabec K. Low-dose glucose-insulin-potassium is ineffective in acute myocardial infarction: results of a randomized multicenter Pol-GIK trial. Cardiovasc Drugs Ther 1999;13:191–200.

95. van der Horst ICC, Zijlstra F, van't Hof AWJ, Doggen CJM, de Boer M-J, Suryapranata H, Hoorntje JCA, Dambrink J-HE, Gans ROB, Bilo HJG. on behalf of the Zwolle Infarct Study Group. Glucose-insulin-potassium infusion in patients treated with primary angioplasty for acute myocardial infarction. The Glucose-Insulin-Potassium Study: a randomized trial. J Am Coll Cardiol 2003;42:784–791.

96. Apstein CS. The benefits of glucose-insulin-potassium for acute myocardial infarction (and some concerns). J Am Coll Cardiol 2003;42:792–795.

97. Malmberg K, Ryden L, Efendic S, Herlitz J, Nicol P, Waldenstrom A, Wedel H, Welin L. Randomized trial of insulin-glucose infusion followed by subcutaneous insulin treatment in diabetic patients with acute myocardial infarction (DIGAMI study): effects on mortality at 1 year. J Am Coll Cardiol 1995;26:57–65.

98. Antithrombotic Trialists' Collaboration. Collaborative meta-analysis of randomised trials of antiplatelet therapy for prevention of death, myocardial infarction, and stroke in high risk patients. Br Med J 2002;324:71–86.

99. CAPRIE Steering Committee. A randomised, blinded, trial of clopidogrel versus aspirin in patients at risk of ischemic events (CAPRIE). Lancet 1996;348:1329–1339.

100. Bhatt DL, Marso SP, Hirsch AT, Ringleb PA, Hacke W, Topol EJ. Amplified benefit of clopidogrel versus aspirin in patients with diabetes mellitus. Am J Cardiol 2002;90:625–628.

101. The Clopidogrel in Unstable Angina to Prevent Recurrent Events Trial Investigators. Effects of clopidogrel in addition to aspirin in patients with acute coronary syndromes without ST-segment elevation. N Engl J Med 2001;345:494–502.

102. Mehta SR, Yusuf S, Peters RJG, Bertrand ME, Lewis BS, Natarajan MK, Malmberg K, Rupprecht H-J, Zhao F, Chrolavicius S, Copland I, Fox KAA. for the Clopidogrel in Unstable angina to prevent Recurrent Events trial (CURE) Investigators. Effects of pretreatment with

clopidogrel and aspirin followed by long-term therapy in patients undergoing percutaneous coronary intervention: the PCI-CURE study. Lancet 2001;358:527–533.

103. Freemantle N, Cleland J, Young P, Mason J, Harrison J. Blockade after myocardial infarction: systematic review and meta regression analysis. Br Med J 1999;318:1730–1737.

104. The CAPRICORN Investigators. Effect of carvedilol on outcome after myocardial infarction in patients with left-ventricular dysfunction: the CAPRICORN randomised trial. Lancet 2001; 357:385–1392.

105. Malmberg K, Herlitz J, Hjalmarson A, Rydén L. Effects of metoprolol on mortality and late infarction in diabetics with suspected acute myocardial infarction: retrospective data from two large studies. Eur Heart J 1989;10:423–428.

106. Kjekshus J, Gilpin E, Cali G, Blackey AR, Henning H, Ross J. Diabetic patients and beta-blockers after acute myocardial infarction. Eur Heart J 1990;11:43–50.

107. Lowel H, Koenig W, Engel S, Hormann A, Keil U. The impact of diabetes mellitus on survival after myocardial infarction: can it be modified by drug treatment? Results of a population-based myocardial infarction register follow-up study. Diabetologia 2000;43: 218–226.

108. Gottlieb SS, McCarter RJ, Vogel RA. Effect of beta-blockade on mortality among high-risk and low-risk patients after myocardial infarction. N Engl J Med 1998;339:489–497.

109. Chen J, Marciniak TA, Radford MJ, Wang Y, Krumholz HM. Beta-blocker therapy for secondary prevention of myocardial infarction in elderly diabetic patients. Results from the National Cooperative Cardiovascular Project. J Am Coll Cardiol 1999;34:1388–1394.

110. Malmberg K, Rydén L, Hamsten A, Herlitz J, Waldenström A, Wedel H. Mortality prediction in diabetic patients with myocardial infarction: experiences from the DIGAMI study. Cardiovasc Res 1997;34:248–253.

111. Younis N, Burnham P, Patwala A, Weston PJ, Vora JP. Beta blocker prescribing differences in patients with and without diabetes following a first myocardial infarction. Diabet Med 2001;18:159–161.

112. ACE Inhibitor Myocardial Infarction Collaborative Group. Indications for ACE inhibitors in the early treatment of acute myocardial infarction: systematic overview of individual data from 100,000 patients in randomized trials. Circulation 1998;97:2002–2012.

113. Ambrosioni E, Borghi C, Magnani B. for the Survival of Myocardial Infarction Long-term Evaluation (SMILE) Investigators. The effect of the angiotensin-converting-enzyme inhibitor zofenopril on mortality and morbidity after anterior myocardial infarction. N Engl J Med 1995;332:80–85.

114. Zuanetti G, Latini R, Maggioni AP, Franzosi M, Santoro L, Tognoni G. on behalf of the GISSI-3 Investigators. Effect of the ACE-inhibitor lisinopril on mortality in diabetic patients with acute myocardial infarction: the data from the GISSI-3 study. Circulation 1997;96: 4239–4245.

115. Gustafsson I, Torp-Pedersen C, Køber L, Gustafsson F, Hildebrandt P. on behalf of the TRACE Study Group. Effect of the angiotensin-converting enzyme inhibitor trandolapril on mortality and morbidity in diabetic patients with left ventricular dysfunction after acute myocardial infarction. J Am Coll Cardiol 1999;34:83–89.

116. Heart Outcomes Prevention Evaluation (HOPE) Study Investigators. Effects of ramipril on cardiovascular and microvascular outcomes in people with diabetes: results of the HOPE study and MICRO-HOPE substudy. Lancet 2000;355:253–259.

117. Urata H, Healy B, Stewart RW, Bumpus FM, Husain A. Angiotensin II-forming pathways in normal and failing human hearts. Cir Res 1990;66:883–890.

118. Roig E, Perez-Villa F, Morales M, Jimenez W, Orús J, Heras M, Sanz G. Clinical implications of increased plasma angiotensin II despite ACE inhibitor therapy in patients with congestive heart failure. Eur Heart J 2000;21:53–57.

119. Awan NA, Mason DT. Direct selective blockade of the vascular angiotensin II receptors in therapy for hypertension and severe congestive heart failure. Am Heart J 1996;131:177–185.

120. Dickstein K, Kjekshus J. and the OPTIMAAL Steering Committee. Effects of losartan and captopril on mortality and morbidity in high-risk patients after acute myocardial infarction: the OPTIMAAL randomised trial. Lancet 2002;360:752–760.

121. Pfeffer MA, McMurray J, Leizorovicz A, Maggioni AP, Rouleau J-L, Van de Werf F, Henis M, Neuhart E, Gallo P, Edwards S, Sellers MA, Velazquez E, Califf RM. for the VALIANT Investigators. Valsartan in Acute Myocardial Infarction (VALIANT): rationale and design. Am Heart J 2000;140:727–734.

122. Goldberg RB, Mellies MJ, Sacks FM, Moyé LA, Howard BV, Pfeffer MA, Braunwald E. for the CARE Investigators. Cardiovascular events and their reduction with pravastatin in diabetic and glucose-intolerant myocardial infarction survivors with average cholesterol levels. Subgroup analyses in the Cholesterol And Recurrent Events (CARE) Trial. Circulation 1998;98:2513–2519.

123. Pyörälä K, Pedersen TR, Kjekshus J, Faergeman O, Olsson AG, Thorgeirsson G. the Scandinavian Simvastatin Survival Study (4S) Group. Cholesterol lowering with simvastatin improves prognosis of diabetic patients with coronary heart disease. A subgroup analysis of the Scandinavian Simvastatin Survival Study (4S). Diabetes Care 1997;20:614–620.

124. Keech A, Colquhoun D, Best J, Kirby A, Simes RJ, Hunt D, Hague W, Beller E, Arulchelvam M, Baker JAT. for the LIPID Study Group. Secondary prevention of cardiovascular events with long-term pravastatin in patients with diabetse or impaired fasting glucose. Results from the LIPID trial. Diabetes Care 2003;26:2713–2721.

125. Heart Protection Study Collaborative Group. MRC/BHF Heart Protection Study of cholesterol-lowering with simvastatin in 5963 people with diabetes: a randomised placebo-controlled trial. Lancet 2003;361:2005–2016.

126. Gray RP, Yudkin JS, Patterson DL. Enzymatic evidence of impaired reperfusion in diabetic patients after thrombolytic therapy for acute myocardial infarction: a role for plasminogen activator inhibitor?. Br Heart J 1993;70:530–536.

127. Strenestrand U, Wallentin L. for the Swedish Register of Cardiac Intensive Care (RIKS-HIA). Early statin treatment following acute myocardial infarction and 1-year survival. JAMA 2001;285:430–436.

128. Schwartz GG, Olsson AG, Ezekowitz MD, Ganz P, Oliver MP, Waters D, Zeiher A, Chaitman BR, Leslie S, Stern T. for the Myocardial Ischemia Reduction with Aggressive Cholesterol Lowering (MIRACL) Study Investigators. Effects of atorvastatin on early recurrent ischemic events in acute coronary syndromes. JAMA 2001;285:1711–1718.

129. Aronow HD, Topol EJ, Roe MT, Houghtaling PL, Wolski KE, Lincoff AM, Harrington RA, Califf RM, Ohman EM, Kleiman NS, Keltai M, Wilcox RG, Vahanian A, Armstrong PW, Lauer MS. Effect of lipid-lowering therapy on early mortality after acute coronary syndromes: an observational study. Lancet 2001;357:1063–1068.

130. Dupuis J, Tardif JC, Cernacek P, Théroux P. Cholesterol reduction rapidly improves endothelial function after acute coronary syndromes: the RECIFE (Reduction of Cholesterol in Ischemia and Function of the Endothelium) study. Circulation 1999;99:3227–3233.

131. Ridker PM, Cushman M, Stampfer MJ, Tracy RP, Hennekens CH. Inflammation, aspirin, and the risk of cardiovacular disease in apparently healthy men. N Engl J Med 1997;336:973–979.

132. Koenig W, Sund M, Fröhlich M, Fischer H-G, Löwel H, Döring A, Hutchinson WL, Pepys MB. C-reavctive protein, a sensitive marker of inflammation, predicts future risk of coronary heart disease in initially healthy middle-aged men. Results from the MONICA (Monitoring Trends and Determinants in Cardiovascular Dsiease) Augsburg Cohort Study, 1984 to 1992. Circulation 1999;99:237–242.

133. Ridker PM, Hennekens CH, Buring JE, Rifai N. C-reactive protein and other markers of inflammation in the prediction of cardiovascular disease in women. N Engl J Med 2000;342:836–843.

134. Morrow DA, Rifai N, Antman EM, Weiner DL, McCabe CH, Cannon CP, Braunwald E. C-reactive protein is a potent predictor of mortality independently of and in combination with troponin T in acute coronary syndromes: a TIMI 11A substudy. Thrombolysis in Myocardial Infarction. J Am Coll Cardiol 1998;31:1460–1465.

135. Heeschen C, Hamm CW, Bruemmer J, Simoons ML. Predictive value of C-reactive protein and troponin T in patients with unstable angina: a comparative analysis. CAPTURE Investiga-

tors. Chimeric c7E3 AntiPlatelet Therapy in Unstable angina REfractory to standard treatment trial. J Am Coll Cardiol 2000;35:1535–1542.

136. Lindahl B, Toss H, Siegbahn A, Venge P, Wallentin L. for the Fragmin during Instability in Coronary Artery Disease (FRISC) Study Group. Markers of myocardial damage and inflammation in relation to long-term mortality in unstable coronary artery disease. N Engl J Med 2000;343:1139–1147.

137. James SK, Armstrong P, Barnathan E, Califf R, Lindahl B, Siegbahn A, Simoons ML, Topol EJ, Venge P, Wallentin L. for the GUSTO-IV-ACS Investigators. Troponin and C-reactive protein have different relations to subsequent mortality and myocardial infarction after acute coronary syndrome: a GUSTO-IV substudy. J Am Coll Cardiol 2003;41:916–924.

138. Mueller C, Buettner HJ, Hodgson JM, Marsch S, Perruchoud AP, Roskamm H, Neumann FJ. Inflammation and long-term mortality after non-ST elevation acute coronary syndrome treated with a very early invasive strategy in 1042 consecutive patients. Circulation 2002; 105:1412–1415.

139. Danesh J, Whincup P, Walker M, Lennon L, Thomson A, Appleby P, Gallimore R, Pepys MB. Low grade inflammation and coronary heart disease: prospective study and updated meta-analyses. Br Med J 2000;321:199–204.

140. Danenberg HD, Szalai AJ, Swaminathan RV, Peng L, Chen Z, Seifert P, Fay WP, Simon DI, Edelman ER. Increased thrombosis after arterial injury in human C-reactive protein-transgenic mice. Circulation 2003;108:512–515.

141. Ridker PM, Rifal N, Rose L, Buring JE, Cook NR. Comparison of C-reactive protein and low-density lipoprotein cholesterol levels in the prediction of first cardiovascular events. N Engl J Med 2002;347:1557–1565.

142. Pradhan AD, Ridker PM. Do atherosclerosis and type 2 diabetes share a common inflammatory basis? Eur Heart J 2002;23:831–834.

143. Ridker PM, Buring JE, Cook NR, Rifai N. C-reactive protein, the metabolic syndrome, and risk of incident cardiovascular events: an 8-year follow-up of 14 719 initially healthy American women. Circulation 2003;107:391–397.

144. Ferreiros ER, Boissonnet CP, Pizarro R, Merletti PF, Corrado G, Cagide A, Bazzino OO. Independent prognostic value of elevated C-reactive protein in unstable angina. Circulation 1999;100:1958–1963.

145. Kinlay S, Schwartz GG, Olsson AG, Rifai N, Leslie SJ, Sasiela WJ, Szarek M, Libby P, Ganz P. for the Myocardial Ischemia Reduction with Aggressive Cholesterol Lowering (MIRACL) Study Investiagors. High-dose atorvastatin enhances the decline in inflammatory markers in patients with acute coronary syndromes in the MIRACL Study. Circulation 2003;108:1560–1566.

146. Chew DP, Bhatt DL, Robbins MA, Penn MS, Schneider JP, Lauer MS, Topol EJ, Ellis SG. Incremental prognostic value of elevated baseline C-reactive protein among established markers of risk in percutaneous coronary intervention. Circulation 2001;104:992–997.

147. Lindmark E, Diderholm E, Wallentin L, Siegbahn A. Relationship between interleukin 6 and mortality in patients with unstable coronary artery disease: effects of an early invasive or noninvasive strategy. JAMA 2001;286:2107–2113.

148. de Winter RJ, Koch KT, van Straalen JP, Heyde G, Bax M, Schotborgh CE, Mulder KJ, Sanders GT, Fischer J, Tijssen JG, Piek JJ. C-reactive protein and coronary events following percutaneous coronary angioplasty. Am J Med 2003;115:85–90.

149. Zairis MN, Ambrose JA, Manousakis SJ, Stefanidis AS, Papadaki OA, Bilianou HI, DeVoe MC, Fakiolas CN, Pissimissis EG, Olympios CD, Foussas SG. for the Global Evaluation of New Events and Restenosis After Stent Implantation Study Group. The impact of plasma levels of C-reactive protein, lipoprotein (a) and homocysteine on the long-term prognosis after successful coronary stenting: The Global Evaluation of New Events and Restenosis After Stent Implantation Study. J Am Coll Cardiol 2002;40: 1375–1382.

150. Chan AW, Bhatt DL, Chew DP, Reginelli J, Schneider JP, J TE, Ellis SG. Relation of inflammation and benefit of statins after percutaneous coronary interventions. Circulation 2003;107:1750–1756.

151. Schönbeck U, Libby P. CD40 signaling and plaque instability. Circ Res 2001;89: 1092–1103.

152. Aukrust P, Müller F, Ueland T, Berget T, Aaser E, Brunsvig A, Solum NO, Forfang K, Frøland SS, Gullestad L. Enhanced levels of soluble and membrane-bound CD40 ligand in patients with unstable angina. Possible reflection of T lymphocyte and platelet involvement in the pathogenesis of acute coronary syndromes. Circulation 1999;100:614–620.

153. Varo N, de Lemos JA, Libby P, Morrow DA, Murphy SA, Nuzzo R, Gibson CM, Cannon CP, Braunwald E, Schonbeck U. Soluble CD40L: risk prediction after acute coronary syndromes. Circulation 2003;108:1049–1052.

154. Marx N, Imhof A, Froehlich J, Siam L, Ittner J, Wierse G, Schmidt A, Maerz W, Hombach V, Koenig W. Effect of rosiglitazone treatment on soluble CD40L in patients with type 2 diabetes and coronary artery disease. Circulation 2003;107:1954–1957.

155. Varo N, Vicent D, Libby P, Nuzzo R, Calle-Pascual AL, Bernal MR, Fernandez-Cruz A, Veves A, Jarolim P, Varo JJ, Goldfine A, Horton E, Schonbeck U. Elevated plasma levels of the atherogenic mediator soluble CD40 ligand in diabetic patients: a novel target of thiazolidinediones. Circulation 2003;107:2664–2669.

156. Park L, Raman KG, Lee KJ, Lu Y, Ferran LJ, Chow WS, Stern D, Schmidt AM. Suppression of accelerated diabetic atherosclerosis by the soluble receptor for advanced glycation endproducts. Nat Med 1998;4:1025–1031.

157. Schmidt AM, Yan SD, Wautier JL, Stern D. Activation of receptor for advanced glycation end products: a mechanism for chronic vascular dysfunction in diabetic vasculopathy and atherosclerosis. Circ Res 1999;84:489–97.

158. Bucciarelli LG, Wendt T, Qu W, Lu Y, Lalla E, Rong LL, Goova MT, Moser B, Kislinger T, Lee DC, Kashyap Y, Stern DM, Schmidt AM. RAGE blockade stabilizes established atherosclerosis in diabetic apolipoprotein E-null mice. Circulation 2002;106:2827–2835.

159. Cipollone F, Iezzi A, Fazia M, Zucchelli M, Pini B, Cuccurullo C, De Cesare D, De Blasis G, Muraro R, Bei R, Chiarelli F, Schmidt AM, Cuccurullo F, Mezzetti A. The receptor RAGE as a progression factor amplifying arachidonate-dependent inflammatory and proteolytic response in human atherosclerotic plaques. Role of glycemic control. Circulation 2003;108:1070–1077.

160. Goldner MG, Knatterud GL, Prout TE. Effects of hypoglycemic agents on vascular complications in patients with adult-onset diabetes. 3. Clinical implications of the UGDP results. JAMA 1971;218:1400–1410.

161. United Kingdom Prospective Diabetes Study Group. Effect of intensive blood-glucose control with metformin on complications in overweight patients with type 2 diabetes (UKPDS 34). Lancet 1998;352:854–865.

162. United Kingdom Prospective Diabetes Study Group. Intensive blood-glucose control with sulphonylureas or insulin compared with conventional treatment and risk of complications in patients with type 2 diabetes (UKPDS 33). Lancet 1998;352:837–853.

163. Morice M-C, Serruys PW, Sousa JE, Fadajet J, ban Hayashi E, Perin M, Colombo A, Schuler G, Barragan P, Guagliumi G, Molnàr F, Falotico R. for the RAVEL Study Group. A randomized comparison of a sirolimus-eluting stent with a standard stent for coronary revascularization. N Engl J Med 2002;346:1773–1780.

164. Colombo A, Drzewiecki J, Banning A, Grube E, Hauptmann K, Silber S, Dudek D, Fort S, Schiele F, Zmudka K, Guagliumi G, Russell ME. for the TAXUS II Study Group. Randomized study to assess the effectiveness of slow- and moderate-release polymer-based paclitaxel-eluting stents for coronary lesions. Circulation 2003;108:788–794.

165. Grabe E TAXUS VI Trial Insights into Diabetics: Highlights. In Paris Course on Revascularization 2004; Paris, France 2004.

166. Stone GW. TAXUS IV: the Pivotal Trial in Perspective. In. Transcatheter Therapeutics 2003. Washington. DC, 2003.

167. Fajadet J, Perin M, Hayashi E, Colombo A, Schuler G, Barragan P, Bode C, Sousa JE, Morice MC, Serruys PW. 210-day follow-up of the RAVEL Study: a randomized study with the sirolimus-eluting Bx Velocity™ balloon-expandable stent in the treatment of

patients with de novo native coronary artery lesions (abstract). J Am Coll Cardiol 2002; 39:20A.

168. Leon MB, Moses JW, Popma JJ, Kuntz RE, Fitzgerald P. for the SIRIUS Investigators. SIRIUS: Prospective randomized evaluation of the sirolimus-eluting stent in patients with de novo coronary lesions. In. Transcatheter Therapeutics 2002. Washington. DC, 2002.

169. Lemos PA, Lee C-H, Degertekin M, Saia F, Tanabe K, Arampatzis CA, Hoye A, van Duuren M, Sianos G, Smits PC, de Feyter P, van der Giessen WJ, van Domburg RT, Serruys PW. Early outcome after sirolimus-eluting stent implantation in patients with acute coronary syndromes. Insights from the Rapamycin-Eluting Stent Evaluated At Rotterdam Cardiology Hospital (RESEARCH) Registry. J Am Coll Cardiol 2003;41:2093–2099.

# 26

# Cardiac Rupture: Pathobiology, Diagnosis, Medical Management, and Surgical Intervention

**Richard C. Becker**
*Duke University Medical Center*
*Durham, North Carolina, U.S.A*

**Thomas A. Pezzella**
*University of Massachusetts Medical School*
*Worcester, Massachusetts, U.S.A*

## INTRODUCTION

Cardiac rupture is a well-recognized complication of acute myocardial infarction that is responsible for 10% to 15% of all in-hospital deaths. Written descriptions of this life-threatening event, which most often involves the left ventricular free wall and less frequently the interventricular septum, papillary muscle, right ventricular free wall, and atrium, have appeared in the medical and surgical literature for centuries. William Harvey (1647) is credited with the initial report [1], followed some years later by a detailed account of cardiac rupture found within the autopsy notes from King George II (1727).

The anatomist Morgagni collected 10 cases of cardiac rupture in 1765 [2]. In 1859 Malmsten reported a case of cardiac rupture and for the first time described "softening of the myocardium" within the involved area due to occlusive coronary artery thrombosis [3,4]. By 1925, Krumbhaar and Crowell [5] had collected 632 cases of rupture from the literature and added 22 cases of their own, emphasizing its association with coronary artery disease and acute myocardial infarction. Despite increasing insight, there are many unanswered questions regarding the pathobiology, prevention, diagnosis, medical management, and surgical intervention of cardiac rupture.

## CARDIAC RUPTURE

### Epidemiology

Autopsy series serve as the basis for determining the overall incidence of rupture associated with myocardial infarction (Table 1) [6–40]. Several large series are commonly cited. Malmo General Hospital (Sweden) reported 2477 myocardial infarctions between 1935

**Table 1** Cardiac Rupture in Acute Fatal Myocardial Infarction: Historic Time Line of Necropsy-Based Series

| Authro(s) | Year | Cases of fatal myocardial infarction | Cases of cardiac rupture | |
|---|---|---|---|---|
| | | | Total | % |
| Parkinson and Bedford | 1928 | 51 | 5 | 9.8 |
| Levine | 1929 | 46 | 9 | 19.6 |
| Bean | 1938 | 114 | 17 | 14.9 |
| Mallory | 1939 | 72 | 8 | 11.0 |
| Edmondson and Hoxie | 1942 | 865 | 72 | 8.3 |
| Friedman and White | 1944 | 105 | 10 | 9.5 |
| Mintz and Katz | 1947 | 46 | 5 | 10.4 |
| Wartman and Hellerstein | 1948 | 111 | 6 | 5.5 |
| Selzer | 1948 | 95 | 8 | 8.4 |
| Diaz-Rivera and Miller | 1948 | 53 | 5 | 9.4 |
| Foord | 1948 | 264 | 33 | 12.5 |
| Wang | 1948 | 267 | 23 | 8.6 |
| Howell and Turnbull | 1950 | 111 | 8 | 7.2 |
| Zinn and Cosby | 1950 | 430 | 34 | 7.9 |
| Oblath | 1952 | 1,026 | 91 | 8.9 |
| Wessler | 1952 | 256 | 14 | 6.0 |
| Waldron | 1954 | 545 | 40 | 7.5 |
| Goetz and Gropper | 1954 | 145 | 14 | 9.6 |
| McDonnieal | 1955 | 144 | 12 | 8.0 |
| Lee | 1956 | 500 | 25 | 5.0 |
| Maher | 1956 | 183 | 21 | 11.5 |
| Aarseth | 1958 | 1,229 | 89 | 7.3 |
| Zeman and Rodstein | 1960 | 81 | 16 | 19.7 |
| Griffith | 1961 | 3,103 | 215 | 6.9 |
| Spiekerman | 1962 | 87 | 21 | 24.0 |
| Ross and Young | 1963 | 606 | 43 | 7.0 |
| Sievers | 1964 | 811 | 104 | 12.8 |
| London and London | 1965 | 1,001 | 47 | 5.0 |
| Lautsh | 1967 | 585 | 43 | 7.3 |
| Sugiura | 1968 | 129 | 17 | 15.0 |
| Sahebjamin | 1969 | 933 | 37 | 3.8 |
| Lewis | 1969 | 1,228 | 106 | 8.6 |
| Beutler | 1970 | 250 | 20 | 8.0 |
| Meurs | 1970 | 34 | 8 | 23.5 |
| Gjol | 1972 | 440 | 51 | 12.0 |
| Naeim | 1972 | 989 | 44 | 4.0 |
| Hammer | 1972 | 47 | 7 | 15.0 |
| Havig | 1973 | 122 | 14 | 11.5 |
| Total | | 17,109 | 1,342 | 7.8 |

and 1959. One-third of the events were fatal, and autopsies performed in 95% of cases revealed cardiac rupture with pericardial tamponade in 12.5% of patients [41]. An overview of 1326 patients suffering either in-hospital or out-of-hospital death in Rochester, MN (1947–1959), cited a 24% rupture rate (from 691 patients autopsied) among persons older than 20 years of age [42]. The most common cause of cardiac rupture is acute myocardial infarction; other, less common causes include infective endocarditis, myocardial abscesses, aortic dissection, myocarditis, tuberculosis, echinococcal cysts, trauma (blunt or penetrating, with or without pericardial rupture), and malignancy (primary or metastatic).

## Site of Involvement

Rupture associated with acute myocardial infarction can involve the ventricular free wall, ventricular septum, papillary muscles, multiple sites, and, rarely, the atrium (Fig. 1).

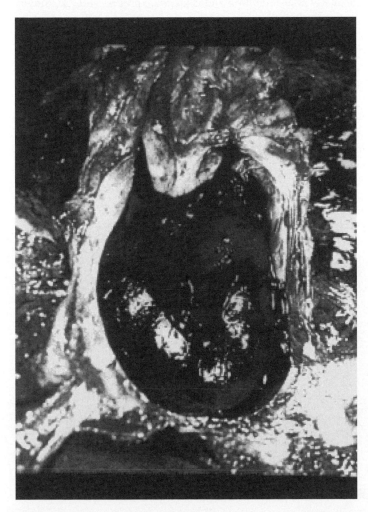

**Figure 1** Gross specimen of the heart in situ with a layer of fresh blood on its surface and within the pericardial space resulting from acute myocardial (free wall ) rupture.

*Ventricular Free Wall Rupture*

Rupture of the ventricular free wall is the most common variety of rupture. According to descriptions offered in the era before the use of reperfusion, left ventricular free wall rupture can occur at any time between 1 day and 3 weeks after infarction, but most develop between days 3 and 5 (Fig. 2). Overall, left ventricular rupture is 7 times more frequent than right ventricular rupture and typically involves the anterior and lateral walls. Among 1048 patients enrolled in the international SHOCK trial registry [43], 28 (2.7%) had free wall rupture or tamponade. They were less likely to have pulmonary edema, diabetes mellitus, or prior infarction than patients who had not experienced rupture; however, they were more likely to have new Q waves. The in-hospital mortality was 60%.

The myocardial tear is commonly identified near the junction of infarcted tissue and adjacent healthy muscle. The following classification of rupture into 3 types was proposed by Becker and Van Mantgem [44].

**Type I Rupture.** Type I rupture is characterized by an abrupt tear in the left ventricular wall. In most cases, there is no appreciable decrease in wall thickness, suggesting that type I rupture occurs early after infarction and is an *acute* process (Fig. 3). Single-vessel disease is present in a majority of cases.

**Type II Rupture.** Type II rupture is characterized by an advanced but well-localized loss of myocardium and an area of erosion blended with thrombus and necrotic tissue. These features suggest that type II rupture is a *subacute* process in which overt rupture is preceded by myocardial erosion (Fig. 4). Multivessel disease is present in a majority of cases.

**Type III Rupture.** Type III rupture occurs in areas of extensive myocardial thinning and aneurysmal bulging and is consistent with a subacute *or* chronic process (Fig. 5). Rupture is almost always localized to the aneurysm's central portion. The extent of coronary artery disease varies.

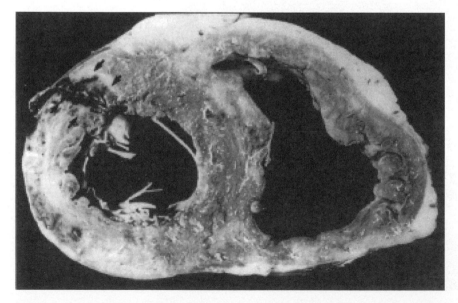

**Figure 2**   Acute left ventricular free wall rupture (*arrows*) causing cardiac tamponade and death. A serpiginous path leading from the endocardium to the epicardial surface is evident.

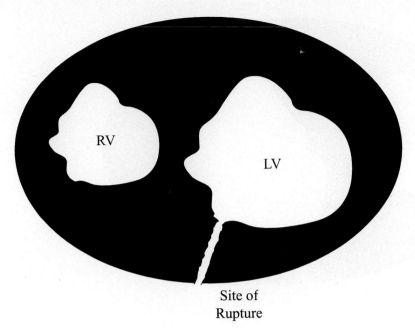

**Figure 3** Type I cardiac rupture is an acute process characterized by a "slit-like" tear through the myocardium.

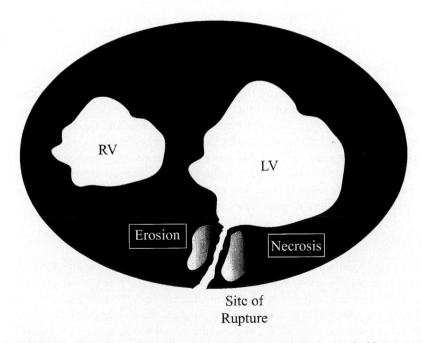

**Figure 4** Type II cardiac rupture is a subacute process preceded by myocardial necrosis and erosion.

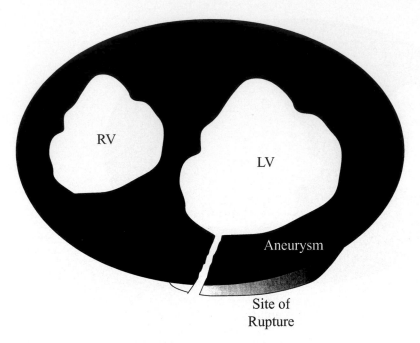

**Figure 5**    Type III cardiac rupture is a chronic process that occurs in an area of myocardial thinning and aneurysmal bulging.

The age of infarction, determined histologically, differs considerably among the 3 types of myocardial rupture. In general, hearts with type I rupture exhibit the most recent infarcts with nearly 50% being younger than 24 hours old. In contrast, type II and type III ruptures show a much wider age range, averaging 8 and 21 days, respectively.

*Ventricular Septal Rupture*

Rupture of the ventricular septum occurs in 1.0% to 3.0% of individuals with acute myocardial infarction (one-tenth the incidence of ventricular free wall rupture) (Fig. 6) (31,45-46). It is reported to be more common in the elderly and among women, and typically occurs within 7 days of infarction. An anterior site of infarction is most common.

In the SHOCK trial registry [47], 55 patients experienced acute ventricular septal rupture a median of 16 hours from myocardial infarction onset. Patients with septal rupture tended to be older, were more often female, and less often had prior infarction, diabetes mellitus, or severe coronary artery disease. The inhospital mortality was 81%.

*Papillary Muscle Rupture*

Complete rupture of the papillary muscle causing sudden and torrential mitral insufficiency is a rare but often fatal complication of acute myocardial infarction. It occurs in less than 1% of all patients; however, papillary muscle rupture carries an 80% mortality (Fig. 7). Rupture of the posteromedial papillary muscle is 5 to 10 times more common than rupture of the anterolateral papillary muscle owing to its single-vessel blood supply. Rupture of the right ventricular papillary muscle is rare but can cause tricuspid insufficiency and right-sided heart failure.

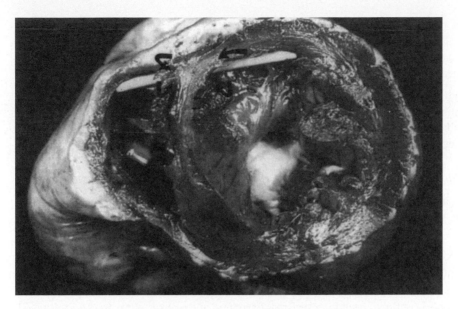

**Figure 6**  Acute rupture of the posteromedial papillary muscle (arrows) causing torrential mitral insufficiency, cardiogenic shock, and death.

Partial papillary muscle rupture is more common than complete rupture and can often be addressed surgically. Like ventricular free wall and septal ruptures, papillary muscle rupture typically occurs within the first week of an acute myocardial infarction.

The SHOCK trial registry included 98 patients with severe mitral regurgitation who developed cardiogenic shock a median of 12.8 hours from infarct onset. Patients with severe mitral insufficiency were more likely to have experienced non–ST-segment eleva-

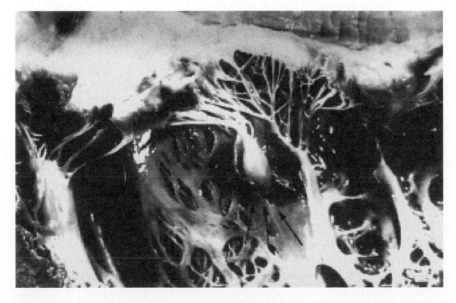

**Figure 7**  Acute rupture of the interventricular septum (*large arrows, marker*). A zone of infarction extends from the anterior wall to the septum (*small arrows*).

tion MI involving the inferior or posterior walls than those experiencing shock in the absence of severe mitral insufficiency. The inhospital mortality was 61% [48].

### Combined Rupture

Although the incidence rates for rupture vary by site, the pathobiologic substrates share similarities. As a result, multiple ruptures (ventricular septal rupture and left ventricular free wall rupture [49] and ventricular septal rupture and papillary muscle rupture [50]) while uncommon are not rare.

### Atrial Rupture

Despite involvement of the atria in some instances of myocardial infarction, the low-pressure chambers rarely rupture.

### Intramyocardial/Dissecting Hematoma

Sealed free wall rupture with an intact epicardium (dissecting hematoma) has been described in patients following an acute myocardial infarction [51]. While the natural history remains poorly defined, pseudoaneurysmal formation and overt rupture are a concern [52].

## PATHOBIOLOGY OF CARDIAC RUPTURE

Between 1936 and 1950 a total of 1641 autopsies were performed at the Beth Israel Hospital in Boston [21]. Overall there were 19 cases (1.2%) of spontaneous cardiac rupture (7.0% of all myocardial infarction cases). In each instance, there was evidence of a recent infarction. A group of 104 hearts with fresh infarction but without cardiac rupture were examined for comparison. All ruptures were limited to the left ventricle and septum; 6 involved the anterior and 9 the posterior walls, and there was considerable variability in size and shape. Some were described as ragged with gaping holes, whereas others were linear slits. Tears on the epicardial surface were easily found and varied in length from 3.0–30.0 mm. In contrast, the endocardial rents were often small and hidden behind ventricular trabeculae. Old coronary occlusions antedating the acute infarction were present in one-third of hearts with rupture, compared to three-fourths of nonruptured hearts. There was a high incidence of fresh coronary artery occlusions (100%) in hearts with rupture; however, a well-developed collateral circulation was uncommon. There was minimal myocardial fibrosis within the infarct zone and site of rupture. The overall size of the infarct zone did not differ significantly between hearts with rupture and those without; however, transmural infarction was always present in hearts with cardiac rupture. In most instances, the path of rupture traversed an area of recent infarction that was free of fibrosis. These observations suggest that the major pathologic findings among hearts with cardiac rupture are: a) fresh coronary artery occlusion, b) recent infarction, c) transmural necrosis, d) poorly developed collateral circulation, and e) minimal or absent myocardial fibrosis.

One of the largest published autopsy series [53] consisted of 9109 autopsies and was performed at Temple University between 1945 and 1963. This series reported a 6.4% incidence of rupture in men and 9.1% in women. Several pathologic characteristics of the hearts that contained rupture were notable: a) there was extensive necrosis and neutrophil infiltration; b) intramural hemorrhage was not marked nor was there evidence of intramural hematoma; and c) the plane of rupture was invariably through the most necrotic zone. With regard to the tears themselves, 65% contained thrombus, suggesting progression rather than a sudden event. Ruptures were not observed in areas with completed (healed) infarction.

A total of 3416 consecutive autopsies performed at the Miami Heart Institute and Mt. Sinai Hospital contained 1001 cases of acute myocardial infarction, including 47 cases of rupture [54]. The average age of patients with fatal rupture was 69 years, supporting the association between advanced age and mechanical complications of myocardial infarction. The majority of deaths (rupture, nonrupture) occurred within the first 3 days.

## MECHANISMS: MECHANICAL AND CELLULAR

While a model for studying cardiac rupture has not yet been developed, hypotheses based on pathological descriptions have been proposed. They are as follows.

### Pressure Theory

The development of an endocardial tear may result either from increased or sustained intracavitary pressure or from forces generated by the contracting heart directed toward the infarct zone. The ''pull'' of contracting healthy muscle on an adjacent zone of softened necrotic muscle could produce the initial tear, widening with subsequent systolic contractions. In addition, healthy muscle could conceivably produce paradoxical pulsations within the infarcted area (because of differences in elasticity). These actions, coupled with a sustained increase in diastolic pressure at the endocardial surface commonly observed in myocardial ischemia and infarction, could create the ''pressure substrate'' for rupture, particularly at the junction of normal and abnormal (necrotic) tissue (Fig. 8).

The pressure theory has been extended further to include a transient, acquired dynamic outflow tract obstruction with systolic anterior motion of the mitral valve leaflets in the setting of acute anterior wall myocardial infarction. The focal increase in end-systolic wall stress could facilitate rupture in areas of ''vulnerable'' myocardium (Fig. 9)

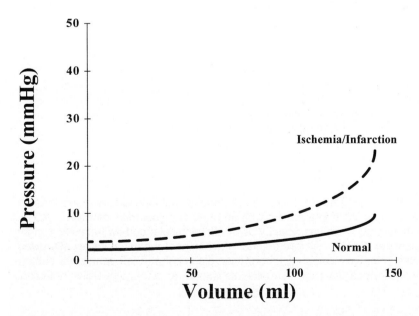

**Figure 8** In the setting of myocardial ischemia and infarction, a greater increase in left ventricular end-diastolic pressure is generated (steep pressure-volume relationship) in response to a given ventricular volume when compared to a healthy (compliant) heart.

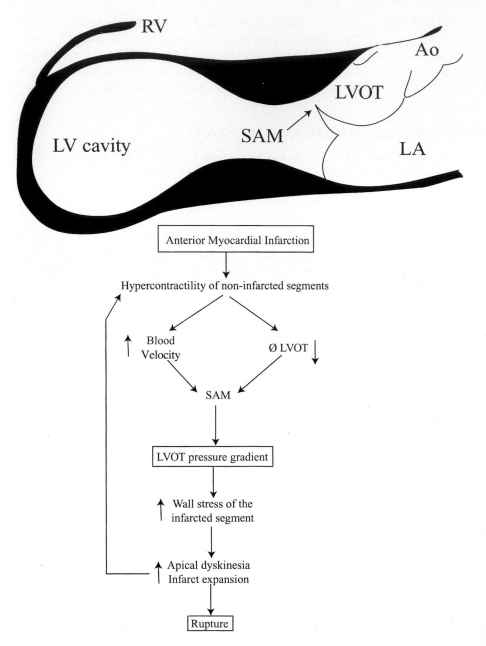

**Figure 9** (**Top**) Schematic representation of a 2-dimensional longitudinal plane through the left ventricle during systole in a patient with an anterior myocardial infarction. (AO = aorta; LA = left atrium; LV = left ventricle; LVOT = left ventricular outflow tract; RV = right ventricle; Ø = diameter; SAM = systolic anterior movement of the mitral valve). (**Bottom**) Cascade of events potentially contributing to the development of a left ventricular outflow tract gradient and to myocardial rupture in patients with an anterior myocardial infarction. (From Ref. 55)

[55]. Lastly, the important contribution of wall stress ''surges'' to myocardial rupture is supported by reported events during dobutamine stress testing [56].

## Collagen Matrix Theory

Although increased intracavitary pressure may play an important role in myocardial rupture, the event itself in all likelihood requires a ''vulnerable'' myocardium. In other words, the myocardium must be weakened, even if only in a small, well-localized region, for the effects of increased pressure to have important pathologic consequences. Indeed, areas of rupture are often heavily infiltrated by neutrophils, proteolytic enzymes, and a poorly developed supporting collagen framework (Fig. 10). The importance of a strong matrix

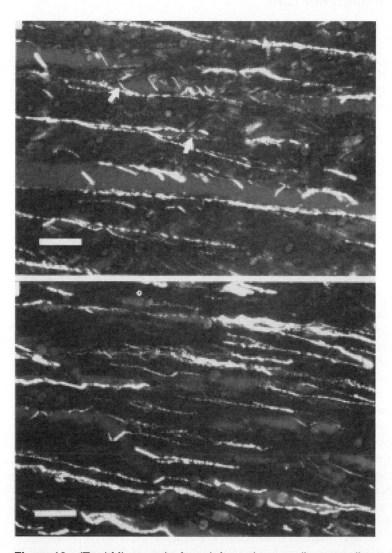

**Figure 10** (**Top**) Micrograph of non-infarcted myocardium revealing normal collagen fibers. (**Bottom**) Micrograph of infarcted myocardium 3 days after coronary artery occlusion. Fewer collagen fibers are present and their internal supporting structure has been altered. (From Ref. 64)

scaffold for infarct healing is highlighted by the protection from myocardial rupture observed in mice given a plasminogen-activator inhibitor or matrix metalloproteinase inhibitor after coronary artery ligation [57].

## Patient Characteristics and Cardiac Rupture

The major demographic and clinical features associated with cardiac rupture, as determined by necropsy series performed in the prereperfusion era, include advanced age (60 years or older), female sex, first infarction, and hypertension (in the acute phase of infarction).

# GENOMICS OF CARDIAC RUPTURE

Local concentration and generation of angiotensin II as well as the number of angiotensin II receptors are increased in infarcted regions. Of the major angiotensin II receptor isoforms, AT2 has been investigated for its fibrogenetic effects during wound healing. Transgenic mice lacking the AT2 receptor Agtr2-/γ frequently die of cardiac rupture following coronary ligation. mRNAs of collagen I, collagen III, and fibronectin are significantly reduced compared with wild-type mice, and the extent of fibrosis within the infracted region is decreased markedly [58].

Mice lacking urokinase-type plasminogen activator (u-PA -1-) are protected from cardiac rupture, whereas those with deficiency of gelatinase-β are partially protected. These observations suggest that administration of plasminogen activator or matrix metalloproteinase inhibitors may offer protection against cardiac rupture [59].

# REPERFUSION ERA

## Pathological Features

*Animal Models*

Coronary ligation experiments designed to investigate the pathologic and histologic features of myocardial infarction following reperfusion have been conducted in animals and nonhuman primates. NcNamara and colleagues [60] documented hemorrhagic infarction in all hearts (nonhuman primates) with coronary occlusion followed by reperfusion (releasing an occlusive clamp). Hemorrhage within the infarct zone was greatest with reperfusion after 4 or more hours of occlusion. Similar observations were made by Vander Salm [61] and Higginson [62], who also found that hemorrhage after reperfusion occurred predominantly in zones of severe myocardial necrosis. The impact of fibrinolytic agents on myocardial hemorrhage has been investigated by Kloner and Alker [63], who randomly assigned anesthetized, open-chest dogs to reperfusion alone (release of an occlusive clamp) or reperfusion plus intracoronary streptokinase. All animals had 3 hours of occlusion followed by 3 hours of reperfusion. There were no differences in the extent of gross hemorrhage or the calculated intramyocardial hemoglobin concentrations between the two experimental groups.

Stunned myocardium (ischemia followed by reperfusion) exhibits increased collagenase activity and procollagenase activation. Following permanent coronary occlusion (with or without reperfusion), collagen degradation can be observed within 24 hours of infarction. The fewer the number of collagen fibers, the greater the degree of subsequent infarct expansion [64]. Coronary ligation followed by reperfusion leads to myocardial necrosis with a hemorrhagic component and a loss of the collagen-supporting framework.

*Necropsy-Based Experience in Humans with Acute Myocardial Infarction*

Myocardial hemorrhage has been observed in humans following coronary reperfusion. In a report by Mathey [65], 6 of 101 patients with myocardial infarction whose coronary arteries were initially recanalized using intracoronary streptokinase (average time to recanalization 2.9 hours) subsequently died in the ensuing weeks (range 1–18 days). Hemorrhagic infarction was identified in 3 patients and was confined to areas of necrosis. Similar observations were made by Fujiwara based on an autopsy study of 30 patients who had received intracoronary urokinase [66]. In 5 patients, myocardial hemorrhage was observed in the absence of reperfusion. Marked focal hemorrhage was not identified in patients dying within 4 hours of receiving fibrinolytic therapy.

A necropsy-based series by Waller [67], including 19 patients who underwent either pharmacological (fibrinolytic) or mechanical (predominantly balloon coronary angioplasty) reperfusion, reported a 74% rate of hemorrhagic infarction. Each of the patients with hemorrhagic infarction had received fibrinolytic therapy (or a combination of lytics and angioplasty). In contrast, anemic infarctions were found in patients undergoing mechanical reperfusion.

A study was done of 23 patients with suspected myocardial infarction and 17 received fibrinolytic therapy to determine the effects of plasmin generation on collagen breakdown [68]. Amino terminal propeptide of type III procollagen and carboxy-terminal propeptide of type I procollagen were assayed. During a streptokinase infusion, serum concentrations of both type I and type III procollagen increased rapidly by 50%, suggesting that fibrinolytics, by generating the nonspecific protease plasmin from its inactive precursor plasminogen, stimulate collagen breakdown.

The hearts of 52 TIMI II study patients (age $67 \pm 11$ years) who died between 5 hours and 260 days (median 2.7 days) after myocardial infarction were examined [69]. A total of 38 patients received tissue plasminogen activator (without coronary angioplasty or bypass surgery). A comparison of 23 patients with hemorrhagic infarction and 20 patients with nonhemorrhagic infarction revealed a) similar frequencies of myocardial rupture—26% of patients with rupture had hemorrhagic infarction whereas 25% did not; b) similar infarct size; and c) similar extent of coronary artery disease.

Observations from necropsy studies suggest that myocardial hemorrhage and collagen breakdown are hallmarks of reperfusion therapy in humans.

## Proposed Mechanisms for Myocardial Rupture

There is evidence that transmural infarction is an absolute prerequisite for cardiac rupture. Although hemorrhagic infarction could conceivably weaken the supporting framework, few studies have shown that hemorrhage extends beyond the zone of myocardial necrosis. Thus, based on the available information, the critical factor in rupture appears to be disruption of the myocardial connective tissue matrix [70].

Areas of infarction have diminished collagen density [71], and hearts with rupture have a virtual absence of collagen at the involved site [72]. Fibrinolytic therapy, by generating plasmin, activates latent tissue collagenases, thereby contributing to early collagen breakdown [68]. The added feature of increased endocardial pressure within ischemic/infarcted regions is likely an important contributor.

## CLINICAL EXPERIENCE: RANDOMIZED CLINICAL TRIALS AND LARGE-SCALE REGISTRIES

### Prereperfusion Era

The incidence of cardiac rupture was determined among 849 patients enrolled in the Multicenter Investigation of Limitation of Infarct Size (MILIS) study [73]. Although there were only 14 cases (1.7%) of rupture, rupture accounted for 14% of all in-hospital deaths. The following characteristics were associated with a near 10-fold increase of cardiac rupture events: a) no prior history of angina or myocardial infarction; b) presence of electrocardiographic ST-segment elevation or the development of Q waves; and c) a peak creatine kinase >150 IU/L (Table 2).

### Reperfusion Era

A total of 9720 patients participating in the GISSI-2 study [74] who had experienced their first myocardial infarction were analyzed. The in-hospital mortality was 1.9% for patients younger than 40 years of age, but increased to 31.9% among those older than 80 years. Autopsies were performed in 20% of 772 patients dying in-hospital. The frequency of cardiac rupture was 19% in patients younger than 60 years of age, increasing to 86% (72 out of a total of 84 patients) for those older than 70 years. Approximately half of all deaths occurred within the initial 48 hours of infarction. The findings suggest that cardiac rupture is a particularly common cause of early death in older patients.

**Table 2**  Infarct-Related Features Among Patients With Subsequent Rupture: Prereperfusion Era

| Characterization | Free wall rupture (N = 8) | Ventricular septal rupture (N = 8) | No rupture (N = 831) | P value |
|---|---|---|---|---|
| Location of MI | | | | |
|   Anterior | 5 | 3 | 389 | .79[a] |
|   Inferior | 3 | 3 | 376 | |
|   Lateral or other | 0 | 0 | 65 | |
| Peak MB-CK (IU/L) | | | | |
|   Sample size | 8 | 6 | 830 | |
|   Mean | 312 | 210 | 145 | .01[b] |
| Infarct size index by MB-CK (CK-g-eq/m$^2$) | | | | |
|   Sample size | 4 | 5 | 713 | |
|   Mean | 56 | 21 | 17 | .01[b] |
| % Dyskinetic segments on admission RVG | | | | |
|   Sample size | 7 | 4 | 731 | |
|   Mean | 20 | 4.5 | 3.9 | .01[b] |
| LVEF on admission RVG | | | | |
|   Sample size | 7 | 4 | 718 | |
|   Mean | 26 | 42 | 46 | .01[b] |

MI = myocardial infarction; RVG = radionuclide ventriculogram; LVEF = left ventricular ejection fraction.
*P* values reported are from chi-square test of homogeneity or analysis of variance.
[a] Chi-square test may be invalid because of the limited size of the simple in certain groups.
[b] *P* <.05 when the three groups were tested with one another.
(From Ref. 73)

The TIMI II study included a total of 3534 patients with suspected myocardial infarction. From this overall cohort, 23 patients had cardiac rupture verified at either autopsy or surgery, and an additional 10 patients died following an episode of pulseless electrical activity (PEA) (without preceding pump heart failure, ventricular tachycardia, or ventricular fibrillation). The incidence of cardiac rupture was 0.95%. In a subset of patients undergoing protocol-directed coronary angiography, complete occlusion of the infarct-related coronary artery was more common among patients with rupture compared with the overall study population (40% vs. 11%, $P = .03$). Advanced age and female sex were independent predictors of cardiac rupture (Currier JW: personal communication).

Of 350,755 patients enrolled in phase 1 of the National Registry of Myocardial Infarction (NRMI), 122,243 received fibrinolytic therapy, and 228,512 did not [75]. The in-hospital mortality rate was 10.4% for the overall patient population, 12.9% for patients not treated with fibrinolytics, and 5.9% for those who received fibrinolytic therapy. Cardiogenic shock from primary pump failure was the most common cause of death in each patient group. Even though there was a low overall incidence rate of cardiac rupture. (<1.0%), it was responsible for an increasing proportion of hospital deaths: 7.3% of patients in the overall population; 6.1% of patients not treated with fibrinolytics, and 12.1% of patients treated with fibrinolytic therapy. Death from cardiac rupture also occurred earlier with fibrinolytic treatment (Table 3). Despite the early occurrence of rupture among fibrinolytic-treated patients, death rates were lower for this group during each of the first 30 post-infarction days (Figs. 11 and 12). By multivariable analysis, older age, female sex, and fibrinolytic therapy were associated with early myocardial rupture.

The GISSI-1 trial [76], in which patients were enrolled up to 12 hours from symptom onset, reported an increased incidence of myocardial rupture among late-entry patients treated with fibrinolytics. An overview of 4 clinical trials which included a total of 1638 patients (58 cases of myocardial rupture) [77] identified a correlation between increasing time to treatment and rupture. However, these data are not conclusive. A prospectively designed ancillary study including a total of 5711 patients randomly assigned to fibrinolytic therapy or placebo 6–24 hours from symptom onset [78] revealed no evidence of increased rupture events with treatment beyond 12 hours.

**Table 3**   National Registry of Myocardial Infarction: Timing of In-Hospital Death

| Hospital | All MI patients | No fibrinolytic therapy | Fibrinolytic therapy | $P$ value[a] |
|---|---|---|---|---|
| Time from presentation to death, mean ± SEM (n) | 6.1 ± 0.0 days (35,442) | 6.3 ± 0.1 days (28,488) | 4.9 ± 0.1 days (6,954) | <.001 |
| Subanalysis Rupture/EMD: yes mean ± SEM (n) | 3.4 ± 0.1 days (2,621) | 3.7 ± 0.1 days (1,762) | 2.7 ± 0.1 days (859) | <.001 |
| Rupture/EMD: no mean ± SEM (n) | 6.3 ± 0.0 days (32,821) | 6.5 ± 0.1 days (26,726) | 5.2 ± 0.1 days (6,095) | <.001 |
| $P$ value[b] | <.001 | <.001 | <.001 | |

[a] Patients with versus those without fibrinolytic therapy.
[b] Patients with versus those without myocardial rupture/electromechanical dissociation (EMD).
The Wilcoxon test was used to compare time intervals.
MI = myocardial infarction.
(From Ref. 75)

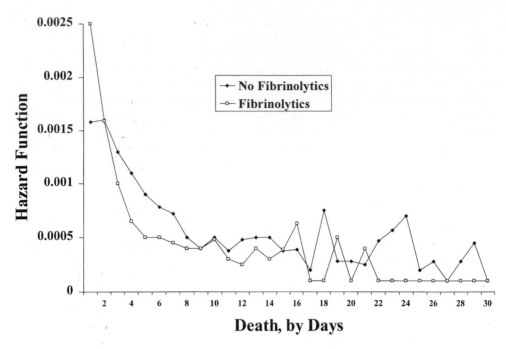

**Figure 11** Hazard function for death due to myocardial rupture in patients enrolled in the National Registry of Myocardial Infarction (Phase 1). Rupture was a more common cause of early death among fibrinolytic-treated patients. (From Ref. 72)

## Fibrinolytic Therapy and the Risk of Cardiac Rupture

Although fibrinolytic therapy represents an established means to reduce mortality in the setting of myocardial infarction, some clinicians remain concerned that its use is accompanied by an ''early hazard'' attributable to cardiac rupture. A comparison of studies carried out during the prereperfusion era does not reveal a major increase in events, which suggests that reperfusion itself is less likely to be a cause of cardiac rupture. In addition, the incidence of rupture also has not differed between groups in placebo-controlled fibrinolytic therapy trials. There is clear evidence that reperfusion reduces the extent of transmural injury and necrosis [79], still considered a prerequisite for rupture. Accordingly, successful thrombolysis should reduce the overall occurrence of mechanical events that are themselves the end result of extensive myocardial necrosis [80]. The low incidence of ventricular septal defects in GUSTO-1 coupled with the observation that a majority of patients with this mechanical event had an occluded infarct-related coronary artery support the ''closed artery hypothesis'' for cardiac rupture [81].

The most common cause of death among patients dying within 18 hours of enrollment in TIMI II was pump failure [82]. In a separate report by the GUSTO Investigators [83], early death (within the first 4 hours) was not influenced by coronary arterial patency status. This observation has several important implications. First, it suggests that very early death may not be preventable even with the restoration of coronary blood flow (at least not with current treatment strategies). Second, deaths occurring between 6 and 24 hours may, because of a predominant ischemic component, be preventable by means of reestablishing coronary blood flow. Lastly, the available evidence does not support the contention that cardiac rupture is a manifestation or form of ''reperfusion injury.''

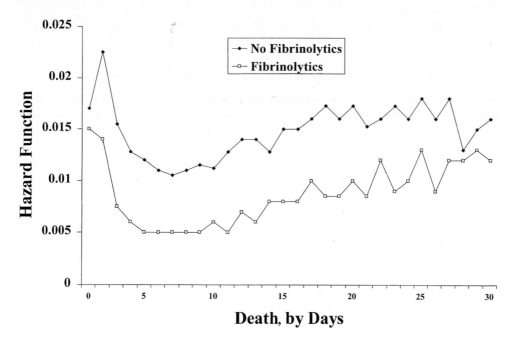

**Figure 12** Hazard function for deaths (all causes) among patients enrolled in the National Registry of Myocardial Infarction (Phase 1). Despite having an increased number of early myocardial rupture-related events, patients treated with fibrinolytics experienced a lower overall mortality than those not treated with fibrinolytics. (From Ref. 75)

The very low incidence of mechanical complications following primary angioplasty suggests strongly that reperfusion (or reperfusion injury) is not a cause of rupture [84]. An overview of the PAMI I and PAMI II trials (1295 patients undergoing primary angioplasty) reported a 0.31% combined incidence of acute mitral insufficiency and ventricular septal defects.

## Choice of Fibrinolytic Agent and the Risk of Cardiac Rupture

There is limited clinical and pathologic information that permits a direct comparison of fibrinolytic agents. However, based on the proposed mechanistic algorithm for rupture, one would anticipate a higher incidence of mechanical defects with agents (strategies) that yield relatively low patency rates (reduced myocardial salvage) and higher circulatory concentrations of plasmin. In the GUSTO-1 study, the incidence of rupture (mitral insufficiency/ventricular septal defect) correlated inversely with early TIMI grade 3 flow.

## Does Fibrinolytic Therapy Accelerate Cardiac Rupture?

When specific causes of death are being investigated, the beneficial impact of reperfusion therapy on overall patient outcome must never be overlooked. Indeed, as the mortality from early pump failure and malignant ventricular arrhythmias declines with the use of more effective reperfusion and adjunctive therapies, the contribution attributable to early rupture could increase. This "shift" may also be influenced by a reduced number of late ruptures—a direct reflection of myocardial preservation, reduced infarct expansion, and limited substrate for aneurysm development.

An acceleration of cardiac rupture, typically within the initial 24–48 hours, was appreciated in the TIMI II study, the LATE study [78], GUSTO-1 [81], and NRMI-1 [75].

Although there is limited information on the subject, it is conceivable that fibrinolytic therapy, through plasmin generation, accelerates type I and possibly type II ruptures.

### Does Antithrombotic Therapy Increase the Risk of Cardiac Rupture?

Anticoagulant therapy, either as a primary form of treatment or used adjunctively with fibrinolytics or primary angioplasty, is commonly utilized in the management of myocardial infarction. The association between anticoagulation and cardiac rupture has been examined; however, much of the information is based on observational studies.

From a series of 47 cases of cardiac rupture [31], 45% of patients had received either intravenous unfractionated heparin or oral anticoagulants. A comparative group of patients with fatal myocardial infarction (nonrupture) had a similar proportion of anticoagulant use. Among patients with rupture who were given anticoagulants, the majority received subtherapeutic levels (determined by the prothrombin time or Lee White clotting time). The investigators concluded that anticoagulant therapy did not affect the likelihood of cardiac rupture. Similar observations were made by Maher [85]; however, somewhat differing conclusions have been drawn by other investigators [86–88], who found a 3-fold increase in cardiac rupture and/or hemopericardium (with or without rupture) with anticoagulant use, particularly when the level of systemic anticoagulation was excessive. Considering all of the available information (964 patients in 5 moderate-size case series), the likelihood of cardiac rupture with and without anticoagulation was 4.2% and 3.7%, respectively.

The discrepant findings are difficult to explain; however, methodologic limitations within existing studies must be considered. First, anticoagulant therapy was not administered in a randomized fashion. Second, it is likely that heparin (and warfarin) was given to patients with larger infarctions. Lastly, several studies reporting an association between anticoagulant use and rupture compared patients from different time periods, introducing potentially important confounding variables.

Anticoagulant therapy is not known to have an adverse effect on myocardial healing following infarction, nor does it increase the extent of hemorrhage within the necrotic zone [89]. In the TIMI 9 study [90], hirudin, a potent and direct thrombin antagonist, when given adjunctively with either streptokinase or tPA did not increase the likelihood of rupture compared with heparin (Table 4). Hirudin also did not accelerate rupture events.

**Table 4**  Independent Predictors of Myocardial
Rupture: TIMI 9B Trial

| Variable | Odds ratio | value |
|---|---|---|
| Age >70 yrs | 4.96 | .0001 |
| Female sex | 3.59 | .0005 |
| Streptokinase | 1.69 | .10 |
| Hypertension | 1.32 | .42 |
| Q-wave MI | 1.28 | .52 |
| Smoker | 1.19 | .64 |
| Prior MI | 1.06 | .90 |
| Systolic BP >160 mm Hg | 0.94 | .01 |
| Hirudin | 0.79 | .48 |
| Diabetes | 0.65 | .38 |
| Fibrinolytic therapy >6 hr from symptom onset | 1.00 | 0.98 |

(From Ref. 90)

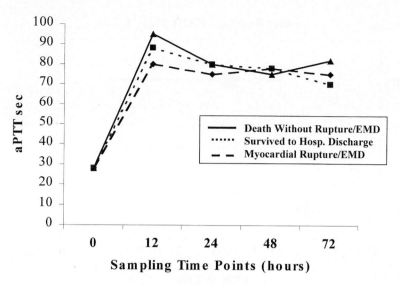

**Figure 13** Serial coagulation measurements (activated partial thromboplastin times, aPTT) for patients with and without cardiac rupture-related death and those surviving to hospital discharge. There were no differences in the intensity of anticoagulation at the 12-, 24-, 48-, and 72-hr sampling time points. (From Ref 90)

Although there was a clear relationship between the intensity of anticoagulation (as determined by the activated partial thromboplastin time) and the incidence of major hemorrhage, no correlation was found with myocardial rupture (Fig. 13).

## Do Platelet GPIIb/IIIa Antagonists Influence the Risk for Cardiac Rupture?

The available evidence derived from clinical trials of medically treated patients with acute coronary syndromes, those undergoing percutaneous coronary interventions, and combination low-dose fibrinolytic/intravenous GPIIb/IIIa receptor antagonists studies have not uncovered an increased occurrence of cardiac rupture.

## Age and Sex as Contributing Factors for Cardiac Rupture

In the TIMI 9 study [90] age older than 70 years, female sex, and prior angina were associated independently with cardiac rupture (Fig. 14a). Nonrupture-related death was associated with age older than 70 years, initial pulse more than 100 beats per minute, and prior myocardial infarction; female sex was not an independent predictor (Fig. 14b). Thus, cardiac rupture-related death may be responsible for the high early-mortality rates experienced by older women.

## DIAGNOSING CARDIAC RUPTURE

### Acute Free Wall Rupture

The primary obstacle to preventing death following acute free wall rupture is the limited time available to secure a diagnosis and rapidly proceed to the operating room for definitive

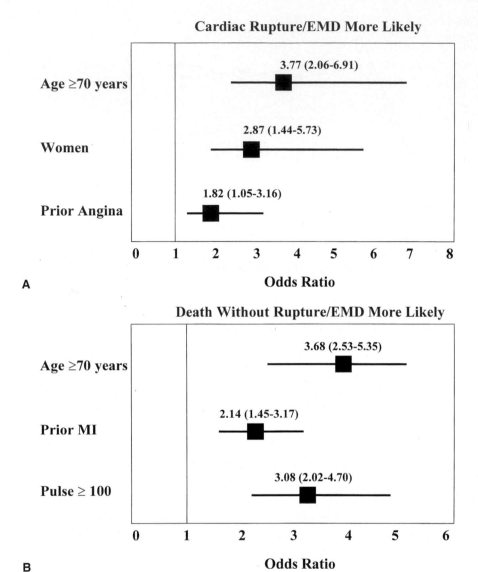

**Figure 14** (**A**) Multivariable analysis of patients experiencing myocardial rupture or electromechanical dissociation (EMD) identified age (70 years, female gender, and prior angina as independent predictors of an in-hospital event. (**A**) Multivariable analysis of patients with nonrupture-related death. Female sex was not associated with deaths unrelated to cardiac rupture.

treatment. Although free wall rupture most often causes progressive clinical deterioration, characterized by hypotension, electromechanical dissociation [91], and ultimately death, there are several preceding clinical features that may herald its occurrence. The clinical course and evolutionary electrocardiographic changes in 70 consecutive patients with cardiac rupture were described by Oliva and colleagues [92]. Patients experiencing rupture had increased incidence of pericarditis, repetitive emesis, restlessness, and agitation compared with patients without rupture. A deviation from the normal ST and T-wave evolutionary

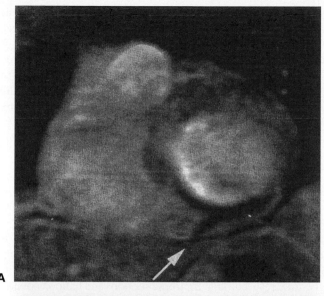

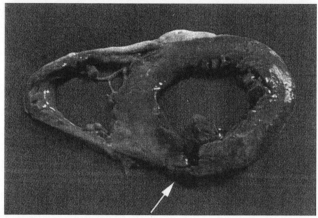

**Figure 15** (**A**) Cardiac MRI of acute myocardial infarction. Gradient-echo fast low-angle shot (2D-FLASH) sequence after gadolinium dethylene triamine pentaacetic acid injection; note in the infarcted area, a systolic hypoenhancement signal proceeding from the endocardium to the epicardium, suggesting impending rupture (*arrow*). (**B**) Cardiac rupture in middle portion of infarcted posterior wall (*arrow*). (From Ref. 94)

pattern (persistent ST elevation or upright T-waves) following infarction was observed in a majority of patients. An abrupt but transient period of hypotension and bradycardia was experienced by nearly one-quarter of patients within 24 hours after rupture. Free wall rupture may be the presenting manifestation of acute myocardial infarction in diabetic patients [93].

Magnetic resonance imaging could potentially be used to identify patients with impending cardiac rupture [94] (Fig. 15).

## Subacute Free Wall Rupture

In some cases, free wall rupture can progress over a 24- to 48-hour period—starting as a small endocardial tear followed by an intramyocardial hematoma that subsequently dissects to the myocardial surface. The sensitivity and specificity of clinical, hemodynamic, and electrocardiographic variables in diagnosing subacute free wall rupture were prospectively studied in 1247 consecutive patients with acute myocardial infarction, including 33 patients with rupture diagnosed at the time of surgery. The incidence of syncope, recurrent chest pain, hypotension, pulseless electrical activity, cardiac tamponade, pericardial effusion, echocardiographic right atrial or right ventricular wall collapse, and hemopericardium (demonstrated by pericardiocentesis) was significantly higher among patients with rupture than among those without [95].

## Ventricular Septal Rupture

Rupture of the ventricular septum causes less abrupt hemodynamic deterioration than free wall rupture and should be suspected in patients with unexplained hemodynamic deterioration, particularly in the presence of a new holosystolic murmur. The diagnosis can be strengthened by echocardiographic findings and confirmed by the presence of an oxygen ''step up'' at the level of the right ventricle. Progressive hemodynamic deterioration represents the combined effects of decreased left ventricular stroke volume and right ventricular failure. Accordingly, fluid resuscitation, inotropic support, and balloon counterpulsation represent the therapeutic mainstays that are designed to provide initial stabilization followed by definitive surgical intervention [96]. The use of intrapulmonary balloon counterpulsation should be considered a perioperative management option for patients undergoing surgical repair.

## SURGICAL INTERVENTION OF CARDIAC RUPTURE

The surgical approach to cardiac rupture has historically been individualized and approached on a case-by-case basis. Since the natural history of subacute or ''delayed'' rupture is largely unknown, emergent or urgent surgery is warranted if the patient is deemed an operative candidate. Attempts to optimize comorbid conditions must be factored against progressive hemodynamic deterioration or sudden death. The goals of surgery are: a) relief of tamponade, b) cardiac resuscitation, c) repair or containment of the defect, and d) concomitant myocardial revascularization.

Repair of the infarcted area ranges from wide debridement of infarcted myocardial muscle and linear buttressed closure or patch closure around a pledgeted base. The current technique, which includes placing a prosthetic or bovine pericardial patch over the unresected area, is expedient and technologically appealing; however, long-term follow-up of this technique is incomplete.

## Surgical History of Cardiac Rupture Repair

Lillehei in 1969 [97] is credited with the first attempt at surgical repair of cardiac rupture. In March 1968, a 50-year-old man underwent repair 10 days after an acute myocardial infarction. He died 37 days postoperatively. In 1971, Friedman reported an unsuccessful attempt to repair a posterior rupture without cardiopulmonary bypass. FitzGibbon [98] successfully repaired a cardiac rupture developing 21 days after a large anteroseptal myocardial infarction.

The early cases, while considered anecdotal by current standards, were nonetheless vital to the development of surgical techniques [97–126]. The majority of patients were male and had either mixed anterior or posterior sites of infarction, surgical infarctectomy, debridement, and buttressed repair. Few patients underwent concomitant myocardial revascularization; however, cardiopulmonary bypass did play a pivotal role in the initial resuscitation of patients who survived the operation (35 of 49; 70%). The reports, however, focused solely on short-term outcome and offered little diagnostic or investigative follow-up.

There are several case studies that have included complex ruptures and at least 2 published reports of cardiac rupture following myocardial revascularization. Charnvechai [127] reported 7 patients with rupture of the left ventricular free wall following internal mammary artery implantation (Vineberg procedure). Few details were provided, yet false passage to the subepicardial area is a potential explanation. Fortunately, this procedure is rarely performed today. Bojar [128] reported successful left ventricular free wall rupture repair in a patient 5 days after bypass surgery.

Myocardial cardiac rupture does occur in association with left ventricular true or false aneurysms. Abel in 1976 [106] observed a rupture at the junction of a left ventricular aneurysm and normal myocardium. This observation is in conflict with the findings of Vlodaver [129], who reported that fibrous left ventricular aneurysms rarely rupture. There is little question, however, that false aneurysms do rupture. Yaku in 1995 [130] reported the successful repair of an early false aneurysm (less than 10 days).

Recent advances in surgery have focused on an aggressive approach to patients with subacute cardiac rupture, including patients with dissection, hematoma, or "concealed" ruptures. Pliam reviewed 12 cases from 1944 to 1991 [131–142]. All 5 surgical cases survived while only one of 7 patients receiving medical management did so. The appealing features of the surgery are omission of cardiopulmonary bypass and avoidance of resection/debridement. Instead, biological glues buttressed with pericardial or synthetic patches are used. Although the short-term results are dramatic, long-term data regarding survival or pseudoaneurysm formation is incomplete. The role of concomitant myocardial revascularization is also unknown. We recommend preoperative coronary angiography if the clinical status of the patient permits.

Advances in the surgical approach to cardiac rupture were highlighted by Padró in 1989 [143]. A 62-year-old woman underwent emergency surgery 7 days after an acute myocardial infarction. A large anterolateral transmural infarction was found with several epicardial bleeding points and a large volume of blood in the pericardium. Without the institution of cardiopulmonary bypass, the bleeding points were controlled with butyl-2-cyanoacrylate glue. A large Teflon patch was then placed over the entire area. The patient was alive at 15-month follow-up. Zogno [144] applied the same technique successfully. During cardiopulmonary bypass, a 2-cm linear anterolateral tear was coated with fibrin glue. A glutaraldehyde-stiffened patch of autologous pericardium was then placed over the area and sewn to surrounding normal myocardium with a running 5-0 polypropylene suture. Padró [145] summarized his surgical experience with myocardial rupture in 1993. For 13 patients with rupture, repair was done with cyanoacrylate glue and Teflon patch. Only 1 patient (with a posterior wall rupture) required cardiopulmonary bypass. All patients survived surgery. At follow-up (26 months), there was 100% survival. Five patients had transthoracic echocardiography performed at 3–7 months without evidence of psuedoaneurysm development. A similar result was reported by Almdahl [146].

Coletti and colleagues [147] reported 3 cases of cardiac rupture repaired with fibrin glue (2 cases) and gelatin-resorcinol-formol (GRF) biological glue (1 case) covered by an autologous glutaraldehyde-stiffened pericardial patch and fixed with running sutures on the adjacent healthy myocardium. Echocardiography performed serially to 3 months did not reveal evidence of pseudoaneurysm formation.

## Current Considerations for Surgical Repair

The natural history of cardiac rupture that includes 50% mortality within 5 days and 87% within 2 weeks of infarction justifies the urgency of surgical repair. Traditional methods of repair including infarctectomy, debridement, and buttressed linear or patch closure has been challenged in recent years. The employment of biological glues with patch reinforcement has provided encouraging short-term results. It should be stressed that preoperative use of intraaortic balloon counterpulsation and pericardiocentesis are temporizing modalities. Although the use of cardiopulmonary bypass is not universally accepted, supporters point out that a more precise repair, concomitant myocardial revascularization, and optimization of resuscitative efforts are more successfully accomplished while the patient is on bypass.

In emergent or urgent situations, the presence of cardiac tamponade following acute myocardial infarction indicates left ventricular free wall rupture until proven otherwise. Immediate echocardiography followed by surgery is the best chance for survival. According to López-Sendón [95], based on a series of 33 operative cases, 25 (76%) survived after an aggressive approach was undertaken. A series by Cheriex [148] in 1995 showed 9 of 12 patients (75%) surviving myocardial rupture after aggressive treatment. The trend toward rapid diagnosis and aggressive surgical intervention has yielded a greater than 70% chance of survival.

## Percutaneous Strategies for Cardiac Rupture

Although surgical intervention represents the standard of care for patients with free wall myocardial rupture in whom aggressive intervention is deemed appropriate, percutaneous strategies have been investigated as a means of achieving rapid stabilization. A recent report outlined the potential use of intrapericardial fibrin glue following pericardial drainage as a therapeutic option [149].

## SUMMARY

Cardiac rupture is an infrequent but well-recognized and typically fatal complication of acute myocardial infarction that can involve the left ventricular free wall, ventricular septum, papillary muscle, right ventricular free wall, and atrium. Although typically occurring between 4–7 days after infarction, cardiac rupture can manifest within the first 24–48 hours, particularly among patients receiving fibrinolytic therapy. Older women are at increased risk for cardiac rupture, possibly due to unique features of reparative processes, collagen matrix, proteolytic enzymes, and wall stress, defining the genomic profile of patients at risk for cardiac rupture in an area of investigation. Early β-blockade and ACE inhibitor therapy do offer protective effects.

The diagnosis of cardiac rupture begins with a high index of suspicion and must be considered strongly in the setting of sudden or rapidly progressive hemodynamic compromise. Prompt diagnosis and stabilization achieved with pericardiocentesis, intravenous fluid administration, and hemodynamic support followed by definitive surgical intervention are the keys to a favorable clinical outcome.

## REFERENCES

1. Harvey W. Complete Works. London: Syndenham Society, 1847.
2. Morgagni JB. The Seats and Causes of Disease Investigated by Anatomy: In Five Books, Containing a Great Variety of Dissections with Remarks. Millar A&, Cadell T, Eds. Vol. 1. London: Translated by B. Alexander, 1769 Letter 27:830.

3. Malmsten T, Cited by Benson RL, Hunter WC, Manlove CH. Spontaneous rupture of heart: report of 40 cases in Portland, Oregon. Am J Pathol 1933;9:295–328.

4. Benson RL, Hunter WC, Manlove CH. Spontaneous rupture of heart: report of 40 cases in Portland, Oregon. Am J Pathol 1933;9:295–328.

5. Krumbhaar EB, Crowell C. Spontaneous rupture of heart: clinicopathologic study based on 22 unpublished cases and 632 from literature. Am J Med Sci 1925;170:828–856.

6. Parkinson J, Bedford DE. Cardiac infarction and coronary thrombosis. Lancet 1928;1:4–11.

7. Levine SA. Coronary thrombosis: its various clinical features. Medicine 1929;8:245–418.

8. Bean WB. Infarction of heart. III. Clinical course and morphological findings. Ann Intern Med 1938;12:71–94.

9. Mallory GK, White PD, Sahedo-Salgar J. The speed of healing of myocardial infarction. Am Heart J 1939;18:647–671.

10. Edmondson HA, Hoxie HJ. Hypertension and cardiac rupture. Am Heart J 1942;24:719–733.

11. Friedman S, White PD. Rupture of the heart in myocardial infarction. Ann Intern Med 1944; 21:778–782.

12. Mintz SS, Katz LN. Recent myocardial infarction: Analysis of 572 cases. Arch Intern Med 1947;80:205–236.

13. Wartman WB, Hellerstein HK. Incidence of heart disease in 2,000 consecutive autopsies. Ann Intern Med 1948;28:41–65.

14. Selzer A. Immediate sequelae of myocardial infarction: their relation to prognosis. Am J Med Sci 1948;216:172–178.

15. Diaz-Rivera RS, Miller AJ. Rupture of heart following acute myocardial infarction: Incidence in public hospital, with five illustrative cases including one of perforation of interventricular septum diagnosed antemortem. Am Heart J 1948;35:126–133.

16. Foord AG. Embolism and thrombosis in coronary artery disease. JAMA 1948;138: 1009–1009.

17. Wang CH, Bland EF, White PD. Note on coronary occlusion and myocardial infarction found postmortem at Massachusetts General Hospital during twenty year period from 1926 to 1945 inclusive. Ann Intern Med 1948;29:601–606.

18. Howell DA, Tumbell GC. Hypertension and effort in cardiac rupture following acute myocardial infarction. Q Bull NWU Med School 1950;24:100–103.

19. Zinn WJ, Cosby RS. Myocardial infarction. I. Statistical analysis of 679 autopsy proven cases. Am J Med 1950;8:169–176.

20. Oblath RW, Levenson DC, Griffith GC. Factors influencing rupture of the heart after myocardial infarction. JAMA 1952;149:1276–1281.

21. Wessler S, Zoll PM, Schlesinger MI. The pathogenesis of spontaneous cardiac rupture. Circulation 1952;6:334–351.

22. Waldron BR, Fennel RH, Castelman B, Bland EF. Myocardial rupture and hemopericardium associated with anticoagulant therapy. A postmortem study. N Engl J Med 1954;251:892–894.

23. Goetz AA, Gropper AN. Perforation of interventricular septum. Am Heart J 1954;48:130–140.

24. Mcdonniael SH, Humbrecht M, Voorhies NW. Cardiac rupture. J Louisiana Med Soc 1955; 107:171–177.

25. Maher JF, Mallory GK, Laurenz GA. Rupture of the heart after myocardial infarction. N Engl J Med 1956;255:1–10.

26. Zeman F, Rodstein M. Cardiac rupture complicating myocardial infarction in the aged. Arch Intern Med 1960;105:431–433.

27. Griffith GC, Hedge B, Oblath RW. Factors in myocardial rupture. An analysis of 204 cases at Los Angeles County Hospital between 1924–1959. Am J Cardiol 1961;8:792–798.

28. Friedberg CK. General treatment of acute myocardial infarction. Circulation 1969;39(40: Suppl IV):IV–252–260.

29. Ross RM, Young JA. Clinical and necropsy findings in rupture of the myocardium. A review of 43 cases. Scott Med J 1963;8:222–226.

30. Sievers J. Cardiac rupture in acute myocardial infarction. Geriatrics 1966;21:125–130.

31. London RE, London SB. Rupture of the heart. A critical analysis of 47 consecutive autopsy cases. Circulation 1965;31:202–208.

32. Sugiura M, Okada R, Morii T, Hiraoka K, Shimada H, Nakanishi A. A clinicopathological study on the cardiac rupture following myocardial infarction in the aged. Jpn Heart J 1968; 9:265–280.

33. Sahebjaml H. Myocardial infarction and cardiac rupture. Analysis of 37 cases and a brief review of the literature. South Med J 1969;62:1058–1063.

34. Lewis JL, Burchell HB, Titus JL. Clinical and pathologic features of postinfarction cardiac rupture. Am J Cardiol 1969;23:43–53.

35. Beutler SM, Toscano M. Cardiac rupture in the University of Chicago. Personal observations. Am Heart J 1942;23:455–467.

36. Meurs AAH, Vos AK, Verhey JB, Gerbrandy J. Electrocardiogram during cardiac rupture by myocardial infarction. Br Heart J 1970;32:232–235.

37. Gjol N. Cardiac rupture and acute myocardial infarction. Geriatrics 1972;26:126–137.

38. Naeim F, de al Maza LM, Robbins SL. Cardiac rupture during myocardial infarction: a review of 44 cases. Circulation 1972;45:1231–1239.

39. Hammer J, Fabian J, Pavlovic J, Smid J. Myocardial rupture in acute myocardial infarction. Cor Vasa 1972;14:180–187.

40. Havig O. Cardiac rupture in recent myocardial infarction. Acta Pathol Microbiol Scand [A] 1973;81:501–506.

41. Sievers J. Cardiac rupture in acute myocardial infarction:. Geriatrics 1996;21:125–130.

42. Spiekerman RE, Brandenburg JT, Achor RWP. The spectrum of coronary artery disease in a community of 30,000. A clinicopathologic study. Circulation 1962;25:57–65.

43. Slater J, Brown RJ, Antonelli TA, Menon V, Boland J, Col J, Dzavik V, Greenberg M, Menegus M, Connery C, Hochman JS. Cardiogenic shock due to cardiac free-wall rupture or tamponade after acute myocardial infarction: a report from the SHOCK Trial Registry. Should we emergently revascularize occluded coronaries for cardiogenic shock? J Am Coll Cardiol; 2000;36(3 Suppl A):1117–1122.

44. Becker AE, van Mantgem JP. Cardiac tamponade. A study of 50 hearts. Eur J Cardiol 1974; 3/4:349–358.

45. Kassis E, Vogelsang M, Lyngborg K. Cardiac rupture complicating myocardial infarction. A study concerning early diagnosis and possible management. Dan Med Bull 1981;48:164–167.

46. Matsui K, Kay JH, Mendez M. Ventricular septal rupture secondary to myocardial infarction. Clinical approach and surgical results. JAMA 1981;245:1537–1539.

47. Menon V, Webb JG, Hillis LD, Sleeper LA, Abboud R, Dzavik V, Slater JN, Forman R, Monrad ES, Talley JD, Hochman JS. Outcome and profile of ventricular septal rupture with cardiogenic shock after myocardial infarction: a report from the SHOCK Trial Registry. Should we emergently revascularize Occluded Coronaries in cardiogenic shock? J Am Coll Cardiol 2000; Vol. 36:1110–1116.

48. Thompson CR, Buller CE, Sleeper LA, Antonelli TA, Webb JG, Jaber WA, Abel JG, Hochman JS. Cardiogenic shock due to acute severe mitral regurgitation complicating acute myocardial infarction: a report from the SHOCK Trial Registry. Should we use emergently revascularize Occluded Coronaries in cardiogenic shock. J Am Coll Cardiol; 2000;36(3 Suppl A): 1104–1109.

49. Figueras J, Cortadellas J, Soler-Soler J. Comparison of ventricular septal and left ventricular free wall rupture in acute myocardial infarction. Am J Cardiol 1998;81(4):495–497.

50. Srichai MB, Casserly IP, Lever HM. Cardiac tamponade masking clinical presentation and hemodynamic effects of papillary muscle rupture after acute myocardial infarction. J Am Soc Echocardiography 2002;15(9):1000–1003.

51. Vargas-Barron J, Roldan FJ, Romero-Cardenas A, Espinola-Zavaleta N, Keirns C, Gonzalez–Pacheco H. Two- and three-dimensional transesophageal echocardiographic diagnosis of intramyocardial dissecting hematoma after myocardial infarction. J Am Soc Echocardiography 2001;14(6):637–640.

52. Harpaz D, Kriwisky M, Cohen AJ, Medalion B, Rozenman Y. Unusual form of cardiac rupture: sealed subacute left ventricular free wall rupture, evolving to intramyocardial dissecting hematoma and to pseudoaneurysm formation—a case report and review of the literature. J Am Soc Echocardiography 2001;14(3):219–227.

53. Lautsch EV, Lanks KW. Pathogenesis of cardiac rupture. Arch Path 1967;84:264–271.

54. London RE, London SB. The electrocardiographic signs of acute hemopericardium. Circulation 1962;25:780–786.

55. Bartunek J, Vanderheyden M, De Bruyne B. Dynamic left ventricular outflow obstruction after anterior myocardial infarction. Eur Heart J 1995;16:1439–1442.

56. Reisenhofer B, Squarcini G, Picano E. Cardiac rupture during dobutamine stress test. Ann Int Med 1998;128:605.

57. Heymans S, Luttun A, Nuyens D, Theilmeier G, Creemers E, Moons L, Dyspersin GD, Cleutjens JPM, Shipley M, Angellilo A, Levi M, NüBaker A, Keshet E, Lupu F, Herbert J–M, Smits JFM, Shapiro SD, Baes M, Borgers M, Collen D, Daemen MJAP, Carmeliet P. Inhibition of plasminogen activators or matrix metalloproteinases prevents cardiac rupture but impairs therapeutic angiogenesis and causes cardiac failure. Nature Med 1999;5:1135–1142.

58. Ichihara S, Senbonmatsu T, Prices E, Ichiki T, Gaffney FA, Inagami T. Targeted deletion of angiotensin II type 2 receptor caused cardiac rupture after acute myocardial infarction. Circulation 2002;106(17):2244–2249.

59. Heymans S, Luttun A, Nuyens D, Theilmeier G, Creemers E, Moons L, Dyspersin GD, Cleutjens JP, Shipley M, Angellilo A, Levi M, Nube O, Baker A, Keshet E, Lupu F, Herbert JM, Smits JF, Shapiro SD, Baes M, Borgers M, Collen D, Daemen MJ, Carmeliet P. Inhibition of plasminogen activators or matrix metalloproteinases prevents cardiac rupture but impairs therapeutic angiogenesis and causes cardiac failure. Nature Medicine 1999;5(10):1135–42.

60. McNamara JJ, Lacro RV, Yee M, Smith GT. Hemorrhagic infarction and coronary reperfusion. J Thorac Cardiovasc Surg 1981;81:498–501.

61. Vander Salm TJ, Pape LA, Price J, Burke M. Hemorrhage from myocardial revascularization. J Thorac Cardiovasc Surg 1981;82:768–772.

62. Higginson LAJ, White F, Heggtveit HA, Sanders TM, Bloor CM, Covell JW. Determinants of myocardial hemorrhage after coronary reperfusion in the anesthetized dog. Circulation 1982;65:62–69.

63. Kloner RA, Alker KJ. The effect of streptokinase on intramyocardial hemorrhage, infarct size, and the no-reflow phenomenon during coronary reperfusion. Circulation 1984;70:513–521.

64. Whittaker P, Boughner DR, Kloner RA. Role of collagen in acute myocardial infarct expansion. Circulation 1991;84:2123–2134.

65. Mathey DG, Schofer J, Kuck K-H, Beil U, Klöppel G. Transmural, haemorrhagic myocardial infarction after intracoronary streptokinase. Clinical, angiographic, and necropsy findings. Br Heart J 1982;48:546–551.

66. Fujiwara H, Onodera T, Tanaka M, Fujiwara T, Wu DJ, Kawai C, Hamashima Y. A clinicopathologic study of patients with hemorrhagic myocardial infarction treated with selective coronary thrombolysis with urokinase. Circulation 1986;73:749–757.

67. Waller BF. The pathology of acute myocardial infarction: Definition, location, pathogenesis, effects of reperfusion, complications and sequelae. Cardiol Clin 1988;6:1–28.

68. Peuhkurinen KJ, Risteli L, Melkko JT, Med C, Linnaluoto M, Jounela A, Risteli J. Thrombolytic therapy with streptokinase stimulates collagen breakdown. Circulation 1991;83: 1969–1975.

69. Gertz SD, Kalan JM, Kragel AH, Roberts WC, Braunwald E. and the TIMI Investigators. Cardiac morphologic findings in patients with acute myocardial infarction treated with recombinant tissue plasminogen activator. Am J Cardiol 1990;65:953–961.

70. Whittaker P. Unravelling the mysteries of collagen and cilatrix after myocardial infarction. Cardiovasc Res 1996;31:19–26.

71. Charney RH, Takahashi S, Zhao M, Sonnenblick EH, Eng C. Collagen loss in the stunned myocardium. Circulation 1992;85:1483–1490.

72. Factor SM, Robinson TF, Dominitz R, Cho S. Alterations of the myocardial skeletal framework in acute myocardial infarction with and without ventricular rupture. A preliminary report. Am J Cardiovasc Pathol 1986;1:91–97.

73. Pohjola-Sintonen S, Muller JE, Stone PH, Willich SN, Antman EM, Davis VG, Parker CB, Braunwald E. and the MILIS study group. Ventricular septal and free wall rupture complicat-

ing acute myocardial infarction: Experience in the multicenter investigation of limitation of infarct size. Am Heart J 1989;117:809–816.

74. Maggioni AP, Maseri A, Fresco C, Franzosi MG, Mauri F, Santoro E, Tognoni G. on behalf of the Investigators of the Gruppo Italiano per lo Studio della Sopravvivenza nell 'Infarto Miocardico (GISSI-2). Age-related increase in mortality among patients with first myocardial infarctions treated with thrombolysis. N Engl J Med 1993;11:1442–1448.

75. Becker RC, Gore JM, Lambrew C, Weaver WD, Rubison RM, French WJ, Tiefenbrunn AJ, Bowlby LJ, Rogers WJ. A composite view of cardiac rupture in the United States National Registry of Myocardial Infarction. J Am Coll Cardiol 1996;27:1321–1326.

76. Mauri F, DeBiase AM, Franzosi MD, Pampallona S, Foresti A, Gasparini M. GISSI analisis cause di morte intraspedaliera. G Ital Cardiol 1987;17:37–44.

77. Honan MB, Harrell FE, Reimer KA, Califf RM, Mark DB, Pryor DB, Hlatky MA. Cardiac rupture, mortality and the timing of thrombolytic therapy: a meta-analysis. J Am Coll Cardiol 1990;16:359–367.

78. Becker RC, Charlesworth A, Wilcox RG, Hampton J, Skene A, Gore JM, Topol EJ. Cardiac rupture associated with thrombolytic therapy: Impact of time to treatment in the late assessment of thrombolytic efficacy (LATE) study. J Amer Coll Cardiol 1995;25:1063–1068.

79. Correale E, Maggioni AP, Romano S, Ricciardiello V, Battista R, Salvarola G, Santoro E, Tognoni G. on behalf of the Gruppo Italiano per lo Studio della Sopravvivenza nell'Infarto Miocardico (GISSI). Am J Cardiol 1993;71:1377–1381.

80. Nakamura F, Minamino T, Higashino Y, Ito H, Fujii K, Fujita T, Nagano M, Higaki J, Ogihara T. Cardiac free wall rupture in acute myocardial infarction: Ameliorative effect of coronary reperfusion. Clin Cardiol 1992;15:244–250.

81. Crenshaw BS, Granger CB, Birnbaum Y, Pieper KS, Morris DC, Kleiman NS, Vahanian A, Califf RM, Topol EJ. Risk factors, angiographic patterns, and outcomes in patients with ventricular septal defect complicating acute myocardial infarction. GUSTO-I (Global Utilization of Streptokinase and TPA for Occluded Arteries) Trial Investigators. Circulation 2000; 101(1):27–32.

82. Kleiman NS, Terrin M, Mueller H. and the TIMI Investigators. Mechanisms of early death despite thrombolytic therapy: Experience from the TIMI II Study. J Am Coll Cardiol 1992; 19:1129–1135.

83. Kleiman NS, White HD, Ohman EM. for the GUSTO Investigators. Mortality within 24 hours of thrombolysis from myocardial infarction: the importance of early reperfusion. Circulation 1994;20:2658–2665.

84. Brodie BR, Stuckey TD, Hansen CJ, Muncy DB, Weintraub RA, Kelly TA, Berry JJ. Timing and mechanism of death determined clinically after primary angioplasty for acute myocardial infarction. Am J Cardiol 1997;79:1586–1591.

85. Maher JF, Mallory GK, Laurenz GA. Rupture of the heart after myocardial infarction. N Engl J Med 1956;255:1–10.

86. Aarseth S, Lange HF. The influence of anticoagulant therapy on the occurrence of cardiac rupture and hemopericardium following heart infarction. I. A study of 89 cases of hemopericardium (81 of them cardiac ruptures). Am Heart J 1958:250–256.

87. Lee KT, O'Neal RM. Anticoagulant therapy of acute myocardial infarction. An evaluation from autopsy data with special reference to myocardial rupture and thromboembolic complications. Am J Med 1956;21:555–559.

88. Capeci NE, Levy RL. The influence of anticoagulant therapy on the incidence of thromboembolism, hemorrhage and cardiac rupture in acute myocardial infarction. Am J Med 1959;26: 76–80.

89. Blumgart HL, Freedberg AS, Zoll PM, Lewis HB, Wessler S. Effect of Dicumarol on heart in experimental acute coronary occlusion. Am Heart J 1948;36:13–27.

90. Becker RC, Hochman JS, Cannon CP, Spencer FA, Ball SP, Rizzo MJ, Antman EM. Fatal cardiac rupture among patients treated with thrombolytic agents and adjunctive thrombin antagonists: Observations from the Thrombolysis and Thrombin Inhibition in Myocardial Infarction 9 Study. J Am Coll Cardiol 1999;33:479–487.

91. Figueras J, Curós A, Cortadellas J, Soler-Soler J. Reliability of electromechanical dissociation in the diagnosis of left ventricular free wall rupture in acute myocardial infarction. American Heart Journal 1996;131:861–864.

92. Oliva PB, Hammill SC, Edwards WD. Cardiac rupture, a clinically predictable complication of acute myocardial infarction: Report of 70 cases with clinicopathologic correlations. J Amer Coll Cardiol 1993;22:720–726.

93. Zahger D, Milgalter E, Pollak A, Hasin Y, Merin G, Beeri R, Gotsman MS. Left ventricular free wall rupture as the presenting manifestation of acute myocardial infarction in diabetic patients. Am J Cardiol 1996;78:681–682.

94. Zoni A, Arisi A, Corradi D, Ardissino D. Images in cardiovascular medicine. Magnetic resonance imaging of impending left ventricular rupture after acute myocardial infarction. Circulation 2003;108(4):498–499.

95. López-Sendón J, González A, López de Sá E, Coma-Canella I, Roldán I, Domínguez F, Maqueda I, Jadraque LM. Diagnosis of subacute ventricular wall rupture after acute myocardial infarction: Sensitivity and specificity of clinical, hemodynamic and echocardiographic criteria. J Amer Coll Cardiol 1992;19:1145–1153.

96. Radford MJ, Johnson RA, Daggett WM, Fallon JT, Buckley MJ, Gold HK, Leinbach RC. Ventricular septal rupture: A review of clinical and physiologic features and an analysis of survival. Circulation 1981;64:545–553.

97. Lillehei CW, Lande AJ, Rassman WR, Tanaka S, Bloch JH. Surgical management of myocardial infarction. Circulation (Suppl. IV) 1969;39:315–333.

98. FitzGibbon GM, Hooper GD, Heggtveit HA. Successful surgical treatment of postinfarction external cardiac rupture. J Thorac Cardiovasc Surg 1972;63:622–630.

99. Hatcher CR, Mansour K, Logan WD, Symbas PN, Abbott OA. Surgical complications of myocardial infarction. Am Surg 1970;36:163–170.

100. Friedman HS, Kuhn LA, Katz AM. Clinical and electrocardiographic features of cardiac rupture following acute myocardial infarction. Am J Med 1971;50:709–720.

101. Löfström B, Mogensen L, Nyquist O, Orinius E, Sjögren A, Werner B. Attempts at emergency surgical treatment. Chest 1972;61:10–13.

102. Montegut FJ. Left ventricular rupture secondary to myocardial infarction. Ann Thorac Surg 1972;14:75–78.

103. Cobbs BW, Hatcher CR, Robinson PH. Cardiac rupture. JAMA 1973;223:532–535.

104. O'Rourke MF. Subacute heart rupture following myocardial infarction. Lancet 1973;2:124–126.

105. Calick A, Kerth W, Barbour D, Cohn K. Successful surgical therapy of ruptured myocardium. Chest 1974;66:188.

106. Abel RM, Buckley MJ, Friedlich AL, Austen WG. Survival following free rupture of left ventricular aneurysm: report of a case. Ann Thorac Surg 1976;21:175–179.

107. Anagnostoupoulos E, Beutler S, Levett JM, Lawrence JM, Lin CY, Replogle RL. Myocardial rupture: major left ventricular infarct rupture treated by infarctectomy. JAMA 1977;238:2715–2716.

108. Eisenmann B, Bareiss P, Pacifico AD, Jeanblanc B, Kretz JG, Baehrel B, Warter J, Kieny R. Anatomic, clinical, and therapeutic features of acute cardiac rupture. J Thorac Cardio Vasc Surg 1978;76:78–82.

109. Kendall RW, DeWood MA. Postinfarction cardiac rupture: surgical success and review of the literature. Ann Thorac Surg 1978;25:311–315.

110. Parr GV, Pae WE, Pierce WS, Zellis R. Cardiogenic shock due to ventricular rupture. J Thorac Cardiovasc Surg 1981;82:889–891.

111. Windsor HM, Chang VP, Shanahan MX. Postinfarction cardiac rupture. J Thorac Cardiovasc Surg 1982;84:755–761.

112. Bashour T, Kabbani SS, Ellertson DG, Crew J, Hanna ES. Surgical salvage of heart rupture: Report of two cases and review of the literature. Ann Thorac Surg 1983;36:209–213.

113. Feneley MP, Chang VP, O'Rourke MF. Myocardial rupture after acute myocardial infarction. Br Heart J 1983;49:550–556.

114. Nunez L, de la Llana R, López-Sendon J, Coma I, Gil-Aguado M, Larrea JL. Diagnosis and treatment of subacute free wall ventricular rupture after infarction. Ann Thorac Surg 1983; 35:525–529.

115. Pifarré R, Sullivan HJ, Grieco J, Montoya A, Bakhos M, Scanlon PJ, Gunnar RM. Management of left ventricular rupture complicating myocardial infarction. J Thorac Cardiovasc Surg 1983;86:441–443.

116. Hochreiter C, Goldstein J, Borer JS, Tyberg T, Goldberg HL, Subramanian V, Rosenfeld I. Myocardial free-wall rupture after acute infarction. Circulation 1982;65:1279–1284.

117. Choo MH, Chia BL, Chia F. Cardiac tamponade from ventricular rupture: value of two-dimensional echocardiography in guiding acute surgical management. Crit Care Med 1985; 13:446–447.

118. McMullan MH, Kilgore TL, Dear HD, Hindman SH. Sudden blowout rupture of the myocardium after infarction: urgent management. J Thorac Cardiovasc Surg 1985;89:259–263.

119. Stiegel M, Zimmern SH, Robicsek F. Left ventricular rupture following coronary occlusion treated by streptokinase infusion: Successful surgical repair. Ann Thorac Surg 1987;44: 413–415.

120. Pierli C, Lisi G, Mezzacapo B. Subacute left ventricular free wall rupture. Chest 1991;100: 1174–1176.

121. Luciani GB, Tappainer E, Pessotto R, Fabbri A, Mazzucco A. Mechanical support for decompression of the left ventricle in repair of ischemic cardiac rupture. J Card Surg 1993;8: 638–640.

122. Komeda M, Mickleborough LL. Concealed rupture of the left ventricle: successful surgical repair. Ann Thor Surg 1994;57:1333–1335.

123. Sakakibana T, Matsuwaka R, Shintani H, Yagura A, Yamaguchi T, Nirayama A, Kodama K. Successful repair of postinfarction left ventricular free wall rupture: New strategy with hypothermic percutaneous cardiopulmonary bypass. J Thorac Cardiovasc Surg 1996;111: 276–276.

124. Sutherland FW, Guell FJ, Pathi VL, Naik SK. Postinfarction ventricular free wall rupture: strategies for diagnosis and treatment. Ann Thorac Surg 1996;61:1281–1285.

125. Reardon MJ, Carr CL, Diamond A, Letsou GV, Safi HJ, Espada R, Baldwin JC. Ischemic left ventricular free wall rupture: Prediction, diagnosis, and treatment. Ann Thorac Surg 1997; 64:1509–1513.

126. Zeebregts CJ, Noyez L, Hensens AG, Skotnicki SH, Lacquet LK. Surgical repair of subacute left ventricular free wall rupture. J Card Surg 1997;12:416–419.

127. Charnvechai C, Effler DB. Postoperative myocardial rupture. Ann Thorac Surg 1972;13: 458–463.

128. Bojar RM, Overton JW, Madoff IM. Successful management of left ventricular rupture following myocardial revascularization. Ann Thorac Surg 1987;44:312–314.

129. Vlodaver Z, Coe JI, Edwards JE. True and false left ventricular aneurysms. Propensity for the latter to rupture. Circulation 1975;51:567–572.

130. Yaku H, Fermanis G, Horton DA, Guy D, Lvoff R. Successful repair of a ruptured postinfarct pseudoaneurysm of the left ventricle. Ann Rhorac Surg 1995;60:1097–1098.

131. Pliam MB, Sternlieb JJ. Intramyocardial dissecting hematoma: an unusual form of subacute cardiac rupture. J Card Surg 1993;8:628–637.

132. Wood A. Perforation of the interventricular septum due to cardiac infarction. Br Heart J 1944;6:191–193.

133. Peel AAF. Dissecting aneurysm of the interventricular septum. Br Heart J 1948;10:239–243.

134. Lewis AJ, Burchell HB, Titus JL. Clinical and pathologic features of postinfarction cardiac rupture. Am J Cardiol 1969;23:43–53.

135. Awan NA, Ikeda R, Olson H, Hata J, DeMaria AN, Vera Z, Miller RR, Amsterdam EA, Mason DT. Intraventricular free wall dissection causing acute interventricular communication with intact septum in myocardial infarction. Chest 1976;69:782–785.

136. Daubert JC, Mattheyses M, Fourdilis M, Pony JC, Gouffault J. L'infarctus du ventricule droit. 2. Incidences pronostiques et therapeutiques. Arch Mal Coeur Vaiss 1977;70:257–264.

137. Stewart S, Huddle R, Stuard I, Schreiner BF, DeWeese JA. False aneurysm and pseudo-false aneurysm of the left ventricle: etiology, pathology, diagnosis, and operative management. Ann Thorac Surg 1981;31:259–265.

138. Hodsden J, Nanda NC. Dissecting aneurysm of the ventricular septum following acute myocardial infarction: diagnosis by real time two-dimensional echocardiography. Am Heart J 1981;101:671–672.

139. Tanimoto M, Iwasaki T, Yamamoto T, Makihata S, Konisiike A, Mihata S, Matsumori Y, Yasutomi N, Koide T, Kawai Y. Two-dimensional echocardiography in ventricular septal rupture after acute myocardial infarction. J Cardiogr 1985;15:625–637.

140. Scanu P, Lamy E, Commeau P, Grollier G, Charbonneau P. Myocardial dissection in right ventricular infarction: two-dimensional echocardiographic recognition and pathologic study. Am Heart J 1986;111:422–425.

141. Kanemoto N, Hirose S, Goto Y, Matsuyama S. Disappearing false aneurysm of the ventricular septum without rupture: a complication of acute inferior myocardial infarction—a case report. Angiology 1988;39:263–271.

142. Savage MP, Hopkins JT, Templeton JY, Goldburgh WP, Goldberg S. Left ventricular pseudo-pseudoaneurysm: angiographic features and surgical treatment of impending cardiac rupture. Am Heart J 1988;116:864–866.

143. Padró JM, Caralps JM, Montoya JD, Cámara ML, Garcia-Picart JG, Arís A. Sutureless repair of postinfarction cardiac rupture. J Card Surg 1988;3:491–493.

144. Zogno M, Lacanna GC, Ceconi C, Ferrari M, Latini L, Lorusso R, Sandrelli L, Alfieri O. Postinfarction left ventricular free wall rupture: original management and surgical technique. J Card Surg 1991;6:396–399.

145. Padró JM, Mesa JM, Silvesre J, Larrea JL, Caralps JM, Cerrón F, Aris A. Subacute cardiac rupture: repair with a sutureless technique. Ann Thorac Surg 1993;55:20–24.

146. Almdahl SM, Hotvedt R, Larsen U, Srlie DG. Postinfarction rupture of left ventricular free wall repaired with a glued-on pericardial patch. Scan J Thor Cardiovasc Surg 1993;27:105–107.

147. Coletti G, Torracca L, Zogno M, LaCanna G, Lorusso R, Pardini A, Alfieri O. Surgical management of left ventricular free wall rupture after acute myocardial infarction. Cardiovasc Surg 1995;3:181–186.

148. Cheriex EC, deSwart H, Dijkman LW, Havenith MG, Maessen JG, Engelen DJ, Wellens HJ. Myocardial rupture after myocardial infarction is related to the perfusion status of the infarct-related coronary artery. Am Heart J 1995;129:644–649.

149. Kyo S, Ogiwara M, Miyamoto N, Tsutsumi H, Asano H, Tanabe H, Ohuchi H, Yokote T, Omoto R. Clinical effect of percutaneous intra-pericardial fibrin-glue infusion therapy for the treatment of rupture of left ventricular free wall following acute myocardial infarction. Circulation 1999;100:I–867.

# 27

# Microcirculatory Dysfunction in Acute Myocardial Infarction: Evaluation, Management, and Treatment

**Michael H. Yen**
*Department of Cardiovascular Medicine Cleveland Clinic Foundation*
*Cleveland, Ohio*

**Eric J. Topol**
*Department of Cardiovascular Medicine Joseph J. Jacobs Center for Thrombosis
and Vascular Biology Cleveland Clinic Foundation*
*Cleveland, Ohio*

## INTRODUCTION

Despite an excellent angiographic result after percutaneous intervention (PCI) or thrombolysis for acute myocardial infarction (MI), there is often a dissociation between the angiographic result and clinical outcome [1]. With the introduction of sophisticated imaging and diagnostic modalities within the last two decades, it has become apparent that embolization and microcirculatory dysfunction (MCD) occur considerably more often than expected [2]. In this chapter, we will review the enhanced imaging and diagnostic assessment of MCD as well as set the foundation for improved pharmacological and mechanical approaches to protect the integrity of the microcirculation in acute MI.

## PATHOPHYSIOLOGY OF MICROCIRCULATORY DYSFUNCTION IN ACUTE MYOCARDIAL INFARCTION

In acute MI, MCD is hypothesized to occur via two mechanisms: microembolization and reperfusion injury. Rupture of the atherosclerotic plaque and subsequent fibrinolysis can lead to dislodgement of platelet aggregates resulting in impairment of flow in the microcirculation. Evidence of platelet and fibrin microthrombi have been found in animal models of myocardial ischemia and in pathological specimens of patients who died from ischemic heart disease [3,4]. Iatrogenic injury to the coronary vasculature and inflammation may further propagate microembolization during PCI in acute MI. Balloon angioplasty and stenting leads to arterial wall fissuring and plaque erosion that predisposes to the formation of microemboli [2]. These microemboli are composed of lipids, platelet and fibrin complexes, macrophage foam cells, cholesterol crystals, and other vessel wall constituents that impair microvascular perfusion directly through occluding capillaries or indirectly through the release of substances that further potentiate vasoconstriction, inflammation, and vascular injury [5]. The embolic material contains increased levels of tissue factor, a key mediator of coagulation [6].

Tissue reperfusion injury after mechanical or pharmacologic reperfusion for acute MI can also lead to MCD. Factors that may play a role in reperfusion injury include myocyte necrosis, microvascular spasm, tissue edema, endothelial dysfunction, oxygen free-radical injury, obstruction of capillaries by neutrophil aggregates, and augmented vessel permeability [7]. Thus, the interaction between embolization, tissue reperfusion injury, and microvascular spasm further propagates MCD in the setting of acute MI.

## ASSESSMENT OF MICROVASCULAR INJURY DURING ACUTE MYOCARDIAL INFARCTION

### Epicardial Perfusion

Assessment of epicardial coronary artery flow in acute MI has traditionally been assessed by Thrombolysis In Myocardial Infarction (TIMI) flow grade, and unfortunately this has been viewed as the reference standard for myocardial reperfusion. The degree and rapidity of epicardial flow after either pharmacological or mechanical revascularization in the infarct-related artery is assessed and compared to a non-infarct related artery [8]. The corrected TIMI frame count provides a more quantitative and continuous assessment of epicardial flow by documenting the number of cineframes that it takes for contrast to traverse to standardized distal coronary vessel landmarks [9].

Although several fibrinolytic [10,11] and PCI trials [12] have shown that the TIMI flow classification can predict clinical outcomes after revascularization for acute MI, its use is limited by a myriad of factors (Fig. 1) [7]. These limitations reflect the inability of

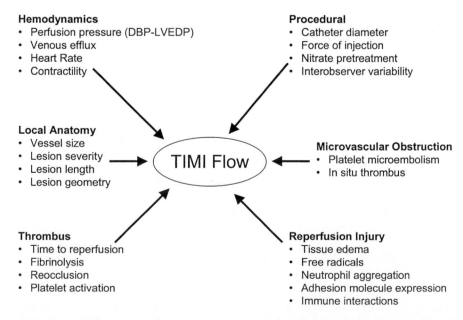

**Figure 1**  Factors that determine thrombolysis in myocardial infarction (TIMI) flow grade. DBP = diastolic blood pressure; LVEDP = left ventricular end-diastolic pressure.(From Ref. 7)

the TIMI flow classification to accurately assess the flow through the microvasculature. Using contrast echocardiography, Ito and associates were the first to show that 1 in 4 patients with TIMI 3 flow had impaired myocardial tissue level perfusion [13]. More recently, Stone et al. showed that despite restoration of TIMI 3 flow by PCI in 94% of 173 consecutive patients with acute MI, only 29% had normal myocardial tissue-level as assessed by the myocardial blush score [14]. Other studies have shown discordance between epicardial flow and microcirculatory flow, establishing a paradigm that restoration of epicardial flow frequently does not imply significant perfusion at the microcirculatory level [15–22].

## TIMI Myocardial Perfusion Grade

The TIMI myocardial perfusion (TMP) grade was developed to provide an angiographic, semiquantitative method of assessing MCD. This technique relies on the interpretation of the washout of myocardial blush that is visualized angiographically as a ground-glass appearance of the myocardium after intracoronary contrast administration [23]. An analysis of the TIMI 10B trial showed that TMP grade at 90 minutes after thrombolytic drug administration was a significant and independent predictor of 30-day mortality (Fig. 2). TMP grade was also able to risk stratify patients who had normal epicardial flow on their angiograms. Among the patients who had TIMI 3 flow after thrombolytic administration, those with a TMP 3 grade had significantly lower 30-day mortality than those with impaired TMP grades [23]. Patients with normal TIMI and TMP grades had significantly reduced mortality compared to patients who had impaired epicardial and microcirculatory perfusion [23]. The ability of TMP grade to predict mortality was sustained at two-year follow-up of the TIMI 10B trial [24]. TMP grade also can predict the degree of myocardial salvage after acute MI [20,25]. Lower TMP grades are independently associated with elevations in troponin T even after adjusting for TIMI flow, thrombus, and prior MI [26]. Lastly,

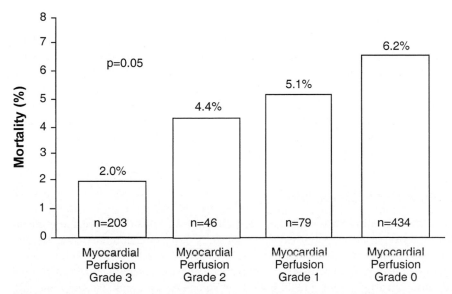

**Figure 2** Association between TIMI myocardial perfusion (TMP) grade and mortality. (From Ref. 23)

improved TMP grades after revascularization have been correlated with smaller infarct size [20].

*Myocardial Blush Grade*

Myocardial blush grade (MBG) relates similarly to TMP, however, it focuses mainly on contrast density in the myocardium rather than washout [27]. Classification of MBG or dye density score was originally described by van't Hof and colleagues on a 0–3 scale with a score of 3 signifying normal myocardial blush or contrast density [27]. In the initial study of MBG in patients who underwent PCI for acute MI, MBG scores were able to predict recovery of left ventricular function after MI, enzyme infarct size, and mortality [27]. As with TMP, the MBG scores correlated with TIMI flow grades, however, 67% of patients with low MBG scores of 0 or 1 had TIMI 3 flow [27]. Lower MBG scores are associated with higher one-year cumulative mortality in patients who had TIMI 3 flow after PCI for acute MI [14]. Henriques et al. further corroborated these results by demonstrating that patients who had poor MBG scores after mechanical revascularization had increased mortality, larger enzymatic infarct sizes, and lower left ventricular ejection fractions at a mean follow-up of 16 months [28].

## ST-segment Resolution

The simplest, least expensive, most readily available modality to evaluate MCD in the setting of acute MI is the degree of ST segment resolution on the electrocardiogram (ECG) after revascularization. Several large substudies of fibrinolytic trials in acute MI have shown a consistent relationship between the degree of ST-segment resolution defined as complete (>70%), partial resolution (<70% − 30%), and no resolution (<30%) at 60–180 minutes with short- and long-term mortality that is independent of TIMI flow (Table 1) [29–36]. Matetzky et al. reported similar findings in 117 patients who underwent PCI for acute MI where greater ST-segment resolution within 30 minutes was associated with significantly improved predischarge ejection fractions, less congestive heart failure, and reduced mortality [37].

ST-segment resolution after either fibrinolysis or mechanical reperfusion correlates with not only mortality, but also with reduced infarct size and greater myocardial salvage as assessed by nuclear scintigraphy (Fig. 3) [38]. Feldman et al. recently validated the use of ST-segment resolution as a marker of MCD in patients who underwent PCI for acute MI [39]. In this study, lack of ST-segment resolution (<50%) 60 minutes after reestablishment of TIMI 3 flow correlated with impaired coronary flow Doppler wire measurements after stent implantation and higher rates of congestive heart failure, larger infarct sizes, and reduced regional and global ventricular function [39].

## Doppler Flow and Pressure Wires

A Doppler flow wire allows assessment of microcirculatory perfusion before and immediately after PCI. Iwakura et al. published the initial study describing coronary flow velocity (CFV) patterns in patients with acute MI and MCD as determined by contrast echocardiography after PCI [40]. Patients with MCD had decreased systolic antegrade flow, abnormal retrograde flow in early systole, and diastolic flow velocities with rapid deceleration [40]. Subsequent studies have defined CFV measurements indicative of severe MCD as a diastolic velocity deceleration time of less than 600 ms and the occurrence of systolic flow

**Table 1** Relationship Between Degree of ST-segment Resolution and Short- and Long-term Mortality after Pharmacologic Reperfusion for Acute Myocardial Infarction

| Trial | Time (Min) | Complete resolution (≥70%) | Partial resolution (>30%–<70%) | No resolution (≤ 30%) | Length of follow-up |
|---|---|---|---|---|---|
| GUSTO V (n=1764) | 60 | 2.0% | 5.2% | 5.5% | 30 days |
| InTIME 2 (n=900) | 60 | 1.7% | 4.5% | 7.7% | 30 days |
| InTIME 2 (n=900) | 60 | 2.7% | 7.5% | 10.7% | 1 year |
| GUSTO III (n=2241) | 90 | 3.8% | 5.8% | 10% | 30 days |
| TIMI 14 (n=444) | 90 | 1.0% | 4.2% | 5.9% | 30 days |
| InTIME 2 (n=764) | 90 | 3.1% | 5.3% | 8.9% | 30 days |
| HIT 4 (n=904) | 90 | 1.8% | 4.2% | 8.6% | 30 days |
| GUSTO III (n=2241) | 90 | 7.4% | 9.6% | 14.9% | 1 year |
| InTIME 2 (n=764) | 90 | 4.7% | 7.4% | 11.3% | 1 year |
| ISAM (n=1516) | 180 | 2.2% | 3.4% | 8.6% | 21 days |
| HIT 4 (n=998) | 180 | 2.8% | 6.0% | 14.3% | 30 days |
| GUSTO III (n=2218) | 180 | 3.6% | 7.7% | 9.8% | 30 days |
| INJECT (n=1398) | 180 | 2.5% | 4.3% | 17.5% | 35 days |
| GUSTO III (n=2218) | 180 | 7.9% | 412.2% | 13.3% | 1 year |
| ISAM (n=1516) | 180 | 8.1% | 13.7% | 20.8% | 2 years |
| ISAM (n=1516) | 180 | 16.4% | 24% | 31% | 5 years |

ISAM = Intravenous Streptokinase in Acute Myocardial Infarction (Ref. 36)
INJECT = International Joint Efficacy Comparison of Thrombolytics (Ref. 33)
GUSTO III = Global Use of Strategies to Open Occluded Coronary Arteries III study (Ref. 30)
HIT 4 = Hirudin for Improvement of Thrombolysis (HIT)-4 (Ref. 35)
InTIME 2 = Intravenous nPA for Treatment of Infarcting Myocardium Early-II (Ref. 32)
GUSTO V = Global Use of Strategies to Open Occluded Coronary Arteries V (Ref. 34)

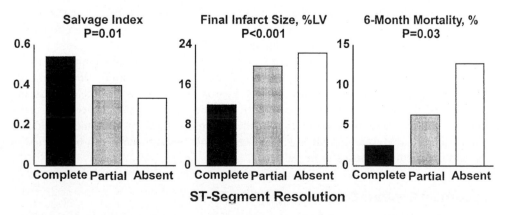

**Figure 3** Relationship between degree of ST-segment resolution after revascularization for acute myocardial infarction and mean myocardial salvage index, mean final infarct size, and 6-month mortality. LV = left ventricle. (From Ref. 38)

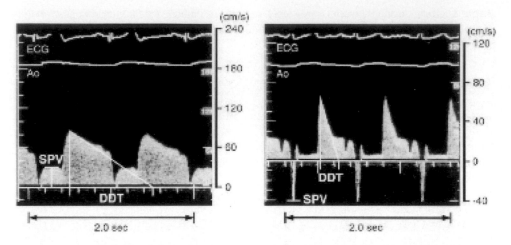

**Figure 4** Differing coronary flow velocity recordings in patients without severe microcirculation impairment after percutaneous intervention (PCI) and with severe microcirculation impairment after PCI. Left, normal velocity pattern after PCI showing dominant antegrade flow during systole or systolic peak velocity (SPV) and normal deceleration of the diastolic peak velocity (DDT). Right, dominant retrograde flow of SPV with decreased antegrade flow and rapid DDT indicative of microcirculation impairment after PCI. (From Ref. 42)

reversal [41]. Using these parameters, measuring CFV after PCI for acute MI has been able to predict short-term adverse outcomes (Fig. 4) [42].

Doppler flow as well as pressure wire measurements allow calculation of coronary flow reserve (CFR) defined as the ratio between coronary flow during maximal hyperemia to baseline coronary flow [43]. Several studies have shown that higher CFR values after PCI for acute MI is associated with an improvement in regional and global left ventricular function [44,45]. In contrast, Claeys et al. showed no correlation between CFR measurements and infarct size or viability [46]. One major limitation of CFR for the assessment of MCD is that it cannot discriminate between epicardial and microcirculatory flow [43]. By using the CFR value in a reference vessel that is angiographically normal, one can calculate the ratio of CFR in the target vessel to the reference vessel (rCFR). In the setting of elective PCI, lower rCFR correlated with higher levels of microvascular embolization and injury as assessed by myocardial biomarkers [47].

Additional refinements to pressure wire technology have enabled simultaneous recording of coronary artery pressure and an estimate of coronary artery flow using the principle of thermodilution. In a swine model, Fearon et al. demonstrated that measuring an index of microcirculatory resistance (IMR) defined as the ratio between the distal coronary artery pressures to the inverse of the hyperemic mean transit time provided a quantitative method to assess MCD [17].Whether IMR measurements can be applied to the acute MI setting remains to be validated.

## Myocardial Contrast Echocardiography

Myocardial contrast echocardiography (MCE) has been used for the last two decades to evaluate the integrity of the microcirculation in the setting of acute MI. Administration of contrast microbubbles and subsequent ultrasonic imaging prior to or after revascularization for acute MI allows the detection of MCD and subsequent perfusion abnormalities

[13]. Use of MCE in the early 1990s demonstrated that perfusion defects in acute MI correlated with impaired TIMI flow. More importantly, these studies conclusively showed that a significant proportion of patients (16–29%) had impaired microvascular perfusion as detected by MCE that correlated with reduced regional and global ventricular function at up to 3 month follow-up despite successful reperfusion and angiographic restoration of TIMI 3 flow [29,48]. MCE can predict myocardial viability early after acute MI [49,50]. Leeper et al. used MCE to evaluate for perfusion defects and ventricular function prior to PCI in 25 patients with acute MI, after 24 hours and at one-month follow-up [16]. Patients who had improved perfusion defects at 24 hours compared to baseline, had a significant improvement in regional wall motion compared to patients who had a persistent perfusion defect (Fig. 5) [16]. The recent development of intravenous contrast agents, intermittent harmonic imaging, and the use of delayed triggered imaging have improved the ease and accuracy of MCE [16,49].

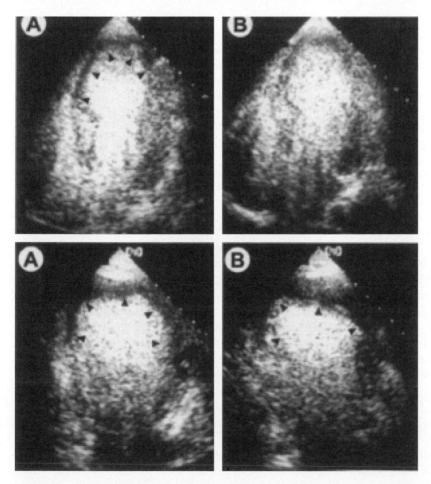

**Figure 5**  Representation of perfusion defects detected by myocardial contrast echocardiography. **Top**, significant reduction in perfusion defect 24 hours after successful percutaneous intervention (PCI) for acute MI. **Bottom**, persistent perfusion defect after 24 hours despite successful reestablishment of epicardial flow by PCI for acute MI. (From Ref. 16)

### Radiological Techniques

Nuclear scintigraphy using either thallium or technetium and single photon emission computed tomography (SPECT) can detect MCD after revascularization for acute MI. Kondo et al. showed in a study of 25 patients thart SPECT had the ability to show perfusion defects after PCI for acute MI despite no angiographic evidence of no-reflow [19]. The main disadvantage of nuclear scintigraphy is that it entails transport of a potentially unstable patient to a radiological suite and the inherent delays of imaging after injection (usually 4–6 hours) that impair the visualization of early changes in microcirculatory perfusion [7]. Other clinical studies have used nuclear scintigraphy to correlate myocardial salvage [25,38] and infarct size [20] with more readily accessible techniques to measure MCD such as TMP, MBG, or ST-segment resolution.

Magnetic resonance imaging (MRI) and positron emission tomography (PET) also have the ability to visualize defects in myocardial tissue perfusion. Animal studies have correlated hypoenhanced regions on MRI with markedly reduced tissue-level perfusion [51]. In a study of 44 patients who predominantly received thrombolysis for acute MI, patients with MRI findings of microvascular obstruction 10 days post infarct had increased morbidity and mortality at a mean follow-up of 16 months [22]. MRI also can provide relatively accurate measurements of infarct size [22]. PET can assess myocardial viability with $^{18}$FDG and myocardial blood flow with the use of $^{13}$NH$_3$. Maes et al. demonstrated that patients who had severe reduction in myocardial tissue flow by PET despite successful thrombolysis (defined by TIMI 3 flow) had persistent perfusion defects at 3 month follow-up with no improvement in ventricular function [21]. The major limitations of MRI and PET are similar as with nuclear scintigraphy, most notably a need for transport and a delay in imaging.

### Summary of Diagnostic Techniques to Measure Tissue-level Perfusion

There are several validated techniques to evaluate the integrity of the microcirculation after revascularization for MI. Nuclear scintigraphy, MRI, and PET probably do not allow a "real-time" assessment of microvasculature perfusion immediately after reperfusion and have inherent logistic constraints and delays in imaging. Doppler flow and pressure wires as well as MCE can provide an immediate assessment of tissue-level perfusion after either thrombolysis or mechanical revascularization when performed by experienced operators. ST-segment resolution and either TMP or MBG scores provide relatively uncomplicated, readily accessible techniques to evaluate the microcirculation without the need for additional equipment or operators. Recent studies have shown that combining ST-segment measurements with MBG scores increases the ability to predict adverse outcomes following revascularization for acute MI (Fig. 6) [52,53].

### TREATMENT OPTIONS FOR IMPAIRED MICROCIRCULATION

In recent years, there has been a development of several potential treatment strategies to protect the microcirculation in the setting of revascularization for acute MI. These treatment modalities have focused on reducing and preventing microembolization as well as the many factors believed to be mediators in reperfusion injury such as oxygen free radical production, neutrophil-mediated obstruction of the microvasculature, interstitial and cellular edema, spasm, vasoconstriction, and endothelial dysfunction.

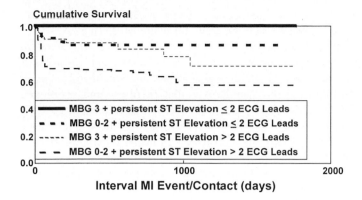

**Figure 6** Cumulative survival in 253 patients after percutaneous intervention (PCI) for acute myocardial infarction stratified by myocardial blush grade and resolution of ST-segments after PCI. (From Ref. 52)

## Pharmacologic

Since platelets plays a key role in the early phases of microembolization, pharmacologic agents such as glycoprotein IIb/IIIa inhibitors which impair their ability to aggregate theoretically should mitigate, at least in part, the formation of emboli and their subsequent impairment of microcirculatory flow. Several studies have shown that the use of abciximab in the setting of acute MI improves myocardial tissue-level perfusion. In a substudy of the TIMI 14 trial, the patients who received the combination of abciximab and reduced-dose tPA had improved resolution of ST-segments at 90 minutes and TIMI flow scores compared to tPA alone [54]. Neumann and colleagues compared Doppler flow wire and global/regional wall motion measurements immediately after revascularization and at 14-day angiographic follow-up in 200 patients randomized to either abciximab or heparin who underwent primary stenting for acute MI [45]. Coronary peak flow velocities induced by papaverine and regional and global ventricular function were significantly improved when compared to baseline in the patients who received abciximab to the heparin control group. The Adjunctive Platelet Glycoprotein IIb/IIIa Receptor Inhibition with Tirofiban before Primary Angioplasty (TIGER-PA) pilot trial recently showed that the benefit of IIb/IIIa inhibitors may be enhanced by earlier administration prior to PCI for acute MI [55]. TIGER-PA randomized 100 patients to either early administration of tirofiban in the emergency room or later administration in the cardiac catheterization laboratory. Patients with earlier administration of tirofiban not only had enhanced epicardial flow as measured by TIMI grade and corrected TIMI frame count, but also improved TMP grades which correlated with a trend towards reduced adverse clinical events at 20 days [55].

These findings of improved microcirculatory perfusion may provide a possible mechanism for the ability of abciximab to improve clinical outcomes. The recently completed Abciximab and Carbostent (ACE) trial randomized 400 patients with acute MI to either stenting alone or stenting with adjunctive abciximab. In the abciximab group (n = 200), there was a significant improvement in the degree of early ST segment resolution as well as a reduction in infarct size at one-month as measured by nuclear scintigraphy. These findings of improved microcirculatory flow translated to a reduction in the composite of death, recurrent MI, and target vessel revascularization at 30 days and 6 months [56]. Use of abciximab resulted in a 46% relative reduction in death, reinfarction, and target vessel revascularization as well as a 34% relative reduction in death or reinfarction at 30 days in a pooled analysis of the five major PCI stenting trials for acute MI [57].

In contrast to the strong evidence favoring the use of abciximab as the standard adjunctive pharmacotherapy for PCI in acute MI, there is scant evidence that vasodilators decrease MCD in the setting of acute MI. Small clinical studies of nicorandil and papaverine in acute MI have shown improvements in microvascular perfusion and ventricular function as assessed by MCE and TIMI flow grade when compared to placebo [58,59]. In animal models, nitroprusside has been shown to be an effective vasodilator in resistance arterioles of the microcirculation [60]. Use of intracoronary administration of nitroprusside (median dose of 200 μg) in PCI cases complicated by impaired or complete cessation of epicardial flow was associated with improved TIMI flow and corrected TIMI frame counts in a retrospective study of 19 patients [61].

Adenosine and verapamil have been more rigorously studied in the setting of acute MI. The initial small studies of adenosine showed that this vasodilator could improve TIMI flow in elective PCI of saphenous vein graft lesions complicated by no-reflow [62]. Assali and colleagues showed in a retrospective study that intracoronary administration of 24–48 μg of adenosine, before and after each balloon inflation, in the setting of acute MI was associated with statistically significant fewer occurrences of no-reflow with a trend towards improved clinical outcomes [63]. Marzilli et al. confirmed these findings in a randomized trial of 54 patients with acute MI who underwent primary PCI and were randomized to either adenosine (4000 μg) administered via the lumen of an inflated balloon or to saline [64]. Patients who received this relative high adenosine dose compared to other trials had significant fewer occurrences of no-reflow, improved ventricular function, and less major adverse events (recurrent angina, nonfatal MI, congestive heart failure, and cardiac death) than the patients in the placebo group [64]. The largest randomized trial of adenosine in acute MI was the Acute Myocardial Infarction Study of ADenosine (AMIS-TAD) which was a prospective, open-label, placebo-controlled trial of 236 patients with acute MI who received thrombolysis and were randomized to a peripheral intravenous infusion of adenosine at 70 μg/kg/min for 3 hours or saline [65]. The AMISTAD subjects with anterior MI had a reduction in infarct size; however, the trial was not powered to show a significant difference in clinical endpoints [65].

Intracoronary verapamil (500 μg) has been shown in a randomized trial of 40 patients with acute MI who underwent primary PTCA to improve microvascular perfusion and ventricular wall motion as measured by MCE [66]. In the setting of elective saphenous vein graft interventions, the randomized Vasodilator Prevention of no-Reflow (VAPOR) pilot trial of 22 patients demonstrated that the administration of intragraft verapamil (200 μg) prior to PCI resulted in a statistically significant improvement in TIMI frame count and a trend towards less no-reflow and improved microvascular perfusion as assessed by TMPG when compared to placebo [67].

In summary, use of adjunctive abciximab protects the integrity of the microvasculature during mechanical revascularization for acute MI resulting in improved clinical outcomes. Intracoronary administration of other vasodilatory agents may be beneficial in not only restoring epicardial flow, but also improving tissue-level perfusion. However, there is a relative paucity of large, prospective, randomized trials of the use of these agents in acute MI. Parikh et al. showed in a randomized trial of 67 patients with acute coronary syndromes that the combination of adenosine and nitroprusside is superior to adenosine alone in improving epicardial flow in PCI cases complicated by no-reflow [68]. The results of larger vasodilator trials will hopefully enable identification of which agent or combination of agents is most effective. Because of the limitations of pharmacological agents in situations where there is a large burden of thrombus or atherosclerotic debris such as in acute MI, studies have begun using mechanical devices to complement pharmacological therapies in preventing or improving microcirculatory flow in acute MI.

## Mechanical

Emboli protection devices can be classified into two main categories, filters and occlusion balloons (Fig. 7). Each class has its own inherent shortcomings and advantages (Table 2). Filter devices such as the AngioGuard filter wire and FilterWire-EX are nonocclusive devices that collect emboli of a certain size based on the diameter of pores in the device (110 μm for FilterWire-EX, 100 μm for AngioGuard) while maintaining antegrade blood flow [69,70]. The PercuSurge GuardWire is the prototypical distal balloon occlusion device that occludes antegrade flow past the lesion of interest, allowing entrapment of embolic debris that occurs during PCI, which is then removed with an aspiration catheter after successful stent deployment [71].

The emboli protection devices were initially developed and for use in saphenous vein graft interventions. Encouraging results from a pilot study of the PercuSurge device [72] prompted the Saphenous vein graft Angioplasty Free of Emboli Randomized (SAFER) Trial. SAFER was a pivotal trial since it was the first large-scale, multicenter, randomized trial of emboli protection [71]. At 30-day follow-up, the primary endpoint (death, MI, emergent bypass, or target lesion revascularization) occurred significantly less with the use of the PercuSurge GuardWire when compared to placebo (9.6% vs. 16.5%; P = 0.004). The reduction in the primary endpoint was predominantly driven by the reduction in periprocedural MI which was defined as a creatine kinase-myocardial band greater than three times the upper limit of normal. There was also significant less occurrence of no-reflow with the use of the PercuSurge GuardWire (Figure 8). Subanalysis of SAFER revealed that the beneficial effects of emboli protection were maintained regardless of whether IIb/IIIa inhibitors were used [71].

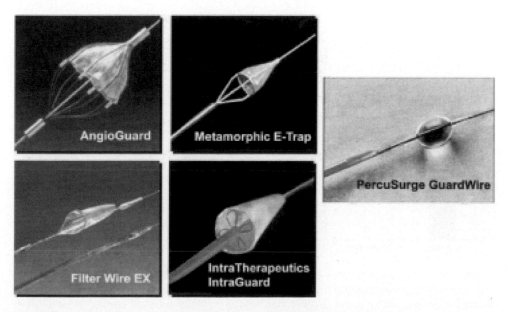

**Figure 7** Examples of distal emboli protection devices. (From Ref. 71a)

**Table 2**  Characteristics of Coronary Emboli Protection Devices

|  | Advantages | Disadvantages |
| --- | --- | --- |
| Filters | Preserves coronary blood flow | Larger, bulkier crossing profile may increase risk of embolization or failure to cross the lesion |
|  | Relative easy to use | Filter could detach from wire and embolize |
|  | Allows complete visualization of the lesion | Filter may get stuck in stent when withdrawn |
|  |  | May have incomplete apposition with vessel wall |
|  |  | Degree of emboli entrapment depends on pore size and model type |
|  |  | Does not allow protection of lesions in distal vessel |
|  |  | Steerability and support of guidewire can be difficult |
|  |  | Directs flow towards side branches |
| Distal Occlusion Balloons | Entrapment of all emboli regardless of size | Ischemia secondary to total occlusion of blood flow |
|  | Allows aspiration of vasoactive factors and cytokines | Difficult to visualize lesion once balloon inflated |
|  | Smaller crossing profile than filters | Does not allow protection of lesions in distal vessel |
|  |  | Steerability and support of guidewire can be difficult |
|  |  | Directs flow towards side branches |

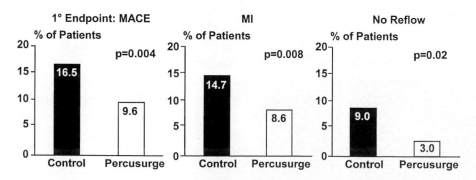

**Figure 8**  Reduction in primary endpoint of major adverse cardiac events with corresponding declines in periprocedural myocardial infarction (MI) and no reflow with the use of the PercuSurge GuardWire in the SAFER trial. MACE = Major adverse cardiac events. MI = Myocardial infarction. TVR = Target vessel revascularization. (From Ref. 71)

The phase II safety trial of the FilterWire EX device for elective saphenous vein graft PCI showed a cumulative adverse event rate of 11.3% [73]. These results led to the FilterWire EX Randomized Evaluation (FIRE), a multicenter, randomized trial of patients undergoing elective, planned stenting of saphenous vein graft lesions comparing the Percu-Surge GuardWire with the FilterWire EX [70]. FIRE included 651 randomized patients with a primary endpoint of 30-day composite major adverse events (MACE) that included death, MI, and target vessel revascularization. MACE events occurred similarly between the two groups (Fig. 9), and the 1-sided test of noninferiority was met with a P = 0.0008. Furthermore, measurements of TIMI flow and periprocedural myonecrosis were also similar among the groups [70].

SAFER and FIRE have conclusively shown that the use of emboli protection devices in saphenous vein graft interventions markedly reduces MACE. However, studies of emboli protection devices in the setting of acute MI currently consist of small patient registries. Belli et al. described the successful use of the PercuSurge GuardWire in acute MI patients who presented with thrombotic occlusion of predominantly proximal, large native coronary vessels [74]. Others have reported using only the aspiration component of the PercuSurge GuardWire device to reduce thrombus and embolic burden prior to PCI for acute MI [75]. Limbruno et al. conducted one of the largest studies with the use of FilterWire Ex in 53 patients with acute MI who had infarct vessels greater than 3.0 mm [69]. When compared to a case-matched control group, use of the FilterWire Ex was associated with significant improved corrected TIMI frame count, MBG, and earlier ST-segment resolution [69]. The Enhanced Myocardial Efficacy and Recovery by Aspiration of Liberalized Debris (EMERALD) is currently enrolling 500 patients with acute MI who will be randomized to either PCI with adjunct PercuSurge GuardWire protection or PCI alone. The primary endpoint of EMERALD will be the incidence of complete ($\geq$ 70% baseline) ST-segment resolution measured 30 minutes after the last angiogram as well as infarct size determined by tc-99m sestamibi imaging at 5–14 days after revascularization.

In summary, the development of distal emboli protection devices represents a promising strategy to decreasing MACE in the setting of PCI for acute MI. However, the roughly 10% rate of major adverse events in both SAFER and FIRE in predominantly elective PCI for saphenous vein graft reinforces the concept that no device is totally effective at reducing embolic burden. Further improvements in device technology, adjunc-

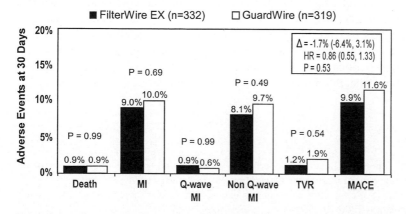

**Figure 9** Comparison between the PercuSurge GuardWire and FilterWire EX according to the primary endpoint of major adverse clinical events at 30 days follow-up. (From Ref. 70)

tive pharmacological strategies, and completion of additional randomized trials powered for relevant clinical endpoints will clarify the optimal use of these devices for acute MI.

## CURRENT RECOMMENDATIONS AND FUTURE INVESTIGATION

On the basis of our current knowledge regarding the microcirculation in acute MI, it is clear that more attention is warranted both clinically and on an investigational basis. Physicians caring for acute MI patients should, at the very least, use a 60 minute ECG in all patients following fibrinolytics, or soon after PCI, to determine whether the ST-segment elevation has resolved by more than 70%. If this has not occurred, it is likely that microcirculatory perfusion has not been adequately restored. Confirmation may be done by MCE at the patient's bedside, and if the infarction is large there should be consideration for emergent transfer to the cardiac catheterization laboratory. If lack of ST-segment resolution is occurring within the catheterization laboratory setting and epicardial flow is fully restored, there should be consideration for administration of vasodilators. The use of MBG or TMP as a visual, angiographic estimate of MCD is clearly useful and should be documented in the catheterization report and patient chart. During PCI, strong consideration should be given for platelet glycoprotein IIB/IIIa inhibition, particularly abciximab since it has been the most rigorously studied in randomized trials. The emboli protection devices are not yet approved for use in acute MI, but in infarct patients with a saphenous vein graft occlusion or large vessels (such as a hyperdominant right coronary artery), their use may be appropriate in select patients as we await the completion of ongoing trials. There is particular uncertainty with respect to whether glycoprotein IIb/IIIa blockade is necessary or additive with emboli protection devices, and if effective platelet receptor blockade with adenosine diphosphate receptor antagonists can substitute for glycoprotein IIb/IIIa inhibitors (or be additive) in this setting.

Further clinical investigation is necessary to determine the links between coronary arterial inflammation, microvasculature injury and inflammatory response to ischemia, infarction, and embolization. Systematic measurements of marker proteins such as sCD40L, myeloperoxidase, and Von Willebrand factor would help characterize the platelet, white cell and endothelial cell response, respectively. Moreover, the assorted limitations of our current assessment techniques including ECG, MCE, angiographic MBG, and TMP support the need for a simple, rapid, inexpensive biomarker that would indicate whether true, tissue level perfusion has been restored. Ultimately, testing potent anti-inflammatory agents in this setting may be guided by such diagnostic tests. Although it has taken decades for the unseen coronary microcirculation to be highlighted for its prognostic importance, it can now be recognized that there should be a heightened awareness in the daily care of acute MI patients and that this represents a major unmet domain of clinical investigation.

## REFERENCES

1. Lincoff AM, Topol EJ. Illusion of reperfusion. Does anyone achieve optimal reperfusion during acute myocardial infarction? Circulation 1993;88:1361–1374.
2. Topol EJ, Yadav JS. Recognition of the importance of embolization in atherosclerotic vascular disease. Circulation 2000;101:570–580.
3. El-Maraghi N, Genton E. The relevance of platelet and fibrin thromboembolism of the coronary microcirculation, with special reference to sudden cardiac death. Circulation 1980;62: 936–944.

4. Minamino T, Kitakaze M, Asanuma H, Tomiyama Y, Shiraga M, Sato H, Ueda Y, Funaya H, Kuzuya T, Matsuzawa Y, Hori M. Endogenous adenosine inhibits P-selectin-dependent formation of coronary thromboemboli during hypoperfusion in dogs. J Clin Invest 1998;101: 1643–1653.

5. Kotani J, Nanto S, Mintz GS, Kitakaze M, Ohara T, Morozumi T, Nagata S, Hori M. Plaque gruel of atheromatous coronary lesion may contribute to the no-reflow phenomenon in patients with acute coronary syndrome. Circulation 2002;106:1672–1677.

6. Penn MS, Topol EJ. Tissue factor, the emerging link between inflammation, thrombosis, and vascular remodeling. Circ Res 2001;89:1–2.

7. Mukherjee D, Moliterno DJ. Achieving tissue-level perfusion in the setting of acute myocardial infarction. Am J Cardiol 2000;85:39C–46C.

8. Group TS. The Thrombolysis in Myocardial Infarction (TIMI) trial. Phase I findings. N Engl J Med 1985;312:932–936.

9. Gibson CM, Cannon CP, Daley WL, Dodge JT, Alexander B, Marble SJ, McCabe CH, Raymond L, Fortin T, Poole WK, Braunwald E. TIMI frame count: a quantitative method of assessing coronary artery flow. Circulation 1996;93:879–888.

10. Investigators TGA. The effects of tissue plasminogen activator, streptokinase, or both on coronary-artery patency, ventricular function, and survival after acute myocardial infarction. N Engl J Med 1993;329:1615–1622.

11. Anderson JL, Karagounis LA, Becker LC, Sorensen SG, Menlove RL. TIMI perfusion grade 3 but not grade 2 results in improved outcome after thrombolysis for myocardial infarction. Ventriculographic, enzymatic, and electrocardiographic evidence from the TEAM-3 Study. Circulation 1993;87:1829–1839.

12. Montalescot G, Barragan P, Wittenberg O, Ecollan P, Elhadad S, Villain P, Boulenc JM, Morice MC, Maillard L, Pansieri M, Choussat R, Pinton P. Platelet glycoprotein IIb/IIIa inhibition with coronary stenting for acute myocardial infarction. N Engl J Med 2001;344: 1895–1903.

13. Ito H, Tomooka T, Sakai N, Yu H, Higashino Y, Fujii K, Masuyama T, Kitabatake A, Minamino T. Lack of myocardial perfusion immediately after successful thrombolysis. A predictor of poor recovery of left ventricular function in anterior myocardial infarction. Circulation 1992;85:1699–1705.

14. Stone GW, Peterson MA, Lansky AJ, Dangas G, Mehran R, Leon MB. Impact of normalized myocardial perfusion after successful angioplasty in acute myocardial infarction. J Am Coll Cardiol 2002;39:591–597.

15. de Lemos JA, Braunwald E. ST segment resolution as a tool for assessing the efficacy of reperfusion therapy. J Am Coll Cardiol 2001;38:1283–1294.

16. Lepper W, Hoffmann R, Kamp O, Franke A, de Cock CC, Kuhl HP, Sieswerda GT, Dahl J, Janssens U, Voci P, Visser CA, Hanrath P. Assessment of myocardial reperfusion by intravenous myocardial contrast echocardiography and coronary flow reserve after primary percutaneous transluminal coronary angioplasty [correction of angiography] in patients with acute myocardial infarction. Circulation 2000;101:2368–2374.

17. Fearon WF, Balsam LB, Farouque HM, Robbins RC, Fitzgerald PJ, Yock PG, Yeung AC. Novel index for invasively assessing the coronary microcirculation. Circulation 2003;107: 3129–3132.

18. Ito H, Maruyama A, Iwakura K, Takiuchi S, Masuyama T, Hori M, Higashino Y, Fujii K, Minamino T. Clinical implications of the 'no reflow' phenomenon. A predictor of complications and left ventricular remodeling in reperfused anterior wall myocardial infarction. Circulation 1996;93:223–228.

19. Kondo M, Nakano A, Saito D, Shimono Y. Assessment of "microvascular no-reflow phenomenon" using technetium-99m macroaggregated albumin scintigraphy in patients with acute myocardial infarction. J Am Coll Cardiol 1998;32:898–903.

20. Angeja BG, Gunda M, Murphy SA, Sobel BE, Rundle AC, Syed M, Asfour A, Borzak S, Gourlay SG, Barron HV, Gibbons RJ, Gibson CM. TIMI myocardial perfusion grade and ST segment resolution: association with infarct size as assessed by single photon emission computed tomography imaging. Circulation 2002;105:282–285.

21. Maes A, Van de Werf F, Nuyts J, Bormans G, Desmet W, Mortelmans L. Impaired myocardial tissue perfusion early after successful thrombolysis. Impact on myocardial flow, metabolism, and function at late follow-up. Circulation 1995;92:2072–2078.

22. Wu KC, Zerhouni EA, Judd RM, Lugo-Olivieri CH, Barouch LA, Schulman SP, Blumenthal RS, Lima JA. Prognostic significance of microvascular obstruction by magnetic resonance imaging in patients with acute myocardial infarction. Circulation 1998;97:765–772.

23. Gibson CM, Cannon CP, Murphy SA, Ryan KA, Mesley R, Marble SJ, McCabe CH, Van De Werf F, Braunwald E. Relationship of TIMI myocardial perfusion grade to mortality after administration of thrombolytic drugs. Circulation 2000;101:125–130.

24. Gibson CM, Cannon CP, Murphy SA, Marble SJ, Barron HV, Braunwald E. Relationship of the TIMI myocardial perfusion grades, flow grades, frame count, and percutaneous coronary intervention to long-term outcomes after thrombolytic administration in acute myocardial infarction. Circulation 2002;105:1909–1913.

25. Dibra A, Mehilli J, Dirschinger J, Pache J, Neverve J, Schwaiger M, Schomig A, Kastrati A. Thrombolysis in myocardial infarction myocardial perfusion grade in angiography correlates with myocardial salvage in patients with acute myocardial infarction treated with stenting or thrombolysis. J Am Coll Cardiol 2003;41:925–929.

26. Wong GC, Morrow DA, Murphy S, Kraimer N, Pai R, James D, Robertson DH, Demopoulos LA, DiBattiste P, Cannon CP, Gibson CM. Elevations in troponin T and I are associated with abnormal tissue level perfusion: a TACTICS-TIMI 18 substudy. Treat Angina with Aggrastat and Determine Cost of Therapy with an Invasive or Conservative Strategy-Thrombolysis in Myocardial Infarction. Circulation 2002;106:202–207.

27. van 't Hof AW, Liem A, Suryapranata H, Hoorntje JC, de Boer MJ, Zijlstra F. Angiographic assessment of myocardial reperfusion in patients treated with primary angioplasty for acute myocardial infarction: myocardial blush grade. Zwolle Myocardial Infarction Study Group. Circulation 1998;97:2302–2306.

28. Henriques JP, Zijlstra F, van 't Hof AW, de Boer MJ, Dambrink JH, Gosselink M, Hoorntje JC, Suryapranata H. Angiographic assessment of reperfusion in acute myocardial infarction by myocardial blush grade. Circulation 2003;107:2115–2119.

29. Porter TR, Li S, Oster R, Deligonul U. The clinical implications of no reflow demonstrated with intravenous perfluorocarbon containing microbubbles following restoration of Thrombolysis In Myocardial Infarction (TIMI) 3 flow in patients with acute myocardial infarction. Am J Cardiol 1998;82:1173–1177.

30. Anderson RD, White HD, Ohman EM, Wagner GS, Krucoff MW, Armstrong PW, Weaver WD, Gibler WB, Stebbins AL, Califf RM, Topol EJ. Predicting outcome after thrombolysis in acute myocardial infarction according to ST-segment resolution at 90 minutes: a substudy of the GUSTO-III trial. Global Use of Strategies To Open occluded coronary arteries. Am Heart J 2002;144:81–88.

31. de Lemos JA, Antman EM, Giugliano RP, McCabe CH, Murphy SA, Van de Werf F, Gibson CM, Braunwald E. ST-segment resolution and infarct-related artery patency and flow after thrombolytic therapy. Thrombolysis in Myocardial Infarction (TIMI) 14 investigators. Am J Cardiol 2000;85:299–304.

32. de Lemos JA, Antman EM, Giugliano RP, Morrow DA, McCabe CH, Cutler SS, Charlesworth A, Schroder R, Braunwald E. Comparison of a 60- versus 90-minute determination of ST-segment resolution after thrombolytic therapy for acute myocardial infarction. In TIME-II Investigators. Intravenous nPA for Treatment of Infarcting Myocardium Early-II. Am J Cardiol 2000;86:1235–1237.

33. Schroder R, Wegscheider K, Schroder K, Dissmann R, Meyer-Sabellek W. Extent of early ST segment elevation resolution: a strong predictor of outcome in patients with acute myocardial infarction and a sensitive measure to compare thrombolytic regimens. A substudy of the International Joint Efficacy Comparison of Thrombolytics (INJECT) trial. J Am Coll Cardiol 1995;26:1657–1664.

34. Cura FA, Roffi M, Pasca N, Wolski KE, Topol EJ, Lauer MS. Predictive value of 60-minute ST segment resolution in electrocardiogram after lytic therapy in patients with acute

myocardial infarction: results from the GUSTO V-RESTART study. J Am Coll Cardiol 2002; 39(Suppl A):202A.

35. Schroder R, Zeymer U, Wegscheider K, Neuhaus KL. Comparison of the predictive value of ST segment elevation resolution at 90 and 180 min after start of streptokinase in acute myocardial infarction. A substudy of the hirudin for improvement of thrombolysis (HIT)-4 study. Eur Heart J 1999;20:1563–1571.

36. Schroder R, Dissmann R, Bruggemann T, Wegscheider K, Linderer T, Tebbe U, Neuhaus KL. Extent of early ST segment elevation resolution: a simple but strong predictor of outcome in patients with acute myocardial infarction. J Am Coll Cardiol 1994;24:384–391.

37. Matetzky S, Novikov M, Gruberg L, Freimark D, Feinberg M, Elian D, Novikov I, Di Segni E, Agranat O, Har-Zahav Y, Rabinowitz B, Kaplinsky E, Hod H. The significance of persistent ST elevation versus early resolution of ST segment elevation after primary PTCA. J Am Coll Cardiol 1999;34:1932–1938.

38. Dong J, Ndrepepa G, Schmitt C, Mehilli J, Schmieder S, Schwaiger M, Schomig A, Kastrati A. Early resolution of ST-segment elevation correlates with myocardial salvage assessed by Tc-99m sestamibi scintigraphy in patients with acute myocardial infarction after mechanical or thrombolytic reperfusion therapy. Circulation 2002;105:2946–2949.

39. Feldman LJ, Coste P, Furber A, Dupouy P, Slama MS, Monassier JP, Tron C, Lafont A, Faraggi M, Le Guludec D, Dubois-Rande JL, Steg PG. Incomplete resolution of ST-segment elevation is a marker of transient microcirculatory dysfunction after stenting for acute myocardial infarction. Circulation 2003;107:2684–2689.

40. Iwakura K, Ito H, Takiuchi S, Taniyama Y, Nakatsuchi Y, Negoro S, Higashino Y, Okamura A, Masuyama T, Hori M, Fujii K, Minamino T. Alternation in the coronary blood flow velocity pattern in patients with no reflow and reperfused acute myocardial infarction. Circulation 1996;94:1269–1275.

41. Akasaka T, Yoshida K, Kawamoto T, Kaji S, Ueda Y, Yamamuro A, Takagi T, Hozumi T. Relation of phasic coronary flow velocity characteristics with TIMI perfusion grade and myocardial recovery after primary percutaneous transluminal coronary angioplasty and rescue stenting. Circulation 2000;101:2361–2367.

42. Yamamuro A, Akasaka T, Tamita K, Yamabe K, Katayama M, Takagi T, Morioka S. Coronary flow velocity pattern immediately after percutaneous coronary intervention as a predictor of complications and in-hospital survival after acute myocardial infarction. Circulation 2002; 106:3051–3056.

43. Kern MJ. Coronary physiology revisited : practical insights from the cardiac catheterization laboratory. Circulation 2000;101:1344–1351.

44. Mazur W, Bitar JN, Lechin M, Grinstead WC, Khalil AA, Khan MM, Sekili S, Zoghbi WA, Raizner AE, Kleiman NS. Coronary flow reserve may predict myocardial recovery after myocardial infarction in patients with TIMI grade 3 flow. Am Heart J 1998;136:335–344.

45. Neumann FJ, Blasini R, Schmitt C, Alt E, Dirschinger J, Gawaz M, Kastrati A, Schomig A. Effect of glycoprotein IIb/IIIa receptor blockade on recovery of coronary flow and left ventricular function after the placement of coronary-artery stents in acute myocardial infarction. Circulation 1998;98:2695–2701.

46. Claeys MJ, Vrints CJ, Bosmans J, Krug B, Blockx PP, Snoeck JP. Coronary flow reserve during coronary angioplasty in patients with a recent myocardial infarction: relation to stenosis and myocardial viability. J Am Coll Cardiol 1996;28:1712–1719.

47. Herrmann J, Haude M, Lerman A, Schulz R, Volbracht L, Ge J, Schmermund A, Wieneke H, von Birgelen C, Eggebrecht H, Baumgart D, Heusch G, Erbel R. Abnormal coronary flow velocity reserve after coronary intervention is associated with cardiac marker elevation. Circulation 2001;103:2339–2345.

48. Ito H, Okamura A, Iwakura K, Masuyama T, Hori M, Takiuchi S, Negoro S, Nakatsuchi Y, Taniyama Y, Higashino Y, Fujii K, Minamino T. Myocardial perfusion patterns related to thrombolysis in myocardial infarction perfusion grades after coronary angioplasty in patients with acute anterior wall myocardial infarction. Circulation 1996;93:1993–1999.

49. Swinburn JM, Lahiri A, Senior R. Intravenous myocardial contrast echocardiography predicts recovery of dysynergic myocardium early after acute myocardial infarction. J Am Coll Cardiol 2001;38:19–25.

50. Ragosta M, Camarano G, Kaul S, Powers ER, Sarembock IJ, Gimple LW. Microvascular integrity indicates myocellular viability in patients with recent myocardial infarction. New insights using myocardial contrast echocardiography. Circulation 1994;89:2562–2569.

51. Judd RM, Lugo-Olivieri CH, Arai M, Kondo T, Croisille P, Lima JA, Mohan V, Becker LC, Zerhouni EA. Physiological basis of myocardial contrast enhancement in fast magnetic resonance images of 2-day-old reperfused canine infarcts. Circulation 1995;92:1902–1910.

52. Haager PK, Christott P, Heussen N, Lepper W, Hanrath P, Hoffmann R. Prediction of clinical outcome after mechanical revascularization in acute myocardial infarction by markers of myocardial reperfusion. J Am Coll Cardiol 2003;41:532–538.

53. Poli A, Fetiveau R, Vandoni P, del Rosso G, D'Urbano M, Seveso G, Cafiero F, De Servi S. Integrated analysis of myocardial blush and ST-segment elevation recovery after successful primary angioplasty: Real-time grading of microvascular reperfusion and prediction of early and late recovery of left ventricular function. Circulation 2002;106:313–318.

54. de Lemos JA, Antman EM, Gibson CM, McCabe CH, Giugliano RP, Murphy SA, Coulter SA, Anderson K, Scherer J, Frey MJ, Van Der Wieken R, Van De Werf F, Braunwald E. Abciximab improves both epicardial flow and myocardial reperfusion in ST-elevation myocardial infarction. Observations from the TIMI 14 trial. Circulation 2000;101:239–243.

55. Lee DP, Herity NA, Hiatt BL, Fearon WF, Rezaee M, Carter AJ, Huston M, Schreiber D, DiBattiste PM, Yeung AC. Adjunctive platelet glycoprotein IIb/IIIa receptor inhibition with tirofiban before primary angioplasty improves angiographic outcomes: results of the TIrofiban Given in the Emergency Room before Primary Angioplasty (TIGER-PA) pilot trial. Circulation 2003;107:1497–1501.

56. Antoniucci D, Rodriguez A, Hempel A, Valenti R, Migliorini A, Vigo F, Parodi G, Fernandez-Pereira C, Moschi G, Bartorelli A, Santoro GM, Bolognese L, Colombo A. A randomized trial comparing primary infarct artery stenting with or without abciximab in acute myocardial infarction. J Am Coll Cardiol 2003;42:1879–1885.

57. Topol EJ, Neumann FJ, Montalescot G. A preferred reperfusion strategy for acute myocardial infarction. J Am Coll Cardiol 2003;42:1886–1889.

58. Sakata Y, Kodama K, Komamura K, Lim YJ, Ishikura F, Hirayama A, Kitakaze M, Masuyama T, Hori M. Salutary effect of adjunctive intracoronary nicorandil administration on restoration of myocardial blood flow and functional improvement in patients with acute myocardial infarction. Am Heart J 1997;133:616–621.

59. Ito H, Taniyama Y, Iwakura K, Nishikawa N, Masuyama T, Kuzuya T, Hori M, Higashino Y, Fujii K, Minamino T. Intravenous nicorandil can preserve microvascular integrity and myocardial viability in patients with reperfused anterior wall myocardial infarction. J Am Coll Cardiol 1999;33:654–660.

60. Myers PR, Banitt PF, Guerra R, Harrison DG. Characteristics of canine coronary resistance arteries: importance of endothelium. Am J Physiol 1989;257:H603–H610.

61. Hillegass WB, Dean NA, Liao L, Rhinehart RG, Myers PR. Treatment of no-reflow and impaired flow with the nitric oxide donor nitroprusside following percutaneous coronary interventions: initial human clinical experience. J Am Coll Cardiol 2001;37:1335–1343.

62. Sdringola S, Assali A, Ghani M, Yepes A, Rosales O, Schroth GW, Fujise K, Anderson HV, Smalling RW. Adenosine use during aortocoronary vein graft interventions reverses but does not prevent the slow-no reflow phenomenon. Catheter Cardiovasc Interv 2000;51:394–399.

63. Assali AR, Sdringola S, Ghani M, Denkats AE, Yepes A, Hanna GP, Schroth G, Fujise K, Anderson HV, Smalling RW, Rosales OR. Intracoronary adenosine administered during percutaneous intervention in acute myocardial infarction and reduction in the incidence of "no reflow" phenomenon. Catheter Cardiovasc Interv 2000;51:27–31; discussion 32.

64. Marzilli M, Orsini E, Marraccini P, Testa R. Beneficial effects of intracoronary adenosine as an adjunct to primary angioplasty in acute myocardial infarction. Circulation 2000;101:2154–2159.

65. Mahaffey KW, Puma JA, Barbagelata NA, DiCarli MF, Leesar MA, Browne KF, Eisenberg PR, Bolli R, Casas AC, Molina-Viamonte V, Orlandi C, Blevins R, Gibbons RJ, Califf RM, Granger CB. Adenosine as an adjunct to thrombolytic therapy for acute myocardial infarction:

results of a multicenter, randomized, placebo-controlled trial: the Acute Myocardial Infarction STudy of ADenosine (AMISTAD) trial. J Am Coll Cardiol 1999;34:1711–1720.

66. Taniyama Y, Ito H, Iwakura K, Masuyama T, Hori M, Takiuchi S, Nishikawa N, Higashino Y, Fujii K, Minamino T. Beneficial effect of intracoronary verapamil on microvascular and myocardial salvage in patients with acute myocardial infarction. J Am Coll Cardiol 1997; 30:1193–1199.

67. Michaels AD, Appleby M, Otten MH, Dauterman K, Ports TA, Chou TM, Gibson CM. Pretreatment with intragraft verapamil prior to percutaneous coronary intervention of saphenous vein graft lesions: results of the randomized, controlled vasodilator prevention on no-reflow (VAPOR) trial. J Invasive Cardiol 2002;14:299–302.

68. Parikh KH, Chag MC, Shah UG, Baxi HA, Chandarana AH, Naik AM, Shah KJ, Goyal RK. Reversal of Slow or No-Reflow During Percutaneous Transluminal Coronary Angioplasty Using Boluses of Intracoronary Adenosine and Sodium Nitroprusside in Combination. J Am Coll Cardiol 2002;39(Suppl A):39A.

69. Limbruno U, Micheli A, De Carlo M, Amoroso G, Rossini R, Palagi C, Di Bello V, Petronio AS, Fontanini G, Mariani M. Mechanical prevention of distal embolization during primary angioplasty: safety, feasibility, and impact on myocardial reperfusion. Circulation 2003;108: 171–176.

70. Stone GW, Rogers C, Hermiller J, Feldman R, Hall P, Haber R, Masud A, Cambier P, Caputo RP, Turco M, Kovach R, Brodie B, Herrmann HC, Kuntz RE, Popma JJ, Ramee S, Cox DA. Randomized Comparison of Distal Protection With a Filter-Based Catheter and a Balloon Occlusion and Aspiration System During Percutaneous Intervention of Diseased Saphenous Vein Aorto-Coronary Bypass Grafts. Circulation 2003;108:548–553.

71. Baim DS, Wahr D, George B, Leon MB, Greenberg J, Cutlip DE, Kaya U, Popma JJ, Ho KK, Kuntz RE. Randomized trial of a distal embolic protection device during percutaneous intervention of saphenous vein aorto-coronary bypass grafts. Circulation 2002;105: 1285–1290.

71a. Bhatt DL, Topol EJ. Periprocedural Myocardial infarction and emboli protection. In: Topol EJ, ed. Textbook of interventional cardiology. Fourth ed. Philadelphia: Saunders, 2003: 251–266. Figures 12–9 to 12–10.

72. Grube E, Schofer JJ, Webb J, Schuler G, Colombo A, Sievert H, Gerckens U, Stone GW. Evaluation of a balloon occlusion and aspiration system for protection from distal embolization during stenting in saphenous vein grafts. Am J Cardiol 2002;89:941–945.

73. Stone GW, Rogers C, Ramee S, White C, Kuntz RE, Popma JJ, George J, Almany S, Bailey S. Distal filter protection during saphenous vein graft stenting: technical and clinical correlates of efficacy. J Am Coll Cardiol 2002;40:1882–1888.

74. Belli G, Pezzano A, De Biase AM, Bonacina E, Silva P, Salvade P, Piccalo G, Klugmann S. Adjunctive thrombus aspiration and mechanical protection from distal embolization in primary percutaneous intervention for acute myocardial infarction. Catheter Cardiovasc Interv 2000;50:362–370.

75. Wang HJ, Kao HL, Liau CS, Lee YT. Export aspiration catheter thrombosuction before actual angioplasty in primary coronary intervention for acute myocardial infarction. Catheter Cardiovasc Interv 2002;57:332–339.

# 28
# Stem Cell Therapy for ACS: The Possibility of Myocardial Regeneration

**Arman T. Askari**
*University Hospitals of Cleveland and Case Western Reserve University*
*Cleveland, Ohio, U.S.A.*

**Marc S. Penn**
*The Cleveland Clinic Foundation*
*Cleveland, Ohio, U.S.A.*

## INTRODUCTION

Acute coronary syndromes (ACS) account for the majority of the morbidity and mortality in patients with coronary artery disease. Despite continued advances, not only in pharmacological and mechanical reperfusion, but also in adjunctive therapies such as β-blockers, angiotensin-converting enzyme inhibitors, HMG CoA reductase inhibitors, and enhanced anti-platelet therapy (e.g., glycoprotein IIb/IIIa inhibitors), a substantial adverse event rate persists for patients who present with ACS [1].

The current, "reperfusion," era for the management of acute coronary syndromes has enjoyed the lowest mortality rate to date through exploitation of an emerging treatment armamentarium of mechanical and pharmacologic reperfusion strategies [2–4]. However, a considerable proportion of patients exist that are either ineligible for these life altering therapies, present days to years after an initial insult with an already established ischemic cardiomyopathy, or undergo reestablishment of antegrade coronary perfusion but achieve sub-optimal left ventricular (LV) preservation. Furthermore, few if any of these recent advances address the need for optimizing or regenerating the damaged myocardial tissue. Born out of this reality is the increasing incidence of congestive heart failure (CHF), a crippling syndrome that will affect greater than 6 million people in the United States by the year 2030 [5].

Congestive heart failure results from ventricular remodeling, a dynamic process of LV cavity dilation and fibrosis, ultimately leading to depressed cardiac function [6,7]. Current therapies for CHF remain limited, and death rates from CHF continue to rise [8]. Furthermore, the definitive therapy for CHF, cardiac transplantation, remains limited in number and often simply trades one set of symptoms for another. This understanding has prompted the search for novel therapies that can attenuate myocardial cell death during MI, minimize pathologic remodeling, and regenerate myocardium.

The burgeoning field of cell therapy has recently shown promise. Initial, preclinical studies have focused on using differentiated cell types ranging from fetal cardiac myocytes

[9,10] to fibroblasts [11], smooth muscle cells [12], and, the most widely studied, skeletal myoblasts (SKMB) [13,14]. Skeletal myoblasts have received the greatest amount of attention largely as a result of their relative resistance to ischemia as well as their in situ regenerative and reparative properties in response to injury [15,16]. In addition, SKMBs have been shown to engraft into injured myocardium and to attenuate LV remodeling resulting in a modest and sustained improvement in ventricular performance [17–21].

These encouraging data prompted the recent phase I clinical trials assessing the efficacy and safety of SKMB transplantation at the time of coronary artery bypass surgery (CABG) [22]. This study revealed the feasibility and relative safety of SKMB transplantation in addition to increased scar thickness and contraction of non-viable segments. Despite the demonstration that SKMBs can engraft into scarred myocardium, attenuate negative LV remodeling, and marginally improve LV function, enthusiasm for SKMB transplantation for the treatment of patients with ACS is significantly dampened by the fact that it takes weeks to isolate and expand a sufficient number of SKMB prior to therapy. Furthermore, the ability to regenerate, not simply replace, functional myocardium has become the major focus of cell therapy for the treatment of ischemic heart disease.

The demonstration that hematopoietic stem cells (HSC) and mesenchymal stem cells (MSC) possess the ability to differentiate into cardiac and vascular structures [23–26] has catapulted these pluripotent stem cells to the forefront of regenerative medicine for cardiac dysfunction. Systemic delivery of bone marrow-derived stem cells [27], direct injection of c-Kit$^+$ positive bone marrow stem cells into the infarct border zone [28], and mobilization of endogenous stem cells with systemically administered growth factors [29] have demonstrated the ability of these cells to attenuate the amount of damage following an MI and the ability to replace a substantial portion of the infarcted wall with regenerated myocardium. The apparent ability of these stem cells to transdifferentiate into both cardiomyocytes and vascular structures was a seminal step forward for regenerative medicine. However, recent data has questioned this observation alluding to the presence of cell fusion [30,31] or regeneration of "lost" myocardium by a resident cardiac stem cell [32] rather than transdifferentiation of bone marrow derived stem cells that "homed" to and regenerated injured tissues as the mechanism of benefit. In addition to these controversies, the optimal timing, mode of delivery, and most beneficial cell type for myocardial regeneration remains undefined. Furthermore, it is distinctly possible that augmentation of the natural myocardial repair process through the delivery of key proteins such as SDF-1 [33] will be sufficient to significantly recover myocardial function and ultimately obviate the need for cell injection. Finally, it needs to be determined if these potential therapeutic strategies can be extrapolated to patients with ACS that have missed the "window" of reperfusion therapy. This chapter will review the research to date involving stem cell therapy for the treatment of acute coronary syndromes as well as the emerging understanding of the mechanisms through which stem cell therapy achieves regeneration of "lost" myocardium. Controversies surrounding the optimal cell type, the route and timing of stem cell delivery, and the mechanisms of benefit will also be discussed.

## SOURCES OF STEM CELLS FOR MYOCARDIAL REGENERATION

The excitement surrounding the use of stem cells for myocardial regeneration is based on the unique biological properties of these cells coupled with their ability to perpetuate their own lineage as well as to replace/regenerate other cells/tissue types [34–38]. Sources of stem cells for myocardial regeneration include, but are not limited to, embryonic stem cells, adult hematopoietic and mesenchymal stem cells, mulitpotent adult progenitor cells (MAPC), and unselected bone marrow stem cells (BMSC) each with their own advantages and disadvantages (Table 1). Although embryonic stem cells are easily harvested from the embryonal blastocyst and are truly totipotent [39,40], the current ethical and political environment has hindered the realization of their true restorative potential. Also, injection of these cells into the native myocardium more often than not leads to teratoma formation, indicating that a substantial amount of work needs to be done so that we can learn to regulate ESC differentiation into cardiac myocytes.

On the other hand, adult HSC are capable of fully reconstituting the hematopoietic system [41,42], and emerging data suggests the potential of HSC to transdifferentiate into nonhematopoietic cell types as well [26,29,43,44]. Mesenchymal stem cells possess the capability to differentiate into cells of all three germ layers. MAPC differentiate, at the single cell level, not only into mesenchymal cells, but also cells with visceral mesoderm, neuroectoderm and endoderm characteristics in vitro [38]. In vivo, single MAPC contribute to most somatic cell types. The value of all of these cell types arises out of their easily accessible state, varying grades of "potency," the ability to use autologous cell populations circumventing the need for immunosuppression, and the lack of ethical objections. The majority of recent studies assessing the utility of stem cell therapy for the treatment of ACS have focused on these cell types.

The use of the cell types discussed so far requires that these cells be selected through various cell processing techniques such as cell sorting and density gradient centrifugation. These processes may potentially limit the applicability of purified populations of stem cells for the treatment of ACS as a result of the time delay. However, the demonstration that MSC and MAPC fail to induce an immune response may allow for the development of stores of "off-the-shelf" stem cells available for injection at the time of MI, essentially eliminating this time delay [37]. In addition, the use of undifferentiated BMSC could eliminate this delay and facilitate a more efficient delivery of cells with regenerative capabilities to patients with acute ischemic syndromes. Nishida et al. assessed the efficacy of unselected BMSC transplantation in a rat hypoperfusion heart model [45]. They demonstrated a significant increase in neoangiogenesis, attenuated LV remodeling and an ensuing improvement in cardiac function. Despite the potential benefit of using unselected bone marrow for the treatment of ACS, the utility for selecting populations of cells to study

**Table 1** Advantages and Disadvantages of Stem Cell Types

| Cell type | Advantages | Disadvantages |
| --- | --- | --- |
| Embryonic stem cells | Pluripotent<br>Easily expanded | Ethical issues<br>Immunogenicity<br>Tendency to form teratomas<br>Lack of identification markers<br>Difficult to isolate |
| Adult stem cells | No ethical issues<br>Easily obtainable<br>Multipotent<br>Nonimmunogenin<br>(autologous)<br>Easily expanded in vitro | Potentially limited differentiation capacity |

affords a more systematic method of understanding the benefits of each cell type and the mechanisms through which they achieve their regenerative capacity.


## EVIDENCE FOR INTRINSIC MYOCARDIAL REPAIR

Several studies have now demonstrated that a normal physiologic response to MI involves mobilization of stem cells, "homing" of stem cells to the damaged myocardium, and differentiation of at least some stem cells into cardiac myocytes [46,47]. In one study, wild-type C57B/6 mice underwent bone marrow transplantation with hematopoietic stem cells from syngeneic Rosa 26 mice. All the cells from these mice express the marker protein LacZ in all their cells and, therefore, any LacZ positive cells in the transplanted wild-type mice had to originate from the donor marrow. Transplanted mice underwent LAD ligation, and their hearts were assessed for LacZ positive endothelium and cardiac myocytes 2 and 4 weeks later. This study clearly demonstrates that, following myocardial infarction, bone marrow derived cells home to the damaged myocardium and differentiate into endothelial cells (frequently) and cardiac myocytes (rarely) [47]. Similarly, human female hearts transplanted into males were found to have cardiac myocytes and vascular structures that stained positive for the Y-chromosome, suggesting that these cells were derived from recipient stem cells [48].

An emerging concept within the field of myocardial regeneration is that of the resident cardiac stem cell (CSC). The traditional dogma asserts that cardiac myocytes are terminally differentiated and that the sole mechanism of cardiac adaptation to injury is via cardiac hypertrophy. However, cells that express the stem cell markers c-kit, MDR1, and Sca-1, but exhibit features consistent with cardiac myocytes have recently been identified within the myocardium. Beltrami et al. demonstrated the ability of cardiac myocytes to divide in myocardium from patients who died of ACS [49]. Furthermore, when these cells were harvested and re-injected into an ischemic heart, they gave rise to cardiac myocytes, smooth muscle cells, and vascular endothelial cells encompassing approximately 70% of the ventricle [44]. Similarly, cardiac stem cells have also been demonstrated to substantially contribute to the increased cardiac mass in response to aortic stenosis [32]. Unfortunately, these studies demonstrate that both stem cell engraftment and differentiation into cardiac myocytes as well as CSC proliferation occurs at a rate that is incapable of resulting in any meaningful regeneration of damaged myocardium. However, these studies suggest that if this natural repair mechanism can be potentiated, clinically significant myocardial regeneration may be achievable.


## PRECLINICAL STUDIES OF STEM CELL THERAPY IN ACS-MYOCARDIAL REGENERATION

The ultimate goal of any therapy for the treatment of acute coronary syndromes is the amelioration of morbidity and mortality associated with myocardial damage. Currently available therapies serve to limit myocardial damage and resultant LV remodeling but are incapable of regenerating damaged myocardium or restoring lost myocardial function. Several studies have suggested that, through the regenerative capabilities of stem cells, the possibility of myocardial regeneration is closer to reality than previously thought. Hematopoietic [27–29], mesenchymal [50–55], and unselected bone marrow stem cells [45] have been shown to possess this regenerative capacity and, in some instances, to almost completely regenerate infarcted myocardium (Table 2). More importantly, the mechanisms by which these cells perform this regenerative function are beginning to be elucidated.

## Hematopoietic Stem Cells in ACS

### Stem Cell Transplantation

The regenerative capacity of HSC was initially demonstrated in a mouse MI model. Three to five hours after LAD ligation a specific sub-population of stem cells, $Lin^-c\text{-}kit^{POS}$, from a mouse whose cells express green fluorescent protein were directly injected into the peri-infarct border zone. Not only did this result in partial regeneration of the infarcted anterior wall, transplanted hearts also exhibited improved function as evident by a lower diastolic pressure with an increased force generating capacity 9 days after MI compared with control animals [28]. This specific population of HSC also revealed their capacity to differentiate into endothelial and smooth muscle cells, resulting in neovascularization, a necessary component of total myocardial regeneration.

Expanding upon the above study, human bone marrow derived CD34 + HSC were systemically delivered via tail vein injection in nude rats 2 days following left anterior descending (LAD) ligation [27]. A significant improvement in cardiac function was realized. Several plausible mechanisms for this improvement included the observed neoangiogenesis, decreased apoptosis of hypertrophied myocytes in the peri-infarct region, salvaged viable myocardium and reduced myocardial fibrosis. Inferred to by Orlic et al. [28] and supported by this study was the concept that circulating stem cells possess the ability to ''home'' to the infarct zone.

Development of a nonsurgical technique of direct HSC delivery to ischemic/infarcted myocardium is on-going. In addition, a technique that would decrease the number of cells required to achieve the maximal regenerative benefit of stem cell transplantation while minimizing any potential untoward effect has yet to be optimally defined. Kawomoto et al. attempted to provide insight into these two concerns [56]. They tested the feasibility and efficacy of percutaneously transplanting autologous CD31 + cells in a pig model of myocardial ischemia, respectively. Utilizing an electromechanical mapping system to localize ischemic zones for cell delivery, isolated CD31 + cells were delivered to ischemic pig myocardium 4 weeks after ischemic insult. In a parallel study to assess efficacy of a lower number of HSC than previous studies, human CD34 + cells were directly delivered into infarcted immunodeficient rat myocardium 10 minutes after LAD ligation. Increased capillary density and improved LV function were observed in both study groups compared to control animals. These data provide support that the use of freshly isolated HSC can be utilized and are effective for the treatment of myocardial ischemia.

### Stem Cell Mobilization

That stem cells possess the ability to home to infarcted myocardium, coupled with the recent demonstration that an intrinsic, albeit inefficient, myocardial repair mechanism exists, prompted a scientifically elegant study by Orlic et al. [29]. They mobilized intrinsic HSC with daily administration of granulocyte colony stimulating factor (G-CSF) and stem cell factor (SCF) for five days before and three days after LAD ligation in rats. The upregulation of HSC using this technique resulted in decreased infarct size (40%) and cavitary dilation (26%). Ejection fraction progressively increased and hemodynamics significantly improved as a consequence of the formation of new myocytes and vasculature. Although intriguing, these results are not clinically useful given the need to predict when

**Table 2** Preclinical Trials of Stem Cell Therapy for ACS

| Study | Animal model | Stem cell type | Source | Timing of stem cell delivery | LV function | Comments |
|---|---|---|---|---|---|---|
| Hematopoietic stem cells | | | | | | |
| Kocher (27) | Rat | CD34+ Cells | Human | 2 days after MI | Improved | CD34+ cells introduced systemically homed to myocardial infarct zone. |
| Orlic (28) | Mouse | Lin⁻c-kit⁺ bone marrow cells | Autologous | 3–5 hours after MI | Improved | Cells injected into infarct border zone almost completely regenerated infarct zone. |
| Orlic (29) | Mouse | Unselected BMSC | Endogenous | 5d prior and 3d post MI | Improved | Mobilized stem cells with daily G-CSF and SCF given 5d before and 3d after LAD ligation. |
| Kawamoto (56) | Pig and rat | CD31+ cells (pig study) CD34+ cells (rat study) | Autologou–pig study Human–rat study | Pig–4 weeks after MI Rat-10 min after MI | Improved in both studies | Intramyocardial transplantation of both CD31+ cells in pigs resulted in increased capillary density within the ischemic regions and improved cardiac function with a substantially smaller number of HSC than previous studies. Furthermore, freshly isolated human CD34+ cells transplanted within 10 minutes of MI in rats increased capillary density and improved LV function. This study further supports the utility of HSC transplantation for the treatment of ACS. |
| Mesenchymal stem cells | | | | | | |
| Tomita (50) | Rat | Bone marrow stromal cells | Autologous | 3 weeks after MI | Improved | Improved function with 5-azacytidine treated cells directly injected 3 weeks following cryoinjury. |
| Wang (58) | Rat | Bone marrow stromal cells | Autologous | No MI | NA | This study demonstrates the integral role of an appropriate microenvironment for differentiation of bone marrow stromal cells. |
| Tomita (51) | Pig | Bone marrow stromal cells | Autologous | 4 weeks after MI | Improved | Improved angiogenesis and LV function with 5-azacytidine treated cells directly injected into the infarct zone 4 weeks following LAD occlusion. |
| Shake (52) | Pig | Mesenchymal stem cells | Autologous | 2 weeks after MI | Improved | MSCs engrafted, differentiated into cardiac muscle expressing cells, and improved LV function. |

| | | | | | | |
|---|---|---|---|---|---|---|
| Yau (53) | Pig | Bone marrow stromal cells | Autologous | 4 weeks after MI | Improved | Direct injection of 5-azacytidine selected bone marrow stromal cells improved perfusion and LV function. These cells demonstrated greater plasticity in vivo than cardiac cells. |
| Kudo (54) | Mouse | Cultured MSC and fresh Lin- BMSC | Autologous | 10 minutes after MI | NA | Transplantation of both MSC and Lin- BMSC revealed their ability to differentiate into cardiac myocytes and endothelial cells as well as resulted in smaller infarct size and less fibrosis. |
| Barbash (55) | Rat | MSC | Autologous | 2 or 10–14 days after MI | NA | MSC delivered by LV cavity infusion resulted in greater engraftment within the infarct zone compared to intravenous delivery by tail vein injection. IV delivery resulted in a substantial proportion of MSC entrapment in the lungs. This study also suggested that an MSC homing mechanism exists for at least 14 days after MI. |
| Wang (59) | Rat | Bone marrow stromal cells | Autologous | 2 weeks after MI | NA | Coronary-infused MSC home to infarcted myocardium and differentiate into cardiac myocytes, fibroblasts and endothelial cells. |

ACS, acute coronary syndrome; BMSC, bone marrow stem cell; G-CSF, granulocyte colony stimulating factor; HSC, hematopoietic stem cell; IV, intravenous; LAD, left anterior descending coronary artery; LV, left ventricular; MSC, mesenchymal stem cells; MI, myocardial infarction; NA, not assessed; SCF, stem cell factor.

an MI would occur. In addition, the safety of a technique that results in a substantial leukocytosis in the peri-infarct period would need to be established before it could be accepted as a viable treatment option in patients presenting with ACS.

The mechanisms of stem cell homing are beginning to be uncovered (discussion following). Stromal cell derived factor (SDF)-1 has been shown to be upregulated early after an MI and to be integral in mediating stem cell homing and myocardial regeneration late after an MI [57]. Schuster et al. sought to optimize the effects of stem cell mobilization with systemic administration of G-CSF or granulocyte-macrophage colony stimulating factor (GM-CSF) coupled with intramyocardial injections of SDF-1 in the peri-MI period. They observed that the combination of systemic stem cell mobilization with intramyocardial injection of SDF-1 resulted in a synergistic effect on neoangiogenesis, attenuation of cardiomyocyte apoptosis and LV function [33]. These data suggest that if the release and targeting of stem cells from the bone marrow following myocardial infarction could be optimized, the possibility of improving LV function by non-invasive means could be realized.

## Mesenchymal Stem Cells in ACS

Mesenchymal stem cells are multipotent cells that can be isolated from adult bone marrow and can be induced in vitro and in vivo to differentiate into a variety of mesenchymal tissues, including bone, cartilage, tendon, fat, and muscle. This marked plasticity of MSC has been demonstrated in several studies to date [34,37]. MSC have also been shown to engraft into normal myocardium and to differentiate into cardiac tissue when placed with the correct milieu [58]. The controversy surrounding the ability of HSC to transdifferentiate makes these cells an attractive option for the purposes of myocardial regeneration. Pertinent to the treatment of ACS, these cells have been shown to be able to engraft into intact and injured myocardium, differentiate into cardiac myocytes and endothelial cells and improve LV function when administered within 4 weeks of the ischemic insult (Table 2).

Shake et al. assessed the efficacy of undifferentiated MSC in a swine ischemia-reperfusion model [52]. Two weeks following MI, labeled MSC were directly injected into the infarct zone. MSC engrafted, demonstrated expression of cardiac muscle specific proteins, attenuated pathologic remodeling and improved LV function supporting the plastic nature of this cell type even when untreated to differentiate into myogenic precursors.

Two questions arise when considering MSC therapy for the treatment of ischemic heart disease. Do MSC possess a similar in vivo regenerative capacity as has been seen with HSC? What is the optimal mode of delivery of MSC? To provide some insight into the first question, Kudo et al. assessed the effects of transplantation of both MSC and Lin- bone marrow cells 10 minutes after MI [54]. MSC migrated to the infarct zone and differentiated into myocytes and endothelial cells within the infarct zone, reducing infarct size and fibrosis. Consistent with prior studies of stem cell therapy for the treatment of MI, Lin-/c-kit+ cells were shown to migrate and differentiate into cardiac phenotypes, supporting the observation that both MSC and HSC possess regenerative capabilities. That one is more optimal than the other has yet to be fully demonstrated.

With respect to the mode of delivery of MSC, effective delivery of MSC has been demonstrated via direct intramyocardial injection. However, this technique would require patients to undergo open heart surgery before they could realize the benefits of MSC therapy. Efficacy of MSC delivery via the coronary or intravenous route would expand the eligibility of this therapy. Wang et al. demonstrated the efficacy of coronary delivery of MSC [59]. MSC delivered by their technique were shown to home to the infarct zone and differentiate into cardiac myocytes, endothelial cells and fibroblasts 2 weeks following

MI. Expanding these data, a recent study demonstrated that infusion of MSC into the LV cavity within 10–14 days of MI was an effective method of delivery [55]. In fact, it was more efficacious than intravenous delivery in part because of the significant lung sequestration seen with the latter technique. The technique that would be most widely applicable to patients with ACS, intracoronary delivery, has not been optimally addressed but is inferred from the prior two studies.

## Unselected Bone Marrow Stem Cells

Demonstration that unselected bone marrow possesses regenerative capabilities would be attractive for the ACS setting given the time constraints of benefit as well as the cell processing delays necessary to select specific subpopulations of the bone marrow. Nishida et al. recently assessed the efficacy of unselected BMSC transplantation in a rat myocardial hypoperfusion model [45]. Local implantation of autologous bone marrow cells induced angiogenesis, improved perfusion of ischemic myocardium, attenuated LV remodeling and improved deteriorated cardiac function caused by myocardial hypoperfusion. The attraction of using unselected BMSC also may arise out of the presence of both MSC and HSC fractions and the substrate to regenerate myocytes and vasculature, respectively, circumventing the transdifferentiation versus cell fusion controversy.

## POTENTIAL MECHANISMS INVOLVED IN MYOCARDIAL REGENERATION

### Stem Cell Mobilization and Homing

A fundamental concept of stem cell therapy for the treatment of ACS that has emerged is that of stem cell homing. Systemic administration of G-CSF mobilized stem cells which were then able to home to and regenerate infarcted myocardium in response to acute injury. Other potential mediators of stem cell mobilization and homing in the peri-infarct period are beginning to be identified. With an enhanced understanding of these signaling pathways, the ability to harness the regenerative capacity of stem cell therapy will be more easily achieved.

In addition to G-CSF, other endogenous (growth factors) and exogenous (pharmacologic) mediators of stem cell mobilization and homing in the cardiovascular arena are becoming more evident. Vascular endothelial growth factor (VEGF) administration has been shown to possess the capacity to mobilize CD34+ HSC from bone marrow and induce them to home to ischemic tissue in mice, promoting augmented neovascularization [60]. Our group has also observed that local delivery of VEGF to remodeled myocardium results significantly increases stem cell engraftment and augments neovascularization (unpublished data). Further supporting the role of VEGF in inducing stem cell mobilization, a recently published clinical study demonstrated that, in response to MI, increased numbers of CD34+ cells in the periphery were seen peaking at 7 days [46]. This peak in circulating CD34+ cells was coincident with the peak in plasma levels of VEGF.

Interestingly, HMG CoA reductase inhibitors (statins) also induce stem cell mobilization, which could be an explanation for the early benefits of statin therapy in patients following an MI. Treatment of mice with these agents significantly increased the levels of circulating endothelial progenitor cells [61]. Furthermore, an increase in the number of circulating endothelial progenitor cells with enhanced functional activity was demonstrated in patients with stable coronary artery disease (CAD) given statins [62]. Despite the encouraging results revealed in the studies above, a better understanding of the safety and efficacy of various stem cell mobilization techniques needs to be achieved before this therapy, one that may be most clinically relevant, can become a reality. Equally important is the underlying mechanism that prompts homing to the injured myocardium.

Although the mechanisms involved are incompletely understood, "homing" of stem cells to injured myocardium is essential as it concentrates BMSC in a milieu conducive for their engraftment, expansion and differentiation. That G-CSF-mobilized stem cells failed to engraft in already remodeled myocardium suggested that whatever the homing signal was which present in the early postinfarct period was gone late after MI. This prompted the search for factors that may possess transient expression profiles early after MI [57]. Using a candidate gene approach, the expression of several factors was shown to be up-regulated after MI. Given its integral role in stem cell trafficking to bone marrow, our group assessed the expression of stromal cell-derived factor-1 (SDF-1) as a function of time after MI. We observed that SDF-1 expression was increased within 1 hour after MI and lasted at least 3 days following and becoming absent by 7 days following MI [57]. We subsequently demonstrated that the expression of SDF-1 could be stimulated with cell transplantation and that chronic over-expression of SDF-1 resulted in stem cell homing to remodeled myocardium, increased angiogenesis, and improved LV function [57].

## Stem Cell Transdifferentiation or Stem Cell Fusion?

As alluded to earlier, both HSC [27–29] and MSC [34,37,58] have been shown to possess the ability to differentiate into cells of different tissues and to contribute to restoration and regeneration of these injured tissues. The capability of BMSC to undergo this process of transdifferentiation has recently come into question. Castro et al. [63] failed to detect neural-like cells in the brains of mice that received purified stem cells derived from bone marrow or unfractionated bone marrow cells. Similarly, after transplanting single hematopoietic stem cells labeled with green fluorescent protein (GFP) into lethally irradiated mice, the contribution of these cells to non-hematopoietic tissues was an extremely rare event [64]. One potential explanation for the discrepant findings could be that an environment conducive for transdifferentiation, one of tissue injury, was not present in these studies. Alternatively, a different mechanism may exist to account for the apparent plasticity seen in the early preclinical trials of tissue regeneration.

A potential explanation for these divergent results is that what was thought to be stem cell transdifferentiation actually represented cell fusion. Several studies have assessed the effect of coculturing labeled embryonal cells with adult BMSC or neural stem cells and demonstrated that within several weeks the labeled cells were found to express protein markers consistent with transdifferentiation [65,66]. However, further analysis revealed cells with a hybrid, polyploid DNA content strongly suggesting cell fusion as the mechanism underlying the apparent transdifferentiation. Confirming these data, two in vivo studies of mice with a fatal metabolic liver disease have provided more evidence that bone marrow cells from normal donors generate healthy hepatocytes by forming hybrid cells that contain both donor and host genes [30,31].

A controversial aspect of the cell fusion hypothesis is that fusion has been shown to be relatively infrequent in vivo, occurring perhaps once in 10,000–100,000 cells. However, transdifferentiation has been reported to occur quite frequently in coculture assays [26]. Therefore, fusion cannot solely account for the regeneration of large amounts of liver [36] and near complete regeneration of myocardium [28] demonstrated in early trials of BMSC delivery. Despite some data to suggest that transdifferentiation is the predominant mechanism for regeneration of tissue [44], the "truth" may actually lie somewhere in between the mechanisms of cell fusion and transdifferentiation as recently suggested [67]. Cell fusion may serve as an ongoing physiologic repair mechanism by which cells deliver healthy and new genes to highly specialized cells to prevent them from dying while transdifferentiation of a larger number of delivered BMSC may ultimately serve in the regenerative capacity envisioned for these cells.

## CLINICAL TRIALS OF STEM CELL THERAPY FOR ACS-MYOCARDIAL REGENERATION

The rapid accumulation of knowledge of stem cell plasticity and the demonstration of benefit in preclinical models has paved the way for clinical trials of stem cell therapy in patients with acute and chronic ischemic heart disease (Table 3). Despite the small size of these trials, the feasibility and safety of stem cell therapy has been demonstrated utilizing both surgical and percutaneous delivery methods.

### Stem Cell Therapy for the Treatment of Ischemic Heart Disease

The feasibility and safety of autologous BMSC transplantation into ungraftable regions of myocardium as an adjunct to CABG surgery in patients with chronic ischemic heart disease was recently demonstrated [68] perfusion in three of the five patients suggesting enhanced collateralization as a result of BMSC transplantation. More importantly, no obvious detrimental effects of cell transplantation were observed during the 1 year of follow-up. However, it is difficult to separate the benefits seen with BMSC transplantation versus those resulting form CABG surgery in this study.

An alternative method of stem cell delivery in vivo that circumvents the risks associated with open heart surgery would be a welcomed avenue for stem cell delivery. Two recent studies evaluated transmyocardial delivery of BMSC, using a percutaneous electromechanical guiding system (NOGA), in patients with ischemic heart disease. Tse et al. assessed the feasibility and safety of percutaneous mononuclear BMSC transplantation in 8 patients with stable angina refractory to maximal medical therapy [69]. Despite a lack of improvement in global left ventricular ejection fraction (LVEF), an improvement in regional wall thickening and a decrease in the percentage of hypoperfused myocardium was observed. This correlated with a significant reduction in weekly anginal episodes. Consistent with the safety of surgical BMSC transplantation, no acute or long-term adverse effects of BMSC were observed.

The utility of this technique for stem cell delivery was also assessed in patients with end-stage ischemic heart disease [70]. An improvement in regional perfusion defects and global LV function was seen as early as 2 months following cell transplantation. This benefit persisted through 4 months of follow-up revealing an improvement in regional and global LV function. Similar to direct cell transplantation at CABG surgery, these studies revealed the safety of BMSC transplantation in patients across the spectrum of chronic ischemic heart disease.

Alternatively, the feasibility of harnessing the regenerative capacity of one's endogenous stem cells could altogether avoid the risks of transplanting exogenous cells into ischemic myocardium. Seiler et al. assessed the effects of stem cell mobilization using GM-CSF [71]. GM-CSF was administered for two weeks to patients with nonrevascularizable CAD and resulted in improved coronary collateral blood flow assessed invasively. Overall, stem cell therapy has the potential to be a safe and effective adjunct to currently available treatments for patients with ischemic heart disease. The suggested benefits, how-

**Table 3** Clinical Trials of Stem Cells for the Treatment of Ischemic Heart Disease

| Study | Number of patients | Cell type | Delivery method | Time after infarct | LV function | Comments |
|---|---|---|---|---|---|---|
| Acute MI Trials | | | | | | |
| Strauer (73) | 10 | Autologous mononuclear BM Cells | Stem cell transplantation (Percutaneous/ Intracoronary) | 5–9 days | Improved | An improvement in LV cavity dimensions and systolic function as well as improved myocardial perfusion were seen at 3-month follow-up. No acute procedure-related complications or long-term complications were seen. |
| Assmus (74) | 20 | BM-derived or circulating blood-derived progenitor cells | Stem cell transplantation (Percutaneous/ Intracoronary) | 4.3 + 1.5 days | Improved | Improved ejection fraction, regional contractile function and increased myocardial viability were seen within the infarct zone at 4 months follow-up. No acute procedure-related complications or long-term complications were seen. |
| Stamm (72) | 6 | BM-derived AC 133$^+$ Cells | Stem cell transplantation (Direct intramyocardial injection at time of CABG) | 10 days-3 months | Unchanged | Pronounced improvement in myocardial perfusion by SPECT imaging at 2 weeks following cell implant. |
| Wollert | 30 | BM cells harvested from iliac crest | Stem cell transplantation (Percutaneous/ Intracoronary) | 3.5 days | Improved | This randomized, controlled trial revealed improved LVEF 6 months after receiving BMC infusions early after presentation for STEMI plus optimal care assessed by MRI. No acute procedure-related complications or long-term complications were seen. |
| Ellis, CCF | 9 | Mobilized BM stem cells | Daily G-CSF for 5 days following reperfusion | < 48 hours from symptom onset | Actively being analyzed | To date, no acute complications were seen with G-CSF administration in an acute MI setting. |

| Trial | n | Cell type | Intervention | Indication | LVEF | Results |
|---|---|---|---|---|---|---|
| CAD Trials Tse (69) | 8 | CD34$^+$ (3.2%) CD3$^+$ (7.6%) CD11b$^+$D15$^+$ (43.7%) 117 CFU-GM per 10$^5$ cells | Stem cell transplantation (NOGA-Guided catheter-based intramyocardial injection) | Stable angina refractory to medical therapy | Unchanged | Despite no change in LVEF, an improvement in target wall thickening and target wall motion was seen by MRI. No acute procedure-related complications or long-term complications were seen. |
| Seiler (71) | 21 | Mobilized BM progenitor cells | Stem cell mobilization (GM-CSF for 2 weeks) | Non-revascularizable CAD | NA | First study of stem cell mobilization to induce angiogenesis as assessed by improved coronary collateral blood flow with 2 weeks of daily GM-CSF administration. |
| Hamano (68) | 5 | Autologous BMC | Stem cell transplantation (Intramyocardial at CABG) | Chronic ischemic heart disease | NA | Demonstrated the feasibility and safety of BMC transplantation into ungraftable areas at the time of CABG. SPECT revealed improved coronary perfusion in 3 of 5 patients. No acute procedure-related complications or long-term complications were seen. |
| Perin (70) | 21 | Autologous BMC | Stem cell transplantation (NOGA-Guided catheter-based intramyocardial injection) | End-stage ischemic cardiomyopathy | Improved | This study demonstrates the relative safety of intramyocardial injections of bone marrow-derived stem cells in patients with severe heart failure. In addition, the potential for improving myocardial blood flow with associated enhancement of regional and global LV function. |

BM, bone marrow; BMC, bone marrow cell; CABG, coronary artery bypass graft surgery; CAD, coronary artery disease; CCF, Cleveland Clinic Foundation; G-CSF, granulocyte colony stimulating factor; GM-CSF, granulocyte-macrophage colony stimulating factor; NA, not assessed; STEMI, ST-elevation myocardial infarction.

ever, need to be corroborated by larger randomized controlled trials before they can be accepted as clinically useful.

## Stem Cell Therapy for the Treatment of ACS

Expanding upon the remarkable findings of preclinical studies, several early trials using cell types ranging from selected stem cells to unselected bone marrow derived and peripheral blood derived mononuclear stem cells have established the feasibility, safety, and utility of this treatment in patients with acute MI, fostering the hope that this therapy will be able to break through the apparent ''ceiling'' of benefit that exists with conventional treatment modalities. As an adjunct to CABG surgery, a recent group transplanted $1 \times 10^6$ AC 133+ stem cells, a subset of mononuclear BMSC with prominent angiogenic potential, into regions of myocardium deemed unsuitable for grafting. This was associated with improved efection fraction in 4 of the 6 patients and a striking improvement in perfusion in 5 of the 6 patients transplanted 10days to 3 months after an acute MI [72]. Furthermore, all six patients experienced an improvement in functional capacity following stem cell transplantation. This study suggests that transplantation of AC 133+ cells promotes angiogenesis with a resultant improvement in global LV function. Furthermore, the safety of transplantation of this quantity of cells has been demonstrated 9 to 16 months following surgery.

Two recent clinical trials of intracoronary, autologous, mononuclear BMSC transplantation for improving LV function and perfusion during the immediate postinfarction period have been reported [73,74]. In the first study, ten previously revascularized patients received additional treatment with intracoronary autologous BMSC infusion of approximately $10^4$ cells five to nine days after percutaneous intervention for acute MI. After 3 months of follow-up a significant decrease in the size of the infarct region and a concomitant improvement in regional cardiac function were appreciated in patients that received BMSC infusions [73]. No acute, procedure-related, or long-term complications were seen with BMSC therapy. Expanding upon these data, the second study assessed the safety and efficacy of both BMSC and peripheral blood progenitor cells (PBSC) in the immediate postinfarction period. Intracoronary infusion of both cell types at a mean of approximately 4 days after MI resulted in a significant increase in global LV function, improved regional function and attenuated LV remodeling 4 months after treatment [74]. In addition, no acute or long-term adverse effects were seen with stem cell therapy. These studies suggest that early, intracoronary delivery of unselected BMSC and PBSC may be a safe and effective adjunct to conventional therapy for acute MI. Similar to the limitations described for adjunctive stem cell therapy for chronic ischemic heart disease, it is difficult to separate the benefits imparted by stem cell therapy from those imparted by prompt revascularization therapy.

The benefits demonstrated by the preceding, predominantly nonrandomized studies, were recently supported in a randomized trial of adjunctive, intracoronary BMSC delivery (Wollert reference). Sixty patients were randomized to receive optimal care versus optimal care plus BMSC infusions 3.5 days after successful PCI for acute MI. A significantly greater improvement in LVEF assessed by MRI was seen at 6 month follow-up. Patients that experienced the longest delays to revascularization also enjoyed the greatest improvement in LVEF with BMSC transplantation. Furthermore, the benefit was seen irrespective of infarct location or gender. Consistent with prior studies, no acute or long-term adverse effects of BMSC transplantation were observed.

Despite the encouraging results of the preclinical and clinical trials to date, a substantial amount of work remains to be performed before we can achieve our goal of improving outcomes in patients with ACS through regenerative medicine.

## FUTURE DIRECTIONS

The demonstration that stem cells can regenerate functional myocardium in preclinical studies and that stem cell transplantation is feasible and safe in clinical studies has set the stage for further development of these therapies for the treatment of ACS. However, many significant challenges remain.

## Mode of Stem Cell Delivery

Although several modes of stem cell delivery have been identified and studied in preclinical and clinical trials, the optimal method has yet to be defined. Perhaps one mode of stem cell delivery will not prove to be better than another overall, but rather the optimal mode of delivery will be dictated by the clinical situation in which stem cell therapy is to be employed. For example, in the acute coronary syndrome setting recent data has revealed substantial upregulation of "homing" factors which may allow for either peripheral or locally infused delivery of stem cells. On the other hand, direct surgical or percutaneous transmyocardial injection of stem cells may result in optimal regenerative capacity late after MI when the expression of "homing" factors has ceased.

### Direct Myocardial Injection

The most invasive technique of stem cell delivery, this technique best suits patients already scheduled to undergo a surgical procedure. Direct visualization of potential target zones makes this technique simple. However, incomplete delivery of stem cells may occur as a result of deficient access to target areas.

The feasibility of transendocardial delivery of stem cells using an eletromechanical mapping system, NOGA, has recently been demonstrated (discussed previously). The benefits to this approach include the ability to precisely deliver stem cells to the regions of interest. The possibility of requiring fewer cells to achieve similar benefit with precise delivery may decrease the risk of arrhythmia that was evident with injection of larger numbers of cells in an early trial of SKMB transplantation.

### Intracoronary Stem Cell Delivery

This technique of stem cell delivery, successful in early clinical trials, allows for delivery of stem cells to a specific coronary territory (discussed previously). However, the optimal pressure of cell infusion, duration of cell delivery and volume of cells infused remains to be determined. In addition, the retention of cells within the region of interest remains a vital issue.

### Intravenous Stem Cell Delivery

The least invasive method of stem cell delivery, this technique relies heavily on the presence of "homing" factors for success. Integral to the utility of this method of stem cell delivery is the demonstration of sequestration of a proportion of the cells within other organs [55] allowing a small number of cells to actually reach the ischemic myocardium. Therefore, optimization of dosing will contribute to this method of stem cell delivery.

A unifying benefit to the above methods of stem cell delivery is the possibility to genetically alter the harvested stem cells to express potential homing or differentiation factors in order to augment the regenerative capacity of these cells. Clearly, a better understanding of these factors is necessary before this approach can be exploited.

*Endogenous Stem Cell Mobilization*

The feasibility and safety of stem cell mobilization with the administration of growth factors has been demonstrated in a recent clinical trial of patients with stable CAD (discussed previously). However, the safety of this approach in the ACS setting remains to be determined. Researchers at the Cleveland Clinic Foundation are exploring the feasibility and safety of G-CSF in patients presenting with acute MI. Further recommendations for the use of this technique are premature at this time.

## Timing of Stem Cell Delivery

The majority of studies to date have focused on the early peri-infarct period. When administered within a few days to 3 months after an MI, stem cell transplantation improved regional perfusion and LV function. The question of whether earlier or later cell delivery can achieve a greater benefit remains to be seen. Of note, the potential to attenuate any benefit of stem cell therapy exists when cells are delivered early after MI perhaps as a result of the extensive acute inflammatory response.

## What is the Optimal Cell Type for the Treatment of ACS?

Although alluded to in the previous sections, the optimal cell type for myocardial regeneration remains to be determined. Both HSC and MSC have shown promise in this regard. Alternatively, some studies have suggested that the use of unselected BMSC may circumvent the need for cell processing and provide a more readily available population of cells that are made up of both HSC and MSC, potentially resulting in more complete myocardial regeneration through lineage dependent differentiation. Randomized studies comparing these cell types as well as others may shed light on which cell type will reign supreme.

## Combined Cell Therapy and Gene Transfer

Gene transfer as a therapeutic modality for the treatment of myocardial ischemia and/or infarction has been proposed as a revolutionary approach to improve collateral circulation, enhance myocardial viability and optimize the healing process. However, direct gene transfer into infarcted myocardium, while feasible, is limited by low transfection efficiency and the inflammatory response to the viral vectors presently being tested [75]. On the other hand, skeletal myoblasts stably transfected expression vectors encoding genes of interest such as transforming growth factor beta-1 (TGFβ-1) or VEGF have been successfully engrafted into the myocardium and lead to neovascularization [76,77]. In addition, our group has demonstrated that SKMB based VEGF delivery results in less inflammation, greater neovascularization, and improved LV function in an ischemic cardiomyopathy model [78].

Similar results have been observed with the transplantation of genetically engineered stem cells into infarcted myocardium [79,80]. In an attempt to enhance MSC engraftment and survival in ischemic myocardium, Mangi et al. transplanted genetically engineered MSC expressing the prosurvival gene Akt1 60 minutes after LAD ligation [80]. Transplantation of $5 \times 10^6$ cells overexpressing Akt1 into ischemic rat myocardium attenuated remodeling by reducing inflammation, collagen deposition and cardiac myocyte hypertrophy. In addition, this combined therapy regenerated 80–90% of lost myocardial volume and almost completely normalized LV function. MSCs transfected with Akt1 restored significantly greater myocardial volume than an equal number of control MSCs transfected with the reporter gene lacZ.

The study by Mangi et al. demonstrates that BMSCs can be genetically engineered to address specific limitations or pathways in order to augment the utility of stem cell therapy for ACS. Our group utilized genetic engineering to address the utility of restoring stem cell homing in already remodeled myocardium [57]. One could envision combining cell therapy with gene transfer to address additional issues integral to myocardial regeneration including targeted stem cell differentiation.

## Quantification of Cell Engraftment

In order to adequately compare potential therapies in vivo noninvasive techniques for quantifying cell engraftment are actively being pursued. With the development of accurate techniques such as MRI and myocardial strain and strain rate assessed by color Doppler tissue imaging, the need to sacrifice study animals in order to assess treatment effects will not persist. Furthermore, the level of engraftment could be correlated with clinical outcomes facilitating a better understanding of the benefits imparted on subjects receiving cell therapy.

## CONCLUSIONS

The potential now exists to break through the "ceiling" of benefit of currently available therapies for patients with ACS. Recent studies have demonstrated that myocardial regeneration is not simply a dream but rather an eminent reality. Through further elucidation of the underlying mechanisms involved in myocardial regeneration, a significant burden imparted upon society, that of the acute coronary syndromes, can be lifted.

## REFERENCES

1. Rogers WJ, Canto JG, Lambrew CT, Tiefenbrunn AJ, Kinkaid B, Shoultz DA, Frederick PD, Every N. Temporal trends in the treatment of over 1.5 million patients with myocardial infarction in the US from 1990 through 1999: the National Registry of Myocardial Infarction 1, 2 and 3. J Am Coll Cardiol. 2000;36:2056–63.
2. Reperfusion therapy for acute myocardial infarction with fibrinolytic therapy or combination reduced fibrinolytic therapy and platelet glycoprotein IIb/IIIa inhibition: the GUSTO V randomized trial. The GUSTO V Investigators. Lancet 2001;357:1905–1914.
3. Efficacy and safety of tenecteplase in combination with enoxaparin, abciximab, or unfractionated heparin: the ASSENT-3 randomised trial in acute myocardial infarction. Lancet 2001; 358:605–13.
4. Keeley EC, Boura JA, Grines CL. Primary angioplasty versus intravenous thrombolytic therapy for acute myocardial infarction: a quantitative review of 23 randomised trials. Lancet 2003; 361:13–20.
5. Robbins MA, O'Connell JB. Economic impact of heart failure. In: Rose EA , Stevenson LW, Eds. Management of End-Stage Heart Disease. Philadelphia: Lippincott-Raven, 1998:3–13.
6. Pfeffer MA, Braunwald E. Ventricular remodeling after myocardial infarction. Experimental observations and clinical implications. Circulation 1990;81:1161–1172.
7. Pfeffer JM, Pfeffer MA, Fletcher PJ, Braunwald E. Progressive ventricular remodeling in rat with myocardial infarction. Am J Physiol 1991;260:H1406–1414.
8. Eriksson H. Heart failure: a growing public health problem. J Intern Med 1995;237:135–141.

9.  Koh GY, Soonpaa MH, Klug MG, Field LJ. Long-term survival of AT-1 cardiomyocyte grafts in syngeneic myocardium. Am. J. Physiol 1993;264:H1727–H1733.

10. Soonpaa MH, Koh GY, Klug MG, Field LJ. Formation of nascent intercalated disks between grafted fetal cardiomyocytes and host myocardium [see comments]. Science 1994;264:98–101.

11. Sakai T, Li RK, Weisel RD, Mickle DA, Jia ZQ, Tomita S, Kim EJ, Yau TM. Fetal cell transplantation: a comparison of three cell types. J Thorac Cardiovasc Surg. 1999;118:715–24.

12. Li RK, Jia ZQ, Weisel RD, Merante F, Mickle DA. Smooth muscle cell transplantation into myocardial scar tissue improves heart function. J Mol Cell Cardiol 1999;31:513–522.

13. Taylor DA, Atkins BZ, Hungspreugs P, Jones TR, Reedy MC, Hutcheson KA, Glower DD, Kraus WE. Regenerating functional myocardium: improved performance after skeletal myoblast transplantation [published erratum appears in Nat Med 1998 Oct;4(10):1200]. Nature Medicine. 1998;4:929–33.

14. Jain M, DerSimonian H, Brenner DA, Ngoy S, Teller P, Edge AS, Zawadzka A, Wetzel K, Sawyer DB, Colucci WS, Apstein CS, Liao R. Cell therapy attenuates deleterious ventricular remodeling and improves cardiac performance after myocardial infarction. Circulation. 2001; 103:1920–7.

15. Campion DR. The muscle satellite cell: a review. Int Rev Cytol 1984;87:225–251.

16. Jennings RB, Reimer KA. Lethal myocardial ischemic injury. Am J Pathol 1981;102:241–255.

17. Murry CE, Wiseman RW, Schwartz SM, Hauschka SD. Skeletal myoblast transplantation for repair of myocardial necrosis. J Clin Invest 1996;98:2512–2523.

18. Chiu RC, Zibaitis A, Kao RL. Cellular cardiomyoplasty: myocardial regeneration with satellite cell implantation. Ann Thorac Surg 1995;60:12–18.

19. Atkins BZ, Hueman MT, Meuchel JM, Cottman MJ, Hutcheson KA, Taylor DA. Myogenic cell transplantation improves in vivo regional performance in infarcted rabbit myocardium. Journal of Heart & Lung Transplantation 1999;18:1173–1180.

20. Atkins BZ, Hueman MT, Meuchel J, Hutcheson KA, Glower DD, Taylor DA. Cellular cardiomyoplasty improves diastolic properties of injured heart. J Surg Res 1999;85:234–42.

21. Ghostine S, Carrion C, Souza LC, Richard P, Bruneval P, Vilquin JT, Pouzet B, Schwartz K, Menasche P, Hagege AA. Long–term efficacy of myoblast transplantation on regional structure and function after myocardial infarction. Circulation. 2002;106:I131–6.

22. Menasche P, Hagege AA, Vilquin JT, Desnos M, Abergel E, Pouzet B, Bel A, Sarateanu S, Scorsin M, Schwartz K, Bruneval P, Benbunan M, Marolleau JP, Duboc D. Autologous skeletal myoblast transplantation for severe postinfarction left ventricular dysfunction. J Am Coll Cardiol. 2003;41:1078–83.

23. Maltsev VA, Wobus AM, Rohwedel J, Bader M, Hescheler J. Cardiomyocytes differentiated in vitro from embryonic stem cells developmentally express cardiac-specific genes and ionic currents. Circ Res 1994;75:233–244.

24. Makino S, Fukuda K, Miyoshi S, Konishi F, Kodama H, Pan J, Sano M, Takahashi T, Hori S, Abe H, Hata J, Umezawa A, Ogawa S. Cardiomyocytes can be generated from marrow stromal cells in vitro. J Clin Invest. 1999;103:697–705.

25. Takahashi T, Kalka C, Masuda H, Chen D, Silver M, Kearney M, Magner M, Isner JM, Asahara T. Ischemia– and cytokine–induced mobilization of bone marrow–derived endothelial progenitor cells for neovascularization. Nat Med. 1999;5:434–8.

26. Badorff C, Brandes RP, Popp R, Rupp S, Urbich C, Aicher A, Fleming I, Busse R, Zeiher AM, Dimmeler S. Transdifferentiation of blood–derived human adult endothelial progenitor cells into functionally active cardiomyocytes. Circulation. 2003;107:1024–1032.

27. Kocher AA, Schuster MD, Szabolcs MJ, Takuma S, Burkhoff D, Wang J, Homma S, Edwards NM, Itescu S. Neovascularization of ischemic myocardium by human bone–marrow–derived angioblasts prevents cardiomyocyte apoptosis, reduces remodeling and improves cardiac function. Nat Med. 2001;7:430–6.

28. Orlic D, Kajstura J, Chimenti S, Jakoniuk I, Anderson SM, Li B, Pickel J, McKay R, Nadal–Ginard B, Bodine DM, Leri A, Anversa P. Bone marrow cells regenerate infarcted myocardium. Nature. 2001;410:701–5.

29. Orlic D, Kajstura J, Chimenti S, Limana F, Jakoniuk I, Quaini F, Nadal–Ginard B, Bodine DM, Leri A, Anversa P. Mobilized bone marrow cells repair the infarcted heart, improving function and survival. Proc Natl Acad Sci U S A. 2001;98:10344–9.

30. Vassilopoulos G, Wang PR, Russell DW. Transplanted bone marrow regenerates liver by cell fusion. Nature 2003;422:901–904.

31. Wang X, Willenbring H, Akkari Y, Limana F, Jakoniuk I, Quaini F, Nadal–Ginard B, Bodine DM, Leri A, Anversa P, Cabuhat ML. Cell fusion is the principal source of bone–marrow–derived hepatocytes. Nature. 2003;422:897–901.

32. Urbanek K, Quaini F, Tasca G, Torella D, Castaldo C, Nadal–Ginard B, Leri A, Kajstura J, Quaini E, Anversa P. Intense myocyte formation from cardiac stem cells in human cardiac hypertrophy. Proc Natl Acad Sci U S A. 2003;100:10440–5.

33. Schuster MD, Witkowski P, Boyle A, Seti T, Kocher AA, Seruya M, Way K, Itescu S. Stromal derived factor (SDF)–1 augments cytokine induced stem cell mobilization and cardiac functional recovery after acute infarction. Circulation. 2003;108:IV–38.

34. Pittenger MF, Mackay AM, Beck SC, Jaiswal RK, Douglas R, Mosca JD, Moorman MA, Simonetti DW, Craig S, Marshak DR. Multilineage potential of adult human mesenchymal stem cells. Science. 1999;284:143–7.

35. Brazelton TR, Rossi FM, Keshet GI, Blau HM. From maroow to brain: Expression of neuronal phenotypes in adult mice. Science 2000;290:1775–1779.

36. Lagasse E, Connors H, Al–Dhalimy M, Reitsma M, Dohse M, Osborne L, Wang X, Finegold M, Weissman IL, Grompe M. Purified hematopoietic stem cells can differentiate into hepatocytes in vivo. Nat Med. 2000;6:1229–1234.

37. Liechty KW, MacKenzie TC, Shaaban AF, Radu A, Moseley AM, Deans R, Marshak DR, Flake AW. Human mesenchymal stem cells engraft and demonstrate site–specific differentiation after in utero transplantation in sheep. Nat Med. 2000;6:1282–6.

38. Jiang Y, Jahagirdar BN, Reinhardt RL, Schwartz RE, Keene CD, Ortiz–Gonzalez XR, Reyes M, Lenvik T, Lund T, Blackstad M, Du J, Aldrich S, Lisberg A, Low WC, Largaespada DA, Verfaillie CM. Pluripotency of mesenchymal stem cells derived from adult marrow. Nature. 2002;418:41–9.

39. Kehat I, Kenyagin–Karsenti D, Snir M, Segev H, Amit M, Gepstein A, Livne E, Binah O, Itskovitz–Eldor J, Gepstein L. Human embryonic stem cells can differentiate into myocytes with structural and functional properties of cardiomyocytes. J Clin Invest. 2001;108:407–14.

40. Min JY, Yang Y, Sullivan MF, Ke Q, Converso KL, Chen Y, Morgan JP, Xiao YF. Long–term improvement of cardiac function in rats after infarction by transplantation of embryonic stem cells. J Thorac Cardiovasc Surg. 2003;125:361–9.

41. Korbling M. Peripheral Blood Stem Cells: A Novel Source for Allogeneic Transplantation. Oncologist 1997;2:104–113.

42. Kondo M, Wagers AJ, Manz MG, Prohaska SS, Scherer DC, Beilhack GF, Shizuru JA, Weissman IL. Biology of hematopoietic stem cells and progenitors: implications for clinical application. Annu Rev Immunol. 2003;21:759–806.

43. Orlic D, Kajstura J, Chimenti S, Bodine DM, Leri A, Anversa P. Transplanted adult bone marrow cells repair myocardial infarcts in mice. Ann N Y Acad Sci 2001;938:221–229; discussion 229–230.

44. Beltrami AP, Barlucchi L, Torella D, Baker M, Limana F, Chimenti S, Kasahara H, Rota M, Musso E, Urbanek K, Leri A, Kajstura J, Nadal–Ginard B, Anversa P. Adult cardiac stem cells are multipotent and support myocardial regeneration. Cell. 2003;114:763–76.

45. Nishida M, Li TS, Hirata K, Yano M, Matsuzaki M, Hamano K. Improvement of cardiac function by bone marrow cell implantation in a rat hypoperfusion heart model. Ann Thorac Surg 2003;75:768–73; discussion 773–774.

46. Shintani S, Murohara T, Ikeda H, Ueno T, Honma T, Katoh A, Sasaki K, Shimada T, Oike Y, Imaizumi T. Mobilization of endothelial progenitor cells in patients with acute myocardial infarction. Circulation. 2001;103:2776–9.

47. Jackson KA, Majka SM, Wang H, Pocius J, Hartley CJ, Majesky MW, Entman ML, Michael LH, Hirschi KK, Goodell MA. Regeneration of ischemic cardiac muscle and vascular endothelium by adult stem cells. J Clin Invest. 2001;107:1395–402.

48. Quaini F, Urbanek K, Beltrami AP, Finato N, Beltrami CA, Nadal–Ginard B, Kajstura J, Leri A, Anversa P. Chimerism of the transplanted heart. N Engl J Med. 2002;346:5–15.

49. Beltrami AP, Urbanek K, Kajstura J, Yan SM, Finato N, Bussani R, Nadal–Ginard B, Silvestri F, Leri A, Beltrami CA, Anversa P. Evidence that human cardiac myocytes divide after myocardial infarction. N Engl J Med. 2001;344:1750–7.

50. Tomita S, Li RK, Weisel RD, et al. Autologous transplantation of bone marrow cells improves damaged heart function. Circulation 1999;100:II247–256.

51. Tomita S, Mickle DA, Weisel RD, Jia ZQ, Tumiati LC, Allidina Y, Liu P, Li RK. Improved heart function with myogenesis and angiogenesis after autologous porcine bone marrow stromal cell transplantation. J Thorac Cardiovasc Surg. 2002;123:1132–40.

52. Shake JG, Gruber PJ, Baumgartner WA, Senechal G, Meyers J, Redmond JM, Pittenger MF, Martin BJ. Mesenchymal stem cell implantation in a swine myocardial infarct model: engraftment and functional effects. Ann Thorac Surg. 2002;73:1919–25; discussion 1926.

53. Yau TM, Tomita S, Weisel RD, Jia ZQ, Tumiati LC, Mickle DA, Li RK. Beneficial effect of autologous cell transplantation on infarcted heart function: comparison between bone marrow stromal cells and heart cells. Ann Thorac Surg. 2003;75:169–76; discussion 176–7.

54. Kudo M, Wang Y, Wani MA, Xu M, Ayub A, Ashraf M. Implantation of bone marrow stem cells reduces the infarction and fibrosis in ischemic mouse heart. J Mol Cell Cardiol 2003; 35:1113–1139.

55. Barbash IM, Chouraqui P, Baron J, Feinberg MS, Etzion S, Tessone A, Miller L, Guetta E, Zipori D, Kedes LH, Kloner RA, Leor J. Systemic delivery of bone marrow–derived mesenchymal stem cells to the infarcted myocardium: feasibility, cell migration, and body distribution. Circulation. 2003;108:863–8.

56. Kawamoto A, Tkebuchava T, Yamaguchi J, Nishimura H, Yoon YS, Milliken C, Uchida S, Masuo O, Iwaguro H, Ma H, Hanley A, Silver M, Kearney M, Losordo DW, Isner JM, Asahara T. Intramyocardial transplantation of autologous endothelial progenitor cells for therapeutic neovascularization of myocardial ischemia. Circulation. 2003;107:461–8.

57. Askari AT, Unzek S, Popovic ZB, Goldman CK, Forudi F, Kiedrowski M, Rovner A, Ellis SG, Thomas JD, DiCorleto PE, Topol EJ, Penn MS. Effect of stromal–cell–derived factor 1 on stem–cell homing and tissue regeneration in ischaemic cardiomyopathy. Lancet. 2003;362: 697–703.

58. Wang J, Shum-Tim D, Galipeau J, Chedrawy E, Eliopoulos N, Chiu R. Marrow stromal cells for cellular cardiomyoplasty: feasibility and potential clinical advantages. J Thorac Cardiovasc Surg 2000;120:999–1005.

59. Wang JS, Shum-Tim D, Chedrawy E, Chiu RC. The coronary delivery of marrow stromal cells for myocardial regeneration: pathophysiologic and therapeutic implications. J Thorac Cardiovasc Surg 2001;122:699–705.

60. Asahara T, Takahashi T, Masuda H, Kalka C, Chen D, Iwaguro H, Inai Y, Silver M, Isner JM. VEGF contributes to postnatal neovascularization by mobilizing bone marrow–derived endothelial progenitor cells. Embo J. 1999;18:3964–72.

61. Dimmeler S, Aicher A, Vasa M, Mildner–Rihm C, Adler K, Tiemann M, Rutten H, Fichtlscherer S, Martin H, Zeiher AM. HMG–CoA reductase inhibitors (statins) increase endothelial progenitor cells via the PI 3–kinase/Akt pathway. J Clin Invest. 2001;108:391–7.

62. Vasa M, Fichtlscherer S, Adler K, Aicher A, Martin H, Zeiher AM, Dimmeler S. Increase in circulating endothelial progenitor cells by statin therapy in patients with stable coronary artery disease. Circulation. 2001;103:2885–90.

63. Castro RF, Jackson KA, Goodell MA, Robertson CS, Liu H, Shine HD. Failure of bone marrow cells to transdifferentiate into neural cells in vivo. Science 2002;297:1299.

64. Wagers AJ, Sherwood RI, Christensen JL, Weissman IL. Little evidence for developmental plasticity of adult hematopoietic stem cells. Science 2002;297:2256–2259.

65. Terada N, Hamazaki T, Oka M, Hoki M, Mastalerz DM, Nakano Y, Meyer EM, Morel L, Petersen BE, Scott EW. Bone marrow cells adopt the phenotype of other cells by spontaneous cell fusion. Nature. 2002;416:542–5.

66. Ying QL, Nichols J, Evans EP, Smith AG. Changing potency by spontaneous fusion. Nature 2002;416:545–548.

67. Oh H, Bradfute SB, Gallardo TD, Nakamura T, Gaussin V, Mishina Y, Pocius J, Michael LH, Behringer RR, Garry DJ, Entman ML, Schneider MD. Cardiac progenitor cells from adult

myocardium: homing, differentiation, and fusion after infarction. Proc Natl Acad Sci U S A. 2003;100:12313–8.

68. Hamano K, Nishida M, Hirata K, Mikamo A, Li TS, Harada M, Miura T, Matsuzaki M, Esato K. Local implantation of autologous bone marrow cells for therapeutic angiogenesis in patients with ischemic heart disease: clinical trial and preliminary results. Jpn Circ J. 2001;65:845–7.

69. Tse HF, Kwong YL, Chan JK, Lo G, Ho CL, Lau CP. Angiogenesis in ischaemic myocardium by intramyocardial autologous bone marrow mononuclear cell implantation. Lancet 2003;361: 47–49.

70. Perin EC, Dohmann HF, Borojevic R, Silva SA, Sousa AL, Mesquita CT, Rossi MI, Carvalho AC, Dutra HS, Dohmann HJ, Silva GV, Belem L, Vivacqua R, Rangel FO, Esporcatte R, Geng YJ, Vaughn WK, Assad JA, Mesquita ET, Willerson JT. Transendocardial, autologous bone marrow cell transplantation for severe, chronic ischemic heart failure. Circulation. 2003; 107:2294–302.

71. Seiler C, Pohl T, Wustmann K, Hutter D, Nicolet PA, Windecker S, Eberli FR, Meier B. Promotion of collateral growth by granulocyte–macrophage colony–stimulating factor in patients with coronary artery disease: a randomized, double–blind, placebo–controlled study. Circulation. 2001;104:2012–7.

72. Stamm C, Westphal B, Kleine HD, Petzsch M, Kittner C, Klinge H, Schumichen C, Nienaber CA, Freund M, Steinhoff G. Autologous bone–marrow stem–cell transplantation for myocardial regeneration. Lancet. 2003;361:45–6.

73. Strauer BE, Brehm M, Zeus T, Kostering M, Hernandez A, Sorg RV, Kogler G, Wernet P. Repair of infarcted myocardium by autologous intracoronary mononuclear bone marrow cell transplantation in humans. Circulation. 2002;106:1913–8.

74. Assmus B, Schachinger V, Teupe C, Britten M, Lehmann R, Dobert N, Grunwald F, Aicher A, Urbich C, Martin H, Hoelzer D, Dimmeler S, Zeiher AM. Transplantation of Progenitor Cells and Regeneration Enhancement in Acute Myocardial Infarction (TOPCARE–AMI). Circulation. 2002;106:3009–17.

75. Leor J, Quinones MJ, Patterson M, Kedes L, Kloner RA. Adenovirus-mediated gene transfer into infarcted myocardium: feasibility, timing, and location of expression. J Mol Cell Cardiol 1996;28:2057–2067.

76. Koh GY, Kim SJ, Klug MG, Park K, Soonpaa MH, Field LJ. Targeted expression of transforming growth factor-beta 1 in intracardiac grafts promotes vascular endothelial cell DNA synthesis. J Clin Invest 1995;95:114–121.

77. Suzuki K, Murtuza B, Smolenski RT, Sammut IA, Suzuki N, Kaneda Y, Yacoub MH. Cell transplantation for the treatment of acute myocardial infarction using vascular endothelial growth factor–expressing skeletal myoblasts. Circulation. 2001;104:I–207–I–212.

78. Askari A, Unzek S, Goldman CK, Ellis SG, Thomas JD, DiCorleto PE, Topol EJ, Penn MS. Cellular, but not direct, adenoviral delivery of vascular endothalial growth factor results in improved left ventricular function and neovascularization in dilated ischemic cardiomyopally J Am Coll Cardial 43.

79. Yang Y, Min JY, Rana JS, Ke Q, Cai J, Chen Y, Morgan JP, Xiao YF. VEGF enhances functional improvement of postinfarcted hearts by transplantation of ESC–differentiated cells. J Appl Physiol. 2002;93:1140–51.

80. Mangi AA, Noiseux N, Kong D, He H, Rezvani M, Ingwall JS, Dzau VJ. Mesenchymal stem cells modified with Akt prevent remodeling and restore performance of infarcted hearts. Nat Med. 2003;9:1195–201.

# 29
# Cardiogenic Shock and Heart Failure Complicating Acute Myocardial Infarction

**Vladimir Dzavik**
*Associate Professor of Medicine, University of Toronto*
*Toronto, Canada*

**Judith S. Hochman**
*Harold Snyder Family Professor of Cardiology, New York University*
*New York*

## OVERVIEW

Pump failure complicates the course of a significant proportion of patients presenting with acute myocardial infarction (MI). The syndrome encompasses a spectrum ranging from mild pulmonary congestion on presentation at one end to a severe shock state secondary to left ventricular (LV) pump failure or a mechanical complication of MI at the other. In this chapter, this spectrum will be discussed, beginning with the more severe form of low output, cardiogenic shock, and then reviewing the characteristics, treatment and outcome of patients with heart failure, an important subset of patients with acute MI whose high risk is largely unappreciated.

## CARDIOGENIC SHOCK

### Introduction

Cardiogenic shock, characterized by systemic hypoperfusion due to low cardiac output despite high filling pressures, complicates approximately 7% of all cases of acute myocardial infarction (AMI), with the majority resulting from LV pump failure. The remaining AMI patients who develop shock do so from mechanical complications such as ventricular septal rupture, mitral regurgitation, tamponade, or other etiologies. While modern therapy, including aggressive revascularization therapy and intra-aortic balloon support, has contributed to an improvement in survival, the overall 30-day mortality associated with this catastrophic complication of AMI remains over 50%.

### Etiologies and Pathophysiology

The most common cause of shock after AMI is predominant LV pump failure, being responsible for 78.5% of cases of shock in the combined SHould We Emergently Revascularize Occluded Coronaries for Cardiogenic Shock (SHOCK) Trial and Registry [1]. In the same database, isolated right ventricular failure was the cause of cardiogenic shock in 2.8%. Mechanical complications are reported to be responsible for 12–20% of cases, with acute severe mitral regurgitation occurring in 7–10%, ventricular septal rupture in less than 4%, and free-wall rupture or tamponade in only 1.4–3% of cases (Fig. 1) [1,2].

Cardiogenic shock is typically related to acute dysfunction of a large amount of left ventricular myocardium. In the classic paradigm described by Hollenberg et al. [3], MI leads to systolic as well as diastolic dysfunction. On the systolic side, this leads to a decrease in cardiac output and stroke volume, hypotension, decreased coronary perfusion pressure, and the ensuing vicious spiral of more ischemia, and subsequently more myocardial dysfunction. The low cardiac output also results in a decrease in systemic perfusion that in the classic paradigm initiates compensatory vasoconstriction, still more myocardial dysfunction, and finally death [3]. Several observations suggest, however, that the mechanisms may be somewhat more complex and that infarction-induced systemic inflammation may play a role. First is the observation that the left ventricular dysfunction in patients with shock secondary to pump failure is only moderately severe. The mean LV ejection fraction of approximately 30% observed in the SHOCK Trial is in fact higher than that of many ambulatory patients with chronic left ventricular dysfunction and the same as minimally symptomatic or asymptomatic patients in a post-MI study of beta blockade [4,5]. Survivors of cardiogenic shock remain in New York Heart Association (NYHA) Class I or II functional status once they have recovered from the acute event. In addition, many patients with cardiogenic shock exhibit a clinically apparent systemic inflammatory response syndrome (SIRS), with fever and an elevated white cell count. Finally, the systemic vascular resistance of patients in cardiogenic shock is generally not elevated—hence there is inadequate vasoconstriction to compensate for low cardiac output and blood pressure—and thus tends to be inappropriately low for the hemodynamic conditions [6].

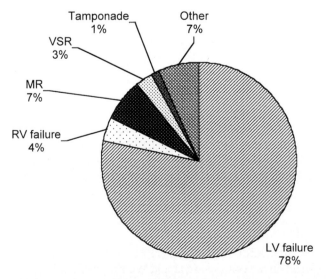

**Figure 1**   Distribution of etiologies of cardiogenic shock in the combined SHOCK Trial and Registry population. (From Ref. 1)

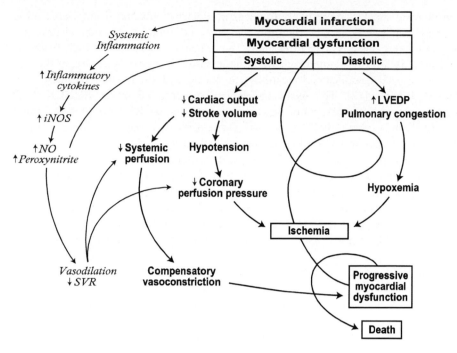

**Figure 2**    The new paradigm of cardiogenic shock complicating acute myocardial infarction. (From Ref. 3 and Ref. 6)

In recognition of these observations, the classical shock paradigm has been expanded to reflect a significant inflammatory component (Fig. 2). The large MI precipitates a response of systemic inflammation, and elevated levels of inflammatory markers are associated with shock and death [7]. The release of inflammatory cytokines results in expression of inducible nitric oxide synthase (iNOS). This in turn generates the release of supraphysiological quantities of nitric oxide (NO) that are oxidized to peroxynitrites. High NO and its oxidation products are deleterious to the myocardium and the integrity of vascular tone, resulting in further myocardial depression and inappropriate vasodilation, further reducing coronary perfusion pressure and systemic perfusion, leading to more ischemia and myocardial dysfunction. The central role of systemic inflammation and iNOS and NO in the pathogenesis of cardiogenic shock has been suggested by the positive results of a study of complement inhibition [8] and two small pilot studies of NOS inhibition in cardiogenic shock, discussed later in this chapter [9,10].

## Epidemiology of Cardiogenic Shock

While the definition of cardiogenic shock is not consistent across investigations, a commonly accepted one [4] includes the following criteria: a) hypotension (systolic blood pressure less than 90mmHg for at least 30 minutes, need for vasopressors, or balloon pump support), b) clinical evidence of end-organ hypoperfusion with confirmation of cardiac index (CI) less than or equal to 2.2 l/min/m$^2$, and c) confirmatory hemodynamic or radiographic features of elevated ventricular filling pressures: pulmonary capillary wedge pressure (PCWP) greater than 15mmHg and or pulmonary congestion on chest X-ray or right atrial (RA) pressure greater than 10mm Hg for RV failure.

Cardiogenic shock is more likely to occur in older patients and women presenting with acute MI [1]. Age is, in fact, the most powerful independent predictor of development of cardiogenic shock [11]. Furthermore, a comparative analysis of data from the GUSTO-I and GUSTO-III randomized trials indicates a significant increase in the age of patients with AMI complicated by cardiogenic shock, with the median age increasing from 68 to 71 years [12]. The mean age of patients enrolled in the SHOCK Trial Registry was almost 69 years, while in the Second National Registry of Myocardial Infarction (NRMI-2), almost half of the patients registered to have cardiogenic shock were 75 years of age or older [13]. Older MI patients are more likely to develop cardiogenic shock due to loss of ischemic preconditioning, which may be partially reversible with prior exercise training, and which predisposes to the development of a more extensive myocardial infarction [14,15]. They more often have severe and extensive coronary artery disease and comorbidities. In addition, mitochondria of senescent cardiac myocytes undergo structural changes in mitochondrial proteins, and are thus more susceptible to reperfusion injury and less likely to recover their respiration activity [16].

Women comprise almost 50% of all patients with cardiogenic shock. In contrast, they make up less than 30% of all patients with AMI. They do not, however, suffer a worse outcome than men with MI complicated by cardiogenic shock [17]. Similarly, diabetics with AMI are more likely than nondiabetic MI patients to develop shock. Their mortality is somewhat higher than that of nondiabetics, with in-hospital mortality in the SHOCK Trial Registry of 67% in patients with diabetes, vs. 59% in those without. After risk-adjustment, diabetes was of borderline significance as an independent predictor of mortality [18].

The GUSTO-I Investigators found age to be the most powerful predictor of development of cardiogenic shock in trial patients treated with thrombolytic therapy [11]. For every 10-year increase in age, there was a 47% increase in the risk of developing shock. Systolic blood pressure, heart rate, and Killip Class II or III on presentation were the three other most important predictors of development of cardiogenic shock. Other important predictors included anterior MI location, presence of diabetes, female sex, prior MI, lower weight, hypertension, a higher diastolic blood pressure, and treatment with streptokinase vs. tPA. These findings underscored the importance of the physical examination in identifying patients at high-risk for developing shock.

## Clinical Presentation

The majority of patients who develop cardiogenic shock during their MI course do so after admission to hospital, with postpresentation shock patients accounting for 60–90% of all cases [13,19]. In the SHOCK experience, half of cardiogenic shock patients had multiple infarct locations on ECG, with anterior location in 55%, inferior in 46%, lateral in 32%, posterior in 19%, apical in 11%, and unknown location in 10% of cases [1]. Clinically, patients with shock are hypotensive, although a subset has been identified with normal blood pressure. The latter maintain blood pressure through peripheral vasoconstriction, but have systemic hypoperfusion with cool extremities and decreased urine output. Tachypnea and evidence of pulmonary edema are often present, unless the shock is due to isolated right ventricular failure or cardiac tamponade. Interestingly, up to 30% of patients with shock due to LV failure have clear lungs on clinical and radiographic examination, despite markedly elevated PCWP [20].

Chest pain or equivalent will generally be present as an element of the AMI presentation. However, there may be delayed onset of shock post-MI, in which case chest pain may be already absent [21,22]. Moreover, the diagnosis may be less apparent in the elderly for several reasons. Elderly patients with an acute MI are more likely to present with a non–ST-elevation MI [23,24], and in general are less likely to have chest pain on presentation. This lack of symptoms and findings delays presentation as well as diagnosis, thus decreasing the effectiveness of administered therapies and ultimately contributing to increased mortality [25].

## Evaluation

All patients with cardiogenic shock should undergo 2-D and Doppler echocardiographic examination in order to rule out potentially reversible mechanical etiologies of shock and to provide valuable information regarding function of the left and right ventricles. Moderate mitral regurgitation (MR) is often present when LV failure causes shock and is an important independent predictor of mortality, as is the LV ejection fraction (Fig. 3) [26]. Swan-Ganz catheterization and pulmonary artery monitoring have always been considered indispensable tools in the diagnosis and management of patients with cardiogenic shock, though echo-Doppler has largely obviated this diagnostic role. Indwelling pulmonary artery pressure monitoring is useful in titrating vasoactive and inotropic agents as well as management of fluids; however, it is unclear whether this type of monitoring improves patient outcome. Risk may be conferred if the information is unreliable due to poor tracings or if inappropriate actions are taken based on the information obtained. Left heart cardiac catheterization with coronary angiography remains a key diagnostic tool for those who are candidates for an invasive strategy, as optimal management includes mechanical revascularization, as discussed later in this chapter.

Cardiac power, the product of mean arterial pressure and cardiac output, is a novel concept that may add valuable prognostic information to the overall assessment of patients with acute MI complicated by cardiogenic shock, as well as those with heart failure (Fig. 4) [27,28].

## Management of Cardiogenic Shock Secondary to Pump Failure

While the overwhelming majority of cases of cardiogenic shock complicating AMI are due to LV failure, shock occurred secondary to a mechanical complication in 12% of patients registered in the SHOCK Trial Registry. Many of the elements of therapy pertain to all etiologies of shock. In this section we will focus on strategies pertinent to pump failure. Figure 5 presents a general management algorithm for cardiogenic shock.

### Ventilatory Care

Although many patients who develop cardiogenic shock during the course of acute MI require ventilatory support, early ventilation has not been utilized as a potentially outcome-altering therapeutic tool in patients with cardiogenic shock. Limited nonrandomized data suggest that routine use of mechanical ventilation may result in significant reduction in failure of weaning from mechanical support. Kontoyannis et al. treated 28 consecutive patients with strictly defined cardiogenic shock with inotropic support and intra-aortic balloon counterpulsation. The first 18 patients were treated with this regimen alone, while the last 10 patients also received continuous mechanical ventilation with positive end-expiratory pressure (PEEP) at 10cm $H_2O$ [29]. Eight of 18 patients in the first group and 9 of 10 in the second group were weaned off balloon pump support (p = 0.04). Ultimately, 8 of 10 patients in group 2, but only 5 of 18 group 1 patients, were discharged from the

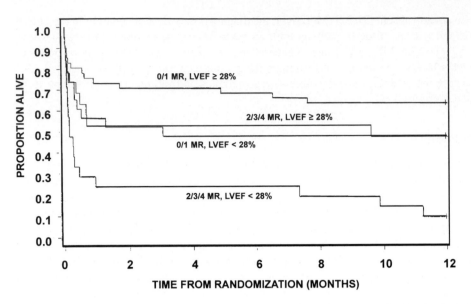

**Figure 3** Kaplan-Meier estimates of survival up to 1 year after randomization for 4 combinations of LVEF and MR (log-rank test P = 0.0001). Total n = 90; MR 0/1 and LVEF 28%, n = 33; MR 0/1 and LVEF <28%, n = 20; MR 2/3/4 and LVEF 28%, n = 16; MR 2/3/4 and LVEF <28%, n = 21. (From Ref. 26)

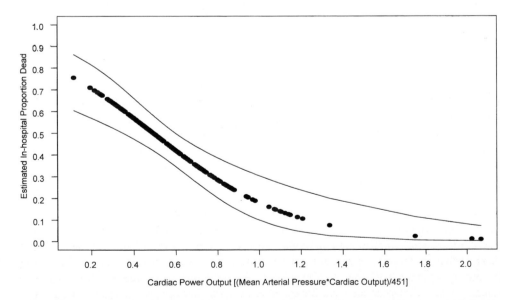

**Figure 4** Relationship between cardiac power output (cardiac output X mean arterial pressure) and estimated in-hospital mortality in the SHOCK Registry. (From Ref. 1. with permission of Elsevier Publishing Group)

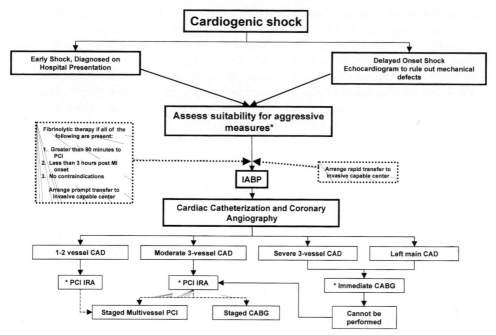

**Figure 5**   Outline of emergency management of patients with cardiogenic shock (CS), acute pulmonary edema (PE) or both. Inotropic/vasopressor agents may be titrated, replaced by other agents, or used in combination, as needed. (From Ref. 32a)

hospital (p = 0.01). While the study was nonrandomized, it suggests a benefit of early mechanical ventilation in patients with cardiogenic shock. This is particularly important prior to coronary angiography. Given the continued high mortality in this setting, a randomized study to confirm this result would be helpful.

The use of continuous positive airway pressure (CPAP) has been studied more in the setting of nonshock acute cardiogenic pulmonary edema [30–32]. However, it may be an attractive early alternative in patients with shock and impending respiratory failure, where intubation may be difficult and/or mechanical ventilation not immediately feasible.

### Inotrope and Vasopressor Support

Administration of inotropes and vasopressors is one of the earliest steps in the management of the patient with AMI and hypotension secondary to left ventricular failure. Experimental evidence suggests that inotropic agents may improve mitochondrial function even in noninfarcted myocardium that becomes deranged during an acute MI complicated by shock [33]. However, administered catecholamines can cause contraction band necrosis, arrhythmias, and an increase in oxygen consumption. Therefore the minimal required doses should be used. Dopamine is generally the first inotropic agent of choice in the management of shock secondary to LV pump failure. However, high-dose dopamine is clearly deleterious, resulting in worsening of hypoxemia, severe vasoconstriction, and ischemia [34]. In contrast, the combination of lower-dose dopamine and dobutamine (approximately 7.5µg/kg/min) has been shown to have a better hemodynamic effect than either agent administered alone at 15 µg/kg/min, and does not result in the worsening of hypoxemia seen with high-dose dopamine therapy. When dopamine/dobutamine therapy fails to improve hemodynamics adequately, or when severe hypotension is present, norepinephrine should be the preferred agent because of the lower adverse effect profile seen with this drug than with epinephrine. The latter can exacerbate lactic acidosis, already a problem in the shock setting. Experimentally, epinephrine has also been shown to exert a prothrombotic effect in coronary vasculature, in contrast to norepinephrine, which appears to have the opposite effect [35]. If epinephrine must be infused, its dose and duration of administration must be minimized as much as possible in order to reduce the possibility of adverse effects. Vasopressin has not been investigated in cardiogenic shock complicating AMI.

*Intra-aortic Balloon Counterpulsation*

Intra-aortic balloon pump (IABP) counterpulsation provides circulatory support while reducing oxygen consumption. Aortic impedance is reduced and coronary perfusion improved, resulting in an augmentation of blood pressure and an increase in cardiac output. It is considered an integral component of management for patients with AMI complicated by cardiogenic shock who are candidates for additional therapies, such as percutaneous coronary intervention (PCI) or coronary artery bypass grafting (CABG), and has a Class I recommendation in the 1999 ACC/AHA guidelines [36]. Nonetheless, IABP utilization rates are low. In the National Registry of Myocardial Infarction (NRMI), 31% of the 23,180 patients with cardiogenic shock received IABP support [37]. In the international Global Registry of Acute Coronary Events (GRACE), utilization rates reported in the 583 patients with AMI complicated by cardiogenic shock varied markedly across regions, with rates as low as 20.6% in Europe ranging to 46.3% in the United States [38]. In the SHOCK Registry the IABP rate was only 42%. In contrast, in the randomized SHOCK Trial, IABP support was given to most patients (86%), as it was suggested by the study protocol [4].

The efficacy of IABP support in cardiogenic shock has not been tested in a randomized controlled trial. However, several large registries have reported on the outcomes associated with IABP use specifically in patients with acute MI complicated by cardiogenic shock [37,39]. Bearing in mind the potential for bias in this type of analysis, the association of IABP use with better outcome is remarkable. In the SHOCK Registry, patients treated with IABP had an in-hospital mortality of 50%, compared with 72% for those not receiving this treatment (p<0.0001) [39]. In the NRMI-2 shock study, IABP use was associated with a significant reduction in mortality, but only in patients treated with thrombolytic therapy (67% without and 49% with IABP) [37]. In this large cohort, IABP use was independently associated with lower in-hospital mortality in patients receiving thrombolysis, but not in those undergoing PCI or CABG as their primary reperfusion modality. In a subsequent analysis, the NRMI-2 investigators found that frequency of hospital use of IABP is an independent predictor of survival in patients in cardiogenic shock, with 150 fewer deaths occurring per 1000 patients treated in the high-volume hospitals (with a median annual volume of 37.4 pumps) compared with those with a low volume (3.4 pumps per year) (Fig. 6) [40].

Recent analysis of the SHOCK population has revealed that early reversal of hypoperfusion with IABP support predicts improved survival, independent of early revascularization and clinical, hemodynamic and angiographic variables [41]. Rapid shock reversal, which is not predicted by the variables noted, may be a marker of viability and myocardial reserve; methods to improve augmentation and the rate of reversal of shock may increase

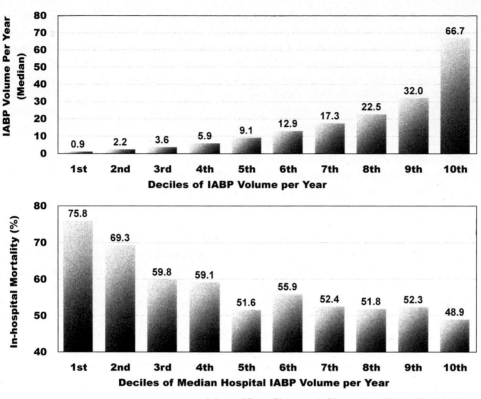

Adapted from Chen et al. Circulation  2003;108:951-957.

**Figure 6**    Annual median hospital IABP volume by deciles (**A**), and in-hospital unadjusted mortality of patients who received IABP by deciles (**B**). (From Ref. 40)

survival. These hypotheses will require further evaluation in prospective studies. Failure to rapidly reverse hypoperfusion may serve as a useful selection criterion for other therapies, including left ventricular assist devices.

*Thrombolytic Therapy*

The efficacy of thrombolytic therapy in reperfusing the acutely occluded infarct-related artery is markedly attenuated once shock has ensued, due to the marked decrease in systemic and coronary perfusion pressure. Experimentally, much of the effect of thrombolytic therapy may be regained by concomitant use of IABP counterpulsation [42]. In the SHOCK Registry, patients who received thrombolytic therapy had significantly lower mortality than those with no thrombolysis (54% vs. 64%; p = 0.005). The patients with the lowest mortality were those who received thrombolytic therapy and IABP support prior to undergoing a revascularization procedure [39].

The NRMI-2 registry similarly reported an association between the utilization of thrombolytic therapy, IABP support, and lower mortality in 23,180 patients registered with cardiogenic shock [37]. The investigators suggested a synergistic effect of the 2 modalities. In-hospital mortality in patients receiving neither thrombolytic therapy nor IABP support was 78%, decreasing to 67% in the group receiving thrombolysis alone, and dropping down to 49% in the group receiving both thrombolysis and IABP support.

However, in both the NRMI-2 and SHOCK registries, patients receiving IABP support were significantly younger than those not treated with an IABP, pointing to a possible clinician treatment bias with respect to treating older patients with aggressive mechanical support. An increased incidence of severe comorbid conditions such as peripheral vascular disease that may also have been more likely to have precluded femoral artery cannulation and mechanical support in older shock patients.

Although definitive evidence is still lacking, an approach of thrombolysis augmented by IABP support as initial therapy may improve survival in patients with cardiogenic shock when percutaneous or surgical revascularization is not readily available, and may be especially lifesaving in the elderly, with their greater burden of preexisting disease and thus much higher risk of mortality. In the SHOCK Trial, thrombolytic administration was associated with improved survival for those who were assigned to initial medical stabilization (discussion following) [43]. The TACTICS trial randomized 57 of planned 538 patients with shock or pre-shock in a trial evaluating the effect of IABP in the context of thrombolysis. There was a trend toward lower mortality in those randomized to IABP with thrombolysis (34% vs. 46%; p = 0.23). In the small subset with classic shock (n = 31), the mortality reduction was significant (39% vs. 80%; p = 0.05) and the major bleeding rate was low (3%) [44]. When an IABP is inserted in a patient receiving thrombolytic therapy, extra care must be taken to reduce the risk of bleeding (anterior puncture only of the femoral artery).

IABP support is not recommended in patients who are not candidates for reperfusion/revascularization therapy or do not have a correctable mechanical cause of shock, as in these extreme settings this aggressive approach is generally futile.

## Mechanical Reperfusion

**Early Evidence.**   Over the past 15 years, a series of small and generally retrospective case studies suggested that in-hospital mortality could be significantly reduced by use of PCI [45–53]. The GUSTO-I investigators similarly showed a higher survival rate with coronary angioplasty in the large subset of 2972 patients who developed shock after fibrinolytic treatment [54]. In most of these analyses, the patients treated with aggressive measures, including mechanical revascularization, were younger, were generally less sick than those who did not undergo mechanical revascularization, and survived long enough to undergo the procedure. In all cases the reports were observational, and were limited in their impact due to their small sample size.

**Randomized Trials.**   Two randomized trials were conducted to test the efficacy of early revascularization suggested by the non-randomized reports (Fig. 7). The Swiss Multicenter Trial of Angioplasty for Shock (SMASH) enrolled only 55 patients and was abandoned due to low enrollment. [54a] Of the 32 patients randomized to immediate angiography and revascularization, 28 were actually revascularized by PCI and one by CABG. At 30 days, mortality was 69% in the revascularization group and 78% in the medical therapy group (relative risk 0.88, 95%CI 0.6, 1.2). The authors concluded that although the trial did not demonstrate a significant benefit of early revascularization, a clinically meaningful benefit from early revascularization may have been missed because the study was grossly underpowered.

In the SHOCK Trial, the efficacy of early revascularization was tested in patients with AMI complicated by shock secondary to predominant LV pump failure and less than 12 hours in duration. Patients assigned to the early revascularization arm of the study were assigned to receive a revascularization procedure within 6 hours of randomization, while those in the initial medical stabilization arm were to undergo no intervention for at least 54 hours after

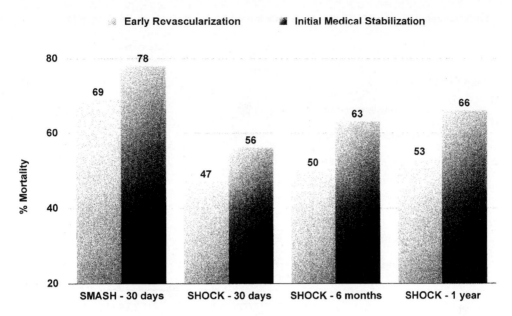

**Figure 7**  Mortality of patients in the early intervention and conservative arms of the SMASH Trial (p = ns) and SHOCK Trial at 30 days (p = .11), 6 months (p<0.03) and one year (p<0.03). (From Ref. 4, Ref. 5, and Ref. 56) [54a]

randomization. The trial showed a non-significant 9% absolute reduction in 30-day mortality, the primary endpoint (p = 0.11). However, this difference increased over time, and by 6 months the reduction in mortality increased to 13% (p = 0.04) [4]. This difference was maintained at 1 year, with 47% of patients in the early revascularization group surviving to 1 year vs. 34% of those randomized to a strategy of initial medical stabilization (p = 0.025) [55]. Functional status at one year was very good, with most patients (more than 80%) being in NYHA Class 1 or 2. In general, all SHOCK patients appeared to benefit, except for one pre-specified age subgroup. Subgroup analysis suggested that only patients aged younger than 75 years benefited from early revascularization; early revascularization appeared to confer no benefit in patients aged older than 75 years. Unfortunately, the entire SHOCK Trial group aged 75 and older consisted of just 56 patients, rendering the trial results inconclusive in elderly patients. The elderly in the initial medical stabilization arm were unusual in that their mortality was no different than that of the younger medical stabilization patients. Subsequent analysis of the SHOCK data revealed that the elderly in the initial medical stabilization arm had significantly higher LV ejection fraction than the elderly assigned to early revascularization (personal communication)

The question then arises as to whether any patients who are 75 years old, or older, should be offered revascularization. Although in general the results of a randomized trial guide management, in this particular case, we must turn to the larger body of registry data. The prospective SHOCK Registry, conducted concurrently with the SHOCK trial, enrolled 277 patients aged older than 75. The in hospital mortality of patients in this age group treated with a revascularization procedure within 18 hours of onset of shock was 48%, in contrast to the 81% mortality in those revascularized later or never (adjusted relative risk 0.46, p<0.002) (Fig. 8) [57]. The outcomes for the elderly selected for early PCI and early CABG were similar. Similar outcomes in elderly patients undergoing PCI

**Early revascularization (< 18 hrs. from shock onset) vs late or no revascularization**

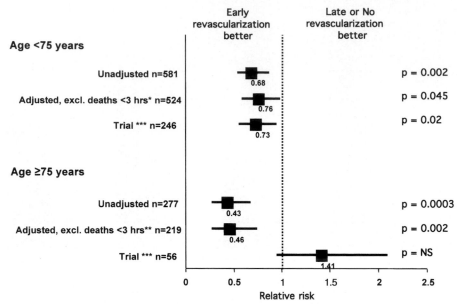

\*    45 patients with death <3 hours from admission and 12 patients with missing baseline data excluded.
     Adjusted for diabetes (p=0.047) and prior CABG (p=0.017)
\*\*   20 patients with death <3 hours from admission and 28 patients with missing baseline data excluded
     Adjusted for transfer status (p=0.002) and inferior MI location (p=0.089)

**Figure 8**   Analysis of covariate relative risk for in-hospital mortality of SHOCK Registry patients who underwent early revascularization ($<18$ h after shock onset) vs. late or no revascularization, stratified by age group. (Ref. 57a)

for cardiogenic shock were reported by both the Worcester Registry and the New England Registry (Table 1) [58,59].

Not all elderly patients with AMI complicated by cardiogenic shock will benefit from an aggressive revascularization strategy. In general, cardiac arrest requiring cardiopulmonary resuscitation is associated with poor outcomes regardless of PCI performance. Functional status prior to the MI event serves as a major influence on the selection of elderly patients for an invasive strategy. The authors recommend that clinicians assess each patient on an individual basis, and that those with a good premorbid status be offered all the aggressive measures afforded to younger patients, including percutaneous or surgical revascularization. These selected patients should do as well as younger patients managed similarly.

The physician must understand the preferences of the patient and ensure that those desiring nonaggressive care be treated with compassionate measures. Advance directives should be clarified very early after hospital arrival, particularly for extremely elderly patients, in order to avoid the potential of treatment in a manner contrary to their wishes.

*New Approaches to Better Outcome*

In spite of significant gains made in recent years in improving the outcome of patients with AMI complicated by shock secondary to pump failure, more than 50% of these

**Table 1**  Characteristics and Outcome of Elderly Patients with Acute MI Complicated by Cardiogenic Shock in Multicenter Registries Comparing Different Reperfusion Strategies

| Author | Study description | Age group | Number | Outcome |
|---|---|---|---|---|
| Berger et al. | Cooperative Cardiovascular Project Database. Only patients with bp < 90 mmHg on presentation and no cardiac arrest; Patients transferred in from other acute care hospitals excluded; Only patients with shock on presentation included (<1% of all patients with acute MI | 65 years | 601 total: 314 admitted to revasc. hospitals; 287 admitted to non-revasc hosp. | 30-day mortality: Revasc. hospital 66%; Non-revasc 74% Adjusted odds ratio 0.83 (95% CI 0.47, 1.45). No difference between patients <75 years and 75 years old |
| Dzavik et al. | SHOCK Registry: All patients with AMI and CS secondary to left or right ventricular failure. Patients who died <3 hours from presentation excluded | 75 years | 257: 44 with early revasc; 213 with no early revasc | 30-day mortality: Early revasc. 48%; Non-early revasc 79%, p=0.001 |
| Dauerman et al. | Worcester metropolitan area. Two cohorts: 1986–91 – reperfusion; 1993–97 reperfusion and PCI | 65 years; subgroup 75 years | 310: Early revasc increased from 2% to 16%; IABP use from 11% to 38% | In-hospital mortality: Early revasc. 56%; Non-early revac 77%, p=0.02. Improved case fatality rate in latter period in patients aged 75 years |

patients die during their index admission. It is likely that little more can be gained by further refinement of revascularization strategies in improving this desperate outcome. To achieve further gains in management of these most critically ill (and for the most part elderly) patients will require a shift to a new paradigm of treatment.

**Metabolic Intervention.** The next major advance in the treatment of patients with extensive AMI complicated by shock will likely be aimed at protecting myocardial metabolism. Two interventions, both linked at least in part to glucose metabolism, have shown promise in early investigations. Treatment with glucose-insulin-potassium (GIK), which shifts energy production away from glycogen and free fatty acids that predominate during ischemia, has already been shown in smaller clinical studies to improve outcome in the acute MI setting, and is currently being evaluated in larger studies [60–63].

In a recent study in a primarily nondiabetic (90%) population treated with primary PCI, GIK infusion improved outcomes only in those with Killip Class I on presentation [64]. Those with Killip Class 2 or greater who were randomized to GIK had a somewhat higher 30-day mortality than similar patients receiving placebo (36% vs. 26.5%, p = ns). To date, the only data suggestive of benefit of GIK in critically ill cardiac patients comes from a small study of 22 patients in the post cardiac surgery setting [65]. Thus, until further data are available, the use of GIK is not recommended for patients in cardiogenic shock. However, intensive insulin therapy to normalize elevated blood glucose was beneficial in acute MI patients in the randomized DIGAMI study, and led to marked survival benefit in ICU patients [66,67]. Therefore, intensive insulin therapy is recommended to treat the hyperglycemic state, particularly for these high-risk patients with pump failure, irrespective of whether the patient is known to be diabetic.

**Nitric Oxide Synthase Inhibition.** Infusion of a nitric oxide (NO) synthase inhibitor has recently shown promise in improving hemodynamics and in-hospital survival in a small, randomized pilot study of patients with cardiogenic shock complicating AMI [10]. During ischemia and reperfusion, inducible NO synthase effects the release of excess NO. This results in production of peroxynitrites, which have a deleterious effect on cell function and contribute to myocyte injury. Excess NO also suppresses glucose metabolism. In addition, patients with cardiogenic shock often have inappropriate vasodilation. These effects are diminished by NO synthase inhibition. A NO synthase inhibitor is now being evaluated in a phase 2 trial in cardiogenic shock, and other, similar strategies will likely follow. Further studies are investigating the effect of inhibition of mediators of the inflammatory response to MI (such as complement C5) on the genesis and persistence of the shock state [8,68]. These may provide hope for improving outcomes, especially in groups with continued high mortality such as the elderly.

**Left Ventricular Assist Therapy.** For patients who are not responding to maximal therapy, including reperfusion/revascularization and IABP, mechanical circulatory assistance as a bridge to cardiac transplantation, or destination therapy may be the only option to avert certain death. There are, however, no randomized data (and a paucity of any data at all) to show that this extremely resource-intensive and costly modality improves outcome in patients in cardiogenic shock. Castells et al. implanted an Abiomed ventricular assist device in 11 patients (mean age 52 years), 12 hours to 4 days after onset of refractory cardiogenic shock [69]. Three patients died while on support, one patient was successfully weaned from the device, and 7 went on to successful transplant. Of these, one died of sepsis. The overall long-term survival was thus 69%. In a study by Entwistle, using the same Abiomed device, only patients with MI and shock secondary to left ventricular failure appeared to have benefit as 8 of 11 such patients who were supported with a LVAD were weaned from the device, and 6 (54%) survived to hospital discharge [70]. In contrast, none of 6 patients with biventricular failure who were supported could be weaned from the BiVAD device, with 2 undergoing cardiac transplant, and only one surviving. Kherani et al. reported on the use of ventricular assist devices in 46 patients with cardiogenic shock, some of whom were treated medically and others by surgical revascularization [71]; overall survival was 56%. This therapy requires evaluation by large randomized trials before routine use can be recommended for patients with AMI complicated by cardiogenic shock. Meanwhile, it may be the only option left and the last resort for the younger patient with good premorbid functional status and without significant comorbidities who has slipped into cardiogenic shock, continues to deteriorate on maximal therapy, and has not yet developed irreversible multiorgan failure. A femoral artery inserted percutaneous support system based on circulation of oxygenated left atrial blood, obtained through transseptal catheter, appears to improve flow and perfusion in a preliminary study and is under investigation [72].

## Summary

Important advances in treatment strategies have markedly improved the poor prognosis for patients with acute MI complicated by shock due to LV pump failure. Early revascularization plays an important role, as does intra-aortic balloon counterpulsation. We recommend this strategy for all patients younger than 75 years unless irreversible multiple end-organ failure has developed, or severe comorbidities with poor life expectancy and functional status. This strategy is recommended for the elderly with good prior functional status when deemed feasible by the treating physician and agreed to by the patient, unless irreversible multiple end-organ failure has developed. When early revascularization is not possible, fibrinolytic therapy with IABP followed by urgent delayed revascularization is recommended, based on the individual clinical setting and judgment of the treating physician. Selected pharmacological approaches aimed at inhibiting inflammation and protecting the metabolic integrity of the myocardium during ischemia and reperfusion show early promise and are now undergoing further evaluation in multicenter randomized trials.

## Cardiogenic Shock Secondary to Acute Mitral Regurgitation

Patients with cardiogenic shock secondary to severe mitral regurgitation present somewhat later than those with shock secondary to left ventricular pump failure, although most develop it within 24 hours of MI onset. Similar to other forms of cardiac rupture (septal and free wall), there is a bimodal distribution with a second peak at 3–5 days post-MI. Women are more likely to be affected. Over half of patients with shock secondary to acute mitral regurgitation in the SHOCK Registry were women, while women comprised only a third of patients with shock secondary to LV pump failure. In contrast to patients with shock secondary to LV pump failure, who are more likely to have an anterior wall location, those who are in shock due to severe acute MR are more likely to have ECG evidence of an acute inferior wall MI [73]. However, a third of patients have an anterior infarct location, while fewer than 50% have ST-segment elevation on ECG. Pathological series reveal that the most common mechanism is rupture of the posteromedial mitral papillary muscle/chordae tendinae. LV function is often better than observed in patients with shock secondary to LV failure; however, associated severe LV dysfunction is common. In the SHOCK Registry, the mean LV ejection fraction was 36.5% in patients with shock secondary to MR who had this parameter measured, compared with 30.0% in patients with LV failure shock [73].

Echocardiography with color flow Doppler is essential to accurate diagnosis, as auscultation may not reveal the presence of severe MR. When the index of suspicion is high, or visualization inadequate, transesophageal echocardiography is indicated because a transthoracic study may miss a localized jet. Initial therapy docs not differ greatly from that recommended for patients with shock secondary to pump failure. Ventilatory support and vasopressor and inotropes support should be utilized as needed in order to improve oxygenation and hemodynamics. Intra-aortic balloon counterpulsation is a key to successful stabilization. Experimentally, this intervention markedly raises cardiac output, blood pressure and cerebral blood flow, and decreases MR. Although overall coronary blood pressure remains unchanged, there is a marked shift toward greater diastolic flow [74]. It is unclear whether IABP support reduces mortality, as randomized data are lacking. In the SHOCK Registry, 68% of patients with shock secondary to MR were managed with IABP. Almost all patients who went on to surgical valve replacement or repair were also managed with IABP counterpulsation, whereas only 43% of those not treated surgically had a balloon pump inserted [73]. Indeed, in the overall severe MR group of 98 patients, in-hospital mortality was significantly lower in the 43 surgically-treated patients at 40%, vs. the 71% mortality in the 51 patients who did not undergo valve surgery. Revascularization only by PCI does not appear to improve survival of patients with acute ischemic MR, although there are no data in the current era of stents and antiplatelet therapy [75]. However, the potential benefit is limited to those with a brief period of reversible ischemia, not those with irreversible infarction or rupture of the papillary muscle or chordae. In those who underwent PCI for LV failure in the SHOCK Trial, the presence of MR was independently associated with death at 30 days [76].

## Cardiogenic Shock Secondary to Ventricular Septal Rupture

It is fortunate that this dire complication is the cause of fewer than 4% of cases of cardiogenic shock, since mortality associated with ventricular septal rupture once shock develops is exceedingly high (>80%). Compared with those with LV failure and shock, patients with shock secondary to ventricular septal rupture (VSR) tend to be older, and are much more likely to be women [77]. Interestingly, they are less likely to have had a prior MI or be diabetic, suggesting that the presence of scarring from prior MI or fibrosis secondary to the diabetes may serve to protect the diabetic patient from this complication.

Transthoracic echocardiography is an important diagnostic tool, as VSR can be difficult to differentiate from MR in the shock patient. In most cases, transesophageal echocardiography is needed to accurately define the anatomy of the rupture when planning definitive therapy. Right heart catheterization can also be helpful, as the presence of left-to-right shunt can be confirmed by measuring oxygen saturations, and the magnitude of the shunt can also be determined. Right ventricular function, assessed by echo or by hemodynamics, is also prognostically important.

As is the case with shock secondary to acute MR, initial treatment consists of inotropic and vasopressor therapy and IABP support. The definitive treatment is surgical, and includes excision of infarcted tissue and subsequent repair of the defect with a Dacron patch [78,79]. An alternate technique that has had some success consists of completely excluding the infarcted myocardium by over-sewing a patch of pericardial tissue to noninfarcted myocardium on the left ventricular side, without excision of the infarcted territory, thus preserving the geometry of the ventricular chambers [80]. Complete surgical revascularization is typically performed concomitantly with the repair of the defect.

Outcome continues to be poor once shock develops post-VSR. Only 13% of the 55 patients in the SHOCK Registry with ventricular septal rupture survived to hospital discharge (Fig. 9) [77]. Of the 31 patients who underwent surgical repair in this multicenter

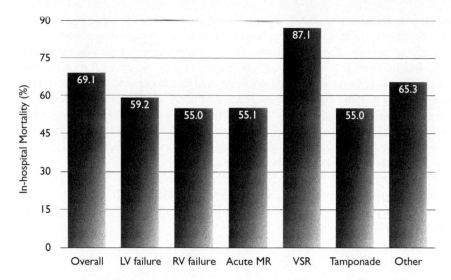

**Figure 9**   In-hospital mortality of patients in the combined SHOCK Trial and Registry patients according to etiology of shock. (From Ref. 1)

experience, 25 (81%) died. This outcome is similar to that reported in some prior single-center case series, while others reported in-hospital mortality as low as 20% [79,81–87].

Use of percutaneous closure devices has been reported in isolated cases. The results have been mixed, and it is as yet unclear whether this approach combined with percutaneous revascularization can be recommended as a reasonable alternative for all patients with ventricular septal rupture and shock, or only as a last resort for those who are deemed to be poor surgical candidates (Fig. 10).

## Pericardial Tamponade and Free-wall Rupture/

Although free-wall rupture or tamponade is diagnosed in fewer than 3% of cases of cardiogenic shock, its true prevalence is likely higher, since free-wall rupture is immediately fatal in a number of patients in whom the complication is never confirmed. Only 28 of the 1190 patients entered in the SHOCK Registry had free-wall rupture and/or tamponade

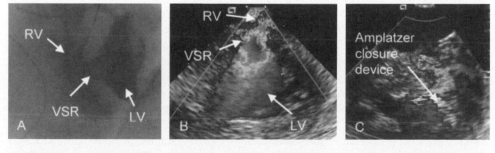

**Figure 10**   A large ventricular septal rupture in an 80-year old woman in cardiogenic shock diagnosed with a contrast LV angiogram (**A**)and with intracardiac ultrasound before (**B**) and after (**C**) percutaneous closure.

[88]. Patients with this complication tend to be somewhat older than other patients with shock. As with other mechanical causes of shock, free-wall rupture or tamponade occurs more frequently in women. The one distinguishing clinical feature of patients with free-wall rupture and tamponade is the lack of pulmonary edema on physical examination. This may indeed be an important early diagnostic feature that may point toward the correct diagnosis, especially as other physical signs, such as pulsus paradoxus or blunted Y descent, are neither sensitive nor specific in this setting. On echocardiography, a pericardial effusion is identified in most patients. A striking finding in the SHOCK Registry was that in none of the 28 cases of shock and free-wall rupture or tamponade was the right coronary artery identified as the culprit infarct-related artery.

Initial treatment consists of immediate pericardiocentesis, while surgical repair of the defect constitutes definitive therapy, essential in almost all cases. In-hospital survival is similar to that of patients with shock secondary to LV pump failure (39.3% in the SHOCK Registry).

## HEART FAILURE COMPLICATING ACUTE MYOCARDIAL INFARCTION

Heart failure without shock complicates the course of 15% to 30% patients suffering an acute myocardial infarction. Although its consequences are not as dire as those of cardiogenic shock, morbidity and mortality remain surprisingly high, creating a tremendous burden on the patient and healthcare system.

### Epidemiology

As is the case with those developing cardiogenic shock, patients whose AMI course is complicated by heart failure are older, more likely to be female, and are more likely to have an anterior infarct location. In an analysis of 190,518 patients with AMI, the NRMI-2 investigators reported that 36,303 (19.1%) presented in Killip Class II (70%) or III (30%) heart failure. The mean age of 72.6 years was similar to patients in the NRMI-2 registry who were previously reported to be developing cardiogenic shock [13]. Similarly, 47% of patients who presented in CHF in this report were women, compared to only 32% of those without heart failure. In an analysis of 61,041 patients enrolled in 4 thrombolytic trials who did not develop shock and whose heart failure status was known, 17,949 (29.4%) developed Killip Class II or III failure at some point during their course [89]. The fact that patients enrolled in thrombolytic trials are highly selected, likely representing a lower-risk group, suggests that the true incidence of heart failure complicating acute MI is higher. In this combined series, fewer than 10% of patients with documented heart failure had it only on presentation, and had early resolution after admission. The majority of patients developed heart failure after presentation, while a somewhat smaller proportion of patients had it both on presentation and persistent failure during their hospitalization. In both of these large datasets, patients with heart failure were also more likely to be diabetic, to be hypertensive, to have had a prior MI, and to have had an anterior MI on presentation.

As is the case with cardiogenic shock, heart failure complicating AMI is not limited to those with ST-elevation MI. A combined analysis of four trials in the setting of non–ST-elevation acute coronary syndromes studied 23,187 patients; of these, 2903 (12.5%) were in Killip Class II or greater at the time of randomization. These patients were older, more likely female, diabetic, hypertensive, and were more likely to have had a history of prior MI, CVA, congestive heart failure, renal insufficiency, peripheral vascular disease and severe chronic obstructive pulmonary disease than those who had no heart failure on presentation.

## Clinical Presentation

Clinical presentation is as defined in the original 1967 manuscript by Killip and Kimball [90]. Patients with heart failure have a more rapid heart rate than those without it. They are typically hypertensive; absence of elevated blood pressure suggests more severe pump failure and the risk of shock. They are tachypneic and have an elevated jugular venous pulse on examination. In addition, they have rales on auscultation of the chest. On cardiac auscultation heart failure is distinguished by the presence of a third heart sound, though in general an S4 may also be present, reflecting the stiffness of the left ventricular muscle due to ongoing ischemia. Radiographic examination of the chest reveals the usual signs of pulmonary congestion, from increased interstitial markings to frank alveolar changes indicating pulmonary edema. Echocardiographically, patients with heart failure are distinguished by a lower LV ejection fraction; interestingly, in the combined thrombolytic trial analysis, the ejection fraction of patients who had heart failure on presentation only was similar to that of patients without heart failure (median 55%) [89]. Only those with either new or persistent heart failure during the index hospitalization had significantly lower ejection fraction (median 45%).

While heart failure in the context of AMI is generally caused by systolic dysfunction, diastolic function is an important modulator of long-term outcome. Specifically, a restrictive filling pattern of diastolic dysfunction has been found to be a significant independent predictor of long-term mortality in patients with a recent acute ST-elevation MI [91]. Furthermore, a subset of patients with heart failure and preserved LV systolic function after AMI has been identified. In a substudy of the Bucindolol Evaluation in Acute Myocardial Infarction trial, almost half of the 1474 patients with heart failure during their acute MI hospitalization were found to have preserved LV systolic function, defined as wall motion index greater than 1.3, corresponding to LV ejection fraction greater than 40%, while 167 patients had a normal wall motion index of greater than or equal to 2.0 [92]. These patients were more likely to have had a history of hypertension and diabetes.

## Management of Heart Failure Complication Acute Myocardial Infarction

### General Measures

Adequate oxygenation is an important element of effective therapy. As is the case with patients in cardiogenic shock, those with severe acute heart failure often develop respiratory distress and require ventilatory support. The use of continuous positive airway pressure (CPAP) ventilation can avert the need for intubation and should be considered in all patients, especially the elderly. In a randomized study of 100 patients with acute cardiogenic pulmonary edema, Lin et al. found that those assigned CPAP had a significantly improved breathing pattern as well as decreased use of intercostals and suprasternal muscles [32]. In addition, they experienced a decrease in intrapulmonary shunt and improvement in PaO2 compared with those treated by mask alone. More importantly, those assigned to CPAP therapy had a significantly lower rate of endotracheal intubation (16% vs. 36%; p<0.01). No difference was noted between the two treatment groups in in-hospital survival, although only 20% of the patients in each arm actually had an acute MI on presentation. In a small, randomized study in patients with pulmonary edema secondary to acute MI specifically, Takeda et al. found a significant reduction in need for intubation (18% vs. 73%; p = 0.03) as well as in-hospital mortality (9% vs. 64%; p = 0.02) in the group randomized to CPAP therapy [31]. Although these studies are small, they strongly suggest that this simple and essentially harmless modality should be considered early in patients with acute MI complicated by heart failure.

*Pharmacotherapy*

Preload and afterload reduction constitute the mainstay of pharmacotherapy in patients with MI and heart failure. The simplest and most rapid method is to utilize sublingual nitroglycerin and intravenous morphine, unless the systolic pressure is low. A diuretic should be administered intravenously when the patient has been assessed to be volume overloaded. Most patients with a first MI are euvolemic; pulmonary congestion results from transudation of fluid from the intravascular to extravascular space.

Studies performed primarily in the 1970s showed the benefit of intravenous nitroglycerin therapy in decreasing afterload, reducing pulmonary capillary wedge pressure, and improving failure [93]. A more recent small randomized trial suggested superiority of isosorbide dintrate infusion compared to high dose diuretics [94].

Nitroglycerin is preferable to nitroprusside, as it reduces ischemia, while the latter may increase it [95]. In fact, Cohn et al. showed no benefit in mortality in a trial of 800 patients with acute MI and elevated left ventricular filling pressures randomized to receive a nitroprusside infusion up to 48 hours or placebo, especially when initiated within 9 hours of onset of chest pain [96]. Thus nitroglycerin, not nitroprusside, should be the agent of choice in this setting. Although nesiritide is efficacious at facilitating a diuresis in volume-overloaded patients with decompensated chronic heart failure, it has not been studied in patients with AMI. It is a potent vasodilator and diuretic and may precipitate hypotension, intravascular depletion, and shock in patients with AMI, who are typically euvolemic as noted earlier.

Early oral vasodilator therapy in the form of angiotensin-converting enzyme (ACE) inhibition in the setting of acute MI has been shown to improve short as well as long-term outcome, and should be instituted on the day of admission. However, caution should be exercised in patients with low blood pressure, in whom it is likely more prudent to withhold ACE inhibitor therapy until they are hemodynamically more stable. Initiation by intravenous route should only be considered in those with severe hypertension [97].

Beta-receptor antagonist therapy is beneficial in the management of patients with acute MI and improves long-term outcome, likely on the basis of increasing parasympathetic tone [98]. There is, however, no direct randomized data on the safety and efficacy of early beta-receptor blockade in patients with heart failure at acute MI presentation. Patients with heart failure were in fact excluded from trials evaluating this class of drugs in the acute MI setting [99,100]. Indeed, the use of early beta-blockers is contraindicated in patients with acute MI and frank pulmonary congestion or signs of low output [36]. In contrast, initiation of beta blockade in the subacute phase prior to hospital discharge is strongly recommended (Class IA) for secondary prevention. The efficacy of early beta blockade in patients with acute MI and mild-to-moderate heart failure has been suggested by post hoc analysis of a small randomized trial of beta blockade in acute MI [101] and by nonrandomized data from the Acute Infarction Ramipril Efficacy (AIRE) trial (Fig. 11) [102]. In AIRE, 2006 patients with mild-to-moderate heart failure were randomized to receive ramipril or placebo from day 2 to day 9 after acute MI. In terms of severity of baseline heart failure, only those with NYHA Class IV were excluded. In a retrospective analysis of the trial, Spargias et al. reported that the use of beta receptor antagonists at

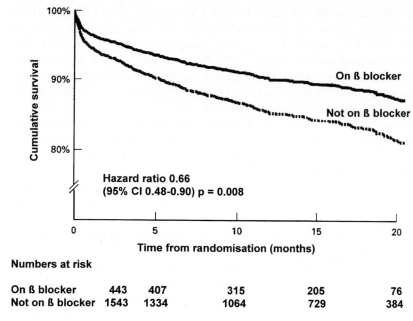

**Figure 11**  Kaplan-Maier survival curve of patients in the AIRE trial who were or were not on beta-blockers at the time of randomization (3–10 days post MI). (From Ref. 102)

baseline was independently associated with a lower risk of in-hospital mortality as well as progression to severe heart failure [102]. Thus, careful initiation and up-titration of beta blockade in patients with acute MI and heart failure should be considered, but only after the acute heart failure and low output state have improved.

There is some controversy whether initiation of beta receptor blockade should be intravenous or oral. While in most trials the initial doses were given intravenously, patients with heart failure were not included except in the Goteborg Metoprolol Trial [101]. Further-more, data from GUSTO-I indicate that this route of administration is associated with an increased risk of heart failure, cardiogenic shock, and need for temporary pacing when compared with oral loading, even in those patients who do not have heart failure at baseline [103]. Thus, in this high-risk group of patients, intravenous loading should be used with extreme caution or avoided altogether. Rather, initiation with a low dose of a beta receptor antagonist once other measures to correct failure have been instituted, and subsequent up-titration to effect with careful monitoring for adverse effects, is the more prudent option. Of the numerous novel drug therapies under recent investigation, glucose-insulin-potassium appears promising for patients with acute MI. Although therapies that have been shown to be of benefit in general tend to benefit those at high risk the most, a subgroup analysis of a recent study of GIK therapy showed no benefit in patients in Killip Class 2 or higher who underwent primary PCI for acute MI [104]. However, there were only 84 patients in the study who were in Killip Class 2 or higher. Nonetheless, the results of GIK administra-tion in this population are of concern, as the authors suggest, probably due to the negative effect of the volume load needed. Thus, this therapy should not be utilized in this high-risk patient population. As is the case with patients in cardiogenic shock, intensive insulin therapy in patients with hyperglycemia is warranted and should be utilized. The goal should be to lower serum glucose to the 80–110 mg/dL range [64].

Mineralocorticoid receptor blockade with spironolactone has been demonstrated to improve survival in a population of patients with chronic CHF, which includes those with remote MI [105]. Spironolactone begun early and in conjunction with initiation of ACE inhibition is another modality that has recently been shown to reduce untoward remodeling better than ACE inhibition alone [106]. As aldosterone stimulates cardiac collagen synthesis and fibroblast proliferation, it likely exerts its benefit by inhibiting local mineralocorticoid receptors, which in turn inhibits collagen synthesis.

In addition, randomized clinical trials have demonstrated that long-term outcome is improved by administration of aldosterone antagonists following MI in patients with heart failure. Epleronone, started 3–14 days post MI for patients with CHF and LVEF less than 40% significantly reduced the risk of death as well as recurrent hospitalizations [107]. ACE inhibitors initiated early should be continued for secondary prevention. As demonstrated in the VALIANT study, an adequate dose of an angiotensin receptor blocker such as valsartan had similar efficacy long-term and is a reasonable alternative, especially for those intolerant of ACE inhibitors [108]. In light of the enormous dataset showing improved outcomes with ACE inhibitors, they are preferred for those who are not intolerant.

Oral warfarin therapy is indicated for patients with extensive wall motion abnormalities and LV dysfunction, which would be the case with many patients with heart failure complicating acute MI [36]. Therapy should be initiated prior to discharge and once all interventions involving central vascular access have been completed. Finally, lipid-modifying therapy is indicated for all patients early after acute MI and should prove especially beneficial in the high-risk patients with heart failure [36]. The pharmacotherapy discussed here as being recommended for patients with acute MI complicated by heart failure is also intended for survivors of cardiogenic shock who will equally benefit.

*Reperfusion/revascularization Therapy*

Patients with heart failure during their hospitalization are less likely to have received reperfusion therapy. Indeed, when heart failure is a factor at presentation, the most timely and effective reperfusion therapy should be offered. Current evidence from randomized trials suggests that primary PCI should be the preferred mode of reperfusion, as it is associated with lower in-hospital mortality and re-infarction rates, as well as a reduced likelihood of intracranial hemorrhage than reperfusion with fibrinolytic therapy [109]. The association of primary PCI and improved outcome has not been observed in large prospective registries, quite likely due to a variety of factors including prolonged door-to-balloon time in the majority of clinical settings, as well as a heterogeneity of operator and institutional experience in acute MI intervention that is less likely to have been present in randomized trials [110,111]. However, for this high-risk group with heart failure, superiority of primary PCI was suggested in an adjusted model of the non-randomized NRMI cohort.

Because primary PCI is rapidly available only to a small minority of patients presenting with acute MI, and time to reperfusion is of utmost importance to the early presenters [112], patients with acute MI and heart failure on presentation should be treated with fibrinolysis unless a door-to-balloon time of 60 minutes or less can realistically be anticipated. However, as is the case with patients in shock, physicians treating acute MI patients complicated by heart failure in non-interventional centers should seek early transfer, as the failure of reperfusion in these patients can be catastrophic. It is reasonable to transfer these patients as soon as possible to a tertiary care center, with a view to immediate coronary angiography and percutaneous intervention. Even if reperfusion has occurred, early cardiac catheterization and PCI is still reasonable based on data from the recently-published ALKK and SIAM studies, in which patients after successful reperfusion by fibrinolysis who had infarct-related artery patency but a significant stenosis did better in the long-term if they underwent PCI than if they were treated conservatively [113,114].

*Novel Therapies*

Recent reports suggestive of efficacy of stem cell therapy early after myocardial infarction have created a wave of excitement and may be particularly useful for patients with large infarcts and heart failure or shock. Clearly, this modality is not ready for general clinical use, and further investigation is needed to refine the technique and evaluate its efficacy in improving long-term outcome.

## Outcome in Patients with Heart Failure Complicating Acute Myocardial Infarction

The NRMI investigators have reported a large series of nonselected patients [115,116]. In a report by Wu et al. of patients presenting within 12 hours of onset of symptoms, 21.4% of the 36,303 patients with Killip class II or III heart failure died during the index hospitalization, compared with 7.2% of patients who had no heart failure on presentation. Similarly, patients with heart failure on presentation were more likely to experience recurrent MI, stroke, sustained ventricular arrhythmias, cardiac rupture, and unexpected sudden death. In a larger series that included 176,158 patients with heart failure either at the time of presentation or developing during hospitalization, Spencer et al. found alarmingly low rates of any reperfusion therapy in heart failure patients. In-hospital mortality was 21% in patients who presented with heart failure and 31% in those who developed it after presentation (Fig. 12) [116]. A similar incremental risk was observed in the four random-

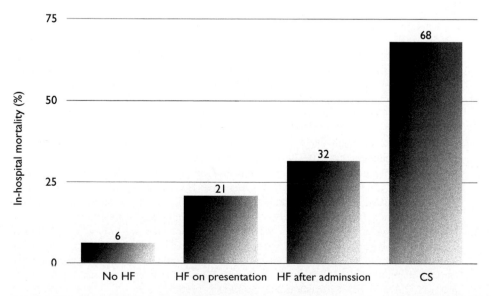

**Figure 12**    In-hospital mortality of patients with acute MI enrolled in NRMI-2 and NRMI-3 based on heart failure (HF) status. Patients with cardiogenic shock (CS) are included for comparison.

ized trials; the 30-day mortality of patients with heart failure was 8%, vs. 2% in those who did not have heart failure at any time during their hospital admission [89]. In this analysis the presence of heart failure was an independent predictor of 30-day mortality, with a relative risk of 1.55 (95% CI 1.38–1.74) vs. those with no heart failure.

Increased long-term mortality is also seen in patients with heart failure and preserved systolic function. In the Bucindolol Evaluation in Acute Myocardial Infarction Trial, 3-year mortality was 13% for patients without heart failure during their acute MI admission, 37% for those with heart failure and preserved systolic function, and 53% when heart failure was associated with systolic dysfunction [92].

*Summary*

Patients with acute MI complicated by heart failure continue to represent a high-risk group, with in-hospital mortality that is between that of patients with uncomplicated MI and those with cardiogenic shock. Their acute management is challenging and to a large extent unsupported by large bodies of research data, as they have been for the most part excluded from randomized trials of therapies in acute MI. However, reperfusion therapy, preferentially primary PCI, is strongly recommended. Inhibition of the renin-angiotensin-aldosterone system and beta-blockers are strongly indicated for secondary prevention, as is antithrombotic therapy. New modalities of therapy show promise but require further study.

## REFERENCES

1. Hochman JS, Buller CE, Sleeper LA, Boland J, Dzavik V, Sanborn TA, Godfrey E, White HD, Lim J, LeJemtel T. Cardiogenic shock complicating acute myocardial infarction—etiologies, management and outcome: a report from the SHOCK Trial Registry. SHould we emergently revascularize Occluded Coronaries for cardiogenic shocK? J Am Coll Cardiol 2000;36: 1063–1070.

2. Hasdai D, Topol EJ, Califf RM, Berger PB, Holmes DR. Cardiogenic shock complicating acute coronary syndromes. Lancet 2000;356:749–756.

3. Hollenberg SM, Kavinsky CJ, Parrillo JE. Cardiogenic shock. Ann Intern Med 1999;131: 47–59.

4. Hochman JS, Sleeper LA, Webb JG, Sanborn TA, White HD, Talley JD, Buller CE, Jacobs AK, Slater JN, Col J, McKinlay SM, LeJemtel TH. Early revascularization in acute myocardial infarction complicated by cardiogenic shock. SHOCK Investigators. Should We Emergently Revascularize Occluded Coronaries for Cardiogenic Shock. N Engl J Med 1999;341:625–634.

5. Coats AJ. CAPRICORN: a story of alpha allocation and beta-blockers in left ventricular dysfunction post-MI. Int J Cardiol 2001;78:109–113.

6. Hochman JS. Cardiogenic shock complicating acute myocardial infarction: expanding the paradigm. Circulation 2003;107:2998–3002.

7. Valencia R, Theroux P, Granger C, Mahaffey K, Gudaye T, Malloy K, Weaver W, Todaro T, Mojcik C, Armstrong P, Hochman J. Congestive Heart Failure and Cardiogenic Shock Complicating AMI Have High Mortality and Are Associated with Intense Inflammatory Response: Results from the CARDINAL Trials. J Am Coll Cardiol 2004:in press.

8. Granger CB, Mahaffey KW, Weaver WD, Theroux P, Hochman JS, Filloon TG, Rollins S, Todaro TG, Nicolau JC, Ruzyllo W, Armstrong PW. Pexelizumab, an anti-C5 complement antibody, as adjunctive therapy to primary percutaneous coronary intervention in acute myocardial infarction: the COMplement inhibition in Myocardial infarction treated with Angioplasty (COMMA) trial. Circulation 2003;108:1184–1190.

9. Cotter G, Kaluski E, Blatt A, Milovanov O, Moshkovitz Y, Zaidenstein R, Salah A, Alon D, Michovitz Y, Metzger M, Vered Z, Golik A. L-NMMA (a nitric oxide synthase inhibitor) is effective in the treatment of cardiogenic shock. Circulation 2000;101:1358–1361.

10. Cotter G, Kaluski E, Milo O, Blatt A, Salah A, Hendler A, Krakover R, Golick A, Vered Z. LINCS: L-NAME (a NO synthase inhibitor) in the treatment of refractory cardiogenic shock: a prospective randomized study. Eur Heart J 2003;24:1287–1295.

11. Hasdai D, Califf RM, Thompson TD, Hochman JS, Ohman EM, Pfisterer M, Bates ER, Vahanian A, Armstrong PW, Criger DA, Topol EJ, Holmes DR. Predictors of cardiogenic shock after thrombolytic therapy for acute myocardial infarction. J Am Coll Cardiol 2000; 35:136–143.

12. Menon V, Hochman JS, Stebbins A, Pfisterer M, Col J, Anderson RD, Hasdai D, Holmes DR, Bates ER, Topol EJ, Califf RM, Ohman EM. Lack of progress in cardiogenic shock: lessons from the GUSTO trials. Eur Heart J 2000;21:1928–1936.

13. Goldberg RJ, Gore JM, Thompson CA, Gurwitz JH. Recent magnitude of and temporal trends (1994–1997) in the incidence and hospital death rates of cardiogenic shock complicating acute myocardial infarction: the second national registry of myocardial infarction. Am Heart J 2001;141:65–72.

14. Abete P, Ferrara N, Cacciatore F, Madrid A, Bianco S, Calabrese C, Napoli C, Scognamiglio P, Bollella O, Cioppa A, Longobardi G, Rengo F. Angina-induced protection against myocardial infarction in adult and elderly patients: a loss of preconditioning mechanism in the aging heart? J Am Coll Cardiol 1997;30:947–954.

15. Abete P, Calabrese C, Ferrara N, Cioppa A, Pisanelli P, Cacciatore F, Longobardi G, Napoli C, Rengo F. Exercise training restores ischemic preconditioning in the aging heart. J Am Coll Cardiol 2000;36:643–650.

16. Lucas DT, Szweda LI. Cardiac reperfusion injury: aging, lipid peroxidation, and mitochondrial dysfunction. Proc Natl Acad Sci USA 1998;95:510–514.

17. Wong SC, Sleeper LA, Monrad ES, Menegus MA, Palazzo A, Dzavik V, Jacobs A, Jiang X, Hochman JS. Absence of gender differences in clinical outcomes in patients with cardiogenic shock complicating acute myocardial infarction. A report from the SHOCK Trial Registry. J Am Coll Cardiol 2001;38:1395–1401.

18. Shindler DM, Palmeri ST, Antonelli TA, Sleeper LA, Boland J, Cocke TP, Hochman JS. Diabetes mellitus in cardiogenic shock complicating acute myocardial infarction: a report from the SHOCK Trial Registry. Should we emergently revascularize Occluded Coronaries for cardiogenic shocK? J Am Coll Cardiol 2000;36:1097–1103.

19. Hasdai D, Holmes DR, Califf RM, Thompson TD, Hochman JS, Pfisterer M, Topol EJ. Cardiogenic shock complicating acute myocardial infarction: predictors of death. GUSTO Investigators. Global Utilization of Streptokinase and Tissue-Plasminogen Activator for Occluded Coronary Arteries. Am Heart J 1999;138:21–31.

20. Menon V, White H, LeJemtel T, Webb JG, Sleeper LA, Hochman JS. The clinical profile of patients with suspected cardiogenic shock due to predominant left ventricular failure: a report from the SHOCK Trial Registry. SHould we emergently revascularize Occluded Coronaries in cardiogenic shocK? J Am Coll Cardiol 2000;36:1071–1076.

21. Lindholm MG, Kober L, Boesgaard S, Torp-Pedersen C, Aldershvile J. Cardiogenic shock complicating acute myocardial infarction; prognostic impact of early and late shock development. Eur Heart J 2003;24:258–265.

22. Webb JG, Sleeper LA, Buller CE, Boland J, Palazzo A, Buller E, White HD, Hochman JS. Implications of the timing of onset of cardiogenic shock after acute myocardial infarction: a report from the SHOCK Trial Registry. SHould we emergently revascularize Occluded Coronaries for cardiogenic shocK? J Am Coll Cardiol 2000;36:1084–1090.

23. Jacobs AK, French JK, Col J, Sleeper LA, Slater JN, Carnendran L, Boland J, Jiang X, LeJemtel T, Hochman JS. Cardiogenic shock with non-ST-segment elevation myocardial infarction: a report from the SHOCK Trial Registry. SHould we emergently revascularize Occluded coronaries for Cardiogenic shocK? J Am Coll Cardiol 2000;36:1091–1096.

24. Hasdai D, Holmes DR, Criger DA, Topol EJ, Califf RM, Harrington RA. Age and outcome after acute coronary syndromes without persistent ST-segment elevation. Am Heart J 2000; 139:858–866.

25. Dorsch MF, Lawrance RA, Sapsford RJ, Durham N, Oldham J, Greenwood DC, Jackson BM, Morrell C, Robinson MB, Hall AS. Poor prognosis of patients presenting with symptomatic myocardial infarction but without chest pain. Heart 2001;86:494–498.

26.  Picard MH, Davidoff R, Sleeper LA, Mendes LA, Thompson CR, Dzavik V, Steingart R, Gin K, White HD, Hochman JS. Echocardiographic predictors of survival and response to early revascularization in cardiogenic shock. Circulation 2003;107:279–284.

27.  Cotter G, Moshkovitz Y, Kaluski E, Milo O, Nobikov Y, Schneeweiss A, Krakover R, Vered Z. The role of cardiac power and systemic vascular resistance in the pathophysiology and diagnosis of patients with acute congestive heart failure. Eur J Heart Fail 2003;5:443–451.

28.  Fincke R, Hochman J, Lowe A, Menon V, Slater J, Webb JG, LeJemtel T, Cotter G. Cardiac Power is the Strongest Hemodynamic Predictor of Mortality in Cardiogenic Shock: A Report from the SHOCK Trial Registry. J Am Coll Cardiol, in press.

29.  Kontoyannis DA, Nanas JN, Kontoyannis SA, Stamatelopoulos SF, Moulopoulos SD. Mechanical ventilation in conjunction with the intra-aortic balloon pump improves the outcome of patients in profound cardiogenic shock. Intensive Care Med 1999;25:835–838.

30.  Kaye DM, Mansfield D, Aggarwal A, Naughton MT, Esler MD. Acute effects of continuous positive airway pressure on cardiac sympathetic tone in congestive heart failure. Circulation 2001;103:2336–2338.

31.  Takeda S, Nejima J, Takano T, Nakanishi K, Takayama M, Sakamoto A, Ogawa R. Effect of nasal continuous positive airway pressure on pulmonary edema complicating acute myocardial infarction. Jpn Circ J 1998;62:553–558.

32.  Lin M, Yang YF, Chiang HT, Chang MS, Chiang BN, Cheitlin MD. Reappraisal of continuous positive airway pressure therapy in acute cardiogenic pulmonary edema. Short-term results and long-term follow-up. Chest 1995;107:1379–1386.

32a. Guidelines 2000 for Cardiopulmonary Resuscitation and Emergency Cardiovascular Care Part 7: The Era of Reperfusion Section 1: Acute Coronary Syndromes (Acute Myocardial Infarctions. Circulation 2000;102(Suppl. I):I-172–216.

33.  Mukae S, Yanagishita T, Geshi E, Umetsu K, Tomita M, Itoh S, Konno N, Katagiri T. The effects of dopamine, dobutamine and amrinone on mitochondrial function in cardiogenic shock. Jpn Heart J 1997;38:515–529.

34.  Richard C, Ricome JL, Rimailho A, Bottineau G, Auzepy P. Combined hemodynamic effects of dopamine and dobutamine in cardiogenic shock. Circulation 1983;67:620–626.

35.  Lin H, Young DB. Opposing effects of plasma epinephrine and norepinephrine on coronary thrombosis in vivo. Circulation 1995;91:1135–1142.

36.  Ryan TJ, Antman EM, Brooks NH, Califf RM, Hillis LD, Hiratzka LF, Rapaport E, Riegel B, Russell RO, Smith EE, Weaver WD, Gibbons RJ, Alpert JS, Eagle KA, Gardner TJ, Garson A, Gregoratos G, Smith SC. 1999 update: ACC/AHA guidelines for the management of patients with acute myocardial infarction. A report of the American College of Cardiology/American Heart Association Task Force on Practice Guidelines (Committee on Management of Acute Myocardial Infarction). J Am Coll Cardiol 1999;34:890–911.

37.  Barron HV, Every NR, Parsons LS, Angeja B, Goldberg RJ, Gore JM, Chou TM. The use of intra-aortic balloon counterpulsation in patients with cardiogenic shock complicating acute myocardial infarction: data from the National Registry of Myocardial Infarction 2. Am Heart J 2001;141:933–939.

38.  Harold L, Dauerman M, Robert J, Goldberg J, Kami White MPH, Joel M, Gore MD, Immad Sadiq MD, Enrique Gurfinkel MD, Andrzej Budaj MD, Esteban Lopez de Sa, Jose Lopez-Sendon. for the GRACE Investigators*. Revascularization, Stenting, and Outcomes of Patients With Acute Myocardial Infarction Complicated by Cardiogenic Shock. Am J Cardiol 2002; 90:838–842.

39.  Sanborn TA, Sleeper LA, Bates ER, Jacobs AK, Boland J, French JK, Dens J, Dzavik V, Palmeri ST, Webb JG, Goldberger M, Hochman JS. Impact of thrombolysis, intra-aortic balloon pump counterpulsation, and their combination in cardiogenic shock complicating acute myocardial infarction: a report from the SHOCK Trial Registry. SHould we emergently revascularize Occluded Coronaries for cardiogenic shocK? J Am Coll Cardiol 2000;36: 1123–1129.

40.  Chen EW, Canto JG, Parsons LS, Peterson ED, Littrell KA, Every NR, Gibson CM, Hochman JS, Ohman EM, Cheeks M, Barron HV. Relation between hospital intra-aortic balloon counter-

pulsation volume and mortality in acute myocardial infarction complicated by cardiogenic shock. Circulation 2003;108:951–957.

41. Ramanathan K, Cosmi H, Harkness S, French J, Farkouh M, Sleeper L, Dzavik V, Hochman J. Reversal of Systemic Hypoperfusion Following Intra-Aortic Balloon Pumping is Associated with Improved 30-Day Survival Independent of Early Revascularization in Cardiogenic Shock Complicating an Acute Myocardial Infarction. Circulation 2003;108:IV-672.

42. Prewitt RM. Thrombolytic therapy in patients where hypotension or cardiogenic shock complicate acute myocardial infarction. Can J Cardiol 1993;9:155–157.

43. French JK, Feldman HA, Assmann SF, Sanborn T, Palmeri ST, Miller D, Boland J, Buller CE, Steingart R, Sleeper LA, Hochman JS. Influence of thrombolytic therapy, with or without intra-aortic balloon counterpulsation, on 12-month survival in the SHOCK trial. Am Heart J 2003;146:804–810.

44. Ohman EM, Mannas J, Stomel RJ, Leesav MA, Nielsen D, Hudson MP, Fraulo B, Shaw LK, Lee LK, O'Dea D, Rogers FJ, Harber D. Thrombolysis and counter pulsation to improve Cardiogenic Shock. Survival (TACTICS): Results of a prospective randomized trial. Circulation. 2000;106:II–600.

45. Mathey D, Kuck KH, Remmecke J, Tilsner V, Bleifeld W. Transluminal recanalization of coronary artery thrombosis: a preliminary report of its application in cardiogenic shock. Eur Heart J 1980;1:207–212.

46. Lee L, Bates ER, Pitt B, Walton JA, Laufer N, O'Neill WW. Percutaneous transluminal coronary angioplasty improves survival in acute myocardial infarction complicated by cardiogenic shock. Circulation 1988;78:1345–1351.

47. Verna E, Repetto S, Boscarini M, Ghezzi I, Binaghi G. Emergency coronary angioplasty in patients with severe left ventricular dysfunction or cardiogenic shock after acute myocardial infarction. Eur Heart J 1989;10:958–966.

48. Yamamoto H, Hayashi Y, Oka Y, Sumii K, Taniguchi C, Maeda Y, Watanabe M, Tsuchiya T. Efficacy of percutaneous transluminal coronary angioplasty in patients with acute myocardial infarction complicated by cardiogenic shock. Jpn Circ J 1992;56:815–821.

49. Seydoux C, Goy JJ, Beuret P, Stauffer JC, Vogt P, Schaller MD, Kappenberger L, Perret C. Effectiveness of percutaneous transluminal coronary angioplasty in cardiogenic shock during acute myocardial infarction. Am J Cardiol 1992;69:968–969.

50. Hibbard MD, Holmes DR, Bailey KR, Reeder GS, Bresnahan JF, Gersh BJ. Percutaneous transluminal coronary angioplasty in patients with cardiogenic shock. J Am Coll Cardiol 1992;19:639–646.

51. Gacioch GM, Ellis SG, Lee L, Bates ER, Kirsh M, Walton JA, Topol EJ. Cardiogenic shock complicating acute myocardial infarction: the use of coronary angioplasty and the integration of the new support devices into patient management. J Am Coll Cardiol 1992;19:647–653.

52. Moscucci M, Bates ER. Cardiogenic shock. Cardiol Clin 1995;13:391–406.

53. Dzavik V, Burton JR, Kee C, Teo KK, Ignaszewski A, Lucas AR, Tymchak WJ. Changing practice patterns in the management of acute myocardial infarction complicated by cardiogenic shock: elderly compared with younger patients. Can J Cardiol 1998;14:923–930.

54. Holmes DR, Bates ER, Kleiman NS, Sadowski Z, Horgan JH, Morris DC, Califf RM, Berger PB, Topol EJ. Contemporary reperfusion therapy for cardiogenic shock: the GUSTO-I trial experience. The GUSTO-I Investigators. Global Utilization of Streptokinase and Tissue Plasminogen Activator for Occluded Coronary Arteries. J Am Coll Cardiol 1995;26:668–674.

55. Hochman JS, Sleeper LA, White HD, Dzavik V, Wong SC, Menon V, Webb JG, Steingart R, Picard MH, Menegus MA, Boland J, Sanborn T, Buller CE, Modur S, Forman R, Desvigne-Nickens P, Jacobs AK, Slater JN, LeJemtel TH. One-year survival following early revascularization for cardiogenic shock. JAMA 2001;285:190–192.

56. Urban P, Stauffer JC, Bleed D, Khatchatrian BN, Anmann W, Bertel O, van den Brand M, Danchin N, Kaufmann U, Meier B, Machecourt J, Pfisterer M. A randomized evaluation of early revascularization to Treat Shock complication acute myocardial infarction. The Swiss Multicenter Trial of Angioplasty for Shock. (SMASH) Eur Heart J 1999;20:1030–1038.

57. Dzavik V, Sleeper LA, Cocke TP, Moscucci M, Saucedo J, Hosat S, Jiang X, Slater J, LeJemtel T, Hochman JS. Early revascularization is associated with improved survival in

elderly patients with acute myocardial infarction complicated by cardiogenic shock: a report from the SHOCK Trial Registry. Eur Heart J 2003;24:828–837.

57a. Carnendran L, Abboud R, Sleeper LA, Gurunathan R, Webb JG, Menon V, Dzavik V, Cocke T, Hochman JS. Trends in cardiogenic shock: report from the SHOCK Study. Should we emergently revascularize occluded coronaries for cardiogenic shock? Eur Heart J 2001;22(6): 472–478.

58. Dauerman HL, Goldberg RJ, Malinski M, Yarzebski J, Lessard D, Gore JM. Outcomes and early revascularization for patients > or = 65 years of age with cardiogenic shock. Am J Cardiol 2001;87:844–848.

59. Dauerman HL, Ryan TJ, Piper WD, Kellett MA, Shubrooks SJ, Robb JF, Hearne MJ, Watkins MW, Hettleman BD, Silver MT, Niles NW, Malenka DJ. Outcomes of Percutaneous Coronary Intervention Among Elderly Patients in Cardiogenic Shock: A Multicenter, Decade-long Experience. J Invasive Cardiol 2003;15:380–384.

60. Rogers WJ, Stanley AW, Breinig JB, Prather JW, McDaniel HG, Moraski RE, Mantle JA, Russell RO, Rackley CE. Reduction of hospital mortality rate of acute myocardial infarction with glucose-insulin-potassium infusion. Am Heart J 1976;92:441–454.

61. Sundstedt CD, Sylven C, Mogensen L. Glucose-insulin-potassium-albumin infusion in the early phase of acute myocardial infarction--a controlled study. Acta Med Scand 1981;210: 67–71.

62. Marano L, Bestetti A, Lomuscio A, Tagliabue L, Castini D, Tarricone D, Dario P, Tarolo GL, Fiorentini C. Effects of infusion of glucose-insulin-potassium on myocardial function after a recent myocardial infarction. Acta Cardiol 2000;55:9–15.

63. Fath-Ordoubadi F, Beatt KJ. Glucose-insulin-potassium therapy for treatment of acute myocardial infarction: an overview of randomized placebo-controlled trials. Circulation 1997;96: 1152–1156.

64. van den Berghe G, Wouters P, Weekers F, Verwaest C, Bruyninckx F, Schetz M, Vlasselaers D, Ferdinande P, Lauwers P, Bouillon R. Intensive insulin therapy in the critically ill patients. N Engl J Med 2001;345:1359–1367.

65. Coleman GM, Gradinac S, Taegtmeyer H, Sweeney M, Frazier OH. Efficacy of metabolic support with glucose-insulin-potassium for left ventricular pump failure after aortocoronary bypass surgery. Circulation 1989;80:I91–96.

66. Malmberg K, Norhammar A, Ryden L. Insulin treatment post myocardial infarction: the DIGAMI study. Adv Exp Med Biol 2001;498:279–284.

67. Gradinac S, Coleman GM, Taegtmeyer H, Sweeney MS, Frazier OH. Improved cardiac function with glucose-insulin-potassium after aortocoronary bypass grafting. Ann Thorac Surg 1989;48:484–489.

68. Mahaffey KW, Granger CB, Nicolau JC, Ruzyllo W, Weaver WD, Theroux P, Hochman JS, Filloon TG, Mojcik CF, Todaro TG, Armstrong PW. Effect of pexelizumab, an anti-C5 complement antibody, as adjunctive therapy to fibrinolysis in acute myocardial infarction: the COMPlement inhibition in myocardial infarction treated with thromboLYtics (COMPLY) trial. Circulation 2003;108:1176–1183.

69. Castells E, Calbet JM, Saura E, Manito N, Miralles A, Fontanillas C, Benito M, Granados J, Rabasa M, Roca J, Rullan C, Flajsig I, Mayosky A, Chevez H, Worner F, Octavio de Toledo MC, Esplugas E. Acute myocardial infarction with cardiogenic shock: treatment with mechanical circulatory assistance and heart transplantation. Transplant Proc 2003;35: 1940–1941.

70. Entwistle IJ, Bolno PB, Holmes E, Samuels LE. Improved survival with ventricular assist device support in cardiogenic shock after myocardial infarction. Heart Surg Forum 2003;6: 316–319.

71. Kherani AR, Cheema FH, Oz MC, Fal JM, Morgan JA, Topkara VK, Wilson DA, Vigilance DW, Garrido MJ, Naka Y. Implantation of a left ventricular assist device and the hub-and-spoke system in treating acute cardiogenic shock: who survives? J Thorac Cardiovasc Surg 2003;126:1634–1635.

72. Thiele H, Lauer B, Hambrecht R, Boudriot E, Cohen HA, Schuler G. Reversal of cardiogenic shock by percutaneous left atrial-to-femoral arterial bypass assistance. Circulation 2001;104: 2917–2922.

73.  Thompson CR, Buller CE, Sleeper LA, Antonelli TA, Webb JG, Jaber WA, Abel JG, Hochman JS. Cardiogenic shock due to acute severe mitral regurgitation complicating acute myocardial infarction: a report from the SHOCK Trial Registry. SHould we use emergently revascularize Occluded Coronaries in cardiogenic shocK? J Am Coll Cardiol 2000;36: 1104–1109.

74.  Dekker AL, Reesink KD, van der Veen FH, van Ommen GV, Geskes GG, Soemers AC, Maessen JG. Intra-aortic balloon pumping in acute mitral regurgitation reduces aortic imped-ance and regurgitant fraction. Shock 2003;19:334–338.

75.  Tcheng JE, Jackman JD, Nelson CL, Gardner LH, Smith LR, Rankin JS, Califf RM, Stack RS. Outcome of patients sustaining acute ischemic mitral regurgitation during myocardial infarction. Ann Intern Med 1992;117:18–24.

76.  Webb JG, Lowe AM, Sanborn TA, White HD, Sleeper LA, Carere RG, Buller CE, Wong SC, Boland J, Dzavik V, Porway M, Pate G, Bergman G, Hochman JS. Percutaneous coronary intervention for cardiogenic shock in the SHOCK trial. J Am Coll Cardiol 2003;42: 1380–1386.

77.  Menon V, Webb JG, Hillis LD, Sleeper LA, Abboud R, Dzavik V, Slater JN, Forman R, Monrad ES, Talley JD, Hochman JS. Outcome and profile of ventricular septal rupture with cardiogenic shock after myocardial infarction: a report from the SHOCK Trial Registry. SHould we emergently revascularize Occluded Coronaries in cardiogenic shocK? J Am Coll Cardiol 2000;36:1110–1116.

78.  Ellis CJ, Parkinson GF, Jaffe WM, Campbell MJ, Kerr AR. Good long-term outcome follow-ing surgical repair of post-infarction ventricular septal defect. Aust N Z J Med 1995;25: 330–336.

79.  Weintraub RM, Wei JY, Thurer RL. Surgical repair of remediable postinfarction cardiogenic shock in the elderly. Early and long-term results. J Am Geriatr Soc 1986;34:389–392.

80.  David TE, Dale L, Sun Z. Postinfarction ventricular septal rupture: repair by endocardial patch with infarct exclusion. J Thorac Cardiovasc Surg 1995;110:1315–1322.

81.  Loisance DY, Cachera JP, Poulain H, Aubry P, Juvin AM, Galey JJ. Ventricular septal defect after acute myocardial infarction: Early repair. J Thorac Cardiovasc Surg 1980;80:61–67.

82.  Daggett WM, Buckley MJ, Akins CW, Leinbach RC, Gold HK, Block PC, Austen WG. Improved results of surgical management of postinfarction ventricular septal rupture. Ann Surg 1982;196:269–277.

83.  Takano T, Saito H, Tanaka K, Endo T, Harada A, Yamauchi S, Osaka S, Ino T, Yamate N, Hayakawa H, et al. [Effects and limitation of intra-aortic balloon pumping in patients with acute myocardial infarction complicated with cardiogenic shock, ventricular septal perfora-tion, and mitral regurgitation]. Nippon Naika Gakkai Zasshi 1984;73:332–340.

84.  Anderson DR, Adams S, Bhat A, Pepper JR. Post-infarction ventricular septal defect: the importance of site of infarction and cardiogenic shock on outcome. Eur J Cardiothorac Surg 1989;3:554–547.

85.  Guzman F, Renzulli MA, Behl PR, D'Onofrio A, Sante P, Naik S. Post infarction ventricular septal defect. Review of 41 surgical cases. Ital J Surg Sci 1989;19:179–185.

86.  Komeda M, Fremes SE, David TE. Surgical repair of postinfarction ventricular septal defect. Circulation 1990;82:IV243–247.

87.  Killen DA, Piehler JM, Borkon AM, Gorton ME, Reed WA. Early repair of postinfarction ventricular septal rupture. Ann Thorac Surg 1997;63:138–142.

88.  Slater J, Brown RJ, Antonelli TA, Menon V, Boland J, Col J, Dzavik V, Greenberg M, Menegus M, Connery C, Hochman JS. Cardiogenic shock due to cardiac free-wall rupture or tamponade after acute myocardial infarction: a report from the SHOCK Trial Registry. Should we emergently revascularize occluded coronaries for cardiogenic shock? J Am Coll Cardiol 2000;36:1117–1122.

89.  Hasdai D, Topol EJ, Kilaru R, Battler A, Harrington RA, Vahanian A, Ohman EM, Granger CB, Van de Werf F, Simoons ML, O'Connor CM, Holmes DR. Frequency, patient characteris-tics, and outcomes of mild-to-moderate heart failure complicating ST-segment elevation acute myocardial infarction: lessons from 4 international fibrinolytic therapy trials. Am Heart J 2003;145:73–79.

90. Killip T, Kimball JT. Treatment of myocardial infarction in a coronary care unit. A two year experience with 250 patients. Am J Cardiol 1967;20:457–64.

91. Moller JE, Poulsen SH, Sondergaard E, Seward JB, Appleton CP, Egstrup K. Impact of early changes in left ventricular filling pattern on long-term outcome after acute myocardial infarction. Int J Cardiol 2003;89:207–215.

92. Moller JE, Brendorp B, Ottesen M, Kober L, Egstrup K, Poulsen SH, Torp-Pedersen C. Congestive heart failure with preserved left ventricular systolic function after acute myocardial infarction: clinical and prognostic implications. Eur J Heart Fail 2003;5:811–819.

93. Armstrong PW, Walker DC, Burton JR, Parker JO. Vasodilator therapy in acute myocardial infarction. A comparison of sodium nitroprusside and nitroglycerin. Circulation 1975;52: 1118–1122.

94. Cotter G, Metzkor E, Kaluski E, Faigenberg Z, Miller R, Simovitz A, Shaham O, Marghitay D, Koren M, Blatt A, Moshkovitz Y, Zaidenstein R, Golik A. Randomised trial of high-dose isosorbide dinitrate plus low-dose furosemide versus high-dose furosemide plus low-dose isosorbide dinitrate in severe pulmonary oedema. Lancet 1998;351:389–393.

95. Chiariello M, Gold HK, Leinbach RC, Davis MA, Maroko PR. Comparison between the effects of nitroprusside and nitroglycerin on ischemic injury during acute myocardial infarction. Circulation 1976;54:766–773.

96. Cohn JN, Franciosa JA, Francis GS, Archibald D, Tristani F, Fletcher R, Montero A, Cintron G, Clarke J, Hager D, Saunders R, Cobb F, Smith R, Loeb H, Settle H. Effect of short-term infusion of sodium nitroprusside on mortality rate in acute myocardial infarction complicated by left ventricular failure: results of a Veterans Administration cooperative study. N Engl J Med 1982;306:1129–1135.

97. Swedberg K, Held P, Kjekshus J, Rasmussen K, Ryden L, Wedel H. Effects of the early administration of enalapril on mortality in patients with acute myocardial infarction. Results of the Cooperative New Scandinavian Enalapril Survival Study II (CONSENSUS II). N Engl J Med 1992;327:678–684.

98. Lampert R, Ickovics JR, Viscoli CJ, Horwitz RI, Lee FA. Effects of propranolol on recovery of heart rate variability following acute myocardial infarction and relation to outcome in the Beta-Blocker Heart Attack Trial. Am J Cardiol 2003;91:137–142.

99. Randomised trial of intravenous atenolol among 16 027 cases of suspected acute myocardial infarction: ISIS-1. First International Study of Infarct Survival Collaborative Group. Lancet 1986;2:57–66.

100. Metoprolol in acute myocardial infarction. Patients and methods. The MIAMI Trial Research Group. Am J Cardiol 1985;56:3G–9G.

101. Herlitz J, Waagstein F, Lindqvist J, Swedberg K, Hjalmarson A. Effect of metoprolol on the prognosis for patients with suspected acute myocardial infarction and indirect signs of congestive heart failure (a subgroup analysis of the Goteborg Metoprolol Trial). Am J Cardiol 1997; 80:40J–44J.

102. Spargias KS, Hall AS, Greenwood DC, Ball SG. beta blocker treatment and other prognostic variables in patients with clinical evidence of heart failure after acute myocardial infarction: evidence from the AIRE study. Heart 1999;81:25–32.

103. Pfisterer M, Cox JL, Granger CB, Brener SJ, Naylor CD, Califf RM, van de Werf F, Stebbins AL, Lee KL, Topol EJ, Armstrong PW. Atenolol use and clinical outcomes after thrombolysis for acute myocardial infarction: the GUSTO-I experience. Global Utilization of Streptokinase and TPA (alteplase) for Occluded Coronary Arteries. J Am Coll Cardiol 1998;32:634–640.

104. van der Horst IC, Zijlstra F, van't Hof AW, Doggen CJ, de Boer MJ, Suryapranata H, Hoorntje JC, Dambrink JH, Gans RO, Bilo HJ. Glucose-insulin-potassium infusion inpatients treated with primary angioplasty for acute myocardial infarction: the glucose-insulin-potassium study: a randomized trial. J Am Coll Cardiol 2003;42:784–791.

105. Pitt B, Zannad F, Remme WJ, Cody R, Castaigne A, Perez A, Palensky J, Wittes J. The effect of spironolactone on morbidity and mortality in patients with severe heart failure. Randomized Aldactone Evaluation Study Investigators. N Engl J Med 1999;341:709–717.

106. Hayashi M, Tsutamoto T, Wada A, Tsutsui T, Ishii C, Ohno K, Fujii M, Taniguchi A, Hamatani T, Nozato Y, Kataoka K, Morigami N, Ohnishi M, Kinoshita M, Horie M. Immedi-

ate administration of mineralocorticoid receptor antagonist spironolactone prevents post-infarct left ventricular remodeling associated with suppression of a marker of myocardial collagen synthesis in patients with first anterior acute myocardial infarction. Circulation 2003; 107:2559–2565.

107. Pitt B, Remme W, Zannad F, Neaton J, Martinez F, Roniker B, Bittman R, Hurley S, Kleiman J, Gatlin M. Eplerenone, a selective aldosterone blocker, in patients with left ventricular dysfunction after myocardial infarction. N Engl J Med 2003;348:1309–1321.

108. Pfeffer MA, McMurray JJ, Velazquez EJ, Rouleau JL, Kober L, Maggioni AP, Solomon SD, Swedberg K, Van de Werf F, White H, Leimberger JD, Henis M, Edwards S, Zelenkofske S, Sellers MA, Califf RM. Valsartan, captopril, or both in myocardial infarction complicated by heart failure, left ventricular dysfunction, or both. N Engl J Med 2003;349:1893–1906.

109. Keeley EC, Boura JA, Grines CL. Primary angioplasty versus intravenous thrombolytic therapy for acute myocardial infarction: a quantitative review of 23 randomised trials. Lancet 2003;361:13–20.

110. Tiefenbrunn AJ, Chandra NC, French WJ, Gore JM, Rogers WJ. Clinical experience with primary percutaneous transluminal coronary angioplasty compared with alteplase (recombinant tissue-type plasminogen activator) in patients with acute myocardial infarction: a report from the Second National Registry of Myocardial Infarction (NRMI-2). J Am Coll Cardiol 1998;31:1240–1245.

111. Danchin N, Vaur L, Genes N, Etienne S, Angioi M, Ferrieres J, Cambou JP. Treatment of acute myocardial infarction by primary coronary angioplasty or intravenous thrombolysis in the ''real world'': one-year results from a nationwide French survey. Circulation 1999;99: 2639–2644.

112. Steg PG, Bonnefoy E, Chabaud S, Lapostolle F, Dubien PY, Cristofini P, Leizorovicz A, Touboul P. Impact of time to treatment on mortality after prehospital fibrinolysis or primary angioplasty: data from the CAPTIM randomized clinical trial. Circulation 2003;108: 2851–2856.

113. Zeymer U, Uebis R, Vogt A, Glunz HG, Vohringer HF, Harmjanz D, Neuhaus KL. Randomized comparison of percutaneous transluminal coronary angioplasty and medical therapy in stable survivors of acute myocardial infarction with single vessel disease: a study of the Arbeitsgemeinschaft Leitende Kardiologische Krankenhausarzte. Circulation 2003;108: 1324–1328.

114. Scheller B, Hennen B, Hammer B, Walle J, Hofer C, Hilpert V, Winter H, Nickenig G, Bohm M. Beneficial effects of immediate stenting after thrombolysis in acute myocardial infarction. J Am Coll Cardiol 2003;42:634–641.

115. Wu AH, Parsons L, Every NR, Bates ER. Hospital outcomes in patients presenting with congestive heart failure complicating acute myocardial infarction: a report from the Second National Registry of Myocardial Infarction (NRMI-2). J Am Coll Cardiol 2002;40: 1389–1394.

116. Spencer FA, Meyer TE, Gore JM, Goldberg RJ. Heterogeneity in the management and outcomes of patients with acute myocardial infarction complicated by heart failure: the National Registry of Myocardial Infarction. Circulation 2002;105:2605–2610.

# 30

# Treatment of Acute Myocardial Infarction: International and Regional Differences

**Louise Pilote**
*McGill University Health Centre*
*Montreal, Quebec, Canada*

## INTRODUCTION

Multiple randomized clinical trials have examined whether aggressive approaches to the treatment of acute myocardial infarction (MI)—using invasive and costly procedures such as angiography in all patients and revascularization in most patients—added a benefit compared with more conservative approaches that use cardiac procedures more selectively [1–9]. The results of these studies have called into question whether there is any clinical advantage to an aggressive approach. Thus, the clinical practice guidelines of authoritative bodies such as the American Heart Association and American College of Cardiology have recommended the use of angiography only in patients who develop complications and show evidence of inducible ischemia after acute MI [10,11]. Despite the results of these studies and the publication of practice guidelines for the use of angiography and revascularization after acute MI, wide international and regional variations in the treatment of acute MI persist.

This chapter describes the results of several studies that examined practice patterns in the treatment of acute MI in different countries and different regions of the United States and Canada, with a particular focus on the use of angiography, revascularization procedures, and cardiac medications for secondary prevention post-acute MI. In addition, this chapter will investigate the impact of these practice variations on clinical outcomes, as well as on quality-of-life measurements and cost of care. Finally, potential reasons for these differences in practice patterns and the determinants of the use of cardiac procedures in clinical practice will be identified and discussed.

## VARIATIONS IN PROCESSES OF CARE

### ST-Segment Elevation Acute MI

The five earliest trials which compared aggressive and conservative management for uncomplicated acute MI exclusively enrolled patients with ST-segment elevation [1]. Correspondingly, the earliest observational studies to report international variations in the treatment of acute MI either focused on patients with ST-segment elevation, or they did not focus on a particular clinical subgroup.

### Variations Between the United States and Canada

The initial studies to report international variations in the treatment of acute MI compared the treatment practices between the US and Canada. Such comparisons are useful in assessing practice patterns in different health care systems; Canada has a universal single-payer health insurance system, whereas the United States has multiple insurance coverage systems. These studies were published at a time when US health care policy makers were looking to Canada for a potential model for changes in the American health care system.

In one of the first studies comparing the treatment of acute MI in the US and Canada, Rouleau et al. studied patients admitted between 1987 and 1990 from 19 Canadian and 93 US hospitals participating in the Survival and Ventricular Enlargement (SAVE) study [12]. Despite the similarity of the United States and Canadian patients participating in the study, coronary angiography was more commonly performed in the United States than in Canada (68% vs. 35%); revascularization procedures were also more common in the US (31% vs. 12%). These differences did not result in any apparent differences in mortality (22% vs. 23%) or reinfarction (14% vs. 13%) incidences over 1 year. However, the incidence of activity-limiting angina was more common in Canada than the United States (33% vs. 27%).

The more intensive use of cardiac procedures such as bypass surgery suggests a more expensive treatment strategy for acute MI in the US than in Canada. Given the absence of significant differences in cumulative mortality and reinfarction incidences, this study raised questions as to whether the frequent use of cardiac procedures after acute MI was in fact cost-effective; the results also raised questions about potential overuse of cardiac procedures in the US and underuse in Canada.

A subsequent study to compare the practice patterns in the US and Canada was a retrospective cohort study performed in two university hospitals: Stanford Medical Center (Palo Alto, CA) and the Royal Victoria Hospital at McGill University (Montreal) [13]. This 1994 study extended the results of Rouleau's study, obtaining more extensive data on patient functional status among consecutive patients treated for ST-segment elevation acute MI over 2 years. The study confirmed findings of a more invasive approach in the US than in Canada, but also found an increased use of noninvasive tests in Canada compared with the US. Reinfarction and mortality cumulative incidences at 1 year were similar at Stanford and McGill. In contrast, angina was reported less commonly at Stanford (33% vs. 40%), and the functional status of Stanford patients was superior to that of McGill patients (Duke Activity Status Index mean: 28.8 and 22.9, respectively).

Additional studies of administrative databases in Canada and in the US have provided population-based analyses of patients with acute MI. These studies have confirmed the findings drawn from secondary analyses of randomized trials. Tu et al. compared elderly Medicare beneficiaries in the US to elderly patients in Ontario, Canada in 1991 [14]. The higher use of cardiac procedures in the US did not appear to affect prognosis, as the 1-year mortality was similar for US and Canadian patients (34.3% vs. 34.4%). Furthermore, Pilote et al. looked at temporal trends in technology use for the treatment of acute MI in the elderly in the US and Quebec, Canada between 1988 and 1994 [15]. Growth in technology use was greater in the US than in Quebec. For example, use of PTCA increased from 7% to 18% in the US compared with 2% to 6% in Quebec. Yet, downward trends in mortality were similar; one-year mortality went from 39.1% to 32.8% in the US and from 37.6% to 32.1% in Quebec.

Finally, a study by Langer et al. has shown that the trends in treatment differences for ST-segment elevation acute MI between the US and Canada have persisted in more recent years [16]. This study compared the treatment and outcomes of US and Canadian patients enrolled in the Coumadin/Aspirin Reinfarction Study (CARS) and found a more aggressive approach to treatment in the US. In contrast to previous studies, the US patients had a lower cumulative incidence of a primary endpoint of cardiovascular deaths, nonfatal MI, and nonfatal ischemic stroke at 1 year (8.0% vs. 11.3%). However, the authors point out that there may have been a selection bias due to enrollment of US patients at low-risk for subsequent clinical events in comparison with Canadian patients. As the approach to care in Canada has become increasingly more aggressive over time [17], newer studies are needed to confirm whether such marked treatment differences between US and Canada persist today.

*Variations Between Countries Other than the US and Canada*

International variations in ST-segment elevation acute MI management have been reported between countries other than the US and Canada. In these studies, the US has consistently been shown to provide a highly aggressive approach to care in comparison to other countries. For example, in an early study making use of the first Global Utilization of Streptokinase and tissue plasminogen activator (t-PA) for Occluded Coronary Arteries (GUSTO-I) trial database, Van de Werf et al. compared the treatment of ST-segment elevation acute MI between the US and 14 other countries [18]. Angioplasty and bypass surgery were used more commonly in the US than elsewhere (angioplasty in 31% of US patients, compared with 10% elsewhere; bypass surgery in 13% compared with 3%). Despite the more aggressive use of cardiac procedures in the US than in the other countries, enrolment in the US was only a marginally significant predictor of improved survival (30-day mortality: 6.8% in the US vs. 7.2% elsewhere).

Among other studies of international variations, Matsui et al. conducted chart reviews for 694 consecutive patients with acute MI admitted in teaching hospitals in the US (Brigham and Women's Hospital), Japan, Brazil, Germany, and Switzerland [19]. They found that the US hospital did not have the highest rates of use for any invasive cardiac procedure. However, length of stay was much shorter and the use of thrombolytic therapy was lowest at the US hospital. These comparisons are limited, however, by variations in case-mix among the 5 hospitals.

Giugliano et al. also found variations using the database provided by the Intravenous nPA for Treatment of Infarcting Myocardium Early (InTIME II) trial to study ST-segment elevation acute MI patients admitted in various countries within Western Europe, Eastern Europe, North America, and Latin America between 1997 and 1998 [20]. The use of cardiac procedures and medical therapy was most intensive in North America.

Finally, Heller et al. surveyed doctors in Australia, Brazil, Chile, India, and Thailand in 1996 and found both between- and within-country variation in the reported use of most cardiac interventions and medications [21].

## Non–ST-segment Elevation Acute MI

Most recent studies of international and regional variations in acute coronary syndrome treatment have focussed on patients with non–ST-segment elevation acute MI or unstable angina. In part, this shift in focus reflects continuing uncertainty as to the appropriate course of management for these acute coronary syndromes. This shift in focus also reflects changes in the pathophysiology of patients with acute coronary syndromes that have resulted from the widespread administration of thrombolytic therapy. Many patients presenting to hospitals with ST-segment elevation acute MI experience coronary reperfusion following administration of thrombolytic therapy [22]. In addition, the increasing use of troponins has shifted the diagnosis of patients presenting to hospital with unstable angina to non–ST-segment elevation acute MI. Thus, the prevalence of patients with non–ST-segment elevation acute MI has increased and is now greater than the prevalence of patients with ST-segment elevation acute MI [23]. There is therefore increasing interest in determining the appropriate course of management for patients presenting with non–ST-segment elevation and unstable angina. Accordingly, the most recent clinical trials have enrolled this clinical subgroup of patients [6–9].

*Variations Between the United States and Canada*

A study by Fu et al. has used the database provided by the GUSTO IIb Trial to compare the treatment and outcomes of MI patients without ST-segment elevation admitted in the US and Canada between 1994 and 1995 [24]. Trends in invasive cardiac procedure use for these patients were similar to those observed for MI patients with ST-segment elevation. For example, twice as many US patients received angiography during the initial hospitalization as compared with Canadian patients (81% vs. 42%). Discharge prescription rates for cardiac medications were similar in the two countries, except US patients were less likely to receive β-blockers than Canadian patients (55% vs. 69%). Also similar to previous studies, 1-year mortality rates were comparable between the two countries (10.5% vs. 10.6%), as were rates of recurrent MI within 6 months postdischarge (9.3% vs. 11.8%).

*Variations Between Countries Other than the US and Canada*

Two studies have used data from large patient registries to compare processes of care and outcomes among MI patients without ST-segment elevation in the United States and other countries. Anderson et al. used data from the Thrombolysis in Myocardial Infarction (TIMI) III registry to examine all consecutive admissions for non–Q-wave MI or unstable angina at 14 US and 4 Canadian tertiary care hospitals between 1990 and 1993 [25]. In this study, rates of use of invasive cardiac procedures were similar for patients admitted in the US and Canada. For example, coronary angiography rates during the index hospitalization were similar in both countries (63.4% in the US vs. 66.9% in Canada). Mortality at 1 year was also similar (10.0% vs. 10.2%).

A later study using registry data found variations in non–ST-segment elevation MI treatment between several different countries. Yusuf et al. used data from the Organization to Assess Strategies for Ischaemic Syndromes (OASIS) registry to examine consecutive patients admitted with unstable angina or MI without ST-segment elevation in the United States and 5 other countries between 1995 and 1996 [26]. Rates of use of angiography within 7 days were highest in the US (58%) and Brazil (60%), lowest in Poland (2%) and Hungary (15%), and intermediate in Canada (35%) and Australia (22%). The higher rate of use of invasive procedures in the United States and Brazil was not associated with differences in mortality between countries with lower rates of use (OR for death or MI 0.91; 95% CI: 0.7–1.1). However, it was associated with a lower rate of refractory angina within 6 months (OR 0.64; 95% CI: 0.56–0.73), but higher rates of stroke (OR 1.6; 95% CI: 1.1–2.4).

## Regional Variations

International variations in care are largely a result of the different health care systems. Whether variations in the treatment of acute MI existed within the United States, that is, within the same health care system is a question addressed by several investigators. Pilote et al. merged the databases of the GUSTO-I trial and the American Hospital Association in order to examine the treatment of ST-segment elevation acute MI among the major census regions in the US between 1990 and 1993 [27]. The proportion of patients undergoing cardiac procedures varied greatly across the US and was lowest in New England. Medication use during the initial hospitalization also varied greatly across regions (Fig. 1), with New England having the greatest use of oral beta-blockers, nitrates and ACE inhibitors, and the lowest use of calcium channel blockers, lidocaine, and digitalis. Thus, compared with other regions, the practice in New England was closer to evidence-based medical practice and, in that way, followed a pattern similar to that among Canadian patients enrolled in the GUSTO-I trial. Finally, differences in the frequency of cardiac procedures were not clearly related to clinical outcomes. Mortality cumulative incidences at 1 year ranged from 8.6% to 10.3%.

Regional variations in the treatment of acute MI within the US have also been observed in other databases. Using the Medicare database, Guadagnoli et al. studied elderly US patients who were admitted to 478 different hospitals during 1990 in the states of Texas and New York for the treatment of acute MI [28]. While coronary angiography was performed more often among patients with acute MI in Texas than in New York, the risk of death at 2 years was lower in New York. Furthermore, in contrast with the findings of other studies, the patient group who underwent the more aggressive approach (Texans) had more angina and more difficulty with performing activities requiring high energy expenditure than the New York patient group.

A series of recent studies describing geographic variation in acute MI treatment across the United States have used the Cooperative Cardiovascular Project (CCP) databases. The CCP is a project of the Health Care Quality Improvement Initiative, implemented in 1992 by the Health Care Financing Administration to improve the quality of care for Medicare beneficiaries.

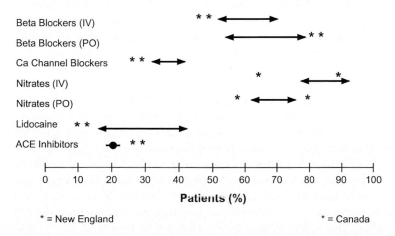

**Figure 1** Comparison across regions of the United States and Canada showing the range in the percentage of patients on any given medication. (From Ref. 27)

O'Connor et al. identified all patients admitted for acute MI between 1994 and 1995 in 50 US states using the Medicare database, and determined whether patients adhered to quality indicators for acute MI treatment as defined by the CCP [29]. These quality indicators included rates of prescription for beta-blockers and angiotensin-converting enzyme inhibitors at discharge. There was considerable variation in quality indicators across the 306 hospital referral regions identified. For example, discharge prescription rates for beta-blockers ranged from 0% to 92%.

Krumholz et al. used the CCP database to determine whether the higher rates of use of recommended treatments observed for acute MI patients admitted between 1994 and 1996 in New England were independent of regional differences in patient, hospital or physician characteristics [30]. After adjusting for patients' clinical characteristics, hospital characteristics (MI volume, teaching status and ownership), as well as state factors (median adjusted income, distance to hospitals, regions), beta-blocker use in New England was higher than in other regions, while the use of aspirin and reperfusion therapy showed less variation. In addition, patients in New England had the lowest adjusted 30-day mortality rates. It is suggested that the aggressive treatment of both ideal and nonideal candidates with recommended therapies in New England could be associated with this improved survival.

Guadagnoli et al. also used data from the CCP to examine whether regional variation in use of coronary angiography between 1994 and 1995 could be ascribed to underuse, overuse or discretionary use of this procedure [31]. It was found that discretionary use of angiography was the biggest contributor to the variation observed. That is, variation was highest among patients for whom angiography was deemed appropriate, but not necessary or uncertain. Variation was lowest among patients deemed unsuitable for angiography.

Even within the same region, marked variations in the use of angiography for acute MI have been reported. For example, Selby et al. found that the rates of angiography in 16 Kaiser Permanente hospitals in Northern California between 1990 and 1992 were inversely related to the risk of heart disease events and death [32]. In hospitals with high frequency of angiography in this study, the use of thrombolysis and of ACE inhibitors was higher than in hospitals with lower angiography rates. Greater use of recommended therapies might explain the lower mortality incidences in hospitals with more frequent use of angiography in this particular study.

Marked variations within the same region have also been demonstrated within Canada. For example, Rodrigues et al. found substantial variation in the use of cardiac medications and procedures across the 16 administrative regions in the province of Quebec [33]. There were significant variations across the administrative regions in the one-year cumulative incidence of cardiac catheterization for patients admitted between 1988 and 1995, ranging from 27% to 40%. In addition, age- and sex-adjusted rates of prescription for beta-blockers within 3 months of discharge for patients aged 65 years and older in Quebec ranged from 32% to 54%. Marked regional variations in these treatments have also been observed in other provinces, such as Ontario [14,34]. More recently, using administrative data on acute MI admissions from 1997 to 1999, widespread variations in post-acute MI outcomes [35] across Canadian provinces have been demonstrated.

In summary, several studies have demonstrated wide geographic variations in the use of cardiac procedures and medications for the treatment of both ST-segment and non–ST-segment elevation acute MI. Several regions in the United States and several countries take an approach to the care of MI patients that is more in accordance with an evidence-based medicine. This approach may be associated with improved clinical outcomes. In contrast, the more frequent use of invasive cardiac procedures among US patients with acute MI does not appear to improve reinfarction and mortality incidences when compared with those rates resulting from a much lower use of these procedures among patients from other countries. The more frequent use of noninvasive cardiac procedures and the longer length of hospital stay in Canada compared with the United States, suggest that the differences in cost of care might not be as large as previously thought. Viewed together, these studies raise questions about the potential benefit of an aggressive approach to the treatment of acute MI in terms of increased functional status and reduced post-MI angina.

## VARIATIONS IN OUTCOMES

### Mortality and Incidence of Reinfarction

*ST-segment Elevation Acute MI*

In all but one study [16] of patients with ST-segment elevation acute MI described thus far, marked variations in practice have not been associated with any clinically significant differences in mortality or incidence of reinfarction (Table 1). This absence of association was present regardless of the duration of follow-up, or the ages of the patients enrolled. This observation is consistent with the findings of randomized controlled trials, in which mortality and reinfarction rates did not differ between patients with ST-segment elevation acute MI managed with the invasive versus the non-invasive approach [1–5]. A limitation of all these studies, however, is that they have not been conducted in the current clinical context. Recent advances in medical therapy and revascularization techniques may now result in improved mortality outcomes for patients managed with the invasive approach. For instance, within the last seven years, cardiac outcomes following invasive cardiac procedures have improved with the advent of stenting and platelet glycoprotein (GP) IIb/IIIa inhibitors [36,37]. CABG techniques and postoperative care have also improved.

*Non–ST-segment Elevation Acute MI*

In each observational study of regional variations in processes of care for non-ST-segment elevation acute MI, mortality was similar for patients admitted in regions adopting aggressive and conservative management (Table 1). In terms of reinfarction outcomes, however, Fu et al. [24] provided evidence to suggest that aggressive management of patients with unstable angina is associated with lower incidence of reinfarction in comparison with a more conservative approach. In addition, Yusuf et al. found that more invasive management was associated with lower rates of readmission for unstable angina, as well as lower rates of refractory angina [26]. These observational studies add to the body of evidence that suggests that the incidence of cardiac complications is lower for patients without ST-segment elevation managed with the aggressive versus conservative approach.

The results from these observational studies are consistent with those of randomized clinical trials. For example, the incidence of reinfarction was significantly lower for patients in the aggressive arm in the FRISC II [9] and TACTICS–TIMI 18 [8] trials, and showed a trend towards being lower in the TIMI III B trial [6]. The investigators of these trials suggest that the advances in available technology and post operative care have contributed to improved clinical outcomes for patients managed with the aggressive approach. Patients not presenting with ST-segment elevation may also benefit more from aggressive management than patients with ST-segment elevation, as they are at greater risk of recurrent cardiac events.

**Table 1** Rates of Use of Invasive Cardiac Procedures, Reinfarction and Mortality in Regions with Invasive (Inv) or Noninvasive (N-Inv) Management

| First Author (Ref.) | Year | Sample size | Cumulative incidence* (%) | | | | | | | | | |
| --- | --- | --- | --- | --- | --- | --- | --- | --- | --- | --- | --- | --- |
| | | | CATH | | PTCA | | CABG | | Reinfarction | | Death | |
| | | | Inv | N-Inv | Inv | N-Inv | Inv | N-Inv | Inv | N-Inv | Inv | N-Inv |
| ST-segment elevation AMI only | | | | | | | | | | | | |
| Pilote (13) | 1994 | 518 | 60.5 | 41.8 | 33.5 | 18.2 | 14.2 | 11.2 | 13.3 | 7.7 | 27.9 | 27.0 |
| Mark (38) | 1994 | 3,000 | 72† | 25† | 29† | 11† | 14† | 3† | 3.7† | 4.5†‡ | 9.3 | 9.7 |
| Van de Werf (18) | 1995 | 41,021 | – | – | 30.6 | 10.4 | 13.1 | 2.8 | 3.7† | 4.3†‡ | 6.8 | 7.2 |
| Pilote (27) | 1995 | 21,772 | 81† | 52† | 34† | 22† | 17† | 9† | 3.9† | 4.1† | 8.6 | 10.1 |
| Langer (16) | 1999 | 8,803 | 85† | 8† | 56† | 3† | – | – | 6.9 | 7.4† | 2.9 | 4.3‡ |
| Giugliano (20) | 2001 | 5,769 | 55† | 14† | 33† | 6† | 10† | 1† | 4.8†† | 3.8†† | 8.0 | 10.9 |
| ST-segment and non-ST-segment elevation AMI | | | | | | | | | | | | |
| Rouleau (12) | 1993 | 2,231 | 78.0 | 48.2 | 26.5 | 11.4 | 21.6 | 12.6 | 13.4 | 14.1 | 22.7 | 22.2 |
| Guadagnoli (28) § | 1995 | 3,689 | 45|| | 30|| | 15|| | 7|| | 15|| | 13|| | – | – | 37 | 36 |
| Tu (14) § | 1997 | 233,702 | 39.5¶ | 10.4¶ | 14.0¶ | 2.8¶ | 14.5¶ | 3.5¶ | – | – | 34.3 | 34.4 |
| Matsui (19) | 1999 | 694 | 86.6† | 52.2† | 61.9† | 33.3† | 10.3† | 5.2|| | – | – | 11.9 | 19.4 |
| Pilote (15) § | 2003 | 236,163 | 45.2|| | 16.9|| | 18.2|| | 6.7|| | 14.5|| | 4.6|| | – | – | 32.9 | 30.4 |
| Krumholz (30) § | 2003 | 17,936 | 38† | 18† | – | – | – | – | – | – | 18.2 | 15.9 |
| Non-ST-segment elevation AMI | | | | | | | | | | | | |
| Anderson (25) | 1997 | 2,375 | 69.0 | 53.1 | 18.0 | 27.9 | 20.9 | 9.8 | 4.7 | 9.7 | 8.8 | 14.3 |
| Fu (24) | 2000 | 3,172 | 81† | 42† | 37† | 16† | 23† | 8.9† | 9.3¶ | 11.8¶ | 10.5 | 10.6 |
| Non-ST-segment elevation AMI and unstable angina | | | | | | | | | | | | |
| Anderson (25) | 1997 | 2,375 | 67.3 | 69.2 | 23.9 | 30.7 | 19.2 | 17.3 | 5.0 | 4.2 | 6.8 | 7.5 |
| Yusuf (26) | 1998 | 7,987 | 69.4 | 39.2 | 23.6 | 12.9 | 25.2 | 14.6 | – | – | 10.5** | 10.8** |
| Unstable angina | | | | | | | | | | | | |
| Anderson (25) | 1997 | 2,375 | 66.7 | 70.4 | 25.9 | 30.8 | 18.7 | 17.8 | 5.2 | 3.8 | 6.3 | 7.1 |
| Fu (24) §§ | 2000 | 3,172 | 77† | 46† | 25† | 14† | 19† | 13† | 5.8¶ | 8.8¶‡ | 6.7 | 7.6 |

– Denotes date not available.

CATH denotes cardiac catheterization, PTCA denotes percutaneous transluminal coronary angioplasty, CABG denotes coronary artery bypass graft surgery. AMI denotes acute myocardial infarction.

* Follow up periods for the studies were as follows: Van der Werf and Krumholz, 30 days; Yusuf, 6 months; Mark, Pilote (1995), Langer, Giugliano, Matsui, Anderson, Fu, Tu, and Pilote (2003) 1 year; Pilote (1994) and Guadagnoli, 2 years; Rouleau, 24 to 60 months.

† denotes cumulative rates during the initial hospitalization. Cumulative incidence rates for the entire follow-up period were not available.

‡ P<0.05 for comparison.

§ Patients ≥ 65 years old.

†† denotes cumulative rates over 30 days after admission. Cumulative incidence rates for the entire follow-up period were not available.

|| denotes cumulative rates over 90 days after admission. Cumulative incidence rates for the entire follow-up period were not available.

¶ denotes cumulative rates over 180 days after admission. Cumulative incidence rates for the entire follow-up period were not available.

** Rates correspond to composite endpoint of cardiovascular disease death and reinfarction.

## Functional Status and Quality of Life

Mortality and reinfarction cumulative incidences are important measurements in any study of cardiovascular diseases. Yet, much of medical care after acute MI is directed at relieving symptoms and improving functional status and quality of life [13]. Although differences in practice patterns may not affect mortality, they may affect the quality of life of surviving patients. A GUSTO-1 substudy investigated the impact of practice variations on medical outcomes including measurement of quality of life and use of medical resources during the year after ST-segment elevation acute MI [38]. The investigators obtained data on US and Canadian patients randomly selected from the GUSTO-I trial. After 1 year, several measures of quality of life suggested that the quality of life of US patients was superior to that of Canadian patients. For example, the prevalence of chest pain and dyspnea at 1 year was higher among the Canadian patients (34% vs. 21% and 45% vs. 29%), and the Canadian patients also had worse functional status than US patients (Fig. 2). The Canadian patients also had more visits to physicians during the follow-up year but fewer visits to specialists. These results suggest that the more frequent use of cardiac procedures and of specialty care in the US may confer a better quality of life in post-MI patients.

A major question raised by this study was whether the differences in quality of life between Canadian and US patients with MI are due to cultural differences rather than to differences in medical care. Given the subjective nature of quality of life questionnaires, cultural differences could theoretically affect responses [39]. In response to this question, Pilote et al. measured quality of life and functional status in patients with acute MI treated within Québec at 5 sites with and 5 sites without angiography [40]. This study lent support to a positive, albeit small, association between early invasive approaches, more commonly used at sites with angiography, and improved quality of life. However, a substudy of these data by Beck et al. found that baseline clinical characteristics and treatments received in-hospital did not strongly affect patients' long-term perceptions of quality of life [41]. Rather, the results suggested that age and psychosocial characteristics at baseline are the most important predictors of quality of life after acute MI.

The study of subjective outcomes brings an added level of uncertainty. While there are outcomes that are easy to measure—such as mortality—other outcomes, such as disa-

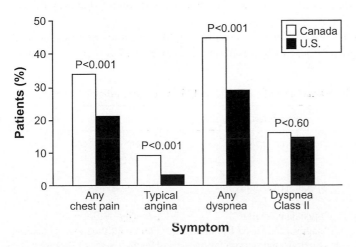

**Figure 2** Status of cardiac symptoms at 1 year in a random sample of Canadian (n = 400) and US (n = 2600) patients who were randomized in the GUSTO I trial. (From Ref. 38)

bility, distress, and dissatisfaction with health care, are more difficult to measure. In fact, most databases used in these types of analyses do not routinely record outcomes relating to functional status and quality of life [42]. More work is needed on outcomes that better describe the burden of illness.

## Cost

Underlying the issues of appropriate care is the issue of cost. To date, there are few studies examining the cost-effectiveness of the invasive versus noninvasive approach to acute MI management. In the TACTICS-TIMI 18 trial, the estimated cost per life-year gained for the invasive strategy ranged from $8371 to $25,739 USD [43]. The investigators concluded that this was a small increase in cost relative to the clinical benefit of reduced cardiac events at 6 months. The TIMI III B and FRISC II trials also provided evidence to suggest that the invasive approach is associated with lower rates of rehospitalization, pointing to an association between the invasive approach and lower levels of health resource utilization. It is not clear whether these findings could be generalized to patients with ST-segment elevation acute MI.

## DETERMINANTS OF THE USE OF CARDIAC PROCEDURES

Wide variations in patterns of care raise questions about the reasons for differing methods of treating patients (Table 2). A number of hypotheses could explain the observed variations in management of acute myocardial infarction [44]. Physicians may remain uncertain about how well clinical guidelines or the findings of a study apply to their patients. The interpretation and applications of the information may be affected by the presence of leading medical centers in a given region or by the ratio of specialists to generalists [45,46]. Physician testing patterns and attitudes and patient preferences may vary across regions, thus affecting treatment selections. Inappropriate use of cardiac procedures may be responsible for some of the variation [47]. Nonclinical factors, including the patient's insurance status and state regulations, may also influence the decision-making process [48]. These wide variations question whether evidence-based medicine is widely and strictly practiced. Thus, the determinants of the use of cardiac procedures and the influences on physicians' behaviors need to be identified in order to promote the practice of medicine that is evidence-based.

Another study used the GUSTO-I database to identify the variables that best predict angiography and revascularization use [49]. Based on this analysis of US patients, younger

**Table 2** Potential Reasons for Variations in Diagnostic and Therapeutic Cardiac Procedures

| Environmental factors | Physician Factors | Patient Factors |
| --- | --- | --- |
| Medical insurance status (fee for service vs. managed care) | Medical uncertainty | Patient preference |
| Availability of needed procedure | Specialist vs. generalist | Demographics |
| Proximity of medical centers with appropriate expertise | Physicians' skills | Severity of illness |
| | Inappropriate use Physicians' beliefs and interpretation of the medical evidence | Patient attitude toward disease |
| | | Heterogeneity of disease expression |
| | | Illness and medical care |

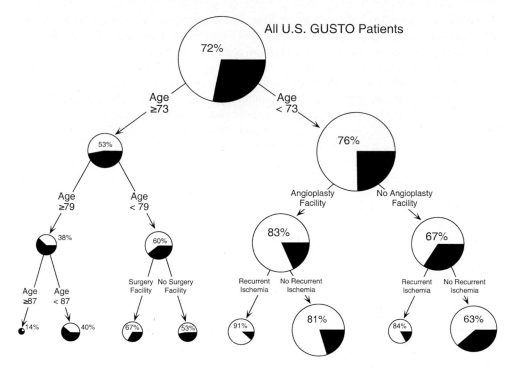

**Figure 3** Classification and regression tree model showing the variables that discriminate between subgroups according to their likelihood of undergoing angiography after thrombosis for acute myocardial infarction. The white area of the pie chart represents the percent use of angiography; the overall area indicates the sample size of the subgroup relative to the total population (From Ref. 49)

age and availability of procedures at the site of admission appear to be the major determinants of angiography, while coronary anatomy largely drives the use and type of revascularization (Fig. 3). In other patient populations, on-site availability of angiography facilities has been shown to be a major determinant of the use of cardiac procedures as well [50,51]. This process of being more aggressive in young patients without complication after acute MI tends to select low-risk patients for a cardiac procedure rather than higher-risk patients, who would most likely benefit from a given procedure.

Finally, more recent studies have suggested that other nonclinical factors, such as socioeconomic status, are important determinants of use of invasive cardiac procedures after acute MI. Pilote et al. found that despite Canada's universal health care system, acute MI patients living in areas of Quebec with low socioeconomic status are less likely to undergo cardiac catheterization than patients in areas with higher socioeconomic status [52]. Alter et al. found a similar association for acute MI patients living in Ontario, Canada [53].

## CONCLUSION

The treatment of acute MI has been the subject of many randomized clinical trials. Despite extensive data on the relative efficacies of the various therapies, extensive regional and international practice variations exist in the treatment of this condition. These geographic variations are not related to severity of illness or clinical presentation. Several studies have failed to relate a more aggressive approach to the treatment of acute MI to a reduction in mortality compared with a more conservative approach. However, the available data suggest that the incidence of cardiac complications is lower for patients with non–ST-segment elevation acute MI treated with the aggressive versus the conservative approach. In addition, the quality of life of patients treated aggressively may be slightly superior to the quality of life of patients treated conservatively. Nonclinical factors, such as availability of cardiac procedures and socioeconomic status, appear to be major determinants of the use of these procedures. Such variations in the treatment of a clinical condition suggest that certain patterns of care for MI patients are inappropriate and might lead to outcomes not commensurate to medical expenses. These variations may also suggest that limited resources may restrict access to cardiac procedures, and might have a negative impact on the quality of life of patients with acute MI. The intensity of the use of cardiac procedures that will optimize outcomes including mortality and quality of life at the lowest level of resource use has yet to be identified.

## REFERENCES

1. Simoons M, Arnold A, Betriu A, de Bono DP, Col J, Dougherty FC, von Essen R, Lambertz H, Lubsen J, Meier B. Thrombolysis with tissue plasminogen activator in acute myocardial infarction: no additional benefit from immediate percutaneous coronary angioplasty. Lancet 1988;i:197–203.
2. Rogers W, Baim D, Gore J, Brown BG, Roberts R, Williams DO, Chesebro JH, Babb JD, Sheehan FH, Wackers FJT, Zaret BL, Robertson TL, Passamani ER, Ross R, Knatterud GL, Braunwald E. Comparison of immediate invasive, delayed invasive and conservative strategies after tissue-type plasminogen activator results of the Thrombolysis In Myocardial Infarction (TIMI) Phase II-A Trial. Circulation 1990;81:1457–1476.
3. SWIFT Trial Study Group. SWIFT trial of delayed elective intervention vs conservative treatment after thrombolysis with anistreplase in acute myocardial infarction. Br Med J 1991;302: 555–560.
4. Williams D, Braunwald E, Knatterud GL, Babb J, Bresnahan J, Greenberg MA, Raizner A, Robertson T, Ross R. One-year results of the Thrombolysis in Myocardial Infarction Investigation (TIMI) Phase II trial. Circulation 1992;85:533–542.
5. Barbash G, Roth AHH, Modan M, Miller HI, Rath S, Zahav YH, Keren G, Motro M, Shachar A, Basan S, Agranat O, Rabinowitz B, Laniado S, Kaplinsky E. Randomized controlled trial of late in-hospital angiography and angioplasty versus conservative management after treatment with recombinant tissue-type plasminogen activator in acute myocardial infarction. Am J Cardiol 1990;66:538–545.
6. Anderson H, Cannon C, Stone P, Williams D, McCabe C, Knatterud GL, Thompson B, Willerson JT, Braunwald E, for the TIMI Investigators. One-year results of the thrombolysis in myocardial infarction (TIMI IIIB) clinical trial. J Am Coll Cardiol 1995;26(7):1643–1650.
7. Boden W, O'Rourke R, Crawford M, Blausten A, Deedwania P, Zoble R, Wexler LF,, Kleiger RE, Pepine CJ, Ferry DR, Chow BK, Lavori PW. for the Veterens Affairs Non-Q-Wave Infarction Strategies in Hospitals (VANQWISH) Trial investigators. Outcomes in patients with acute non-Q wave myocardial infarction randomly assigned to an invasive as compared with a conservative management strategy. N Engl J Med 1998;338(25):1785–1792.
8. Cannon CP, Weintraub WS, Demopoulos LA, Vicari R, Frey MJ, Lakkis N, Neumann FJ, Robertson DH, DeLucca PT, DiBattiste PM, Gibson M, Braunwald E. Comparison of early invasive and conservative strategies in patients with unstable coronary syndromes treated with the glycoprotein IIb/IIIa inhibitor tirofiban. N Engl J Med 2001;344:1879–1887.
9. Wallentin L, Lagerqvist B, Husted S, Kontny F, Stahle E, Swahn E. Outcome at 1 year after an invasive compared with a non-invasive strategy in unstable coronary-artery disease: the FRISC II invasive randomised trial. Lancet 2000;356:9–16.

10.  Ryan TJ, Antman EM, Brooks NH, Califf RM, Hillis LD, Hiratzka LF, Rapaport E, Riegel B, Russell RO, Smith III EE, Weaver WD. 1999 Update: ACC/AHA guidelines for the management of patients with acute myocardial infarction. A report of the American College of Cardiology/American Heart Association Task Force on Practice Guidelines (Committee on Management of Acute Myocardial Infarction). J Am Coll Cardiol 1999; 34:890–911.

11.  Braunwald E, Antman EM, Beasley JW, Califf RM, Cheitlin MD, Hochman JS, Jones RH, Kereiakes DJ, Kupersmith J, Levin TW, Pepine CJ, Schaeffer JW, Smith EE, Steward DE, Theroux P. ACC/AHA 2002 guideline update for the management of patients with unstable angina and non-ST-segment elevation myocardial infarction–summary article. A report of the American College of Cardiology/American Heart Association task force on practice guidelines (committee on the management of patients with unstable angina). J Am Coll Cardiol 2002; 40:1366–1374.

12.  Rouleau J, Moye L, Pfeffer M, Arnold J, Bernstein V, Cuddy T. A comparison of management patterns after acute myocardial infarction in Canada and the United States. The SAVE investigators. N Engl J Med 1993;328:779–784.

13.  Pilote L, Racine N, Hlatky M. Treatment of acute myocardial infarction in the United States and Canada: a comparison of two university hospitals. Arch Intern Med 1994 154:1090–1096.

14.  Tu J, Pashos C, Naylor C, Chen E, Normand S, Newhouse J, McNeil BJ. Use of cardiac procedures and outcomes in elderly patients with myocardial infarction in the United States and Canada. N Engl J Med 1997;337:1008–1009.

15.  Pilote L, Sayina O, Lavoie F, McClellan M. Cardiac procedure use and outcomes in elderly patients with acute myocardial infarction in the United States and Quebec, Canada, 1988 to 1994. Med Care 2003;41:813–822.

16.  Langer A, Fisher M, Califf RM, Goodman S, O'Conner CM, Harrington RA, Fuster V. Higher rates of coronary angiography and revascularization following myocardial infarction may be associated with greater survival in the United States than in Canada. Can J Cardiol 1999; 15(10):1095–1102.

17.  Pilote L, Lavoie F, Ho V, Eisenberg M. Changes in the treatment and outcomes of acute myocardial infarction in Quebec, 1988-1995. Can Med Assoc J 2000;163(1):31–36.

18.  Van der Werf F, Topol E, Lee K, Woodlief LH, Granger CB, Armstrong PW, Barbash GI, Hampton JR, Guerci A, Simes RJ. Variations in patient treatment and outcomes for acute myocardial infarction in the United States and other countries. JAMA 1995;273:1586–1591.

19.  Matsui K, Polanczyk CA, Gaspoz J-M, Theres H, Kleber FX, Sobashima A, Okamatsu S, Viana JM, Ribeiro JP, Emonet S, Lee TH. Management of patients with acute myocardial infarction at five academic medical centers: clinical characteristics, resource utilization, and outcome. J Invest Med 1999;47:134–140.

20.  Giugliano RP, Llevadot J, Wilcox RG, Gurfinkel EP, McCabe CH, Charlesworth A, Thompson SL, Antman EM, Braunwald E. for the In TIME (Intravenous nPA for the Treatment of Infarcting Myocardium Early) II investigators. Geographic variation in patient and hospital characteristics, management, and clinical outcomes in ST-elevation myocardial infarction treated with fibrinolysis. Results from InTIME-II. European Heart Journal 2001;22:1702–1715.

21.  Heller R, O'Connell R, Lim L, Atallah A, Lanas F, Joshi P, Tasanavivat P. Variation in stated management of acute myocardial infarction in five countries. Int J Cardiol 1999;68:63–67.

22.  Topol EJ. Acute Coronary Syndromes. 1 ed.. 0: Marcel Dekker, Inc., 1998.

23.  Furman MI, Dauerman HL, Goldberg RJ, Yarzbeski J, Lessard D, Gore JM. Twenty-two year (1975 to 1997) trends in the incidence, in-hospital and long-term case fatality rates from initial Q-wave and non-Q-wave myocardial infarction: a multi-hospital, community-wide perspective. J Am Coll Cardiol 2001;37(6):1571–1580.

24.  Fu Y, Chang W-C, Mark D, Califf RM, Mackenzie B, Granger CB, Topol EJ, Hlatky M, Armstrong PW. Canadian-American differences in the managment of acute coronary syndromes in the GUSTO IIb trial. One-year follow-up of patients without ST-segment elevation. Circulation 2000;102:1375–1381.

25.  Anderson HV, Gibson RS, Stone PH, Cannon CP, Aguirre F, Thompson B, Knatterud GL, Braunwald E. Management of unstable angina pectoris and non-Q-wave acute myocardial

infarction in the United States and Canada (the TIMI III Registry). Am J Cardiol 1997;79: 1441–1446.

26. Yusuf S, Flather M, Pogue J, Hunt D, Varigos J, Piegas L, Avezum A, Anderson J, Keltai M, Budaj A, Fox K, Ceremuynski L. for the OASIS (Organisation to Assess Strategies for Ischaemic Syndromes) Registry investigators. Variations between countries in invasive cardiac procedures and outcomes in patients with suspected unstable angina or myocardial infarction without initial ST elevation. Lancet 1998;352:507–514.

27. Pilote L, Califf R, Sapp S, Miller D, Mark D, Weaver W, Gore JM, Armstrong PW, Ohman EM, Topol EJ. for the GUSTO investigators. Regional variation across the United States in the treatment of acute myocardial infarction. N Engl J Med 1995;333:565–572.

28. Guadagnoli E, Hauptman P, Ayanian J, Pashos C, McNeil B, Cleary P. Variation in the use of cardiac procedures after acute myocardial infarction. N Engl J Med 1995;333:573–578.

29. O'Connor G, Quinton H, Traven N, Ramunno L, Dodds T, Marciniak T, Wennberg JE. Geographic variation in the treatment of acute myocardial infarction: The Cooperative Cardiovascular Project. JAMA 1999;281:627–633.

30. Krumholz HM, Chen J, Rathore S, Wang Y, Radford MJ. Regional variation in the treatment and outcomes of myocardial infarction: Investigating New England's Advantage. Am Heart J 2003;146:242–249.

31. Guadagnoli E, Landrum MB, Normand SL, Ayanian JZ, Garg P, Hauptman P et al. Impact of underuse, overuse, and discretionary use on geographic variation in the use of coronary angiography after acute myocardial infarction. Med Care 2001;39:446–458.

32. Selby J, Fireman D, Lunstrom R, Swain BE, Truman AF, Wong CC, Froclicher ES, Barron HV, Hlatky MA. Variation among hospitals in coronary angiography practices and outcomes after acute myocardial infarction in a large health maintenance organization. N Engl J Med 1996;335:1888–1984.

33. Rodrigues EJ, Simpson E, Richard H, Pilote L. Regional variation in the management of acute myocardial infarction in the province of Quebec. Can J Cardiol 2002;18:1067–1076.

34. Tu JV, Austin P, Rochon P, Zhang H. Secondary prevention after acute myocardial infarction, congestive heart failure and coronary artery bypass graft surgery in Ontario In: Naylor CD , Slaughter PM, Eds. Cardiovascular Health & Services in Ontario: an ICES Atlas. 0: Institute for Clinical Evaluative Sciences (ICES), 1999:199–238.

35. Tu JV, Austin PC, Filate WA, Johansen H, Brien SE, Pilote L, Alter DA. for the Canadian Cardiovascular Outcomes Research Team. Outcomes of acute myocardial infarction in Canada. Can J Cardiol 2003;19:893–901.

36. The Platelet Receptor Inhibition in Ischemic Syndrome Management in Patients Limited by Unstable Signs and Symptoms (PRISM-PLUS) Study Investigators. Inhibition of the platelet glycoprotein IIb/IIIa receptor with tirofiban in unstable angina and non-Q-wave acute myocardial infarction. N Engl J Med 1998;338:1488–1497.

37. Al Suwaidi, Berger PB, Holmes DR Jr. Coronary artery stents. JAMA 2000;284:1828–1836.

38. Mark D, Naylor C, Hlatky M, Califf R, Topol E, Granger C, Knight JD, Nelson CL, Lee KL, Clapp-Channing N, Pryor DB, Sutherland W, Pilote L, Armstrong PW. Medical resource and quality of life outcomes following acute myocardial infarction in Canada versus the United States: the Canadian – U.S. GUSTO substudy. N Engl J Med 1994;331:1130–1135.

39. Pilote L, Bourassa M, Bacon C, Hlatky M. Better functional status in American than in Canadian patients after acute myocardial infarction: an effect of medical care? J Am Coll Cardiol 1995;26:1115–1120.

40. Pilote L, Lauzon C, Huynh T, Dion D, Roux R, Racine N, Carignan S, Diodati JG, Charbonneau F, Levesque C, Pouliot J, Joseph L, Eisenberg MJ. Quality of life after acute myocardial infarction among patients treated at sites with and without on-site availability of angiography. Arch Intern Med 2002;11:553–559.

41. Beck CA, Joseph L, Belisle P, Pilote L. Predictors of quality of life 6 months and 1 year after acute myocardial infarction. Am Heart J 2001;142:271–279.

42. Naylor C, Guyatt G. for the Evidence-Based Medicine Working Group. Users' Guide to the medical literature. X. How to use and article reporting variations in the outcomes of health services. JAMA 1996;275:554–559.

43. Mahoney EM, Jurkovitz CT, Chu H, Becker ER, Culler S, Kosinski AS, Robertson DH, Alexander C, Nag S, Cook JR, Demopolous LA, DiBattiste PM, Cannon CP, Weintraub WS. for the TACTICS-TIMI 18 investigators. Cost and cost-effectiveness of an early invasive versus conservative strategy for the treatment of unstable angina and non-ST-segment elevation myocardial infarction. JAMA 2002;288:1851–1858.

44. Detsky A. Regional variation in medical care. N Engl J Med 1995;333:589–590.

45. Ayanian J, Hauptman P, Guadagnoli E, Antman E, Pashos C, McNeil B. Knowledge and practices of generalist and specialist physicians regarding drug therapy for acute myocardial infarction. N Engl J Med 1994;331:1136–1142.

46. Jollis J, Delong E, Peterson E, Muhlbaier LH, Fortin DF, Califf RM, Mark DB. Outcome of acute myocardial infarction according to the specialty of the admitting physician. N Engl J Med 1996;335:1880–1887.

47. Leape L, Park R, Solomon D, Chassin M, Kosecoff J, Brook R. Does inappropriate use explain small-area variations in the use of halth care services? JAMA 1990;263:669–672.

48. Wenneker M, Weissman J, Epstein A. The association of payer with utilization of cardiac proedures in Massachusetts. JAMA 1990;264:1255–1260.

49. Pilote L, Miller D, Califf R, Rao J, Weaver W, Topol E. Determinants of the use of coronary angiography and revascularization after thrombolysis for acute myocardial infarction in the United States. N Engl J Med 1996;335:1198–1205.

50. Every N, Larson E, Litwin P, Maynard C, Fihn SD, Eisenberg MS, Hallstrom AP, Martin JS, Weaver WD. The association between on-site cardiac catheterization facilities and the utilization of coronary angiography after acute myocardial infarction. N Engl J Med 1993;329:546–551.

51. Blustein J. High technology cardiac procedures: the impact of service availability on service utilization in New York State. JAMA 1993;270:344–349.

52. Pilote L, Joseph L, Belisle P, Penrod J. Universal health insurance does not eliminate inequities in access to cardiac procedures after acute myocardial infarction. Am Heart J 2003; 146: 1030–1037.

53. Alter DA, Naylor CD, Austin P, Tu JV. Effects of socioeconomic status on access to invasive cardiac procedures and on mortality after acute myocardial infarction. N Engl J Med 1999; 341:1359–1367.

# 31

# Quality of Coronary Disease Report Cards

**Sunil V. Rao and James G. Jollis**
*Duke University Medical Center*
*Durham, North Carolina, U.S.A*

"We know how to measure quality. This is not a knowledge problem. We simply haven't decided we want to expend the necessary resources and political will." Mark Chassin, former health commissioner of New York State, Wall Street Journal October 24, 1996, page R18.

"Today all doctors, hospitals, and health providers are paid federally fixed prices for their services. Injecting a modest incentive for performance based on price and quality will lower cost, improve quality, and enhance the performance of Medicare for many beneficiaries." Thomas A. Scully, Administrator Centers For Medicare & Medicaid Services, United States Senate Finance Committee, June 6, 2003.

Over the past two decades, there have been numerous approaches to lowering cost in the United States health care system including capitated insurance, contracting for services by large purchasers, prospective hospital and outpatient reimbursement, and Medicare physician reimbursement fixed to the growth in the national economy. While these approaches have marginally controlled expenditures, no system is currently in place to assure that health care quality does not suffer as a result of fiscal constraints. This critical need for information about quality, as well as dramatic advances in computerized data, techniques with which to make balanced comparisons among these data, and electronic media have ushered in the "report card era." Beginning with publicly reported comparisons of hospital mortality by the Centers for Medicare and Medicaid Services (CMS) in 1986, a precedent was established whereby medical care providers are scrutinized according to their outcomes. A large number of reports have focused on cardiology, including the New York State Cardiac Surgery and Coronary Angioplasty Reporting Systems, the Pennsylvania Health Care Cost Containment Council's Focus on Heart Attack and Hospital Performance Report, the California Hospital Outcomes Project, the Cooperative Cardiovascular Project (CCP), and the National Acute Myocardial Infarction Project (NAMIP) [1–6]. Provider-specific report cards regarding cardiac care also can be found on the internet including www.Healthscope.org and www.Healthgrades.com. Pharmaceutical sponsored initiatives such as National Registry of Myocardial Infarction (NRMI), and the Can Rapid Risk Stratification of Unstable Angina Patients Suppress Adverse Outcomes with Early Implementation of the American College of Cardiology/American Heart Association guidelines (CRUSADE) combine marketing with quality improvement [7,8]. Since July 1, 2002, the Joint Commission on Accreditation of Healthcare Organizations (JCAHO) has mandated that hospitals collect performance measures for two of four conditions: acute myocardial infarction (MI), heart failure, community-acquired pneumonia, and pregnancy and related conditions. Beginning in 2004, the data will be used by the JCAHO for site evaluations and will be publicly reported on the JCAHO website. Most recently, the US Congress tied hospital reimbursement to the public reporting of quality of care data for acute MI, heart failure, and pneumonia in the Medicare Prescription Drug, Improvement and Modernization Act of 2003.

   With the presentation of these "report cards," interest has intensified among patients, providers, payers, and the general public concerning the validity and implications of such comparisons. Differences between providers identified in current outcome reports can be attributed to at least three factors, differences in the illness severity of patients, differences in the quality and technical abilities of providers, and chance variation. The ideal outcomes system will take into account both illness severity and chance variation, such that providers identified as "outliers" represent better or worse practice. This chapter examines how close current outcomes systems come to this ideal, and identify areas for future improvement to cardiac report cards that will enable them to reliably identify best practice.

## MEASURES OF QUALITY

Outcome comparisons can be viewed as one of at least three perspectives by which to measure quality. Other methods by which to gauge quality include structural measures (e.g., physician credentials and the availability of specialized services), and process measures (e.g., use of medications associated with better outcomes in clinical trails). The inference of systems that measure structure and process is that adherence to such standards will lead to improved outcomes for patients. Measuring quality of care according to outcomes represents the most difficult and resource intensive approach of these alternatives.

## ACUTE MYCARDIAL INFARCTION REPORT CARDS

Three of the most notable regional acute MI report cards are the California Hospital Outcomes Project, the Pennsylvania "Focus on Heart Attack" and Hospital Performance Report, and the National Acute Myocardial Infarction Project (formerly the Cooperative Cardiovascular Project). The California and Pennsylvania systems focus on outcomes, while the NAMIP measures process of care. With the public release of the California and Pennsylvania studies, they are designed to serve as a type of "consumer's report," comparing hospitals, and in the case of Pennsylvania, physicians across the states. A typical report involves a listing of hospitals or physician by region, followed by some indication of whether the outcome measure lies outside of the predicted normal range. The California report rates hospitals according to two different risk models, flagging hospitals for which 30 day death rates are felt to represent outliers (Fig. 1). The California study also published the comments of hospitals and medical staffs regarding the limitations of the study with respect to their specific institution. The Pennsylvania report provides details regarding actual, expected, and risk adjusted rates of death with confidence intervals, and additional comparisons according to costs and length of hospital stay. Both reports include descriptions targeted to the public concerning the potential uses and limitations of the outcomes comparisons. The Cooperative Cardiovascular Project involved elderly Medicare patients

| Report on Heart Attack, 1997 | Model A | Model B |
|---|---|---|
| **Santa Clara County** | | |
| Alexian Brothers Hospital | ☐ | ☐ |
| Columbia Good Samaritan Hospital | ☐ | ☐ |
| Columbia San Jose Medical Center | ☐ | ☐ |
| Columbia South Valley Hospital | ☐ | ☐ |
| Community Hospital of Los Gatos | ☐ | ☐ |
| El Camino Hospital | ☐ | ✪ |
| Kaiser Foundation Hospital-Santa Clara‡ | ☐ | ☐ |
| Kaiser Foundation Hospital-Santa Teresa Community Hospital‡ | ● | ● |
| O'Connor Hospital | ☐ | ☐ |
| Santa Clara Valley Medical Center | ☐ | ☐ |
| St. Louise Hospital | ☐ | ☐ |
| Stanford University Hospital | ✪ | ✪ |
| **Santa Cruz County** | | |
| Dominican Santa Cruz Hospital | ☐ | ☐ |
| Watsonville Community Hospital | ☐ | ☐ |

| | | | |
|---|---|---|---|
| ✪ | Significantly better than expected (p<0.01) | ● | Significantly worse than expected (p<0.01) |
| ☑ | No deaths reported; too few cases for statistical significance | ✕ | Hospital excluded due to data limitations |
| ☐ | Not significantly different than expected | ‡ | Comment letter received from hospital or hospital system |

**Figure 1** California Hospital Outcomes Project Report on Heart Attack. (From Ref. 8a)

treated in 1994 and 1995 in all 50 states, and the findings were presented to individual hospitals through state peer review organizations. Process indicators such as use of thrombolytic therapy or beta-blockers for the individual hospitals were compared to regional rates of use, and hospitals were asked to respond with a plan to address any one deficiency identified by the CCP data. A more recent iteration of the CCP initiated by CMS is the National Acute Myocardial Infarction Project launched in 1999, in response to the continued under use of guideline-based therapies in eligible patients [5,6]. Compared with the original CCP that sampled 200,000 consecutive hospitalizations for acute MI over an 8-month period, the National Acute Myocardial Infarction is considerably smaller in scale. For acute MI indicators, the median number of cases sampled per state ranged from 6 for primary angioplasty to 301 for aspirin. The quality measures identified by CMS are updated from those used in the CCP. The seven measures are: administration of aspirin within 24 hours before or after hospital arrival, administration of beta-blocker within 24 hours of hospital arrival, aspirin prescribed at discharge, ACE inhibitor prescribed at discharge for patients with left ventricular dysfunction, smoking cessation counseling during hospitalization, and timely initiation of reperfusion therapy. Due to the small size of the National Acute Myocardial Infarction Project, data can only be analyzed on a state level, insufficient data are available to consider speed of reperfusion, and no data are available regarding the rate of reperfusion.

Quality improvement initiatives funded through industry include the NRMI and CRUSADE. When quality measures involve the administration of specific medications, particularly those still under patent such as thrombolysis or direct platelet inhibitors, pharmaceutical companies have a financial interest in supporting such initiatives. NRMI, sponsored by Genentech, has undergone four iterations with each one reflecting changes in guideline-based treatment. NRMI 1 was launched in 1990, NRMI 2 in 1994, NRMI 3 in 1998, and NRMI 4 in 2000. Since inception, over 1600 hospitals have participated and data has been collected in over 2 million patients. Each NRMI site collects and submits data on patient demographics, diagnostic procedures, and treatments on a standardized case report form. The information is analyzed and compared with aggregate data from similar hospitals and reported to the site on a quarterly basis. The CRUSADE national quality initiative, initially sponsored by the manufacturer of eptifibatide, focuses specifically on non–ST-segment elevation acute coronary syndromes (NSTE ACS) and reports data to participating sites in a fashion similar to NRMI.

## REVASCULARIZATION REPORT CARDS

A number of report cards focus on coronary revascularization, a key procedure in the treatment of acute coronary syndromes. The prototypical regional angioplasty scorecard is the New York State Coronary Angioplasty Reporting System (Table 1) [9].Since 1991, all hospitals performing percutaneous coronary interventions (PCI) in the state are required to provide demographic, illness severity, complication, and outcome data concerning all procedures. Every three years, the Health Department publishes a brochure that contains hospital specific outcome information including number of procedures and deaths, as well as expected and risk adjusted mortality rates with confidence intervals. As mortality comparisons are limited due to the low death rate associated with PCI, the Health Department attempted to examine procedural myocardial infarctions as a second measure of quality. Recently, mandatory reporting of creatinine phosphokinase-MB measurements was abandoned due to impracticality. A challenge to any report card system including that of New York involves the time delay between data collection and release of the report. There is currently a 2 to 3 year lag in the release of angioplasty comparisons.

**Table 1**  Grading the Scorecards

| Scorecard | Grade | Quality standard | Comments |
|---|---|---|---|
| National Acute Myocardial Infarction Project | D+ | Process of care | Sample size too small to identify better care at the hospital level. |
| Medicare Prescription Drug, Improvement and Modernization Act Hospital Data Release | B+ | Process of care | Likely to include most hospitals in United States. |
| New York Coronary Angioplasty Reporting System | B | Outcome | Detailed clinical data collection supported by state regulation, long delay in publication. |
| California Hospital Outcomes Project | C− | Outcome | Insurance claims-based comparison, best methodology available to consider limited data |
| Pennsylvania Health Care Cost Containment Council | C | Outcome | Proprietary methodology – MediQual, Methodology potentially gives hospitals credit for complications. |
| Michigan Hospital Report | C− | Outcome | Risk adjustment based on "All Patient Refined Diagnosis Related Groups," a proprietary manipulation of claims data. |
| NRMI | B | Process of care | Detailed process indicators identify approaches to improvement. |
| CRUSADE | B− | Process of care | Incorporates American College of Cardiology guidelines, and marketing of platelet inhibitors. |
| Healthscope.org | C− | Outcome | Based on California Hospital Outcomes Project. Consumer focus. |
| Healthgrades.com | D | Outcome | Proprietary claims data comparison. Marketing focus. |

NRMI: National Registry of Myocardial Infarction.
CRUSADE: Can Rapid Risk Stratification of Unstable Angina Patients Suppress Adverse Outcomes with Early Implementation of the American College of Cardiology/American Heart Association guidelines.

## OUTCOME COMPARISONS

The fundamental issue regarding outcomes reporting involves balancing comparisons, or "leveling the playing field." By using mathematical models to account for differences between patients and hospitals, report cards attempt to provide a control group by which outcomes can be compared. Issues regarding data collection as well as model derivation can have substantial influence on outcome estimates. Report cards need to be considered according to their methodology, in order to understand the validity of their findings.

### Insurance Claims Data

Most regional outcomes reporting systems rely on insurance claims data in some part to identify patients, adjust for illness severity, or determine outcome. The typical elements of insurance claims include patient identifiers, dates, diagnoses, procedures, charges, and discharge status. Diagnoses are coded according to the International Classification of

Diseases (ICD) system, and procedures may be coded according to either the ICD system, or Current Procedural Terminology codes [10,11]. This coding system may be used to derive Diagnosis Related Groups (DRG), an illness classification system adopted and modified by the federal government for standard health care billing and reporting. The advantages of insurance claims include their routine collection in a computerized format, and their geographically dispersed, population-based samples. Using patient identifiers and dates, longitudinal records of patient care can be constructed. In fee-for-service healthcare systems, patient bills are often the only available source of information to identify patients who underwent procedures of interest or were hospitalized with conditions of interest. For the California Hospital Outcomes Project, the Pennsylvania Focus on Heart Attack and Hospital Performance Report, the Cooperative Cardiovascular Project, the National Acute Myocardial Infarction Project, and www.HealthGrades.com Hospital Report Cards, patients were identified by hospital claims.

## Comorbidity Vs. Complication

As insurance claims are generated for the purpose of determining reimbursement rather than risk adjustment, they have many limitations in outcomes comparisons. The greatest limitation involves the difficulty in distinguishing comorbid conditions from complications among claims diagnoses. For example, conditions such as congestive heart failure or cardiogenic shock may represent illnesses present on admission, or "predictors," or they may be the result of a complication that occurred during hospitalization, or "postdictors." While a number of approaches have attempted to separate complications from comorbidities, currently there is no reliable way to entirely distinguish between these two entities. By considering complications to represent comorbidities in outcomes comparisons, hospitals and physicians may be given "credit" for complications and assigned a lower mortality estimate. Thus, problems with quality apparent in unadjusted data may be obscured by risk adjustment. The inclusion of complications in risk adjustment models will also enhance the apparent performance characteristics of these models, as they reinforce the tautology that "patients with the most complications have the most complications."

## Other Claims Data Limitations

Other significant limitations of insurance claims data in risk adjustment have been previously documented [12–14]. These include the lack of definitions, under-coding of many conditions, biases in coding such that diagnoses that increase compensation are more likely to be coded, chronic conditions in acutely ill patients are less likely to be coded, and inadequate surveillance of accuracy. Potential approaches to the proper use of claims data include the recognition of these limitations, and a focus on claims data elements that are most likely to be reliable such as age, gender, the performance of higher priced procedures, and mortality [15].

Two studies that use claims data to identify acute MI patients potentially fail to include a substantial portion of complicated patients. Both the National Acute Myocardial Infarction Project and Pennsylvania Focus on Heart Attack rely on a principal diagnosis of acute MI to identify patients. Patients who were assigned a principal diagnosis involving a complication of acute MI such as cardiogenic shock or papillary muscle rupture were excluded from these studies. Using the Medicare database as a reference, we found that patients with complications of acute MI listed as the principal diagnosis represented an additional 21% of patients with 28% in-hospital mortality, compared to the 14% mortality for patients identified according to a principal diagnosis acute MI alone. By excluding these complicated patients, both systems miss the opportunity to identify outcome differences among a high risk group of patients. Studies using claims data to identify acute MI patients should be broadened to include such patients with complications.

## Other Data Sources

In an effort to overcome the limitations of insurance claims data, a number of outcomes systems obtain patient data from additional sources. Both NRMI and CRUSADE identify patients through individual hospital reporting based on a set of predefined inclusion criteria. Enrollment into these initiatives relies on the diligence of the teams designated by each participating site. To satisfy federal regulations regarding health information privacy, patient identifiers are excluded. This lack of identification prohibits the tracking of clinical outcomes following hospital discharge. For the New York State Cardiac Surgery and Coronary Angioplasty Reporting Systems, each hospital submits data to the Health Department following all coronary revascularization procedures according to a standard data collection form that includes definitions of each data element. In Pennsylvania, hospitals are required to submit data according to the MediQual System, a proprietary chart review system that measures illness severity according to the presence of a number of Key Clinical Findings. For the Cooperative Cardiovascular Project, contracted chart abstracters identified over 200 data elements from medical charts. While additional data collection requires substantial resources, the improved data concerning illness severity allow more balanced and meaningful comparisons among patients, hospitals, and physicians that would not be possible with claims data alone.

Report card systems that collect additional data represent a substantial improvement over systems that rely on claims data alone, but they still have some limitations. The MediQual system shares the same limitation as claims data in distinguishing comorbidities from complications. While the exact methodology is not publicly available, the MediQual system assigns an Admission Severity Group among five levels of risk (0–4), and is based on 23 Key Clinical Findings involving vital signs, physical examination, and laboratory studies are identified by chart review. Reviewers are instructed to select the most abnormal value during the first 48 hours of hospitalization, and missing variables are considered to be normal by default. By assigning the most abnormal value during the 48 hour review period, complications may potentially be considered comorbidities. For example, low systolic blood pressure or mechanical ventilation that were the result of complications within the first 48 hours would be included in Admission Severity Group calculation, attributing higher risk to the patient on admission. Other systems for risk adjustment such as All Patient Refined Diagnosis Related Groups used by many insurers and hospitals share the same difficulty in distinguishing comorbidities and complications [16]. To overcome the problem of confusing complications for comorbidities as noted above, illness severity indicators in the MediQual system should be limited to those present on admission, and data elements that may represent complications should be excluded from risk adjustment models whenever possible.

## Potential for Gaming

A limitation of any system that relies on self reporting such as the New York system, NRMI, and CRUSADE is the potential for "gaming." Gaming is defined as the specification of risk factors to achieve the highest estimate of expected mortality. In the case of New York, the prevalence of a number of risk factors increased substantially since the initial public release of provider specific outcomes [17]. Risk factors that are most susceptible to manipulation involve elements that are subjective, or involve broad definitions such as angina class or urgent procedure [18]. To the extent that "gaming" encourages more complete specification of risk, comparisons among providers will improve. However, gaming also carries great potential to skew risk estimates for individual providers. There are a number of approaches to minimize the potential for gaming to confound comparisons. First, whenever possible, risk adjustment models should focus on objective measures of severity. For example, admission systolic blood pressure may represent a more objective measure of circulatory state than cardiogenic shock. Second, precise definitions of risk factors should be specified to the extent possible. Third, risk models should be periodically recalculated on more recent data. Risk factors that become overly reported by all providers will fall in prognostic importance. Fourth, some level of independent data auditing should be routinely applied to all outcomes systems. In addition to identifying potential discrepancies, the "Hawthorne effect" of such an audit is likely to encourage accurate risk factor specification among all providers. In the case of New York, hospitals that were felt to have inaccurately reported procedural data according to independent audit were requested to resubmit their data in a corrected format.

## Missing Data

Missing data is a common occurrence among all of the current scorecard systems. Systems that use MediQual consider missing data to be within normal limits, while systems that rely on insurance claims consider missing diagnoses to signify the absence of such a diagnosis. Risk may be improperly assigned if the biases that led to missing data are also related to the outcome of interest. For example, in MediQual, ejection fraction may be missing for patients who do not survive long enough to undergo ventricular function measurement, and such patients would be expected to have lower ejection fractions on average, rather than the value of 70% assigned by the system [2,19]. For claims data, conditions such as hypertension have been found to be associated with lower mortality, a finding that is counter to clinical intuition [20]. It has been postulated that chronic conditions are associated with lower mortality because they are less likely to be coded for severely ill patients.

To improve risk adjustment, missing data may be accounted for in a number of ways. Characteristics that are missing for a substantial number of patients should be excluded from risk adjustment models. From a statistical approach, missing information can sometimes be imputed from other available data. For example, estimating left ventricular ejection fraction based on other measures of the circulatory state such as Killip class, infarct location, or systolic blood pressure may result in a less biased risk estimate than assuming ejection fraction to be normal. The reliability of insurance claims in identifying a particular disease can be determined by examining a sample of claims for which more detailed clinical data are available. Previous work has shown that more severe illnesses such as acute MI and diabetes were more likely to be identified, while other diagnoses such as tobacco use disorder were less reliable [21]. Finally, routine data checks can be used to identify missing data elements at the point of collection, possibly serving to target efforts at improved collection of such missing items.

## Small Numbers Problem: Low Volume Providers

Report cards are limited in their ability to reliably identify quality of care in the setting of a small number of outcomes. This situation arises for conditions in which outcomes are rare such as death following angioplasty, or situations where providers are infrequently involved with the condition of interest as in the case of low volume angioplasty operators. Due to small numbers, outcomes estimates have wide confidence intervals.

The issue of small numbers takes on particular significance in the debate about angioplasty volume guidelines. In the US, it is estimated that approximately one-half of physicians and one-quarter of hospitals performing coronary angioplasty fail to meet the volume limits proposed by expert panels. There are also consistent findings from regional and national studies that suggest patient treated by low volume operators have worse outcomes. Studies involving California, Medicare, New York State, and Society for Coronary Angiography and Intervention have found higher rates of bypass surgery and death for low volume hospitals, and studies from New York State, Northern New England, Medicare, and an academic registry have found worse outcomes for low volume physicians [22–28]. However, a few reports have failed to find such a relationship regarding physician volume [29,30]. These latter studies were less likely to identify a volume relationship, as they involved relatively few low volume physicians and were conducted in relatively high volume hospitals. While the majority of evidence indicates that low volume physicians and hospitals are associated with worse outcomes on average, some of these low volume operators have mortality and complication rates that are better than the average. The argument against volume limits is that they potentially restrict high quality, low volume operators from practice. Opponents of volume limits believe that individual operators should be judged on the basis of their outcomes, rather than strict volume limits. Proponents of volume limits note that the absence of proof of a difference (outlier status) is not the same as proof of no difference. As low volume operators have worse outcomes on average, and quality low volume operators are difficult to identify due to wide confidence intervals around individual outcome estimates, they believe that adherence to a process measure such as volume limits is the most reliable approach to assuring quality angioplasty.

In order to increase the chances of identifying quality low volume providers, systems will need to incorporate additional outcomes that occur more frequently, can be reliably identified, and are considered to represent negative outcomes. While it is difficult to arrive at consensus as to which outcomes represent significant complications, possible endpoints include bypass surgery prior to discharge, or post angioplasty myocardial infarction. Another approach to reliably identifying quality low volume operators is to combine angioplasty experience over a number of years.

The problem of low volume operators takes on particular significance in the setting of primary percutaneous coronary intervention for acute MI. The preponderance of recent evidence indicates that primary angioplasty is superior to thrombolysis in the treatment of acute MI [31]. Tempering the rush to provide primary angioplasty, studies have also shown worse outcomes for low volume primary PCI hospitals, and better outcomes for primary PCI even when patients require transfer to angioplasty centers [32–34]. Thus, based on current data, it appears that optimal myocardial infarction care involves the rapid administration of primary angioplasty, including transfer of patients to PCI centers for hospitals lacking adequate facilities or experience. The challenge in the US involves organizing systems for rapid triage and transfer similar to those that have demonstrated better efficacy in clinical trials. The time to primary angioplasty in the US for patients who remain in the same hospital approaches 120 minutes, far longer than the 90 minutes recommended in clinical guidelines or achieved in primary PCI trials [6]. Treatment times are likely much longer for patients requiring hospital transfer. The majority of communities in the US, lack the organization, authority, or financial incentives to facilitate hospital transfer and consolidate primary angioplasty. Examples of practical barriers include locally funded ambulance systems that are prohibited from routinely transporting patients to hospitals beyond county limits, and rural hospitals that rely on an adequate patient volume to maintain services and face a financial disincentive in transferring acute MI patients. Quality of care efforts must encourage and measure systems that provide a rapid regional approach to primary PCI. Current systems that measure time to reperfusion therapy including the Joint Commission on Accreditation of Healthcare Organizations and the National Acute Myocardial Infarction Project exclude patients who are either transferred to another hospital, or are received in transfer for acute MI care. To achieve an integrated system of care and transfer, quality measurement initiatives must be expanded to include patients who are transferred in the measurement of reperfusion time. This measurement will allow for the understanding of whether acute MI care achieved in clinical trials can be implemented in general practice, and identify opportunities for improving the provision of reperfusion therapy on a regional basis.

## Identification of providers

One important component of report cards involves the identification of the appropriate physician or hospital involved in a patient's care. Ideally, the physician or hospital most likely to influence a patient's outcome should be examined. In the case of major procedures, the angioplasty operator or surgeon is compared. For acute coronary syndromes where survival may be influenced by early therapeutic decisions, the physician or hospital initially involved in patient care should be examined. Given the complex interactions between health care providers, with the potential for multiple physicians and hospitals to interact in a patient's care, the issue of identifying the responsible provider becomes somewhat confounded.

The greatest potential bias regarding provider identification involves the ''Will Rogers'' effect, based upon the humorous comment that when people migrated from Oklahoma to California, the intelligence quotient of both states increased. In the case of report cards, certain physicians or hospitals may be more likely to be selected for complicated patients, with the potential for such providers to become associated with worse outcomes. The same bias may also overestimate the performance of providers who transfer complicated patients. Such a bias may be present in the Pennsylvania Heart Attack and Hospital Performance studies, where the patients who died after transfer to another hospital were attributed to the receiving hospital and excluded from comparisons involving the transferring hospital. Worse outcomes may have been attributed to the receiving hospital that were actually due to practice issues in the initial hospital such as failure to initiate reperfusion therapy. Thus, such a system misses the opportunity to identify hospitals in which early acute MI treatment could be improved. In order to avoid the biases introduced by the transfer of patients, outcomes systems should include comparisons that attribute care to the earliest provider. This is especially relevant when the clinical situation involves transfer of patients with acute MI for primary PCI as described earlier.

To identify hospitals, most systems rely on hospital identification submitted with hospital claims or mandatory hospital reports. The ideal outcomes system will link all hospitals involved in an episode of care, relying on admission and discharge dates, the admission source and the discharge status. The identification of physicians is somewhat more difficult, partly because a given patient may receive care from a number of physicians involved in a variety of relationships including group practice, consultation, emergency department, and transfers between services. Various state systems rely on state license numbers to identify the physician associated with care. Beginning in 1992, all physicians submitting claims to Medicare were required to include their Unique Physician Identification Number (UPIN) with their bills. Given the prevalence of coronary disease in Medicare patients, most physicians treating acute coronary syndromes outside of Federal and staff-model health maintenance organization hospitals participate in the UPIN system. The Federal initiative to identify providers of care is being extended to physicians in training, nurse practitioners and physician assistants according to a National Provider Identifier. For Medicare patients, there are at least two sources for physician identification. Hospital claims (Part A) identify a procedure physician and an attending physician; the latter defined as "the clinician who is primarily and largely responsible for the care of the patient from the beginning of the hospital episode" [35]. All physician claims (Part B) including claims for initial hospital evaluation, consults, and procedures identify the physician submitting the claim. When the author compared admitting physician according to hospital or physician bills, the author found that the two sources agreed approximately 80% of the time. When the two sources disagreed, it is likely that the physician associated with the majority of care was different than the admitting physician. As noted earlier, to attribute care to the provider most able to influence outcome, as well as to avoid biases involved in transfer, the earliest hospital and physician involved in an episode of care should be identified in outcomes comparisons. This may be accomplished through definitions which include the earliest provider, as well as through the use of physician and hospital bills to identify the earliest provider.

## Risk Adjustment Models

There are a number of statistical approaches to making balanced comparisons. Most current report cards examine dichotomous endpoints such as the occurrence of death or a complication, and use logistic regression models to balance comparisons. Estimated outcomes are subject to wide variation, depending on a number of factors including patient and provider identification, data quality, risk factor and outcome selection, and model development. Regardless of the statistical approach, the most important element of any outcomes comparison involves the concurrent publication of the methodology involved in making the comparison. Such information allows readers to understand whether differences in outcome were due to methodological factors, differences between patients, or differences in the quality of care. Risk adjustment systems that restrict the publication of the underlying methodology represent "black boxes." Given the potential for differences in outcome to be attributable to methodology rather than quality of care, such systems cannot be used to reliably identify "best practice" in a peer reviewed fashion. If the methodology behind comparisons cannot be released due to proprietary considerations, the author believes that resources should be directed to a system that can be fully scrutinized as part of scorecard reporting.

The methodological reports accompanying the California Hospital Outcomes Project and the Pennsylvania Focus on Heart Attack represent excellent examples of the information that should be provided in order to understand scorecard comparisons. These reports included clear descriptions of inclusion and exclusion criteria, prevalence of risk factors across hospitals, unadjusted outcomes, and model derivation and performance. While there is no consensus as to the optimal measure of model performance, standard measures include discrimination, reliability, and validation. Discrimination can be described according to the shape and area of the Receiver Operator Characteristic (ROC) curve, with 1 indicating perfect discrimination among all possible pairs of patients, and 0.5 indicating no discrimination. Most models yield ROC areas in the 0.70 to 0.85 range. Reliability refers to the ability of a model to predict outcomes that closely follow observed outcomes. This can be illustrated by dividing patients into equal sized groups based on their level of estimated risk, and then comparing estimated to observed outcomes within each group. A model with excellent reliability will yield estimated outcomes that are similar to the observed outcomes. "Validation" refers to the ability of a model derived in one population to perform in a different population. Well derived models should show similar performance among populations, while models that contain statistically spurious associations will show a decline in performance in other populations. Common approaches to validating include a split sample approach, where the model may be derived on one-half of the population, and tested on the remaining half. Other approaches include "bootstrapping," a technique whereby the model is repeatedly derived on randomly selected subgroups of the original sample, and performance characteristics are estimated among these smaller samples. Finally, models may be "externally" validated by applying the model to an entirely separate population, such as patients treated in another state or at different time.

## STRUCTURE AND PROCESS MEASURES: PHYSICIAN SPECIALTY AND VOLUME

A common strategy to reduce costs by managed care organizations involved limiting access to specialty care. This shift in medical care represented a fundamental alteration in structure (specialty certification) and process (specialty care). Quality of care is likely to improve to the extent that primary care physicians provide better care to an individual patient across a broad range of illnesses. Costs fell as primary care physicians use fewer resources [36]. If specialists continue to be associated with higher costs in managed care settings, specialty certification may no longer suffice as a measure of quality, unless such care can be shown to favorably influence outcome.

Better outcomes for specialty care are most likely to be seen with severe illnesses, such as acute coronary syndromes. The potential impact of specialty care on acute coronary syndromes has been examined in a number of studies. In a survey of 1,211 physicians in Texas and New York, Ayanian and colleagues reported that family practitioners and internists were less aware of or less certain about effective and life-saving drugs in the treatment of acute MI than cardiologists [37]. As part of the Pennsylvania Focus on Heart Attack, Nash and colleagues reported that in-hospital mortality was lower for acute MI patients cared for by cardiologists [38]. After adjusting for illness severity for all 40,684 hospital admissions for acute MI in Pennsylvania in 1993, cardiology patients had lower adjusted mortality compared to internal medicine (risk ratio 1.26, 95% confidence interval 1.17 to 1.35) or family practitioners (risk ratio 1.29, 95% confidence interval 1.18 to 1.40). The study also found improved survival for physicians who treated 12 or more MI patients per year, regardless of specialty [39]. Specialty and volume were related, as 80% of the higher volume physicians were cardiologists.

Our study also found that Medicare patients admitted by a cardiologist were 12% more likely to survive to 1 year compared to those admitted by a primary care physician, after adjusting for patient and hospital characteristics (p<0.001) [40]. Patients who were admitted by a primary care physician and underwent cardiology consultation had an intermediate survival. We also identified two potential mechanisms for the better survival. Cardiology patients were more likely to be treated with medications associated with improved survival including thrombolytic therapy, beta-blockers, and aspirin. With the increased use of coronary angiography, a greater proportion of cardiology patients were identified to have left main or three-vessel coronary artery disease, and more cardiology patients went on to revascularization.

There are three possible explanations for the relationship between specialty and outcome. First, as suggested by the Ayanian and Medicare studies, specialists are more familiar with the management of acute MI, and their treatment decisions lead to improved

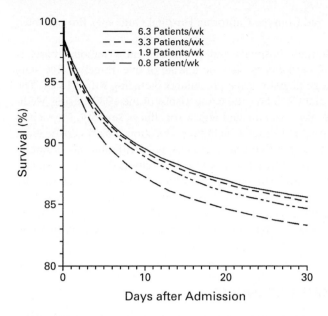

**Figure 2** Relationship between hospital volume and survival after acute myocardial infarction. Crude Kaplan–Meier 30-Day Survival Curves, by quartile, according to hospital volume of Medicare patients with acute myocardial infarction. For each quartile, the median hospital volume of Medicare patients with myocardial infarction per week is shown. (From Ref. 41)

survival. A second explanation may be that patients cared for by specialists have better survival due to lower illness severity. While both the Pennsylvania and Medicare studies adjusted for illness severity in their mortality comparisons, it is possible that factors related to illness severity that were not measured by these observational studies led to the improved survival.

A third explanation is that other factors associated with specialty care lead to better survival, such as hospitals that care for larger numbers of acute MI patients, have emergency room physicians who are more likely to recognize acute MIs and initiate early treatment, and have on-site resources available for the management of complications, such as coronary angioplasty or bypass surgery. For Medicare patients with acute coronary syndromes, Thiemann and colleagues showed that hospitals with more experience treating MI, reflected by their case volume, had lower mortality than low-volume hospitals (Fig. 2). These findings persisted after consideration of physician specialty, availability of invasive procedures, clinical factors and geographic location [41].

## Internet-Based Report Cards

Increased consumer interest and internet access have sparked the emergence of web-based report cards using both structural and outcomes measures. Healthscope.org, supported by a consortium of California employers, compares hospitals, physician groups, and health plans according to consumer surveys, health maintenance organization ratings (The Health Plan Employer Data and Information Set—HEDIS), and California government reports. Viewers are presented with simple menus that provide ready access to a broad array of comparative information including patient satisfaction, waiting time to see a specialist, treatment of hyperlipidemia and hypertension, angioplasty volume, and myocardial infarction mortality comparisons (derived from the California Hospital Outcomes Project noted earlier).

Another internet site that rates hospitals and physicians on a national basis is www.healthgrades.com. Hospital mortality is rated on a scale of one, three, or five stars according to a number of discharge diagnoses and procedures including MI and PCI. The methodology is similar to the initial CMS hospital comparisons of the 1980s, using Medicare ICD-9 discharge data to identify patients and adjust for illness severity. Physicians are rated according to simple structural criteria including education, board certification, governmental disciplinary actions within five years, and hospital affiliations according to Healthgrades rankings. Hospital data are free, and consumers are charged $6 for physician-specific reports. While the site provides a stunning array of hospital and physician specific data, the underlying methodology shares all of the limitations of rudimentary, insurance claims-based outcomes comparisons. As the internet evolves and sites continue to compete for viewers of health-related ''portals,'' the content of internet report cards is likely to substantially improve.

## DO REPORT CARDS IMPROVE OUTCOMES?

The first regional report cards involving bypass surgery were published in 1990, and a number of studies have attempted to gauge their impact according to trends in mortality following their publication. Bypass surgery mortality declined following the reporting of outcomes in New York State and Northern New England, and O'Connor and Hannan have suggested that scorecarding efforts in these regions have been responsible for the improved outcomes [42,43]. A comparison of short-term bypass surgery mortality among Medicare beneficiaries in regions with publicly available hospital report cards identified lower mortality in such regions [44]. Using national Medicare data from 1994 to 1999, Hannan and colleagues found lower adjusted mortality (odds ratio 0.79, 95% confidence interval 0.72–0.85) for patients treated in hospitals participating in New York, Pennsylvania, New Jersey, Northern New England, and Cleveland Health Quality Choice initiatives. While the findings of declining surgical mortality in regions with scorecard systems are intriguing, the impact of outcomes systems cannot be fully understood based on current literature. Comparisons of the relative decline in surgical mortality between regions are hampered by differences in patient population that cannot be resolved with the available data. It is likely that national trends of improved mortality are due to technical enhancements, advancement along the ''learning curve,'' as well local quality improvement efforts. Regional report cards may have also played a role in the improved outcomes. Ghali and colleagues suggested that outcomes systems be evaluated according to a randomized comparison, taking into account the cost of information systems relative to the measured improvement in outcome [45]. Such randomized trials are unlikely to be conducted, and the potential benefits of measuring outcomes would be difficult to fully measure. Regardless of the results of such trials, scorecard systems are likely to proliferate.

## RATING REPORT CARDS

While this chapter highlights opportunities to improve current scorecard systems, it should be noted that all of the current outcomes systems are far superior to systems in which health care is administered without any attempt at measurement or comparison. An appropriate analogy for the latter situation is driving at night without the use of headlights; it is difficult to know where the vehicle is heading, and there is little potential to avoid hazardous situations. Keeping in mind the tenet that any outcome system is better than no outcome system, compares representative scorecarding efforts in coronary disease. Among the current scorecard initiatives, systems that rely on risk adjustment data beyond insurance claims go a long way toward providing meaningful comparisons. Given the potential limitations of all current scorecarding efforts, their findings should only serve to direct additional study and review in identifying best practice.


## FUTURE OF REPORT CARDS

With the growing demand for information about quality of care, governmental and commercial entities are likely to continue to expand efforts to compare providers. The techniques by which to make comparisons among observational data are fairly well established. As outlined in this chapter, we understand how to attribute differences in outcomes to differences in illness severity, differences in care, and chance variation. However, there are a number of obstacles to scorecarding which must be overcome before such efforts can realize their full potential in identifying best practice. The greatest impediment involves the allocation of adequate resources to properly compare outcomes. Current efforts would be greatly enhanced if additional resources were directed toward data collection and validation. Such resources are essential in order to obtain reliable information about patient identification, risk adjustment, and outcomes. A second obstacle to better report cards involves the issue of patient confidentiality. As computer databases expand, there is great concern that confidential health information may be publicly released. Due to this concern, efforts such as federal standards for the privacy of personal health information have led to the removal of patient identifiers from medical databases. Such removal of identifiers actually runs counter to the law that established federal privacy standards, the Health Insurance Portability and Accountability Act of 1996 (HIPAA) [46]. This act actually recognizes the value of maintaining identified patient information to improve medical care, and contains specific provisions that allow for such access with investigational review board oversight. Without patient identifiers, outcomes comparisons are severely restricted. Such identifiers are required to link episodes of care, identify associated health care facilities, characterize socioeconomic status, combine data sources, and track long-term outcomes. Adequate safeguards exist, such as encryption, access barriers, and peer oversight, whereby privacy can be maintained. The author believes that the potential benefit of patient identifiers in improving care far outweighs the potential risk of lost privacy.

A third obstacle involves maintaining active participation among providers to properly execute outcomes comparisons. With any comparison, a number of providers are likely to fall toward the lower end of quality measures, and the potential to be identified as such may motivate some to hinder outcomes comparisons. Over the long term, comparisons among providers will continue to expand, regardless of the willing participation of providers. Private sector initiatives which include internet-based services are not subject to the political process or public scrutiny and is more likely to expand in the absence of public or physician supported systems. The author believes that the best approach to ensuring the long-term success of physicians and hospitals, as well as the best approach to improving patient care, is for physicians and hospitals to actively participate in outcomes comparisons. Active involvement of health care providers will assure that comparisons are properly derived, permit physicians and hospitals to demonstrate their abilities to patients and health care purchasers, and allow physicians to determine best practice.

## REFERENCES

1. Chassin MR, Hannan EL, DeBuono BA. Benefits and hazards of reporting medical outcomes publicly. N Engl J Med 1996;334:394–398.
2. Focus on heart attack in Pennsylvania, the technical report, The Pennsylvania Health Care Cost Containment Council, June 1996.
3. State of California, Office of Statewide Planning and Development, Annual report of the California hospital outcomes project, December 1993.
4. Ellerbeck EF, Jencks SF, Radford MJ, Kresowik TF, Craig AS, Gold JA, Krumholz HM, Vogel RA. Quality of care for Medicare patients with acute myocardial infarction. A four-state pilot study from the Cooperative Cardiovascular Project. J Am Med Assoc 1995;273: 1509–1514.
5. Jencks SF, Cuerdon T, Burwen DR, Fleming B, Houck PM, Kussmaul AE, Nilasena DS, Ordin DL, Arday DR. Quality of medical care delivered to Medicare beneficiaries: a profile at state and national levels. J Am Med Assoc 2000;284:1670–1676.
6. Jencks SF, Huff ED, Cuerdon T. Change in the quality of care delivered to Medicare beneficiaries, 1998–1999 to 2000–2001. J Am Med Assoc 2003;289:305–312.
7. Roe MT, Ohman EM, Pollack CV, Peterson ED, Brindis RG, Harrington RA, Christenson RH, Smith SC Jr, Califf RM, Gibler WB. Changing the model of care for patients with acute coronary syndromes – implementing practice guidelines and altering physician behavior. Am Heart J 2003;146:605–612.
8. Rogers WJ, Canto JG, Lambrew CT, Tiefenbrunn AJ, Kinkaid B, Shoultz DA, Frederick PD, Every N. Temporal trends in the treatment of over 1.5 million patients with myocardial infarction in the US from 1990 through 1999. J Am Coll Cardiol 2000;36:2056–2063.
8a. Zach AP, Romano PS, Luft HS. Report on heart attack 1991–1993 Volume1: user's guide. Sacramento: California Office of Statewide Health Planning and Development, 1997.
9. Percutaneous coronary interventions in New York State, 1998–2000, New York State Department of Healthhttp: //www.health.state.ny.us/nysdoh/reports/pci_1998–2000.pdf., January 2003.
10. International Classification of Diseases, 9th Revision, Clinical Modification. Los Angeles: Practice Management Information Corp., 1991.
11. Physicians' Current Procedural Terminology 1994 Chicago: American Medical Association, 1994.
12. Jenks SF, Williams DK, Kay TL. Assessing hospital-associated deaths from discharge data. J Am Med Assoc 1988;260:2240–2246.
13. Iezzoni LI, Foley SM, Daley J, Hughes J, Fisher ES, Heeren T. Comorbidities, complications, and coding bias. J Am Med Assoc 1992;267:2197–2203.
14. Jollis JG, Ancukiewicz M, DeLong ER, Pryor DB, Muhlbaier LH, Mark DB. Discordance of databases designed for claims payment versus clinical information systems. Implications for outcomes research. Ann Intern Med 1993;119:844–850.
15. Hannan EL, Kilburn H, Lindsey ML, Lewis R. Clinical versus administrative data bases for CABG surgery. Does it matter? Med Care 1992;30:892–907.
16. Iezzoni LI, Ash AS, Shwartz M, Daley J, Hughes JS, Mackiernan YD. Predicting who dies depends on how severity is measured: implications for evaluating patient outcomes. Ann Intern Med 1995;123:763–770.
17. Green J, Wintfeld N. Report cards on cardiac surgeons. Assessing New York State's approach. N Engl J Med 1995;332:1229–1232.
18. Ellis SG, Omoigui N, Bittl JA, Lincoff M, Wolfe MW, Howell G, Topol EJ. Analysis and comparison of operator-specific outcomes in interventional cardiology. From a multicenter database of 4860 quality-controlled procedures. Circulation 1996;93:431–439.
19. Focus on heart attack in Pennsylvania, research methods and results. The Pennsylvania Health Care Cost Containment Council, April 1996.
20. Jenks EJ, Iezzoni LI, Foley SM, Daley J, Hughes J, Fisher ES, Heeren T. Comorbidities, complications, and coding bias. J Amer Med Assoc 1992;267:2197–2203.

21. Jollis JG, Ancukiewicz M, DeLong ER, Pryor DB, Muhlbaier LH, Mark DB. Discordance of databases designed for claims payment versus clinical information systems. Implications for outcomes research. Ann Intern Med 1993;119:844–850.

22. Ritchie JL, Phillips KA, Luft HS. Coronary angioplasty. Statewide experience in California. Circulation 1993;88:2735–43.

23. Jollis JG, Peterson ED, DeLong ER, Mark DB, Collins SR, Muhlbaier LH, Pryor DB. The relationship between hospital volume of coronary angioplasty and short term mortality in patients over age 65 in the United States. N Engl J Med 1994;331:1625–1629.

24. Kimmel SE, Berlin JA, Laskey WK. The relationship between coronary angioplasty procedure volume and major complications. J Am Med Assoc 1995;274:1137–1142.

25. Hannan EL, Racz M, Ryan TJ, McCallister BD, Johnson LW, Arani DT, Guerci AD, Sosa J, Topol EJ. Coronary angioplasty volume-outcome relationships for hospitals and cardiologists. J Am Med Assoc 1997;277:892–898.

26. McGrath PD, Wennberg DE, Malenka DJ, Kellett MA, Ryan TJ, O'Meara JR, Bradley WA, Hearne MJ, Hettleman B, Robb JF, Shubrooks S, VerLee P, Watkins MW, Lucas FL, O'Connor GT. Operator volume and outcomes in 12,998 percutaneous coronary interventions. Northern New England Cardiovascular Disease Study Group. J Am Coll Cardiol 1998;31:570–576.

27. Jollis JG, Peterson ED, Nelson CL, Stafford JA, DeLong ER, Muhlbaier LH, Mark DB. Relationship between physician and hospital coronary angioplasty volume and outcome in elderly patients. Circulation 1997;95:2485–2491.

28. Ellis SG, Weintraub W, Holmes D, Shaw R, Block PC, King SB. Relation of operator volume and experience to procedural outcome of percutaneous coronary revascularization at hospitals with high interventional volumes. Circulation 1997;95:2479–2484.

29. Malenka DJ, McGrath PD, Wennberg DE, Ryan TJ, Kellett MA, Shubrooks SJ, Bradley WA, Hettlemen BD, Robb JF, Hearne MJ, Silver TM, Watkins MW, O'Meara JR, VerLee PN, O'Rourke DJ. The relationship between operator volume and outcomes after percutaneous coronary interventions in high volume hospitals in 1994–1996 - The northern New England experience. J Am Coll Cardiol 1999;34:1471–1480.

30. Grines CL. Thrombolysis or primary angioplasty for acute myocardial infarction. N Engl J Med 1997;336:1102–1103.

31. Keeley EC, Boura JA, Grines CL. Primary angioplasty versus intravenous thrombolytic therapy for acute myocardial infarction: a quantitative review of 23 randomised trials. Lancet 2003; 361:13–20.

32. Canto JG, Every NR, Magid DJ, Rogers WJ, Malmgren JA, Frederick PD, French WJ, Tiefenbrunn AJ, Misra VK, Kiefe CI, Barron HV. The volume of primary angioplasty procedures and survival after acute myocardial infarction. N Engl J Med 2000;342:1573–1580.

33. Grines CL, Westerhausen DR, Grines LL, Hanlon JT, Logemann TL, Niemela M, Weaver WD, Graham M, Boura J, O'Neil WW, Balestrini C, Air PAMI Study Group. A randomized trial of transfer for primary angioplasty versus on-site thrombolysis in patients with high-risk myocardial infarction. J Am Coll Cardiol 2002;39:1713–1719.

34. Andersen HR, Nielsen TT, Rasmussen K, Thuesen L, Kelbaek H, Thayssen P, Abildgaard U, Pedersen F, Madsen JK, Grande P, Villadsen AB, Krusell LR, Haghfelt T, Lomholt P, Husted SE, Vigholt E, Kjaergard HK, Mortensen LS. DANAMI-2 Investigators. A comparison of coronary angioplasty with fibrinolytic therapy in acute myocardial infarction. N Engl J Med 2003;349:733–742.

35. Iezzoni LI. Data sources and implications: administrative data bases. In: Iezzoni LI, Ed. Risk adjustment for measuring health care outcomes. Ann Arbor: Health Administration Press, 1994:122.

36. Greenfield S, Nelson EC, Zubkoff M, Manning W, Rogers W, Kravitz RL, Keller A, Tarlov AR, Ware JE Jr. Variations in resource utilization among medical specialties and systems of care. J Am Med Assoc 1992;267:1624–30.

37. Ayanian JZ, Hauptman PJ, Guadagnoli E, Antman EM, Pashos CL, McNeil BJ. Knowledge and practices of generalist and specialist physicians regarding drug therapy for acute myocardial infarction. N Engl J Med 1994;331:1136–1142.

38. Nash IS, Nash DB, Fuster V. Do Cardiologists Do It Better? J Am Coll Cardiol 1997;29(3): 475–478.
39. Casale PN, Jones JL, Wolf FE, Pei Y, Eby LM. Patients treated by cardiologists have a lower in-hospital mortality for acute myocardial infarction. J Am Coll Cardiol 1997;29(Suppl A): 392A.
40. Jollis JG, DeLong ER, Peterson ED, Muhlbaier LH, Fortin DF, Califf RM, Mark DB. Outcome of acute myocardial infarction according to the specialty of the admitting physician. N Engl J Med 1996;335:1880–1887.
41. Thiemann DR, Coresh J, Oetgen WJ, Powe NR. The association between hospital volume and survival after acute myocardial infarction in elderly patients. N Engl J Med 1999;340: 1640–1648.
42. Hannan EL, Kilburn H, Racz M, Shields E, Chassin MR. Improving the outcomes of coronary artery bypass surgery in New York State. J Am Med Assoc 1994;271:761–766.
43. O'Connor GT, Plume SK, Olmstead EM, Morton JR, Maloney CT, Nugent WC, Hernandez F, Clough R, Leavitt BJ, Coffin LH, Marrin CA, Wennberg D, Birkmeyer JD, Charlesworth DC, Malenka DJ, Quinton HB, Kasper JF. A regional intervention to improve the hospital mortality associated with coronary artery bypass graft surgery. J Am Med Assoc 1996;275: 841–846.
44. Hannan EL, Sarrazin MS, Doran DR, Rosenthal GE. Provider profiling and quality improvement efforts in coronary artery bypass graft surgery: the effect on short-term mortality among Medicare beneficiaries. Med Care 2003;41:1164–1167.
45. Ghali WA, Ash AS, Hall RE, Moskowitz MA. Statewide quality improvement initiatives and mortality after cardiac surgery. J Am Med Assoc 1997;277:379–382.
46. Public Law 104–191, 104th Congress.

# 32

# Cost-Effectiveness of New Diagnostic Tools and Therapies for Acute Coronary Syndromes

**Eric L. Eisenstein and Daniel B. Mark**
*Duke University Medical Center*
*Durham, North Carolina, USA*

## INTRODUCTION

Three 20th century trends have converged to create today's technology-driven health care system [1]. First, increasing life expectancy (49.2 years in 1900 vs. 77.2 years in 2001 for the United States) means that people live long enough to develop more chronic diseases [2]. Second, greater societal wealth permits a larger portion of society's resources to be spent on health care (3% of US gross domestic product in 1900 vs. 13.6% in 1997) [1–3]. Finally the development of medical insurance provides a large pool of funds for medical expenses (paying 0% of US medical expenses in 1900 vs. 83% in 1990) [1]. These trends are particularly important for acute coronary syndrome (ACS) patients who are typically older and whose 30-day medical costs ($17,251 in 1995) [4] are 3.7 times the annual per capita health expenditures in the US [5].

In the past, the incremental value of new acute coronary syndrome (ACS) therapies was not questioned. The introduction of intensive care units, external defibrillators, and CPR in the late 1950s and early 1960s reduced short-term acute myocardial infarction (MI) mortality by 20% (32% to 12%) [6–9]. The addition of thrombolytic and aspirin therapy in the 1980s resulted in a further 5% reduction (12% to 7%). However, recent reperfusion innovations (i.e., tissue plasminogen activator and direct angioplasty) of the 1990s have further reduced short-term acute MI mortality by 2% at best (from 7% to 5%) [10,11]. Thus, past technological successes have limited the ability of new technologies to reduce short-term ACS patient mortality. For this reason, 21st century cardiologists will need to develop more sophisticated means for placing a value on the care they provide.

In this chapter, the authors introduce a framework for evaluating the economic attractiveness of new medical therapies, define its elements (medical costs and health benefits), and compare methods for their measurement. The authors then use this framework to evaluate the economics of new diagnostic tools and therapies for ACS patients.

## CLINICAL ECONOMICS CONCEPTS

Traditional economic value assessment estimates the incremental monetary value of any differences between a new product and its best alternative [12]. However, health care

**723**

differs from other industries in that many benefits of its products (e.g., increased life expectancy, reduced morbidity, or improved quality of life) are not easily translated into monetary terms. Thus, health economists typically use methods that simultaneously compare monetary costs and non-monetary health benefits when evaluating medical goods and services. While most would agree that this is fair, differences frequently arise regarding which costs and health benefits should be included in specific analyses as well as how best to measure them.

## Economic Evaluation Framework

The cost-effectiveness ratio, as shown, compares the incremental cost per incremental unit of health benefit gained by the new therapy versus the standard of care.

$$\left( \frac{C_{New} - C_{Old}}{E_{New} - E_{Old}} \right) \text{ Where C} = \text{Cost and E} = \text{Effectiveness}$$

While the theoretical time frame for assessing costs and health benefits is the patient's lifetime, this approach leads to obvious practical limitations in data collection. Thus, most economic studies measure costs and health benefits to a point at which the differences in strategies become negligible. For ACS patients, the acute period typically lasts 30 to 60 days with sequelae continuing from six to twelve months, after which patients return to a chronic coronary artery disease (CAD) state [13,14]. Thus, economic studies of ACS therapies typically do not measure costs beyond one year and assume there is no difference in costs between treatment strategies after that point. However, the health benefits of ACS therapies may extend well beyond one year and should be accounted for in the analysis.

## Types of Economic Analysis

There are several possible relationships between incremental costs and incremental health benefits in an economic analysis (Fig. 1). When a new patient management strategy reduces health benefits in comparison to usual care, an economic analysis is not performed because the strategy is usually considered clinically irrelevant. When there is no difference in health benefits between patient management strategies, the analysis reduces to a comparison of cost differences ($C_{New} - C_{Old}$). This is called a cost-minimization analysis. When the new

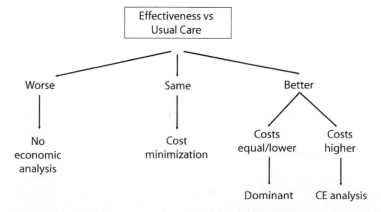

**Figure 1**  Types of economic analyses as a function of outcomes and costs.

patient management strategy has greater health benefits and costs more than the standard of care, a tradeoff is involved between the strategy's greater health benefits and its greater costs, and a cost-effectiveness analysis is required. Finally, when the new patient management strategy has greater health benefits and costs less, it is known as a dominant strategy (better in both cost and health benefit) and no further analysis is required. Although the term "cost effectiveness" has been used colloquially to denote something perceived to be a good economic value, this usage is incorrect [15]. To avoid confusion, this chapter will use the term "economically attractive" when a patient management strategy is dominant or when an economic analysis (cost minimization or cost effectiveness) has a favorable result.

## Economic Attractiveness Criteria

Various criteria have been proposed for assessing the relative economic attractiveness of new medical therapies that improve outcomes but also increase costs. Goldman proposed the most straightforward method, which uses the cost of dialysis for treating end-stage renal disease (now covered by the federal government regardless of patient age) as a benchmark for economic attractiveness [16]. Between 1996 and 2000, Medicare costs per patient year at risk averaged $54,917 for hemodialysis and $46,121 for peritoneal dialysis patients [17]. Using dialysis as a benchmark, most experts consider therapies costing less than $50,000 per year of life saved (YOLS) to be economically attractive, those costing $50,000 to $100,000 per YOLS are considered borderline, and therapies costing more than $100,000 per YOLS are economically unattractive [18].

League tables, which rank health care alternatives by ascending cost-effectiveness ratios, are frequently used to compare the economic attractiveness of therapeutic options (Table 1). It is important to note that the economic attractiveness of a new therapy is not fixed, but a function of both the alternative against which it is being compared as well as the patient population in which it is administered. For example, a therapy will generally be more economically attractive in a higher than in a lower risk population (e.g., secondary vs. primary prevention) and when it is compared against placebo vs. an active therapy. Health care policy makers find league tables attractive guides in resource allocation decisions because of their simplicity [19–21]. However, they oversimplify a complex problem and can mislead decision makers [22]. For example, league tables rarely include the measure of uncertainty around a cost-effectiveness estimate (e.g., confidence intervals), and they do not alert the user when substantially different methods have been used to estimate costs and outcomes. Because of these limitations, league tables should only be used for illustrative purposes and not to guide decision making [22,23].

## Perspective

The perspective is the viewpoint from which an economic analysis is conducted. Although economic analyses have been performed from the patient, employer, payer, and provider perspective, they most often use a societal perspective because it is the most comprehensive [24]. All other perspectives omit certain costs or health benefits from their analyses or count transfer payments between societal members as cash inflows or outflows. The societal perspective accounts for all economic elements including costs associated with the current episode of care (index costs) as well as all down-stream medical costs (follow-up costs). Although insurance and income transfers (e.g., welfare or disability payments) are frequently the most important cash flows for patients, payers, employers, and providers, they are not included in analyses performed from the societal perspective because they are not

**Table 1**  Example "League Table" of Different Cardiovascular Therapies

| New technology | Existing technology | Patient population | Cost/ YOLS | Reference |
|---|---|---|---|---|
| Beta-blockers | No therapy | Myocardial infarction survivors | $1,000 | Wilhelmsson (1981) |
| CABG | Medical therapy | Left main coronary artery disease | $6,700 | Weinstein (1982) |
| PTCA | Medical therapy | Men age 55 with severe angina | $8,900 | Wong (1990) |
| Hypertension screening | No screening | Asymptomatic men age 60 | $13,200 | Littenberg (1990) |
| Exercise stress test | No testing | Age 60 with mild pain and no left ventricular dysfunction | $15,600 | Lee (1988) |
| Beta-blockers | No therapy | Hypertensive age 35–64, no heart disease, and ≥95 mmHg | $16,800 | Edelson (1990) |
| Lovastatin | No therapy | Men age 55–64 with heart disease and <250 mg/dL | $24,000 | Goldman (1991) |
| t-PA | Streptokinase | Anterior myocardial infarction, age 61–75 | $24,800 | Mark (1995) |
| Lovastatin | No therapy | Men age 45–54 with no heart disease and ≥300 mg/dL | $40,900 | Goldman (1991) |
| t-PA | Streptokinase | Anterior myocardial infarction, age 41–60 | $60,000 | Mark (1995) |
| CABG | Medical therapy | Two-vessel coronary artery disease | $90,200 | Weinstein (1982) |
| Hypertension screening | No screening | Asymptomatic women age 20 | $104,600 | Littenberg (1990) |
| PTCA | Medical therapy | Men age 55 with mild angina | $132,200 | Wong (1990) |

Costs adjusted to 1998 dollars using the consumer price index.

costs of care. However, they should be included when analyses are performed from any other perspective [25].

## MEDICAL COSTS

As shown earlier, the perspective of an analysis also determines which economic elements are included. The remainder of this section will discuss the measurement of those elements and will be limited to analyses conducted from the societal perspective.

### Medical Cost Terminology

Cost accountants use different cost classification systems for different types of analyses. Product costing systems seek to identify all costs involved with providing specific medical goods and services (e.g., primary angioplasty) to patients whereas marginal analysis systems are concerned with the relationship between changes in patient volume and changes in costs (e.g., how costs in chest pain units increase as the number of patients increases) [24]. In marginal analysis, costs varying in direct proportion with the number of patients seen are called variable costs (e.g., contrast medium and catheters in a catheterization laboratory) whereas costs that remain stable regardless of changes in patient volume are called fixed costs (e.g., equipment and facilities in a catheterization laboratory). Fixed costs are always defined for a specific capacity (e.g., number of beds in a chest pain unit), thus all costs will necessarily become variable in the long run with extreme variation in patient volume. Some costs are hybrids and exhibit characteristics of both variable and fixed costs. Semivariable costs have both fixed and variable components (e.g., utilities in which there is a fixed connection fee and a variable fee based upon volume used). Semifixed costs, the other type of hybrid cost, vary in a semifixed (stepwise) way with changes in patient volume (e.g., nursing middle management staffing which varies with the number of nurses).

*Medical Cost Calculation*

Three cost calculation methods are used for estimating medical costs: bottom-up, top-down, and imputation models. Bottom-up methods estimate the costs of individual components and then sum them to arrive at a cost for the whole episode; top-down methods estimate aggregate costs from aggregate charges; and imputation models use patient characteristics and resource utilization as inputs for cost estimation models.

Three bottom-up methods have been used in previous economic analyses. Microcosting (the gold standard) uses industrial engineering techniques to estimate the unit cost of each resource used and sums them to yield total case costs. The advantage of microcosting is its precision; the disadvantage is the cost of collecting and maintaining this level of data. Modern hospital cost accounting systems typically combine industrial engineering techniques with expert opinion to estimate the average costs for resources. Although not as precise as microcosting, hospital cost accounting systems yield results that are close approximations and have lower data collection costs. The third bottom-up method, ''big ticket'' costing, assigns fixed costs to major health care resources (e.g., coronary artery bypass graft [CABG], percutaneous transluminal coronary angiography [PTCA], ICU room day) and uses them to estimate case costs. The advantage is the low cost of data collection; its disadvantage is its lack of detail (e.g., ability to differentiate among various stent and pacemaker procedures).

Two top-down methods have been used in US economic analyses: ratio of cost to charge (RCC) and Medicare standard costs. The RCC method estimates costs from the line item charges on the patient's bill using conversion factors (typically aggregate ratios for institutional departments). The advantage of this method is its ease of use because all US hospitals treating Medicare patients file annual cost reports that contain department level cost conversion factors. The disadvantage of RCC is that it sacrifices some of the accuracy of microcosting. Several studies have used Medicare Diagnosis Related Groups (DRG) and/or Physician Fee Schedule reimbursements as surrogates for costs. Again, the advantage in these methods is the ease of data collection. The disadvantage of the DRG approach is its lack of detail (e.g., all CABG surgeries without catheterization are assigned the same costs). Since Medicare reimburses physicians at the current procedural terminology (CPT) code level, these reimbursements are a reasonable estimate of physician costs.

Two studies compared bottom-up and top-down costing methods. In a single institution study of CABG and PTCA costs, Lipscomb and colleagues found that average case costs were approximately the same when using results from a hospital cost accounting system and the RCC method, but costs at the department level varied [26]. In a study of

14 hospitals with automated bottom-up cost accounting systems, Ashby found that the average case costs across 40 DRGs were 4.4% higher using the top-down methods than they were using a bottom-up method [27]. However, the differences in average cost between methods varied by DRG. Because the reported differences between hospital cost accounting and RCC methods are relatively small, most experts consider the results comparable.

Various imputation models have also been used to estimate costs in economic analyses. The two principal approaches are the use of case mix-adjusted cost functions [28] and the use of resource-based regression equations [29]. The advantage to these methods is that they don't require the collection of detailed cost data. The disadvantages relate to imprecision of the estimates due to differences between the patient population under study and that represented in the database used to create the model.

The results of an economic analysis will be sensitive to the costing method used. For example, when it is anticipated that the difference in costs between two patient management strategies will be driven by differences in the rates of rehospitalization, a general costing method which does not require the collection of detailed costing data may be satisfactory. However, when it is anticipated that cost differences in the analysis will be driven by the utilization of specific resources (e.g., balloons or stents within the catheterization laboratory), a more detailed costing method will be required.

## Health Benefits

Measuring health benefits is even more difficult than measuring costs [30], because there is no universal clinical outcome that can be used in all economic analyses. An additional difficulty is the inherent variability in many clinical outcome measurements [30,31]. While survival is an easily identifiable clinical outcome, many commonly used medical therapies have no effect on patient life expectancy. Even when therapies do increase patient life expectancy, the gains are typically modest [32–34]. Table 2 shows differences in incremental life expectancy associated with prevention of and treatment for CAD. Although exercising and quitting smoking both produce modest gains in life expectancy for 35-year-old patients at average risk, life expectancy gains in higher risk patients are much greater. This is because these therapies are targeted to patients who will benefit whereas the benefits of therapies in lower risk patients are averaged across those who will and will not benefit. Interestingly, life expectancy gains in patients with CAD are modest at best and decline significantly when the comparison is between therapies (e.g., t-PA versus streptokinase) rather than between therapy and placebo (e.g., thrombolysis with t-PA vs. placebo). Because of this, quality-adjusted life years (QALYs) have been adopted as a standard measure of effectiveness. QALYs assign a weight to a patient's life expectancy representing their health-related quality of life (with 1 denoting perfect health and 0 denoting death). This adjustment allows all life expectancy estimate comparisons to be made from the same base (i.e., deviations from life years in perfect health). The rationale behind using QALYs is that therapies may improve the patient's overall quality of life without affecting longevity.

*Adjusting for Differences in Timing*

Patient management strategies often require different resources and produce different health benefits over time. For example, in a comparison of CABG surgery versus percutaneous coronary interventions (PCI) for patients with multivessel CAD, CABG patients typically will incur higher index costs and greater short-term mortality whereas PCI patients will incur greater follow-up costs and long-term mortality. Discounting (the reverse

**Table 2** Gains In Life Expectancy

| Treatment/prevention strategy | Patient population | Gains in life expectancy (years added) | |
|---|---|---|---|
| | | Men | Women |
| **Average-risk patients** | | | |
| Exercise consuming 2000 kcal/wk for 30 yrs | 35-year-old men | 0.517 | — |
| Quitting cigarette smoking | 35-year-olds | 0.833 | 0.667 |
| **High-risk patients** | | | |
| Reduction of diastolic bp to 88 mm Hg | 35-year-olds with: | | |
| | Diastolic bp of 90–94 mm Hg | 1.083 | 0.917 |
| | Diastolic bp >105 mm Hg | 5.333 | 5.667 |
| Reduction of cholesterol to 200 mg/dL | 35-year-olds with: | | |
| | Cholesterol level of 200–239 mg/dL | 0.500 | 0.417 |
| | Cholesterol level of >300 mg/dL | 4.167 | 6.333 |
| Reduction of weight to ideal level | 35-year-olds: | | |
| | <30% over their ideal weight | 0.667 | 0.500 |
| | ≥30% over their ideal weight | 1.667 | 1.083 |
| **Patients with established disease** | | | |
| Revascularization with CABG or PTCA | Men with 2 VD | 0.333 | — |
| | Men with 3 VD | 0.750 | — |
| Routine beta blocker therapy | 55-year-old male AMI survivor with: | | |
| | Low risk of recurrence | 0.100 | — |
| | Medium risk of recurrence | 0.342 | — |
| | High risk of recurrence | 0.467 | — |
| Thrombolysis with t-PA | Men or women w/ suspected AMI | 1.250 | 1.250 |
| t-PA versus streptokinase | Men or women w/ suspected AMI: | | |
| | Inferior | 0.163 | 0.163 |
| | Anterior | 0.196 | 0.196 |
| Heart transplant | Men or women with end-stage heart failure | 5.417 | 5.417 |

Data from Refs. 33, 55, 129–133.

of compound interest) is used to adjust for cost and health benefits that occur at different times and treats all costs and health benefits as if they occurred at baseline. Although various discount rates have been used, a 3% rate has become the standard when making comparisons using a societal perspective [25].

*Cost-Effectiveness Calculations*

Table 3 shows the cost-effectiveness ratio calculations for comparing two patient management strategies. The new therapy has higher index costs but lower follow-up costs than

**Table 3**  Cost-Effectiveness Computations

|                                              | New therapy | Usual care |
|----------------------------------------------|-------------|------------|
| Index costs                                  | $45,000     | $30,000    |
| Follow-up costs:                             |             |            |
|   Year 1                           | $ 0         | $ 3,000    |
|   Year 2                           | $ 0         | $12,000    |
| Cumulative costs                             | $45,000     | $45,000    |
| Discounted costs:                            |             |            |
|   Year 1                           | $ 0         | $ 2,913    |
|   Year 2                           | $ 0         | $11,310    |
| Present value                                | $45,000     | $44,223    |
| Cost difference                              | $ 777       |            |
| Life expectancy                              | 10 Years    | 10 Years   |
| Discounted life expectancy                   | 8.530 LY    | 8.530 LY   |
| Quality of life                              | 0.92        | 0.85       |
| Discounted quality-adjusted life expectancy  | 7.7 QALY    | 7.3 QALY   |
| QALY difference                              | 0.4 QALY    |            |
| Cost per QALY (cost-effectiveness ratio)     | $1822       |            |

the usual care strategy, but their cumulative costs at two years are identical. (For the purpose of this analysis, assume that there is no difference in follow-up costs after two years.) After discounting, the new therapy has $777 higher cumulative costs since the timing of its cash flows were earlier than those for usual care. Although both strategies yield identical life expectancies (10 years undiscounted and 8.53 years discounted), the new therapy produces a slightly higher quality of life for its patients (7.7 vs. 7.3 QALY). Thus, there is a 0.4 QALY benefit for the new therapy versus usual care. Although usual care costs $777 less, the new therapy is favored because it produces greater quality of life at an acceptable cost of $1822 per QALY, well below the accepted threshold for economic attractiveness.

## ECONOMIC STUDIES OF ACUTE CORONARY SYNDROMES

### General Considerations

Acute coronary syndromes typically resolve within 30 to 60 days [13,14]. Nonetheless, treatment decisions made by health care professionals during this period will account for 35–40% of the total medical costs these patients will incur over the next 10 years [29]. Conceptually, ACS medical costs can be divided into five major resource utilization components (Fig. 2).

### Prehospital Phase

*Preadmission Evaluation*

Annually, 5 to 6 million acute chest pain patients are evaluated in U.S. emergency departments (ED) at a total cost of more than $6 billion [35,36]. Most will be admitted to a hospital where they will stay for an average of 1.9 days and incur $4135 in charges [37]. Ultimately, 15% will be identified as having acute myocardial infarction, 45% unstable angina or nonacute CAD, and 40% chest pain without an underlying coronary etiology

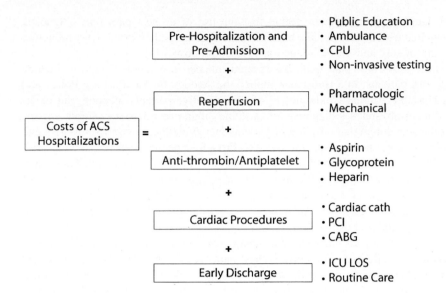

**Figure 2** Economic components of ACS hospitalization.

[38]. The annual cost for those found to be free of acute disease is $600 million [38]. At the same time, 5% of chest pain patients will have an undiagnosed MI and be inappropriately discharged [39,40].

*Chest Pain Units*

For the ED physician, one of the benefits of chest pain units is that they delay the hospital admission decision and provide an alternative to either discharging patients prematurely or admitting the patient and committing expensive cardiac care unit resources. Several studies have demonstrated the safety and economic viability of chest pain units (Table 4)[41–45]

**Table 4** Chest Pain Unit Reductions in Length of Stay and Costs

| Publication | | Reduction | |
|---|---|---|---|
| Study | year | LOS | Average costs |
| Gaspoz et al. | 1994 | | |
| CCU | | 4.0 | $7,274 |
| Step-down | | 2.0 | $2,104 |
| Wards | | 3.0 | $2,785 |
| Gomez et al. | 1996 | 0.5 | $ 981 |
| Newby | 1996 | 2.3 | $1,765 |
| Mikhail | 1997 | ND | $1,470 |
| Roberts | 1997 | 0.5 | $ 567 |

ND = No data recorded.
Reduction in LOS and costs are for initial hospitalization except for
  Gaspoz, which includes follow-up through 6 months.
(From Ref. 45)

In the Duke program, Newby found that the use of a chest pain unit diagnostic strategy compared with conventional admission and rule-out resulted in a 2.3 day reduction in mean length of stay and a 47% reduction in hospital costs [45].

The success of chest pain units has created interest in extending them to include intermediate-risk patients. In a study that applied the Agency for Health Care Policy and Research's Unstable Angina Guidelines to 457 consecutive patients receiving an emergency department physician's diagnosis of unstable angina or rule-out unstable angina, Katz and colleagues found that only 6% of patients met guideline criteria for low-risk and were suitable for direct home discharge [46,47]. Fifty-four percent met intermediate-risk criteria and 40% met high-risk criteria requiring intensive care unit admission. Thus, there remains great potential to expand the use of chest pain units to include the majority of chest pain patients, those at intermediate-risk, who were excluded by earlier protocols.

Farkouh and colleagues randomized 424 intermediate-risk Mayo Clinic patients to chest pain unit or standard hospital admission [40]. After six hours, 60 of the 212 patients randomized to the chest pain unit were admitted because of positive creative kinase-MB (CK-MB) assays or symptoms of recurrent chest pain. The remaining patients underwent stress testing (either exercise treadmill or pharmacologic) after which 55 were admitted. Ninety-seven patients had a negative stress test and were discharged to their homes with outpatient follow-up within 72 hours. The use of selected cardiac tests and procedures and cardiac rehospitalizations was greater in patients randomized to initial hospital admission through six months follow-up (p = 0.003). During the 6-month study duration, patients randomized to initial hospital admission incurred 61% more costs (measured with cumulative cost weights) than patients randomized to the chest pain unit. This study's 38% reduction in cost from use of a chest pain unit versus standard care diagnostic strategy is similar to results from the studies reported in Table 4.

Cardiac-specific troponins are the preferred risk stratification biomarkers for patients suspected of ACS [48]. While clinical studies have shown that cardiac troponins can provide additional prognostic information in chest pain patients over that available from assays CK alone, their incremental value has not been assessed in randomized studies [49–51]. Two observational studies tested the hypothesis that routine cardiac troponin testing may improve diagnostic accuracy and lead to reduced lengths of stay in chest pain patients [52]. Heeschen and colleagues performed troponin testing on 812 consecutive patients at emergency admission and 4 hours later [53]. When admission decisions were based upon clinical symptoms, echocardiograph (ECG) findings, and CK-MB results, 65% of patients were admitted for 4.2 days average length of stay. However, no patients with negative troponin tests and ECGs without ST-T changes experienced cardiac events during 30 days follow-up. These researchers estimated that had hospital admission been restricted to patients with positive troponin tests and ST-T changes on ECGs, total costs of care would be reduced by 14%. These results were confirmed in a similarly designed US study that found routine troponin testing was associated with shorter lengths of stay and reduced costs (variable and total) in lower risk patients [54]. While troponin use may improve efficiency of ED evaluation of chest pain patients, its use in low probability patients as a screening tool for acute coronary syndrome may lead to inappropriate CCU admissions and increased costs. The extent to which such overuse negates the benefits of appropriate use needs to be determined.

## Reperfusion Therapies

*Pharmacological Reperfusion*

Although earlier studies modeled the economic attractiveness of reperfusion therapies, the GUSTO-I economics and quality of life study was the first to compare the incremental economic attractiveness of tissue plasminogen activator (t-PA) versus streptokinase in ST-elevation acute MI patients using prospectively collected resource utilization information [55]. Mark and colleagues found that cumulative 1-year inpatient costs exclusive of thrombolysis were similar for patients in both study arms. However, because of the disparity in thrombolytic agent costs (AWP of streptokinase $320; t-PA $2750) [56], the incremental 1-year cost of the t-PA treatment strategy was $2845 greater than streptokinase. These investigators estimated a 0.09 year discounted survival advantage for t-PA versus streptokinase patients, with a resulting cost-effectiveness ratio of $32,678 per YOLS. Since GUSTO-I, two other recombinant thrombolytics have been introduced that are mutants of the t-PA molecule (reteplase and tenecteplase) [11,57]. However, as their costs and efficacy are similar to that of t-PA, it is generally felt that all three agents have similar economic attractiveness [58].

Attempts to improve the clinical effectiveness and safety of pharmacologic reperfusion has led to the combination of thrombolytic agents with glycoprotein IIb/IIIa platelet inhibitors and low-molecular-weight heparin [59,60]. The ASSENT 3 investigators compared three treatment regimens: tenecteplase plus enoxaparin; half-dose tenecteplase plus low-dose unfractionated heparin and abciximab; and tenecteplase plus unfractionated heparin [60]. Both the enoxaparin and abciximab regimens reduced acute MI complications when compared with the unfractionated heparin regimen [60]. Recently, Kaul and colleagues performed an economic analysis using data from the ASSENT 3 study [61]. They found that resource consumption patterns (readmissions, cardiac procedure use, and lengths of stay) were similar among all three treatment regimens and that cost differences were largely driven by differences in study medication costs. At 30-days follow-up, enoxaparin was the least costly regimen ($410 less than costs for unfractionated heparin patients). The enoxaparin regimen proved to be cost saving versus the unfractionated heparin regimen in 80% of bootstrap samples.

*Mechanical Reperfusion*

Initial studies concluded that primary angioplasty was economically neutral versus pharmacological reperfusion [62–66]. However, these findings were predicated upon the presumption that facilities and personnel to do these procedures were already in place. A recent decision analysis found that primary angioplasty could be cost saving versus thrombolytic therapy in a hospital with an existing catheterization laboratory, night/weekend staffing coverage, and admitting more than 200 MI patients annually. However, primary angioplasty would not be economically attractive in a lower volume institution particularly when new laboratories needed to be constructed and new personnel hired [67]. These issues prompted studies such as AIR-PAMI and DANAMI 2 to investigate a patient management strategy of transfer for emergency angioplasty versus onsite thrombolytic therapy [68–70]. Recently, the CAPTIM study compared treatment strategies involving prehospital thrombolysis with transfer to an interventional facility. Unfortunately, none of the studies comparing patient transfer for intervention with thrombolytic therapy (inhospital or prehospital) have reported prospective economic substudies that evaluated the incremental costs of emergency transportation versus the reported reduction in cardiac events. The DANAMI group has an economic analysis in preparation. The Stenting versus Thrombolysis in Acute myocardial infarction Trial (STAT) randomized 62 acute MI patients to primary stenting and 61 to accelerated t-PA at a single center in Ontario Canada between 1997 and 1999 [71]. The primary finding of the trial was a significant reduction in the composite primary event rate for the stenting arm. A cost analysis of the trial was published recently [72]. The stent arm had a $1500 lower hospital cost (p < 0.05) due to a combination of lower reperfusion therapy/invasive therapy costs and shorter length of stay (6.7 days for stent arm versus 8.7 for t-PA). In this small study, 64% of the t-PA arm underwent in-hospital catheterization on the basis of perceived clinical need (not protocol-driven).

Clinical trials have demonstrated significant clinical benefits for primary stenting versus primary angioplasty [73–75]. In a randomized study of 227 patients, Suryapranata and colleagues found a significant reduction in 6-month event-free survival (95% vs. 80%, p = 0.012 for death, re-MI, subsequent CABG, or target vessel revascularization (TVR) [74]. In this trial's economic substudy, van't Hof and colleagues compared resource utilization and costs through 12 months of follow-up and observed that in-hospital costs were lower for patients treated with primary angioplasty ($15,322 vs. $17,508). However, 1-year costs were similar between patient groups (primary angioplasty $22,107 vs. primary stenting $21,418) due to higher follow-up rates of re-MI, re-PTCA, and CABG for primary angioplasty patients [76]. In the PAMI-STENT study, 900 ST-elevation MI patients were randomized to primary stent versus balloon angioplasty [77]. At 6-month follow-up 12.6% of primary stent and 20.1% of balloon angioplasty (p < 0.01) had reached the composite cardiovascular endpoint. However, the decrease in events was entirely attributable to a reduced need for target-vessel revascularization. Cohen and colleagues conducted a prospective economic analysis and found that while stenting increased baseline procedure costs ($6538 vs. $4561, p < 0.001), these patients had significantly fewer revascularizations and rehospitalizations [77]. At one year, cumulative costs for stent patients were approximately $1000 greater; however, with current stent technology and pricing, this difference was projected to fall to less than $350. Assuming primary stenting did not increase 1-year mortality by more than 0.2%, its cost utility versus balloon angioplasty was estimated at less than $50,000 per quality-adjusted life year gained.

While several studies have investigated the use of abciximab in conjunction with primary intervention (with and without stents), CADILLAC is the only study with a prospective economic analysis [78–81]. CADILLAC randomized AMI patients to four interventional strategies: PTCA alone, PTCA plus abciximab, stent alone, and stent plus abciximab. Primary stenting (with or without abciximab) was clinically superior to PTCA (with or without abciximab) at six months follow-up [79]. Bakhai and colleagues performed a cost-effectiveness analysis of US patients enrolled in the CADILLAC study, comparing stent versus PTCA and abciximab versus no abciximab [81]. These investigators found that stent use increased initial hospitalization costs by $1384 (p = 0.001); however, this cost difference was reduced to $169 (p = 0.75) at one year follow-up. The cost-effectiveness ratio for stent versus PTCA was $11,237 per QALY (based upon quality of life differences assigned to repeat revascularizations). Although abciximab increased procedural costs, its use was associated with a 0.6 day reduction in length of stay. Initial hospitalization costs were only $413 greater with abciximab use (p = 0.13); however, cumulative costs at one-year were $1244 greater for the abciximab-treated patients (p = 0.02) with no difference in quality of life. Thus, standard anticoagulation (i.e., no abciximab) was cost saving when compared with routine abciximab use.

## Antithrombin and Antiplatelet Therapies

Unfortunately, neither the most commonly used antithrombin (unfractionated heparin) nor antiplatelet (aspirin) therapies have been the subject of a formal economic analysis. Thus, while there is strong belief among practitioners that aspirin is cost saving and that heparin may be economically attractive in certain populations, there is no evidence to substantiate these beliefs [82]. In this section, the authors will review the results from economic studies of newer direct antithrombin (low-molecular-weight heparin) and antiplatelet (clopidogrel and glycoprotein [GP] IIb/IIIa platelet inhibitor) therapies in non–ST-elevation ACS patients.

Recent research in antithrombins has focused on novel anticoagulants (e.g., direct antithrombins and low-molecular-weight heparins) in non–ST-elevation ACS patients. Although the early benefits of the direct thrombin hirudin were shown to diminish over time, the low-molecular-weight heparin enoxaparin has demonstrated a durable treatment effect versus unfractionated heparin [83–88]. The ESSENCE clinical trial reported an initial 16% relative reduction (16.6% vs. 19.8%, p = 0.019) in the composite endpoint of death, MI, or recurrent angina at 14 days which was sustained at 30 days (19.8% vs. 23.3%, p = 0.016) for patients receiving low-molecular-weight heparin versus those receiving unfractionated heparin [86]. A prospective economic analysis using US patients enrolled in ESSENCE examined whether the increased cost of enoxaparin versus unfractionated heparin ($155 vs. $80 per patient) would be offset by cost savings in the initial 30 days after treatment [87]. During the index hospitalization, patients receiving enoxaparin consumed fewer medical resources than patients receiving heparin (e.g., PTCA 15% vs. 20%, p = 0.04) and had lower inpatient (hospital and physician) costs ($11,857 vs. $12,620, p = 0.18). Through 30 days follow-up the trend toward less medical resource consumption with enoxaparin persisted (e.g., diagnostic catheterization 57% vs. 63%, p = 0.04 and ICU days 2.4 vs. 2.8, p = 0.05) resulting in significantly lower cumulative inpatient costs for enoxaparin-treated patients ($13,155 vs. $14,357, p = 0.04). Since the enoxaparin treatment strategy demonstrated both a clinical and an economic ($1202 cost-saving) benefit versus unfractionated heparin, it was considered a dominant strategy [87].

Although the economic attractiveness of GP IIb/IIIa platelet inhibitors has been demonstrated in decision-analytic and other economic models, PURSUIT is the only clinical trial to include a prospective economic analysis in its design (4,89–91). The PURSUIT clinical trial randomized ACS patients (unstable angina or non–Q-wave myocardial infarction) to eptifibatide therapy or placebo and observed a 1.5% absolute reduction (15.7% vs. 14.2%, p = 0.042) in the composite endpoint of death or MI at 30 days for patients treated with eptifibatide [92]. In the US PURSUIT economic analysis, no significant difference in average inpatient costs (hospital plus physician) was detected between eptifibatide-treated and placebo patients exclusive of the cost of eptifibatide (index hospitalization $14,729 vs. $14,957, p>0.10; cumulative 6-month costs $18,456 vs. $18,828, p >0.10). Thus, the only cost difference between treatment strategies was that of the drug itself ($1217) [91]. Using the 6-month PURSUIT follow-up data, the PURSUIT investigators estimated that the life expectancy for patients receiving eptifibatide would be 15.96 years (vs. 15.85 years for patients receiving placebo), resulting in a cost-effectiveness ratio of $16,491 per YOLS. Since ACS survivors rated their health at 0.84 on a 0 (death) to 1 (excellent health) utility scale, the corresponding cost-utility ratio was $23,449 per QALY.

Two large clinical trials have established the benefits of clopidogrel therapy for secondary prevention in ACS patients. The CAPRIE trial found that long-term administration of clopidogrel was more effective than aspirin in reducing cardiac events (vascular death, ischemic stroke, or myocardial infarction) (5.3% vs. 5.8% per year, p = 0.043) [93], while the CURE trial reported that clopidogrel plus aspirin was more effective than aspirin alone in reducing cardiac events (cardiovascular death, stroke, or MI) (9.3% vs. 11.4%, relative risk 0.80) at less than 6 months average follow-up [94]. Although neither trial has published a formal economic analysis, Gaspoz et al. simulated the application of these results to the US population using the Coronary Heart Disease Policy Model and found that the use of clopidogrel for aspirin-intolerant patients cost less than $11,000 per QALY; however, the routine use of clopidogrel was not economically attractive (cost

>$130,000 per QALY) [95]. The difficulty with this analysis is that it assumed that patients were on lifetime clopidogrel therapy. In contrast, patients in the CURE trial continued therapy for an average of 9 months. An economic analysis by the CURE investigators using the shorter duration of therapy is ongoing [96].


## Cardiac Procedures

The use of cardiac procedures and longer hospital lengths of stay are the two most expensive decisions that clinicians make and thus have been the focus of several important cost management studies. Calvin and colleagues used four variables from the Braunwald unstable angina classification system along with patient age and history of diabetes to predict the occurrence of major in-hospital cardiac complications in unstable angina patients [97,98]. Although these clinical variables accurately predicted major complications, collectively they explained only 4.7% of the variance in these patients' total hospital costs. In contrast, the use of cardiac procedures alone explained an additional 32.9% of the variance [99]. When these researchers compared resource utilization across four risk groups defined by their probability of major complication (i.e., ≤2.0%, 2.1%–5.0%, 5.1%–15.0%, and ≥15.1%), they found that more than half of the patients in each group were admitted to the CCU, but there were no differences in the use of coronary angiography and percutaneous coronary interventions among risk groups. The principal risk-based resource use difference was that higher risk patients were more likely to undergo CABG surgery than lower risk patients. These results confirm that treatment-related factors (i.e., cardiac procedures and lengths of stay) rather than patient-related factors are the primary determinants of ACS patient costs (29,100,101).

Coronary angiography has received a great deal of attention from those seeking to control ACS patient costs because it functions as a gatekeeper for the more expensive cardiac revascularization procedures [102]. Although large variances in the use of coronary angiography have been well documented, higher usage rates have not been associated with better patient outcomes [103–106], but appear to be directly related to the availability of coronary angiography facilities in a given geographic area [107–110].

The TIMI IIIB clinical trial investigated the relative effectiveness of an early invasive versus an early conservative patient management strategy in patients with unstable angina and non-Q-wave myocardial infarction and found no difference in cardiac event rates (i.e., death and nonfatal MI) between patient management strategies [111]. More recently, the TACTICS-TIMI 18 investigators reported that the use of an early invasive strategy (i.e., routine catheterization within 4 to 48 hours with revascularization as appropriate) versus a more conservative strategy (i.e., selectively invasive) reduced the incidence of six month death, nonfatal MI, or rehospitalization for ACS in unstable angina and non–ST-elevation MI patients treated with GP IIb/IIIa platelet inhibitor therapy (15.9% vs. 19.4%, p = 0.025) [112]. Mahoney and colleagues examined the economic attractiveness of this study's findings [113]. Although initial hospitalization costs were higher for the early invasive versus the more conservative strategy ($1667 difference, 95% confidence interval, $387–$3091), much of this difference was offset during the 6 month follow-up period. When lost productive costs were included, the incremental 6-month costs for the early invasive strategy were $586 (95% confidence interval, −$1087 to $2486). When lost productivity costs were excluded, the difference was $670 (95% confidence interval, −$1035 to $2321). The estimated cost per year of life gained was $12,739 with the aggressive versus conservative strategy.

## Early Discharge

Reductions in length of stay (ICU and regular room) have been a primary focus of many ACS patient management strategies [114]. For example, lengths of stay at Duke University Medical Center for acute MI patients were reduced from 10.6 days in 1986 to 7.8 days in 1997 and those for unstable angina patients were reduced from 11.7 to 4.7 days during that period (E. Eisenstein unpublished data).

Newby and colleagues used clinical data from GUSTO-I to investigate the potential for early discharge in acute MI patients who were uncomplicated at 96 hours [115]. Early discharge criteria included the absence of death, reinfarction, ischemia, stroke, shock, heart failure (Killip class >1), CABG surgery, balloon pumping, emergency catheterization, or cardioversion/defibrillation in the first four days. Patients meeting these criteria had 1.0% mortality at 30 days and 3.6% mortality at one year. Using these risk-stratification criteria, 57.3% of GUSTO-I patients were "uncomplicated" and eligible for discharge on day four; their actual mean length of stay was 8.9 days [116]. Eisenstein and colleagues used information from the GUSTO-I economic substudy to simulate the cost effects of Newby's early discharge criteria [116]. Average costs for US uncomplicated patients were $15,825 vs. $24,582 for complicated patients before implementing Newby's early discharge criteria. Assuming uncomplicated AMI patients were discharged on day four, their average index hospitalization costs could be reduced by 26.5% to $11,624.

In a subsequent analysis, Newby estimated the cost effectiveness of the fourth hospital day for uncomplicated acute MI patients [117]. This analysis was based on GUSTO-I data and assumed that the only preventable in-hospital deaths were patients who had VT/VF on day four. The incremental cost of a regular room with telemetry and physician care was $624 and the life expectancy benefit of the fourth hospital day was 0.006 years yielding a cost-effectiveness ratio of $105,629 per YOLS for the fourth hospital day in uncomplicated acute MI patients. However, this analysis assumed that all required testing and patient education can be completed by 72 hours, and most hospitals in the US would be unable to achieve this level of efficiency at present.

### Quality Management

The American College of Cardiology and the American Heart Association have jointly produced ischemic heart disease management guidelines to assist physicians in defining the optimal range of practice [118–120]. Recently, Chen and colleagues compared care for acute myocardial infarction patients provided by "America's Best Hospitals," as defined by U.S. News and World Report, with that offered in other hospitals [121]. These researchers found that admission to "America's Best Hospitals" was associated with greater aspirin and beta blocker use, less use of reperfusion therapy, and lower adjusted 30-day mortality (p = 0.05). However, this survival advantage diminished after adjusting for treatment received (e.g., aspirin and beta blockers) (p = 0.38). Recently, the CRU-SADE registry compared rates of ACC/AHA guideline adherence with adjusted in-hospital mortality in 44,158 non-ST elevation ACS patients treated at 400 medical centers [122,123]. These researchers found an inverse relationship between guideline adherence and mortality, ranging from 3.6% mortality in hospitals with more than 80% adherence to 5.9% mortality in hospitals with less than 65%. Thus, hospitals with less than 65% adherence have the potential to achieve greater in-hospital mortality reductions through increased guideline adherence than has been reported for most ACS therapies.

Several studies investigated factors associated with greater/lesser guideline adherence among physicians and hospitals [122,124–127]. Generally, hospitals with greater adherence have: shared goals for improvement, substantial administrative support, strong physician leadership, and use credible data feedback. In a recent meta-analysis of ACS quality improvement initiatives in randomized trials and observational studies, Chen and Scott found that the audit and feedback mechanism was associated with improvements in time to reperfusion; aspirin, beta blocker, and ACE inhibitor use; and 30-day mortality [127]. While many of these quality improvement interventions appear to be economically attractive, there have been no systematic economic studies that assessed cost versus health benefit and highlighted those techniques that were associated with greater overall value.

## CONCLUSION

It is now clear that the short-term effect of managed care expansion has ended, and current projections are that health expenditures will increase to 15.5% of the US Gross Domestic Product in 2007 [128]. Thus, at a time when we are receiving ever-diminishing clinical returns from successive investments in new medical technologies, our society's willingness to fund these technologies may be diminishing. In this environment, questions of value in health expenditures and how to achieve it (e.g., new technology investment versus guideline implementation) will likely become even more important.

## ACKNOWLEDGMENT

We acknowledge the editorial assistance of Maqui Ortiz and Melanie Daniels.

## REFERENCES

1.  Getzen TE. Health economics: fundamentals and flow of funds. New York: John Wiley & Sons, 1997.
2.  CDC Faststats A-Z. Centers for Disease Control National Center for Health Statistics, 2003.
3.  Jacobs E, Shipp S. How family spending has changed in the United-States. Mon Labor Rev 1990;113:20–27.
4.  Eisenstein EL, Peterson ED, Jollis JG, Tardiff BE, Califf RM, Knight JD, Mark DB. Evaluating the potential 'economic attractiveness' of new therapies in patients with non-ST elevation acute coronary syndrome. Pharmacoeconomics 2000;17:263–272.
5.  Health United States 1998. Health Care Financing Administration. In: http://www.cdc.gov/nchs/fastats/pdf/hu98t119.pdf. Accessed March 06, 2000.
6.  Day HW. An intensive coronary care area. Dis Chest 1963;44:423–427.
7.  Koch EB, Reiser SJ. Critical care: historical development and ethical considerations. In: Fein IA , Strosbers MA, Eds. Managing the clinical care unit. Rockville. MD: Aspen, 1987:3–20.
8.  Hilberman M. The evolution of intensive care units. Crit Care Med 1975;3:159–165.
9.  Reiser SJ. The intensive care unit. The unfolding ambiguities of survival therapy. Int J Technol Assess Health Care 1992;8:382–394.
10. Weaver WD, Simes RJ, Betriu A, Grines CL, Zijlstra F, Garcia E, Grinfeld L, Gibbons RJ, Ribeiro EE, DeWood MA, Ribichini F. Comparison of primary coronary angioplasty and intravenous thrombolytic therapy for acute myocardial infarction: a quantitative review. JAMA 1997;278:2093–2098.
11. The ASSENT-2 Investigators. Single-bolus tenecteplase compared with front-loaded alteplase in acute myocardial infarction: the ASSENT-2 double-blind randomised trial. Assessment of the Safety and Efficacy of a New Thrombolytic Investigators. Lancet 1999;354:716–722.
12. Nagle TT, Holden RK. The strategy and tactics of pricing: a guide to profitable decision making, Upper Saddle River, Prentice Hall. 2002.

13. Mark DB, Topol EJ. Chronic coronary artery disease. In: Talley JD, Mauldin PD, Becker ER, Eds. Cost effective diagnosis and treatment of coronary artery disease. Baltimore. MD: Williams & Wilkins, 1997:168–177.

14. Califf RM, Eisenstein EL. Cost-effectiveness of therapy for acute ischemic heart disease. In: Talley JD, Ed. Cost-effective diagnosis and treatment of coronary artery disease, Igaku-Shoin. 1997:139–167.

15. Doubilet P, Weinstein MC, McNeil BJ. Use and misuse of the term "cost effective" in medicine. N Engl J Med 1986;314:253–256.

16. Goldman L, Weinstein MC, Goldman PA, Williams LW. Cost-effectiveness of HMG-CoA reductase inhibition for primary and secondary prevention of coronary heart disease. JAMA 1991;265:1145–1151.

17. US Renal Data System. USRDS 2002 Annual Data Report. Bethesda, MD: NIH, National Institutes of Diabetes and Digestive and Kidney Diseases, 2002.

18. Mark DB. Medical economics in cardiovascular medicine. In: Topol EJ, Ed. Textbook of cardiovascular medicine. New York. NY: Lippincott-Raven, 1997:1033–1062.

19. Hadorn DC. Setting health care priorities in Oregon. Cost-effectiveness meets the rule of rescue. JAMA 1991;265:2218–2225.

20. Eddy DM. Oregon's methods. Did cost-effectiveness analysis fail? JAMA 1991;266: 2135–2141.

21. Leichter HM. Oregon's bold experiment: whatever happened to rationing? J Health Polit Policy Law 1999;24:147–160.

22. Mason J, Drummond M, Torrance G. Some guidelines on the use of cost effectiveness league tables. Br Med J 1993;306:570–572.

23. Glassman PA, Model KE, Kahan JP, Jacobson PD, Peabody JW. The role of medical necessity and cost-effectiveness in making medical decisions. Ann Intern Med 1997;126:152–156.

24. Finkler SA. Cost accounting for health care organizations. Rockville. MD: Aspen Publishers, 1994.

25. Gold MR, Siegel JE, Russell LB, Weinstein MC. Cost-effectiveness in health and medicine. New York. NY: Oxford University Press, 1996.

26. Lipscomb J, Mark DB, Cowper PA. Comparison of hospital costs derived from cost-to-charge ratios and from a detailed cost accounting system for patients undergoing cardiac procedures. Associated Health Services Research Conference, 1994.

27. Ashby JL. The accuracy of cost measures derived from Medicare cost report data. Hospital (Rio J) 1992;3:1–8.

28. Barnett PG. Research without billing data. Econometric estimation of patient-specific costs. Med Care 1997;35:553–563.

29. Eisenstein EL, Shaw LK, Anstrom KJ, Nelson CL, Hakim Z, Hasselblad V, Mark DB. Assessing the clinical and economic burden of coronary artery disease: 1986–1998. Med Care 2001;39:824–35.

30. Detsky AS. Using cost-effectiveness analysis for formulary decision making: from theory into practice. Pharmacoeconomics 1994;6:281–288.

31. Hornberger JC, Redelmeier DA, Petersen J. Variability among methods to assess patients' well-being and consequent effect on a cost-effectiveness analysis. J Clin Epidemiol 1992; 45:505–512.

32. Naimark D, Naglie G, Detsky AS. The meaning of life expectancy: what is a clinically significant gain? J Gen Intern Med 1994;9:702–7.

33. Tsevat J, Weinstein MC, Williams LW, Tosteson AN, Goldman L. Expected gains in life expectancy from various coronary heart disease risk factor modifications. Circulation 1991; 83:1194–1201.

34. Wright JC, Weinstein MC. Gains in life expectancy from medical interventions--standardizing data on outcomes. N Engl J Med 1998;339:380–386.

35. Barish RA, Doherty RJ, Browne BJ. Reengineering the emergency evaluation of chest pain. J Healthc Qual 1997;19:6–12.

36. National Center for Health Statistics. National Hospital Ambulatory Medical Care Survey: 1995 Emergency Department Survey. Advance data from vital health statistics. Hyattsville. MD: Public Health Service, 1997.

37. The DRG handbook: comparative clinical and financial standards. Baltimore. MD: HCIA, 1997.
38. Newby LK, Gibler WB, Christenson RH, Ohman EM. Serum markers for diagnosis and risk stratification in acute coronary syndromes. In: Cannon CP, Ed. Contemporary cardiology: management of acute coronary syndromes. Totowa. NJ: Humana Press Inc, 1998:147–217.
39. Jesse RL, Kontos MC. Evaluation of chest pain in the emergency department. Curr Probl Cardiol 1997;22:149–236.
40. Farkouh ME, Smars PA, Reeder GS, Zinsmeister AR, Evans RW, Meloy TD, Kopecky SL, Allen M, Allison TG, Gibbons RJ, Gabriel SE. A clinical trial of a chest-pain observation unit for patients with unstable angina. Chest Pain Evaluation in the Emergency Room (CHEER) Investigators. N Engl J Med 1998;339:1882–1888.
41. Gomez MA, Anderson JL, Karagounis LA, Muhlestein JB, Mooers FB. An emergency department-based protocol for rapidly ruling out myocardial ischemia reduces hospital time and expense: results of a randomized study (ROMIO). J Am Coll Cardiol 1996;28:25–33.
42. Gaspoz JM, Lee TH, Weinstein MC, Cook EF, Goldman P, Komaroff AL, Goldman L. Cost-effectiveness of a new short-stay unit to ''rule out'' acute myocardial infarction in low risk patients. J Am Coll Cardiol 1994;24:1249–1259.
43. Mikhail MG, Smith FA, Gray M, Britton C, Frederiksen SM. Cost-effectiveness of mandatory stress testing in chest pain center patients. Ann Emerg Med 1997;29:88–98.
44. Roberts RR, Zalenski RJ, Mensah EK, Rydman RJ, Ciavarella G, Gussow L, Das K, Kampe LM, Dickover B, McDermott MF, Hart A, Straus HE, Murphy DG, Rao R. Costs of an emergency department-based accelerated diagnostic protocol vs. hospitalization in patients with chest pain: a randomized controlled trial. JAMA 1997;278:1670–1676.
45. Newby LK, Califf RM. Identifying patient risk: the basis for rational discharge planning after acute myocardial infarction. J Thromb Thrombolysis 1996;3:107–115.
46. Braunwald E, Mark DB, Jones RHet al. Unstable angina: diagnosis and management.Agency for Health Care Policy and Research. Pamphlet #94–0682. Rockville. MD: U.S. Department of Health and Human Services, 1994.
47. Katz DA, Griffith JL, Beshansky JR, Selker HP. The use of empiric clinical data in the evaluation of practice guidelines for unstable angina. JAMA 1996;276:1568–1574.
48. Braunwald E, Antman EM, Beasley JW, Califf RM, Cheitlin MD, Hochman JS, Jones RH, Kereiakes D, Kupersmith J, Levin TN, Pepine CJ, Schaeffer JW, Smith EE, Steward DE, Theroux P, Gibbons RJ, Alpert JS, Eagle KA, Faxon DP, Fuster V, Gardner TJ, Gregoratos G, Russell RO, Smith SC. ACC/AHA guidelines for the management of patients with unstable angina and non-ST-segment elevation myocardial infarction: executive summary and recommendations. A report of the American College of Cardiology/American Heart Association task force on practice guidelines (committee on the management of patients with unstable angina). Circulation 2000;102:1193–1209.
49. Green GB, Beaudreau RW, Chan DW, DeLong D, Kelley CA, Kelen GD. Use of troponin T and creatine kinase-MB subunit levels for risk stratification of emergency department patients with possible myocardial ischemia. Ann Emerg Med 1998;31:19–29.
50. Tucker JF, Collins RA, Anderson AJ, Hauser J, Kalas J, Apple FS. Early diagnostic efficiency of cardiac troponin I and Troponin T for acute myocardial infarction. Acad Emerg Med 1997; 4:13–21.
51. Hamm CW, Goldmann BU, Heeschen C, Kreymann G, Berger J, Meinertz T. Emergency room triage of patients with acute chest pain by means of rapid testing for cardiac troponin T or troponin I. N Engl J Med 1997;337:1648–1653.
52. Collinson PO. Troponin T or troponin I or CK-MB (or none?). Eur Heart J 1998;19(Suppl N):N16–N24.
53. Heeschen C, Hamm CW, Goldmann BU, Moeller RH, Meinertz T. [Cost-effectiveness of a rapid test for troponin in emergency admissions]. Dtsch Med Wochenschr 1998;123: 1229–1234.
54. Anderson FP, Fritz ML, Kontos MC, McPherson RA, Jesse RL. Cost-effectiveness of cardiac troponin I in a systematic chest pain evaluation protocol: use of cardiac troponin I lowers length of stay for low-risk cardiac patients. Clin Lab Manage Rev 1998;12(2):63–69.

55. Mark DB, Hlatky MA, Califf RM, Naylor CD, Lee KL, Armstrong PW, Barbash G, White H, Simoons ML, Nelson CL. Cost effectiveness of thrombolytic therapy with tissue plasminogen activator as compared with streptokinase for acute myocardial infarction. N Engl J Med 1995; 332:1418–1424.

56. 1994 drug topics red book. Montvale. NJ: Medical Economics Data, 1994.

57. Topol EJ, Ohman EM, Armstrong PW, Wilcox R, Skene AM, Aylward P, Simes J, Dalby A, Betriu A, Bode C, White HD, Hochman JS, Emanuelson H, Vahanian A, Sapp S, Stebbins A, Moliterno DJ, Califf RM. Survival outcomes 1 year after reperfusion therapy with either alteplase or reteplase for acute myocardial infarction: results from the Global Utilization of Streptokinase and t-PA for Occluded Coronary Arteries (GUSTO) III Trial. Circulation 2000; 102:1761–1765.

58. Mark DB. Ecomomics of therapy for acute coronary syndromes. In: Weintraub WS, Ed. Cardiovascular health care economics. Totowa. NJ: Humana Press, 2003:173–185.

59. Topol EJ. Reperfusion therapy for acute myocardial infarction with fibrinolytic therapy or combination reduced fibrinolytic therapy and platelet glycoprotein IIb/IIIa inhibition: the GUSTO V randomised trial. Lancet 2001;357:1905–1914.

60. The ASSENT 3 Investigators. Efficacy and safety of tenecteplase in combination with enoxaparin, abciximab, or unfractionated heparin: the ASSENT-3 randomised trial in acute myocardial infarction. Lancet 2001;358:605–613.

61. Kaul P, Armstrong PW, Cowper PA, Eisenstein EL, Granger CB, Van de Werf F, Mark DB. Economic analysis of the assessment of the ssafety and efficacy of a new thrombolytic regimen (ASSENT-3) study: costs of reperfusion strategies in acute myocardial infarction. Am Heart J 2004:in press.

62. Reeder GS, Bailey KR, Gersh BJ, Holmes DR, Christianson J, Gibbons RJ. Cost comparison of immediate angioplasty versus thrombolysis followed by conservative therapy for acute myocardial infarction: a randomized prospective trial. Mayo Coronary Care Unit and Catheterization Laboratory Groups. Mayo Clin Proc 1994;69:5–12.

63. de Boer MJ, van Hout BA, Liem AL, Suryapranata H, Hoorntje JC, Zijlstra F. A cost-effective analysis of primary coronary angioplasty versus thrombolysis for acute myocardial infarction. Am J Cardiol 1995;76:830–833.

64. Zijlstra F, de Boer MJ, Hoorntje JC, Reiffers S, Reiber JH, Suryapranata H. A comparison of immediate coronary angioplasty with intravenous streptokinase in acute myocardial infarction. N Engl J Med 1993;328:680–684.

65. Stone GW, Grines CL, Rothbaum D, Browne KF, O'Keefe J, Overlie PA, Donohue BC, Chelliah N, Vlietstra R, Catlin T, O'Neill WW. Analysis of the relative costs and effectiveness of primary angioplasty versus tissue-type plasminogen activator: the Primary Angioplasty in Myocardial Infarction (PAMI) trial. The PAMI Trial Investigators. J Am Coll Cardiol 1997; 29:901–907.

66. Beatt KJ, Fath-Ordoubadi F. Angioplasty for the treatment of acute myocardial infarction. Heart 1997;78(Suppl 2):12–15.

67. Lieu TA, Gurley RJ, Lundstrom RJ, Ray GT, Fireman BH, Weinstein MC, Parmley WW. Projected cost-effectiveness of primary angioplasty for acute myocardial infarction. J Am Coll Cardiol 1997;30:1741–1750.

68. Grines CL, Westerhausen DR, Grines LL, Hanlon JT, Logemann TL, Niemela M, Weaver WD, Graham M, Boura J, O'Neill WW, Balestrini C. A randomized trial of transfer for primary angioplasty versus on-site thrombolysis in patients with high-risk myocardial infarction: the Air Primary Angioplasty in Myocardial Infarction study. J Am Coll Cardiol 2002; 39:1713–1719.

69. Andersen HR, Nielsen TT, Vesterlund T, Grande P, Abildgaard U, Thayssen P, Pedersen F, Mortensen LS. Danish multicenter randomized study on fibrinolytic therapy versus acute coronary angioplasty in acute myocardial infarction: rationale and design of the DANish trial in Acute Myocardial Infarction-2 (DANAMI-2). Am Heart J 2003;146:234–241.

70. Cannon CP, Baim DS. Expanding the reach of primary percutaneous coronary intervention for the treatment of acute myocardial infarction. J Am Coll Cardiol 2002;39:1720–1722.

71. Le May MR, Labinaz M, Davies RF, Marquis JF, Laramee LA, O'Brien ER, Williams WL, Beanlands RS, Nichol G, Higginson LA. Stenting versus thrombolysis in acute myocardial infarction trial (STAT). J Am Coll Cardiol 2001;37:985–991.

72. Le May MR, Davies RF, Labinaz M, Sherrard H, Marquis JF, Laramee LA, O'Brien ER, Williams WL, Beanlands RS, Nichol G, Higginson LA. Hospitalization costs of primary stenting versus thrombolysis in acute myocardial infarction: cost analysis of the Canadian STAT Study. Circulation 2003;108:2624–2630.

73. Steinhubl SR, Topol EJ. Stenting for acute myocardial infarction. Lancet 1997;350:532–533.

74. Suryapranata H, van't Hof AW, Hoorntje JC, de Boer MJ, Zijlstra F. Randomized comparison of coronary stenting with balloon angioplasty in selected patients with acute myocardial infarction. Circulation 1998;97:2502–2505.

75. Grines CL, Cox DA, Stone GW, Garcia E, Mattos LA, Giambartolomei A, Brodie BR, Madonna O, Eijgelshoven M, Lansky AJ, O'Neill WW, Morice MC. Coronary angioplasty with or without stent implantation for acute myocardial infarction. Stent Primary Angioplasty in Myocardial Infarction Study Group. N Engl J Med 1999;341:1949–1956.

76. van 't Hof AW, Suryapranata H, de Boer MJ, Hoorntje JC, Zijlstra F. Costs of stenting for acute myocardial infarction. Lancet 1998;351:1817.

77. Cohen DJ, Taira DA, Berezin R, Cox DA, Morice MC, Stone GW, Grines CL. Cost-effectiveness of coronary stenting in acute myocardial infarction: results from the stent primary angioplasty in myocardial infarction (stent-PAMI) trial. Circulation 2001;104:3039–3045.

78. Brener SJ, Barr LA, Burchenal JE, Katz S, George BS, Jones AA, Cohen ED, Gainey PC, White HJ, Cheek HB, Moses JW, Moliterno DJ, Effron MB, Topol EJ. Randomized, placebo-controlled trial of platelet glycoprotein IIb/IIIa blockade with primary angioplasty for acute myocardial infarction. ReoPro and Primary PTCA Organization and Randomized Trial (RAPPORT) Investigators. Circulation 1998;98:734–741.

79. Stone GW, Grines CL, Cox DA, Garcia E, Tcheng JE, Griffin JJ, Guagliumi G, Stuckey T, Turco M, Carroll JD, Rutherford BD, Lansky AJ. Comparison of angioplasty with stenting, with or without abciximab, in acute myocardial infarction. N Engl J Med 2002;346:957–966.

80. The ADMIRAL Investigators:Montalescot G, Barragan P, Wittenberg O, Ecollan P, Elhadad S, Villain P, Boulenc JM, Morice MC, Maillard L, Pansieri M, Choussat R, Pinton P. Platelet glycoprotein IIb/IIIa inhibition with coronary stenting for acute myocardial infarction. N Engl J Med, 2001.

81. Bakhai A, Stone GW, Grines CL, Murphy SA, Githiora L, Berezin RH, Cox DA, Stuckey T, Griffin JJ, Tcheng JE, Cohen DJ. Cost-effectiveness of coronary stenting and abciximab for patients with acute myocardial infarction: results from the CADILLAC (Controlled Abciximab and Device Investigation to Lower Late Angioplasty Complications) trial. Circulation 2003;108:2857–2863.

82. Krumholz HM. Cost-effectiveness analysis and the treatment of acute coronary syndromes. In: Cannon CP, Ed. Contemporary cardiology: management of acute coronary syndromes. Totowa. NJ: Human Press, 1998:601–610.

83. Antman EM. Hirudin in acute myocardial infarction. Thrombolysis and Thrombin Inhibition in Myocardial Infarction (TIMI) 9B trial. Circulation 1996;94:911–921.

84. Antman EM, Handin R. Low-molecular-weight heparins: an intriguing new twist with profound implications. Circulation 1998;98:287–289.

85. The GUSTO IIb Investigators. A comparison of recombinant hirudin with heparin for the treatment of acute coronary syndromes. The Global Use of Strategies to Open Occluded Coronary Arteries (GUSTO) IIb investigators. N Engl J Med 1996;335:775–782.

86. Cohen M, Demers C, Gurfinkel EP, Turpie AG, Fromell GJ, Goodman S, Langer A, Califf RM, Fox KA, Premmereur J, Bigonzi F. A comparison of low-molecular-weight heparin with unfractionated heparin for unstable coronary artery disease. Efficacy and Safety of Subcutaneous Enoxaparin in Non-Q-Wave Coronary Events Study Group. N Engl J Med 1997;337:447–452.

87. Mark DB, Cowper PA, Berkowitz SD, Davidson-Ray L, DeLong ER, Turpie AG, Califf RM, Weatherley B, Cohen M. Economic assessment of low-molecular-weight heparin (enoxaparin)

versus unfractionated heparin in acute coronary syndrome patients: results from the ESSENCE randomized trial. Efficacy and Safety of Subcutaneous Enoxaparin in Non-Q wave Coronary Events [unstable angina or non-Q-wave myocardial infarction]. Circulation 1998;97: 1702–1707.

88. Fox KA. Implications of the Organization to Assess Strategies for Ischemic Syndromes-2 (OASIS-2) study and the results in the context of other trials. Am J Cardiol 1999;84: 26M–31M.

89. McElwee NE, Johnson ER. Potential economic impact of glycoprotein IIb-IIIa inhibitors in improving outcomes of patients with acute ischemic coronary syndromes. Am J Cardiol 1997; 80:39B–43B.

90. Szucs TD, Meyer BJ, Kiowski W. Economic assessment of tirofiban in the management of acute coronary syndromes in the hospital setting: an analysis based on the PRISM PLUS trial. Eur Heart J 1999;20:1253–1260.

91. Mark DB, Harrington RA, Lincoff AM, Califf RM, Nelson CL, Tsiatis AA, Buell H, Mahaffey KW, Davidson-Ray L, Topol EJ. Cost-effectiveness of platelet glycoprotein IIb/IIIa inhibition with eptifibatide in patients with non-ST-elevation acute coronary syndromes. Circulation 2000;101:366–371.

92. The PURSUIT Investigators. Inhibition of platelet glycoprotein IIb/IIIa with eptifibatide in patients with acute coronary syndromes. The PURSUIT Trial Investigators. Platelet Glycoprotein IIb/IIIa in Unstable Angina: Receptor Suppression Using Integrilin Therapy. N Engl J Med 1998;339:436–443.

93. The CAPRIE Steering Committee. A randomised, blinded, trial of clopidogrel versus aspirin in patients at risk of ischaemic events (CAPRIE). CAPRIE Steering Committee. Lancet 1996; 348:1329–1339.

94. Yusuf S, Zhao F, Mehta SR, Chrolavicius S, Tognoni G, Fox KK. Effects of clopidogrel in addition to aspirin in patients with acute coronary syndromes without ST-segment elevation. N Engl J Med 2001;345:494–502.

95. Gaspoz JM, Coxson PG, Goldman PA, Williams LW, Kuntz KM, Hunink MG, Goldman L. Cost effectiveness of aspirin, clopidogrel, or both for secondary prevention of coronary heart disease. N Engl J Med 2002;346:1800–1806.

96. Lindgren P, Jonsson B. Modeling the cost effectiveness of clopidogrel in acute coronary syndromes without ST-segment elevation in Sweden. J Am Coll Cardiol 2003;41:540A.

97. Calvin JE, Klein LW, VandenBerg BJ, Meyer P, Condon JV, Snell RJ, Ramirez-Morgen LM, Parrillo JE. Risk stratification in unstable angina. Prospective validation of the Braunwald classification. JAMA 1995;273:136–141.

98. Braunwald E. Unstable angina. A classification. Circulation 1989;80:410–414.

99. Calvin JE, Klein LW, VandenBerg BJ, Meyer P, Ramirez-Morgen LM, Parrillo JE. Clinical predictors easily obtained at presentation predict resource utilization in unstable angina. Am Heart J 1998;136:373–381.

100. Spertus JA, Weiss NS, Every NR, Weaver WD. The influence of clinical risk factors on the use of angiography and revascularization after acute myocardial infarction. Myocardial Infarction Triage and Intervention Project Investigators. Arch Intern Med 1995;155: 2309–2316.

101. Mark DB. Implications of cost in treatment selection for patients with coronary heart disease. Ann Thorac Surg 1996;61:S12–S15.

102. Wennberg DE, Kellett MA, Dickens JD, Malenka DJ, Keilson LM, Keller RB. The association between local diagnostic testing intensity and invasive cardiac procedures. JAMA 1996;275: 1161–1164.

103. Guadagnoli E, Hauptman PJ, Ayanian JZ, Pashos CL, McNeil BJ, Cleary PD. Variation in the use of cardiac procedures after acute myocardial infarction. N Engl J Med 1995;333: 573–578.

104. Pilote L, Califf RM, Sapp S, Miller DP, Mark DB, Weaver WD, Gore JM, Armstrong PW, Ohman EM, Topol EJ. Regional variation across the United States in the management of acute myocardial infarction. GUSTO-1 Investigators. Global Utilization of Streptokinase and

Tissue Plasminogen Activator for Occluded Coronary Arteries. N Engl J Med 1995;333: 565–572.

105. McClellan M, McNeil BJ, Newhouse JP. Does more intensive treatment of acute myocardial infarction in the elderly reduce mortality? Analysis using instrumental variables. JAMA 1994; 272:859–866.

106. Marrugat J, Sanz G, Masia R, Valle V, Molina L, Cardona M, Sala J, Seres L, Szescielinski L, Albert X, Lupon J, Alonso J. Six-month outcome in patients with myocardial infarction initially admitted to tertiary and nontertiary hospitals. RESCATE Investigators. Recursos Empleados en el Sindrome Coronario Agudo y Tiempos de Espera. J Am Coll Cardiol 1997; 30:1187–1192.

107. Gatsonis CA, Epstein AM, Newhouse JP, Normand SL, McNeil BJ. Variations in the utilization of coronary angiography for elderly patients with an acute myocardial infarction. An analysis using hierarchical logistic regression. Med Care 1995;33:625–642.

108. Every NR, Fihn SD, Maynard C, Martin JS, Weaver WD. Resource utilization in treatment of acute myocardial infarction: staff-model health maintenance organization versus fee-for-service hospitals. The MITI Investigators. Myocardial Infarction Triage and Intervention. J Am Coll Cardiol 1995;26:401–406.

109. Pilote L, Miller DP, Califf RM, Rao JS, Weaver WD, Topol EJ. Determinants of the use of coronary angiography and revascularization after thrombolysis for acute myocardial infarction. N Engl J Med 1996;335:1198–1205.

110. van Miltenburg-van Zijl AJ, Simoons ML, Bossuyt PM, Taylor TR, Veerhoek MJ. Variation in the use of coronary angiography in patients with unstable angina is related to differences in patient population and availability of angiography facilities, without affecting prognosis. Eur Heart J 1996;17:1828–1835.

111. The TIMI IIIB Investigators. Effects of tissue plasminogen activator and a comparison of early invasive and conservative strategies in unstable angina and non-Q-wave myocardial infarction. Results of the TIMI IIIB Trial. Thrombolysis in Myocardial Ischemia. Circulation 1994;89:1545–1556.

112. Cannon CP, Weintraub WS, Demopoulos LA, Vicari R, Frey MJ, Lakkis N, Neumann FJ, Robertson DH, DeLucca PT, DiBattiste PM, Gibson CM, Braunwald E. TACTICS (Treat Angina with Aggrastat and Determine Cost of Therapy with an Invasive or Conservative Strategy). Comparison of early invasive and conservative strategies in patients with unstable coronary syndromes treated with the glycoprotein IIb/IIIa inhibitor tirofiban. N Engl J Med 2001;344:1879–1887.

113. Mahoney EM, Jurkovitz CT, Chu H, Becker ER, Culler S, Kosinski AS, Robertson DH, Alexander C, Nag S, Cook JR, Demopoulos LA, DiBattiste PM, Cannon CP, Weintraub WS. Cost and cost-effectiveness of an early invasive vs conservative strategy for the treatment of unstable angina and non-ST-segment elevation myocardial infarction. JAMA 2002;288: 1851–1858.

114. Newby LK, Califf RM, Guerci A, Weaver WD, Col J, Horgan JH, Mark DB, Stebbins A, Van de Werf F, Gore JM, Topol EJ. Early discharge in the thrombolytic era: an analysis of criteria for uncomplicated infarction from the Global Utilization of Streptokinase and t-PA for Occluded Coronary Arteries (GUSTO) trial. J Am Coll Cardiol 1996;27:625–632.

115. Newby LK, Califf RM. Identifying Patient Risk: The Basis for Rational Discharge Planning After Acute Myocardial Infarction. J Thromb Thrombolysis 1996;3:107–115.

116. Eisenstein EL, Newby LK, Knight JD, Shaw LJ, Califf RM, Topol EJ, Mark DB. Cost avoidance through early discharge of the uncomplicated acute myocardial infarction patient. J Am Coll Cardiol 330A;27.

117. Newby LK, Eisenstein EL, Califf RM, Thompson TD, Nelson CL, Peterson ED, Armstrong PW, Van de WF, White HD, Topol EJ, Mark DB. Cost effectiveness of early discharge after uncomplicated acute myocardial infarction. N Engl J Med 2000;342:749–755.

118. Gibbons RJ, Chatterjee K, Daley J, Douglas JS, Fihn SD, Gardin JM, Grunwald MA, Levy D, Lytle BW, O'Rourke RA, Schafer WP, Williams SV, Ritchie JL, Cheitlin MD, Eagle KA, Gardner TJ, Garson A, Russell RO, Ryan TJ, Smith SC. ACC/AHA/ACP-ASIM guidelines

for the management of patients with chronic stable angina: a report of the American College of Cardiology/American Heart Association Task Force on Practice Guidelines (Committee on Management of Patients With Chronic Stable Angina). J Am Coll Cardiol 1999;33: 2092–2197.

119. Braunwald E, Antman EM, Beasley JW, Califf RM, Cheitlin MD, Hochman JS, Jones RH, Kereiakes D, Kupersmith J, Levin TN, Pepine CJ, Schaeffer JW, Smith EE, Steward DE, Theroux P, Alpert JS, Eagle KA, Faxon DP, Fuster V, Gardner TJ, Gregoratos G, Russell RO, Smith SC. ACC/AHA guidelines for the management of patients with unstable angina and non-ST-segment elevation myocardial infarction. A report of the American College of Cardiology/American Heart Association Task Force on Practice Guidelines (Committee on the Management of Patients With Unstable Angina). J Am Coll Cardiol 2000;36:970–1062.

120. Ryan TJ, Antman EM, Brooks NH, Califf RM, Hillis LD, Hiratzka LF, Rapaport E, Riegel B, Russell RO, Smith EE, Weaver WD, Gibbons RJ, Alpert JS, Eagle KA, Gardner TJ, Garson A, Gregoratos G, Smith SC. 1999 update: ACC/AHA Guidelines for the Management of Patients With Acute Myocardial Infarction: Executive Summary and Recommendations: A report of the American College of Cardiology/American Heart Association Task Force on Practice Guidelines (Committee on Management of Acute Myocardial Infarction). Circulation 1999;100:1016–1030.

121. Chen J, Radford MJ, Wang Y, Marciniak TA, Krumholz HM. Do ''America's Best Hospitals'' perform better for acute myocardial infarction? N Engl J Med 1999;340:286–292.

122. Ohman EM, Peterson E. Implications and challenges using practice guidelines for chronic angina. Ann Intern Med 2001;135:527–529.

123. CRUSADE investigation. http: //www.millenium.com/clinicians/cardiovascular/crusade/index.asp. Accessed, 2003.

124. Bradley EH, Holmboe ES, Mattera JA, Roumanis SA, Radford MJ, Krumholz HM. A qualitative study of increasing beta-blocker use after myocardial infarction: Why do some hospitals succeed? JAMA 2001;285:2604–2611.

125. Jamtvedt G, Young JM, Kristoffersen DT, Thomson O'Brien MA, Oxman AD. Audit and feedback: effects on professional practice and health care outcomes. Cochrane Database Syst Rev, 2003; CD000259.

126. Roe MT, Ohman EM, Pollack CV, Peterson ED, Brindis RG, Harrington RA, Christenson RH, Smith SC, Califf RM, Gibler WB. Changing the model of care for patients with acute coronary syndromes. Am Heart J 2003;146:605–612.

127. Chen V, Scott I. Systematic review of quality improvement interventions on inpatient management of acute coronary syndromes. Barcelona: XI Cochrane Colloquium, 2003.

128. National Health Expenditures. Health Care Financing Administration. In: www.hcfa.gov/stats/NHE-OAct./tables/t1.htm. Accessed March 07, 2000.

129. Hatziandreu EI, Koplan JP, Weinstein MC, Caspersen CJ, Warner KE. A cost-effectiveness analysis of exercise as a health promotion activity. Am J Public Health 1988;78:1417–1421.

130. Wong JB, Sonnenberg FA, Salem DN, Pauker SG. Myocardial revascularization for chronic stable angina. Analysis of the role of percutaneous transluminal coronary angioplasty based on data available in 1989. Ann Intern Med 1990;113:852–871.

131. Goldman L, Sia ST, Cook EF, Rutherford JD, Weinstein MC. Costs and effectiveness of routine therapy with long-term beta-adrenergic antagonists after acute myocardial infarction. N Engl J Med 1988;319:152–157.

132. Levin LA, Jonsson B. Cost-effectiveness of thrombolysis--a randomized study of intravenous rt-PA in suspected myocardial infarction. Eur Heart J 1992;13:2–8.

133. O'Brien BJ, Buxton MJ, Ferguson BA. Measuring the effectiveness of heart transplant programmes: quality of life data and their relationship to survival analysis. J Chronic Dis 1987; 40(suppl 1):137S–158S.

# Index